This book is to be returned on or before
the last date stamped below.

LIBREX —

Volume II

Pediatric Otolaryngology

Edited by

CHARLES D. BLUESTONE, M.D.

Professor of Otolaryngology
University of Pittsburgh
School of Medicine
Director, Department of Otolaryngology
Children's Hospital of Pittsburgh

and

SYLVAN E. STOOL, M.D.

Professor of Otolaryngology and Pediatrics
University of Pittsburgh
School of Medicine
Director of Education, Department of Otolaryngology
Children's Hospital of Pittsburgh

SANDRA K. ARJONA, B.A.

Associate Editor

1983

W. B. SAUNDERS COMPANY
Philadelphia London Toronto Mexico City Rio de Janeiro Sydney Tokyo

W. B. Saunders Company: West Washington Square
Philadelphia, PA 19105

1 St. Anne's Road
Eastbourne, East Sussex BN21 3UN, England

1 Goldthorne Avenue
Toronto, Ontario M8Z 5T9, Canada

Apartado 26370—Cedro 512
Mexico 4, D.F., Mexico

Rua Coronel Cabrita, 8
Sao Cristovao Caixa Postal 21176
Rio de Janeiro, Brazil

9 Waltham Street
Artarmon, N.S.W. 2064, Australia

Ichibancho, Central Bldg., 22-1 Ichibancho
Chiyoda-Ku, Tokyo 102, Japan

Library of Congress Cataloging in Publication Data

Main entry under title:

Pediatric otolaryngology.

1. Pediatric otolaryngology.   I. Bluestone, Charles D.
II. Stool, Sylvan E.   III. Arjona, Sandra K. [DNLM:
1. Otorhinolaryngologic diseases—In infancy and childhood.
WV 100 P3703]

RF47.C4P38   618.92′09751   78–64698
ISBN 0–7216–1758–1 (set)
ISBN 0–7216–1761–1 (v. 1)
ISBN 0–7216–1762–X (v. 2)

Volume I ISBN   0–7216–1761–1
Volume II ISBN   0–7216–1762–X
SET ISBN   0–7216–1758–1

Pediatric Otolaryngology

Last digit is the print number: 9   8   7   6   5   4   3   2   1

CONTENTS

VOLUME I

Chapter 17

INTRATEMPORAL COMPLICATIONS AND SEQUELAE OF OTITIS MEDIA 513

Charles D. Bluestone, M.D., and Jerome O. Klein, M.D.

VOLUME II

Section IV

THE MOUTH, PHARYNX, AND ESOPHAGUS

Chapter 38

EMBRYOLOGY AND ANATOMY

Vincent G. Caruso, M.D.
Eberhardt K. Sauerland, M.D.

INTRODUCTION

The anatomy of the mouth, pharynx, and esophagus is the result of a developmental process that begins in the fertilized ovum and continues, though at a slower rate, through infancy, childhood, and adulthood. This chapter will review the developmental anatomy of the mouth, pharynx, and esophagus and stress the anatomy in the newborn.

MOUTH

Roof of the Mouth

Primary Palate. Since the mouth is formed by the development and differentiation of the embryological facial primordia, we will begin with a review of the embryology of the face. Figure 38–1 illustrates the anatomy of the face in the embryo of 3.5 weeks. Notice the frontonasal elevation and maxillary and mandibular growth areas (processes). The maxillary and mandibular growth areas are derivatives of the first branchial arch. The stomodeum, which at this stage is a superficial surface depression, lies between the first

branchial arch derivatives bilaterally and below the frontonasal elevation. By the fifth week of development, nasal placodes begin to develop as bilateral paired thickenings of the frontonasal ectoderm dorsolateral to the stomodeum. Invagination of the nasal placode forms the nasal sac. This invagination continues posteriorly until it reaches the epithelium of the stomodeum as noted in Figure 38–2, in an embryo of 5.5 weeks. During the seventh week of gestation, the oronasal membrane at the junction of the stomodeum and the nasal sac disappears, producing the primitive posterior nares, or choanae, that open directly into the anterior part of the stomodeum or primitive oral cavity. Posterior to the primitive choanae, the nasal and oral cavities share a common vault. This same arrangement is seen in amphibians and some reptiles.

A horseshoe-shaped elevation surrounds each nasal placode. The part of this elevation lying medial to the nasal placode is called the medial nasal elevation, and the part lying lateral to the nasal placode is called the lateral nasal elevation. The groove between the lateral nasal elevation and the maxillary elevation is called the nasolacrimal groove. This anatomy, as seen in the embryo of about 4.5

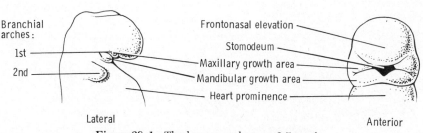

Figure 38–1 The human embryo at 3.5 weeks.

865

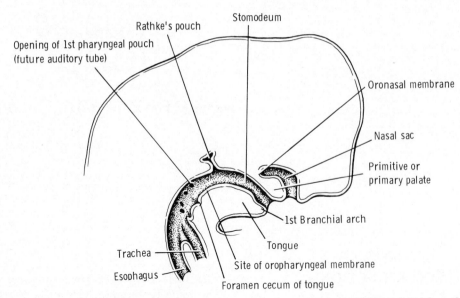

Figure 38–2   Facial structures. Midsagittal section of the human embryo at 5.5 weeks. (Adapted from an original painting by Frank H. Netter, M.D., from Clinical Symposia, copyright CIBA Pharmaceutical Co., Division of CIBA-GEIGY Corp.)

weeks, is illustrated in Figure 38–3. The medial nasal elevations form the premaxilla, including the medial part of the upper lip called the philtrum, the middle portion of the upper jaw, and the primary palate. The lateral nasal elevations form the nasal alae, and the maxillary elevations form the lateral aspect of the upper lip. Mesoderm proliferates, filling in the groove between the medial nasal elevation and the maxillary elevation and causing an apparent fusion at this site. Evidence suggests that there is no actual breakdown of epithelium or fusion at this site, and at no time during normal embryological development is a cleft lip apparent (Davies, 1973). The posterior edges of the primary palate are the medial palatine processes, as illustrated in Figure 38–4.

Secondary Palate.   The lateral palatine processes begin growing downward from the lateral walls of the oral cavity during the seventh week of gestation (Fig. 38–4). Initially, these extend inferomedially to lie under the lateral surface of the tongue, but eventually they rise to lie above the tongue. Posteriorly, they meet and fuse in the midline with each other and with the nasal septum. Anteriorly, they fuse with the medial palatine process of the primary palate. The nasal septum, which has grown from the roof of the nose inferiorly, reaches and joins the lateral palatine processes as they fuse. The process of palatal fusion is completed by about the 12th week of gestation. The two incisive foramina lie adjacent to each other in the midline at the junction of the medial and lateral palatine processes. These foramina, which lead to the incisive canals, transmit the nasopalatine nerves. The portions of the lateral palatine processes that fuse, but do not contact the nasal septum, form the soft palate. The portion of the nasal septum that does not contact the lateral nasal processes forms the posterior edge of the nasal septum.

The roof of the mouth in a fetus of 9 weeks

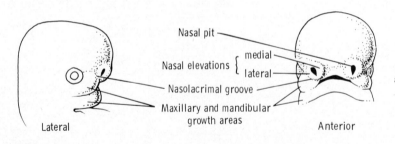

Figure 38–3   The human embryo at 4.5 weeks.

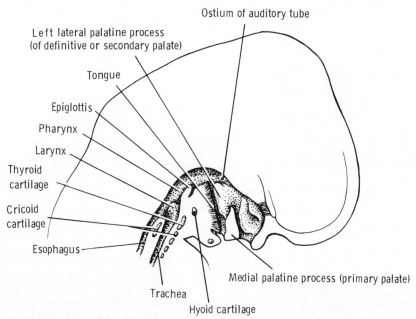

Figure 38–4   Facial structures. Sagittal section of the human embryo at 7.5 weeks. (Adapted from an original painting by Frank H. Netter, M.D., from Clinical Symposia, copyright CIBA Pharmaceutical Co., Division of CIBA-GEIGY Corp.)

is illustrated in Figure 38–5. At this time, the fusion of the various components of the roof of the mouth is complete, and the anatomy, as illustrated, closely resembles that seen in the normal newborn. This unique anatomy (the completed primary and secondary palate) was developed as reptiles evolved into mammals. If the lateral palatine processes do not fuse with each other and with the nasal septum, the result is a cleft palate, which may involve only the secondary palate or both the secondary and the primary palates.

An ectodermal ingrowth along the edge of

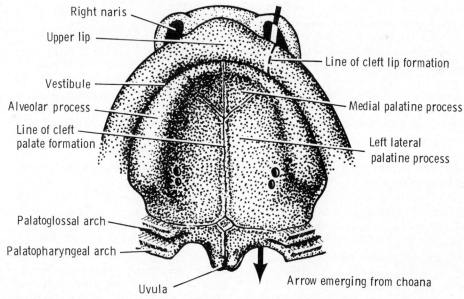

Figure 38–5   Roof of oral cavity of the human embryo at 9 weeks as seen from below. Note the lines of cleft lip and cleft palate formation. (Adapted from an original painting by Frank H. Netter, M.D., from Clinical Symposia, copyright CIBA Pharmaceutical Co., Division of CIBA-GEIGY Corp.)

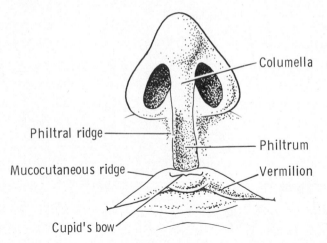

Figure 38–6 Anatomy of the structures derived from the primary palate.

the upper jaw is called the labiodental lamina. The center of this epithelial band breaks down, leaving a cavity that forms the vestibule of the mouth. It lies between the lips and teeth. In the midline, the cavity is incomplete, forming the frenulum. The shelves created are called the anterior labiodental lamina and the posterior dental lamina. The anterior labiodental lamina becomes the upper lip, and the posterior dental lamina becomes the alveolar process (Fig. 38–5).

Lip and Palate of the Newborn. The upper lip (Fig. 38–6) contains the *orbicularis oris* muscle, which is innervated by the facial nerve. Sensation is supplied by the inferior orbital nerve. The blood supply is provided mainly by the paired superior labial arteries, which lie beneath the mucous membrane. The vermilion, which is red because of the highly vascular connective tissue papillae lying beneath the surface, is covered by non-keratinizing squamous epithelium. The junction between the skin and the vermilion is called the mucocutaneous ridge. This thick white line is important because it must be carefully approximated when lacerations that extend across its border are closed. The arch of the mucocutaneous ridge is broken by the slight concavity of the so-called "Cupid's bow." Extending from this region to the columella, there is a vertical depression called the philtrum. Lateral to the philtrum are philtral ridges. The slight projection of the vermilion below "Cupid's bow" is the tubercle. These landmarks are important in the evaluation and surgical correction of congenital and traumatic lip deformities.

The hard palate of the normal newborn is short, wide, and only slightly arched (Crelin, 1973). It usually contains five or six trans-verse ridges that are thought to aid the infant in holding the nipple when sucking. Sensation to the palate is supplied by the greater and lesser palatine nerves via the greater and lesser palatine canals and by the nasopalatine nerves via the incisive foramina. These nerves originate in the maxillary division of the trigeminal nerve. Generally, the infant's tongue fills the oral cavity and lies against the roof of the mouth, with the oral cavity being a potential space. The completed palatal structures provide the newborn with velopharyngeal competence and the ability to breathe through his nose while he is sucking with his mouth. Cleft palate deformities or a shortened soft palate result in velopharyngeal incompetence and marked feeding problems in the infant.

Floor of the Mouth

Tongue. The anterior region of the floor of the mouth, like the palate, is derived from the mandibular or first branchial arch (Figs. 38–7 and 38–8). This area, which forms the anterior two thirds of the tongue, includes the lateral lingual swellings bilaterally and the tuberculum impar centrally. The lateral lingual swellings eventually meet in the midline to form the tongue with its poorly vascularized median raphe. The *foramen cecum* is located posterior to the first branchial arch derivatives in the floor of the mouth. This foramen, a blind depression, lies in the midline at the apex of the V-shaped line of circumvallate papillae (Fig. 38–8). The *sulcus terminalis* extends across the entire base of the tongue along the line of circumvallate papil-

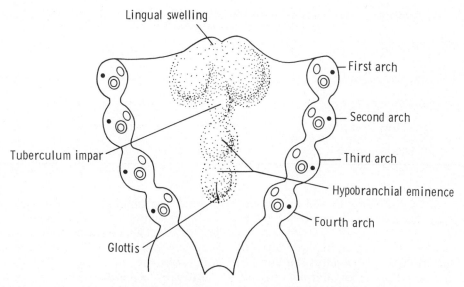

Figure 38–7 Development of the tongue in the human embryo at 5 weeks.

lae. The foramen cecum and the sulcus terminalis lie between the first and third branchial arch derivatives. The sulcus marks the site of the original oropharyngeal membrane in the floor of the mouth. The site of the original oropharyngeal membrane on the lateral wall of the pharynx is represented by the palatoglossal fold. Posterior to these structures, the epithelium is derived from the primitive foregut. The thyroid gland originates at the foramen cecum and migrates inferiorly. For this reason, thyroid tissue may be found anywhere along a tract from the foramen cecum to the lower neck (thyroglossal duct). Indeed, should the thyroid gland fail to migrate inferiorly, it may be located in the base of the tongue. A persistent sinus or cyst along this tract may be seen as a thyroglossal duct sinus or cyst. Anterior to the foramen cecum and the sulcus terminalis, the epithelium is derived from the first branchial arch. Accordingly, the mucosa of this region

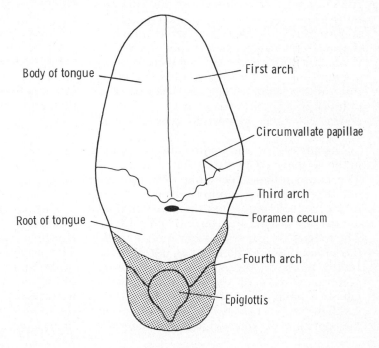

Figure 38–8 Development of the adult human tongue. Note the absence of the second arch mesoderm.

Table 38–1   IMPORTANT BRANCHIAL (PHARYNGEAL) ARCHES
AND THEIR NERVE SUPPLY

First pharyngeal arch	Mandibular nerve (V_3)
Second pharyngeal arch	Facial nerve (VII)
Third pharyngeal arch	Glossopharyngeal nerve (IX)
Fourth pharyngeal arch	Superior laryngeal branch of vagus (X)
Sixth pharyngeal arch	Recurrent laryngeal branch of vagus (X)

is innervated by the nerve of the first branchial arch, the mandibular nerve (V_3) (Table 38–1).

The muscles of the tongue are derived from mesodermal tissue, which is not part of the first branchial arch but migrates to the tongue area under the epithelium of the first branchial arch from myotomes of the occipital somites. Therefore, the tongue muscles are supplied by their own specific cranial nerve, the hypoglossal nerve (XII). The tongue is a complex organ containing a variety of intrinsic and extrinsic muscles. Of the extrinsic muscles, the bilateral *genioglossi* are of considerable importance, since they alone are capable of protruding the tongue. Bilateral loss of genioglossus function (e.g., during deep general anesthesia or as a consequence of a central neurological lesion) leads to a relapse of the tongue against the posterior pharyngeal wall, with the attendant risk of upper airway obstruction and suffocation. Thus, the normally functioning genioglossi can be considered as "safety muscles" that aid in the patency of the upper airway. It is now known that the genioglossus muscles are innervated with each inspiration and that this important muscle activation can become defunct in certain patients with the sleep apnea syndrome (Sauerland and Harper, 1976).

The anatomy of the oropharyngeal region in the newborn differs from that in the adult. The entire tongue, including the posterior one third, is located within the mouth of the newborn. It descends into the pharynx during the first 4 years after birth (Crelin, 1973). The tongue is located farther forward, while the larynx is located higher than in the adult. In the newborn, the epiglottis reaches the posterior surface of the soft palate to establish a nasal airway for respiration while suckling (Sasaki et al., 1977). Milk flows along the dorsum of the tongue and laterally

around the epiglottis to enter the pharynx without spilling into the elevated larynx (Crelin, 1973). The newborn is an obligate nose breather and may suffocate if the nasal airway is obstructed.

Salivary Glands. The major salivary glands are ectodermal derivatives, originating in the floor of the mouth as epithelial buds between the sixth and eighth weeks of fetal life. They grow as a branching system of solid ducts ending in acini. Secondarily, by the sixth fetal month, the ducts become hollow and the acini are partially differentiated. Although differentiation of the acini is not completed until after birth, saliva is secreted by the fetus (Arey, 1965). The cells of the parotid gland are all serous, while those of the submaxillary and sublingual glands are a combination of serous and mucous cells. Salivary secretion, which occurs constantly and spontaneously, is augmented by reflex stimulation. Parasympathetic and sympathetic nerve fibers supply the glands and surrounding vasculature to regulate secretion. The composition of the saliva varies according to the proportion secreted by each gland and according to the nature of the stimulus. Minor salivary glands are found throughout the mouth and pharynx.

PHARYNX

Oropharynx

The anatomy of the pharynx is usually considered in three parts: the oropharynx, nasopharynx, and hypopharynx (Fig. 38–9). The oropharynx is the posterior continuation of the oral cavity beyond the palatine arches or tonsillar pillars. The anterior palatine arch is formed by the palatoglossus muscle, and the posterior palatine arch by the palatopharyngeus muscle. Between these two

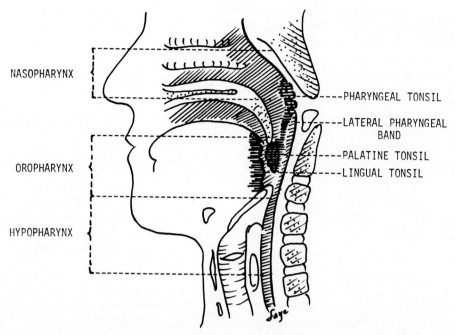

NASOPHARYNX

OROPHARYNX

HYPOPHARYNX

PHARYNGEAL TONSIL

LATERAL PHARYNGEAL BAND

PALATINE TONSIL

LINGUAL TONSIL

Figure 38–9   Relationships of the nasopharynx, oropharynx, and hypopharynx.

arches, and on either side of the passageway between the mouth and the oropharynx, are the palatine tonsils. The oropharynx extends superiorly to the line of contact between the soft palate and the posterior pharyngeal wall and inferiorly to the tip of the epiglottis.

The most striking features of the oropharynx are the base of the tongue and vallecula. The base of the tongue and larynx descend inferiorly during the first 4 years after birth. By age 4 years, the base of the tongue forms part of the anterior wall of the oropharynx and contains the lingual tonsil. Between the tongue and the epiglottis lies a median mucosal fold, the glossoepiglottic fold. Two lateral mucosal folds extend from the junction of the tongue and the lateral pharyngeal wall to the epiglottis. These are called the pharyngoepiglottic folds. Between these pharyngoepiglottic folds is the epiglottic vallecula. The roof of the oropharynx is formed by the soft palate.

Histologically, the oropharynx and hypopharynx are both lined with stratified squamous epithelium supported by a dense network of elastic fibers. The lamina propria contains connective tissue and is penetrated by stratified squamous papillae. It contains numerous seromucinous glands and numerous polymorphonuclear cells, lymphocytes, and plasma cells. Sensation to the oropharyngeal mucosa, including the dorsal

third of the tongue, tonsillar pillars, and adjacent soft palate, is supplied by the glossopharyngeal nerve. The superior laryngeal branch of the vagus nerve also supplies the mucosa of the base of the tongue and epiglottis.

Nasopharynx

The nasopharynx lies above the soft palate and posterior to the choanae (Fig. 38–9). It communicates with the nasal cavities, eustachian tube, and oropharynx. the junction between the nasopharynx and the oropharynx is the pharyngeal isthmus. It is bounded anteriorly by the free edge of the soft palate, posteriorly by the posterior pharyngeal wall, and laterally by the palatopharyngeal arches. In the newborn, the pharynx is about 4 cm in length (including all three parts), and follows a gentle curve, whereas by puberty the nasopharynx and oropharynx form an angle of almost 90 degrees (Crelin, 1973) (Fig. 38–9). The superior constrictor supports the lateral walls of the nasopharynx. Closure of the nasopharynx during speech is accomplished through the combined function of the superior constrictor, palatopharyngeus, salpingopharyngeus, and levator veli palatini muscles (Hollinshead, 1968). In addition, the tensor veli palatini aids in closure during swallowing. The sphenoid and occipital bones support the roof of the nasopharynx, while the first three cervical vertebrae support the posterior wall. The adenoids (pharyngeal tonsil) are located in the roof of the nasopharynx and are considered in detail later. Located on the lateral walls of the nasopharynx, lateral to the bulk of adenoid tissue and slightly above the floor of the nasopharynx, lie the openings of the eustachian (auditory) tube. The torus tubarius, a prominent cartilaginous projection, marks the posterior edge of the tubal opening. The nasopharynx is similar in histologic structure to the nose, its surface being covered with respiratory epithelium.

Hypopharynx

The hypopharynx (laryngeal pharynx) extends from the tip of the epiglottis superiorly to the level of the cricopharyngeus muscle inferiorly (Fig. 38–9). These locations correspond roughly with the level of the hyoid bone superiorly and the cricoid cartilage inferiorly. The posterior and lateral walls are supported by the middle and inferior constrictors. The lateral walls extend anteriorly within the shield-like thyroid cartilage as the piriform sinuses. The anterior wall consists of the laryngeal structures, the cuneiform, corniculate, and arytenoid cartilages; the aryepiglottic folds; the posterior lamina of the cricoid cartilage; and the laryngeal inlet. At the inferior extent of the pharynx, the oblique fibers of the inferior constrictor end and the horizontal fibers of the cricopharyngeus muscle begin. The cricopharyngeus muscle has no median raphe as do the constrictors. It is in a state of tonic contraction, thereby functioning as a pharyngoesophageal sphincter. It prevents reflux of gastric contents during straining and keeps air from being swallowed during breathing. It relaxes during deglutition to make possible the passage of the bolus of food into the esophagus below. Killian's dehiscence is an area of weakness in the pharyngeal wall between the inferior constrictor above and the cricopharyngeus muscle below. It is a common site of pharyngeal diverticula. The mucosa of the hypopharynx, just above the cricopharyngeus, is very thin and is vulnerable to injury and perforation from foreign bodies and the passage of endoscopy instruments.

Lymphoid Tissue

A ring of lymphoid tissue (Waldeyer's tonsillar ring) encircles the beginning of the respiratory and alimentary tracts. Waldeyer's tonsillar ring is composed of three large masses of tonsillar tissue: the lingual, pharyngeal (adenoids), and faucial (palatine) tonsils. They appear during the fifth month of fetal life. They are unique in that they contain only efferent and no afferent lymphatic circulation (Koburg, 1968). Smaller aggregates of lymphoid tissue in this area are included in Waldeyer's ring by some authors. These are the "tubal tonsils," lateral "pharyngeal bands," "pharyngeal granulations," and lymphoid tissue within the laryngeal ventricle (Ash and Raum, 1949).

The pharyngeal tonsil tissue, located in the roof of the nasopharynx, increases rapidly in size during the first year and usually atrophies by puberty. It may be large enough to fill the nasopharynx, causing nasal airway and eustachian tube obstruction. The pharyngeal tonsil is a single, lobulated mass of tissue, in contradistinction to the palatine tonsils, which are paired. Invagination of surface epithelium produces crypts that may be very prominent. The surface epithelium is the typical respiratory epithelium that normally covers the nasopharynx. However, it may eventually undergo metaplasia from columnar to stratified squamous type. In addition, the crypts may be filled with squamous, keratin-like debris and white blood cells. Germinal centers are located immediately below the epithelium. The tonsillar epithelium is structured loosely, permitting passage of cells and antigens.

The two palatine tonsils are oval, prominent lymphoid masses located between the anterior and posterior tonsillar pillars (the palatoglossal and the palatopharyngeal arches). At birth, the palatine tonsils are about 5 mm in anteroposterior diameter and 3.5 mm in vertical diameter (Crelin, 1973). During childhood, the palatine tonsils descend within their fossae, as their vertical diameter grows faster than their anteroposterior diameter. In contrast to the lingual and pharyngeal tonsils, the palatine tonsils have a capsule that is formed from the pharyngobasilar fascia. From this fascia, septa extend into the tonsils. The capsule is separated from the underlying musculature by loose connective tissue. The glossopharyngeal nerve and styloid process descend nearly vertically on the lateral surface of this musculature. The dorsal lingual, ascending pharyngeal, lesser palatine, facial, ascending palatine, and internal and external carotid arteries are located beneath the musculature in this fossa. The palatine tonsils contain from 10 to 20 crypts which penetrate the surface to reach various depths. The crypts may penetrate the entire tonsil to reach the fibrous capsule. Unlike the surface of the pharyngeal tonsil, the surface epithelium is stratified squamous epithelium. It follows the crypts and blends imperceptibly with the mesenchymal structures. Migratory leukocytes are seen infiltrating the surface epithelium (Ash and Raum, 1949).

The lingual tonsils, at the base of the tongue, develop later than the other tonsils and usually persist into adult life.

The tonsils are active in the synthesis of humoral immunoglobulins such as IgG, IgM, and IgA, and they produce lymphocytes in a complete sequence of lymphopoiesis, being related immunologically to the gut-associated lymphoid system in man. The tonsils are the first lymphoid aggregates to encounter pathogens that enter the host via the upper respiratory and gastrointestinal tracts. Hence, they may play a role in host immunity to pathogens (Sprinkle and Veltri, 1976).

ESOPHAGUS

Embryology

The esophagus develops from the primitive foregut between the respiratory diverticulum and the gastric dilatation. It is recognizable as a tubular structure by the third week of gestation (Botha, 1962) and elongates to accommodate the growth of the neck, heart, and lungs. Surrounding mesoderm differentiates into circular musculature by the sixth week, longitudinal musculature by the eighth week, and *muscularis mucosae* by the tenth week (Botha, 1962). By the fifth month of fetal life, the ciliated epithelium of the esophagus is replaced by stratified squamous epithelium, beginning in the middle of the esophagus and extending superiorly and inferiorly (Johns, 1952). At birth, some patches of ciliated epithelium may still exist. Although most deeper glands develop after birth (Arey, 1965), superficial mucosal glands are present by the fifth month of gestation.

Anatomy

The esophagus is the passageway from the hypopharynx to the stomach. It is a thin, distensible muscular tube with large, longitudinal folds that become "ironed out" with the passage of a bolus of food. The length of the esophagus increases from birth so that the distance from the incisor teeth to the cardia (including the mouth, pharynx, hypopharynx, and esophagus) averages about 18 cm in neonates, 22 cm in 3 year olds, and 27 cm in 10 year olds (Fransen and Valembois, 1974). Four areas of narrowing are recognized. These are at (1) the entrance at the level of the cricoid cartilage (C-6), (2) the thoracic inlet (T-1), (3) the level at which the aorta (T-4) or left main bronchus (T-6) crosses it, and (4) the diaphragmatic aperture (T-11).

The esophagus is intimately related to many important structures in its course through the neck and thorax. As it descends, it veers to the left behind the cervical trachea and back to the midline behind the aortic arch. It veers to the left and anteriorly as it reaches the diaphragm. In the neck, it lies anterior to the cervical vertebrae, posterior to the trachea, and between the carotid arteries. The retropharyngeal space is a potential space that lies behind the esophagus and communicates with the mediastinum. Instrumental perforations of the posterior wall of the esophagus may contaminate this space, leading to mediastinitis. The recurrent laryngeal nerves lie on either side of the esophagus in the tracheoesophageal groove. The left lobe of the thyroid gland lies anterior to the esophagus. The trachea, left main bronchus, thoracic duct, aortic arch, pericardium, and esophageal nerves and vessels all lie in close proximity to the thoracic esophagus. The esophageal hiatus, through which the esophagus traverses the diaphragm, lies anterior to the aortic hiatus and posterior and to the left of the inferior vena caval foramen. The esophagus extends 1 to 2.5 cm beyond the hiatus to end in the stomach.

The esophagus is supplied by the inferior thyroid arteries, esophageal branches of the descending aorta and right intercostal arteries, left gastric branch of the celiac artery, and left inferior phrenic branch of the abdominal aorta. Venous drainage is into the inferior thyroid veins from the upper third, the azygos vein from the middle third, and the coronary (left gastric) vein from the lower third. The coronary vein of the stomach communicates with the portal circulation. The esophagus receives both sympathetic and parasympathetic fibers. The intrinsic nervous sytem consists of Meissner's and Auerbach's plexuses, which lie between the inner circular and outer longitudinal musculature.

The wall of the esophagus is composed of four layers: *tunica mucosa, submucosa, muscularis,* and *adventitia.* Unlike the lower digestive tract, the esophagus has no layer of serosa. Perforations of the esophageal wall lead to contamination of deep neck and mediastinal spaces.

Vascular Compression and Atresia

The close anatomic relationship between the esophagus and the derivatives of the dorsal and ventral aorta explain the congenital vascular anomalies that cause tracheoesophageal difficulties in children. The aberrant right subclavian artery, double aortic arch, and right-sided aortic arch, which are the most common anomalies, present as vascular rings compressing the esophagus. A thorough treatment of this subject is beyond the scope of this chapter but is available in other sources (Lasher, 1958; Klinkhamer, 1969).

Vascular compression has also been suggested as a cause of congenital esophageal atresia by local pressure. However, the theory that epithelial occlusion is the cause for esophageal atresia is more widely held. This theory explains atresia as an arrest of revacuolization and recanalization after the phase of solid development of the esophagus. This process of differentiation of the esophagus occurs in normal embryos of 21 to 32 days. The final tracheoesophageal septum forms inferiorly to superiorly, ending at the larynx. It is postulated that failure of complete formation of the septum results in a tracheoesophageal fistula. The incidence of esophageal atresia is increased in the presence of hydramnios during pregnancy, prematurity in the child and other congenital malformations (especially vascular and gastrointestinal).

Six different types of esophageal atresia and tracheoesophageal fistula are recognized (Fig. 38–10). The most common is atresia of the esophagus with a fistula from the distal

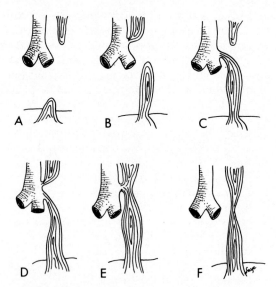

Figure 38–10 Diagrammatic representation of six combinations of esophageal atresia and tracheoesophageal fistula. *A* represents simple esophageal atresia. *B,* Esophageal atresia with a tracheoesophageal fistula from the proximal stump. *C,* Esophageal atresia with a tracheoesophageal fistula from the distal stump. *D,* Esophageal atresia with proximal and distal fistulas. *E,* H-type tracheoesophageal fistula. *F,* Atresia of esophageal lumen.

segment to the trachea. Congenital esophageal atresia is to be differentiated from congenital esophageal stenosis. In congenital esophageal stenosis, a submucosal band of collagen constricts the esophageal lumen at the level of the junction of the middle and lower thirds of the esophagus (Bluestone, Kerry, and Sieber, 1969).

SELECTED REFERENCES

Crelin, E. S. 1973. Functional Anatomy of the Newborn. New Haven, Yale University Press.
    Dr. Crelin's text provides the most complete review of newborn anatomy available.

Crelin, E. S. 1976. Development of the Upper Respiratory System. Summit, N.J., CIBA Pharmaceutical Co., Clinical Symposia, Vol. 28, no. 3.
    This beautifully illustrated review of the developmental anatomy of the upper respiratory system is well worth studying.

Davies, J. 1973. Embryology and anatomy of the head and neck; Embryology and anatomy of the face, palate, nose and paranasal sinuses; Embryology and anatomy of the larynx, respiratory apparatus, diaphragm and esophagus. *In* Paparella, M. M., and Shumrick, D. A. (Eds.): Otolaryngology, Vol. 1, Philadelphia, W. B. Saunders Co., Chaps. 2, 3, and 4, pp. 111–185.
    Dr Davies, an anatomist, gives an excellent, in-depth review of head and neck embryology in these three chapters

REFERENCES

Arey, L. B. 1965. Developmental Anatomy: A Textbook and Laboratory Manual of Embryology. 7th ed. Philadelphia, W. B. Saunders Co., pp. 213–247.

Ash, J. E., and Raum, M. 1949. An Atlas of Otolaryngologic Pathology, 4th ed. The American Academy of Ophthalmology and Otolaryngology. The American Registry of Pathology, The Armed Forces Institute of Pathology, New York, Roskin Photo Offset Co.

Bluestone, C. D., Kerry, R., and Sieber, W. K. 1969. Congenital esophageal stenosis. Laryngoscope, 9:1095–1104.

Botha, G. S. M. 1962. The Gastro-Oesophageal Junction: Clinical Applications to Oesophageal and Gastric Surgery. Boston, Little, Brown & Co., Chap. 5, pp. 48–58.

Crelin, E. S. 1973. Functional Anatomy of the Newborn. New Haven, Yale University Press.

Crelin, E. S. 1976. Development of the Upper Respiratory System. Summit, N.J. CIBA Pharmaceutical Co., Clinical Symposia, Vol. 28, no. 3.

Davies, J. 1973. Embryology and anatomy of the face, palate, nose and paranasal sinuses. In Paparella, M. M., and Shumrick, D. A. (Eds.): Otolaryngology, Vol. 1. Philadelphia, W. B. Saunders Co., Chap. 3, pp. 150–178.

Fransen, G., and Valembois, P. 1974. Anatomy and embryology. In Vantrappen, G., and Hellemens, J. (Eds.): Diseases of the Esophagus. New York, Springer-Verlag, pp. 1–16.

Hollinshead, W. H. 1968. Anatomy for Surgeons, Vol. 1. 2nd ed. New York, Harper & Row, Chap. 8, pp. 440–500.

Johns, B. A. E. 1952. Developmental changes in the oesophageal epithelium in man. J. Anat., 86:431–442.

Klinkhamer, A. C. 1969. Esophagography in Anomalies of the Aortic Arch System. Baltimore, Williams & Wilkins Co.

Koburg, E. 1968. Cell production and cell migration in the tonsil. In Cottier, N., et al. (Eds.): Germinal Centers in the Immune Response. New York, Springer-Verlag, p. 176.

Lasher, E. P. 1958. Types of tracheal and esophageal constriction due to arterial anomalies of the aortic arch, with suggestion as to treatment. Am. J. Surg., 96:228–233.

Sasaki, C. T., Levine, P. A., Laitman, J. T., and Crelin, E. S. 1977. Postnatal descent of the epiglottis in man: A preliminary report. Arch. Otolaryngol., 103:169–171.

Sauerland, E. K., and Harper, R. M. 1976. The human tongue during sleep: Electromyographic activity of the genioglossus muscle. Exp. Neurol., 51:160–170.

Sprinkle, P. M., and Veltri, R. W. 1976. Microbiology of the Head and Neck. In English, G. M. (Ed.): Otolaryngology, Vol. V. New York, Harper & Row, Chap. 15 N, pp. 1–7.

Vantrappen, G., and Hellemans, J. (Eds.): 1974, Diseases of the Esophagus. New York, Springer-Verlag.

Chapter 39

PHYSIOLOGY

Timothy J. Reichert, M.D.

INTRODUCTION

The human's most basic functions are respiration and nutrition, which require the proper working of the mouth, pharynx, and esophagus. Ideally, the respiratory and alimentary tracts should be able to operate independently, and indeed they do so in lower mammals — for example, a deer can drink from a pond while constantly scenting the air for danger. In humans, that ability has been lost, and the respiratory and alimentary tracts cross at the pharynx, requiring a complex breathing–swallowing mechanism. However, humans also have the ability to communicate with a complex variety of sounds, which are produced within the respiratory tract but are modified and articulated in the pharynx and mouth. Thus, although some functions are lost as a result of the communication of the respiratory and alimentary tracts in humans, this lack of independence has led to our development of speech.

The mouth, pharynx, and esophagus may be considered separately or as a functional anatomic unit. The mouth is a portal for nutriments and the site of origin for endogenous secretions, and the pharynx and esophagus are conduits for these elements. In speech, however, the esophagus has no role, whereas the pharynx and mouth function together. The physiology of these anatomic areas will be described separately, and then their cooperative functions will be reviewed in the discussion of suck, taste, swallowing, and speech.

MOUTH

The mouth is a cavity bounded anteriorly by the lips and posteriorly by the oropharynx. It functions with its contents, the teeth and tongue, to masticate and move food, liquids, and secretions to the pharynx. The teeth are divided into two types: those that tear and those that crush. The front teeth, the incisors, are sharp and serve to divide food into sizes appropriate for chewing. In infants the gums are also used in conjunction with the lips in sucking to roll milk from the nipple. More mature patterns of biting and chewing develop later in the first year of life with the appearance of the teeth. The infant is able to bite at approximately seven months of age with the appearance of the incisors and can chew when the molars appear at approximately one year (Bosma, 1973). In young children the incisors are small and have small roots since ripping and tearing are not necessary. The mouth is also a communicating organ that is used with the velum to articulate sounds.

The tongue is used in mastication, deglutition, and speech. The extrinsic muscles of the tongue serve to protrude (genioglossus), retract (styloglossus), and flatten (hyoglossus). The intrinsic muscles — the muscle fibers interlacing within the tongue and connecting to its fibrous septae — produce changes in the shape of the tongue. Such changes produced by the intrinsic musculature are useful, for example, in swallowing when producing a channel in the dorsum to direct liquids into the pharynx.

Saliva is produced primarily by the six major salivary glands — the parotids, submandibular, and sublingual glands. The secretory units of these glands are the acini, the intercalated ducts, and the striated ducts. The acini may be serous, mucoid, or mixed. Secretions are controlled by physical and psychic stimulation mediated through the autonomic nervous system. Physical stimuli from the oral cavity and psychic stimuli from the taste, smell, and sight centers are relayed to the salivary nuclei. The superior salivatory nucleus innervates the parotid gland, and the inferior salivatory nucleus innervates the sublingual and submandibular glands. The superior cervical sympathethic ganglion provides sympathetic innervation by way of the sympathetic nerves carried along the carotid artery.

Saliva has multiple physical and biochemical characteristics that aid in oral function. The mucus protects the mucosa from irritation and aids in lubrication and speaking as well as in swallowing. The minerals it contains — calcium, bicarbonate, and phosphate — may be useful in preventing tooth dissolution by plaque and may also have some antibacterial activity (Rice, 1973). Secretory IgA is produced by the plasma cells around the intralobular ducts and has antibacterial and antiviral activities. Lastly, salivary lysozymes, lactoferrin, and lactoperoxidase inhibit bacterial proliferation. A bacteriolytic substance has also been detected in the saliva and has been found in increased levels in caries-free people (Green, 1959).

PHARYNX AND ESOPHAGUS

The pharynx and esophagus are primarily conduits. The pharynx, however, also acts as an intersection, directing air to enter the respiratory tract and food to enter the alimentary tract. The velum in the pharynx aids in directing air and sound through the nose or mouth; thus, the pharynx also has an active function in speech.

Pharyngeal walls contract in concert with the soft palate. In the resting position, the soft palate is depressed against the tongue by the palatoglossus, palatopharyngeus, and salpingopharyngeus muscles. In swallowing and speech when nasal escape is to be prevented, the levator palatini and uvulus muscles act with the superior pharyngeal constrictor to elevate the palate and close the nasopharynx. In swallowing the tongue is elevated higher and more posteriorly to aid in occlusion and separation of the oropharynx from the nasopharynx. Such tongue mobility also aids the child with a cleft palate in swallowing because the tongue is used to occlude the nasopharynx and prevent reflux. Superior pharyngeal constrictor activity, however, must

also be present to close the lateral and posterior parts of the nasopharynx. In some children, pharyngeal function seems to be delayed (Ardran, 1970), and in such cases stimulation of the pharynx and palate may improve their function with time. This improvement would seem to indicate that they are governed by different areas of coordination in the brain stem; or perhaps the tensor veli palatini muscle, innervated through the fifth cranial nerve, can be stimulated to improve function and contribute to palatal closure.

The pharynx, composed of the pharyngeal sphincters, acts to begin a peristaltic wave to push material into the alimentary tract. Deep to the pharyngobasilar fascia, attached to the base of the skull and to a median raphe and inserting on the pterygomandibular raphe and the hyoid and thyroid cartilages, the constrictors form the posterior and lateral walls of the pharynx. The most inferior part of the inferior constrictor is not attached to the median raphe but instead forms a complete sphincter (the cricopharyngeus muscle) circling the entrance to the esophagus. At rest (in the nonswallowing state), the cricopharyngeus muscle remains contracted, and its tone increases with inspiration and decreases with expiration to prevent air from entering the esophagus (Parish, 1968). Its tone also increases with reflux esophagitis (Hunt et al., 1970) regardless of the cause (hiatus hernia or incompetent gastroesophageal sphincter); presumably this increase in tone prevents refluxing gastric secretions from entering the pharynx and possibly the airway. The exact innervation of the cricopharyngeus muscle is unclear. In dogs there is a separate nerve innervating the muscle (Lund, 1965), but no such nerve has been identified in humans. Innervation could not be directly from the vagus nerve, as vocal cord paralysis is not associated with cricopharyngeus dysfunction. Innervation, therefore, must be a combination of parasympathetic (vagal) and sympathetic (superior cervical ganglion and pharyngeal plexus).

The pharyngeal constrictors are composed of striated muscle, which allows for rapid passage of material. Peristalsis proceeds at approximately 4 to 8 cm per second. Pharyngeal pressures in swallowing may be as great as 200 cm of H_2O, while at rest the pressure exerted by the pharyngeus muscle is 15 to 40 cm H_2O. After swallowing, the cricopharyn-

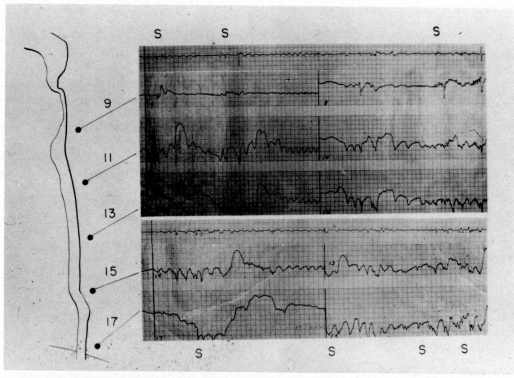

Figure 39-1 An example of a secondary wave. There is no relaxation at a point 9 cm from the nose (the cricopharyngeus muscle) after swallows (marked by S). Positive pressure spikes are seen at 11, 13, 15, and 17 cm as noted and are temporally related to swallows. These secondary waves are important in this example in conducting the bolus through the esophagus, since the primary wave is not conducted through the cricopharyngeus muscle.

geus pressure increases to and remains at approximately 100 cm H₂O for one to two seconds.

Esophageal contractions proceed by stimulation in the pharyngeal phase of swallowing, as seen in Chapter 54, Figure 54–1. Primary and secondary peristaltic waves, innervated through the myenteric plexus, proceed to the stomach. The esophageal submucosa also contains racemose glands, the secretions of which help lubricate food particles during their descent. Primary waves of contraction are those that arise in the pharynx and continue along the entire length of the esophagus. Secondary waves begin in the body of the esophagus, as shown in Figure 39–1, and continue to the stomach. The secondary waves are initiated by esophageal distention. Tertiary waves are localized areas of spasm and are not considered part of the normal physiologic function of the esophagus. In the normal person, however, 10 per cent of the esophageal waves may be of the disordered secondary or tertiary variety. The gastroesophageal junction is an area of increased

muscle thickening at the distal 4 cm of the esophagus. It is not readily seen from inside the esophagus via endoscopy but is easily identified by esophageal manometry. The mean pressure of this high-pressure zone is 30 to 50 cm H₂O. Relaxation begins ½ to 2½ seconds after swallowing is initiated and continues for approximately 10 seconds. This sphincter is under neurogenic and endocrine control. The neurogenic control is the reflex relaxation and constriction of peristalsis, and the endocrine influences are from the stomach and duodenum: when the stomach fills, gastrin is secreted and the pressure increases, and when the duodenum is filled, secretin is produced and the pressure decreases.

SUCK AND TASTE

In infancy the mouth and pharynx are arranged more horizontally and relatively higher in the head and neck than they are in the adult. Such positioning allows for a closed oral cavity and facilitates sucking as the tongue may then act as a piston in sucking milk from the nipple. After the nipple is introduced into the mouth, fluid is obtained by closing the mandible on the nipple and simultaneously applying oral suction. The tongue tip is rolled up to express milk from the teat and then depressed to suck more milk into the mouth. When the bolus of milk is of sufficient quantity it is moved into the pharynx and deglutition begins. Sucking is present in fetuses as young as 24 weeks. In premature infants sucking is present but occurs at a slower rate than in mature infants. With maturation sucks occur at a rate of approximately 2 per second with as many as 30 sucks in a "burst" and are well-coordinated with swallowing (Gryboski, 1965). As the face elongates with growth of the child, the oral cavity becomes open, decreasing the ability to suck and increasing the ability to take food into the mouth for mastication.

Respirations continue during sucking, but when swallowing is begun respirations are stopped by way of a coordinating center in the medulla. A sucking center has been located in the medulla adjacent to the trigeminal nucleus — infants with little organized cranial material above the medulla have been observed to have normal sucking ability (Bosma, 1973).

Sucking may be analyzed in terms of coarse and fine elements. The coarse elements are response bursts — the number of bursts per unit of time and the length of pauses between bursts are measured. The fine elements are the number of sucks within a burst. Measurements of such characteristics have shown marked differences between non-nutritive and nutritive sucking. Non-nutritive sucking has a more marked burst and pause rhythm, and the pauses are shorter than has been observed in nutritive sucking (Wolf, 1968).

The types of fluid provided seem definitely to affect the characteristics of nutritive sucking as well as the facial expressions that occur in response to the type of fluids provided. Sweet fluids, such as a 15 per cent sucrose solution, lead to a sucking pattern that is slower and with fewer pauses, although the number of sucks is relatively the same, than does a less sweet solution. Distilled water results in significantly less sucking (Crook, 1977). The gustofacial response to different types of fluids has also been noted and seems to be coordinated in the midbrain. Infants exhibit a relaxed, pleased expression in response to sweet fluids, whereas sour fluids

produce lip pursing and bitter fluids result in an elevation of the upper lip, angling of the mouth, and protruding of the tongue — an appearance of disgust. Such responses have been noted in anencephalic infants (Steiner, 1977). The tastes of sweet and salty foods are better discriminated on the tongue, whereas bitter and sour tastes are discriminated on the palate. Taste also seems to be related to a variety of other factors — heredity, the time of day, the patient's age, and diseases present. Taste buds have been noted in the pharynges of infants but not in those of adults. Diseases such as rickets and familial dysautonomia result in markedly diminished taste sensations.

An interesting response of the chorda tympani nerves of hamsters and squirrel monkeys to different tastes has been measured. In the past it was assumed that every nerve fiber would respond to every stimulus, but careful observation seems to contradict this classical theory. Measuring single-fiber responses has shown that there is a much greater response to sweet solutions than to solutions that are salty, bitter, or acidic (Frank, 1977).

It may be seen that taste contributes to the development of infants and children. Taste is organized at the bulbar level and is integrated with the sucking response and other functions, such as salivary secretion. Evidence seems to indicate that human neurons are oriented to the sweet taste. Taste is also organized at the cortical level: Voluntary facial expressions occur as a result of certain taste experiences. The effect of taste on cerebral development is uncertain.

SWALLOWING

Swallowing is initiated in the oral cavity by voluntary action. The tongue sweeps the bolus of food or liquid over the dorsum posteriorly toward the oropharynx. Material is prevented from spilling over the sides of the tongue by the buccal muscles laterally sealing themselves against the rigid tongue. (Rigidity of the tongue is created by the intrinsic muscles.) The tongue is aided in its posterosuperior rolling motion by the mylohyoid, geniohyoid, and digastric muscles, which contract and elevate the floor of the mouth.

The soft palate is then elevated above the level of the hard palate and is shortened and thickened dorsally. Then the base of the

Table 39–1   SPEECH PRODUCTION

Manner of Articulation	Site of Articulation				
	Bilabial	Labiodental	Alveolar	Velar	Glottal
Plosive	p, b		t, d	k, g	
Affricative			tr, dr		
Fricative		f, u	s, z		h
Nasal	m		n		
Lateral			l		
Semivowel			r	w	

Modified from Whetnal, E., and Fry, D. B. 1971. The Deaf Child. London, Heineman.

tongue is elevated against the soft palate and the posterior pharyngeal walls by the styloglossus and hyoglossus muscles. The peristaltic wave begins at the level of the Passavant ridge as the tongue is elevated and moved dorsally.

Respiration ceases as the larynx closes. As the tongue is elevated against the soft palate, the larynx is pulled anteriorly and superiorly to create a space for the bolus in the hypopharynx. The epiglottis tilts posteriorly to cover the laryngeal inlet, although this function is probably more vestigial than physiologically significant.

Once the bolus has entered the esophagus it is carried with a single wave to the stomach. "Stripping" waves follow through the esophagus and aid in emptying it. Esophageal activity in humans is only cranial to caudal in direction. Regurgitation or belching does not involve reverse peristalsis.

SPEECH

Speech is defined as the use of voice to convey ideas. Voice is produced in the larynx with characteristic rhythm and intonation and is then given its linguistic and communicative value by the mouth and pharynx (Fry, 1976).

The principal articulator of vowel and consonant sounds is the tongue. Vowels are modified by the tongue and are classified as front, back, open, or closed vowel sounds. Consonants are more complex, involving lip, tongue, dental, velar, and even glottal control, as can be seen from Table 39–1.

The nasal sounds of language are controlled by the velopharyngeal port. Movement of the soft palate is the major component of the velopharyngeal mechanism. The roles of the superior constrictor muscle and the Passavant ridge in speech production are controversial, and they may not be important in normal speakers (Fritzell, 1976) (Chap. 82).

In English the m, n, and ng sounds are the only true nasal speech sounds. However, the soft palate may remain partially open during the creation of some speech sounds to provide a greater nasal quality (nasal resonance) in speech.

SUMMARY

The physiology of the mouth, pharynx, and esophagus is indeed very complex. Simply eating and breathing normally require the complex interaction of many anatomic structures.

As development progresses, anatomic changes aid in modifying normal physiologic function to suit the needs of the maturing child. Such changes are easily seen in the first year of life when the mouth changes from a sucking to a masticating organ. Also, because of the intersection of the alimentary tract and the respiratory tract, challenging and complex dysfunctions must occur. Management of such problems requires an understanding of the fundamentals of normal function.

SELECTED REFERENCES

Bosma, J. 1973. Physiology of the throat. In Otolaryngology. Philadelphia, W. B. Saunders Co.
   Dr. Bosma provides an excellent discussion of various functions of the mouth, pharynx, and esophagus.

The author wishes to thank Beverly Gestring and Pamela Alvarado for their help in the preparation of this manuscript.

Fry, D. B. 1976. Voice and speech. *In* Scientific Foundations of Otolaryngology. London, Heineman.

Dr. Fry provides a detailed analysis of speech and its various components with discussions of sound and anatomic and physiologic aspects.

REFERENCES

Ardran, G. 1970. Some important factors in the assessment of oropharyngeal function. Dev. Med. Child Neurol., *12*:158.

Bosma, J. 1973. Physiology of the throat. *In* Paparella, M. M., and Shumrick, D. A. (Eds.) Otolaryngology. Philadelphia, W. B. Saunders Co.

Crook, C. K. 1977. Taste and the temporal organization of sucking. *In* Taste and Development. Bethesda, MD, Dept. of Health, Education, and Welfare.

Frank, M. 1977. The distinctiveness of responses to sweet in the chorda tympani nerve. *In* Taste and Development. Bethesda, MD, Dept. of Health, Education, and Welfare.

Fritzell, B. 1976. Palatal function. *In* Scientific Foundations of Otolaryngology. London, Heineman.

Fry, D. B. 1976. Voice and speech. *In* Scientific Foundations of Otolaryngology. London, Heineman.

Green, G. E. 1959. A bacteriolytic agent in salivary globulins of caries-immune human beings. J. Dent. Res., *28*:265.

Gryboski, J. 1965. The swallowing mechanism of the neonate. Pediatrics, *35*:445.

Hunt, P. S., Connel, A. M., and Shirley, T. B. 1970. The cricopharyngeal sphincter in gastroesophageal reflux. Gut, *11*:303.

Lund, W. S. 1965. A study of cricopharyngeal sphincter in man and in the dog. Ann. R. Coll. Surg. Engl., *37*:225.

Parish, R. M. 1968. Cricopharyngeus dysfunction and acute dysphagia. Can. Med. Ann. J., *99*:1167.

Rice, D. H. 1973. Salivary gland physiology. Otolaryngol. Clin. North Am., *6*:273.

Steiner, J. E. 1977. Facial expressions of the neonate infant indicating the hedonics of food related chemical stimuli. *In* Taste and Development. Bethesda, MD, Dept. of Health, Education, and Welfare.

Whetnal, E., and Fry, D. B. 1971. The Deaf Child. London, Heineman.

Wolf, P. H. 1968. The serial organization of sucking in the young infant. Pediatrics, *42*:943.

Chapter 40

METHODS OF EXAMINATION

William P. Potsic, M.D.
Steven D. Handler, M.D.

INTRODUCTION

The examination of the oral cavity and pharynx in a child may be a traumatic experience for the patient and examiner alike if there has not been adequate preparation. The child is usually being examined in an unfamiliar environment by a stranger and frequently has unpleasant objects placed in his mouth and nose. To prevent the child from interpreting the examination as an attack, the practitioner needs to establish rapport with his patient during the interview. Children are used to being touched or patted for reassurance, and touching the child while talking to him will frequently relax him.

An explanation of the examination while it is being carried out may help to assure the patient that there will be no unexpected maneuvers or painful surprises. Use of familiar examining aids such as fingers, wooden tongue blades, and flashlights first will promote continued cooperation as unfamiliar instruments are employed. These should be introduced with a simple explanation of their use. Uncomfortable or potentially disquieting portions of the oropharyngeal examination (which may cause gagging) should be reserved until the end of the examination.

The oropharyngeal examination should be performed with the child in a secure position that allows mobility for the patient and exam-

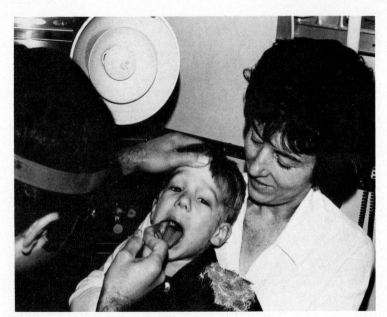

Figure 40–1 Young child being examined while on his mother's lap.

iner — usually in a standard examining chair or, for very young children, on a pediatric examining table. Children may be examined in the lap of a parent, which gives the child a feeling of security and allows the parent to assist in the examination (Fig. 40–1). Visualization of the oral cavity requires good light, directed along the line of sight. This may be provided with a flashlight or with a head mirror, which leaves the examiner's hands free to move the patient and handle instruments.

ORAL CAVITY AND OROPHARYNX

Examination of the oral cavity begins with a general inspection of the face, which can reveal much about a child's emotional and physical state. The examiner may sense anxiety or note an expression of pain in the relationship of the child's mouth to the rest of his face. A careful and thorough examination will permit detection of even the most subtle lesions (Fig. 40–2). Observation of lip color may indicate anemia (pallor) or cardiopulmonary disease (cyanosis). The parched, dry appearance of dehydration or the copious drooling of neuromuscular disorders, oropharyngeal infection, or esophageal foreign bodies may be noted. The mouth that is open to breathe may indicate nasopharyngeal obstruction or generalized air hunger. The odor from the oral cavity should not be ignored for it can be an early sign of metabolic disorders. Inability of the child to open his mouth for the examination may indicate lack of cooperation, dysfunction of the fifth cranial nerve, trismus secondary to a lesion (neoplastic or inflammatory) involving the parapharyngeal space, or a subcondylar

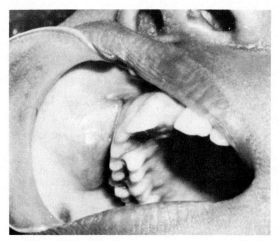

Figure 40–3 Hemangioma of buccal mucosa, seen only by retracting the lip.

mandibular fracture. Asymmetrical pursing of the lips is seen in seventh cranial nerve paralysis.

The primary method of examination of the oral cavity and pharynx is inspection (Becker et al., 1970). The mouth is opened and exposure obtained with the use of a wooden tongue blade, an instrument familiar to all children. A careful and systematic inspection of the oral cavity is performed; this includes an assessment of the teeth, gingiva, buccal mucosa, under-surface of the tongue, palate, and orifices of the salivary glands. The tongue blade facilitates retraction of the lips to expose the entire buccal mucosal surface. Failure to do so may result in the overlooking of significant pathology (Fig. 40–3).

Examination of the teeth and gingiva will give the observer an idea of the child's general hygiene as well as clues to the detection of systemic disorders (e.g., the notched teeth of congenital syphilis, gingival alterations with vitamin deficiencies or drug ingestion) (Fig. 40–4).

The child is then asked to extend his tongue, thus exposing both lateral borders and frequently bringing the posterior third of the tongue forward and into view. In some children the epiglottis may also be visualized at this time. During tongue extension the neuromuscular function of the tongue (twelfth cranial nerve) can be assessed. Fasciculation, atrophy, or deviation of the tongue may be noted. The full range of tongue mobility can be observed; limitation may occur when a very short frenulum or a neuromuscular disorder is present. Tongue

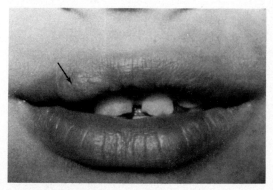

Figure 40–2 Hemangioma of the lip (arrow) that may be missed by a careless examiner.

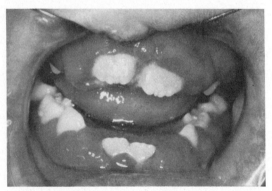

Figure 40–4 Dilantin-induced gingival hypertrophy.

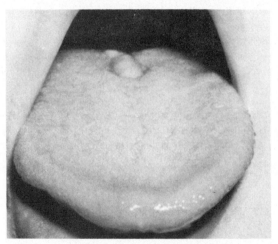

Figure 40–6 Median rhomboid glossitis.

strength can be assessed by opposing pressure with a finger against the patient's cheek when the tongue projects onto the buccal surface.

Inspection of the palate is facilitated by extension of the head. The child is asked to say the familiar "ah," providing an opportunity to evaluate the neuromuscular function of the palate (cranial nerves nine and ten). The careful palate examination may detect a bifid uvula, asymmetrical retraction, or palatomaxillary deformity such as a high-arched palate, torus palatini, or cleft palate. Anesthesia of the palate can be a sign of a destructive process involving the fifth cranial nerve at the foramen rotundum.

Inspection of the oropharynx is facilitated by depression of the tongue inferiorly and anteriorly. Care should be taken to place the tongue blade on the anterior two-thirds of the tongue to avoid the gag reflex. With this maneuver the posterior border of the palate, uvula, tonsils, and posterior pharyngeal wall

can be seen. Tonsillar symmetry as well as surface appearance can be assessed. Care should be taken to place the child's head in the midline position because head turning tenses the parapharyngeal muscles on the same side, displacing the tonsil medially. This may give a false impression of asymmetry, thus mimicking a unilateral tonsillar disease such as abscess or lymphoma (Fig. 40–5).

A complete examination of the oral cavity and pharynx includes palpation. Children usually accept palpation without difficulty, because their own fingers are familiar objects to their mouths. Palpation of the tongue with a gloved finger will offer valuable information about pathology deep within its substance (lymphangioma) or surface anomalies (median rhomboid glossitis) (Fig. 40–6). Palpation of the palate is essential to detect submucous clefts; palpation of the posterior

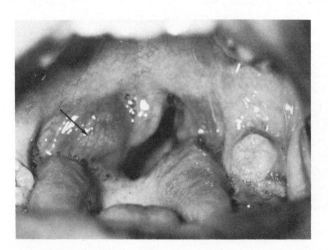

Figure 40–5 Lymphoma of the tonsil (arrow) presenting as tonsillar asymmetry.

third of the tongue may reveal a lingual thyroid.

Bimanual palpation with a finger in the oral cavity and the opposite hand against the cheek permits evaluation of the quality and size of the parotid and submandibular salivary glands. Massage of the gland toward the duct orifice will usually cause clear fluid to flow. A cloudy or sandy suspension is evidence of stasis and usually of inflammation. Salivary fluid can be collected, cultured, and examined microscopically. Immunoelectrophoresis may detect a rare secretory immunoglobulin deficiency. The rate of submandibular salivary flow may also be used to assess salivary disease or salivary gland innervation. Cannulation of the submandibular ducts (rarely done in the unanesthetized child under six years of age) permits evaluation of salivary flow on each side independently. Decreased flow is thought to be an early sign of neuronal degeneration in traumatic and idiopathic facial paralysis (May and Harvey, 1971). Scintillation sialography may also help in evaluating salivary gland disease (Cummings et al., 1971). The sensitivity of the anterior two-thirds of the tongue to taste stimuli (seventh cranial nerve function) may be assessed by chemical and electrical means; however, lack of good clinical correlation with disease states makes these tests of questionable value (Alford et al., 1974). Biopsy specimens of the oral cavity and oropharynx may be obtained with local anesthesia in the cooperative child, but general anesthesia may be required for young children.

Since the oral cavity and oropharynx are accessible to examination by direct visualization and palpation, radiographic techniques are seldom used in their evaluation. However, a lateral neck radiograph permits evaluation of the base of the tongue, and radioisotopic scanning with iodine[131] is also used when a lingual thyroid is suspected. Contrast cineradiography may outline masses or foreign bodies and can be used to assess the oropharyngeal phases of deglutition. While spot radiographs of the palate may be helpful in assessing velopharyngeal competence, cineradiography probably provides the most useful information. The dynamic evaluation of cineradiography in the lateral and base projections during phonation is of great value in assessing movement of both the palate and the lateral pharyngeal walls, and provides a permanent record of function to guide therapeutic intervention.

NASOPHARYNX

Examination of the nasopharynx is most frequently accomplished by indirect visualization. Several techniques have been developed; the one most often used employs a nasopharyngeal mirror held behind the palate while the tongue is displaced downward with a tongue blade (Fig. 40–7). A strong head light or head mirror is required to visualize the nasopharyngeal structures. With the mirror, the eustachian tube, adenoids, posterior nasal septum, and posterior edges of the nasal turbinates can be seen. The examination is limited by the need to use a small mirror in children and by their occasionally poor cooperation during this part of the examination. However, many children over two years of age can be examined in this way.

Telescopic visualization of the nasopharynx with either a flexible (Fig. 40–8) or rigid (Fig. 40–9) instrument provides a panoramic view of the nasopharynx (Fig. 40–10) and may be done in the awake child (Ward et al., 1974). The rigid telescope is inserted into the mouth and advanced into the oropharynx (Fig. 40–11). Topical anesthesia is usually not

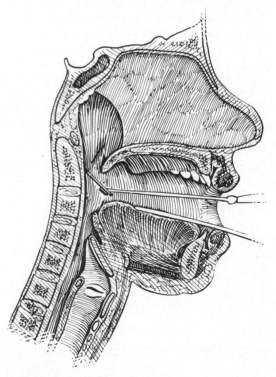

Figure 40–7 Indirect mirror examination of the nasopharynx is accomplished with the tongue depressed and a warmed mirror held posterior to the uvula.

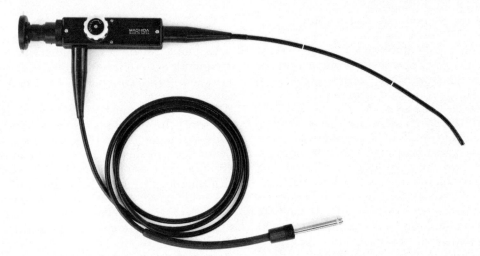

Figure 40–8   Flexible nasopharyngolaryngoscope (available from Machida America, Inc., Norwood, NJ).

necessary. The instrument may be rotated to look at the nasopharynx or hypopharynx, and biopsy specimens can be obtained under direct telescopic vision in cooperative children. The flexible telescope may be inserted into either the nose (Fig. 40–12) or the mouth. A topical anesthetic and vasoconstricting agent (such as cocaine) is usually necessary if the nasal route is selected. Still or cinephotography can be obtained with either of these instruments. In this way, progression or regression of disease can be documented on the patient's record. Teaching attachments are available for each instrument that enable several examiners to view the patient at the same time.

Direct examination of the nasopharynx may be made by utilizing some type of palate retraction. A palate retractor or small rubber catheters passed through the nose and mouth (Fig. 40–13) can be used to expose the nasopharynx. While older children may only need local or topical anesthesia for this, smaller children will usually require a general anesthetic.

Palpation of the nasopharynx is difficult and probably barbaric in the awake patient but provides valuable information and may be performed when the child is anesthetized. Assessment of the adenoids, choanae, and

eustachian tube region as well as visualization of tumors arising in or extending into the nasopharynx can be made. A biopsy specimen from the nasopharynx may be obtained through the nose or the mouth.

Radiographic techniques play a large role in the evaluation of the nasopharynx. Lateral neck radiographs (Fig. 40–14), xeroradiography, and polytomography may all give extensive information about this relatively inaccessible area. Recently, computed tomography (CT) has added a new dimension to examination of the nasopharynx. CT provides information regarding the size, location, and extension of nasopharyngeal masses near the base of the skull (Fig. 40–15). Intracranial communications such as nasopharyngeal encephaloceles may be detected by CT, and contrast injection may show a vascular tumor as an enhanced area of uptake. Arteriography, however, is still required to define the specific blood supply of such a tumor prior to instituting therapy.

Contrast radiography is occasionally used to outline the nasopharynx, to evaluate nasopharyngeal stenosis following adenoidectomy, or to diagnose choanal atresia (Fig. 40–16). Reflux of radiopaque material into the eustachian tube orifice has been used to evaluate tube patency and function, but its

Text continued on page 890

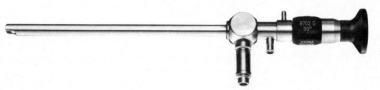

Figure 40–9   Berci-Ward indirect laryngonasopharyngoscope (rigid). (Available from Karl Storz Endoscopy-America, Inc., Los Angeles, CA.)

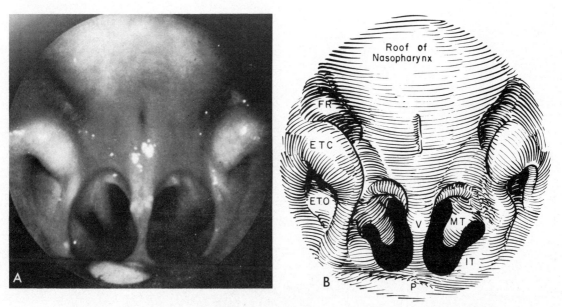

Figure 40–10 *A*, Panoramic view of nasopharynx is obtained by fiberoptic telescope. *B*, FR, fossa of Rosenmuller; ETC, eustachian tube cushion; ETO, eustachian tube orifice; V, vomer; MT, middle turbinate; IT, inferior turbinate; P, palate.

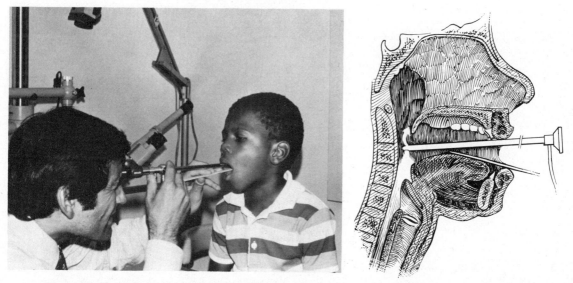

Figure 40–10 *A*, Panoramic view of nasopharynx is obtained by Berci-Ward telescope. *B*, FR, fossa of the nasopharynx or the hypopharynx.

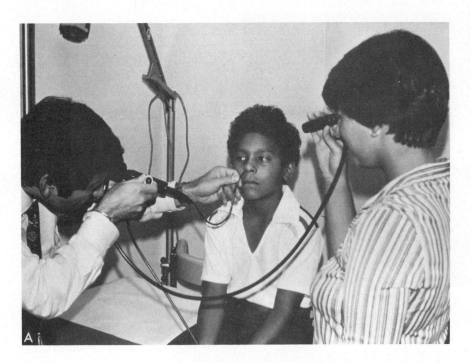

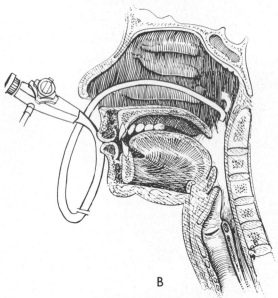

Figure 40–12.   Flexible nasopharyngolaryngoscope can be inserted into the nose (as pictured) or into the mouth. The distal tip can be deflected to view the nasopharynx or the larynx. Teaching attachment allows an additional person to examine the patient.

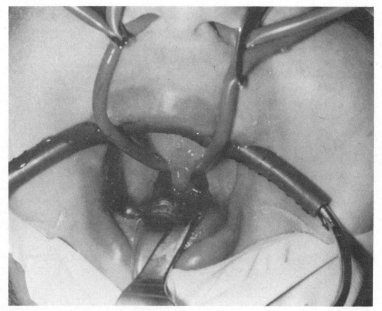

Figure 40–13 Rubber catheters in place retracting the palate to allow visualization of the nasopharynx.

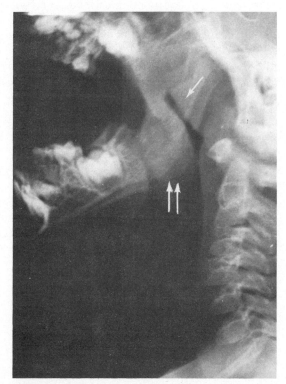

Figure 40–14 Lateral neck radiograph demonstrating enlarged adenoid pad (arrow) and tonsils (double arrows).

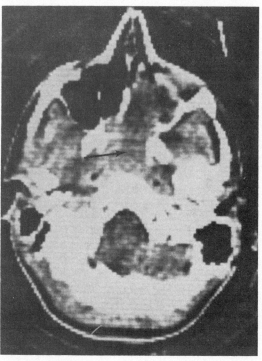

Figure 40–15 CT scan of angiofibroma of nasopharynx (arrow) with extension into the nasal cavity and right maxillary sinus.

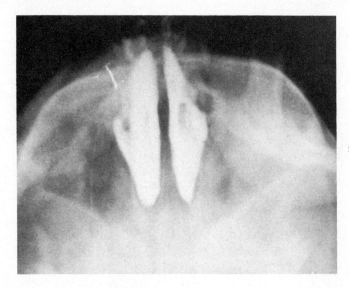

Figure 40–16　Contrast study demonstrating bilateral choanal atresia.

HYPOPHARYNX

reliability and correlation with function is limited (Bluestone et al., 1972).

Indirect examination of the hypopharynx is performed with a mirror held in the oropharynx above the tongue, while the tongue is held forward by the examiner's hand (Fig. 40–17). Telescopic visualization with either a rigid or a flexible telescope provides a panoramic view of the hypopharynx, allows for documentation by photography, and may be used with a side arm for teaching observation. Cinephotographic recording can also be done but is of more value in the evaluation of the larynx than of the hypopharynx.

Direct visualization of the hypopharynx is usually done in conjunction with direct laryngoscopy in the operating room. While this may be done with the patient restrained and without anesthesia in the neonate, general anesthesia is most often used as it allows for a complete examination of the hypopharynx and adjacent structures and also for the re-

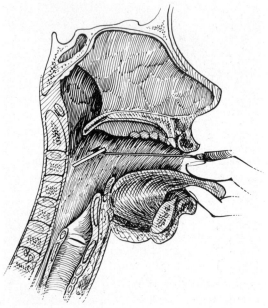

Figure 40–17　Indirect mirror examination of the hypopharynx is accomplished by retracting the tongue and placing a warmed mirror beneath the uvula.

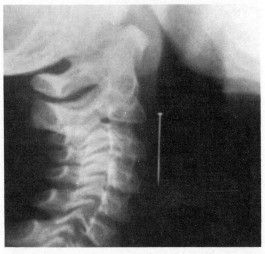

Figure 40–18　Lateral neck radiograph showing straight pin perforating the mucosa of the hypopharynx.

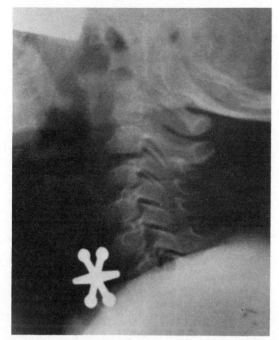

Figure 40–19 Lateral neck radiograph with foreign body obvious in the hypopharynx.

moval of biopsy specimens. Palpation of the hypopharynx should not be performed in the awake child, since this is very uncomfortable, and laryngeal structures can be injured or foreign bodies forced into the mucosa, with subsequent perforation (Fig. 40–18).

Radiographic evaluation is very useful, and lateral neck radiographs (Fig. 40–19), xeroradiography, and laminography, as well as CT, may yield valuable information. Contrast cineradiography may be especially helpful to demonstrate masses, neuromuscular dysfunction in deglutition, and reflux from the hypopharynx into the nasopharynx.

ESOPHAGUS

The definitive method of examination of the esophagus is esophagoscopy; however, radiography of the esophagus should precede endoscopic evaluation in nearly all cases, as the endoscopist is at a great advantage when he has radiographic studies to help determine the nature and location of the pathology to be evaluated. This is especially true in patients with esophageal foreign bodies, strictures, congenital anomalies, or surgically produced anatomic variations (e.g., colon interposition). Careful radiographic

evaluation prior to esophagoscopy can prevent serious complications such as esophageal perforation.

In the child, posterior-anterior neck and chest views are used to demonstrate the esophagus. These projections permit the evaluation of the esophagus in the neck and mediastinum as well as evaluation of its relationship to surrounding structures. In small children the entire length of the esophagus may be included in a single film. Radiopaque foreign bodies (Fig. 40–20), subcutaneous emphysema from perforation, and displacement of structures may be seen with plain films.

Contrast cineradiography of the esophagus is particularly valuable because the esophagus can be outlined easily with varying thicknesses of barium. This allows for the evaluation of the mucosa, outlining of intrinsic masses, and demonstration of compression by external masses (Fig. 40–21). The barium examination is well accepted by children, and the young child will frequently drink the contrast medium from a bottle quite readily.

The esophagram is performed with the child in the prone position and with a slight rotation of the body to the right. In this manner, the transit time of the contrast medium is slowed to allow a careful assessment of motility as the esophagus is projected away from the overlying vertebral column. The

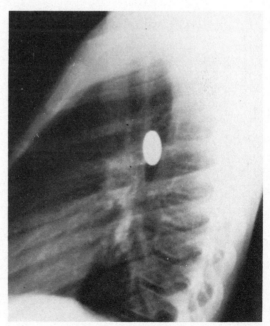

Figure 40–20 Chest radiograph demonstrating foreign body in the thoracic esophagus.

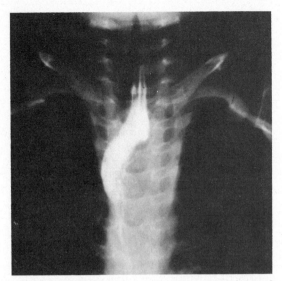

Figure 40–21 Contrast study showing extraluminal compression of esophagus.

normal esophagus has five areas of constriction where foreign bodies can become lodged. Most foreign bodies come to rest at the cricopharyngeal area (C6) or in the hiatal region (T10–T11). Other narrowed regions occur at the thoracic inlet (T1), the aortic arch (T4), and the tracheal bifurcation (T6), where the left main bronchus crosses the esophagus (Fig. 40–22) (Atkins and Atkins, 1974). Abnormal strictures may be seen following esophageal surgery, especially after repaired esophageal atresia (Fig. 40–23). These patients are particularly prone to food impaction at the site of stricture. The stricture may be improved by esophageal dilation (Fig. 40–24) under direct vision with an esophageal dilator.

Cinefluoroscopy using barium provides a qualitative evaluation of the neuromuscular function of the esophagus and should be

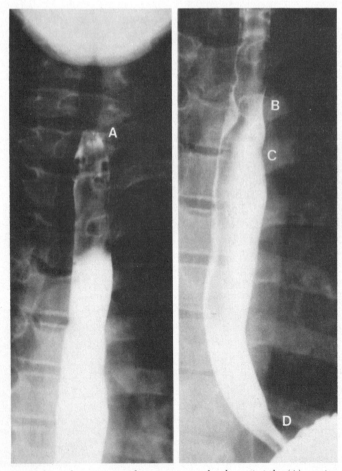

Figure 40–22 Normal esophagogram with narrowing at the thoracic inlet (A), aortic arch (B), take-off of left mainstem bronchus (C), and gastroesophageal junction (D).

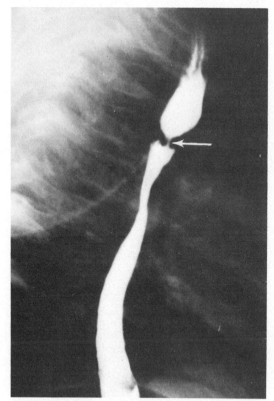

Figure 40-23 Esophageal stricture (arrow) following repair of esophageal atresia.

performed in all patients with suspected esophageal disease. The serial pictures also provide a permanent record to follow the progress of disease and therapeutic responses. When a clinical history of aspiration suggests a communication between the esophagus and the respiratory tract, water-miscible contrast material should be used. Quantitative evaluation of neuromuscular-esophageal function must be made by esophageal manometry.

Esophagoscopy in children is almost always carried out in the operating room under general anesthesia, when muscle relaxants may be used to decrease the risk of esophageal perforation. In the neonate, the procedure may be performed without anesthesia, but this does not always permit an adequate or safe examination of the esophagus. Lack of esophageal relaxation increases the risk of perforation, and the tracheal lumen may be compressed by the pressure of the esophagoscope against the cartilage-free common wall between the esophagus and trachea. In addition, the infant must be restrained securely to prevent musculoskeletal injury. Local anesthesia is not often used for esophagoscopy in

children, as their greater sensitivity to the toxicity of the local anesthetic agents makes this method potentially dangerous. However, if one elects to use a local anesthetic, the pharynx may be sprayed with small amounts of a topical agent such as lidocaine or tetracaine. As the child swallows, topical anesthesia of the oral cavity, pharynx, and esophagus is obtained (Snow, 1977).

Esophagoscopy should be performed after a sufficient period of fasting (usually eight hours) to insure an empty stomach, thereby decreasing the chance of aspiration.

Two types of esophagoscopes are presently available: a rigid (Fig. 40–25) and a flexible (Fig. 40–26) instrument. Both are available in sizes appropriate for pediatric patients, utilize fiberoptic light sources, and have teaching attachments available. If the flexible instrument is chosen, the patient is placed supine on the operating room table. A lubricating agent such as mineral oil is applied to the shaft of the endoscope. The instrument is inserted into the oral cavity and advanced

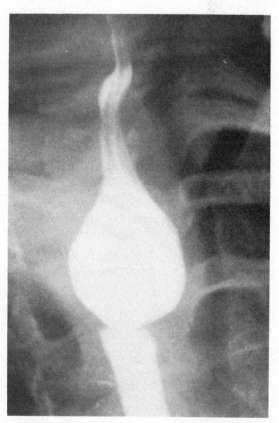

Figure 40–24 Esophageal stricture (same patient as Fig. 40–23) improved after multiple endoscopic dilatations.

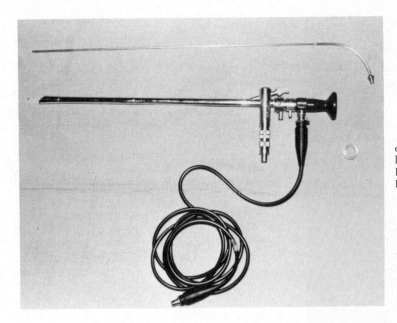

Figure 40–25 Rigid, open-end esophagoscope (with Hopkins rod lens telescope). (Available from Karl Storz Endoscopy-America, Inc., Los Angeles, CA.)

while the examiner observes through the eyepiece (Fig. 40–27). The advancing end of the esophagoscope may be deflected in any direction to facilitate passage through the cricopharyngeus muscle and advancement through the esophageal lumen. Air is insufflated through one of the channels to balloon the esophagus out in front of the advancing esophagoscope. The whole esophagus may be examined, as well as the stomach, if desired. Aspiration and biopsy can be performed through this esophagoscope; however, the size of the operating channel may limit the adequacy of the tissue obtained.

Similarly, the retrieval of foreign bodies using this instrument may be hampered by the size of the forceps. In addition, the foreign body cannot be drawn up into the esophagoscope (as can be done in the rigid open esophagoscope) to protect the esophageal mucosa as the instrument and foreign body are withdrawn.

For esophagoscopy utilizing the rigid esophagoscope, the patient is placed supine on the operating table with a large towel rolled under his shoulder or with his head extending over the edge of the table (Fig. 40–28). This permits the complete freedom

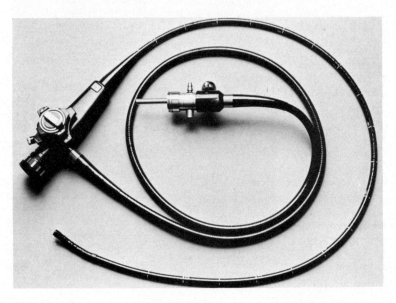

Figure 40–26 Nine mm gastrointestinal fiberscope. (Available from Olympus Corp., New Hyde Park, NY.)

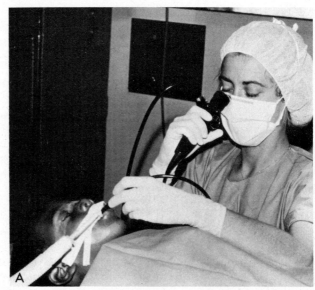

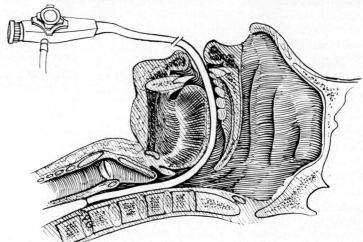

Figure 40–27 Flexible esophagoscope is inserted into the mouth and advanced through the esophagus while controlling the deflection of the distal tip.

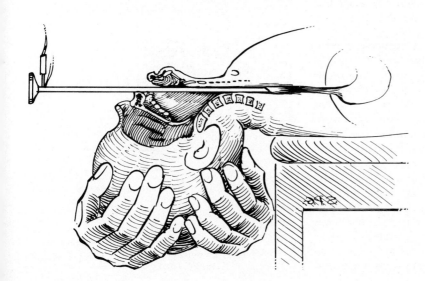

Figure 40–28. The rigid esophagoscope is inserted as the child's head position is controlled by the assistant.

of movement of the patient's head that is necessary for proper introduction and advancement of the instrument. The assistant holds the head extended and the neck flexed, thus placing the oral cavity and the esophageal inlet in a straight, almost vertical line. The patient's mouth is opened by the endoscopist's left hand and a moistened gauze sponge is placed over the upper lip and teeth to prevent them from being injured by the esophagoscope. The proximal end of the instrument is grasped like a pencil with the right hand. The esophagoscope (with its distal shaft lubricated) is held almost vertically and inserted into the mouth on the right side, displacing the tongue to the left. The left hand is held near the patient's mouth to steady and support the instrument while separating the patient's lips and teeth from the esophagoscope. The esophagoscope is advanced slowly and carefully while the oropharyngeal structures are visualized in a sequential fashion. As the epiglottis is visualized in the hypopharynx, the esophagoscope is moved to the midline. The head is gently lowered to the same level as the rest of the body, and the flared and beveled edge of the tip of the esophagoscope is placed posterior to the cricoid cartilage. The thumb of the left hand applies gentle pressure anteriorly to permit opening of the cricopharyngeus muscle and entry into the esophagus. It is at this site that perforation of the esophagus most commonly occurs. If passage of the instrument is difficult, a soft filiform dilator or lumen finder may be inserted through the esophagoscope and into the esophagus. The esophagoscope is then advanced following the dilator under direct vision. If a cuffed endotracheal tube is used, the balloon should be deflated briefly to permit passage. Air may be insufflated to balloon the mucosa out in front of the esophagoscope and to aid in identifying the lumen. The esophagoscope is never advanced unless the lumen is in view. The instrument is gently advanced, never forced, through the thoracic esophagus and, in some patients, into the cardia of the stomach. Since the distal esophagus turns to the left and anteriorly before entering the stomach, the patient's head and shoulders must be lowered below the rest of the body and the the head turned slightly to the right to allow the esophagoscope to enter the stomach. As the stomach is entered, gastric juice and rugal folds are seen in the lumen of the tube. The esophagus is examined again as the esophagoscope is withdrawn. Aspiration, biopsy, and retrieval of foreign bodies can be performed through the open esophagoscope with a variety of special instruments (Chap. 56).

After esophagoscopy, the patient is maintained on intravenous fluids for eight hours and observed for signs of esophageal perforation. Fever, chest or back pain, cervical emphysema, and leukocytosis can all signal the complication of esophageal perforation with cervical or mediastinal involvement. If perforation is suspected, the diagnosis may be confirmed by chest and neck radiographs that demonstrate cervical emphysema, pneumomediastinum, or pleural effusion. The site of the perforation may be localized by having the patient swallow a water-miscible, radiopaque dye. Small, cervical perforations without large tracts or pockets respond well to restricted oral intake and intravenous antibiotics. Larger tears and gross mediastinal involvement may require surgical drainage. The catastrophe of esophageal perforation is best prevented by careful and cautious esophagoscopy. However, if perforation does occur, prompt recognition and treatment are key factors in preventing the significant morbidity and mortality that can accompany this complication.

CONCLUSION

The examination of the oral cavity, pharynx, and esophagus utilizes basic physical diagnostic techniques, radiography, endoscopy, and a variety of other maneuvers to identify disease states. Proper evaluation of these areas requires the physician to be skilled both in the performance of these methods of examination and in the interpretation of their results.

SELECTED REFERENCES

Becker, W., Buckingham, R., Holinger, P., et al. 1970. Atlas of Otorhinolaryngology and Bronchoesophagology. Philadelphia, W. B. Saunders Co.
  Excellent pictorial presentation of disease states of the aerodigestive tract.

Snow, J. 1977. Esophagology. In Ballinger, J. J. (Ed.): Diseases of the Nose, Throat and Ear, 12th ed. Philadelphia, Lea and Febiger.
  Excellent, concise treatise on all aspects of esophagology.

Ward, P., Berci, G., and Calcaterra, T. 1974. Advances in endoscopic examination of the respiratory system. Ann. Otol. Rhinol. Laryngol., *83*:754.

Good description of the recent advances. Historical background as well as the physics of the new systems are well explained.

REFERENCES

Alford, B., Jerger, J., Coats, A., et al. 1974. Diagnostic tests of facial nerve function. Otolaryngol Clin North Am, 7(2):331–342.

Atkins, J. P., Sr., and Atkins, J. P., Jr. 1974. *In* English, G. M. (Ed.) Otolaryngology, Vol. 5, Chap. 1. New York, Harper and Row, Inc.

Becker, W., Buckingham, R., Holinger, P., et al. 1970. Atlas of Otorhinolaryngology and Bronchoesophagology, Philadelphia, W. B. Saunders Co.

Bluestone, C., Wittel, R., Paradise, J., et al. 1972. Eustachian tube function as related to adenoidectomy for otitis media. Trans. Amer. Acad. Ophthalmol. Otolaryngol., 76:1325–1339.

Cummings, N., Schall, G., Asofsky, R., et al. 1971 Sjögren's syndrome — newer aspects of research, diagnosis and therapy. Ann. Int. Med., 75:937–950.

May, M., and Harvey, J. 1971. Salivary flow: A prognostic test for facial paralysis. Laryngoscope, 81:179–182.

Snow, J. 1977. Esophagology. *In* Ballinger, J. J. (Ed.): Diseases of the Nose, Throat and Ear, 12th ed. Philadelphia, Lea and Febiger.

Ward, P., Berci, G., and Calcaterra, T. 1974. Advances in endoscopic examination of the respiratory system. Ann. Otol. Rhinol. Laryngol., 83:754.

Chapter 41

SORE THROAT IN CHILDHOOD: DIAGNOSIS AND MANAGEMENT

David W. Teele, M.D.

Infections of the upper respiratory tract account for a majority of visits for illness to any pediatrician's office. Children from one to ten years old experience an average of between five and eight such infections each year (Badger et al., 1953). Since many of these infections include inflammation of the pharynx, the frequency of the complaint of sore throat demands a rational, expeditious approach to diagnosis and management. This chapter will suggest a plan for diagnosis and management of illnesses of childhood characterized chiefly by sore throat. Inflammatory diseases of the pharynx are discussed in detail in Chapter 47.

PRINCIPLES AND GOALS

Most children complaining of sore throat have a self-limited, presumably infectious illness for which there is now no effective therapy (Dingle et al., 1953; Glezen et al., 1967; Kaplan et al., 1971; Moffet et al., 1968). Only infections of the pharynx due to *Corynebacterium diphtheriae*, *Neisseria gonorrhoeae*, and *Streptococcus pyogenes* (group A) have significant morbidity and are susceptible to antimicrobial therapy. These organisms cause a minority of cases of pharyngitis. Some serious illnesses may have a sore throat as a prominent symptom; illnesses as uncommon as tularemia (Tyson, 1976) may present as pharyngitis.

Goals for the practitioner should include exclusion of serious illness presenting as simple pharyngitis; diagnosis of and therapy for those infections due to *C. diphtheriae*, *N. gonorrhoeae*, and *S. pyogenes* (group A); and provision of relief for those illnesses not susceptible to antimicrobial therapy.

The practitioner must take a history guided by knowledge of illnesses currently prevalent in the community; for example, streptococcal infections are common in some communities (Zimmerman et al., 1962) or populations (Wannamaker, 1972) and relatively uncommon in others (Dingle et al., 1953). Additionally, the practitioner should seek a history of similar illnesses in members of the household as well as any past rheumatic fever in either patient or household member.

While examining the patient, the practitioner should search carefully for stigmata of past rheumatic fever and for findings suggestive of systemic illnesses, which may include pharyngitis; for example, splenomegaly may be a clue to the diagnosis of infectious mononucleosis. Examination of the pharynx must include the entire pharynx and related structures. Thus, examination should reveal both generalized illnesses with an element of pharyngitis and those conditions, such as peritonsillar abscess, requiring immediate therapy.

DIAGNOSTIC METHODS

No physician, however astute, should rely upon history and physical examination alone to determine the cause of a sore throat. Except perhaps during epidemic disease, even the most experienced physician is unable to diagnose accurately streptococcal pharyngitis (Wannamaker, 1972). The microbiologic diagnosis of the cause of a sore throat is made best by culturing oropharyngeal secretions. Most such cultures are taken in an attempt to diagnose infections due to group A streptococci. Many guidelines have been proposed to reduce the numbers of cultures taken; all such guidelines are imperfect. Honikman and Massell (1971) suggested guidelines that would diagnose in a population of 5 to 16 year old children 88.1 per cent of symptomatic streptococcal infections capable of causing rheumatic fever. They suggested taking a culture from the throat of any child with either an illness characterized purely or predominantly by sore throat and an oral temperature greater than or equal to 37.3° C or any other illness with an oral temperature of 38.3° C or above. Patterns of infection, however, may vary from one community to another. Additionally, streptococcal infection in young children may present somewhat differently. Group A streptococci appear to cause rather uncommonly exudative pharyngitis in children aged less than three years (Alpert et al., 1966; Kaplan et al., 1971). Young infants may have a syndrome caused by group A streptococci that includes an indolent course, low fever, persistent nasal discharge, and excoriations at the nares.

Cultures from the oropharynx should be taken with a dry, cotton-tipped swab which is passed over both posterior pharyngeal wall and tonsils (or tonsillar beds). A single such culture will detect approximately 90 percent of children infected with group A streptococci (Kaplan et al., 1971).

When the practitioner suspects either diphtheritic or gonococcal infection, the microbiology laboratory must be alerted, as routine processing of oropharyngeal cultures will not detect most infections due to *C. diphtheriae* and *N. gonorrhoeae*. Diagnosis and management of these infections is discussed in Chapter 47.

Serologic methods have been used to determine the cause of pharyngitis and have proved useful in epidemiologic investigations. These methods cannot be used to guide antimicrobial therapy for suspected or proved streptococcal infections. Children colonized with group A streptococci may have preexisting antibodies, such as antistreptolysin O (ASO), but the titer does not rise. Once a rise occurs, the child is at risk for rheumatic fever, and antimicrobial therapy is of little use (Catanzaro et al., 1954). Thus, serologic methods cannot determine which child harboring group A streptococci requires antimicrobial therapy.

Rapid, inexpensive tests are available to diagnose infectious mononucleosis: the Monophile (Bio-Diagnostic Systems Industry, Plainsboro, NJ) and others (Hoff, 1965). Assays for antibodies against other viral agents known to cause pharyngitis require both acute and convalescent specimens, and, as no antiviral therapy is currently available, their use is limited to epidemiologic investigations.

Other diagnostic procedures, such as determination of the white blood cell count (Zimmerman et al., 1962) and C-reactive protein (Moffet et al., 1968), have not been useful in distinguishing infections of the pharynx due to group A streptococci from infections due to other microorganisms.

THERAPY

Symptomatic therapy is appropriate for most patients with much discomfort. Aspirin and acetaminophen appear to be most effective; each is an analgesic and antipyretic. These drugs are equally effective as antipyretics (Tarlin et al., 1972). Other therapies, such as lozenges and gargles, are of uncertain efficacy, and their use should be restricted to teenagers and adults who believe that these agents produce important relief.

Antimicrobial therapy is required and useful only for pharyngitis due to group A streptococci, *C. diphtheriae*, and *N. gonorrhoeae*. Therapy for the latter two infections is discussed in Chapter 47.

Some principles to guide therapy for streptococcal pharyngitis follow.

1. The vast majority of pharyngitides are not due to group A streptococci, and no physician can diagnose accurately those that are without a culture from the patient's oropharynx (Wannamaker, 1972).

2. Suppurative complications of streptococcal pharyngitis are uncommon; the primary goal of antimicrobial therapy is to prevent rheumatic fever. This complica-

tion may be averted in most cases if therapy with appropriate antimicrobial agents is started within nine days after onset of illness (Catanzaro et al., 1954; Siegel et al., 1961). No data exist to show that therapy at any time will prevent the development of poststreptococcal glomerulonephritis (Weinstein and LeFrock, 1971).

3. The natural history of streptococcal pharyngitis (Moffet et al., 1964) together with a comparison of the efficacy of therapy with either placebo or penicillin G (Denny, 1953) suggest that antimicrobial therapy may have only a limited effect on the signs and symptoms.

4. No test is currently available to select at first visit those children infected with group A streptococci who are or who will be at risk for rheumatic fever.

5. Children who have had rheumatic fever are likely to relapse if infected again with group A streptococci; such relapses can usually be prevented with appropriate antimicrobial therapy (Kuttner and Reyersbach, 1943).

6. Oral antimicrobial therapy must be given for 10 days to eradicate group A streptococci and to prevent rheumatic fever (Stollerman, 1954).

7. Most studies of compliance with regimens requiring administration of medications for 10 days show that many patients will not complete therapy (Charney et al., 1967).

8. Many physicians (especially those who prescribe oral antimicrobial agents), upon completion of 10 days of therapy,

obtain a second culture from the throat. Additional therapy is required for those children who are still infected with group A streptococci.

These principles suggest that there are but few indications for prescribing antimicrobial agents for children with sore throat prior to knowledge of results of culture. Such presumptive therapy should be restricted to those children with suppurative complications, such as otitis media or pneumonia, or with a past history of rheumatic fever or with household members who have had rheumatic fever. Antimicrobial therapy not guided by results of cultures is destined unnecessarily to expose large numbers of children to expensive and potentially toxic agents.

Few antimicrobial agents have been shown both to eliminate group A streptococci from the pharynx and to prevent rheumatic fever. Since its use avoids problems of compliance, the drug of choice is benzathine penicillin G given as a single intramuscular dose. Acceptable alternatives include oral administration of buffered penicillin G, penicillin V (phenoxymethyl penicillin), and erythromycin. Each of these latter agents must be given for 10 days, and their efficacy is reduced markedly by the poor compliance of many patients. Table 41–1 shows the dose for each agent (Kaplan et al., 1977).

Antimicrobial agents that are unacceptable for the treatment of pharyngitis due to group A streptococci include tetracyclines (owing to staining of teeth and the existence of many resistant strains of streptococci) (Kensit, 1977) and sulfa compounds, which do not reduce the attack rate of rheumatic fever

Table 41–1   THERAPY FOR PHARYNGITIS DUE TO GROUP A STREPTOCOCCI

Agent	Dose
Drug of choice	
Benzathine penicillin G°	For children weighing <60 lb
	600,000 units, intramuscularly, once
	For children weighing >60 lb
	1,200,000 units, intramuscularly, once
Acceptable alternatives	
Buffered penicillin G†	200,000 to 250,000 units, by mouth, four times daily for 10 days
Penicillin V (phenoxymethyl penicillin)	200,000 to 250,000 units, by mouth, four times daily for 10 days
Erythromycin§	40 mg per kg per day given daily, by mouth in divided doses for 10 days

°Preparations containing both procaine penicillin G and benzathine penicillin G should not be used unless they contain benzathine penicillin G in the dose listed.
†Least expensive of oral agents
§Drug of choice for patients allergic to penicillin

(Catanzaro, 1954), and trimethoprim-sulfamethoxazole. Other agents, including some cephalosporins and clindamycin, can eliminate group A streptococci from the pharynx and hence — presumably — can prevent rheumatic fever. However, none actually has been shown to prevent rheumatic fever. Each of these agents is likely to be more expensive and more toxic than either penicillin or erythromycin.

In summary, children with sore throats should have cultures obtained from the oropharynx according to the suggested guidelines. In the absence of suppurative complications or signs suggesting serious systemic illness masquerading as simple pharyngitis, such children should be given only therapy for discomfort. Antimicrobial therapy should be withheld pending results of culture.

Certain children complain of recurrent sore throat. These few children account for a disproportionately large share of diagnostic problems. The physician should remember that children have many (up to 10) upper respiratory infections each year and that a sore throat may be part of many of these infections. Thus, the physician must first decide if the child truly has an unusual number of sore throats. Additionally, the child's history of prior sore throats may be misleading, and the physician must be confident of the true frequency of pharyngitis. Finally, few episodes of pharyngitis produce any permanent sequelae. Nonetheless, some children do have recurrent pharyngitis without apparent explanation. Cultures from these children's throats usually yield no streptococci. These children present a peculiarly perplexing problem.

Physicians have marshalled a wide variety of explanations for recurrent sore throat, including allergy, low humidity, mouth breathing, chronic adenoiditis, passive or active smoking, and polluted air. Currently none of these can be incriminated with certainty. Simple, inexpensive, and safe remedies should be tried to relieve discomfort, e.g., increasing humidity in the child's bedroom or eliminating smoking, but more vigorous therapy, such as tonsillectomy, chronic use of antimicrobial agents, or evaluations for allergies, should be withheld until data become available supporting their usefulness. Tonsillectomy, in particular, must be viewed with suspicion until results are available from a current prospective study of its utility.

SELECTED REFERENCE

Wannamaker, L. W. 1972. Perplexity and precision in the diagnosis of streptococcal pharyngitis. Am. J. Dis. Child, *124*:352.

  Wannamaker has written a superb summary of present knowledge of pharyngitis due to group A streptococci. He has skillfully outlined the vexing problems posed by a disease about which we believe we know so much.

REFERENCES

Alpert, J. J., Pickering, M. R., and Warren, R. J. 1966. Failure to isolate streptococci from children under the age of 3 years with exudative tonsillitis. Pediatrics, *38*:663.

Badger, G. F., Dingle, J. H., Feller, A. E., et al. 1953. A study of illness in a group of Cleveland families. II. Incidence of the common respiratory diseases. Am. J. Hyg., *58*:31.

Catanzaro, F. J., Stetson, C. A., Morris, A. J., et al. 1954. The role of the streptococcus in the pathogenesis of rheumatic fever. Am. J. Med. *17*:749.

Charney, E., Bynum, R., Eldredge, D., et al. 1967. How well do patients take oral penicillin? A collaborative study in private practice. Pediatrics, *40*:188.

Denny, F. W., Wannamaker, L. W., and Hahn, E. O. 1953. Comparative effects of penicillin, aureomycin and terramycin on streptococcal tonsillitis and pharyngitis. Pediatrics, *11*:7.

Dingle, J. H., Badger, G. F., Feller, A. E., et al. 1953. A study of illness in a group of Cleveland families. I. Plan of study and certain general observations. Am. J. Hyg., *58*:16.

Glezen W. P., Clyde, W. A., Jr., Senior, R. J., et al. 1967. Group A streptococci, mycoplasmas, and viruses associated with acute pharyngitis. J.A.M.A., *202*:119

Hoff, G., and Bauer, S. 1965. A new rapid slide test for infectious mononucleosis. J.A.M.A., *194*:351.

Honikman, L. H., and Massell, B. F. 1971. Guidelines for the selective use of throat cultures in the diagnosis of streptococcal respiratory infection. Pediatrics, *48*:573.

Kaplan, E. L., Bisno, A., Derrick, W., et al. 1977. Prevention of rheumatic fever. Circulation, *55*:1.

Kaplan, E. L., Top, F. H., Jr., Dudding, B. A., et al. 1971. Diagnosis of streptococcal pharyngitis: differentiation of active infection from the carrier state in the symptomatic child. J. Infect. Dis., *123*:490.

Kensit, J., Farrell, W., Evans, S., et al. 1977. Tetracycline resistance in pneumococci and group A streptococci. Report of an ad-hoc study group on antibiotic resistance. Br. Med. J., *1*:131.

Kuttner, A. G., and Reyersbach, G. 1943. The prevention of streptococcal upper respiratory infections and rheumatic recurrences in rheumatic children by the prophylactic use of sulfanilamide. J. Clin. Invest., *22*:77.

Moffet, H. L., Siegel, A. C., and Doyle, H. K. 1968. Nonstreptococcal pharyngitis. J. Pediatr., *73*:51.

Moffet, H. L., Cramblett, H. G., and Smith, A. 1964. Group A streptococcal infections in a children's home. II. Clinical and epidemiologic patterns of illness. Pediatrics, *33*:11.

Siegel, A. C., Johnson, E. E., and Stollerman, G. H. 1961.

Controlled studies of streptococcal pharyngitis in a pediatric population. 1. Factors related to the attack rate of rheumatic fever. N. Engl. J. Med. *265*:559.

Stollerman, G. H. 1954. The use of antibiotics for the prevention of rheumatic fever. Am. J. Med., *17*:757.

Tarlin, L., Landrigan, P., Babineau, R., et al. 1972. A comparison of the antipyretic effect of acetaminophen and aspirin. Am. J. Dis. Child., *124*:881.

Tyson, H. K. 1976. Tularemia: an unappreciated cause of exudative pharyngitis. Pediatrics, *58*:864.

Wannamaker, L. W. 1972. Perplexity and precision in the diagnosis of streptococcal pharyngitis. Am. J. Dis. Child., *124*:352.

Weinstein, L., and LeFrock, J. 1971. Does antimicrobial therapy of streptococcal pharyngitis or pyoderma alter the risk of glomerulonephritis? J. Infect. Dis., *124*:229.

Zimmerman, R. A., Siegel, A. C., and Steele, C. P. 1962. An epidemiological investigation of a streptococcal and rheumatic fever epidemic in Dickinson, North Dakota. Pediatrics, *30*:712.

Chapter 42

DIFFICULTY WITH SWALLOWING

Seymour R. Cohen, M.D.

INTRODUCTION

Difficulty with swallowing, or dysphagia, is defined as any defect in the intake or transport of endogenous secretions and nutriments necessary for the maintenance of life. Swallowing is the process by which food is transmitted to the stomach and digestive organs.

Understanding the swallowing mechanism in the neonate enhances the ease with which a differentiation of the etiology of dysphagia can be made in older children; therefore, the basis for discussion of dysphagia is the swallowing mechanism as seen in the neonate and infant.

Swallowing in the infant consists of three components: (1) the suck reflex, which is the delivery system and which includes the orobuccal phase of deglutition, (2) the collecting system, which is the oropharynx, and (3) the transport system, which is the esophagus (Bosma, 1972).

Different causes of dysphagia lead to varying symptoms, but the most serious problem is aspiration. Starvation is a delayed concomitant of the swallowing dysfunction, but aspiration and starvation will ultimately lead to death if not corrected. A normal, functioning swallowing mechanism is essential if the respiratory tract is to be spared contamination, and a normal functioning respiratory tract is necessary for normal deglutition. These facts are especially important to consider in dealing with the neonate and young infant. It is of interest to note that just as the respiratory and alimentary tracts arise from common embryologic origin, they remain dependent upon one another for normal function

throughout life. Defects of development common to both systems create functional problems of swallowing and of the maintenance of a normal airway.

The physician who is confronted by a child suffering from dysfunction of the swallowing mechanism is presented with a complex and often challenging problem. In some instances the dysphagia is temporary, being due either to immaturity or a temporary central nervous system aberration that spontaneously subsides. However, a relentless search for the cause is necessary in all cases in order to make a specific diagnosis so that medical management or surgical intervention may be instituted early and thus prevent serious complications. While searching for a specific cause of the swallowing problem, alternative methods of feeding the child, i.e., by nasogastric feeding tubes, gastrostomy, or hyperalimentation, may be necssary. The urgency to establish a diagnosis of difficulty in swallowing is enhanced by the fact that delay can lead to severe pulmonary disease. This is most likely to occur in the very young infant, in whom a poor cough mechanism leads to aspiration and bacterial contamination of the respiratory tract with obstruction of the airway and possible irreversible lung disease.

Dysphagia is almost always due to one or a combination of the factors listed in Table 42–1. Emotional problems, rumination, and failure to acquire normal patterns of intake and swallowing are excluded from this discussion. Table 42–2 gives a fuller outline of these problems, which are discussed at greater length later in this chapter.

The premature infant may be unable to take feedings normally, requiring assistance

Table 42–1 CLASSIFICATION OF ETIOLOGY OF DYSPHAGIA

Prematurity
Upper airway obstruction
Acquired anatomic defects
Congenital defects of larynx, trachea, and esophagus
Neuropathologic deficiencies

with both respiration and feedings (Gryboski, 1969). However, dysphagia due to prematurity is usually temporary and usually subsides with growth and development. During the neonatal period, however, alternative methods of feeding the premature infant (gavage, gastrostomy, or hyperalimentation) may be necessary. The premature infant with a weak suck reflex and who fatigues easily tends to aspirate and should not be fed by nipple. Respirations are paced with suckling in established feeding in a ratio of 1:1 or 1:2 (Halverson, 1944). Irregularities in timing are useful clues to immaturity or an acquired impairment of central neurologic regulation of feeding and respirations (Pieper, 1963).

The child with upper airway obstruction, whether nasal, oropharyngeal, or laryngeal, tends to have a poorly coordinated suck–breathe–swallow rhythm with consequent choking and aspiration and the subsequent development of lower airway disease. When the child with airway obstruction attempts to feed, he or she chokes, sputters, gasps, becomes stridorous, develops cyanosis, and may develop respiratory arrest.

The infant with airway obstruction usually has a normal arousal reflex and may suck eagerly, accept feedings, and swallow quite well for a very short period of time but will fatigue. Whereas maintenance of a patent nasal and nasopharyngeal airway is of utmost importance in the neonate and young infant, it becomes less important in older children. With severe nasal obstruction, such as is seen in bilateral choanal atresia, feeding is impossible, but when the airway obstruction is not severe the infant will feed well except when too eager or when fed too rapidly; however, fatigue will soon cause symptoms of aspiration (stridor, coughing, choking, and cyanosis).

The child with a congenital defect of the larynx, trachea, or esophagus usually has a normal arousal response, sucks eagerly and

---

Table 42–2. DIFFERENTIAL DIAGNOSIS IN DYSPHAGIA

I. **Prematurity**
   Usually infants of short gestation whose birth weight is less than 1500 gm
II. **Upper Airway Obstruction**
   A. Nasal and Nasopharyngeal
      Choanal atresia, stenosis, septal deflections, septal abscess, infections, tumors, and sinusitis
   B. Oropharynx
      Defects of lips and alveolar processes, cerebral palsy, hypopharyngeal stenosis, Pierre Robin syndrome, craniofacial defects, Crouzon or Treacher-Collins syndrome, microstomia, macrostomia (Goldenhar syndrome), and cleft palate
   C. Laryngeal
      Laryngoptosis, stenosis, clefts, and paralysis
III. **Congenital Defects of Larynx, Trachea, and Esophagus**
   A. Laryngotracheoesophageal cleft
   B. Tracheoesophageal fistula (H-type) with associated atresia
   C. Open paralysis of the larynx
   D. Esophageal anomalies, atresia, and strictures
   E. Vascular anomalies
      1. Aberrant right subclavian artery
      2. Double aortic arch
      3. Right aortic arch with left ligamentum
IV. **Acquired Anatomic Defects**
   A. Trauma

External, intubation, endoscopic, and foreign body
   B. Chemical ingestion
      Acids, alkalies, catalysts
   C. Tumors
V. **Neuropathologic Deficiencies**
   A. Central nervous system disease
      1. Head trauma
      2. Hypoxia and anoxia
      3. Cortical atrophy, hypoplasia, agenesis
      4. Infections (meningitis, brain abscess)
   B. Peripheral nervous system
      1. Trauma
      2. Congenital defects
   C. Neuromuscular
      1. Amyotonia (myotonic muscular dystrophy)
      2. Myasthenia gravis
      3. Guillain-Barré syndrome
      4. Poliomyelitis (bulbar paralysis)
   D. Anatomic defects
      1. Cricopharyngeal dysfunction
      2. Nonsphincteric esophageal spasm
      3. Chalasia
      4. Achalasia
      5. Riley-Day syndrome (dysautonomia)
      6. Paralysis of esophagus (atony)
      7. Associated atresia – tracheoesophageal fistula nerve defects

effectively, and has a normal suck–breathe–swallow rhythm. However, swallowing leads to gagging, choking, airway obstruction, and ultimately cyanosis. Stridor becomes prominent, and rales will be heard in the chest. A radiograph of the chest will show pneumonitis. The voice may be normal unless laryngeal clefts, webs, cysts, or adductor paralysis are present, and in some children the airway may be clear except for stridor that develops during and after feedings. If the airway and esophagus are both involved, as with the presence of vascular rings, bronchogenic cysts, or compression by a tumor, a to-and-fro stridor is aggravated by feedings. In some vascular abnormalities or compressive lesions, feeding in early infancy may be normal, but dysphagia develops when solid foods are added to the diet. In these cases esophageal obstruction or dysfunction produces vomiting, but this may also happen when severe coughing spasms due to aspiration occur during or soon after feedings.

The clinical picture in a child with an acquired anatomic defect varies with the site of the problem. When the lips, mouth, face, and oropharynx are involved, the suck reflex may be seriously impaired. When the lesion is in the larynx, trachea, or esophagus, dysphagia presents as described in the section discussing congenital lesions. In cases in which a foreign body or tumor causes obstruction, fluids may be tolerated without difficulty, yet solid foods may produce choking, vomiting, or both. In this category, the most important diagnostic factor will be the history of exposure to chemicals, foreign body ingestion, or intubation trauma. Dysphagia that starts with solid foods and progresses to difficulty with liquids suggests a contracting stricture, progressive obstruction by an enlarging tumor, or a collagen disease.

Neuropathologic deficiencies may create diagnostic problems in early infancy. Since the behavior of the infant at birth is largely a result of reflex activity, it is difficult to evaluate central nervous system development in the neonate (Potter, 1952). Dysphagia may be one of the earliest signs of a neurologic deficiency. The neurologically defective infant, particularly one with central nervous system disease, has poor suck and arousal reflexes and may show other evidence of neurologic disease, such as poor muscular tone, poor head support, and a poor gag reflex. Excessive saliva in the mouth or oropharynx and drooling are evidences of swallowing defects and are prominent symptoms in neurogenic dysphagia. As previously mentioned, there is a loss of the normal 1:1 or 1:2 suck-and-breathe ratio.

THE NORMAL SWALLOWING MECHANISM

To understand the causes and effects of the problem of dysphagia better, it is important to have a thorough knowledge of the normal swallowing pattern.

Swallowing is not new or unknown to the neonate; in the fetus it may start as early as the twelfth week of pregnancy (Davis and Potter, 1946). "Birth is only a stormy episode in what should otherwise be a smooth, continuous transition from aquatic to terrestrial life" (Brans, 1976). That swallowing and digestion may be important to fetal nutrition is suggested by the frequency of intrauterine growth retardation among fetuses who cannot swallow because of alimentary tract obstruction or neurologic damage (Wagner et al., 1968; Brans, 1976).

Approximately 5 ml per kg body weight per hour, or up to a total of 850 ml, are swallowed daily by the fetus (Pritchard, 1966). The normal infant has an arousal response when stimulated for feeding; with depression of the lower lip, the tongue comes forward (Ardran et al., 1972). This response will be found in normal infants unless they have been fed recently or are extremely fatigued and is most important in initiating feeding.

Sucking and swallowing are functions that are vital to the newborn infant (Gryboski, 1965). Both functions are established prenatally but are not fully developed until after birth. In the newborn suckling infant, respirations and swallowing are intimately related to function and rhythmicity (Warner, 1975). Swallowing inhibits respiration. Sucking is a purely reflexive process and acquires complexity and conscious control as other functions emerge and mature (Bosma, 1972). Suckling reflexly initiates swallowing in the infant. Bosma (1972) likens the tongue in infants to a piston within a cylinder. The tongue, lips, and mandible move synergistically as a composite motor organ (Warner, 1977). The mouth is solely concerned with suckling, approximating, and orienting the nipple it encloses (Bosma, 1972).

The mouth later acquires various new

functions, and the tongue, lips, and mandible achieve the independent functions of biting, chewing, moving food, and forming a bolus. All of these new functions demand that new motor patterns be learned. Sucking is a reflex initiated by stimulation of the lips and deeper parts of the oral cavity. The mandible and maxilla (upper gums, lip, palate, and cheeks) are all necessary for compression of the nipple and expression of its contents.

Any defect of the lips, tongue, palate, mandible, maxilla, or cheeks will create problems for the first phase of deglutition, the delivery system of swallowing (Logan et al., 1967); in older children this varies only by being manually delivered by nurse, parents, or self. While suckling reflexly initiates swallowing in the infant, the composite suckling and swallowing processes are subcortically controlled. As new oral skills such as biting and chewing enlist cortical levels for control, the initial phases of swallowing become voluntary. Successively acquired representations of the mouth are integrated with the maturing environmental orientation, intelligence, and motion of the growing child (Bosma, 1972).

The collecting system or buccopharyngeal phase of swallowing is under voluntary control (Cohen, 1955; Ardran and Kemp, 1970; Ardran et al., 1972; Bosma, 1972; Brans, 1976). Food is pushed onto the dorsum of the tongue by muscular action of the tongue and is rolled backwards to lie in front of the fauces. The oral, nasal, and laryngeal orifices are closed by lips, tongue, and soft palate as the larynx moves upward. The mylohyoid muscle contracts and presses the tongue against the hard palate. This movement pushes the bolus downward into the pharynx as the larynx returns to its normal position.

The buccopharyngeal phase occurs as a reflex reaction to stimulation of the sensory areas, which are scattered over the mucosa of the base of the tongue, the soft palate, and the posterior wall of the pharynx. Stimulation of the receptor organs by contact with oral contents causes afferent stimuli to be carried over the glossopharyngeal nerve, the second division of the fifth nerve, and the superior laryngeal nerve to the swallowing center in the floor of the fourth ventricle. Anesthetizing these receptors makes swallowing virtually impossible. Destruction of the central nerves by any neurologic disorder involving this area may result in difficulty with swallowing.

The esophageal phase follows reflexly with relaxation of the cricopharyngeal sphincter and the esophagus as a whole. Liquids drop immediately by gravity to the ampullary end, whereas solids pass by coordinated peristalsis, reaching the distal esophagus at the end of this phase. Even though liquids are thrown down the esophagus without regard to peristalsis, the peristaltic wave, which starts at the onset of the esophageal phase, continues in its usual manner. Peristalsis, at least over the lower two thirds of the esophagus, is an autonomous function of the esophagus initiated voluntarily in the pharynx and completed by the intrinsic myenteric plexus. The reflex continues to function normally even after all central nervous system connections are severed, as long as the intramural plexuses remain intact.

In humans, two types of peristaltic waves are noted. The primary wave travels without interruption towards the distal esophagus and is the propelling force for the bolus. It is initiated by the buccopharyngeal phase. The second peristaltic wave depends on intraesophageal distention for adequate stimulation. Studies suggest that the stimulation of the vagal nerves causes contraction of the circular muscle bundles and at the same time causes relaxation of the longitudinal muscle bundles. Stimulation of the sympathetic nerves produces just the opposite reaction.

The cardiogastric phase begins as swallowed material reaches the ampulla. Here there is a pause and a change in the rhythm as the closing mechanism of the esophagus, just proximal to the stomach, relaxes in quick periods to permit gushes of food to enter the stomach. At the cardia there appears to be a rhythmic mechanism for emptying of the ampulla. The diaphragm appears to have little or no control except that on deep inspiration there is a temporary slowing of the flow of food into the stomach.

There is a very fine correlation between normal peristaltic activity and the release of the closing mechanism at the cardia. The tone of the cardia is inhibited by mild stimulation of the gastric mucosa and by the sensory impulses arising in the mouth and the pharynx. This tone increases as digestion proceeds. Any local irritation at the cardia produces hypertonicity. The vagus nerve is responsible for degrees of tone at the cardia, at least in the normal, resting, terminal esophagus. Sympathetic stimulation invariably causes contraction of the ampullary end of the esophagus. The vagus nerve increases the tonicity of the esophagus at the same time as it relaxes the cardiac end.

THE PROBLEM-ORIENTED APPROACH TO DYSPHAGIA

The differential diagnosis of the innumerable causes of dysphagia requires a detailed history, review of symptomatology, a complete physical examination, and thorough evaluation of laboratory findings.

History

The history of a child with dysphagia should include details of the mother's pregnancy, a family history to uncover possible familial or genetic disorders, and a history of the child's birth. Details of the pregnancy that are important include maternal infections, bleeding, toxemia, intake of drugs, thyroid dysfunction, polyhydramnios, or fetal irradiation.

The birth history may direct the physician's attention to an anomaly or a causative factor for airway obstruction. it is important to document whether respirations and cry were spontaneous or whether resuscitation with or without intubation was required, whether a meningomyelocele was repaired, or whether a ventriculoperitoneal shunt was necessary. Important features of the preceding history may lead to conclusions regarding causes for the swallowing problem.

Maternal ingestion of drugs during pregnancy may obtund the infant's sensorium or cause nasal obstruction. (Antihypertensive drugs in particular may cause this problem.) Polyhydramnios frequently is associated with esophageal anomalies and neurologic deficiencies (Wagner et al., 1968; Pritchard, 1966). Traumatic deliveries may be associated with central nervous system trauma and laryngeal paralysis, a cause for airway obstruction. If a meningomyelocele was repaired or a shunt operation was necessary, it may indicate possible laryngeal and/or other cranial nerve paralysis. Where intubation was performed, airway obstruction from trauma to the larynx and trachea may have occurred, or the child may have suffered hypoxia or anoxia. Intubation trauma to the hypopharynx or upper esophagus may produce severe dysphagia by the production of a pseudodiverticulum (Lynch et al., 1974).

Neurologic problems in the family or the mother will alert the examiner to the possibility of the infant's having a similar disease, e.g., myotonic dystrophy or myasthenia gravis.

In older infants and children, the history should include the age of onset of dysphagia, whether acute (sudden) or chronic, and whether the symptoms are periodic or constant. It is important to look for a history of ingestion of a foreign body or corrosive substance; if the onset of the swallowing difficulty is sudden, accidental ingestion of a large foreign body should be suspected. If dysphagia is progressive, starting with solid foods and progressing to difficulty with liquids, a tumor or foreign body of long standing should be suspected. Also, progressive stricturing from reflux esophagitis, hiatal hernia, corrosive substance ingestion, or a collagen disease should be considered. A history of chalasia with prolonged vomiting and dysphagia suggests a stricture from acid reflux creating chronic esophagitis.

Symptoms

Dysphagia is associated with a number of symptoms. Excessive salivation is rarely due to hypersecretion and should alert the physician to a swallowing problem. The normal infant can root, suck, breathe, swallow, gasp, and gag. The absence of any of these normal abilities indicates a potential problem with the swallowing mechanism. However, the absence of a gag reflex does not necessarily indicate a palatal or pharyngeal paralysis.

Attempts to feed a child who has dysphagia from any cause may produce a choking spell with coughing, gagging, drooling, and flooding of the oral cavity, leading to cyanosis. Death may occur from drowning if persistent efforts are made to force the infant to feed as these symptoms progress. It is important to stress that the only evidence of a swallowing problem may be the development of stridor during or after feeding. The stridor is usually expiratory but may be to-and-fro or wheezing in character. Aspiration ultimately causes recurrent or persistent bronchitis and pneumonia. The airway problem may be so dramatic that it may divert the physician's attention from the primary cause, the swallowing defect.

Vomiting is an important symptom of dysphagia when it occurs soon after or during feeding. Nasopharyngeal regurgitation or contamination may be early indicators of a neurologic deficiency such as cerebral palsy or an obstructive lesion in the upper alimentary tract (Chap. 58).

Physical and Laboratory Examination

By the time the otolaryngologist is consulted, usually so that the child may have an endoscopic examination, a complete history and pediatric examination will have been performed. This does not relieve the otolaryngologist of the responsibility to do a complete history and head and neck examination, including a cranial nerve survey. The difficulties in determining the exact etiology of dysphagia in infants makes this problem a multidisciplined project. A thorough evaluation is necessary prior to endoscopic examination in order to prepare the surgeon to deal with any one of a number of possible causes for the problem. This includes watching the infant feed.

The evaluation of the infant and child varies somewhat from that of the adult. Head size and shape, facial configuration, and the pressure and size of the fontanel or its premature closure may be important clues in the cause of an infant's swallowing problems. Laryngeal paralysis and other cranial nerve palsies are not infrequently associated with increased intracranial pressure following meningomyelocele repair. Low-set ears indicate genetic defects and/or craniofacial and mandibulofacial disproportions. These syndromes produce dysphagia because of defects of the oral cavity, facial structures, or palate, a diminutive hypopharynx, and disproportion of the tongue, mouth, and mesopharynx.

A very careful examination of the nasal airway to determine patency is essential (a No. 8 French catheter should easily pass through the nose into the nasopharynx in the normal, full-term infant). A careful examination of facial development and function, oral cavity anatomy, and neurologic function (lips, tongue, palate, and pharynx) is necessary since these are all important parameters for normal deglutition.

Radiologic examination should include a lateral radiograph of the airway, including the skull, nasopharynx, oropharynx, hypopharynx, laryngopharynx, and tracheal airway. The radiographic study may possibly diagnose an obstructive lesion in one of these areas. Radiographic films of the chest will diagnose bronchial and pulmonary infections and may show the presence of congenital heart disease or a mass lesion in the mediastinum, which may produce airway or esophageal obstruction contributing to the swallowing problem.

An esophagram is essential in evaluating these children and should be obtained with a nipple to determine the effectiveness of oropharyngeal function and laryngeal competence. The recording of an esophagram with a tube can obscure function of vital areas necessary to determine the site of the swallowing defect. When the child refuses to nipple-feed, pharyngeal function can be studied by intranasal instillation of the radiopaque medium into the pharynx. Esophageal anatomy and function can be studied once the competence of the oral, buccal, and pharyngeal components of the swallowing mechanism have been studied. When an unusual or difficult to demonstrate lesion is suspected (H-type fistula), a cine-esophagram can be helpful. A normal esophagram does not necessarily rule out a stricture of the esophagus. In those cases where progressive dysphagia occurs, endoscopy is essential. Endoscopic procedures, such as laryngoscopy, bronchoscopy, and esophagoscopy, either individually or in combination, may be indicated in any specific problem. The procedure may be therapeutic as well as diagnostic.

Motility studies may aid in the diagnosis of the cause of dysphagia where there are neuromuscular abnormalities and sphincter function is faulty (see Chapter 54).

DIFFERENTIATING THE PROBLEM

As the physician's exposure to and experience with swallowing problems in children increases, he or she is more likely to make a tentative diagnosis on the basis of clinical observation, making the diagnosis more accurate and involving a minimum of laboratory studies.

Having obtained from the history all necessary information and having examined the child thoroughly, the physician will then observe the child feed. A discussion with the nurse regarding his or her observations of the child during and after feedings will be extremely helpful at this point. The problem then can be placed into one of the five categories discussed in Tables 42–1 and 42–2.

The Premature Infant

The premature infant whose dysphagia persists in spite of growth and development should undergo an intensive search for another cause of the swallowing problem. The airway is a frequent source of defects of swallowing. Stridor in an infant indicates airway obstruction. The site of any airway obstruction must be rapidly recognized, as correcting the obstruction may correct the swallowing problem. In an infant who develops stridor after feedings, the airway obstruction is probably not the primary problem. In these cases airway obstruction is usually secondary to dysphagia.

Nasopharyngeal Obstruction

It is not within the province of this chapter to give a complete outline of the causes of nasal and nasopharyngeal obstruction, but a few may be mentioned. Problems with the airway in this area can be caused by malformations of the nose, ranging from absence to atresia or stenosis. Tumors rarely obstruct the nasal or nasopharyngeal areas sufficiently to produce dysphagia. Infection in the neonate or older child can produce serious airway obstruction, and a specific bacteriologic cause should be determined by cultures of secretions so that specific therapy can be instituted (Chap. 26).

Bilateral choanal atresia produces serious airway obstruction, and normal feeding is virtually impossible without first establishing an appropriate airway. Unilateral atresia rarely produces airway or swallowing problems unless the normal side is obstructed by infection or other causes. Trauma to the nose with septal deflection rarely produces dysphagia unless very severe, when correction becomes mandatory. Allergic rhinitis is rarely a cause of dysphagia in the neonatal period.

Oropharyngeal Obstruction

Defects of the oropharyngeal area, such as deformities of the lips, alveolar processes, tongue, mandible, and hard and soft palate, produce problems for the normal "piston in the cylinder" sucking reflex that initiates swallowing. Thus, cleft lips, microstomia, macrostomia (Goldenhar syndrome), cleft palate, aglossia, microglossia, macroglossia, ankyloglossia, and tumors of the tongue can create varying degrees of dysphagia. For ex-

ample, both airway and swallowing problems are evident in infants with Pierre Robin syndrome (Chap. 43).

In other craniofacial and mandibulofacial disproportions (Treacher-Collins, Crouzon, and Apert syndromes), airway obstruction and mandibular dysfunction produce dysphagia. Adenoidal and tonsillar hypertrophy are not infrequent causes for feeding problems because of associated airway obstruction. Deep neck infections are uncommon in infants, but just as in older children they can cause severe dysphagia and need to be diagnosed and treated early (Chap. 79).

Obstructions of the Larynx, Trachea, Bronchi, and Esophagus

The larynx is an important area to be considered in problems of dysphagia. Airway obstruction produced by webs, cysts, subglottic stenosis, midline paralysis, or tumors must be treated early. Defects of the larynx, such as clefts, with or without involvement of the tracheoesophageal septum, are causes for aspiration. Neurologic defects produce aspiration when associated with either abductor or bilateral adductor vocal cord paralysis or anesthesia of the larynx produced by superior laryngeal nerve involvement from peripheral or central origin.

Infections in the larynx, especially supraglottic disease (epiglottitis), create dysphagia and represent a serious problem in which early diagnosis and therapy are mandatory. Trauma to the larynx and surrounding areas, when associated with dysphagia, can be indicative of potential serious airway problems.

Congenital defects of the trachea and esophagus produce swallowing problems because of obstruction of the airway, abnormal opening between the tracheobronchial tree and the esophagus, obstruction within the esophagus, compressive lesions involving the trachea and/or esophagus, and neurologic disturbance of motility of the esophagus. The lesions to be considered are clefts of the larynx and tracheoesophageal septum, tracheoesophageal fistula, tracheal stenosis, vascular rings, bronchogenic cysts, duplications of the esophagus, atresia, and stricture of the esophagus (Chap. 66B). In many instances involving congenital defects, airway obstruction is aggravated by swallowing of endogenous secretions and feedings. Congenital bronchobiliary fistula produces reflux into the lung from the biliary tract during feedings, particularly when fatty foods are given. Surgical correction of this condition is essential to preserve life (Weitzman et al., 1968).

Esophageal atresia, with or without tracheoesophageal fistula, represents a challenge to the pediatric surgeon and otolaryngologist (Holder and Ashcraft, 1970). Early diagnosis and correction may be followed by airway obstruction, paralysis of the larynx, strictures of the esophagus, reflux esophagitis, hiatal hernia, and many other disorders. The tracheal stenosis and abnormalities of the tracheobronchial tree are well documented. The neurogenic problem of the lower segment of the esophagus is well documented and is a cause for foreign body obstruction and dysphagia. Endoscopic dilatations and removal of foreign bodies are frequently necessary in children who have had esophageal atresias with tracheoesophageal fistula repairs.

Other esophageal lesions that cause swallowing problems are cricopharyngeal lesions, stenosis or achalasia, congenital strictures of the esophagus, and reflux esophagitis. Reflux may be associated with a hiatal hernia and can lead to stricture formation. Congenital strictures produce swallowing problems and may be associated with recurrent bronchitis and pneumonia. Dysphagia in some children with congenital strictures may not occur until solid foods are given. A foreign body may be the first evidence of a congenitally strictured esophagus.

Tumors of the esophagus are rare in children but can produce dysphagia as they enlarge. Angiomatous tumors (hygromas) may involve the neck and extend into the peritracheal and periesophageal area, causing defects of the swallowing mechanism.

Foreign body obstruction is a common cause for dysphagia even in very young infants (Chap. 56). Ingestion of corrosive substances is self-evident when seen early, but when the physician is confronted with a child with progressive dysphagia, strictures due to this type of ingestion must be considered even in the absence of a positive history. Mediastinal disease, either infection or tumor, may compress the esophagus and cause swallowing problems.

Neuropathologic Problems

It is not within the purview of this chapter to review in detail the neurologic problems causing dysphagia. When an anatomic or acquired defect has been ruled out, a neurologic cause is all that remains to be considered, and one can be fairly certain that a central nervous system, peripheral nerve, neuromuscular, or autonomic defect is the cause of the swallowing problem. The physician, who is usually in search of an anatomic defect as the cause of swallowing problems, must include an evaluation of the child's neurologic status in the search for the cause of dysphagia.

The child with a poor suck reflux and an absent arousal reflex who aspirates secretions and who cannot feed normally can be considered to have a central nervous system defect from trauma, hypoxia, dysgenesis of the brain, infection, or one of a number of neurologic deficiencies.

Defects of swallowing may occur in association with amyotonia (Werdnig-Hoffmann syndrome), myotonic muscular dystrophy, myasthenia gravis, Guillain-Barré syndrome, and bulbar poliomyelitis. A neurologic consultation will usually aid in arriving at the specific diagnosis. Therapy will be directed toward the protection and support of the airway and the use of alternative methods of feeding.

Of great interest to the physician are the autonomic defects involving the esophagus. In many defects in this category, the oral and buccopharyngeal phases of the swallowing mechanism will be normal. However, problems arise once secretions and feedings enter the esophagus, resulting in retention of secretions and food, esophagitis, megaesophagus, and vomiting. In cricopharyngeal dysfunction, food cannot enter the esophagus, and immediately after swallowing (i.e., at the end of the buccopharyngeal phase) the child aspirates or regurgitates.

In nonsphincteric spasm of the esophagus, the feeding enters the esophagus but fails to pass, and regurgitation occurs. In chalasia, regurgitation is frequently seen after feeding, particularly when the child is recumbent, but is relieved by smaller feedings and an upright position. In achalasia, the swallowing mechanism is normal, but with failure of the esophagus to empty, dilatation occurs and vomiting is common. In familial dysautonomia, dysphagia is associated with hypersecretion, recurrent bronchopneumonia from aspiration associated with disordered swallowing from delay in opening of the cricopharyngeus, and marked changes in the motility of the esophagus with improper relaxation of the lower esophageal sphincter (Margulies et al., 1968).

SELECTED REFERENCES

Bosma, J. F., (Ed.) 1972. Third Symposium on Oral Sensation and Perception. Springfield, Ill., Charles C Thomas.

This symposium, edited by an experienced anatomist, physiologist, and researcher, is suggested reading for those interested in the development, physiology, and anatomy of the problems of deglutition.

Holder, T. M., and Ashcraft, K. W. 1970. Esophageal atresia and tracheoesophageal fistula. Ann. Thorac. Surg., 9:415.

For the reader interested in this anomaly, this very extensive review of this subject in this paper gives details of history, medical and surgical management, and personal experiences with atresia. It also lists complications and follow-up care of patients after correction.

Wagner, M. L., et al, 1968. Neonatal defects associated with abnormalities of the amniotic fluid. Radiol. Clin. North Am., 54(6):279.

This is an excellent review of prenatal physiology of the fetal swallowing defects related to anomalies causing abnormal accumulation of amniotic fluid.

REFERENCES

Ardran, G. M., and Kemp, F. H. 1970. Some important factors in assessment of oropharyngeal function. Dev. Med. Child. Neurol., 12:158.

Ardran, G. M., Harker, P., and Kemp, F. H. 1972. Tongue size in Down's syndrome. Ment. Defic. Dis., 16:160.

Bosma, J. F. (Ed.) 1972. Third Symposium on Oral Sensation and Perception, Springfield, Ill., Charles C Thomas.

Brans, Y. 1976. Neonatal nutrition, an overview. Postgrad. Med., 60:113.

Cohen, S. R. 1955. Congenital dysphagia — neurogenic consideration. Laryngoscope, 65:515.

Davis, M. E., and Potter, E. L. 1946. Intrauterine respirations of the human fetus. J.A.M.A., 131:1194.

Gryboski, J. D. 1965. The swallowing mechanism of the neonate. Pediatrics, 35:445.

Gryboski, J. D. 1969. Suck and swallow in the premature infant. Pediatrics, 43:96.

Halverson, H. M. 1944. Mechanisms of early infant feeding. J. Genet. Psychol., 64:185–223.

Holder, T. M., and Ashcraft, K. W. 1970. Esophageal atresia and tracheoesophageal fistula. Ann. Thorac. Surg., 9:415.

Logan, W. J., and Bosma, J. F. 1967. Oral and pharyngeal dysphagia in infancy. Pediatr. Clin. North Am., 14:47.

Lynch, F. P., Coran, A. G., Cohen, S. R., et al. 1974. Traumatic esophageal pseudodiverticula in the newborn. J. Pediatr. Surg., 9(5):675–681.

Margulies, S. I., Brunt, S. W., Donner, M. W., et al. 1968. Familial dysautonomia. Radiology, 90:107.

Peiper, A. 1963. Cerebral function in infancy and childhood. New York, Consultants Bureau.

Potter, E. L. 1952. Pathology of the Fetus and the Newborn. Chicago, Year Book Medical Publ.

Pritchard, J. A. 1966. Fetal swallowing and amniotic fluid volume. Obstet. Gynecol., 28:606.

Wagner, M. L., Rudolph, A. J., and Singleton, E. B. 1968. Neonatal defects associated with abnormalities of the amniotic fluid. Radiol. Clin. North Am., 54(6):279.

Warner, R. A. 1975. Deglutition. Int. J. Orthodont., 13:19.

Weitzman, J. J., Cohen, S. R., Woods, L. O., Jr., et al. 1968. Congenital bronchobiliary fistula. J. Pediatr., 73(3):329–334.

Chapter 43

CONGENITAL MALFORMATIONS OF THE MOUTH AND PHARYNX

James L. Parkin, M.D., M.S.

INTRODUCTION

It is imperative for the physician evaluating congenital malformations of the mouth and pharynx to have an understanding of the normal embryology, anatomy, and physiology of this area. This knowledge not only has academic value in the description of a specific malformation but also is important in the planning and timing of treatment for the individual patient. The reader is referred to Chapters 1, 2, 38, and 39 for more complete discussions of embryology, anatomy, and physiology.

The major portion of embryonic development of the mouth and pharynx occurs in the fourth to eighth weeks of intrauterine life. The formation of the mouth begins in the early part of this period by the development of a depression on the ventral surface of the embryo cephalad to the first branchial arches. This depression is lined with ectoderm and is termed the stomodeum. The entodermal-lined primitive gut extends to the stomodeum and these two structures are separated by the oropharyngeal membrane, which ruptures to allow an oropharyngeal communication. The tongue forms from the lateral tubercles and tuberculum impar, which are covered with ectoderm. The maxillary and mandibular processes extend above and below the stomodeum to form the supportive structures of the mouth and lower face (Smith and Ware, 1972).

The bony framework of the mouth is formed by the maxilla, mandible, and pala-tine bones. The soft tissues include the lips, tongue, soft palate, external facial muscles, mastication muscles, and the lymphoid tissue of Waldeyer's ring. These important anatomical relationships have been covered in Chapter 38, and the reader is strongly encouraged to review this material.

The mouth and pharynx play important roles in life-sustaining functions of the individual, including respiration and intake of food and water. Obviously, severe disturbance of these functions is not compatible with life and must be treated promptly and appropriately. Additional functions of the oral cavity and pharynx are taste and speech.

CONGENITAL SYNDROMES INVOLVING THE MOUTH AND PHARYNX

A large number of congenital and hereditary syndromes involve oropharyngeal structures. This section covers the most common syndromes the physician will encounter and also some of the less common ones. Many of the associated functional as well as the cosmetic problems are best managed by the otolaryngologist on the maxillofacial team (Chap. 4).

Craniofacial Dysostosis (Crouzon Syndrome)

"Dysostosis" refers to a defect in the normal ossification process of the developing fetus. Craniofacial dysostosis has a pattern of autosomal dominant transmission. The syndrome involves premature craniosynostosis, most commonly involving the coronal, sagittal, and lambdoid sutures. The cranial shape depends on the extent and timing of suture involvement. The midface demonstrates the results of maxillary hypoplasia, with a short upper lip, parrot-beak nose, relative mandibular prognathism, and hypertelorism.

The maxillary hypoplasia results in obvious intraoral problems, manifested mainly in the dental occlusion. Class III malocclusion is most commonly encountered, with crowding of the upper teeth, a high, arched palate, and crossbite.

Mental deficiency may be seen in some cases. This is possibly related to the increased intracranial pressure that frequently occurs in this syndrome. Conductive deafness has also been reported as occurring secondary to associated atresia of the external auditory canal and anomalies of the middle ear structures.

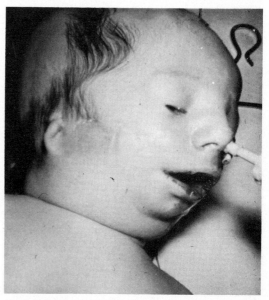

Figure 43–1   Treacher Collins syndrome.

Cleft Palate, Micrognathia, and Glossoptosis (Pierre Robin Syndrome)

This syndrome may occur as an isolated problem or may be associated with other congenital syndromes such as Stickler syndrome (cleft palate, retinal detachment, and hereditary arthro-ophthalmopathy), cerebrocostomandibular syndrome (microcephaly, hypoplastic or absent ribs, and vertebral anomalies), campomelic syndrome (ocular hypertelorism, flat face, and vertebral, scapular, and extremity anomalies), and persistent left superior vena cava syndrome. The Pierre Robin anomaly causes early respiratory embarrassment because the micrognathia and glossoptosis result in pharyngeal airway obstruction.

In mild cases, the airway problems are often managed by placing the infant in a prone position most of the time. Gavage feedings may be required temporarily.

Surgical correction requires anterior displacement of the tongue or tracheostomy. Anterior glossopexy may be accomplished by a suture passed through the anterior arch of the mandible to the base of the tongue, across the base of the tongue, and back to the anterior mandible. The suture is passed through a rubber catheter across the base of the tongue and through a second rubber catheter placed anteriorly to prevent suture damage to the soft tissues. Other suggested

techniques have included the formation of a lingual-labial flap (Hawkins and Simpson, 1974).

Severe cases often will not respond to positioning or glossopexy; in these instances, performance of a tracheostomy is indicated. The child in Figure 43–1, with Treacher Collins syndrome, had marked mandibular hypoplasia. Glossopexy was performed but did not provide an adequate pharyngeal airway, and a tracheostomy was necessary. The tracheostomy remained in place approximately one year.

As the child matures, the mandible increases its dimensions. The glossopexy procedure should be reversible so that normal anatomical relationships can be reestablished following the growth and development of the mandible. Surgical reversal of the glossopexy procedure or closure of the tracheostomy can usually be done before the child's first birthday.

Mandibulofacial Dysostosis (Treacher Collins Syndrome)

The inheritance pattern of this syndrome is autosomal dominant with variable expressivity. Major involvement occurs in those structures that derive from the first branchial arch, groove, and pouch. Unlike Crouzon syndrome, the cranial bones are essentially normal. The midface is involved with abnormal development of the malar bones, nonfusion of the zygomatic arches, defective orbital margins, and small or absent paranasal sinuses. The mandible is also hypoplastic. The ear canals and pinnas are usually malformed, with severe auricular deformities and, frequently, absence of the external auditory canals, with or without ossicular defects resulting in conductive deafness.

The combination of these anomalies results in a characteristic facial appearance with depressed cheek bones, deformed pinnas, downward-sloping, palpebral fissures, a large, fishlike mouth, and receding chin. Dental malocclusion is common, and there is a high frequency of associated high, arched palate or cleft palate. Mental retardation is reportedly present in less than 10 per cent of patients.

Mandibular hypoplasia with relative glossoptosis can result in early pharyngeal respiratory embarrassment in these patients, similar to the problems encountered in patients with Pierre Robin syndrome. Surgical procedures often required include glossopexy, tracheostomy, reconstruction of the external and middle ear, and desired facial cosmetic surgery.

Mongolism (Trisomy 21, Down Syndrome)

There are many different syndromes with basic chromosomal abnormalities and resultant orofacial manifestations. Down syndrome is the most common example of this group of abnormalities and reportedly accounts for approximately 15 per cent of all patients institutionalized for mental deficiency. The incidence of Down syndrome is reportedly one in every 600 to 700 births.

These children commonly have associated cardiorespiratory, gastrointestinal, musculoskeletal, and cutaneous abnormalities. As a complete discussion of the associated anomalies is beyond the scope of this book, only the oral manifestations of this disease will be emphasized (Cohen and Cohen, 1971).

The lips are normal in size at birth; however, progressive enlargement of the lips is the usual clinical course. The tongue is enlarged; this enlargement may be a true macroglossia or a relative macroglossia secondary to a small oral cavity. Most Down syndrome patients will develop fissuring of the tongue by age five years. The palate is high and tends to be narrow. Occasionally, bifid uvula and cleft lip and palate may be seen. The nasopharynx is narrow and adenotonsillar hypertrophy is

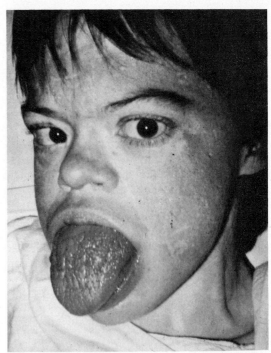

Figure 43–2 Macroglossia seen with Down syndrome. This patient also had an abscess at the base of the tongue with increased apparent macroglossia.

frequently seen, which probably contributes to the chronic open-mouthed appearance of Down syndrome patients. Figure 43–2 shows a mongoloid patient with macroglossia.

There is a lower than average incidence of dental caries in mongoloids; however, there is a high incidence of periodontal disease, a situation probably related to the poor oral hygiene frequently encountered in these patients. Retarded dental eruption is observed in both deciduous and permanent dentition, and missing teeth and small teeth are common in Down syndrome patients. In addition, their lingual papillae are often hypertrophied.

The middle third of the face is often hypoplastic, producing a relative mandibular prognathism and flattened facial appearance. The characteristic appearance includes brachycephaly, short neck, slanted, widespread eyes, short nose, and abnormal ear lobes. Mental retardation, which may be severe, is common.

Acrocephalosyndactyly (Apert Syndrome)

It has been suggested that this syndrome is caused by a defect in the tissues important in bone development before the fifth to sixth week of embryonic life (Park and Powers,

1920). Most cases have occurred sporadically and appear to be associated with increased parental age at the time of conception. Some hereditary patterns suggest autosomal dominant transmission.

Early obliteration of the cranial sutures results in the characteristic brachycephalic and/or oxycephalic appearance. The maxilla is hypoplastic with hypertelorism, and proptosis usually is present. The underdevelopment of the maxilla results in a relative prognathism of the mandible. The nose is small and underdeveloped. Frequently there is a high, arched palate that is constricted and may have a marked median furrow. A soft palate cleft is encountered in 25 to 30 per cent of patients. Again, severe occlusion problems are encountered, with dental crowding and Class III malocclusion. Retarded dental eruption is also a common finding.

Mental retardation may be encountered, although it usually is not as severe as that seen in Down syndrome. The associated deformities of the extremities include syndactyly of digits two, three, and four. Occasionally digits one and five may be involved. The upper extremities are short. Joint involvement may be seen at the elbow, shoulder, and hip.

Arachnodactyly (Marfan Syndrome)

Photographs and medical records of Abraham Lincoln suggest that he might have had Marfan syndrome. The major problem appears to be a defect in protein synthesis at the cellular level, especially involving collagen and elastin. The disorder is transmitted as an autosomal dominant trait with high penetrance and variable expressivity. The typical adult appearance is that of a tall, thin person with scoliosis, pectus excavatum, long fingers and toes, and subluxation of the ocular lenses. Sudden death may occur as a result of inherent dissecting aneurysm due to defects of the wall of the aorta.

Oral manifestations include a high palatal vault, occasionally a cleft palate or bifid uvula, dental malocclusion, and long, narrow teeth. Mandibular prognathism is also frequently associated with this syndrome.

Osteogenesis Imperfecta (Ekman Syndrome)

This condition was early described as "brittle bone disease." The most common form of the disorder is the "tarda" form, which is inherited as an autosomal dominant trait with a wide range of expressivity and incomplete penetrance. The basic defect appears to be a failure of collagen maturation.

The maxillofacial manifestations of this disease have recently been described (Bergstrom, 1977). These findings included condylar deformity, prognathic mandible, frequent mandibular dislocation, hypoplastic hemimandible, depressed zygoma, and dentinogenesis imperfecta. Bergstrom also pointed out that the facial bones are apparently more resistant to fractures than the long bones, which can be attributed to the greater amount of elastic fiber content in facial bones. Fifty to 60 per cent of patients with the tarda form of this syndrome have otosclerosis with stapedial fixation and resultant conductive hearing loss. Sensorineural hearing loss has also been reported in this disorder.

Facial Hemihypertrophy (Curtius or Steiner Syndrome)

This syndrome has a large degree of etiologic heterogeneity. It has been associated with chromosomal abnormalities, vascular or lymphatic abnormalities, central nervous system lesions, and endocrine abnormalities. The hemihypertrophy may be restricted to a single anatomic area such as unilateral facial enlargement or involvement of a single limb or digit. The syndrome may also include involvement of the entire half of the body. It occurs more frequently in males, and the right side of the body appears to be more frequently involved. Asymmetry may be noted at birth but becomes more prominent as growth and development occur. The syndrome has been reported to occur sporadically. The unilateral facial enlargement involves the tongue as well as the musculoskeletal structures of the face.

Hemifacial Atrophy (Romberg Syndrome)

This condition has also been known as *progressive facial hemiatrophy*. Involvement is usually restricted to the facial structures, although in a small percentage of patients the entire half of the body may be involved. Most cases occur sporadically and, again, there are various theories of etiology, with trauma apparently playing a role in some patients. There may be some relationship between this disorder and scleroderma.

The condition is often not obvious at birth, but with the growth and development of the child it becomes apparent within the first decade of life. The development of the hemiface is retarded, and atrophy occurs in the cartilaginous and musculoskeletal structures of the face resulting in facial distortion, unilateral enophthalmos, and maxillary and mandibular abnormalities with resultant dental problems. Hemiatrophy of the tongue also occurs.

Congenital Facial Diplegia (Möbius Syndrome)

This condition consists of congenital bilateral cranial nerve palsies. The sixth and seventh cranial nerves are most commonly involved; however, nearly every cranial nerve can be affected. Facial nerve involvement may be asymmetric and the lower divisions may be spared. The mouth is small. The tongue may demonstrate atrophy, fasciculation, or paralysis. Difficulty with feeding and speech are frequently important clinical aspects of this syndrome. Limb anomalies, chest wall defects, and mental retardation may be associated. Occurrence has been sporadic.

Dwarfism (Turner Syndrome)

Whereas Down syndrome is an example of an autosomal chromosome abnormality, Turner syndrome or gonadal dysgenesis is an example of a sex chromosome abnormality. Klinefelter syndrome would be another example of an abnormality in sex chromosomes.

Patients with Turner syndrome characteristically have mandibular hypoplasia and a high palate. Eruption of the permanent molars may occur prematurely. Cleft palates occur in these patients with a higher than normal frequency.

Achondroplasia

This is another form of dwarfism, which includes the appearance of a large head. Most cases occur sporadically, although some association has been reported with increased parental age at conception. Familial incidence seems to indicate an autosomal dominant pattern of inheritance. These individuals have hypoplasia of the maxilla with resultant depression of the nasal bone. Malocclusion is seen with dental crowding, crossbite, and Class III malocclusive problems. Palatal and pharyngeal maldevelopment contribute to poor eustachian tube function, which often results in frequent otitis media during early childhood.

Mucopolysaccharidosis I-H (Hurler Syndrome or Gargoylism)

Multiple inherited disorders of mucopolysaccharide metabolism have been described. Hurler syndrome is a severe form of mucopolysaccharide abnormality and was one of the first described. The syndrome is inherited as an autosomal recessive trait.

The characteristic facial appearance begins to develop in the first three to six months of life and is usually apparent by the age of three years. The large head exhibits a flattened, small nose, prominent forehead, thick lips, and thick ear lobes. The mouth is usually held open, with the tongue protruding. Lip and tongue enlargement is progressive. The mandible is short and broad. Motion at the temporomandibular joint may be limited because of condylar abnormality.

Cleidocranial Dysostosis (Cleidocranial Dysplasia)

This syndrome consists of clavicular aplasia or hypoplasia, delayed ossification of the fontanels, and exaggerated development of the cranium. Autosomal dominance is the type of transmission. The palate is highly arched and may have a submucous cleft or even a complete cleft. Nonunion of the mandibular symphysis has been reported.

The apparent lack of teeth seen in patients with this syndrome has been shown to be due to delay or failure of eruption of both the deciduous and permanent teeth. Maxillary and mandibular radiographs will demonstrate this. Premaxillary development has also been noted to be poor.

Cutaneous and Mucosal Pigmentation Associated with Gastrointestinal Polyposis (Peutz-Jeghers Syndrome)

This syndrome is representative of a group of syndromes with associated mucosal and cutaneous lesions. Its inheritance is autosomal dominant. The gastrointestinal polyposis component of the syndrome causes most clinical problems. Approximately 50 per cent of these patients have brown to bluish-black maculae present on the skin, particularly periorally, perinasally, or periorbitally. The oral mucosa may demonstrate similar maculae, which are usually 1 to 12 mm in size but which may be confluent. Their pigmentation is similar to the pigmentation of the cutaneous lesions. The tongue and floor of the mouth are rarely involved. There is no correlation between the degree of mucocutaneous pigmentation and the severity of the gastrointestinal polyposis.

Oculoauriculovertebral Dysplasia (Goldenhar Syndrome)

This syndrome involves the structures formed from the first and second branchial arches, in conjunction with vertebral abnormalities. The majority of the cases occur sporadically; however, familial incidence has been reported with different modes of inheritance. In addition to auricular deformity with agenesis of the external auditory canals, severe oral deformities are seen. The condition is often asymmetric, with one side of the face more severely involved than the other. The degree of the mandibular involvement is highly variable, ranging from minimal condylar abnormality to aplasia of the mandibular ramus. There may be associated macrostomia, agenesis of the ipsilateral parotid gland, salivary gland fistulae, lingual hypoplasia, and cleft lip or palate.

Other Congenital Syndromes

Of course there are many other congenital syndromes involving the mouth and pharynx, including whistling face syndrome (Freeman-Sheldon syndrome), lingual malformations seen in Mohr syndrome, the aglossia-adactylia syndrome, and many others. The reader is referred to the book by Gorlin et al. (1976), for more extensive discussions of the syndromes involving the mouth and pharynx.

MANAGEMENT OF CONGENITAL SYNDROMES

The team approach to patients with multiple congenital abnormalities of the head and neck is most likely to result in an accurate assessment, a correct diagnosis, a rational plan of management, and an optimum prognosis. This team should include the pediatrician, otolaryngologist, neurologist, plastic surgeon, geneticist, and dental specialists. Other specialists may be required depending upon the individual patient problems.

When a patient is first seen with a "head and neck syndrome," it is important not to reach a premature diagnostic decision. Radiographs of the skull and facial bones should be obtained. Special neurological assessment of hearing, sight, facial motion, deglutition, etc., is necessary. It may be beneficial to obtain chromosome studies to aid in the diagnosis and also to help provide a basis for parental genetic counseling. Each case needs to be compared with literature descriptions in order to identify the syndrome correctly. This can be accomplished only after a careful, accurate physical examination.

Once the diagnosis has been made, it is important to formulate and pursue an orderly, comprehensive plan of action. With the team approach, it is necessary that one member of the team be responsible for the coordination of therapeutic events. The pediatrician is the logical choice for this role, as he will be providing the child with continuing medical care throughout the period of growth and development.

The "syndrome patient" needs to have his various malformations individualized and corrected by the best-qualified member of the care team. The timing of correction is determined in a triage fashion, with the most serious, life-threatening problems being corrected first. Some malformation corrections may be delayed for several years but require special supportive care in the interim to enhance the ultimate prognosis. An example of this would be the child with bilateral external auditory canal atresia. The planned reconstruction would occur at age four to six years; however, during infancy and prior to the time of correction, the child should be fitted with a hearing aid to facilitate speech and language development.

The ultimate prognosis is dependent on the sum of the expected results of treatment for the specific problems. The skills of the individual team members are important. The rehabilitative facilities and expertise available also contribute greatly to the ultimate prognosis. The concern and follow-through of the physician team members and especially of the parents are of crucial importance. Finally, the parents and doctors must face problems realistically. A patient with severe mental retardation will obviously have a different social and vocational prognosis than a patient with normal mental capabilities. Institutional care may be necessary early in the course of treatment in some patients. It is important to be realistic in expectations but always to provide the parents with hope for the future.

The parents and other family members should not be forgotten in the care of the malformed child. Parents experience anxiety, apprehension, guilt, discouragement, and anger over the problems of their child. The parents need to be counseled, given support, and helped to understand their role in the care process. Social adjustments are often necessary to reduce the trauma the parents and siblings feel in coping with a malformed child. The psychiatrist, psychologist, and social worker can be beneficial in this regard.

ISOLATED CONGENITAL ORAL AND PHARYNGEAL ABNORMALITIES

Maxillofacial clefts are among the most frequent congenital malformations. These may occur in isolation or in conjunction with other syndromes discussed earlier in this chapter. Maxillofacial clefts are more common in males and are also found more commonly on the left side. Cleft lip occurs as an embryonic failure of the premaxilla to fuse with the alveolus. A cleft palate results from a lack of fusion of the horizontal palatal segments. These clefts may occur in association with each other or independently; the degree of cleft is highly variable. The reader is referred to Chapters 1 and 3 for a more complete description of the embryology and development of this area. This understanding is mandatory in appreciating the genesis of the cleft lip and palate.

Lips

The apparent double lip, which is seen when the lips are parted, particularly in smiling, is due to a redundancy of the mucosal lining. This deformity may occur in isolation or as a component of Ascher syndrome (double lip, blepharochalasis, and nontoxic thyroid enlargement).

Cleft lips were referred to previously. These clefts may be paramedian, median,

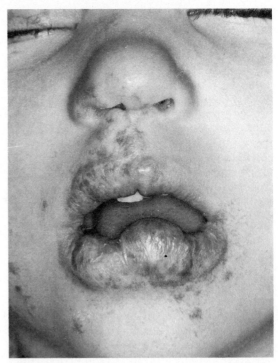

Figure 43–3 Congenital hemangiomata of the face and lips.

oblique, or transverse. Small mucosal sinus tracts or pits may also occur, usually symmetrically in the vermilion of the lower lip. They are often associated with maxillofacial clefts. They communicate with minor salivary glands and simple excision is the treatment of choice.

There is a great deal of individual variability in the size of the oral opening; however, an abnormally large mouth (macrostomia) or abnormally small mouth (microstomia) may be diagnosed. Macrostomia probably represents a form of lateral facial cleft and can be seen in isolation or in conjunction with mandibulofacial dysostosis and oculoauriculovertebral dysplasia.

Congenital tumors can also present in the lips. Figure 43–3 illustrates a patient with multiple congenital hemagiomata and a subglottic hemangioma. The patient had extensive nasal septal hemangiomata as well as the obvious hemangiomata of the lip. A tracheostomy was required to relieve airway obstruction. As the nasal septal hemangiomata have resolved, the nasal septum has essentially disappeared, leaving a large perforation with retraction of the columella. The lip lesions have become significantly less obvious.

Tongue

Variations in the size of the tongue are seen from individual to individual and from one ethnic group to another. Congenital macroglossia is seen in association with other syndromes such as Down syndrome, or it may be isolated and idiopathic. Lymphangioma or hemangioma of the tongue can result in macroglossia.

Maldevelopment of the lingual frenulum will result in mandibular ankyloglossia or tongue-tie. This is a relatively common condition that frequently comes to the attention of the physician for evaluation (Fig. 43–4). The condition may be a cause of poor articulation in children. If it is to be corrected, it should be done prior to speech development (Catlin and DeHann, 1971).

The clinical evaluation of the child with tongue-tie should indicate the necessity for correction. Physical findings indicative of a need for surgical intervention include: notching of the protruding tongue tip, inability of the tongue tip to contact the maxillary alveolar ridge, restriction of lateral tongue motion, or restriction of tongue protrusion beyond the mandibular alveolus (Fletcher and Daly, 1974).

Surgical correction depends upon the extent of the malformation. Occasionally, the short lingual frenulum is a thin, filmy membrane which can simply be clipped under local anesthesia with little incidence of recurrence. However, in most cases the membrane is thickened and requires frenuloplastic surgery in order to give the child adequate lingual mobility and prevent recurrent ankyloglossia. Surgical correction may be achieved by Z plasty, V-Y plasty, or horizontal-to-vertical plasty. The last method has been found to be a simple, effective way of correcting the problem. These techniques may be seen in Figures 43–5A, B, and C, and 43–6.

Other congenital anomalies of the tongue include bifid tongue (Fig. 43–7), fissured or scrotal tongue (Fig. 43–8), geographic tongue (Fig. 43–9), and median rhomboid glossitis. The fissured tongue is seen in nearly all children with Down syndrome. This condition also occurs as an isolated finding with a positive familial incidence. Median rhomboid glossitis is a result of faulty posterior lingual development with papilla-free tissue appearing in the posterior medial aspect of the tongue in the region of the embryonic tuberculum impar.

A mass lesion in the midline of the posterior tongue may represent a lingual or undescended thyroid gland. Embryologically, the thyroid develops from the floor of the primitive pharynx and migrates anteriorly and inferiorly to reach its final adult location. Abnormality of this descent process can result in the development of a thyroglossal duct and cyst or, less commonly, in an undescended thyroid at the base of the tongue or superficial to the hyoid bone.

The lingual thyroid mass usually increases in size as the child becomes older because of the effect of thyroid stimulating hormone on this marginally functioning thyroid tissue. The common symptoms are dysphagia, dysphonia, dyspnea, and occasionally pain.

The lingual thyroid may be the patient's only functioning thyroid tissue. Thyroid scanning with radioactive isotopes is necessary to make the diagnosis and evaluate the amount of active thyroid tissue present in order to plan the management. There is also an increased incidence of thyroid carcinoma in lingual thyroid tissue.

Management considerations include functional, metabolic, and cosmetic factors. If the patient is euthyroid and without functional or cosmetic problems, then no therapy — with

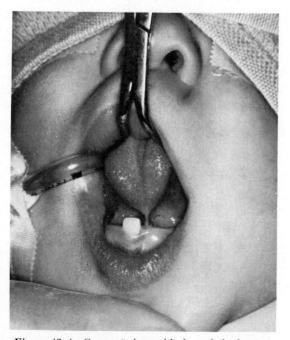

Figure 43–4   Congenital mandibular ankyloglossia.

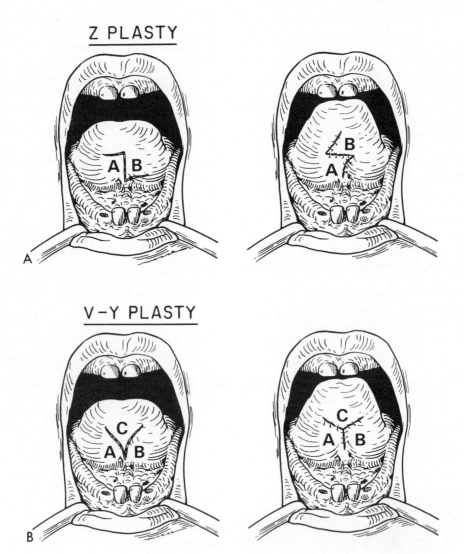

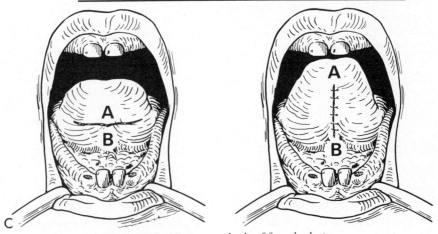

Figure 43–5   Various methods of frenuloplasty.

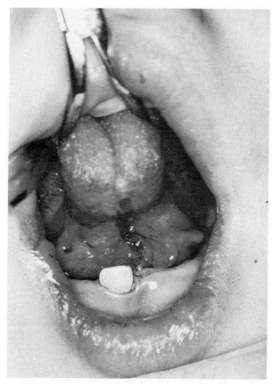

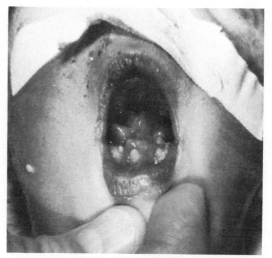

Figure 43–7 Bifid tongue.

Figure 43–6 Mandibular ankyloglossia corrected by horizontal-to-vertical plasty. The same patient as in Figure 43–4.

careful follow-up — is acceptable. If the patient is euthyroid or hypothyroid with functional and/or cosmetic problems, suppressive thyroid hormone therapy should be initiated. If adequate regression of the mass occurs, this therapy can be continued; otherwise, surgical treatment is in order. Excision with

subsequent thyroid hormone replacement or autotransplantation of the thyroid tissue to the neck or abdominal wall are the surgical techniques utilized (Wertz, 1974).

Tongue size, development, and habits have a definite influence on the development of the jaws and the position of the teeth (Austermann and Machtens, 1974). Tongue thrust is an example of an abnormal tongue movement which plays a significant role in subsequent anterior dental occlusion problems.

Maxilla and Mandible

The development of the maxilla is related to airflow through the nose. Conditions caus-

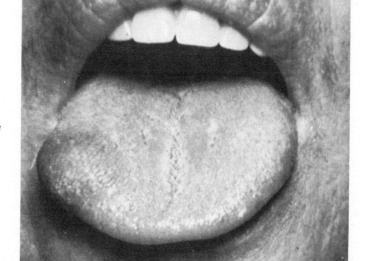

Figure 43–8 Hemangioma of the tongue.

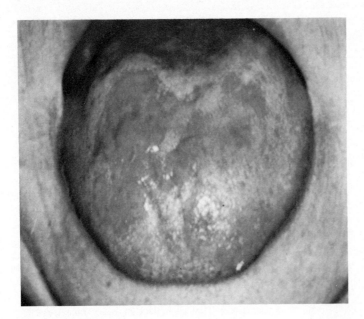

Figure 43–9 Geographic tongue.

ing chronic nasal airway obstruction can result in underdevelopment of the maxilla with a high, arched, narrow palate resulting in occlusion problems such as crossbite. High, arched palates are also seen in many of the previously discussed congenital syndromes. The arching of the palate tends to become more marked as the child grows and develops. Often the palate may appear normal at birth and develop a high arch in the first four to five years of life. The cleft palate problem is the most significant congenital anomaly of the palate and has been previously discussed (Fig. 43–10).

The soft palate may be congenitally short. This can result in velopharyngeal insufficiency with hypernasal speech and leakage of foods and liquids into the nose with swallowing. The short palate is often seen in patients with Down syndrome. It also occurs in otherwise normal children.

It is important to recognize a short palate in children prior to adenoidectomy. Velopharyngeal closure may be adequate with a short palate and the adenoid mass in place but following excision of the adenoids, velopharyngeal insufficiency develops. The parents then become concerned about the resultant hypernasal speech. In most cases the hypernasal speech can be corrected in four to six months with speech therapy. Mild cases resolve spontaneously and more severe cases require pharyngeal or palatal flap surgery. Waiting 9 to 12 months is recommended before this is considered. Prevention is, of course, the best treatment. Conservative or partial adenoidectomy should be considered in the patient with a short palate.

Congenital asymmetries of the mandible and maxilla are uncommon as isolated findings. They may develop secondary to trauma or in relationship to other syndromes previously discussed such as facial hemihypertrophy or hemifacial atrophy.

Torus palatinus and tori mandibularis are rarely seen in the newborn but develop as the patient matures. There are bony exostoses on the center of the hard palate (palatinus) or on the lingual table of the mandible at the level

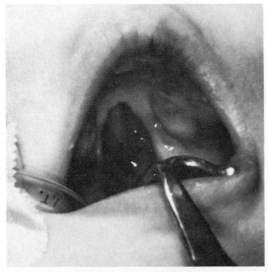

Figure 43–10 Cleft palate.

of the canine and first premolar teeth (mandibularis). Their appearance is characteristic and their removal is not necessary except possibly for the improvement of denture fitting.

Various cysts of the maxilla can be seen during the developmental years. These cysts are rarely congenital and usually present in young adults. They occur mainly in the embryological fusion lines of the premaxilla and maxilla. Examples of these cysts include the globulomaxillary, nasoalveolar, nasopalatine, and palatine cysts.

Pharynx

Posterior choanal atresia and persistence of the buccopharyngeal membrane result in lack of communication between the nose and pharynx. Rare cases have been reported with a failure of communication between the oral cavity and the pharynx. These conditions must be recognized and treated early for the newborn to survive. Congenital tumors may also present in the pharynx. Examples of these include Thornwaldt cyst, branchial cleft cyst, teratomas, chordomas, craniopharyngiomas, cystic hygromas, and hemangiomas (Parkin and Thomas, 1974).

Frequently during indirect laryngoscopy, small, yellowish, thin-walled cysts are seen in the vallecula and hypopharynx. These usually require no therapy. Occasionally, a large vallecular cyst can result in dysphonia, dysphagia, and dyspnea requiring surgical treatment. Recurrence after needle aspiration indicates the need to treat these by marsupialization of the cyst, which is done by excising the protruding wall of the cyst.

SELECTED REFERENCE

Gorlin, R. J., Pindborg, J. J., and Cohen, M. M., Jr. 1976. Syndromes of the Head and Neck, 2nd ed. New York, McGraw-Hill Book Co.
    This book represents a comprehensive, well organized review of syndromes affecting the structures of the head and neck. It is an excellent reference text explaining etiologies, associated malformations, and manifestations of various syndromes.

REFERENCES

Austermann, K. H., and Machtens, E. 1974. The influence of tongue asymmetries on the development of jaws and the position of teeth. Int. J. Oral surg., 3:261.

Bergstrom, L. 1977. Osteogenesis imperfecta: Otologic and maxillofacial aspects. Laryngoscope, 87:Suppl. 6.

Catlin, F. I., and DeHann, V. 1971. Tongue-tie. Arch Otolaryngol, 94:548.

Cohen, M. M., Sr., and Cohen, M. M., Jr. 1971. The oral manifestations of trisomy G_1 (Down syndrome). Birth Defects, 7:241.

Fletcher, S. G., and Daly, D. A. 1974. Sublingual dimensions in infants and young children. Arch Otolaryngol., 99:292.

Gorlin, R. J., Pindborg, J. J., and Cohen, M. M., Jr. 1976. Syndromes of the Head and Neck, 2nd ed. New York, McGraw-Hill Book Co.

Hawkins, D. B., and Simpson, J. V. 1974. Micrognathia and glossoptosis in the newborn. Clin. Pediatr., 13:1066.

Park, E. A., and Powers, G. F. 1920. Acrocephaly and scaphocephaly with symmetrically distributed malformations of the extremities. Am, J. Dis. Child., 20:235.

Parkin, J. L., and Thomas, G. K. 1974. Benign masses of the pharynx. Rocky Mt. Med. J., 71:34.

Smith, L., and Ware, J. L. 1972. Embryology, applied anatomy and physiology. *In* Ferguson, C. F., and Kendig, E. L. (Eds.): Pediatric Otolaryngology, 2nd ed. Philadelphia, W. B. Saunders Co.

Wertz, M. L. 1974. Management of undescended lingual and subhyoid thyroid glands. Laryngoscope, 84:507.

Chapter *44*

PRIMARY CARE OF INFANTS AND CHILDREN WITH CLEFT PALATE

Jack L. Paradise, M.D.

From birth onward the child with a cleft palate faces a diversity of medical and medically related problems, and presents substantial challenges to the physicians and other health professionals involved in his or her care (Paradise et al., 1974). Initially it is the child's parents who, upon learning of the deformity, require understanding and support as they experience reactions that may range from dismay, to grief, guilt, or resentment. Their questions about prognosis must be answered in detail, even though the prognosis may be in some respects uncertain.

Feeding difficulties of some degree are experienced by almost all infants with cleft palate, while those with associated mandibular hypoplasia and glossoptosis (Pierre Robin syndrome) may suffer, in addition, from episodic or chronic upper airway obstruction that in extreme instances may be life-threatening or actually lethal. In all patients with cleft palate, middle ear disease accompanied by some degree of hearing impairment persists, unless treated surgically, throughout infancy and often beyond, and there is risk that chronic otic infection, permanent impairment of hearing, or both will develop. For all patients, periods of hospitalization associated with one or more reconstructive surgical procedures are inevitable. Various instructions received from professionals of various disciplines in the course of frequent visits to hospitals and clinics must be coordinated and incorporated into family scheduling. Finally, some patients will experience continuing difficulties to some extent or other involving cosmesis, speech, language,

cognition, or emotional status. The assiduousness and skill with which all these medical, surgical, and habilitative problems are managed during infancy and childhood can be important determinants of adult attainment and adjustment; sophisticated management can be expected usually to result in gratifyingly good overall outcomes, whereas neglect or inept management may have opposite effects.

This chapter will focus on three areas of particular importance to physicians responsible for the primary or general care — as distinct from reconstructive surgical care — of infants and young children with cleft palate: (1) feeding and nutrition, (2) glossoptotic airway obstruction in the Pierre Robin syndrome, and (3) otologic and audiologic problems.

FEEDING AND NUTRITION

Nature and Extent of the Problem

Feeding difficulty is encountered to some degree or other by most infants with cleft palate, especially during the first few weeks of life, and usually for the first several months. Sucking efficiency is impaired as a consequence of the deficient palate's relative inability to seal off the nasal cavity and nasopharynx from the oral cavity and oropharynx. Nasal regurgitation epidoses due to aspiration of milk into the respiratory tract and choking further disrupt the feeding process. As a result, individual feedings often

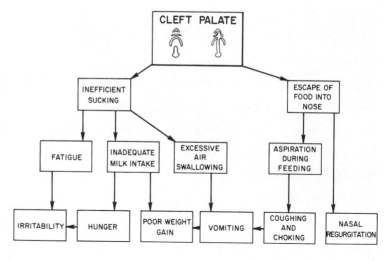

Figure 44–1 Elements of the feeding problem and their interrelationships in infants with cleft palate. (From Paradise, J. L., and McWilliams, B. J. 1974. Simplified feeder for infants with cleft palate. Pediatrics, 53:566. Copyright American Academy of Pediatrics, 1974.)

are laborious and time-consuming, and ingested volume often is inadequate. Both the parent and the infant are deprived of the usual physical and emotional gratifications of the feeding process; the parent may be frustrated, disappointed, and anxious, and the infant hungry and inadequately nourished. The elements of the feeding problem and their interrelationships in infants with cleft palate are shown schematically in Figure 44–1.

Although standard pediatric textbooks have tended to minimize these feeding problems (Parkins and Barbero, 1975; Schaffer and Avery, 1971), various authors (Zickefoose, 1957; Tisza and Gumpertz, 1962; Drillien et al., 1966) have noted their frequent occurrence; in one study of 124 infants, 91 (73 per cent) experienced moderate or severe difficulty in feeding. Beyond descriptive accounts, however, data regarding weight gain during the early months of life have been scant. At the University of Pittsburgh Cleft Palate Center, most infants when first seen, unless specific intervention as described in the next section had been undertaken, have failed to gain weight adequately (Paradise and McWilliams, 1974). Histories of laborious feedings, often lasting an hour or longer, are commonplace.

Management

Since inability to generate effective oral suction is the major cause of the difficulty in feeding, compensation should be attempted through the use of one of various devices that permit direct expression of milk into the infant's mouth. One such device, the Beniflex Cleft Lip/Palate Nurser,* functions satisfactorily for most infants with cleft palate, but its cost as a disposable unit for a single feeding is relatively high. Equally satisfactory is a simple, much less expensive compressible feeder (Fig. 44–2) consisting of a rigid plastic shell

*Mead Johnson Laboratories, Evansville, IN 44721

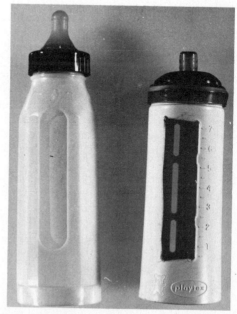

Figure 44–2 Plastic nursing shells that permit feeding from compressible, disposable bags. (From Paradise, J. L., and McWilliams, B. J. 1974. Simplified feeder for infants with cleft palate. Pediatrics, 53:566. Copyright American Academy of Pediatrics, 1974.)

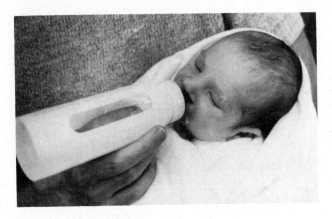

Figure 44–3   Mother feeding infant with cleft palate, using compressible feeder. (From Paradise, J. L., and McWilliams, B. J. 1974. Simplified feeder for infants with cleft palate. Pediatrics, 53:566. Copyright American Academy of Pediatrics, 1974.)

(several types are available commercially) into which is placed a disposable plastic bag (available commercially in convenient, tear-off rolls) to serve as a container for milk, and onto which a conventional nipple-carrying cap is screwed. With a pocket knife or similar tool, slots wide enough to permit inserting a finger are cut into opposite sides of the shell. Through the slot, gentle pressure can then easily be applied to the bag of milk throughout the feeding process (Fig. 44–3). With all feeders, soft rubber ("premie") nipples with cross-cuts are usually preferable to standard nipples with either standard or enlarged holes; however, cross-cut nipples generally require the limbs of the X to be lengthened slightly with a razor blade before initial use in order to achieve effective flap-valve function.

Using this type of compressible feeder, adequate amounts of milk can be fed to most infants with cleft palate in 15 to 20 minutes. In our experience, adoption of a compressible feeder for infants previously using standard bottles not only has greatly facilitated the feeding process but also has generally resulted in prompt upturns of weight toward normal.

The compressible feeding device described here does nothing to prevent either aspiration or nasal regurgitation of milk. These problems usually can be avoided or minimized by keeping the infant in an upright position during feedings, avoiding excessive pressure on the compressible bag, and being alert to early signs of distress in the infant.

Alternatively by way of management, some authors (Zickefoose, 1957; Tisza and Gumpertz, 1962; Drillien et al., 1966; Lifton, 1956; Burston, 1958; Williams et al., 1968; Malson, 1969) have advocated the use of prosthetic feeding appliances that obturate the palatal cleft. Supporting data, however, have not been reported. In our experience, prostheses when fitted early have in some instances seemed effective but in others have been unacceptable to the infant and therefore unsuccessful. The palatal prosthesis seems especially attractive as a potential facilitator of breast-feeding, since unaided breast-feeding of infants with cleft palate generally proves unsuccessful.

"Ducky," lamb's, or other special nipples are also sometimes advised, but parents usually find them no more effective than standard nipples or actually disadvantageous.

THE PIERRE ROBIN SYNDROME

The Pierre Robin syndrome consists of (1) mandibular hypoplasia (commonly but less properly termed micrognathia), (2) glossoptosis, and, virtually always, (3) a midline posterior cleft of the palate. Although the etiology of the syndrome is obscure, all its elements probably result pathogenetically from a primary deficiency early in fetal life of mandibular development (Smith, 1970). Usually the Pierre Robin syndrome occurs as an isolated triad of abnormalities, but occasionally it constitutes part of more complex clinical entities, such as the trisomy 18 and Stickler syndromes.

Airway Obstruction

Infants with mild forms of the Pierre Robin syndrome present no special problems, but those with more severe forms encounter more difficulty and are at greater risk during the first few months of life than infants with much more extensive palatal clefts but no mandibular hypoplasia. Because of the small mandible in the Pierre Robin syndrome, the tongue lies in an abnormally posterior position. It thereby becomes unusually susceptible to the negative-pressure forces of both deglutition and inspiration and tends easily to become aspirated and held in the hypopharynx in ball-valve fashion, effectively obstructing the upper airway (Goldberg and Eckblom, 1962; Fletcher et al., 1969; Mallory and Paradise, 1979). Infants so affected may die suddenly of asphyxia or, more commonly, suffer from chronic, partial obstruction with in some cases cor pulmonale (Mallory and Paradise, 1979; Jeresaty et al., 1969; Cogswell and Easton, 1974; Greenwood et al., 1977) or even congestive heart failure (Mallory and Paradise, 1979; Shah et al., 1970).

Feeding and Nutritional Problems

In severely affected infants with the Pierre Robin syndrome, the feeding and nutritional problems otherwise expected as a consequence of the palatal cleft are compounded by the glossoptotic airway obstruction. Choking episodes during feeding, with aspiration of milk, may in turn further jeopardize respiration. Faced with increased energy needs imposed by the work of labored breathing, infants frequently fail to gain weight or even lose weight and may become progressively enfeebled.

Conservative Management

Because even severe airway obstruction in the Pierre Robin syndrome almost always resolves spontaneously or at least improves markedly by four to six months of age, the cornerstone — indeed the sine qua non — of management for infants with obstruction of any appreciable degree is to assiduously maintain them in the prone position during the first few months in an effort to "buy time." The prone position exploits the influence of gravity on the tongue, so that it tends to fall forward out of the airway, thus becoming less susceptible to being aspirated. If the infant's condition permits, the supine position may be attempted for short periods in order to facilitate diapering, dressing, bathing, and the like, but in the most severe cases all these functions are best carried out with the infant prone. Feeding can in some cases be satisfactorily accomplished in the prone position using a compressible feeder as described earlier, but often attempts at oral feeding not only are more or less unsuccessful but also result in increased respiratory distress. Under such circumstances, gavage feeding via nasogastric tube must be resorted to on a continuing basis. To institute and satisfactorily maintain this regimen, relatively long periods of hospitalization are sometimes necessary, but once the regimen has been successfully instituted, parents usually can be taught quickly to continue it at home.

Surgical Intervention

When, despite maintenance of the infant in the prone position, unacceptable respiratory distress persists, tracheostomy usually must be performed (Pruzansky and Richmond, 1954; Pielou, 1967). Alternative measures, such as nasogastric or nasoesophageal intubation (Stern et al., 1972) or glossopexy (lip-tongue adhesion) (Oeconomopoulos, 1960) in our experience have generally proved ineffective in severe cases, leading to speculation that the reported success of these measures had been achieved in infants who in fact had not been so severely affected and who might have fared equally well with a scrupulously executed conservative regimen.

Mechanism of Spontaneous Resolution of Airway Obstruction

Resolution of airway obstruction in infants with Pierre Robin syndrome who survive the first few months of life has been generally attributed to gradual forward movement of the base of the tongue, assumedly due in turn to progressive mandibular growth (Pruzansky and Richmond, 1954). More likely, however, the underlying event responsible is the infants' acquisition, as a normal developmental phenomenon, of progressively increasing control of tongue musculature (Mallory and Paradise, 1979).

OTOLOGIC AND AUDIOLOGIC PROBLEMS

Almost a century ago (in 1893), Gutzmann first reported that hearing impairment was a significant problem in about half the cleft palate population, and the proportion appears to have remained relatively constant since then (Bluestone, 1971). If patients with relatively minor hearing losses were to be added to the count, the proportion would probably be considerably higher than 50 per cent (Pannbacker, 1969; Walton, 1973). Matching these observations regarding hearing, significant abnormalities of the tympanic membrane have been reported to occur in approximately three quarters of older children and adults with cleft palate (Skolnik, 1958; Aschan, 1966). Those abnormalities have consisted mainly of scarring, distortion of normal architecture, adhesions, perforation, and cholesteatoma. Moreover, otologic difficulties in cleft palate patients appear not to be limited to the middle ear; sensorineural losses also can be found not uncommonly (Bennett, 1972).

Universality of Otitis Media in Affected Infants

In 1966 it was first observed that otitis media with middle ear effusion is present in virtually all infants under two years of age with unrepaired clefts of the palate (Stool and Randall, 1967; Paradise et al., 1969), an observation that has been confirmed in a number of subsequent studies (Paradise and Bluestone, 1974; Paradise 1979; Koch et al., 1970; Møller, 1973; Soudyn and Huffstadt, 1973). Presumably sterile, inflammatory effusions of varied viscosity are found in most infants (Lupovich et al., 1971), but frank suppuration also occurs frequently. Following surgical repair of the palate, the occurrence of otitis media is reduced (Paradise and Bluestone, 1974), but for most patients middle ear disease remains an important problem well into later life.

Pathogenesis of Otitis Media in Patients With Cleft Palate

Investigators interested in the pathogenesis of otitis media in patients with cleft palate have consistently focused on the eustachian tube. The hypothesis that middle ear inflammation develops and persists because the tube, although patent anatomically, is unable to open properly and ventilate the middle ear, has found support in investigations over the past two decades involving anatomic studies (Holborow, 1962, 1969), impedance measurements (Paulsen, 1964) and roentgenographic (Bluestone, 1971; Bluestone et al., 1972), and air pressure studies (Bluestone et al., 1972). This presumed impairment of the opening mechanism of the eustachian tube may be a consequence of greater than normal compliance of the tubal wall. Another possible factor in the pathogenesis of otitis media in patients with cleft palate is defective velopharyngeal valving, which may result in disturbed aerodynamic and hydrodynamic relationships in the nasopharynx and proximal portions of the eustachian tubes.

Implications of Middle Ear Disease

It seems reasonable to infer that some of the structural middle ear damage and associated conductive hearing losses noted in older cleft palate patients might be the end result of chronic middle ear inflammation in earlier life. That the sensorineural losses also found in some cleft palate patients (Bennett, 1972) might similarly have originated from early, chronic otitis media is suggested by the observation that inflammation in the middle ear may lead to pathologic changes in the inner ear (Paparella et al., 1972).

Further, it seems reasonable to assume, both on acoustic grounds and on the basis of audiometric findings in older children and adults with middle ear effusions, that the persistent effusions of infants with cleft palate are accompanied by conductive hearing losses of variable degree. Should that be the case, unless these effusions are somehow relieved, it can be assumed that many infants with cleft palate experience persistent hearing impairment of some degree throughout infancy.

Finally, certain evidence suggests the possibility that mild, sustained hearing loss or fluctuating hearing loss during infancy and early childhood may affect adversely the development of speech, language, and cognitive function. While this evidence is far from conclusive (Paradise, 1980), it seems reasonable to speculate that the restrictions of language skill and the various psychological problems often found in older children with cleft palate (McWilliams et al., 1973) might be at least in part traceable to hearing loss consequent to persistent otitis media during their infancy and early childhood.

Management of Otitis Media in Infants With Cleft Palate

Rational management of presumably non-suppurative middle ear effusion, as distinct from episodes of infection, is limited to one of two opposite approaches: (1) watchful waiting, having advised parents to take into account, in child care, that the effusion may interfere with hearing; or (2) early myringotomy, aspiration of the effusion, and insertion of tympanostomy tubes. The latter approach has produced reasonably satisfactory short-term results, as judged by relief of discomfort and improvement in hearing, and therefore has been advocated in recent years (Paradise and Bluestone, 1974). However, it remains uncertain whether these benefits sufficiently offset the difficulties and complications of the treatment regimen, namely, the necessity of frequent examination to determine whether tympanostomy tubes are in place and patent, the necessity to carry out repeat myringotomy on infants whose tubes have been extruded, the frequent occurrence of purulent otorrhea that is often fairly resistant to treatment, and the frequent development of seemingly significant eardrum scarring (Paradise, 1976).

Until further data are available from long-term studies currently in progress (Paradise, 1979), it seems reasonable to recommend that infants with cleft palate receive myringotomy and tympanostomy tube insertion at a relatively early age (within the first six months or so), especially if hearing acuity seems impaired or if discomfort or frequent bouts of infection are occurring. Two to three months may be a convenient age for infants who also have cleft lip, since at that age lip repair is often undertaken, and the two operations can then be accomplished with a single administration of anesthesia. Once the tubes have been extruded, as is inevitable eventually, myringotomy and tube insertion should be repeated if middle ear effusion recurs and remains persistent. The degree of aggressiveness of surgical management may be guided by the severity of the symptomatology, particularly hearing impairment and recurrent infection. Further discussion of this problem may be found in Chapter 16.

REFERENCES

Aschan, G. 1966. Hearing and nasal function correlated to postoperative speech in cleft palate patients with velopharyngoplasty. Acta Otolaryngol., *61*:371.

Bennett, M. 1972. The older cleft palate patient (a clinical otologic-audiologic study). Laryngoscope, *82*:1217.

Bluestone, C. D. 1971. Eustachian tube obstruction in the infant with cleft palate. Ann. Otol. Rhinol. Laryngol., *80*(Suppl. 2):1.

Bluestone, C. D., Paradise, J. L., Beery, Q. C., et al. 1972. Certain effects of cleft palate repair on eustachian tube function. Cleft Palate J., *9*:183.

Bluestone, C. D., Wittel, R. A., and Paradise, J. L. 1972. Roentgenographic evaluation of eustachian tube function in infants with cleft and normal palates. Cleft Palate J., *9*:93.

Burston, W. R. 1958. The early orthodontic treatment of cleft palate conditions. Dent. Pract., *9*:41.

Cogswell, J.J., and Easton, D. M. 1974. Cor pulmonale in the Pierre Robin syndrome. Arch. Dis. Child., *49*:905.

Drillien, C. M., Ingram T. T. S., and Wilkinson, E. M. 1966. The Causes and Natural History of Cleft Lip and Palate. Baltimore, Williams and Wilkins Co., 1966, pp. 102–140.

Fletcher, M. M., Blum, S. L., and Blanchard, C. L. 1969. Pierre Robin syndrome: Pathophysiology of obstructive episodes. Laryngoscope, *79*:547.

Goldberg, M. H., and Eckblom, R. H. 1962. The treatment of the Pierre Robin syndrome. Pediatrics, *30*:450.

Greenwood, R. D., Waldman, J. D., Rosenthal, A., et al. 1977. Cardio-vascular abnormalities associated with Pierre Robin anomaly. Pediatr. Dig., *19*(11):31.

Gutzmann, H. 1893. Zur Prognose und Behandlung der Angeborenen Gaumendefekte. Mschr. Sprachheilk.

Holborow, C. A. 1962. Deafness associated with cleft palate. J. Laryngol. Otol., *76*:762.

Holborow, C. A. 1969. The assessment of eustachian function. J. Otolaryngol. Soc. Aust., *2*:18.

Jeresaty, R. M., Huszar, R. J., and Basu, S. 1969. Pierre Robin syndrome. Am. J. Dis. Child., *117*:710.

Koch, H. F., Neveling, R., and Hartung, W. 1970. Studies concerning the problems of ear diseases in cleft palate children. Cleft Palate J., *7*:187.

Lifton, J. C. 1956. Methods of feeding infants with cleft palate. J. Am. Dent. Assoc., *53*:22.

Lupovich, P., Bluestone, C. D., Paradise, J. L., et al. 1971. Middle ear effusions: Preliminary viscometric, histologic and biochemical studies. Ann. Otol. Rhinol. Laryngol., *80*:342.

Mallory, S. B., and Paradise, J. L. 1979. Glossoptosis revisited: On the development and resolution of airway obstruction in the Pierre Robin syndrome. New observations from a case with cor pulmonale. Pediatrics, *64*:946.

Malson, T. S. 1969. Prosthesis for the newborn. J. Prosth. Dent., *21*:384.

McWilliams, B. J., Morris, H. L., Shelton, R. L., et al. 1973. Speech, language, and psychological aspects of cleft lip and cleft palate: The state of the art. ASHA, *9*:1.

Møller, P. 1973. Otopathology and hearing loss in cleft palate patients during the first 15 years of life. Presented at the Second International Congress on Cleft Palate, Copenhagen, August 30, 1973.

Oeconomopoulos, C. T. 1960. The value of glossopexy in Pierre Robin syndrome. N. Engl. J. Med., *262*:1267.

Pannbacker, J. 1969. Hearing loss and cleft palate. Cleft Palate J., *6*:50.

Paparella, M. M., Oda, M., Hiraide, F., et al. 1972. Pathology of sensorineural hearing loss in otitis media. Ann. Otol. Rhinol. Laryngol., *81*:632.

Paradise, J. L. 1976. Management of middle ear effusion in infants with cleft palate. Ann. Otol. Rhinol. Laryngol., *85*(Suppl. 25):285.

Paradise, J. L. 1979. Otitis media in infants with cleft palate. *In* Wiet, R. J., and Coulthard, S. W. (Eds) Proceedings of the Second National Conference on Otitis Media, Columbus, Ohio, Ross Laboratories, pp. 62–66.

Paradise, J. L. 1980. Review article: Otitis media in infants and children. Pediatrics, *65*:917.

Paradise, J. L., and Bluestone, C. D. 1974. Early treatment of the universal otitis media of infants with cleft palate. Pediatrics, *53*:48.

Paradise, J. L., and McWilliams, B. J. 1974. Simplified feeder for infants with cleft palate. Pediatrics, *53*:566.

Paradise, J. L., Bluestone, C. D., and Felder, H. 1969. The universality of otitis media in 50 infants with cleft palate. Pediatrics, *44*:35.

Paradise, J. L., Alberti, P. W. R. M., Bluestone, C. D., et al. 1974. Pediatric and otologic aspects of clinical research in cleft palate. Clin. Pediatr., *13*:587.

Parkins, F. M., and Barbero, G. J. 1975. The oral cavity. *In* Vaughan, C. V., III, and McKay, R. N. Nelson Textbook of Pediatrics, 10 ed. Philadelphia, W. B. Saunders Co., p. 796.

Paulsen, J. W. 1964. Studies on the hearing and the tubal function in a series of children with cleft palates. Acta Otolaryngol., *188*(Suppl.) (Stockh):36.

Pielou, W. D. 1967. Nonsurgical management of Pierre Robin syndrome. Arch. Dis. Child., *42*:20.

Pruzansky, S., and Richmond, J. B. 1954. Growth of mandible in infants with micrognathia. Am. J. Dis. Child., *88*:29.

Schaffer, A. J., and Avery, M. E. 1971. Diseases of the Newborn, 3rd ed. Philadelphia, W. B. Saunders Co., p. 722.

Shah, C. V., Pruzansky, S., and Harris, W. S. 1970. Cardiac malformations with facial clefts. Am. J. Dis. Child., *119*:238.

Skolnik, E. M. 1958. Otologic evaluation in cleft palate patients. Laryngoscope, *68*:1908.

Smith, D. W. 1970. Recognizable Patterns of Human Malformation. Philadelphia, W. B. Saunders Co., p. 2.

Soudyn, E. R., and Huffstadt, A. J. C. 1973. Routine micro ear examination in cleft palate babies. Abstracts of the Second International Congress on Cleft Palate, Copenhagen, August 26–31, 1973.

Stern, L. M., Fonkalsrud, E. W., Hassakis, P., et al. 1972. Management of Pierre Robin syndrome in infancy by prolonged nasoesophageal intubation. Am. J. Dis. Child., *124*:78.

Stool, S. E., and Randall, P. 1967. Unexpected ear disease in infants with cleft palate. Cleft Palate J., *4*:99.

Tisza, V. B., and Gumpertz, E. 1962. The parents' reaction to the birth and early care of children with cleft palate. Pediatrics, *30*:86.

Walton, W. K. 1973. Audiometrically "normal" conductive hearing losses among the cleft palate. Cleft Palate J., *10*:99.

Williams, A. C., Rothman, B. N., and Seidman, I. H. 1968. Management of a feeding problem in an infant with cleft palate. J. Am. Dent. Assoc., *77*:81.

Zickefoose, M. 1957. Feeding problems of children with cleft palate. Children, *4*:225.

Chapter 45

DENTAL AND GINGIVAL DISORDERS

Robert Rapp, D.D.S., M.S., F.R.C.D.(C)

The oral cavity can serve as a barometer of a child's general health. Despite the accessibility of the oral soft and hard tissues, however, examination of the tongue, teeth, gingiva, mucosa, and palate is frequently neglected. This simple and important part of the physical examination should never be neglected, as a knowledge of dental and gingival disorders and their identification will assist the pediatrician in evaluating the status of the child's health. In addition, as many systemic infections and syndromes show manifestations in the mouth and teeth, failure to examine these structures could mislead the diagnostician.

THE TEETH

Dental Development

A tooth consists of three calcified tissues: enamel, dentin, and cementum. A specialized connective tissue, the dental pulp, is located within the tooth surrounded by dentin (Fig. 45–1). Formation of the first primary tooth, the mandibular central incisor, begins during the third month of fetal life, and the tooth erupts into the oral cavity when the infant is an average of 7.5 months old (Kraus and Jordan, 1965; Meredith, 1943; Robinow et al., 1942). The primary dentition consists of 10 teeth in the maxilla and 10 in the mandible and persists until approximately six years of age, at which time the first permanent molar usually erupts. Between six and 12 years of age, the child has a mixed dentition, characterized by the presence of both primary and permanent teeth. By approximately 12 years of age, with exfoliation of the last primary

tooth (the second primary molar) and eruption of the remaining permanent teeth (with exception of the third molars — the wisdom teeth), the child is considered to have the permanent dentition (Table 45–3). This dentition is completed at approximately 17 to 21 years of age by eruption of the third molars (Logan and Kronfeld, 1933).

Life Cycle of a Tooth

Each tooth, primary or permanent, passes through recognized stages of development, frequently designated as its life cycle (Table 45–1). Interference with any of these sequential stages of development by trauma, introduction of foreign substances, nutritional deficiencies, or excessive or deficient development can produce characteristic and recognizable defects in the tooth.

Chronology of Dental Development

The chronologic development of the primary and permanent teeth is shown in Tables 45–2 and 45–3. It should be recognized that relating aspects of tooth development to a specific chronologic age is a precarious practice, as growth proceeds according to its own schedule and not always in agreement with tables of average values. Instead these tables of average values should assist the physician in the initial assessment of a child's dental development. A more accurate appraisal of a child's dental chronology may be made by calculating the dental calcification age; comparison of the degree of calcification of a permanent tooth, as seen on a dental radio-

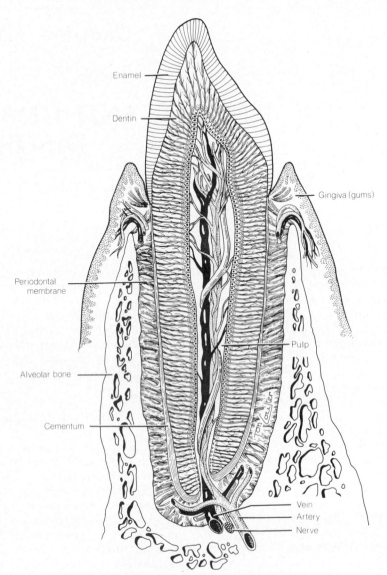

Enamel

Dentin

Gingiva (gums)

Periodontal
membrane

Alveolar bone

Cementum

Pulp

Vein
Artery
Nerve

Figure 45-1 A diagrammatic representation of a tooth and its surrounding tissues. Note the enamel of the crown, dentin, and cementum on the root. The dental pulp, containing blood vessels (arteries and veins) and nerves, is located within the crown and root. Openings at the end of the root, the apical foramina, allow entry and exit of the blood vessels and nerves. The periodontal membrane attaches the root of the tooth to the alveolar bone. Branches of the blood vessels that supply the tooth also supply the periodontal membrane and gingival tissue. Note the attachment of the gingiva to the tooth at the enamel-cementum junction as well as a space between the enamel and gingiva — the gingival sulcus.

graph, to that seen in a series of 10 drawings of normally developing maxillary and mandibular teeth (Table 45–4) allows the physician to determine the percentage of development of a specific tooth relative to the norm. By referring to Tables 45–5 (girls) and 45–6 (boys), which show the percentage of calcification of specific teeth at certain chronologic ages, the physician can estimate the child's physiologic age (Nolla, 1960).

Eruption of Teeth

Of greater clinical significance than the times at which teeth erupt into the oral cavity is the sequence in which they erupt (Moyers, 1973). Sequence of eruption influences tooth position in the dental arch (Fig. 45–2). Less variation occurs in the sequence of eruption of primary teeth than occurs with eruption of the permanent teeth (Moyers, 1973).

Text continued on page 937

Table 45-1 GROWTH STAGES AND ASSOCIATED ANOMALIES OF HUMAN TEETH*

	Growth →							
	Initiation →	Prolifera-tion →	Histo-differentiation →	Morpho-differentiation →	Apposition →	Calcification →	Eruption →	Attrition
Character of Disturbance	*Abnormal Number*		*Atypical Structure*	*Atypical Forms and Sizes*	*Abnormal Amount*	*Abnormal Hardness*	*Abnormal Eruption*	*Abnormal Wearing*
Deficient development	Anodontia – partial or complete Congenital absence of lateral incisors, third molars, bi-cuspids, etc.		Amelogenesis imperfecta (ameloblasts) Dentinogenesis imperfecta (odontoblasts) Vitamin A deficiency (odontogenic epithelium)	Peg teeth Hutchinson's incisor Mulberry molars Microdontia	Hypoplasias – systemic or local Chronologic enamel hypoplasia Localized enamel pits Dentin hypoplasia (pulpal inclusions)	Hypocalcification Mottled (chalky) enamel Malocotic enamel Interglobular dentin	Delayed eruption of teeth single or multiple Submerged denture Submerged teeth (ankylosis) Impacted teeth Malposed teeth	Deficient wear Restricted lateral excursion
Excessive development	Epithelial rests ──→ Odontogenic epithelium ──→ Cysts; Adamantinomas; Odontocoeles ──→ Odontomes ──→ Enamel nodules; Simple, compound and complex odontomes			Extra cusps and roots Dens in dente Macrodontia Supernumerary teeth		Sclerotic dentin resulting from age, injury, or caries	Malocclusions Excessive mesial and occlusal drift of teeth Supraocclusion of teeth	Excessive wear Night grinding (bruxism)

*From Schour and Massler, 1940.

Table 45–2   CHRONOLOGY OF DEVELOPMENT OF THE PRIMARY TEETH*

Tooth	Initiation of Hard Tissue Formation (weeks in utero)	Calcification of Tooth Begins (weeks in utero)	Amount of Enamel at Birth	Crown Completed (month)	Eruption (month)	Root Completed (year)	Root Resorption Begins (year)	Tooth Shed (year)
Maxilla and Mandible								
Central incisor	7	14 (13–16)	3/5–5/6	1–3	6–8	1½–2	5–6	6–7
Lateral incisor	7	16 (14½–16½)	3/5–2/3	2–3	7–9	1½–2	5–6	7–8
Canine	7½	17 (15–18)	1/3	9	16–18	2½–3¼	6–7	9–12
First molar	8	15½ (14½–17)	Cusps united	6	12–14	2–2½	4–5	9–11
Second molar	9	18½ (16–23½)	Cusp tips still isolated	10–12	20–24	3	4–5	10–12

*From Logan and Kronfeld, 1933; Schour and Massler, 1940; and Lunt and Law, 1974.

Table 45-3 CHRONOLOGY OF DEVELOPMENT OF THE PERMANENT TEETH*

Tooth	Initiation (month)	Calcification Begins	Amount of Enamel at Birth	Crown Completed (year)	Eruption (year)	Root Completed (year)
Maxilla:						
Central incisor	5–5¼ *in utero*	3–4 months	Sometimes a trace	4–5	7–8	10
Lateral incisor	5–5¼ *in utero*	1 year		4–5	8–9	11
Canine	5½–6 *in utero*	4–5 months		6–7	11–12	13–15
First premolar	Birth	1½–1¾ years		5–6	10–11	12–13
Second premolar	7½–8	2–2¼ years		6–7	10–12	12–14
First molar	3½–4 *in utero*	Birth		2½–3	6–7	9–10
Second molar	8½–9	2½–3 years		7–8	12–13	14–16
Third molar	3½–4 (yr)	7–9 years		12–16	17–21	18–25
Mandible:						
Central incisor	5–5¼ *in utero*	3–4 months		4–5	6–7	9
Lateral incisor	5–5¼ *in utero*	3–4 months		4–5	7–8	10
Canine	5½–6 *in utero*	4–5 months		6–7	9–11	12–14
First premolar	Birth	1¾–2½ months		5–6	10–12	12–13
Second premolar	7½–8	2¼–2½ years		6–7	11–12	13–14
First molar	3½–4 *in utero*	Birth		2½–3	6–7	9–10
Second molar	8½–9	2½–3 years		7–8	11–13	14–15

*From Logan and Kronfeld, 1933; Schour and Massler, 1940; Lunt and Law, 1974.

Table 45–4 STAGES OF DEVELOPMENT OF PERMANENT TEETH*

Mandible	Maxilla	Percentage of Tooth Calcification
Growth Stage	Growth Stage	
		100. Apical end of root completed
		90. Root almost completed, open apex
		80. Two thirds of the root completed
		70. One third of the root completed
		60. Crown completed
		50. Almost completed crown
		40. Two thirds of the crown completed
		30. One third of the crown completed
		20. Initial calcification
		10. Presence of the crypt
		Absence of the crypt

*From Nolla, 1960. Drawings of the amount (percentage) of tooth calcification, as seen on radiographs. Stage 20 shows the initial trace of calcification. Stage 60 shows completion of enamel calcification (completion of the tooth crown). Stage 100 shows completion of root formation (tooth is completely formed). Compare these percentages of formation to specific teeth, as seen in Tables 45–5 (girls) and 45–6 (boys) to obtain the physiologic age of the child.

Table 45–5 MATURATION OF PERMANENT TEETH — GIRLS*

Mandibular Teeth (Growth Stage) (Percentage)								Maxillary Teeth (Growth Stage) (Percentage)						
Central Incisor	Lateral Incisor	Cuspid	1st Bi-cuspid	2nd Bi-cuspid	1st Molar	2nd Molar	Age (Yrs.)	Central Incisor	Lateral Incisor	Cuspid	1st Bi-cuspid	2nd Bi-cuspid	1st Molar	2nd Molar
11	22	33	44	55	66	77		11	22	33	44	55	66	77
53	47	34	29	17	50	16	3	43	37	33	26	20	45	18
66	60	44	39	28	62	28	4	54	48	43	36	30	57	28
76	72	54	49	38	73	39	5	65	58	53	46	40	69	38
85	81	63	58	48	81	50	6	74	67	62	56	49	79	47
93	89	72	67	57	87	59	7	83	76	70	65	58	87	56
98	95	80	75	66	93	67	8	90	84	78	73	66	93	65
100	99	87	83	74	97	74	9	96	91	85	81	74	97	72
	100	92	89	81	100	81	10	100	96	91	87	81	100	79
		97	94	86		86	11		100	95	93	87		85
		100	97	91		91	12			98	97	93		90
			100	94		95	13			100	100	97		95
				97		97	14					100		97
				100		98	15							98
						100	16							100

*From Nolla, 1960.

Table 45–6 MATURATION OF PERMANENT TEETH – BOYS*

Mandibular Teeth (Growth Stage) (Percentage)							Age (Yrs.)	Maxillary Teeth (Growth Stage) (Percentage)						
Central Incisor	Lateral Incisor	Cuspid	1st Bicuspid	2nd Bicuspid	1st Molar	2nd Molar		Central Incisor	Lateral Incisor	Cuspid	1st Bicuspid	2nd Bicuspid	1st Molar	2nd Molar
11	22	33	44	55	66	77		11	22	33	44	55	66	77
52	45	32	26	11	50	7	3	43	34	30	20	10	42	10
65	57	42	35	22	62	20	4	54	45	39	30	20	53	20
75	68	51	44	33	70	30	5	64	55	48	40	30	64	30
82	77	59	52	43	77	40	6	73	64	56	49	40	74	40
88	85	67	60	53	84	50	7	82	72	63	57	49	82	50
93	91	74	68	62	90	59	8	88	80	70	65	58	89	58
97	95	80	75	70	95	67	9	94	87	77	72	66	94	65
100	98	86	82	77	98	74	10	97	93	84	79	73	97	72
		91	88	83	99	79	11	99.5	97	88	86	80	98	78
		96	94	89		84	12		99.5	92	92	87		83
		98	97	94		89	13			96	96	93		88
		100	100	97		93	14			98	98	96		93
				100		97	15			99	99	99		96
						100	16.5							100

* From Nolla, 1960.

The sequence in which permanent teeth erupt has a profound effect on dental occlusion. The sequence of eruption of permanent teeth that produces the highest rate (45 to 68 per cent) of normal occlusion is shown in Figure 45–2 (Lo and Moyers, 1953; Moyers, 1973). Eruption of the maxillary first permanent molar before the mandibular first molar is prognostic of developing malocclusion in which the upper arch is positioned anteriorly to the lower. More serious alterations in the normal sequence of eruption of permanent

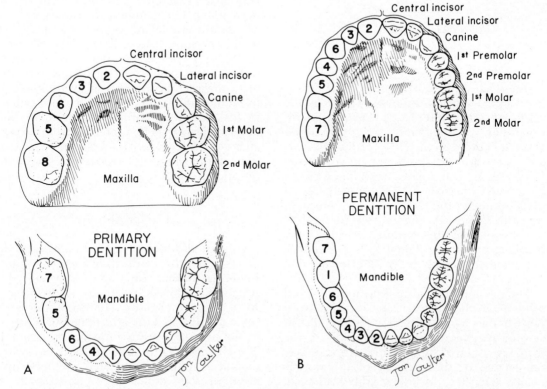

Figure 45–2 A, The most frequent eruption sequence of the primary teeth. B, The sequence of eruption of the permanent teeth most likely to produce normal occlusion.

Table 45-7 NUMBER OF PRIMARY TEETH ERUPTED ACCORDING TO AGE*

Age	Percentage of Children	Number of Teeth Erupted	
		Range	Mean
6 mos.	33	1 or more	—
9 mos.	80	1–6	3
12 mos.	50	4–8	6
18 mos.	85	9–16	12
24 mos.	60	15–18	16
30 mos.	70	20	19

*From Hatton, 1955 and Meredith, 1943.

teeth may occur in the mixed dentition stage of development. Eruption of the second permanent molar before the cuspid in the maxilla can cause shortening of arch length, which leads to impaction of the cuspid. Eruption of the second permanent molar in the mandible before the second bicuspid will push the first molar forward, impacting the bicuspid. Further problems of eruption are discussed later in this chapter.

When examining a child's mouth, the number of teeth present at a given age should also be assessed (Table 45–7) (Hatton, 1955; Meredith, 1943).

DENTAL DISORDERS

Dental Caries

Dental caries is regarded as being the most prevalent disease of humans. Caries is the result of three interacting factors: microorganisms (predominantly *Streptococcus mutans*), susceptible teeth, and a readily fermentable carbohydrate (predominantly sucrose) (Finn, 1973). The organisms, acting within a gelatinous adhesive material called dental plaque, convert the sucrose to acid, which, in turn, decalcifies the enamel to create a carious lesion, or cavity. Removal of plaque by brushing and using dental floss can reduce or eliminate dental decay (McDonald and Avery, 1978).

Topical applications of fluoride gels and solutions to the teeth will increase the resistance of the enamel to acid dissolution. Provision of systemic fluoride, preferably in the drinking water or by pills and drops, is recommended by the majority of the world's health agencies, including the American Medical Association and the American Academy of Pediatrics (Newbrun, 1972). Diets

should be analyzed for their quantities of cariogenic types of food, and excessive amounts of these foods should be reduced or eliminated. All carious lesions should be removed and replaced by appropriate materials to restore the integrity and function of the tooth (Cohen and Hooley, 1977).

Nursing Bottle Caries

Of particular interest to pediatricians is a form of rampant dental decay frequently seen in infants and children who have been kept on a nursing bottle beyond the usual age of weaning. The mandibular primary incisors are usually free of caries, but the remaining teeth develop carious lesions on all their surfaces (Fig. 45–3). This devastating form of decay results from constant exposure of the teeth to sweetened liquids or even milk kept in the nursing bottle, which the child retains in his mouth for prolonged periods. The lower incisors may be protected from carious attack by a labioglossal seal created by protrusion of the tongue to contact the lower lip (Rapp and Winter, 1979).

Alveolar Abscess

Untreated dental caries, unsuccessful dental pulp therapy, or death of the dental pulp following trauma may lead to pulp necrosis. An alveolar abscess frequently follows necrosis of the dental pulp. The acute abscess is often painful, and the affected tooth is usually sensitive to pressure during mastication. The chronic stage of the abscess can be asymptomatic in spite of an infected, inflamed, and often necrotic dental pulp. Destruction of alveolar bone about the root apices is a frequent radiologic finding in permanent teeth,

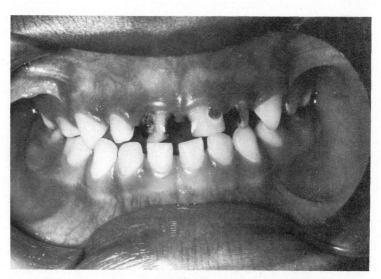

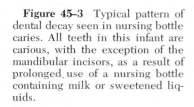

Figure 45–3 Typical pattern of dental decay seen in nursing bottle caries. All teeth in this infant are carious, with the exception of the mandibular incisors, as a result of prolonged use of a nursing bottle containing milk or sweetened liquids.

whereas radiolucency in the root bifurcation-trifurcation areas is seen with primary molars. Unerupted permanent teeth lying beneath the involved primary teeth may become infected, producing a brownish discoloration on the forming enamel of the permanent teeth (Finn, 1973). Formation of a "gum boil" or fistulous opening in the gingival tissue is an indication of pulpal necrosis and drainage of pus from the root canals (Fig. 45–4) (Rapp and Winter, 1979). The involved tooth, especially before pus escapes through the periosteum, often causes intense, throbbing pain, feels slightly elevated, is sensitive to pressure, and appears to be slightly mobile. Extraoral drainage of the abscess onto the face, while not as prevalent as intraoral drainage, is occasionally seen and can leave a facial scar

(Finn, 1973; Rapp and Winter, 1979). Frequently associated with an alveolar abscess is drainage of accumulating pus along fascia and fascial planes, manifesting itself in a facial cellulitis involving the cheek and often the eye (Fig. 45–5). In such a condition, the teeth should be examined closely for large, untreated carious lesions, restorations, excessive mobility, and inflamed gingival tissue. Infection from an abscessed tooth may spread via the lymphatics to regional lymph nodes, which then become swollen, palpable, and tender (Finn, 1973). Treatment of an abscessed permanent tooth consists of administration of systemic antibiotics to control inflammation and infection, followed by endodontic therapy in which the root canals are drained, cleansed, and filled. Primary teeth

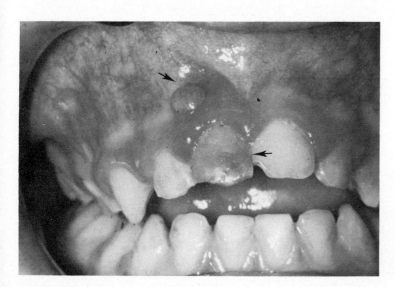

Figure 45–4 A gum boil or draining periapical alveolar abscess (arrow) located above the root of a traumatized discolored, nonvital, right primary central incisor (arrow) on a three year old boy.

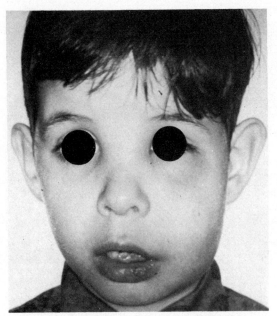

Figure 45–5   Facial cellulitis, arising from an infected tooth and alveolar abscess, involving the left cheek and extending to the left eye. Antibiotic administration followed by removal of the carious tooth will control the infection and inflammation.

may be treated in a similar manner but are more likely to be extracted if root canal therapy appears to be complicated or if the tooth is grossly decayed.

DENTAL CHARACTERISTICS

Shape of Teeth

Although primary and permanent teeth have characteristic morphologic forms, deviations from these forms may occur. A geminated tooth, originating from a single tooth germ, has a bifid crown situated on a single root. Fused teeth originate from two tooth germs, have separate pulp chambers, and are joined at the dentin. Dental decay is frequently found along the fusion line in the crowns of fused teeth (Law et al., 1969). Congenital syphilis may manifest itself through malformed permanent incisors and molars. A notched incisal (biting) edge and screwdriver shape are pathognomonic of Hutchinson disease, as is a pebbly or mulberry appearance on the occlusal surface of affected first permanent molars (Rapp and Winter, 1979). A dilacerated tooth, which forms from trauma to the tooth bud before completion of calcification, has its root abnormally angulated to the crown. Cusps of teeth often assume abnormal shapes, sizes, or even locations. Maxillary central incisors can develop an exaggerated cingulum or supernumerary cusp. Such structures are harmless unless they provide pathways for organisms to enter the pulp chamber. Dental abrasion, often a result of excessively vigorous toothbrushing, is seen as a V-shaped erosion of the cementum and dentin along the border of the gingiva. Dental attrition, in which the occlusal surfaces become worn and flattened, may be seen in children who react adversely to stress (Rapp and Winter, 1979).

Tooth Size

The size of teeth, which is genetically controlled, is a factor in the development of occlusal irregularities (Moyers, 1973; Rapp and Winter, 1979). A child inheriting small facial size in combination with large teeth can be expected to have crowded dental arches or a malocclusion. Aside from teeth that are generally large (macrodontia) or those that

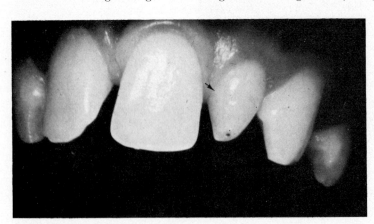

Figure 45–6   An abnormally small, peg-shaped permanent left lateral incisor (arrow). This tooth can be restored to normal shape by use of a dental crown.

Table 45–8 COLOR CHANGES OF TEETH

	Color	Location	Etiology	Population
Extrinsic Colors (descending order of frequency)	Green	Labial surface of upper, lower incisors and canines	Bacterial (?) Poor hygiene	Mainly children
	Brown	Posterior teeth parallel to gingival margins	Bacterial (?)	Children
	Orange	Labial, buccal surfaces of anterior and posterior teeth	Bacterial (?) Poor hygiene	Children
	Black	Labial, buccal surfaces of anterior and posterior teeth	Bacterial (?) Poor hygiene	Children
Intrinsic Colors	Yellow	Entire tooth	Tetracycline medication Jaundice, premature birth Amelogenesis imperfecta	Children, adolescents
	Brown	Entire tooth	Tetracycline medication Amelogenesis imperfecta Dentinogenesis imperfecta Premature birth Cystic fibrosis Porphyria	Children, adolescents
	Blue, blue-green	Entire tooth	Erythroblastosis fetalis	Children
	White	Entire tooth	Amelogenesis imperfecta (hereditary enamel hypoplasia)	Children, adolescents
	White	Localized areas	Amelogenesis imperfecta (hereditary enamel hypocalcification)	Children, adolescents
	Reddish-brown	Entire tooth	Porphyria	Children
	Gray-brown	Entire tooth	Dentinogenesis imperfecta	Children, adolescents

are small (microdontia), a single tooth may be excessively oversized or undersized. An undersized tooth is said to be "pegged" (Fig. 45–6).

Color of Teeth

Primary teeth are whiter in color than are the more beige-yellow colored permanent teeth, a fact that frequently causes parental concern when both tooth types are present in the oral cavity at the same time. There are, however, color changes of the teeth that are abnormal. Tooth discoloration is either extrinsic, arising from a staining agent deposited on the external surfaces of the enamel, or intrinsic, due to a discoloring factor having been incorporated into the enamel and dentin. (Table 45–8). Extrinsic stains occur most frequently on the maxillary primary incisors and canines, along the edges of the gingiva. The stains, which may be green, brown, orange, or black, are usually deposited on roughened enamel surfaces and tend to be somewhat tenacious (Law et al., 1969). The etiology of extrinsic stains is unknown, although poor oral hygiene, bacteria, and iron-containing medications are suspected to be factors. Removal is accomplished by abrasive polishing agents.

Calculus (tartar) is a mineralized deposit that, when it forms on teeth, can create extrinsic discoloration. It is seen infrequently in young children, more commonly in adolescents and adults. Calculus is usually creamy-white in color and is unsightly when severe. It should not be allowed to accumulate, as it may lead to gingivitis and periodontitis (Baer and Benjamin, 1974) (Fig. 45–7).

Intrinsic stains or pigmentation of teeth may be varied in color and are due to a variety of causes, including disintegrating blood pigments within the dental pulp, drugs, or a genetic propensity to develop such discoloration. A yellow or brown pig-

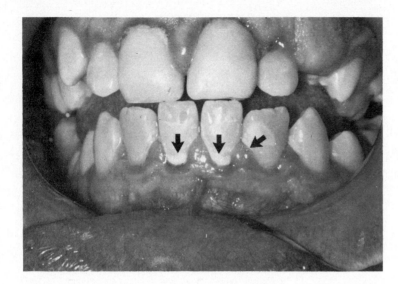

Figure 45–7 Calculus (tartar) can be seen forming on the mandibular central incisors (arrows) of a young boy who is not maintaining proper oral hygiene. Besides being unsightly, calculus can cause gingival inflammation (arrow).

mentation of the enamel of primary teeth is often associated with premature birth. Erythroblastosis fetalis produces a characteristic blue-green color of the primary teeth as a result of bile pigments (bilirubin or biliverdin) being absorbed into the dentin (Finn, 1973; McDonald and Avery, 1978).

Congenital porphyria produces a reddish-brown discoloration of the primary and permanent teeth. Fluorescence of the teeth and fingernails during exposure to ultraviolet light, because of porphyrins in the forming dentin and enamel, is characteristic of this condition (Law et al., 1969). The teeth of children with cystic fibrosis range in color from yellow to gray to dark brown.

Tetracycline antibiotics produce a discoloration of primary and permanent teeth when administered during calcification of the enamel and dentin. Color changes can range from yellow to brown to gray. The intensity of color appears to be related to dosage and type of drug used (McDonald and Avery, 1978). The use of tetracycline drugs while teeth are forming should be avoided (Fig. 45–8).

Dental fluorosis or mottled enamel occurs when the fluoride content of the drinking water greatly exceeds 1 ppm. The characteristic mottling of the enamel ranges from white spots to yellow-brown areas to dark brown patches (Fig. 45–9).

Figure 45–8 Intrinsic, bluish-gray staining of the primary incisor (arrows) as a result of tetracycline administration for the treatment of rubella. (Courtesy of Dr. J. H. Guggenheimer.)

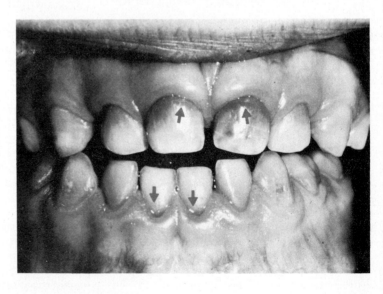

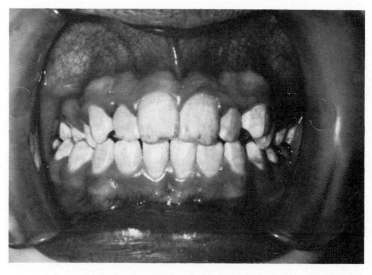

Figure 45–9 Mottled enamel (dental fluorosis) occurring in a 12 year old girl who drank water containing fluoride in excess of 1 ppm. Note the chalky striations on the teeth.

Structure of Teeth

Hereditary interferences with developing teeth produce structural defects, the nature being dependent upon the stage of growth and the cells affected. Amelogenesis imperfecta (hereditary enamel hypoplasia) is one variety of defective enamel in which the principal fault lies in a defect of the ameloblast cells. It is characterized by several different forms of enamel, which can be thin, hard, and discolored (yellow to orange-brown) and smooth, pitted, wrinkled, or grooved on its external surface (Fig. 45–10) (Law et al., 1969; Rapp and Winter 1979). While the enamel is affected, the dentin and pulpal chamber will appear to be normal in a radiograph. The incidence of amelogenesis imperfecta has been reported to be 1 in 14,000 to 1

in 16,000 (Withop, 1959). Another form of amelogenesis imperfecta (hereditary enamel hypocalcification) represents a defect in which an interference occurring during calcification leads the enamel to become softened and abraded. Tooth color in this condition can range from yellow to gray-brown to dull white or to the formation of "snow-capped" areas (Fig. 45–11) (Law et al., 1969; Rapp and Winter, 1979).

An inherited defect of dentin, dentinogenesis imperfecta, causes the teeth to have a blue-gray to brown appearance. The incidence of this condition has been reported to be 1 in 8000 (Law et al., 1969). The teeth abrade rapidly to the level of the gingiva as a result of the enamel chipping off of the dentin (Fig. 45–12). The root canals and pulp chamber become obliterated by accelerated

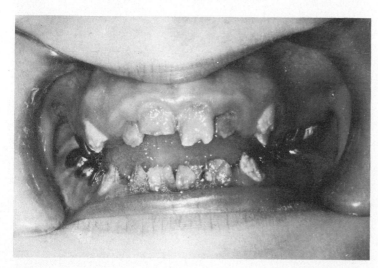

Figure 45–10 An 11 year old girl with hereditary amelogenesis imperfecta (enamel hypoplasia). The enamel of the permanent teeth is discolored, pitted, and hard. Note the use of crowns to protect the posterior teeth from abrasion.

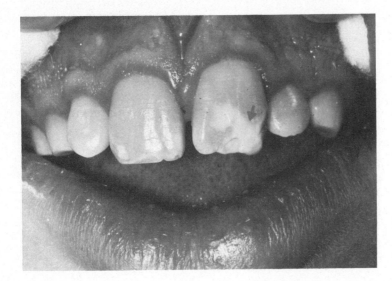

Figure 45–11 Hereditary amelogenesis imperfecta (enamel hypocalcification) is seen on the central incisors (arrow) of this 10 year old boy. Defective calcification of the enamel has produced a "snow-capped" appearance.

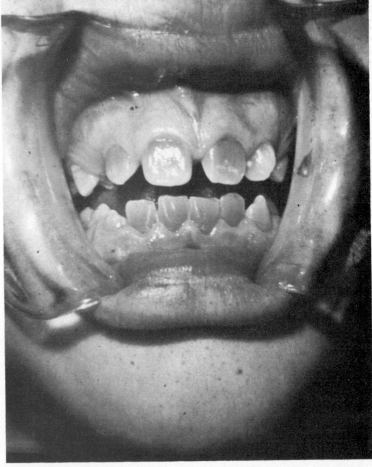

Figure 45–12 A 10 year old child with hereditary dentinogenesis imperfecta. The teeth, which have a blue-gray opalescent appearance, abrade rapidly. The teeth of individuals with osteogenesis imperfecta are similar in appearance.

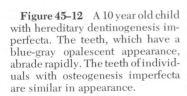

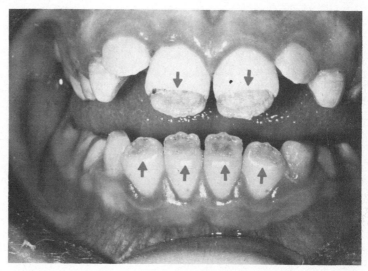

Figure 45–13 Defective enamel (localized enamel hypoplasia) on the maxillary central and mandibular incisors (arrows) of an 8 year old patient who had a history of high fever. Note that the maxillary lateral incisors are not affected as a result of having calcified at a later time.

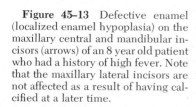

deposition of dentin. Treatment of both dentinogenesis and amelogenesis imperfecta consists of covering the teeth with crowns to prevent additional attrition and pulp death. Localized forms of enamel hypoplasia produce isolated, circumscribed color and structural defects on the surfaces of the tooth crowns. These disturbances can result from fever (during rubella), trauma to the primary teeth, prenatal disturbances, hypoparathyroidism, vitamin D deficiency, and localized infections (Fig. 45–13) (McDonald and Avery, 1978; Rapp and Winter, 1979).

Problems of Eruption

Tooth eruption is the emergence of a developing tooth from its crypt in the alveolar bone into the oral cavity, where it finally contacts its opposing member in the opposite arch (Moyers, 1973). The mechanism of the eruptive process is unknown. Eruption cysts and hematomas may develop as the teeth pass through the gingiva (Fig. 45–14) but do not require treatment, as these tissue enlargements disappear with the appearance of the erupting teeth (McDonald and Avery, 1978; Rapp and Winter, 1979).

Hormonal imbalances such as cretinism, juvenile myxedema, and hypopituitarism, are associated with failure of teeth to erupt. Failure of eruption is also associated with cleidocranial dysostosis, mongolism (Down syndrome) and epidermolysis bullosa (Gorlin et al., 1976; McDonald and Avery, 1978; Shklar and McCarthy, 1976).

In normal children, exfoliating, loose pri-

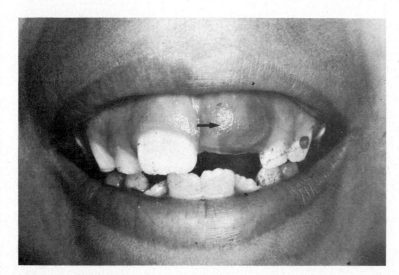

Figure 45–14 An eruption hematoma (arrow) overlying the emerging maxillary left permanent central incisor. The bluish swelling of the gingiva will disappear upon appearance of the tooth.

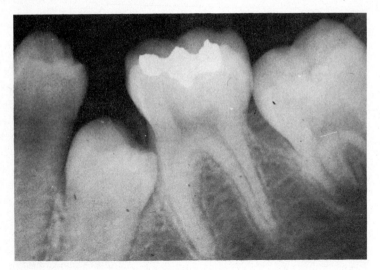

Figure 45–15 Radiograph showing impaction with failure of eruption of a mandibular permanent second bicuspid. The primary molar was extracted prematurely, and a space maintainer was not inserted. As a result, the first molar drifted forward. Insertion of a space maintainer at the time of extraction would have prevented this problem.

mary teeth should usually be left in place unless they are painful or impede mastication. Such teeth should be removed from handicapped children, however, to prevent possible ingestion or aspiration. It is also a common practice to remove exfoliating or otherwise intact teeth from individuals with Lesch-Nyhan syndrome to reduce self-mutilation through biting.

Failure of primary teeth to exfoliate concomitant with failure of permanent teeth to erupt should be evaluated in light of the child's overall development; a slowly growing individual may have late-erupting teeth. If it seems that a child's permanent dentition is slow to develop, metabolic or hormonal disturbances should first be eliminated, as causative factors and then time should be allowed for the child to grow and for the teeth to erupt (Shklar and McCarthy, 1976). Primary teeth should not be removed solely to facilitate eruption of permanent teeth until sufficient time has elapsed, as indicated by available standards, to eliminate normal but slow eruption as the cause. It has been determined that a tooth begins its migration toward the oral cavity upon completion of coronal calcification (Nolla, stage 6). Approximately four to five years are required for a tooth to contact its opposing member following its emergence from the gingival tissues (Shumaker and El Hadary, 1960). Thus, if primary teeth are removed prematurely, a long period of time could elapse before the permanent teeth are in proper position to function in both mastication and maintenance of the arch space.

Eruption of teeth may be delayed by local causes. An ectopically erupting tooth, one which erupts away from its usual position and becomes impacted against a neighboring tooth, usually emerges late. Maxillary first permanent molars and mandibular permanent canines exhibit the greatest tendency to erupt ectopically. Dental arch length may shorten when a primary tooth is prematurely lost, since neighboring teeth will drift into the resulting space. The unerupted permanent tooth, in such a situation, may be prevented from continuing its eruption (Fig. 45–15). A prematurely lost primary tooth, especially a primary molar, should be replaced with a space-maintaining appliance, which will preserve arch length.

A primary molar may become attached to surrounding bone through a calcific union of its root with the bone. Such an ankylosed tooth may fail to erupt, and shortening of the arch length often results. The ankylosed tooth appears to "submerge" beneath the level of neighboring teeth (Fig. 45–16). Diagnosis of an ankylosed tooth is confirmed by percussion to detect a "solid" sound unlike that obtained from other teeth. Radiographs are of limited value in establishing a diagnosis of ankylosis, as the calcific union may not be visible. Following a period of observation to determine if the roots of the ankylosed teeth are not being resorbed, surgical removal is recommended.

An extra (supernumerary) tooth can interfere with eruption, particularly if the supernumerary tooth is itself unerupted and is located in the anterior region of the maxilla or mandible. Supernumerary teeth should be removed only when the surgical procedure will not devitalize neighboring teeth. Permanent maxillary canines occasionally develop

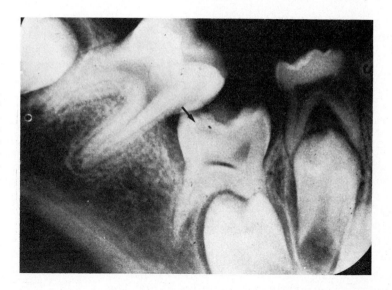

Figure 45–16 Ankylosis and "submergence" of the second primary molar (arrow). Note the forward tipping of the first permanent molar. The ankylosed tooth should have been extracted earlier, and a space maintainer placed to hold the first permanent molar back. (Courtesy of Dr. A. I. Klein.)

high in the palatal vault and will not erupt unassisted. Surgical exposure of their crowns followed by attachment of orthodontic wires can guide such teeth to a normal arch position. While most primary teeth exfoliate prior to eruption of their permanent successors, on occasion this orderly exchange fails to occur, especially in the mandibular anterior region. A condition of "double eruption" is seen if the mandibular permanent incisors erupt lingually to retained primary incisors (Fig. 45–17). The primary teeth should be removed, especially if their roots have not undergone appreciable resorption.

Natal teeth are present at birth, while neonatal teeth erupt during the first month following parturition. The incidence of neonatal teeth has been reported to be 1 per 2000

births and usually involves the lower incisor region (Law et al., 1969; Rapp and Winter, 1979). If the prematurely erupted tooth is supernumerary, it should be removed. Of clinical significance are the dangers of aspiration of a loose natal or neonatal tooth, irritation of the infant's tongue by the tooth, or interference with breast feeding.

THE GINGIVA

Characteristics of the Gingiva

The gingiva surrounds each tooth and extends toward and merges with the alveolar mucosa. Normal gingival tissues of children and adolescents fill the interproximal spaces

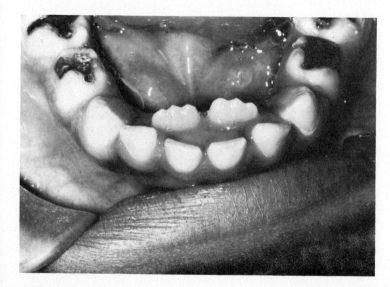

Figure 45–17 Failure of exfoliation of the primary incisors before eruption of the permanent incisors led to the condition of "double eruption." The primary incisors should be removed to allow the permanent incisors to take a more normal position in the dental arch.

**Table 45–9 A CLASSIFICATION
OF PERIODONTAL DISEASE***

Inflammatory
  Gingivitis (inflammation of the gingiva)
  Periodontitis (destruction of the supporting tissues of
    the tooth)

Degenerative
  Noninflammatory diseases of the deeper supporting
    tissues (periodontal and occlusal trauma, gingivo-
    sis, and periodontosis)

Neoplastic
  Neoplastic (tumorous) diseases affecting the perio-
    dontal tissues

*American Academy of Periodontology, 1972.

between the teeth. Healthy gingiva is pale pink in color and somewhat less firm in consistency than that of young adults. The gingival surface also tends to be less stippled than that of adults (Baer and Benjamin, 1974), a feature that tends to increase with age (Finn, 1973). A space, the gingival sulcus, lies between the crown of the tooth and the free margin of the gingiva. The normal sulcus is approximately 1 mm in depth. Periodontal disorders involve the gingiva, periodontal membrane, and alveolar process. A classification of periodontal disease is presented in Table 45–9.

DISORDERS OF THE GINGIVA

Gingivitis

Most children will exhibit some mild, localized gingivitis, but severe forms of gingival inflammation in children are relatively rare (McDonald and Avery, 1978). The most prevalent form of gingivitis is soft tissue inflammation that occurs along the gingival margins and at the gingival papillae, usually in response to poor oral hygiene (Finn, 1973; McDonald and Avery, 1978). Marginal gingivitis can occur at all ages.

Passage of permanent teeth through the gingival tissue is often accompanied by eruption gingivitis, which subsides upon completion of eruption; "teething" in infants is accompanied by an early form of eruption gingivitis. In spite of reports to the contrary, there is no scientific evidence that fever, malaise, or diarrhea results from infant teething.

Acute herpetic gingivostomatitis, an infection caused by the herpes simplex virus, can affect the gingiva of young children, especially those without prior contact and antibody development (Fig. 45–18). The gingiva becomes angry red, and the child usually complains of associated headache, has a high temperature, malaise, excessive salivation, is irritable, and suffers pain, especially after eating citrus fruits (McDonald and Avery, 1978). Treatment should be directed at the relief of symptoms. Owing to the communicability of this condition, the infected individual should be separated from young children. A topical application of tetracycline (Aureomycin) to ulcerated areas to control secondary infection and use of an antihistaminic drug to make the child more comfortable, drowsy, and able to rest have been recommended (McDonald and Avery, 1978). Children with herpes simplex infections frequently develop associated infections of the hands and genitalia through transmission of the virus from lesions on the lips or from saliva (Ravn, 1968).

Acute Necrotizing Ulcerative Gingivitis (ANUG)

Frequently called Vincent infection, acute necrotizing ulcerative gingivitis is seen in older children and young adults, especially when oral hygiene has been neglected (Fig. 45–19). The organisms *Borrelia vincentii* and a fusiform bacillus are believed to be the etiologic agents. A characteristic of necrotizing ulcerative gingivitis is destruction of the interproximal gingival papillae associated with formation of a pseudomembrane over the necrotic tissue. The gingival tissue is inflamed, extremely painful, and hemorrhagic. Patients have a high fever, suffer from general malaise, and have particularly fetid breath. Treatment should consist of antibiotic therapy and removal of oral debris. Oxidizing oral rinses are helpful (Baer and Benjamin, 1974; McDonald and Avery, 1978; Shafer et al., 1974).

Puberty Gingivitis

Males and females in prepubertal and pubertal periods of maturation may develop a characteristic gingivitis (Fig. 45–20). Gingival enlargements of the marginal type occur in the anterior regions of the mouth and are usually larger than those associated with local

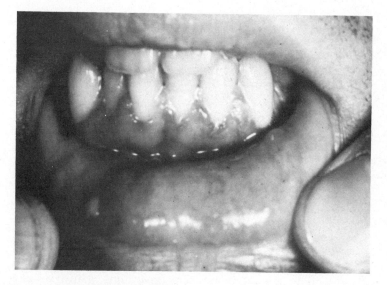

Figure 45–18 Acute herpetic gingivostomatitis in a young patient. The gingiva is red, swollen, and painful, especially with eating. Salivation is excessive. Children with this condition are usually quite ill. (Courtesy of Dr. J. H. Guggenheimer.)

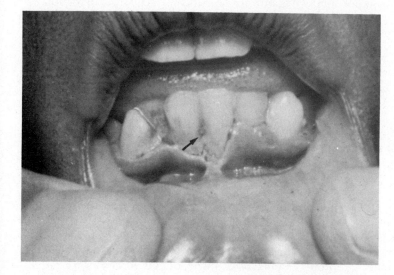

Figure 45–19 Acute necrotizing ulcerative gingivitis (arrow) (Vincent infection), in an adolescent. Note the loss of interproximal gingival papillae, poor oral hygiene, and gingivitis. A high frenum, extending from the oral mucosa to the gingiva, is also present. (Courtesy of Dr. J. H. Guggenheimer.)

Figure 45–20 Bulbous gingival enlargements (arrows) are seen in the maxillary anterior region of this adolescent at the time of puberty. The condition, referred to as "puberty gingivitis," should be treated by surgery if sufficiently severe. (Courtesy of Dr. M. M. Cohen, Sr.)

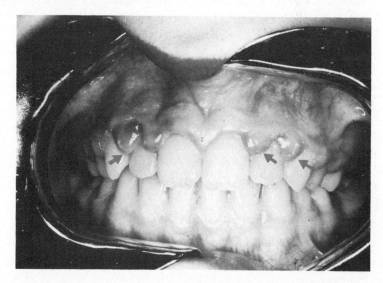

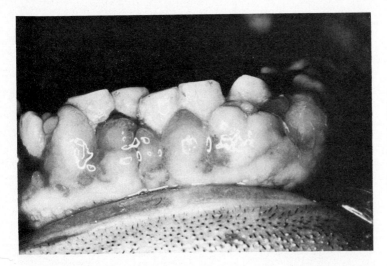

Figure 45–21 Fibrous hyperplasia of the gingiva of an epileptic patient being treated with diphenylhydantoin sodium (Dilantin). Surgical removal of the enlarged tissues, followed by strict oral hygiene procedures, is the frequently recommended treatment. The gingival enlargement commonly recurs. (Courtesy of Dr. M. M. Cohen, Sr.)

irritants. The lingual tissues are rarely involved. Treatment consists of provision and maintenance of excellent oral hygiene (Baer and Benjamin, 1974; McDonald and Avery, 1978; Shklar and McCarthy, 1976).

Dilantin Gingival Hyperplasia

Gingival hyperplasia is frequently seen in children who, for prolonged periods of time, receive diphenylhydantoin sodium (Dilantin) medication for epilepsy. Initially, the gingival tissues are inflamed. Eventually, the tissues become hyperplastic and may enlarge until the crowns of the teeth become covered (Baer and Benjamin, 1974; McDonald and Avery, 1978; Shafer et al., 1974). Surgical removal of the hyperplastic gingiva followed by strict oral hygiene practices remains the accepted method of control, although the problem may recur (Fig. 45–21).

Scorbutic Gingivitis

A rare form of gingivitis, characterized by excessive hemorrhage from the margins and interproximal papillae, may occur when vitamin C intake is deficient. Administration of up to 500 mg of ascorbic acid daily will lead to rapid recovery of gingival health (McDonald and Avery, 1978; Shafer et al., 1974).

Mouthbreathing Gingivitis

Children who breathe through the mouth because of large adenoids or tonsils, nasal blockage, or poor lip muscle tone often demonstrate red, inflamed labial gingival tissues about the maxillary incisors. Correction of the mouthbreathing habit will improve the health of the gingiva.

ORAL TRAUMA

Traumatic injury to the teeth occurs with sufficient frequency to be considered an "occupational hazard" of growing. It has been shown that the incidence of injury to the primary dentition is greater than 18 per cent at six years of age (Andreasen, 1972). During the mixed dentition period, the incidence increases, probably as a result of the child's increasing participation in sports. By the end of the adolescent period, the incidence of oral trauma declines to approximately 10 per cent. Boys incur dental injuries more than twice as often as girls, with the maxillary incisors, especially the centrals, being injured more often than their mandibular counterparts (Ellis and Davey, 1970). Eichenbaum, in 1963, identified an "accident-prone dental profile" in which children with protruding maxillary incisors experience a greater frequency of dental injuries than do those with normal amounts of protrusion and coverage of the teeth by the lips (Chap. 57).

Etiology

The etiology of traumatic injuries to the teeth is associated with the child's stage of growth (Andreasen, 1972).

Infants. Injuries to the teeth, gingiva, and oral mucosa of the infant occur with greater frequency while the child develops greater neuromuscular ability. Falls, such as those from a high chair or during early attempts at walking, produce fractured crowns, gingival lacerations, and intrusions of teeth into their sockets.

School-Age Children. The majority of dental accidents during this period of growth are related to playground activities. Fractures of the incisor crowns, displacement of anterior teeth from their sockets, and injuries to the lips and chin are seen with disconcerting frequency in school-age children.

Teenagers. Injuries to the permanent teeth of teenagers are frequently associated with sporting activities, such as football, baseball, and hockey. Car-related injuries also become more frequent, although the preschool child may also experience car-related injuries to the incisors, lips, and chin through traumatic contact with a dashboard as he sits or stands without safety belts on a seat.

Battered Children. Young children who are physically abused by emotionally unstable parents frequently have a variety of oral injuries, including fractured teeth, lacerated mucosa of the upper lip, and injury to the gingivae (Andreasen, 1972). Associated with these intraoral injuries may be multiple injuries and bruises covering other areas of the body, many in different stages of healing (Kempe and Helfer, 1972). Radiologic examination may also reveal fractures of the long bones, skull, or ribs, again in various stages of healing. Discrepancies between the clinical findings and a history supplied by the parents may be indicative of a battered child problem.

Nature of Traumatic Injuries to Teeth

While similar traumatic injuries may occur to both primary and permanent anterior teeth, anatomic features of the primary incisors and their surrounding alveolar bone predispose them to their own spectrum of damage. The short height of the crowns of primary incisors reduces the incidence of coronal fractures of these teeth. In addition, the short, conical shape of primary incisor roots, as well as the lack of organization of the surrounding bone, reduces the ability of these teeth to withstand impact. Thus, luxations and displacements of the primary incisors are more common than are such injuries to the permanent incisors (Andreasen, 1972; McDonald and Avery, 1978).

Classification of Traumatic Injuries to Teeth

Hargreaves and Craig (1970), Ellis and Davey (1970), and Andreasen (1972) have classified injuries to primary and permanent teeth. Traumatized teeth are described on the basis of a variety of fractures of the crown or root as well as a variety of displacements of the entire tooth, including its loss from the socket.

Injuries to the soft tissues and bone frequently accompany trauma. The gingiva and mucosal tissues should be inspected carefully for tears or buried foreign bodies. The lips should be palpated, even radiographed, if a crown has been fractured; it is not uncommon to locate a portion of a fractured crown embedded within the orbicularis oris muscle (Andreasen, 1972). The tongue may be bitten if the traumatic impact has violently forced the mandible upwards (Ellis and Davey, 1970). In most instances of traumatic injury to the teeth, the periodontal membrane may be injured. If the tooth shows abnormal mobility, immobilization by splinting may be required.

Examination of an Injured Tooth

A thorough examination consisting of four steps is recommended following traumatic injury to the oral tissues. Steps 3 and 4 are best conducted by the dentist.

Step 1: Clinical Inspection. Following a carefully obtained history in which information such as age of the patient and where, when, and how the injury occurred, the tissues are cleaned so that assessment can be made of the type and extent of the injuries. A dental or otolaryngologic mirror and a bright light are used. Teeth are examined for fractures of the enamel and dentin as well as for displacements or avulsions. Oral soft tissues are inspected for lacerations. Damage to the temporomandibular joint and jaws is assessed by having the patient open and close his mouth while checking for mandibular displacements and irregular occlusion.

Step 2: Mobility of Teeth. An injured tooth should be compared to a noninjured antimere to detect excessive mobility, which may be indicative of a root fracture or fractured alveolar (socket) wall.

Step 3: Radiographs. This portion of the examination is best performed by the dentist.

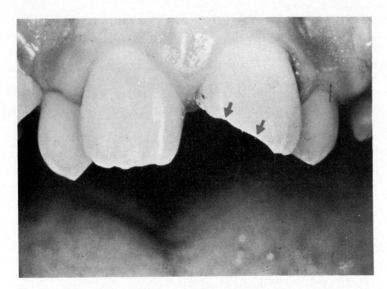

Figure 45–22 A fractured permanent left central incisor of an eight year old boy in which the dentin was exposed (arrows). Such fractures should receive immediate dental care to prevent infection and loss of vitality of the dental pulp. (Courtesy of Dr. J. O. Andreasen.)

Intraoral radiographs are essential for the detection and assessment of crown and root fractures as well as for intrusive, extrusive, and lateral luxations. The radiograph will assist in determining the amount of root formation in the permanent tooth or resorption in a primary tooth, in addition to the proximity of primary tooth roots to developing permanent teeth.

Step 4: Vitality Tests.   Tests to determine whether the dental pulp has retained its vitality are best carried out several weeks following the trauma. Immediate testing often provides inconclusive results as well as psychological trauma to an already apprehensive patient. Such tests involve electrical and thermal (hot and cold) applications to the injured tooth to test for sensitivity.

Treatment of Injured Teeth and Oral Soft Tissues

While treatment of traumatically injured teeth and adjacent soft tissues should be managed by the dentist, much can and should be done by the pediatrician. Management of such injuries is in three stages: emergency, intermediate, and final. As both hard and soft tissues are frequently involved and the range of injuries broad, a variety of treatment procedures may be required.

Emergency Treatment.   It is important that the child be seen by the dentist or pediatrician immediately following the injury (Hargreaves and Craig, 1970). The child and parents may be considerably agitated and require reassurance. Tetanus prophylaxis is recommended for dental, intraoral soft tissue, and facial wounds, especially when contamination is suspected. Saline rinses are effective in removing intraoral hemorrhage to permit examination of the teeth and oral mucosa. Antiseptic mouth rinses are also beneficial. Lacerations of the lips, tongue, or mucosa can be sutured with No. 3-0 silk and a fine, half-inch needle. Facial wounds should be thoroughly debrided and cleansed with antiseptic solutions. Antibiotic therapy is recommended.

Fractures of the Crown.   Fractures of the crown range from chipping of the enamel to exposure of dentin and pulp (Fig. 45–22). To prevent bacterial contamination of the dental pulp either by passage of organisms through the dentinal tubules or by contact with saliva, the crown should be dressed as quickly as possible. The goal of therapy is retention of the vitality of the dental pulp (Andreasen, 1972; Ellis and Davey; 1970; Hargreaves and Craig, 1970).

Fractures of the Root.   Teeth that show excessive mobility and radiographic evidence of a fractured root should be immobilized by means of a splint. A variety of dental splints exist.

The short height of the primary incisor crown, in contrast to that of the permanent incisors, makes these teeth difficult to splint. The recently introduced acid-etch, ultraviolet light composite bonding technique is proving effective for splinting both primary and permanent teeth (Neaverth and Goerig, 1980).

Partial Displacement.   Partially displaced

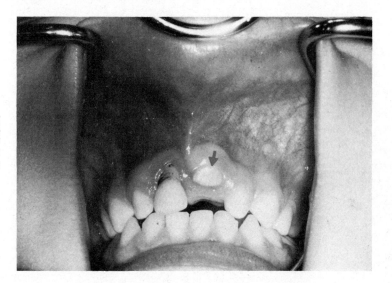

Figure 45–23 An intruded left primary central incisor (arrow) caused by trauma. Such intruded primary teeth should be removed to prevent potential injury to the underlying permanent incisor.

teeth should be examined to determine the nature and degree of injury. Laterally displaced teeth may be associated with fractured labial and lingual alveolar bone. Displaced teeth should be repositioned in their sockets by the application of finger pressure simultaneously on the mucosa over the apical areas and on the cervical portions of the crowns (Andreasen, 1972; Hargreaves and Craig, 1970). Partially extruded teeth should be repositioned in their socket by application of finger pressure on the biting edges. Firm fixation of partially extruded primary teeth is essential, but even when they have been repositioned, the prognosis for pulp vitality is poor.

Primary teeth are more frequently intruded than are permanent teeth (Fig. 45–23). An entire crown may be forced beneath the gingiva with the root apex protruding through the labial alveolar bone. As intruded teeth will tend to re-erupt (Ravn, 1968), a nonintervention policy of allowing the teeth to regain their former height in the arch has been suggested. It has been noted, however, that an intruded primary tooth, because of the close proximity of its root apex to the developing permanent tooth germ, may cause a hypoplastic enamel defect on the labial surface of the permanent tooth (Ravn, 1968). For this reason, some dentists prefer to extract intruded primary incisors and insert a space maintainer to restore function and aesthetics and to maintain arch space. In those instances in which the intruded teeth are allowed to re-erupt, the pulp tissue will usually become necrotic and will require endodontic treatment.

Complete Displacement. Emergency care of completely displaced primary and permanent teeth is frequently similar. An avulsed tooth, free from crown or root fracture, dental caries, and dirt contamination and kept moist and clean can be replanted within its undamaged socket. Andreasen and Hjorting-Hansen (1966) have indicated that failures of permanent tooth replantations as a result of resorption of the root can be reduced by shortening the time the tooth remains out of its socket. These same investigators have also shown that replantation of exarticulated teeth having incompletely formed roots (and open apices) within a period of two hours can increase the probability of tooth retention and pulp vitality. When informed that a patient has lost a tooth through an accident, give instructions to locate the tooth quickly, to wrap it in clean, moist tissue, and to come to the office immediately. The tooth should be placed in a sterile gauze pad without damaging the periodontal fibers on the root surface. The socket should be cleansed of blood clots by irrigation and examined for alveolar bone fractures. The tooth may then be replanted and aligned with its neighbors. The child is requested to bite gently on a gauze pad until the dentist can construct a splint and obtain a postreplantation radiograph. The splint is usually retained for a period of three to six weeks. Tetanus prophylaxis and short-term penicillin therapy should be administered. Root canal therapy, if necessary, can be per-

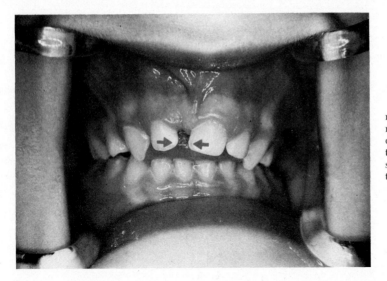

Figure 45–24 Loss of the right primary central incisor as a result of trauma. Note the closure of arch space due to movement of the neighboring teeth (arrow). A space maintainer should have been inserted to prevent this loss of space.

formed once the dental splint has been removed.

A lower rate of success attends the replanting of primary incisors than of permanent teeth as a result of the difficulty in establishing firm fixation of the primary teeth.

Subsequent Treatment. Intermediate and final stages of treatment of oral trauma consist of establishing the status of pulp vitality and selecting the appropriate method of restoring the crown of the fractured permanent incisor. Several intermediate crowns may be used before the final crown is made. An intermediate crown constructed of gold and porcelain or composite resin will cover a fractured tooth during active eruption and until the patient is 18 to 21 years of age. The final crown, constructed of porcelain, can be expected to provide service well into adult life.

Consequences of Traumatic Injury to Teeth

Traumatic injuries to the primary incisors may cause undesirable effects on their permanent successors because of their close proximity (Smith and Rapp, 1980). Localized areas of enamel hypoplasia on the crowns of permanent incisors from intrusion injuries to their primary predecessors present an aesthetic problem to the patient (Ravn, 1968). Dilaceration of a permanent incisor as a result of trauma to the primary incisor could lead to its loss. Another injury that permanent incisors may suffer as a consequence of trauma to primary incisors is cessation of root growth; while the permanent tooth continues its eruption, growth of the root stops (Worth, 1963).

Figure 45–25 A space maintainer containing two false teeth (arrows) has been inserted to replace the maxillary central incisors, which were lost owing to trauma.

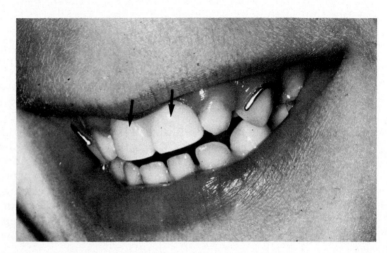

Avulsion of a primary incisor as a result of trauma can lead to loss of the space in the dental arch that the eventually erupting permanent successor requires (Fig. 45–24). Since space closure may occur within a few months following the premature loss of the primary tooth, a space maintainer should be inserted rapidly (Fig. 45–25). The type of space maintainer used will be influenced by the age of the child, his ability to retain the appliance within his mouth, and the specific tooth or teeth that were lost.

An unfortunate source of trauma may be encountered in the hospital operating room. Avulsion of a primary or permanent incisor may occur when a laryngoscope is rested upon a maxillary tooth during anesthetic intubation procedures. The leverage effect of this rather heavy instrument on a tooth, often with incompletely developed roots, is sufficient to cause its loss. Impairment of the patient's appearance, interference with mastication and proper speech, and the long-term nature of the ensuing treatment make such an injury serious; it must be avoided whenever possible.

REFERENCES

American Academy of Periodontology, Dental Health Plan Committee. 1972. Current Procedural Terminology for Periodontics. Chicago, American Academy of Periodontology.

Andreasen, J. O. 1972. Traumatic Injuries of the Teeth. Copenhagen, Munksgaard.

Andreasen, J. O., and Hjorting-Hansen, E. 1966. Replantation of Teeth. II. Histological study of 22 replanted anterior teeth in humans. Acta Odont. Scand., *24*:287.

Baer, P. M., and Benjamin, S. P. 1974. Periodontal Disease In Children and Adolescents. Philadelphia, J. B. Lippincott Co.

Cohen, M. M., Jr., and Hooley, J. R. 1977. Oral Disorders. *In* Smith, D. W. Introduction To Clinical Pediatrics, 2nd ed. Philadelphia, W. B. Saunders Co.

Eichenbaum, I. W. 1963. A correlation of traumatized anterior teeth to occlusion. J. Dent. Child., *30*:229.

Ellis, R. G., and Davey, K. W. 1970. The Classification and Treatment of Injuries to the Teeth of Children. Chicago, Year Book Medical Publishers.

Finn, S. B. 1973. Clinical Pedodontics, 4th ed. Philadelphia, W. B. Saunders Co.

Gorlin R. J., Pindborg, J. J., and Cohen, M. M., Jr. 1976. Syndromes of the Head and Neck, 2nd ed. New York, McGraw-Hill.

Hargreaves, J. A., and Craig, J. W. 1970. The Management of Traumatized Anterior Teeth of Children. Edinburgh, Churchill-Livingstone.

Hatton M. 1955. A measure of the effects of heredity and environment on eruption of the deciduous teeth. J. Dent. Res., *34*:392.

Kempe, D. H., and Helfer, R. E., 1972. Helping the Battered Child and His Family. Philadelphia, J. B. Lippincott Co.

Kraus, B. S., and Jordan, R. E. 1965. The Human Dentition Before Birth. Philadelphia, Lea and Febiger.

Law, D. B., Lewis, T. M., and Davis, J. M. 1969. An Atlas of Pedodontics. Philadelphia, W. B. Saunders Co.

Lo, R. T., and Moyers, R. E. 1953. Studies in the etiology and prevention of malocclusion. I. The sequence of eruption of the permanent dentitions. Am. J. Orthodont., *39*:460.

Logan, W. H. G., and Kronfeld, R. 1933. Development of the human jaws and surrounding structures from birth to the age of 15 years. J. Am. Dent. Assoc., *20*:379.

Lunt, R. C., and Law, D. B. 1974. A review of the chronology of calcification of the deciduous teeth. J. Am. Dent. Assoc., *89*:599.

McDonald, R. E., and Avery, D. R. 1978. Dentistry for the Child and Adolescent, 3rd ed. St. Louis, The C. V. Mosby Co.

Meredith, H. V. 1943. Order and eruption for the deciduous dentition. J. Dent. Res., *25*:43.

Moyers, R. E., 1973. Handbook of Orthodontics, 3rd ed. Chicago, Year Book Medical Publishers, Chap. 6.

Moyers, R. E., and Kopel, H. 1973. Facial Growth and Dentition. *In* Lawrey, G. H. Growth and Development of Children, 6th ed. Chicago, Year Book Medical Publishers.

Neaverth, E. J., and Goerig, A. C. 1980. Technique and rationale for splinting. J. Am. Dent. Assoc., *100*:56.

Newbrun, E. 1972. Fluorides and Dental Caries. Springfield, Charles C Thomas.

Nolla, C. M. 1960. The development of the permanent teeth. J. Dent. Child., *27*:254.

Potter, R. H. Y. 1976. The Genetics of Tooth Size. *In* Stewart, R. E., and Prescott, G. H. Oral Facial Genetics, St. Louis, The C. V. Mosby Co.

Rapp, R., and Winter, G. B. 1979. Color Atlas of Clinical Conditions in Pedodontics. Chicago, Year Book Medical Publishers.

Ravn, J. J. 1968. Sequelae of acute mechanical trauma in the primary dentition. J. Dent. Child., *35*:281.

Robinow, M., Richards, T. W., and Anderson, M. 1942. The eruption of deciduous teeth. Growth, *6*:127.

Schour, I., and Massler, M. 1940. Studies in tooth development. The growth pattern of human teeth. J. Am. Dent. Assoc., *27*:1918.

Shafer, W. G., Hine, M. K., and Levy, B. M. 1974. A Textbook of Oral Pathology, 3rd ed. Philadelphia, W. B. Saunders Co.

Shklar, G., and McCarthy, P. C. 1976. The Oral Manifestations of Systemic Disease. Boston, Butterworth.

Shumaker, D. B., and El Hadary, M. S. 1960. Roentgenographic study of eruption . J. Am. Dent. Assoc., *61*:535.

Smith, R. J., and Rapp, R. 1980. A cephalometric study of the developmental relationship between primary and permanent maxillary and central incisor teeth. J. Dent. Child., *47*:36.

Withop, C. J., Jr. 1959. Genetics and dentistry. Eugenica Quart., *5*:15.

Worth, H. M. 1963. Principles and Practice of Oral Radiologic Interpretation. Chicago, Year Book Medical Publishers.

Chapter 46

ORTHODONTIC PROBLEMS IN CHILDREN

David J. Hall, D.D.S., M.Sc.O.
Donald W. Warren, D.D.S., Ph.D.

GROWTH OF THE CRANIOFACIAL COMPLEX

The face of the infant is usually wide and short, and in proportion, the cranium appears to be quite large. Later, as the midface begins to grow more rapidly, the characteristics of the adult face become more apparent. According to Hellman (1935), the contrast between the infant and the adult face is the result of the different parts growing at different rates at different times. Under the influence of genetic and environmental factors, growth is generally completed first in the calvarium, then in the width of the face, and finally in the length of the face. Postnatal craniofacial growth is also described in Chapter 2.

Contrasting Theories of Growth

Two basic types of bony movements appear to be involved in craniofacial growth. One is deposition and resorption on the surface of bones, which produces cortical drift and results in overall enlargement as well as remodeling (Enlow, 1968).

The other type of movement involves the "displacement" or "translation" of contiguous bones growing away from each other under forces provided by the surrounding soft tissues and, presumably, also by the growth of the separate bones themselves whenever intervening cartilage is present. As groups of bones enlarge, each becomes repositioned as a unit away from the others as all continue to grow and remodel by deposition and resorption.

Certain regions — such as the synchondroses of the cranial base, the nasal septal cartilage, the mandibular condylar cartilages, and the sutures — are often considered to be sites of special importance in determining total skull growth. These regions are assumed to function as growth centers that regulate the rate and amount of growth occurring at sites elsewhere (Moore, 1975). The remodeling processes are considered to be secondary to growth at the centers. This view of skull growth emphasizes that intrinsic growth factors are present in the cartilage and periosteum. Sutural growth is secondary and influenced by synchondrosis proliferation. This contrasts with the traditional theory of Sicher (1952), which suggests that intrinsic genetic factors are most important and modeling changes occur secondary·to the influences of function and environmental factors.

Another popular theory, proposed by Moss (1968), is that all growth of bone is secondary and that growth changes in bone reflect the growth and function of the tissue systems associated with the bones. He calls these functional units *matrices*. Moss distinguishes periosteal from capsular matrices: periosteal include muscles and teeth, while capsular matrices include the volumes enclosed within the skull.

Recently, Limborgh (1970) concluded that none of the present theories on control of bone growth is entirely satisfactory and listed the essential elements of our current knowledge as follows:

1. Chondrocranial growth is controlled mainly by intrinsic genetic factors.

2. Desmocranial growth is controlled by only a few intrinsic genetic factors.

3. Growing skull cartilages are growth centers.

4. Sutural growth is controlled mainly by influences originating from the skull cartilages and from other adjacent head structures.

5. Periosteal growth is controlled mainly by influences originating from adjacent head structures.

6. Sutural growth and periosteal growth are additionally governed by local, nongenetic influences, muscle forces inclusive.

Moyers (1975) has added a seventh point with respect to control of mandibular condylar growth, stating that mandibular condylar growth is controlled, to some extent, by local, nongenetic environmental influences.

The Cranial Base

Growth of the cranial base occurs through sutural growth, elongation at synchondroses, and direct cortical drift and remodeling. This combination allows growth of the contours of the cranial base and maintains the housing for vessels and nerves. The growth sites include the spheno-occipital, intersphenoid, and sphenosphenoid synchondroses. The cartilage growth of these synchondroses follows the neural growth curve primarily, but also partially follows the general growth curve (Fig. 46–1).

The spheno-occipital synchondrosis has been traditionally regarded as the principal growth site in the cranial base during the postnatal period. This synchondrosis closes at 13 to 16 years in males and at 11 to 14 years in females. Activity of the other synchondroses disappears either at birth or shortly thereafter.

Cranial Vault

The cranial vault grows primarily by proliferation and ossification of the sutural connective tissues, in conjunction with relatively small surface deposits on both the ectocranial and endocranial surfaces. Over 90 per cent of calvarium development is achieved by the fifth year of life. Vault growth is directly influenced by the developing brain.

Maxilla

The developing facial skeleton is influenced by the growing cranial base and moves downward and forward in relation to it. The maxilla actually grows in a variety of directions (Fig. 46–2). Addition of bone to the orbital surfaces and the supramaxillary sutures provides downward movement, and additions at the maxillary tuberosity provide forward displacement. Thus, the maxilla is "relocated" or "transposed" as well as enlarged by the growth processes. Sutural connective tissue proliferations, ossification, surface apposition, resorption, and translation are the mechanisms for maxillary growth.

The zygomatic process is constantly moved posteriorly in relation to the maxilla by remodeling. Since it is also anchored to the maxilla and the cranial base, it is consequently lengthened by bone deposition at the sutures.

The midface does not have an endochondral mechanism for growth and, apparently, the nasomaxillary region expands in a forward and downward direction by the interstitially enlarging cartilaginous nasal septum.

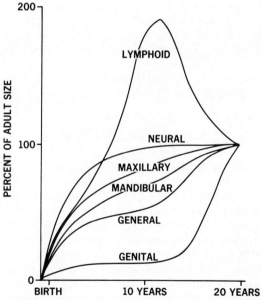

Figure 46–1 Differential growth rate for different body tissues. The mandible follows the general growth curve and the neurocranium follows the neural growth curve. The maxilla falls between the general and neural curves. (Modified from Scammon, R. E., The Measurement of Man. Minneapolis, University of Minnesota Press.)

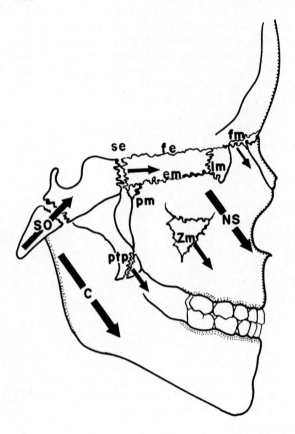

Figure 46–2 Growth directions of the cranial base and facial sutures. Surface apposition and resorption are shown by stippled area. (From Cohen, S. E.: Growth and Class II Treatment. Am. J. Orthod, 52:5–26, 1966.)

Mandible

The mandible appears to "grow" in a forward and downward manner, but actually growth takes place in a number of directions. Vertical movement of the mandible is determined to a great extent by the growing condyle, although some growth also occurs on the superior and inferior borders of the body. Condylar growth is generally upward and backward, which serves to translate the mandible in an anterior-inferior direction. The ramus is subjected to resorption on its anterior border and to deposition on its posterior border. This pattern of resorption and deposition serves to lengthen the body of the mandible. The changes in mandibular position complement the changes occurring simultaneously in the maxilla.

INTRODUCTION TO ORTHODONTIC CONCEPTS

Definition of Orthodontics

Orthodontics is the specialty area of dentistry concerned with the growth and development of the dentofacial complex and with the correction of dentofacial abnormalities. Present-day orthodontic therapy may involve growth redirection and guidance with orthopedic forces, early guidance of tooth eruption, repositioning of teeth for function and aesthetics, and management of orthognathic surgical cases.

Goal of Orthodontic Treatment

The goal of orthodontic treatment is to position the teeth and jaws so as to obtain for each patient the optimal combination of masticatory function and dentofacial aesthetics. The concept of "optimal combination" is important, for it is not always possible to obtain both ideal function and ideal aesthetics for every patient. Thus, ideal occlusion with all teeth present, as shown in Figure 46–3, is not usually a treatment possibility and seldom occurs naturally (Kelly et al., 1973).

A second concept fundamental to an understanding of orthodontics is the differentiation between normal occlusion and abnormal or malocclusion. Graber (1966) states that "normal in physiology is always a range,

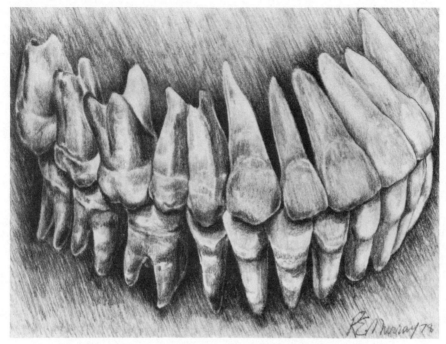

Figure 46–3   Ideal alignment and occlusion of all 32 permanent teeth.

never a point." Normal occlusion and malocclusion should not be thought of as being opposite ends of the spectrum, but rather as overlapping frequency distributions. Malocclusion represents a range of normal human variation and should be used to describe only those occlusion problems that need correction. Normal occlusion would be that which, while not necessarily ideal, requires no orthodontic treatment to improve function or aesthetics. Assessment of the variables that determine the need for orthodontic treatment is the essence of orthodontic diagnosis and will be considered in subsequent sections.

Angle's Classification of Malocclusion

Implicit in the concept of optimal masticatory function is the need to evaluate the teeth from a dynamic viewpoint as the teeth function within the entire stomatognathic system. Indeed, such an evaluation must be made in order to diagnose and treat any orthodontic problem properly. However, for simplicity in describing various types of malocclusions and for ease of communication among professionals, static descriptions are useful.

The most commonly used system of classification in orthodontics is that devised by Edward Angle (1907) at the beginning of the twentieth century. Angle described his various classifications according to the occlusal relationship between the maxillary and mandibular first permanent molars. He defined three general classifications, Class I, Class II, and Class III, which are demonstrated in Figure 46–4.

Class I.   Normal or Class I occlusion is defined as the relationship in which the mesiobuccal cusp of the maxillary first permanent molar articulates in the mesiobuccal groove of the mandibular first permanent molar (Fig. 46–4A). If these teeth are in this Class I relationship and if the remaining teeth are all present, are aligned with proper contacts, and are of the proper size relationships, an ideal occlusion as seen in Figure 46–3 will result.

Class II.   Angle's Class II or disto-occlusion is defined as occurring when the mesiobuccal groove of the mandibular first molar is distal to the mesiobuccal cusp of the maxillary first molar (Fig. 46–4B). This distal positioning of the mandibular first molar relative to the corresponding maxillary molar may be the result of any combination of maxillary skeletal or dental protrusion, or mandibular skeletal or dental retrusion.

Since there are several types of skeletal or dental displacement possibilities in a Class II relationship, these cases are further subdivid-

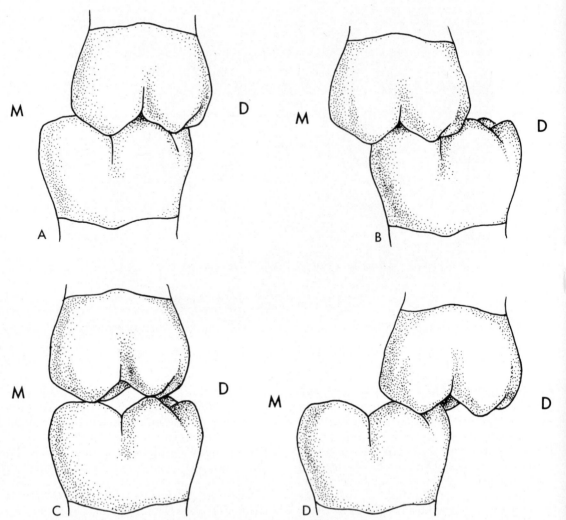

Figure 46–4 Angle's classification of molar occlusion. **M,** mesial, the side of the tooth toward the midline following the curve of the dental arch; **D,** distal, away from the midline following the curve of the dental arch. *A,* Class I. *B,* Class II. *C,* End-to-end. *D,* Class III.

ed into Division 1 or 2. In a Class II Division 1 malocclusion, the molars are in a Class II relationship, and the maxillary incisors are flared forward in a protrusive position (Fig. 46–5). This is the classic "buck tooth" appearance, which frequently demonstrates spacing between the maxillary incisors and an abnormally deep bite.

In a Class II Division 2 malocclusion the molars are in a Class II relationship, but the maxillary central incisors are tipped lingually, usually contacting the mandibular incisors (Fig. 46–6). The maxillary lateral incisors often protrude and may appear to "wrap around or across" the maxillary central incisors. The mandibular teeth are usually very upright and bite depth is usually excessive.

As seen in Figure 46–4C, the permanent first molars may occlude in a position that is actually halfway between the Class I and Class II relationship; this is termed an "end-to-end" relationship. In children in the mixed dentition stage of dental development, before the loss of the primary molars, this relationship is normal. However, it is not normal in the permanent dentition and may be considered as a less severe form of a Class II malocclusion.

Class III. Angle's Class III or mesiocclusion occurs when the mesiobuccal groove of the mandibular first molar is anterior to the mesiobuccal cusp of the maxillary first molar (Fig. 46–4D). In this situation, the lower incisors are usually forward of the upper incisors

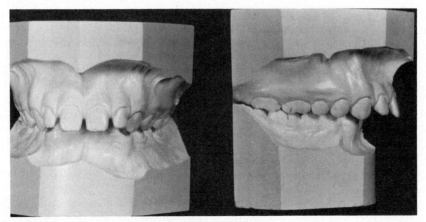

Figure 46–5   Study models of a patient with a Class II Division I malocclusion. Teeth are in a Class II relationship and the maxillary incisors are flared forward and spaced.

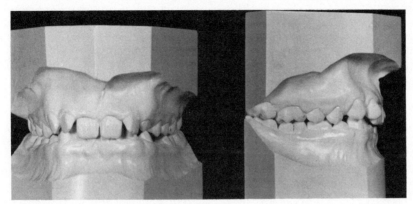

Figure 46–6   Study models of a patient with a Class II Divison II malocclusion. The molars are in an end-to-end relationship, the maxillary central incisors are tipped palatally, and the maxillary lateral incisors protrude facially.

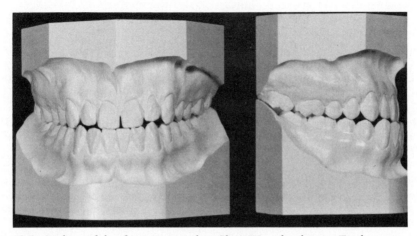

Figure 46–7   Study models of a patient with a Class III malocclusion. Teeth are in a Class III relationship and an anterior crossbite exists.

and an anterior crossbite or negative overjet results (Fig. 46–7). A Class III malocclusion may be the result of any combination of maxillary skeletal or dental retrusion, or mandibular skeletal or dental protrusion.

Classification of Skeletal Types and Patterns of Growth

When he devised his classification system, Angle assumed that the maxillary arch and the teeth within it were relatively stable in relation to the cranium. By relating the teeth to each other, he intended also to relate the maxilla to the mandible. We know today that Angle's assumptions are not always true, and that variations in the positions of the jaws or positions of individual teeth within either jaw may occur. It is true, however, that teeth generally reflect underlying skeletal relationships. For this reason, orthodontists have extended the Angle classification to imply the skeletal pattern usually found with a particular occlusion relationship. Thus, a patient with mandibular prognathism may be said to have a Class III skeletal relationship. Similarly, the Angle classification may also be extended to imply the pattern of growth by which any skeletal relationship developed, for example, "a Class III growth pattern."

ORTHODONTIC DIAGNOSIS

Diagnosis and treatment planning are dependent upon the accumulation of adequate diagnostic data from which to generate a problem list and treatment solutions. Angle's system is simple and well accepted, but is incomplete. It fails to consider dental and skeletal relationships in the transverse and vertical planes of space — considering only the anterior-posterior (sagittal) plane. In addition, it does not consider how the relationship of the teeth to the face affects the aesthetics of the face.

Recently, Ackerman and Proffit (1969) proposed a method of assessing and classifying malocclusions by which five characteristics and their interrelationships are systematically evaluated. Using their method assures the evaluator that all relevant factors are considered, with as little complication as possible.

In sequence, one should examine and describe the alignment and symmetry of the dental arches. Next, facial aesthetics, especially the influence of the teeth and chin position upon the profile, are assessed. Finally, the teeth are related to each other and described in the three planes of space (sagittal, transverse, and vertical), and a differentiation between skeletal and dental problems is made. In the following sections, analyses of these five parameters will be discussed.

Analysis of Alignment

First, the alignment and symmetry of the dental arches are evaluated by quantifying the presence of any crowding or spacing and by describing individually any severely malpositioned teeth. Usually the question to be answered is "Is there enough space to accommodate all the teeth?" The amount of crowding in the permanent dentition can be determined by measuring and comparing the size of the teeth with space available. In the mixed dentition stage methods can be used to estimate the size of the unerupted teeth (Hixon and Oldfather, 1958; Moyers, 1975; Nance, 1947).

Facial Form Analysis

The second step in the systematic description is to assess the patient's facial aesthetics, giving special attention to a description of his profile. The judgments desired in profile analysis are exactly the same as those desired from an analysis of a lateral cephalometric headfilm. What we wish to determine is the relationship of the parts of the face, the jaws, and the teeth to one another.

The patient should be examined with his head held in the "natural head position" (Moorrees and Kean, 1958), the position of natural head posture. A patient will naturally assume this position when he stands relaxed and looks off at the horizon or into his own eyes in a mirror. Ideal facial proportions are illustrated in Figure 46–8 and serve as a model with which to compare any particular patient.

It is helpful in profile analysis to separate a patient's face mentally into five separate anatomical units as illustrated in the schematic face in Figure 46–9. In the ideal face, the cranium and cranial base (1), the skeletal maxilla (2), the maxillary teeth (3), the mandibular teeth (4), and the skeletal mandible

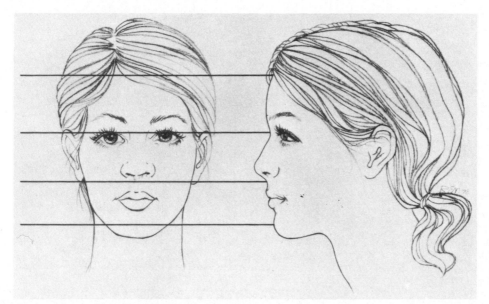

Figure 46–8 Full-face and profile views of ideal facial proportions. The face is divided into equal thirds vertically, and all facial features are in good proportion and balance.

(5) all appear in a relatively straight line. The analysis can then concentrate upon the relationships of these five anatomical segments and can describe the deviation of any segment.

In particular, in a profile analysis, three areas of special focus are important: (1) anterior-posterior position of the chin, (2) degree of lip protrusion, and (3) vertical height of the anterior face, especially the

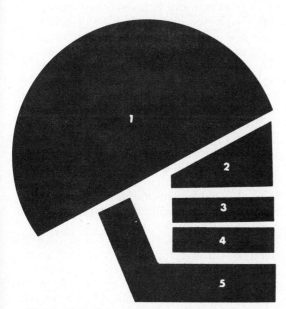

Figure 46–9 Schematic illustration of an ideal arrangement of the dentofacial and craniofacial structures. In the ideal face, the cranium and cranial base (**1**), the skeletal maxilla (**2**), the maxillary teeth (**3**), the mandibular teeth (**4**), and the skeletal mandible (**5**), all align in a relatively straight line.

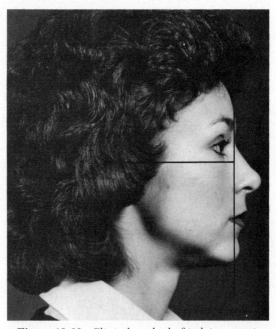

Figure 46–10 Clinical method of judging anterior-posterior position of the mandible. The chin should fall approximately on a vertical line drawn from the soft tissue nasion perpendicular to the Frankfort horizontal (ear-eye plane.)

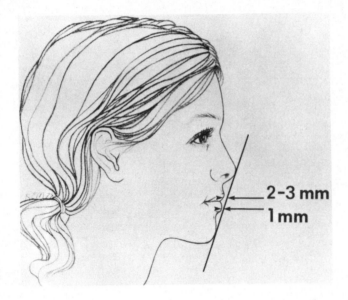

2-3 mm
1 mm

Figure 46–11   Ideal position of the lips relative to the chin and nose.

lower one third. The judgments required in determining the anterior-posterior position of the chin are those involved in relating the chin to a vertical reference line as illustrated in Figure 46–10. If one mentally projects such a reference line (a perpendicular to the Frankfort horizontal from the soft tissue nasion) onto the patient's face, it is easy to look at the relationships of the profile points (Figure 46–10). Angle's terminology is extended to describe the skeletal relationships determined by this analysis. Thus, a patient with an absolute or relative retrusion of the mandible would be said to have a Class II skeletal relationship. Only by separating the face into its five basic components can these differential judgments be made.

Since the soft tissue thickness tends to be relatively constant over the face, lip contour (and especially the degree of lip protrusion) tends to reflect accurately the support provided by the incisor teeth. Specifically, teeth that are positioned forward in the face cause increased lip protrusion, while those positioned more posteriorly offer less support and consequently a more retruded lip profile.

The amount of lip protrusion that is desirable is affected by definite racial and ethnic considerations: for instance, blacks and Orientals normally show a greater degree of protrusion in comparison to whites (Altemus 1960, 1963). For patients of northern European ancestry, a good guide for judging lip position is the aesthetic or "e" line illustrated in Figure 46–11 (Ricketts, 1957). The "e" line, which extends from the tip of the nose to the most anterior point of the chin, describes the acceptable anterior limits of the lips in profile. By mentally projecting this line onto the patient's face, a determination of lip position can be made. Ideally, the lower lip position should range from on the line to 1 mm behind it. The upper lip should be approximately 2 to 3 mm behind the line.

In an ideally proportioned face, the profile can be divided into approximately equal vertical thirds (see Fig. 46–8). The upper third, from the hairline to the bridge of the nose between the eyes (soft tissue nasion), is variable with the hairline and not subject to orthodontic modification. The middle third extends from the soft tissue nasion to directly under the nose (anterior nasal spine) and can be affected by orthodontic treatment, although it is not the area at which treatment is primarily directed. The lower third, from the anterior nasal spine to the chin, contains the alveolar-dental structures and is the area most affected by orthodontic treatment. Consequently, the vertical deviations most significant to orthodontics are seen in the lower third and should be noted as an increase or decrease in facial height. Such deviations influence anterior-posterior relationships of the teeth and jaws, as well as the amount of overbite or open bite. Cephalometric analysis may be used to quantitate any vertical discrepancy observed.

Although orthodontists have typically placed more emphasis upon profile analysis, analysis of facial proportions from a full

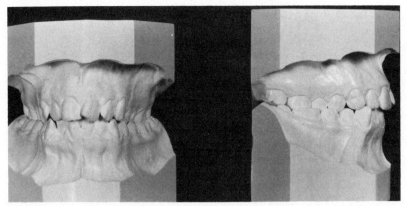

Figure 46-12 Study models of a patient illustrating a bilateral posterior crossbite. Note that the maxillary posterior teeth are positioned palatally and occlude inside the mandibular posterior teeth.

frontal view is equally important. Without special effort patients do not see themselves from a profile view; however, they are usually very aware of their appearance in a full-face view.

The analysis of full-face aesthetics takes into account relationships and proportions in the vertical and transverse planes. In the vertical plane the ideal face can again be divided into approximately equal thirds, just as was done in the profile analysis (see Fig. 46–8). Deviations in vertical balance should be noted and should agree with the assessment made in the profile analysis. A second important vertical determination to make is the relationship of the maxillary incisors to the upper lip. Normally about 1 to 2 mm of incisor tooth may be exposed with the lips slightly apart. In a full smile all of the incisor crown will be exposed, along with perhaps a millimeter or two of gingiva. Excessive vertical exposure of the maxillary incisors at rest, or of the teeth and gingival tissue during a smile, usually results in an unaesthetic appearance and smile line, and may indicate an excessively large vertical dimension of the maxilla with increased lower facial height. Excessive prominence of the maxillary incisors due to horizontal maxillary excess and the relative impact of each upon facial aesthetics must be assessed.

Another important determination to be made from a frontal aspect is transverse or left-right symmetry. The bridge of the nose, tip of the nose, philtrum of the upper lip, center of the lower lip, and center of the chin should all lie on the same vertical line. Assessment of transverse symmetry is concerned with describing any deviation of any of these facial features from this vertical reference line. If a mandibular asymmetry is noted it must be determined whether a true skeletal asymmetry exists or whether the patient is merely shifting his mandible to one side as he closes his teeth together. In the case of a shift the face will appear more symmetrical when the mandible is slightly depressed and the teeth are apart.

Analysis of the Transverse Plane

Abnormalities of the dental arches with respect to the transverse plane of space are referred to as posterior crossbites. Normally, the buccal surfaces of the maxillary posterior teeth lie outside the corresponding surfaces of the mandibular posterior teeth. When the mandibular teeth are in the buccal or outside position, a posterior crossbite exists (Fig. 46–12). In addition, the situation in which the palatal surface of a maxillary tooth lies outside the buccal surface of a mandibular tooth is also termed a crossbite.

Crossbites may be caused by any combination of maxillary or mandibular skeletal or dental deviation and may be either a unilateral or a bilateral problem. Crossbites may involve a single tooth, groups of teeth, or the entire dental arch. Frequently, crossbites can cause a lateral deviation of the mandible as the patient shifts to a more comfortable occlusion position — which is termed a "convenience bite." A diagnosis pinpointing the cause of the crossbite and differentiating between skeletal or dental etiologies is necessary for its treatment.

OVERJET   **OVERBITE**   **OPENBITE**

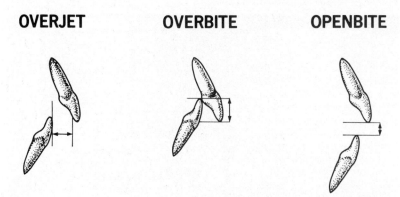

Figure 46–13 Schematic illustration of the terms overjet, overbite, and open bite. Overjet is the horizontal projection of the upper incisors in front of the lower incisors. Overbite is the extent to which the upper anterior teeth overlap the lower in a vertical direction. Open bite is the vertical distance between the upper and lower incisors when they do not overlap.

Analysis in the Sagittal Plane

The Angle classification of occlusion is used to describe the dental arches with regard to the sagittal plane of space. In addition, a determination of whether the problem is skeletal, or dental, or a combination of skeletal and dental, is made. Information gained from the profile analysis will aid in this skeletal-dental differentiation.

Analysis in the Vertical Plane

Finally, the dental arches are viewed with regard to the vertical plane of space (Fig. 46–13). The term used to describe the vertical overlapping of teeth, especially the incisors, is overbite. Overbites are frequently quantitated as the per cent of the crown height of the lower incisor that is overlapped. A normal variation in overbite may include an overlap that covers up to one third of the crown of the mandibular incisors. A complete lack of any vertical overlap of the incisors is termed an open bite. Any degree of open bite is not considered to be normal occlusion.

Cephalometrics

A cephalometric radiograph is actually a lateral skull radiograph taken under highly standardized conditions. The distance from the radiograph source to the patient's midsagittal plane is 5 feet. The midsagittal plane is positioned parallel to and 11 cm from the film. Finally, the patient's head is positioned so that his Frankfort horizontal plane (ear-eye plane) is oriented parallel to the floor. Worldwide use of this standard technique permits comparison of cephalometric films with reasonable accuracy.

Cephalometric analyses are used to assess and compare the size and positional relationships of the various components of the craniofacial and dentofacial complexes. These comparisons may be used as an aid in treatment planning by describing a patient's skeletal and dental relationships at one point in time. In addition, by using serial cephalographs, the magnitude and direction of any dentofacial changes due to growth over a period of time can be determined. Finally, serial cephalographs can be used to evaluate changes in the positions of the jaws or teeth as a response to treatment.

Basically, cephalometric analyses are used to make either linear or angular measurements and comparisons between the following five relationships, both in the vertical and the sagittal planes of space:

1. maxilla to cranial base
2. mandible to cranial base
3. maxilla to mandible
4. maxillary dentition to maxilla
5. mandibular dentition to mandible

Numerous cephalometric analyses have been devised to assess these relationships (Downs, 1952; Moorrees and Lebret, 1962; Ricketts, 1961; Steiner, 1953, 1962) and compilations of mean cephalometric values have been published (Riolo et al., 1974).

When to Refer Children for Orthodontic Treatment

The question frequently arises among health professionals treating children, "When is the best time to refer a child for orthodontic treatment?" Since there is such variation among patients and problems, no definite rule concerning time or age can be made. Most orthodontists will agree, however, that the child should be referred for evaluation as soon as a problem is identified, and they generally like to see patients for an initial examination after the eruption of the permanent incisor teeth — approximately ages 7 to 8 years. No treatment may be indicated at this early age, but since the orthodontist will have the ultimate responsibility for the final correction of any malocclusion, he should be allowed the opportunity to make the decision concerning proper treatment sequencing and timing.

As a general rule, functional problems, such as a mandibular deviation caused by a posterior crossbite, are treated as soon as they are recognized. Similarly, problems involving skeletal growth discrepancies are frequently treated at earlier ages, since treatment may involve growth redirection and guidance with orthopedic forces.

In children in the primary dentition stage, little orthodontic treatment is justified except for space maintenance and the elimination of functional problems. In the mixed dentition stage, correction of functional problems and space maintenance are again indicated. In addition, treatment to correct skeletal discrepancies may begin in the later mixed dentition stage — ages 9 to 11 years.

Most orthodontic treatment cannot be completed until all of the permanent teeth erupt. Treatment should begin earlier only when such early treatment will either eliminate a problem entirely or else significantly reduce its severity, allowing better and faster final correction later on.

Airway Obstruction and Malocclusion

There have been many attempts to establish a causal relationship between dentofacial deformities and nasal airway inadequacy. The most prevalent view has been that mouth breathing resulting from an inadequate nasal airway is often associated with such deformities as retrognathic mandible; protruding maxillary anterior teeth; high palatal vault; constricted, V-shaped maxillary arch; flaccid and short upper lip; flaccid perioral musculature; and a somewhat dull appearance due to a constant, open-mouthed posture.

Angle (1907), in a statement concerning Class II Division 1 malocclusion, noted that "this form of malocclusion is always accompanied and, at least in its early stages, aggravated, if indeed not caused by mouth breathing due to some form of nasal obstructions." Allergists have expressed similar views in their concern for the allergic rhinitis patient and for the patient with enlarged adenoids. Mouth breathing is a common finding in these cases and there are reports of protruding maxillary anterior teeth or a constricted maxillary arch, as well as other dental deformities.

Hunter (1971), however, did not find a relationship between allergic rhinitis and malocclusion. His data did demonstrate that frequency of mouth breathing increases as nasal airway resistance increases. Eighty-three per cent of his subjects were classified as mouth breathers.

Several investigators (Tully, 1966; Linder-Aronson and Aschan, 1963; Linder-Aronson, 1970) have described a special facial type as characteristic of persons with enlarged adenoids and/or mouth breathing. Generally referred to as "adenoid facies," this facial type reportedly is marked by a long, narrow face with pinched nostrils, a short upper lip, prominent maxillary incisors, and a lips-apart posture.

Joshi (1964) suggested that dropping the mandible during mouth breathing may produce an exaggerated distal relationship between the mandible and maxilla by allowing overdevelopment of maxillary posterior alveolar processes. Moffatt (1963) related protrusion of the maxillary incisors to mouth breathing. When the mouth is open, the lower lip tends to fall between the upper and lower incisors and in this retruded position an anterior force is exerted on the upper incisors. Linder-Aronson and Backstrom (1960), however, found no relationship between mouth breathing and either inclination of the upper incisors or overjet.

Similarly Harvold et al. (1973) have drawn attention to a possible association between palatal anatomy and impaired nasal breathing. These researchers simulated hypertrophied adenoids in primates with acrylic blocks and found that the palatal vault increased in vertical height, creating an anterior open bite in 9 to 15 months. Harvold believes that an open, clear nasal airway is a prerequisite to normal facial form and function.

On the other hand, Korkhaus (1960) suggested that maxillary arch form is a primary factor in determining nasal cavity size and, hence, breathing mode. His studies indicated that alterations of the maxilla due to inhibition of growth or deformation is not a local symptom but rather characteristic of a complex anomaly that usually extends beyond the immediate region, and that includes the nose and sinuses.

Further complicating our understanding are findings which demonstrate dentofacial deformities without airway inadequacy and airway inadequacy without dentofacial deformities. For example, Derichsweiler (1956) argued against nasal obstruction as a primary etiologic factor in dentofacial deformity based on three cases of choanal atresia with normally developed jaws and dentition. Similarly, Watson et al. (1968) measured nasal airway resistance in orthodontic patients and noted that, when resistance was high, mouth breathing invariably resulted but skeletal deformity did not always occur. Interestingly, they noted that 23 per cent of the mouth breathers did so out of habit rather than from physiologic need.

Apparently, individuals with a high, narrow palate and posterior dental crossbite often breathe through their mouths (Hershey et al., 1976). This type of malocclusion is often associated with high nasal airway resistance. Treatment of such patients with orthodontic appliances to expand the maxillary arch corrects not only the malocclusion, but also, in many instances, significantly reduces the nasal stenosis as well.

The only conclusion that can be drawn from these many conflicting views is that malocclusion may or may not be associated with an inadequate nasal airway. Whether upper airway obstructions produce dentofacial deformities or whether the deformities produce airway impairment is still unclear in cases in which both problems are present. Certain types of malocclusion, such as a high palatal vault and constricted maxilla, do seem to be associated with nasal impairment, but which causes what cannot be determined from the present data. The only positive statement that can be made is that nasal abnormalities, such as a deviated septum or a small nasal airway due to a constricted maxillary arch, or enlarged adenoids will usually result in a mouth breathing pattern.

SPEECH AND MALOCCLUSION

The relationship between speech and malocclusion is complex and complicated by the many factors that have to be considered in connection with speech disorders. In addition to malocclusion, such elusive considerations as intelligence, hearing acuity, motivation, and, in particular, an individual's ability to compensate may influence speech performance (Rathbone, 1965). For example, even in severe malocclusion, speech may be perfectly normal, as a result of compensatory adjustments of the articulatory structures. In another instance, even a slight malocclusion may be related to a speech problem because of an inability to compensate, as Benediktsson (1954) pointed out.

Although there have been many attempts to explain the relationship between speech and dental disorders, the results are inconclusive. As Jensen (1968) notes, there is general agreement that except in the case of open bite malocclusion there is probably no direct relationship between malocclusion and defective speech articulation. Studies supporting such a relationship generally reflect clinical impressions rather than objective data.

It is certainly possible that while a particular malocclusion is not necessarily the cause of defective speech, it is a factor which can influence sound production. For example, Klechak et al. (1976) saw evidence that the size of the opening in the anterior part of the mouth for sibilant production is modified in the presence of an open bite.

Speech performance does appear to be affected by malocclusion in the presence of cleft palate. Counihan (1956) found that cleft palate patients with narrow maxillary arches do not perform as well as those with normal arches. Similarly Claypoole et al. (1974) report that anterior malocclusion and spacing also appear to affect speech performance in cleft palate patients.

Although the relationship between speech performance and the dentition is not precise, it is obvious that very few patients demonstrate a malocclusion severe enough to prevent them from acquiring adequate sound productions. The speech articulators have the potential to adapt to conditions in the oral cavity. Only severe open bite seems to affect articulation, and this is usually limited to sibilant sounds. Apparently, when articula-

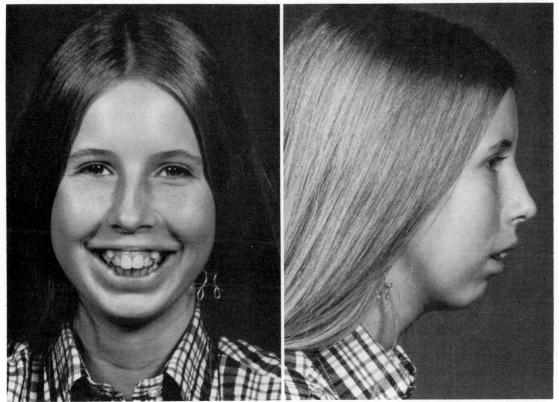

Figure 46–14   Pretreatment full face and profile views which indicate a high lip line, increased lower facial height, retrognathia, and retrogenia.

tion is distorted by a defect in the dentition, there is usually some other physical or psychological factor involved.

CASE REPORT

The following case report will illustrate the use of the diagnostic procedures presented in this chapter and will demonstrate the type of treatment result which can be obtained for a patient with a severe dentofacial deformity.

Patient L. P. was seen for evaluation at the age of 13 years and 8 months. Her chief complaints at that time were protruding maxillary teeth and an inability to incise and chew properly.

Facial Examination

Full-face examination indicated that facial features were symmetrical except that her nasal tip deviated to the right. Lip closure was incompetent and approximately 7 mm of maxillary central incisor crown was exposed when the lips were in the resting position; in a broad smile she had a very high upper lip line, exposing 5 mm of gingival tissue. The lower third of her face was noted to be excessively long (Fig. 46–14).

Facial examination of the patient's profile indicated that she had a severely retrusive mandible, increased lower anterior facial height, and incompetent lip closure with a deeply rolled lower lip (Fig. 46–14).

The intraoral examination revealed poor oral hygiene and generalized dental caries with severe involvement of the mandibular first molars. Her dentition was in a Class II relationship with a 12 mm overjet and a 5 mm anterior open bite. Both the maxillary and mandibular arches had 4 to 5 mm of crowding (Fig. 46–15).

Radiographic examination showed generalized shortening of root structures, especially in the maxillary incisors. Cephalometric analysis supported the clinical impression of a patient who had mandibular retrognathism, a severe skeletal open bite with excessive verti-

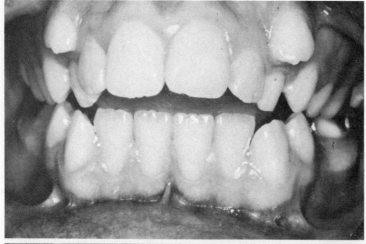

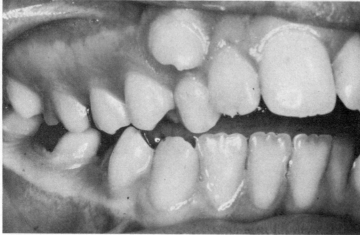

Figure 46–15 Pretreatment dental relationships demonstrating a Class II malocclusion with an anterior open bite, maxillary constriction and arch length deficiency.

cal maxillary development, increased lower anterior facial height, and maxillary and mandibular dental protrusion.

Problem List

From the results of the clinical examination and analysis of the diagnostic records the following problem list was generated:

(1) poor oral hygiene and dental caries with possible pulpal involvement of the mandibular first molars;

(2) maxillary vertical excess causing a downward and backward rotation of the mandible, resulting in a subsequent anterior open bite, mandibular retrognathism, and a long lower facial height;

(3) maxillary and mandibular dental protrusion;

(4) bilateral maxillary constriction;

(5) maxillary and mandibular crowding;

(6) retrogenia.

Treatment Plan

This patient's facial aesthetic and malocclusion problems were judged to be too severe to be corrected with routine orthodontic treatment, and a combination orthodontic-surgical treatment plan was initiated.

The initial phase of orthodontic treatment involved:

(1) elimination of dental caries and extraction of both mandibular first permanent molars;

(2) full banding of both arches;

(3) closure of the mandibular extraction sites and correction of crowding and rotations;

(4) alignment of the maxillary arch;

(5) vertical alignment of the maxillary teeth in three segments.

The goal of the initial orthodontic treatment was to position the teeth in the proper relationship to the basal bone of their respective

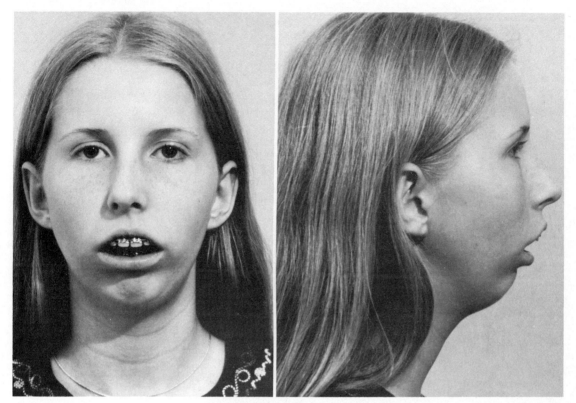

Figure 46–16   Presurgical full face and profile view after initial orthodontic preparation.

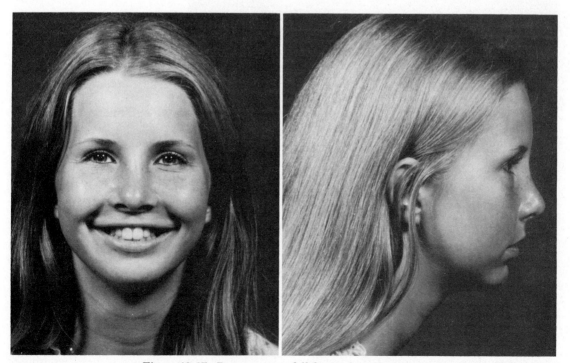

Figure 46–17   Post-treatment full face and profile views.

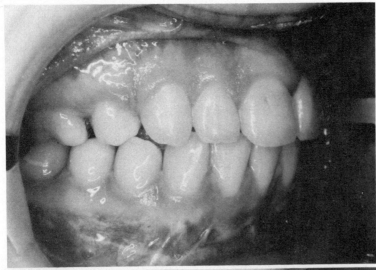

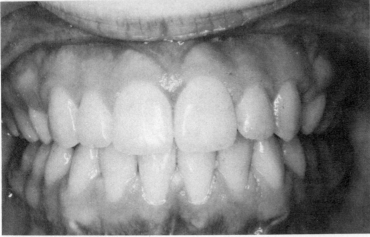

Figure 46–18 Post-treatment dental relationships.

arches. It was realized that following initial orthodontics the patient's teeth would not occlude as well as they had previously and that facial aesthetics would be made worse. The patient was warned to expect these changes initially (Fig. 46–16).

The surgical treatment plan included:

(1) extraction of the maxillary first premolar teeth;

(2) total maxillary osteotomy and ostectomy, mobilizing the maxilla in three segments. The two posterior segments were superiorly repositioned and expanded laterally. The anterior segment was superiorly repositioned and retracted into the premolar extraction sites;

(3) advancement genioplasty.

Cephalometric predictions indicated that this treatment plan would result in a closure of the open bite, correction of the maxillary

protrusion, improvement of the tooth-to-lip relationship, and shortening of the anterior facial height by mandibular rotation. The genioplasty was necessary to eliminate the retrogenic appearance, enhancing the aesthetic result.

Under general anesthesia the osteotomies were performed and a portion of the nasal septum was resected to allow passive, superior repositioning of the maxillary segments. Surgical fixation was maintained by direct wiring of the segments and intermaxillary fixation. Mandibular function was resumed after a six-week period of immobilization. Final orthodontic positioning of the teeth was accomplished in an additional four months.

Postsurgical facial and occlusal photographs (Figs. 46–17 and 46–18) show the improved aesthetic and functional result that was obtained from the combined orthodontic-surgical treatment of this patient. Pre- and postoperative quantitative evaluation of nasal airway resistance revealed an increased capacity for nasal respiration as a result of surgical management of the nasal septal deviation.

REFERENCES

Ackerman, J. L., and Proffit, W. R. 1969. The characteristics of malocclusion: A modern approach to classification and diagnosis. Am. J. Orthod., 56:443–454.

Altemus, L. A. 1960. A comparison of cephalofacial relationships. Angle Orthod., 30:223–239.

Altemus, L. A. 1963. Comparative integumental relationships. Angle Orthod., 33:217–221.

Angle, E. H. 1907. Treatment of Malocclusion of the Teeth, 7th ed. Philadelphia, S. S. White.

Benediktsson, E. 1954. Variations in tongue and jaw position in /S/ sound production in relation to the front teeth occlusion. Am. J. Orthod., 40:149–150.

Claypoole, W. H., Warren, D. W., and Bradley, D. P. 1974. The effects of cleft palate on oral port constriction during fricative productions. Cleft Palate J., 11:95–104.

Counihan, D. T., 1956. A clinical study of the speech efficiency and structural adequacy of operated adolescent and adult cleft palate person. Ph.D. dissertation, Northwestern University.

Derichsweiler, H. 1956. Gaumennahrterweiterung. Munich, Karl Hanser.

Downs, W. B. 1952. The role of cephalometrics in orthodontic case analysis and diagnosis. Am. J. Orthod., 38:162–182.

Enlow, D. H., 1968. The Human Face. New York, Harper and Row, Hoeber Medical Division.

Graber, T. M. 1966. Orthodontics, Principles and Practice, 2nd ed. Philadelphia, W. B. Saunders.

Harvold, E. P., Vargervik, K., and Chierici, G. 1973. Primate experiments on oral sensation and dental malocclusions. Am. J. Orthod., 63:494–508.

Hellman, M. 1935. The face in its developmental career. D Cosmos., 77:685–699.

Hershey, H. G., Stewart, B. L., and Warren, D. W. 1976. Changes in nasal airway resistance associated with rapid maxillary expansion. Am. J. Orthod., 69:274–284.

Hixon, E. H., and Oldfather, R. E. 1958. Estimation of the sizes of unerupted cuspid and bicuspid teeth. Angle Orthod., 28:236–240.

Hunter, B. M. 1971. Nasal airway resistance, breathing patterns and dentofacial characteristics. M. S. thesis, University of North Carolina.

Jensen, R. 1968. Anterior teeth relationship and speech. Acta Radiol., (Suppl) 276:1–69.

Joshi, M. R. 1964. A study of dental occlusion in nasal and oronasal breathers in Maharashtrian children. J. All-India Dent. Assoc., 36:219–239.

Kelly, J. E., Sanchez, M., and Van Kirk, L. E. 1973. An assessment of the occlusion of teeth of children. Data from the National Health Survey. National Center for Health Sciences, U.S. Public Health Service. DHEW Publication No. (HRA)74-1612.

Klechak, T. L., Bradley, D. P., and Warren, D. W. 1976. Anterior open bite and oral port constriction. Angle Orthod., 46:232–242.

Korkhaus, G. 1960. Present orthodontic thought in Germany: Jaw widening with active appliances in cases of mouth breathing. Am. J. Orthod., 46:187–206.

Limborgh, J. V. 1970. A new view on the control of the morphogenesis of the skull. Acta Morph. Neer-Scand.. 8:143–160.

Linder-Aronson, S., 1970. Adenoids: Their effect on mode of breathing and nasal airflow and their relationship to characteristics of the facial skeleton and the dentition. Acta Otolaryngol. (Stockh.) (Suppl.) 265:1–132.

Linder-Aronson, S., and Aschan, G. 1963. Nasal resistance to breathing and palatal height before and after expansion of the median palatine suture. Orthod. Revy., 14:254–270.

Linder-Aronson, S., and Backstrom, A. 1960. A comparison between mouth and nose breathers with respect to occlusion and facial dimensions. Orthod. Revy., 11:343–376.

Marks, M. B. 1965. Allergy in relation to orofacial dental deformities in children: A review. J. Allergy, 36:293–302.

Moffatt, J. B. 1963. Habits and their relation to malocclusion. Aust.Dent. J., 8:142–149.

Moore, W. F. 1975. Bone growth and remodeling: In Applied Physiology of the Mouth. Bristol, John Wright & Sons Ltd., pp. 83–85.

Moorrees, C. F. A., and Kean, M. R. 1958. Natural head position, a basic consideration in the interpretation of cephalometric radiographs. Am. J. Phys. Anthropol., 16:213–234.

Moorrees, C. F. A., and Lebret, L. 1962. The mesh diagram in cephalometrics. Angle Orthod., 32:214–231.

Moss, M. L. 1968. The primacy of functional matrices in orofacial growth. Dent. Pract. Dent. Rec., 19:65–73.

Moyers, R. E. 1975. Handbook of Orthodontics for the Student and General Practitioner, 3rd ed. Chicago, Year Book Medical Publishers, Inc.

Nance, H. N. 1947. The limitations of orthodontic treatment. Parts I & II. Am. J. Orthod., 33:177–223, 253–301.

Rathbone, J. S. 1965. Appraisal of speech defects in dental anomalies. Angle Orthod., 25:42–48.

Ricketts, R. M. 1957. Planning treatment on the basis of the facial pattern and an estimate of its growth. Angle Orthod., 27:14–37.

Ricketts, R. M. 1961. Cephalometric analysis and synthesis. Angle Orthod., 31:141–156.

Riolo, M. L., Moyers, R. E., McNamara, J. A., and Hunter, W. S. 1974. An atlas of craniofacial growth: cephalometric standards from the University School of Growth Study. The University of Michigan, Craniofacial Growth Series, Number 2, 321–330.

Sicher, H. 1952. Oral Anatomy. St. Louis, The C. V. Mosby Co.

Steiner, C. C. 1953. Cephalometrics for you and me. Am. J. Orthod., 39:729–755.

Steiner, C. C. 1962. Cephalometrics as a clinical tool. In Riedel, R. A. (Ed.) Vistas in Orthodontics. Philadelphia, Lea & Febiger.

Tully, W. J. 1966. Abnormal functions of the mouth in relation to the occlusion of the teeth. In Walther, R. P. (Ed.) Current Orthodontics. Baltimore, Williams and Wilkins.

Watson, R. M., Warren, D. W., and Fischer, N. D. 1968. Nasal resistance, skeletal classification, and mouthbreathing in orthodontic patients. Am. J. Orthod., 54:367–379.

Chapter 47

INFLAMMATORY DISEASES OF THE MOUTH AND PHARYNX

David W. Teele, M. D.

INTRODUCTION

Chapter 41 suggested an approach to treatment of the child with a sore throat; this chapter will discuss in detail inflammatory diseases of the oropharynx. Most such diseases have an infectious etiology; some do not. Many have a predilection for one part of the oropharynx, but most can appear in all parts. This chapter has been arranged according to the usual location of the inflammatory process. Certain uncommon diseases of uncertain etiology affecting chiefly oral mucosa are discussed in detail in Chapter 50.

INFLAMMATORY DISEASES INVOLVING CHIEFLY THE ORAL CAVITY

Herpetic Stomatitis

Two variants of herpes simplex virus exist, types 1 and 2, each with differing biologic and epidemiologic characteristics. Type 1 virus causes most infections of the oral cavity; type 2 causes most infections of the genitals. Most primary infections with herpes simplex virus are asymptomatic, although some cause significant illness such as stomatitis. Once the virus infects an individual, it persists, quiescent, usually in the ganglia of the infected dermatome. Certain stimuli, such as fever, ultraviolet light, wind, or menses, cause recrudescent disease. After such a stimulus, virus travels down the axon from a ganglion and reappears in the area infected originally. Such relapses may be either symptomatic or asymptomatic. These data explain the frequent isolation of herpes simplex virus both from persons who are well and from those who are ill (Juel-Jensen, 1973; Nahmias and Roizman, 1973).

Primary infection in the oral cavity causes a spectrum of disease ranging from no evident illness accompanied by serologic evidence of infection to a severe stomatitis. The latter may be so severe as to preclude eating or drinking and to require hospitalization of the child to prevent dehydration.

Herpetic stomatitis usually includes an ulcerovesicular enanthem involving lips, gums, buccal mucosa, and tongue. Most children are ill, with high fever and malaise; cervical adenopathy is common. A limited number of other diseases masquerade as herpetic stomatitis, and an accurate diagnosis usually may be made clinically. Hand, foot, and mouth syndrome includes often a vesicular eruption on hands and feet. Herpangina (see below) causes intraoral ulcers, but characteristically the lesions involve the posterior pharynx. By contrast, herpetic ulcers are confined almost always to the anterior part of the mouth (Parrott, 1954).

Diagnosis of recurrent disease due to herpes simplex virus usually presents few problems; the patient often knows the diagnosis. Vesicles in recurrent disease tend to be smaller and more tightly grouped than those in primary disease. Additionally, unless another illness, such as pneumonia, has triggered the recrudescence, the patient is not ill. Recurrent herpetic disease usually involves the angle of the mouth; intraoral lesions are rare. When recurrent herpetic disease does occur in the mouth, the lesions are confined to mucosa overlying periosteum, i.e., the hard palate and gums (Weathers and Griffin, 1970).

The diagnosis of disease due to herpes simplex virus may be made by isolation of virus from an unruptured vesicle. Because asymptomatic children may shed virus, isolation of virus from the oropharynx is only suggestive evidence. When available, staining with fluorescent antibody directed against herpes simplex virus will provide a rapid, specific diagnosis.

When a clinical virology laboratory is unavailable, a rapid diagnosis may be made if an unruptured vesicle remains. Unroofing the vesicle and bluntly scraping the base produces cells with characteristic cytopathology due to herpes simplex virus (Tzanck test). This material is spread on a slide and allowed to dry. Stains such as hematoxylin and eosin will allow visualization of intranuclear inclusions, but in most cases these stains are not needed. Virtually any stain, such as Wright stain, will allow visualization of multinucleated giant cells, cells caused only by herpes simplex and varicella-zoster viruses. Clinical information should allow the practitioner to choose between herpetic disease and that due to varicella-zoster.

With the notable exceptions of herpetic disease of the eye or central nervous system, no effective antiviral therapy is available. Herpetic stomatitis almost invariably is a self-limited disease; thus, therapy is directed at relief of pain and assurance of an adequate intake of fluid. Rarely, children require hospitalization and intravenous administration of fluids. Most children can be managed at home.

Therapy should provide enough local analgesia to allow drinking. Many different preparations have been suggested; each has drawbacks. Some physicians prescribe a viscous preparation of a local anesthetic such as lidocaine. These agents are effective and often allow a child to drink, but potential toxicity is considerable and includes seizures, lethargy, dizziness, and cardiac dysrhythmias. Few data exist to determine accurately a toxic dose, but it is suggested that toxicity may appear after the topically applied dose exceeds 25 to 33 per cent of the maximal dose used for infiltration (Ritchie and Cohen, 1975). Such dosages may be approached easily with repeated application. For this reason, most physicians are extremely cautious when prescribing these agents, usually prescribing limited use only to prevent hospitalization for dehydration.

Recently, pediatricians have started to use diphenhydramine, an antihistamine with efficacy as a topical anesthetic. Doses prescribed are equal to or less than those routinely prescribed for relief of allergic symptoms. Currently this topical usage of diphenhydramine is based on anecdotal data, and further study is required to determine both safety and efficacy.

Rarely, primary herpetic infections involve more than the oral cavity, with spread to remote organs, such as the liver or brain. Much more commonly, herpes simplex virus is inoculated through breaks in the skin. Small children, especially those who suck their thumbs, often produce vesicular disease on the thumb and fingers. Such painful lesions should be recognized easily when seen together with stomatitis. More difficult to recognize are these infections of the fingers when they occur without stomatitis — usually in medical personnel. These lesions mimic bacterial infections, but usually the vesicular component gives a clue to the diagnosis. The diagnosis may be confirmed by the Tzanck test outlined previously, thus avoiding futile administration of antimicrobial agents and surgery.

Hand, Foot, and Mouth Syndrome

Hand, foot, and mouth syndrome appears frequently, often in small epidemics during the summer. The disease usually includes an ulcerovesicular enanthem, involving both posterior pharynx (as in herpangina) and the anterior pharynx (as in herpetic stomatitis). A characteristic papulovesicular exanthem on the hands and feet frequently appears at the same time. This exanthem causes little discomfort and may be overlooked easily. Systemic signs of illness, such as fever and malaise, are common.

Outbreaks of this syndrome have been reported from many parts of the United States; almost all occurred during summer and early fall. Children are usually the victims, but persons of any age may be infected. Hand, foot, and mouth syndrome has been linked firmly to an enterovirus; thus, it may be assumed that it is spread by either the fecal–oral route or by droplets of oropharyngeal secretions. Coxsackievirus A 16 appears to be the causative agent; several studies have recovered this virus regularly from children with this syndrome. Concomitant serologic evidence of infection was present.

This syndrome is mild and self-limited, and children should require no more than routine care. Coxsackievirus A 16 can cause more severe disease, such as aseptic meningitis, but such involvement of other organs is rarely part of this syndrome (Magoffin et al., 1961; Cherry and Jahn, 1966).

Aphthous Stomatitis

Aphthous stomatitis, recurrent canker sores, affects up to 20 per cent of the population of the United States. For most, this disease is a recurrent, self-limited annoyance. For a few, severe disease can make life miserable, interfering with eating, drinking, and talking. For the physician, aphthous stomatitis is peculiarly annoying; its etiology is unclear, and its treatment is unsatisfactory.

Patients frequently give a family history of aphthous stomatitis. No seasonal or geographic factors appear important. Persons of all ages are affected.

The origin of recurrent canker sores remains obscure; a wide variety of stimuli, both physical and emotional, may trigger recurrences. In 1963 investigators reported the isolation of cell-wall defective forms of *alpha*-hemolytic streptococci from blood of patients with aphthous ulcers (Graykowski and Barile, 1963). Additionally, these investigators reported efficacy of tetracycline, a drug effective against this type of bacteria. The significance of this report remains unclear.

An aphthous ulcer begins as a red, intraoral papule that evolves rapidly, first into a vesicle and then into an ulcer. Any part of the oral mucous membranes may be involved, although the lips rarely are. Multiple ulcers are commonly present. The ulcers are painful, and pain lasts until healing occurs spontaneously one to two weeks later. The differential diagnosis includes all ulcerovesicular enanthems described in this chapter. Each of these is likely to be accompanied by systemic signs of illness, signs notably lacking in aphthous stomatitis. Recrudescent herpetic disease, which also lacks systemic signs, almost always involves the lips.

No therapy is required for most patients; the disease, although recurrent, is self-limited. Rarely, a patient may require topical anesthetics for relief to allow eating and drinking; such agents must be used with caution (see discussion of herpetic stomatitis). A bewildering variety of other therapies has been used; currently no specific therapy of documented efficacy exists.

Vincent Infections

Vincent infections include acute, necrotizing gingivitis (trench mouth), stomatitis, and tonsillitis (Vincent angina). Whenever large numbers of young people are drawn together, as in armies or in schools, these diseases afflict them frequently. Children are affected uncommonly, as the disease has a predilection for teenagers and young adults. The well-known association of trench mouth with life on a battlefield obscures the frequent appearance of these diseases in more normal situations and implies, often unfairly, that the victim has followed substandard hygienic practices (Bloom, 1964).

The origin of Vincent infections remains uncertain. Over a century ago, the disease was attributed to fusiform bacilli and spirochetes, organisms readily demonstrable in the lesions. Currently these bacteria and others are thought to act in concert, perhaps acting on tissue in some way compromised by those circumstances in which the disease is seen so often. These bacteria are normally resident in the mouth, and some other factor must allow the disease to begin. Anaerobic bacteria undoubtedly contribute to the characteristic fetid odor of the breath (Gorbach and Bartlett, 1974).

The infection usually evolves rapidly; initial involvement often appears on interdental papillae, but tonsils may be affected as well. Untreated, the disease spreads to include large areas of the labial and lingual gingivae. Further involvement may include buccal or lingual mucosa (Vincent stomatitis). The natural history of this infection includes spontaneous remission and relapse, but also considerable destruction of the gingivae, ultimately threatening loss of teeth. In addition to a characteristic foul odor to the breath, *fetor oris*, a characteristic membrane is noted.

Greyish-white and loosely bound, its removal causes bleeding. Systemic signs are usually minimal, although severe disease can produce fever, pain, and malaise. Few illnesses masquerade as Vincent infection, although the practitioner should remember that necrotizing gingivitis may be either a presenting symptom of or a complication of hematologic malignancy, notably leukemia.

Most cases respond promptly to regular rinses of the mouth with hot water containing peroxides. The rare patient with severe disease will respond even more quickly with the addition of penicillin G, a drug uniformly active against bacteria of the mouth. Patients should seek regular dental care to help prevent recurrences and loss of teeth.

Ludwig Angina

In 1836 von Ludwig described a gangrenous cellulitis of the sublingual and submaxillary spaces. Most of these infections appear to begin from a focus within the mouth, either traumatic or infectious. Ludwig angina is an uncommon infection of childhood, but it has occurred in infants as young as 12 days old (Steinhauer, 1967; Meyers et al., 1972; Barkin et al., 1975).

Initially, the patient has a tender swelling of the floor of the mouth. Untreated, the swelling spreads rapidly, pushing the tongue up and out. Extensive disease can obstruct the airway and spread inferiorly and laterally into the neck. Pathologic examination reveals a gangrenous cellulitis, spreading along fascial planes; pus does not accumulate.

Properly performed microbiologic studies have implicated a wide variety of bacteria, both aerobic and anaerobic, reflecting species resident in the victim's mouth. In the absence of prior therapy with antimicrobial agents or of an underlying disease that interferes with resistance of the host, usual causative bacteria are the normal residents of the mouth, i.e., fusobacteria, peptostreptococci, and spirochetes (Gorbach and Bartlett, 1974). Ludwig angina occurring in patients whose normal bacterial flora has been supplanted by opportunistic, gram-negative bacilli or fungi may be due to these organisms.

Since no significant amounts of pus accumulate, there is little place for surgery. Rather, therapy should be supportive, including especially maintenance of the airway and antimicrobial therapy directed against causative bacteria. Since many different bacteria cause Ludwig angina, therapy should be guided by results of needle aspiration of the infected space. To avoid contamination by bacteria of the mouth, such an aspiration, if possible, should be performed via a hypopharyngeal approach. Initial therapy should be selected based upon an examination of a gram-stained sample of such an aspirate, and continued therapy should be revised, if necessary, based on results of microbiologic cultures.

Oral Candidiasis

Pediatricians commonly must treat newborn infants for oral candidiasis (thrush); older children may develop this infection while being treated with antimicrobial agents. For most, oral candidiasis is an annoyance; for a few it may be the focus for disseminated disease.

Candida species, particularly *C. albicans*, reside commonly in the maternal genital tract; presumably newborns are infected at or shortly after birth. Many neonates are colonized with *Candida*; *Candida* may also be found commonly on older individuals. Oral candidiasis afflicts up to four per cent of otherwise healthy neonates (Kozinn et al., 1958); beyond this age, in the absence of predisposing factors, disease due to *Candida* is rare. Predisposing factors include therapy with antimicrobial agents and systemic disease that interferes with the defenses of the host (for example, malignancy such as leukemia).

Oral candidiasis appears as adherent white plaques on any or all parts of oral mucosa. Removal of these patches by scraping does not cause bleeding. Patients old enough to talk will complain of a very sore mouth. *Candida* may be identified readily by microscopic examination of scrapings and grown easily on Sabouraud's agar. These diagnostic procedures are required rarely; few other infections mimic candidiasis.

Untreated, oral candidiasis is self-limited, although it may last for weeks. Nystatin, applied directly to oral lesions, will promptly eliminate most infections. Usual dosage for neonates is 100,000 to 200,000 units applied four times each day; therapy is continued for several days after disappearance of plaques. For older children and adults, dosage is increased to 500,000 units four times each day. Nystatin is tolerated well, has few side effects,

Table 47-1   ETIOLOGY OF PHARYNGITIS IN CHILDHOOD

Agent Isolated	Chapel Hill, 1964–1965[°]		Chicago, 1964–1966[°°]	
	Diseased	Controls	Diseased	Controls
Bacteria				
Group A streptococci	263/715 (37)#	39/206 (19)	not done	not done
Viruses				
Adenoviruses	17/258 (6.5)	0/69 (0)	35/154 (23)	5/95 (5.2)
Enteroviruses	2/258 (0.7)	1/69 (1.4)	9/154 (5.8)	6/95 (6.3)
Herpes simplex viruses	2/258 (0.7)	1/69 (1.4)	13/154 (8.4)	0/95 (0)
Parainfluenza viruses	7/258 (2.7)	0/69 (0)	0/154 (0)	0/95 (0)
Rhinoviruses	2/258 (0.7)	0/69 (0)	1/154 (0)	0/95 (0)
Total with viral isolate	30/258 (11.6)	2/69 (2.9)	57/154 (37)	11/95 (11.6)
Mycoplasmas				
M. pneumoniae	22/715 (3.1)	2/206 (0.9)	3/174 (1.7)	not done
M. hominis	0/715 (0)	0/206 (0)	1/174 (0.6)	not done

[°]Glezen, W. P., Clyde, W. A., Jr., Senior, P. J., et al. 1967. Group A streptococci, mycoplasmas, and viruses associated with acute pharyngitis. J.A.M.A., *202*:119.

[°°]Moffet, H. L., Siegel, A. C., and Doyle, H. K., 1968. Nonstreptococcal pharyngitis. J. Pediatr., *73*:51.

$\dfrac{\text{No. children with isolate}}{\text{No. children cultured}}$ (per cent)

and is not absorbed. This agent has replaced gentian violet in the treatment of oral candidiasis, as application of the latter, although effective, was exceedingly messy. An occasional patient who cannot be cured with nystatin will respond to gentian violet.

INFLAMMATORY DISEASES AFFECTING CHIEFLY THE PHARYNX

Pharyngitis, a common disease of childhood, poses numerous problems of diagnosis and management. While most physicians assume that pharyngitis has an infectious etiology, in fact, approximately half of all cases cannot be associated with any microorganism. Imperfect techniques used for isolation of bacteria and viruses may account for some of this deficit, but noninfectious causes probably include smoking, allergy, atmospheric pollution, and excessively low humidity.

The prevalence in the pharynges of asymptomatic individuals of many microorganisms, viral and bacterial, considered "pathogenic" hampers efforts to determine the cause of pharyngitis. Any study of etiology must include either asymptomatic controls or serologic studies or both. Table 47–1 presents the results of several such studies. These studies suggest that some cases are due to viruses, including adenoviruses, herpes simplex virus, and enteroviruses, and that many are due to group A streptococci.

Certain other bacteria cause pharyngitis, notably *Neisseria gonorrhoeae* and *Corynebacterium diphtheriae*. Other pathogenic bacteria, such as *Staphylococcus aureus*, *Streptococcus pneumoniae*, and *Haemophilus influenzae*, are isolated frequently from the pharynges of children with sore throat, but they can be isolated with equal frequency from the pharynges of children who are well (Box, 1961). Thus, these latter organisms appear to cause pharyngitis rarely, if ever.

Viral Agents Causing Recognizable Syndromes

Despite the somewhat discouraging results of most studies of the causes of pharyngitis, certain viruses have been associated firmly with syndromes that include pharyngitis as a prominent finding. Herpangina is a self-limited viral illness characterized chiefly by fever, sore throat, and a vesicular enanthem in the posterior pharynx (Parrott et al., 1954). First described in 1920, herpangina has been associated with many enteric viruses, including most coxsackie A viruses, coxsackie B viruses 1–5, and numerous ECHO viruses. Reports of large outbreaks of herpangina often include sporadic instances of involvement of organs other than the pharynx, such as with aseptic meningitis (Huebner et al., 1951; Cherry and Jahn, 1965).

The syndrome of acute lymphonodular pharyngitis includes sore throat, fever, malaise, and headache. Characteristic raised, solid, white-yellow lesions appear in the posterior pharynx. All signs and symptoms resolve spontaneously within 4 to 14 days. Virologic and serologic studies have implicated a coxsackie A virus (Steigman et al., 1962).

Pharyngoconjunctival fever is a self-limited illness featuring fever (90 per cent of cases), sore throat (70 per cent), and conjunctivitis (66 per cent). Virologic studies have attributed this syndrome to an adenovirus (Bell et al., 1955).

Infection with the Epstein-Barr virus (EB virus) may cause pharyngitis in older children and young adults. While younger children often have serologic evidence of infection, most such infections are asymptomatic (Henle, 1970). Thus, most reports of disease due to EB virus include only older children and young adults. In these patients infection with EB virus may produce infectious mononucleosis, a syndrome characterized by cervical adenopathy (92 to 100 per cent of cases), sore throat (75 to 76 per cent), pharyngeal exudate (23 to 39 per cent), fever over 38.3° C (32 to 61 per cent), splenomegaly (38 per cent), and jaundice (eight per cent) (Hoagland, 1960; Evans, 1960). Palatine petechiae and rashes are noted frequently but may be seen often in other illnesses as well. Infectious mononucleosis is generally a self-limitied illness, although it may last for weeks before subsiding.

Infections due to EB virus may be diagnosed either by culture, a method not generally available, or serologically. Culturing virus alone may be misleading as virus may be isolated long after resolution of illness and decline in levels of antibody (Niederman et al., 1976). Thus, although not perfect, serologic methods offer the best means for the diagnosis. The classic test, the Paul-Bunnel heterophil agglutination test, is positive in more than half of those with infectious mononucleosis. This test has been supplanted largely by simpler tests performed on slides (Hoff, 1965). In younger children these tests may be negative; thus, when the diagnosis must be made with certainty, paired sera should be sent to a reference laboratory.

Examination of peripheral blood may provide additional suggestive evidence to support the diagnosis of infectious mononucleosis; the presence of 10 to 25 per cent of large, atypical lymphocytes strongly suggests the diagnosis. The total peripheral white blood cell count may be elevated but may also be normal or low.

As for all viral pharyngitides, only symptomatic therapy is available. Children with splenomegaly — which may last for months — are at increased risk for splenic rupture and must be excluded from activities likely to produce trauma to the spleen.

Infection with cytomegalovirus may mimic infectious mononucleosis, with fever, malaise, myalgia, sore throat, and hepatitis. While this syndrome occurs commonly in patients who have received many transfusions of blood, it occurs also in young, previously healthy individuals. The physician should suspect this infection when confronted with a patient with an illness resembling infectious mononucleosis but lacking serologic evidence of infection with EB virus. Infections due to cytomegalovirus can be documented by isolation of the virus together with serologic evidence of recent infection (Jordan et al., 1973).

Many other viruses cause pharyngitis but lack the ability to produce a characteristic syndrome. Thus, these illnesses must be diagnosed by culture and serologically.

Although herpes simplex virus can be isolated with some frequency from asymptomatic children (see Table 47–1), it does cause pharyngitis. Most infections due to herpes simplex virus appear as stomatitis, but involvement during a primary infection may extend to, or be confined to, the pharynx. Recurrent herpetic disease appears to cause pharyngitis rarely, if at all.

Adenoviruses commonly cause pharyngitis. These viruses may be particularly troublesome in closed populations of susceptible individuals, e.g., military recruits (van der Veen and Dijkman, 1962). Most studies of endemic pharyngitis include some cases due to adenoviruses (see Table 47–1). Pharyngitis due to adenoviruses is a self-limited illness accompanied by fever, sore throat, cough, nasal discharge, and headache. Pneumonia has been reported to occur simultaneously in a few patients.

In summary, numerous viruses produce a sore throat; a few cause recognizable syndromes. Currently no effective antiviral therapy is available, and the practitioner must exclude bacterial causes of pharyngitis and offer the patient symptomatic relief.

Bacterial Agents Causing Pharyngitis

Few bacteria have been shown convincingly to cause pharyngitis. For practical purposes, only groupable streptococci (groups A, C, and G), *N. gonorrhoeae*, and *C. diphtheriae* cause pharyngitis. Other bacteria may cause sore throat as part of a generalized illness such as tularemia (Tyson, 1976), but discussion of these diseases is beyond the scope of this chapter.

Streptococcal Pharyngitis

Since World War II, a huge volume of literature has been written about streptococcal pharyngitis. Despite the abundance of research, much of it elegantly performed, the day-to-day management of this illness remains a perplexing problem.

Suppurative complications of streptococcal pharyngitis include otitis media, mastoiditis, cervical adenitis, parapharyngeal abscesses, pneumonia, septic arthritis, bacteremia, and meningitis. Fortunately, for reasons that are not entirely clear, such complications have become much less common. This declining frequency preceded to some extent the introduction of antimicrobial agents. For these reasons, research into streptococcal disease has concentrated largely on nonsuppurative complications, rheumatic fever, and post-streptococcal glomerulonephritis.

Microbiology

In 1933 Lancefield showed that β-hemolytic streptococci could be classified immunologically into groups. She based this classification on carbohydrates found in the wall of the streptococcal cell.

Subsequent research has shown that group A streptococci can be classified further according to other constituents of the cell wall, M and T proteins. More than 60 M-types exist, and while immunity results from antibodies that develop against the infecting M-type, immunity is not cross-protective. Thus, repeated streptococcal infections are common. The M-protein accounts also for the virulence of group A streptococci. As virulent strains age or dry they lose both virulence and M-protein. The T-protein (and other proteins) of the wall of the cell allows typing of strains that lack M-protein. While T-protein is antigenic, antibodies thus raised do not protect against disease.

Streptococci other than group A are important pathogens for humans and animals. Group B streptococci are now the leading cause of neonatal sepsis and meningitis.

Groups C and G cause pharyngitis sporadically and have caused epidemic pharyngitis (Hill et al., 1969a).

Streptococci are gram-positive, facultatively anaerobic cocci. Microscopically, they grow in chains (*strepto*-twisted chain and *coccus*-berry). Streptococci will grow on many enriched media, but their growth on infusion agar containing ovine erythrocytes is used by most microbiologists to allow a presumptive classification. When grown on this agar, more than 90 per cent of group A streptococci cause complete (*beta*) hemolysis. Such hemolysis is not confined to group A streptococci, but morphologic differences should allow an experienced microbiologist to exclude groups other than A, C, or G. (Clinicians tempted to perform their own tests in the office should remember that other bacteria also cause *beta*-hemolysis.) Perfectly accurate assignment to group requires immunologic methods as described by Lancefield (1933); these methods are both expensive and tedious. Fortunately, isolates may be classified accurately by noting their sensitivity to bacitracin (Maxted, 1953): of 2468 strains of group A streptococci, 99.5 per cent were sensitive to bacitracin, a false negative rate of 0.5 per cent. False positives are more common, usually resulting in classification of strains as A when in fact they belong to group C or G (Pollock and Dahlgren, 1974). Despite these drawbacks, sensitivity to bacitracin allows an accurate presumptive classification, one suitable for guiding the practitioner.

When available, use of fluorescent-antibodies directed against group A streptococci allows rapid, accurate grouping of clinical isolates (Ayoub and Wannamaker, 1964).

These data suggest that group A streptococci might be identified readily by clinicians using simple equipment. Indeed, many practitioners now "read their own plates." If a physician has proper training and maintains a quality control program, such a practice can save both time and money (Rosenstein et al., 1970; Battle and Glasgow, 1971). However, some researchers feel that bacteriology in the office can be dangerously misleading, resulting in the frequent misdiagnosis of streptococcal pharyngitis (Mondzac, 1967).

Epidemiology

Streptococcal pharyngitis occurs most often in children of school age, although individuals of any age are affected. Rates of

Table 47–2   INCIDENCE OF CARRIAGE OF GROUP A STREPTOCOCCI AMONG
YOUNG SCHOOL CHILDREN°

Location (years)	Per Cent Infected	Range	Cumulative Incidence
Miami (1953–55)	11	2.5–17%	30–40%
Nashville (1953–58)	18	1.7–32%	up to 86%
Bismarck, ND (1960–61)	17	12–21%	56%
Dickinson, ND (1961–62)	24	17–35%	58%

°After Peter, G., and Smith, A. L., 1977. Group A streptococcal infections of the skin and pharynx. N. Engl. J. Med., 297:311.

disease due to group A streptococci increase with crowding and other features associated with lower socioeconomic classes (Peter and Smith, 1977). In situations that crowd together large numbers of young people, such as schools and military camps, streptococci may cause epidemic pharyngitis. When caused by a virulent strain, the attack rate for rheumatic fever following these epidemics may be extraordinarily high.

In temperate climates streptococcal pharyngitis is a seasonal disease, occurring most commonly in winter and early spring.

Studies performed using military recruits (notably at Warren Air Force Base) documented clearly how streptococcal pharyngitis spreads. Neither streptococci-laden dust from floors of barracks, heavily infected blankets, nor dried, infected pharyngeal secretions produced infection, even when inoculated directly into the pharynx of a susceptible recruit. Only fresh, wet secretions could infect volunteers (Perry et al., 1957a, 1957b; Rammelkamp et al., 1958). Additionally, spread of infection could be related directly to the distance between the cot of an infected recruit and the cot of a susceptible recruit (Wannamaker, 1954). Thus, transmission of streptococcal disease is due to close contact with infected persons, allowing ready spread of infected secretions. Occasional outbreaks are caused by infected food (Hill, 1969b; McCormick et al., 1976). In these situations virulent streptococci multiply rapidly in contaminated food, and the large inoculum quickly causes disease in most persons.

Outside of closed populations, streptococci are harbored by children of school age. Rates of carriage vary somewhat, usually peaking in late winter and early spring. The cumulative yearly incidence of pharyngeal carriage of group A streptococci may exceed 50 per cent. Table 47–2 shows rates of carriage by young children from different parts of the United States. Such large reservoirs of organisms allow ready spread into households and make prospects for eradication dim. In a study of respiratory illness in Cleveland, an asymptomatic carrier of streptococci infected nine per cent of members of the family, while a symptomatic child infected 25 to 50 per cent of the family (James et al., 1960). These high rates of carriage and secondary infection pose problems for the physician, especially when coupled with knowledge that up to one third of all victims of rheumatic fever lack an antecedent pharyngitis.

Goals for the Practitioner

Appropriate antimicrobial therapy has little effect on the clinical illness, either in military recruits or in children (Brink et al., 1951; Denny et al., 1953; Merenstein and Rogers, 1974). Patients treated immediately may have some slight symptomatic benefit during the first day or two, benefits that may be exceeded by those of salicylates.

Suppurative complications, once common, are now uncommon. How much of this reduction in frequency is due to biologic changes in humans or in the streptococci and how much is due to effective therapy remains uncertain. In any case, prevention of these complications cannot justify indiscriminate use of antimicrobial agents.

Poststreptococcal glomerulonephritis may follow a pharyngeal infection with group A streptococci. Unfortunately, no data exist to show convincingly that antimicrobial therapy will prevent this complication (Weinstein and LeFrock, 1971).

On the other hand, there is abundant evidence that appropriate antimicrobial therapy will prevent development of rheumatic fever. While the manner in which damage is produced in the heart, joints, and central ner-

Table 47–3 RHEUMATIC FEVER IN RECUITS WITH STREPTOCOCCAL PHARYNGITIS°

Therapy	Episodes of Rheumatic Fever	
None	17/804†	(2.1)
Penicillin	2/798	(0.3)

°Denny, F. W. et al., 1950. Prevention of rheumatic fever. Treatment of the preceding streptococci infection. J.A.M.A., *143*:151.

† $\dfrac{\text{No. with rheumatic fever}}{\text{No. with pharyngitis}}$ (per cent).

vous system remains obscure, much is known about prevention.

In epidemics in closed populations, the attack rate of rheumatic fever following untreated streptococcal pharyngitis has averaged three per cent (Catanzaro et al., 1958). During endemic disease the attack rate has remained relatively constant at somewhat less than 0.5 per cent (Siegel et al., 1961). Differences in attack rates are due partially to differences in virulence of infecting strains and partially to socioeconomic factors (Brownell and Bailen-Rose, 1973).

Appropriate therapy for epidemic disease dramatically reduces the attack rate for rheumatic fever (Table 47–3). In civilian populations with a lower attack rate, the effectiveness of therapy is less obvious. Nonetheless, "comprehensive-care" programs, which include the diagnosis and treatment of streptococcal pharyngitis, do reduce the attack rate of rheumatic fever in civilian children (Gordis, 1973).

Additionally, clear evidence exists to show that the delay of several days required to process a culture from the throat does not increase the attack rate of rheumatic fever (Catanzaro et al., 1954).

Thus, the goals for the practitioner should be to identify children likely to have streptococcal pharyngitis, to obtain a culture, to provide symptomatic relief, and finally to treat with an effective antimicrobial agent those harboring group A streptococci.

Diagnosis

Numerous investigators have sought some combination of signs, symptoms, and findings to diagnose accurately streptococcal pharyngitis. None has succeeded. Classical streptococcal pharyngitis includes fever, chills, sore throat, headache, and abdominal pain. Many

children with "classic" disease, however, have nonstreptococcal pharyngitis. Diagnostic difficulties are compounded by knowledge that during endemic disease only about half of all children with sore throat and a culture yielding group A streptococci have serologic evidence of infection. The balance have nonstreptococcal pharyngitis and are carriers of streptococci. This latter group is at no risk for rheumatic fever. Since no tests exist to determine at first visit which child with sore throat and group A streptococci has disease and requires therapy, practitioners must rely exclusively on results of microbiologic culture (Wannamaker, 1972).

A single swab obtained from the posterior pharynx and tonsils (or tonsillar beds) will detect upwards of 90 per cent of children with group A streptococci (Kaplan et al., 1971). Thus a single swab will exclude reliably streptococcal pharyngitis. Many investigators have suggested guidelines to minimize the number of such cultures required; all such guidelines are imperfect. Obtaining a culture from any child with either an illness characterized by sore throat and any degree of fever or any illness with a temperature greater than 38.3° C will detect 88.1 per cent of clinical illnesses capable of causing rheumatic fever (Honikman and Massell, 1971). Streptococcal infections capable of causing rheumatic fever but not pharyngitis generally remain undetected.

Therapy

Appropriate antimicrobial therapy will promptly eliminate group A streptococci from the pharynx and prevent rheumatic fever (Kaplan et al., 1977). Only those patients in whom the organisms persist are at risk for developing rheumatic fever.

Despite over three decades of intensive exposure to penicillin, group A streptococci remain universally sensitive to this agent. Penicillin may be given parenterally (benzathine penicillin G) or orally (penicillin G or V). Table 47–4 shows dosages for this drug as well as acceptable alternatives discussed later. The physician's estimate of the probability that the patient will take a drug for 10 days in the face of an illness that lasts but three or four days dictates the choice of a therapeutic regimen. Studies have shown repeatedly that many patients will not complete a 10 day course of therapy (Charney et al., 1967; Colcher and Bass, 1972). Table 47–5 shows

Table 47–4 THERAPY OF PHARYNGITIS DUE TO GROUP A STREPTOCOCCI

Agent	Dose
Drug of Choice	
Benzathine penicillin G°	For children weighing <60 lb
	600,000 units, intramuscularly, once
	For children weighing >60 lb
	1,200,000 units, intramuscularly, once
Acceptable Alternatives	
Buffered penicillin G†	200,000 to 250,000 units, by mouth, 4 times daily for 10 days
Penicillin V (phenoxymethyl penicillin)	200,000 to 250,000 units, by mouth, 4 times daily for 10 days
Erythromycin§	20–40 mg per kg per day given daily, by mouth in divided doses for 10 days

° Preparations containing both procaine penicillin G and benzathine penicillin G should not be used unless they contain benzathine penicillin G in the dose listed.
† Least expensive of oral agents
§ Drug of choice for patients allergic to penicillin

results of varying the duration of therapy with penicillin; maximal reduction of the attack rate for rheumatic fever requires 10 days of therapy. For these reasons many physicians administer a single injection of benzathine penicillin G, as this preparation will produce effective levels of penicillin for two to four weeks. Benzathine penicillin G is clearly the drug of choice when compliance is likely to be poor or where the attack rate for rheumatic fever is high. If given faithfully for 10 days, oral preparations are nearly as effective, but when given sporadically they are distinctly inferior. Thus, practitioners who prescribe oral therapy must do so with knowledge that the attack rate for rheumatic fever will not be reduced maximally. Physicians who routinely give penicillin orally are protected to a degree by the relatively low attack rate of rheumatic fever in most civilian populations. Patients intolerant of penicillin require an alternative drug. Erythromycin is currently the drug of choice for such patients. Other agents, such as amoxicillin, ampicillin, clindamycin, and cephalexin have been shown to eliminate group A streptococci from the pharynx, and hence, presumably, to prevent rheumatic fever. Each of these agents is likely to be more expensive and more toxic than either penicillin or erythromycin.

Certain antimicrobial agents are not satisfactory. Tetracyclines not only stain teeth of young children but they are also frequently inactive against group A streptococci (Kensit et al., 1977). Sulfa drugs, although effective as prophylaxis against recurrent rheumatic fever, will not prevent a primary attack when used, to treat streptococcal pharyngitis (Catanzaro et al., 1958). Trimethoprim-sulfamethoxazole frequently fails to eradicate streptococci.

Even appropriate antimicrobial therapy never will eliminate rheumatic fever completely; up to one third of those affected never have an antecedent clinical illness, and many who are ill with pharyngitis never visit a physician.

Table 47–5 EFFECT OF DURATION OF THERAPY WITH PENICILLIN FOR STREPTOCOCCAL PHARYNGITIS°

Agent and Duration of Therapy	Day of Second Culture	Percentage with Streptococci at Time of Second Culture
Penicillin, orally, <5 days	10	50
Penicillin, orally, 5–7 days	10	24
Penicillin, orally, 7 days	10	11
Benzathine penicillin, I.M. × 1	21	4

°Mohler, D. N., et al. 1956. Studies in the home treatment of streptococcal disease. II. A comparison of the efficacy of oral administration of penicillin and intramuscular injection of benzathine penicillin in the treatment of streptococcal pharyngitis. N. Engl. J. Med., 254:45.

Problems of Management

Physicians frequently are uncertain how to manage children whose pharynges continually yield group A streptococci, despite administration of appropriate antimicrobial therapy. Many of these "persistent" infections are in fact due to reinfection from other members of the household or to new infections with different strains of streptococci. Some, however, are truly persistent infections. Several explanations have been offered, but supporting data for these explanations are either scanty or conflicting. Organisms other than streptococci present in the nasopharynx may protect streptococci by inactivating penicillin, e.g., penicillinase-producing staphylococci (Kundsin and Miller, 1964; Rosenstein et al., 1968). Group A streptococci may survive hidden in tonsillar tissue where levels of penicillin are inadequate (Kaplan et al., 1974). Most of these persistent infections are subclinical; most can be cured by a second course of antimicrobial therapy, either with a penicillinase-resistant penicillin or penicillin G in higher doses. Currently no firm recommendations based on adequate data may be made.

Management of members of the family of a child with streptococcal pharyngitis poses a problem. Should "contacts" be cultured? Should contacts infected with streptococci be treated? Certain data have shown that symptomatic children with group A streptococci in their pharynges are likely to infect members of their family (James et al., 1960; Levine et al., 1966). On the other hand, if these newly infected persons remain asymptomatic they are probably at very low risk for rheumatic fever. Thus, in most cases physicians should obtain cultures only from symptomatic contacts and treat only those who are infected. Exceptions to this recommendation include households in which rheumatic fever has already occurred and situations where the attack rate of rheumatic fever is unusually high (Zimmerman et al., 1966).

DIPHTHERIA

Despite the availability for over 50 years of a simple, safe, effective vaccine, diphtheria continues to be a problem in certain parts of the United States and a major problem in many other nations. Each year 200 to 300 cases occur in the United States, the great majority (94 per cent in 1968) in southern states. Despite a major decline since 1920 in incidence and mortality rates for diphtheria, the case fatality rate has remained relatively constant at about 10 per cent (Center for Disease Control, 1969). Thus, a preventable disease continues to occur and

to kill persons who should have been protected. The high case fatality rate requires the physician to maintain a high index of suspicion and to treat after only a presumptive diagnosis.

Diphtheria attacks people of all ages, but about two thirds of cases and most deaths occur in children less than 10 years old. A second peak of disease occurs in older adults whose immunity has lapsed. Except among children less than four years old, there is a slight predominance among females, a trend that becomes pronounced in adults. Diphtheria in the United States affects chiefly non-white populations: from 1959 to 1970 the attack rate for American Indians was 20 times that for whites, and the attack rate for blacks was three times that for whites. Diphtheria occurs most commonly in autumn. Recently the incidence of diphtheria has risen in southern states, while it has continued to decline in the rest of the United States.

Most patients with diphtheria have never been immunized. Of 3462 patients with diphtheria, 68 per cent had never received toxoid; 13 per cent had received one or two injections; and only 19 per cent had received three or more injections (Brooks et al., 1974).

The causative bacterium, *Corynebacterium diphtheriae*, grows aerobically as a pleomorphic, gram-positive bacillus. Intracellular metachromatic granules may appear as polar bodies. Bacilli often grow in clusters resembling "Chinese letters." This characteristic appearance may allow an experienced microbiologist to make a presumptive diagnosis based on examination of material from the base of a suspected lesion. This organism grows well on ordinary media; an alert microbiologist may make a diagnosis not suspected by the clinician. However, one cannot rely on such serendipity. From suspected cases, contacts, or carriers, swabs should be obtained from both nasopharynx and oropharynx and inoculated onto blood agar, Loeffler agar, and a medium with potassium tellurite, such as cystine tellurite, Tinsdale medium. *C. diphtheriae* has several cultural biotypes: *gravis*, *intermedius*, and *mitis*. Characteristic colonial morphology may be an adequate criterion for identification when a laboratory is diagnosing diphtheria frequently as during an outbreak. Usually further characterization is required using both biochemical tests and tests for production of toxin. Table 47–6

Table 47-6 BIOCHEMICAL CHARACTERISTICS OF SOME SPECIES OF *CORYNEBACTERIUM**

Substrate	C. diphtheriae	C. ulcerans	C. xerosis	C. hofmanii
Glucose	+	+	+	−
Maltose	+	+	+	−
Sucrose	−†#	−	+	−
Starch	+/−	+	−	−

*Intended as a guide only. Isolates whose identity and toxigenicity remain uncertain should be submitted to a reference laboratory. (After Hermann, G. J., and Bickham, S. T., 1974. Corynebacterium. *In* Manual of Clinical Microbiology, 2nd ed. Washington, D.C., American Society for Microbiology, p. 130.)

†Isolates from the U.S.A. rarely ferment sucrose.

#Only the *gravis* biotype ferments sucrose.

shows some biochemical characteristics of certain species of *Corynebacterium* (Hermann and Bickham, 1974).

Only after infection with a bacteriophage do diphtheria bacilli become capable of producing toxin. Toxigenic strains cause diphtheria; nontoxigenic strains are of uncertain significance. Some nontoxigenic strains may cause skin lesions. Their role in the epidemiology of diphtheria is unknown; however, it is clear that they may be converted to toxigenic strains.

Both *in vivo* and *in vitro* tests for production of toxin exist. Each relies on either neutralization or precipitation of toxin by equine antitoxin. Occasionally both types of test may be needed to characterize certain isolates. *Gravis* and *mitis* strains are usually toxigenic, while *intermedius* strains vary in toxigenicity. Tests for toxigenicity, if positive, identify with virtual certainty an isolate as *C. diphtheriae*; only *C. ulcerans*, a rare species, also produces a toxin neutralized by antitoxin (Hermann and Bickham, 1974).

C. diphtheriae invades only minimally skin and mucous membranes. Toxin carried in the blood damages distant organs. Pappenheimer and Gill (1973) have reviewed the molecular basis of the pathogenesis of diphtheria.

As toxigenic organisms multiply, toxin causes local inflammation, exudate, and cellular necrosis, producing the characteristic tenacious membrane. While this membrane can kill by obstructing the airway, most damage is caused by toxin. Larger membranes produce more toxin and more severe disease. Diphtheritic toxin appears to cause cellular death by blocking synthesis of protein. Extraordi-

narily low concentrations of toxin (200 to 300 molecules per cell) can kill mammalian cells. (Pappenheimer, 1965).

Following a short incubation period of two to four days (the range is one to six), patients develop an illness characterized chiefly by sore throat, fever, and toxemia out of proportion to clinically apparent disease. The location of the diphtheritic membrane determines, to a considerable degree, signs and symptoms. Thus, nasal diphtheria may appear as rhinitis or a nasal foreign body, while pharyngeal diphtheria usually presents a more classic picture with an obvious membrane, toxemia, and marked cervical adenitis. Laryngeal diphtheria may present a picture dominated by signs of obstruction of the airway. Infection may involve any or all of these regions singly or simultaneously; thus, there is no pathognomonic presentation. Some features of diphtheria are listed in Table 47-7.

Other regions of the body, such as the umbilicus or external ear, may be affected first. Infections of the skin, uncommon in temperate climates, are common in tropical regions. Such infections often produce only an ulcer without toxemia, although on occasion, damage to distant organs may kill (Bray et al., 1972).

Prompt diagnosis of diphtheria is essential; delay may be literally fatal, as Table 47-8 shows. It is apparent that one must not await a microbiologic diagnosis. Smears of material from the base of the membrane may be helpful if viewed by a microbiologist familiar

Table 47-7 CLINICAL FEATURES OF DIPHTHERIA*

Features	San Antonio, 1970 (134)†	Austin, 1967–1969 (80)†
Sore throat	85%#	90%#
Fever	86%	84%
Pain with swallowing	23%	
Nausea, vomiting, or both	25%	15%
Headache	18%	
Edema of neck	18%	
Chills	10%	
Tender neck	4%	
Nasal discharge	2%	
Earache	0.7%	

*After McCloskey, R. V., Eller, J. J., Green, M., et al. 1971. The 1970 epidemic of diphtheria in San Antonio. Ann. Intern. Med., 75:495.

†Location of outbreak, year (number of patients).

#Percent of patients with this feature.

Table 47–8   EFFECT OF DELAY IN
THERAPY OF DIPHTHERIA*

Antiserum given on:	Case fatality rate
Day 1	0 %
Day 2	4.2%
Day 3	11.1%
Day 4	20.3%

*After Pappenheimer, A. M., Jr., 1965. The diphtheria bacilli and the diphtheroid. *In* Dubos R. and Hirsch, J. G. (Eds.) Bacterial and Mycotic Infections of Man. Philadelphia, J. B. Lippincott Co., p. 468.

with diphtheria, but most practitioners must rely on clinical grounds alone. The differential diagnosis includes exudative pharyngitis due to group A streptococci and other microorganisms, infectious mononucleosis, and Vincent angina. The diphtheritic membrane is grey or white (green or black if bleeding has occurred) and tenacious. Removal causes bleeding, a finding not seen commonly with other causes of pharyngitis. Laryngeal diphtheria may mimic croup, epiglottitis, manifestations of a foreign body, or parapharyngeal abscess. Nasal infections may mimic a nasal foreign body (Krugman et al., 1977).

The major goal of therapy is neutralization of unbound toxin; antitoxin will not neutralize toxin already bound to cells. Currently available antitoxin is of equine origin and frequently produces severe allergic reactions. Doses are empiric and must be administered intravenously. Currently recommended doses are as follows: for pharyngeal diphtheria of less than 48 hours duration, 20,000 to 40,000 units; for nasopharyngeal diphtheria, 40,000 to 60,000 units; for extensive disease of more than 48 hours duration or with a "bull neck," 80,000 to 120,000 units. Patients must be tested first for sensitivity to horse serum, and, if sensitive, they must be desensitized. Antimicrobial agents are useful as adjunctive therapy but are no substitutes for antitoxin. Penicillin and erythromycin are the agents of choice (Committee on Infectious Diseases, 1977).

Patients require additional supportive therapy, often including intubation or tracheostomy, artificial ventilation for those with paretic diaphragms, and strict bedrest for those with myocarditis. These latter patients may die suddenly, deaths apparently provoked by physical activity.

In addition to those complications that may affect any critically ill patient, some complications are peculiar to diphtheria. Myocarditis is the leading cause of death and usually appears toward the end of the second week of illness. Of 46 Iranian children with diphtheria, 21 had biochemical and electrocardiographic evidence of myocarditis. Most myocarditis appeared within 12 days of onset of illness (Tahernia, 1969). Diphtheritic neuritis may appear somewhat later, usually three to seven weeks after onset. While any nerve may be affected, certain nerves are involved more frequently. Neurologic sequelae of diphtheria include paralysis or paresis of the diaphragm, soft palate, and extraocular muscles. Paralysis of the extremities may mimic Guillain-Barré syndrome or poliomyelitis. Most victims of diphtheritic neuritis recover completely.

Passive immunity may be induced with antitoxin but is ephemeral. Long-lasting immunity may be produced easily with toxoid (toxin treated with formalin). Such immunity is highly protective; while carriage of virulent organisms may not be prevented, disease is. Immunization of most members of a community will reduce markedly rates of carriage of *C. diphtheriae*. Immunization procedures vary with age, and physicians should follow the latest recommendations of public health authorities (Committee on Infectious Diseases, 1977).

Injection intradermally of a minute amount of diphtheritic toxin is called the Schick test. Immune persons neutralize the toxin and should have no reaction. Susceptible persons will have local redness and induration. In practice, interpretation of this test may be difficult; immune children may have allergic reactions to either the toxin or impurities in the preparation (Pappenheimer, 1965).

Physicians must determine the status of immunization of each contact of a case of diphtheria and must obtain cultures from the nasopharynx and oropharynx. Fully immune persons whose cultures yield *C. diphtheriae* should receive either penicillin or erythromycin to eradicate carriage. Management of unimmunized contacts is controversial. Many recommend both antimicrobial therapy and antitoxin. Others, disturbed by the frequency and severity of reactions to antitoxin, urge antimicrobial therapy combined with daily observation for a week. Patients who then develop diphtheria are treated with antitoxin. Most agree that if a contact is unlikely to comply with either regimen, then both benzathine penicillin G and antitoxin should be given on the first day. All nonimmune patients should be immunized. Finally, *C. diphtheriae* may persist in the pharynx despite therapy, and treated patients should be recultured to document the end of carriage.

GONOCOCCAL PHARYNGITIS

Gonococcal pharyngitis is to a large extent a problem managed by clinics specializing in the treatment of venereal diseases. However, with the continually increasing rate of gonococcal disease in all populations, the pediatrician and general practitioner must be prepared to recognize and treat gonococcal pharyngitis. Certain features of this infection must be kept in mind. First, most infections of the pharynx do not cause sore throat. Second, even asymptomatic infections have the potential to cause disseminated gonococcemia (bacteremia and arthritis). Finally, gonococcal infections of the pharynx may be more difficult to eradicate than the more common infections of the cervix or urethra.

N. gonorrhoeae is a gram-negative diplococcus belonging to a genus many of whose members are normally resident in the oropharynx. A detailed treatment of the microbiologic characteristics and requirements for growth is beyond the scope of this chapter, but certain facts should be kept in mind. First, routine processing of swabs from the oropharynx does not reliably detect gonococcal infections. These failures are due to several factors: poor growth on blood agar incubated without CO_2, overgrowth by more vigorous species, and confusion with other species of *Neisseria* found normally on such plates. Second, routine processing of cultures from the pharynx using methods adequate for cultures from the urethra or cervix results in classification of species other than *N. gonorrhoeae* as gonococci. Thus, when the practioner suspects gonococcal infection of the pharynx, the microbiologist must be alerted. Forewarned, the laboratory will be able to diagnose such infections accurately.

Studies of the epidemiology of gonococcal pharyngitis have come from clinics specializing in treatment of venereal diseases. Thus, infections in other populations may have a different epidemiology. Isolated cases of exudative pharyngitis attributed to gonococci have included one in a child as young as four years (Wiesner et al., 1973). In studies from clinics treating venereal disease, gonococci are found frequently in the pharynx of individuals with gonococcal infection in other organs. In Seattle the prevalence of pharyngeal infection in persons attending such a clinic was 6.0 per cent in women, 1.4 per cent in men, and 9.8 per cent in homosexual men. Gonococci were found in the pharynx only in 4.2 per cent of those who practiced fellatio. Fellatio was correlated significantly with pharyngeal infection and with sore throat. Sore throat, however, was not correlated significantly with pharyngeal infection. Thus, in this population, gonococci did not appear to cause pharyngitis commonly.

Diagnosing gonococcal infections of the pharynx is of more than academic interest, as these infections not only may cause disseminated gonococcal infections but also may be difficult to eradicate with regimens adequate for gonococcal cervicitis or urethritis. Wiesner and colleagues (1973) report that spectinomycin, a drug used commonly to treat patients intolerant of penicillin, frequently failed to eradicate gonococci from the pharynx. Conventional doses of penicillin or tetracycline appeared to be more effective. The practitioner should select a therapeutic regimen based on the most current recommendations of public health authorities.

INFECTIONS OF THE PERITONSILLAR SPACE

Although young children may be affected, infections of the peritonsillar space occur more commonly in older children and adults. Most patients have had "tonsillitis" — which may have subsided — before developing severe sore throat, difficulty swallowing, and high fever.

Knowledge of involved anatomic structures facilitates understanding the pathogenesis, complications, and signs and symptoms of a peritonsillar infection. The fibrous capsule of the pharyngeal tonsil forms the medial wall of the peritonsillar space, while the superior constrictor muscle forms the lateral wall. The anterior and posterior tonsillar pillars form the anterior and posterior walls, respectively. Lymphatics draining the pharyngeal tonsil traverse the peritonsillar space and penetrate the superior constrictor muscle. Most infections appear to originate in the tonsil and to gain access to the peritonsillar space either via lymphatics or by direct extension through the tonsillar capsule (Levitt, 1969).

Cellulitis or abscess in the peritonsillar space causes a number of signs and symptoms, any one of which should suggest strongly the proper diagnosis. Swelling produces medial displacement of both tonsil and uvula; inflammation produces swelling of the anterior pillar and uvula. Patients usually have a muffled or "hot potato" voice and severe pain often referred to the ipsilateral ear. Irritation of the internal pterygoid muscle lying adjacent to the superior constrictor muscle causes marked trismus.

Complications include sepsis, thrombosis of great vessels of the neck, and extension into the neck and mediastinum (Rubinstein et al., 1974).

Distinguishing peritonsillar abscess from peritonsillar cellulitis requires determination of the presence or absence of accumulated pus. Certain findings indicate the presence of an abscess, such as drainage, pointing, or fluctuance on palpation; however, absence of such findings does not exclude an abscess. Thus, many physicians routinely aspirate all such infections.

Patients with peritonsillar abscess require surgical drainage of the abscess in addition to antimicrobial therapy. In a cooperative patient drainage may be performed using local anesthesia only. In very young children or in uncooperative patients intubation and general anesthesia are required to prevent aspiration of pus.

Patients with peritonsillar cellulitis often respond satisfactorily to antimicrobial therapy alone. Careful, frequent examinations assure the physician that an abscess has not developed despite antimicrobial therapy.

Inadequate data exist to determine with certainty how often different bacteria cause peritonsillar infections. Group A streptococci, common residents of the pharynx, are indicted correctly by most authors. However, many studies of the cause of peritonsillar infections have used methods inadequate to isolate more fastidious bacteria. Those that used such methods find, in addition to group A streptococci, many other organisms, including staphylococci (aerobic and anaerobic), *alpha* streptococci, peptostreptococci, fusobacteria, *Bacteroides* species (usually other than *B. fragilis),* and others. In short, bacteria isolated from peritonsillar abscesses are those commonly resident in or on the tonsil (Flodström and Hallander, 1976).

These microbiologic data have important implications for selection of appropriate antimicrobial agents. Virtually all incriminated organisms, with the exception of *S. aureus*, remain very sensitive to penicillin G. Therefore, a suggested approach includes obtaining cultures of blood, aspirating the affected area to obtain material for gram stain and culture, and starting therapy with large doses of penicillin G given parenterally. If review of the gram stain strongly suggests involvement by *S. aureus*, a different agent effective against penicillinase-producing staphylococci may be indicated. Many other antimicrobial agents are available, but few are appropriate therapy for peritonsillar infections. Ampicillin possesses activity against organisms of the pharynx that is similar to that of penicillin G, but rashes are far more frequent with use of ampicillin than with use of penicillin G; thus, ampicillin has little to recommend it for treatment of these infections. The penicillinase-resistant penicillins, e.g., methicillin, nafcillin, and oxacillin, probably should not be used as drugs of first choice; inadequate data exist to show their *in vivo* efficacy against anaerobic organisms. For patients who are allergic to penicillins, the physician has few acceptable alternatives. Clindamycin possesses excellent activity against both aerobic and anaerobic organisms, including *S. aureus*, causing peritonsillar infections, and currently it appears to be the drug of choice for patients unable to take penicillin. The cephalosporins, such as cephalothin, have activity with a spectrum similar to that of penicillin G, but on a weight basis are much less active and hence not indicated. Some newer cephalosporins have excellent activity against anaerobic bacteria and have considerable potential. Currently their routine use is not justified, because they are not superior to penicillin G for infections of the pharyngeal spaces. At concentrations achievable by the oral route, erythromycin has only erratic activity against likely pathogens. With intravenous use this agent may be effective, but parenteral administration of erythromycin has many attendant problems. Tetracyclines no longer have predictable efficacy and should not be used. Finally, the aminoglycosides, such as kanamycin or gentamicin, have little activity against either group A streptococci or anaerobes (Gorbach and Bartlett, 1974). Initial therapy should be continued or revised based on results of cultures.

Considerable controversy exists concerning

the need for tonsillectomy following treatment of peritonsillar infections. Some physicians believe that tonsillectomy, performed after resolution of the acute illness, prevents recurrence of peritonsillar infections. Others point to the relative infrequency of recurrences and do not perform tonsillectomy. Still others believe that abscess formation is a much stronger indication for tonsillectomy than is peritonsillar cellulitis. Currently, inadequate data exist to resolve the controversy, and resolution must await properly performed trials.

INFECTIONS OF THE RETROPHARYNGEAL SPACE

Cellulitis and abscess in the retropharyngeal space share many features with peritonsillar infections. Thus, this section will highlight the differences and, when appropriate, refer the reader to the preceding section.

Infections of the retropharyngeal space tend to occur in younger children than do peritonsillar infections. Most afflicted children are under five years old, and most present with rather sudden onset of fever, difficulty swallowing, a rigid neck, and noisy breathing. Many are unable to swallow and drool continually. The presenting signs together with examination of the pharynx usually allow diagnosis to be made readily. While palpating the retropharynx, care should be taken to have suction available and to position the patient to prevent aspiration of pus should rupture of an abscess occur. Retropharyngeal swelling is usually visible, but a lateral radiograph of the neck may be of help in the evaluation of the uncooperative child. One must position the child carefully for such a radiograph, as normal retropharyngeal tissue may buckle and simulate an abscess. Any doubt as to the significance of "swelling" may be resolved speedily with fluoroscopy.

Careful dissection of the retropharyngeal space of a young child reveals two vertical chains of three or four lymph nodes each. These nodes drain the nasopharynx and parts of the oropharynx and auditory canals. Thus, a variety of infections may seed the retropharynx. As children grow older, these nodes become less prominent, which may explain the decreasing frequency with age of retropharyngeal infections. The parallel vertical chains explain also the occasional observation of unilateral swelling. Other predisposing factors include penetrating wounds of the posterior pharyngeal wall, which may be caused by a fishbone or the fingernail of a parent clearing the pharynx of a choking child.

The hypopharynx and esophagus form the anterior wall of the retropharyngeal space, and the middle layer of deep cervical fascia forms the posterior wall. The space extends cephalad to the base of the skull and caudad to the superior mediastinum. In addition to infecting the mediastinum, retropharyngeal infections may penetrate into the "danger space," a space bound anteriorly by the middle layer of deep cervical fascia and posteriorly by the prevertebral deep fascia. This latter space extends from the skull to the diaphragm. Other complications of retropharyngeal infections include thrombosis of the jugular vein, bacteremia, septic emboli, and erosion of a major vein or artery.

As for peritonsillar infection, microbiologic data are inadequate. However, such data as are available suggest that the causative bacteria are similar to those discussed above under peritonsillar infections, i.e., group A streptococci, aerobic and anaerobic residents of the oropharynx, and *S. aureus.*

Antimicrobial agents alone may cure children with retropharyngeal cellulitis or adenitis; however, whenever pus accumulates, surgery is required. To avoid the danger of aspiration of pus, one must position the child carefully in the Rose and Trendelenburg positions (head and body down). To assure control of the airway, to minimize the danger of aspiration, and to assure immobility, the child should receive general anesthesia through an endotracheal tube. One makes an incision at the point of the abscess approximately one cm lateral to the median raphe. This incision may be extended and deepened somewhat with a hemostat. If the abscess is very large, it may first be decompressed with a large-bore needle attached to a syringe. The incision is allowed to heal by secondary intention.

Antimicrobial therapy should follow collection of proper material (blood and pus) for culture and gram stain. Initial therapy ordinarily is large doses of penicillin G given parenterally. For patients allergic to penicillin, clindamycin appears to be the drug of choice. For a detailed discussion of alternative antimicrobial agents, one should consult the preceding section on peritonsillar infections.

REFERENCES

Ayoub, E. M., and Wannamaker, L. W. 1964. Identification of group A streptococci. Evaluation of the use of the fluorescent-antibody technique. J.A.M.A., 187:118.

Barkin, R. M., Bonis, S. L., Elghammer, R. M., et al. 1975. Ludwig angina in children. J. Pediatr., 87:563.

Battle, C. U., and Glasgow, L. A. 1971. Reliability of bacteriologic identification of β-hemolytic streptococci in private offices. Am. J. Dis. Child., 122:134.

Bell, J. A., Rowe, W. P., Engler, J. I., et al. 1955. Pharyngoconjunctival fever. Epidemiological studies of a recently recognized disease entity. J.A.M.A., 157:1083.

Bloom, J. 1964. Vincent's infection. Med. Sci., 15:55.

Box, Q. T., Cleveland, R. T., and Willard, C. Y. 1961. Bacterial flora of the upper respiratory tract. Am. J. Dis. Child. 102:293.

Bray, J. P., Burt, E. G., Potter, E. V., et al. 1972. Epidemic diphtheria and skin infections in Trinidad. J. Infect. Dis., 126:34.

Brink, W. R., Rammelkamp, C. H., Jr., Denny, F. W., et al. 1951. Effect of penicillin and aureomycin on the natural course of streptococcal tonsillitis and pharyngitis. Am. J. Med., 10:300.

Brooks, G. F., Bennett, J. V., and Feldman, R. A. 1974. Diphtheria in the United States, 1959–1970. J. Infect. Dis., 129:172.

Brownell, K. D., and Bailen-Rose, F. 1973. Acute rheumatic fever in children. Incidence in a borough of New York City. J.A.M.A., 224:1593.

Catanzaro, F. J., Stetson, C. A., Morris, A. J., et al. 1954. The role of the streptococcus in the pathogenesis of rheumatic fever. Am. J. Med., 17:749.

Catanzaro, F. J., Rammelkamp, C. H., Jr., and Chamovitz, R. 1958. Prevention of rheumatic fever by treatment of streptococcal infections. II. Factors responsible for failures. N. Engl. J. Med., 259:51.

Center For Disease Control. 1969. Diphtheria Surveillance. Report No. 10, 1968. Summary, December, 1969, Atlanta.

Charney, E., Bynum, R., Eldredge, D., et al. 1967. How well do patients take oral penicillin? A collaborative study in private practice. Pediatr., 40:188.

Cherry, J. D., and Jahn, C. L. 1965. Herpangina: The etiologic spectrum. Pediatr. 36:632.

Cherry, J. D., and Jahn, C. L. 1966. Hand, foot, and mouth syndrome. Report of six cases due to Coxsackie virus, group A, type 16. Pediatr., 37:637.

Colcher, I. S., and Bass, J. W. 1972. Penicillin treatment of streptococcal pharyngitis. A comparison of schedules and the role of specific counseling. J.A.M.A., 222:657.

Committee on Infectious Disease, 1977. Report of the American Academy of Pediatrics.

Denny, F. W., Wannamaker, L. W., Brink, W. R., et al. 1950. Prevention of rheumatic fever. Treatment of the preceding streptococcic infection. J.A.M.A., 143:151.

Denny, F. W., Wannamaker, L. W., and Hahn, E. O. 1953. Comparative effects of penicillin, aureomycin and terramycin on streptococcal tonsillitis and pharyngitis. Pediatr. 11:7.

Flodström, A., and Hallander, H. O. 1976. Microbiological aspects of peritonsillar abscesses. Scand. J. Infect. Dis., 8:157.

Glezen, W. P., Clyde, W. A., Jr., Senior, R. J., et al. 1967.

Group A streptococci, mycoplasmas, and viruses associated with acute pharyngitis. J.A.M.A., 202:119.

Gorbach, S. L., and Bartlett, J. G., 1974. Anaerobic infections. N. Engl. J. Med., 290:1177.

Gordis, L. 1973. Effectiveness of comprehensive-care programs in preventing rheumatic fever. N. Engl. J. Med., 289:331.

Graykowski, E. A., and Barile, M. F. 1963. Bacteria studied as possible cause of canker sore. J.A.M.A., 184:51.

Henle, G., and Henle, W. 1970. Observations on childhood infections with the Epstein-Barr virus. J. Infect. Dis., 121:303.

Hermann, G. J., and Bickham, S. T. 1974. Corynebacterium. In Manual of Clinical Microbiology, 2nd ed. Washington, D.C., American Society for Microbiology, p. 130.

Hill, H. R. Caldwell, G. G., Wilson, E., et al. 1969. Epidemic of pharyngitis due to streptococci of Lancefield group G. Lancet, 2:371.

Hill, H. R., Zimmerman, R. A., Reid, G. V. K., et al. 1969. Food-borne epidemic of streptococcal pharyngitis at the United States Air Force Academy. N. Engl. J. Med., 280:917.

Hoagland, R. J. 1960. The clinical manifestations of infectious mononucleosis: A report of two hundred cases. Am. J. Med. Sci., 240:21–28.

Hoff, G., and Bauer, S. 1965. A new rapid slide test for infectious mononucleosis. J.A.M.A., 194:351.

Honikman, L. H., and Massell, B. F. 1971. Guidelines for the selective use of throat cultures in the diagnosis of streptococcal respiratory infection. Pediatrics, 48:573.

Huebner, R. J., Cole, R. M., Beeman, E. A., et al. 1951. Herpangina. Etiologic studies of a specific infectious disease. J.A.M.A., 145:628.

James, W. E. S., Badger, G. F., and Dingle, J. H. 1960. A study of illness in a group of Cleveland families. N. Engl. J. Med. 262:687.

Jordan, M. C., Rousseau, W. E., Stewart, J. A., et al. 1973. Spontaneous cytomegalovirus mononucleosis. Clinical and laboratory observations in nine cases. Ann. Intern. Med., 79:153.

Juel-Jensen, B. E. 1973. Herpes simplex and zoster. Br. Med. J., 1:406.

Kaplan, E. L., Bisno, A., Derrick, W., et al. 1977. Prevention of rheumatic fever. Circulation, 55:1.

Kaplan, E. L., Top, F. H., Jr., Dudding, B., et al. 1971. Diagnosis of streptococcal pharyngitis: Differentiation of active infection from the carrier state in the symptomatic child. J. Infect. Dis., 123:490.

Kaplan, J. M., McCracken, G. H., Jr., and Culbertson, M. C. 1974. Penicillin and erythromycin concentrations in tonsils. Am. J. Dis. Child., 127:206.

Kensit, J., Farrell, W., Evans, S., et al. 1977. Tetracycline resistance in pneumococci and group A streptococci. Report of an ad-hoc study group on antibiotic resistance. Br. Med. J., 1:131.

Kozinn, P. J., Taschdjian, C. L., Wiener, H., et al. 1958. Neonatal candidiasis. Pediatr. Clin. North Am., 5:803.

Krugman, S., Ward, R., and Katz, S. L. 1977. Infectious Diseases of Children, 6th ed. St. Louis, C. V. Mosby Co.

Kundsin, R. B., and Miller, J. M. 1964. Significance of the Staphylococcus aureus carrier state in the treatment of disease due to group A streptococci. N. Engl. J. Med., 271:1395.

Lancefield, R. C. 1933. A serologic differentiation of human and other groups of hemolytic streptococci. J. Exp. Med., 57:571.

Levine, J. I., Chapman, S. S., Guerra, V., et al. 1966. Studies on the transmission within families of group A hemolytic streptococci. J. Lab. Clin. Med., 67:483.

Levitt, G. W. 1969. Cervical fascia and deep neck infections. Laryngoscope, 36:4.

Magoffin, R. L., Jackson, E. W., and Lennett, E. H. 1961. Vesicular stomatitis and exanthem. A syndrome associated with Coxsackie virus, type A16. J.A.M.A., 175:117.

Maxted, W. R. 1953. The use of bacitracin for identifying group A haemolytic streptococci. J. Clin. Pathol., 6:224.

McCloskey, R. V., Eller, J. J., Green, M., et al. 1971. The 1970 epidemic of diphtheria in San Antonio. Ann. Intern. Med., 75:495.

McCormick, J. B., Kay, D., Hayes, P., et al. 1976. Epidemic streptococcal sore throat following a community picnic. J.A.M.A., 236:1039.

Merenstein, J. H., and Rogers, K. D. 1974. Streptococcal pharyngitis. Early treatment and management by nurse practitioners. J.A.M.A., 227:1278.

Meyers, B. R., Lawson, W., and Hirschman, S. Z. 1972. Ludwig's angina. Case report, with review of bacteriology and current therapy. Am. J. Med., 43:257.

Moffet, H. L., Siegel, A. C., and Doyle, H. K. 1968. Nonstreptococcal pharyngitis. J. Pediatr., 73:51.

Mohler, D. N., Wallin, D. G., Dreyfus, E. G., et al. 1956. Studies in the home treatment of streptococcal disease. II. A comparison of the efficacy of oral administration of penicillin and intramuscular injection of benzathine penicillin in the treatment of streptococcal pharyngitis. N. Engl. J. Med., 254:45.

Mondzac, A. M. 1967. Throat culture processing in the office — a warning. J.A.M.A., 200:1132.

Nahmias, A. J., and Roizman, B. 1973. Infection with herpes-simplex viruses 1 and 2. N. Engl. J. Med., 289:667.

Niederman, J. C., Miller, G., Pearson, H. A., et al. 1976. Infectious mononucleosis. Epstein-Barr-virus shedding in saliva and the oropharynx. N. Engl. J. Med., 294:1355.

Pappenheimer, A. M., Jr. 1965. The diphtheria bacilli and the diphtheroid. In Dubos and Hirsch (Eds.) Bacterial and Mycotic Infections of Man, Philadelphia, J. B. Lippincott Co., p. 468.

Pappenheimer, A. M., Jr., and Gill, D. M. 1973. Diphtheria. Recent studies have clarified the molecular mechanisms involved in its pathogenesis. Science, 182:353.

Parrott, R. H., Wolf, S. I., Nudelman, J., et al. 1954. Clinical and laboratory differentiation between herpangina and infectious (herpetic) gingivostomatitis. Pediatrics, 14:122.

Perry, W. D., Siegel, A. C., Rammelkamp, C. H., Jr., et al. 1957. Transmission of group A streptococci. I. The role of contaminated bedding. Am. J. Hyg., 66:85.

Perry, W. D., Siegel, A. C., and Rammelkamp, C. H., Jr.: 1957. Transmission of group A streptococci. II. The role of contaminated dust. Am. J. Hyg., 66:96.

Peter, G., and Smith, A. L. 1977. Group A streptococcal infections of the skin and pharynx. N. Engl. J. Med. 297:311.

Pollock, H. M., and Dahlgren, B. J. 1974. Distribution of streptococcal groups in clinical specimens with evaluation of bacitracin screening. Appl. Microbiol., 27:141.

Rammelkamp, C. H., Jr., Morris, A. J., Catanzaro, F. J., et al. 1958. Transmission of group A streptococci. III. The effect of drying on the infectivity of the organism for man. Am. J. Hyg., 56:280.

Report of the Committee on Infectious Diseases, 18th ed. 1977. American Academy of Pediatrics, Evanston, IL.

Ritchie, J. M., and Cohen, P. J. 1975. Cocaine, procaine and other synthetic local anesthetics. In Goodman, L. S., and Gilman, A. (Eds.) The Pharmacological Basis of Therapeutics, 5th ed. New York, Macmillian Pub. Co., p. 379.

Rosenstein, B. J., Markowitz, M., Goldstein, E., et al. 1968. Factors involved in treatment failures following oral penicillin therapy of streptococcal pharyngitis. J. Pediatr., 73:513.

Rosenstein, B. J., Markowitz, M., and Gordis, L. 1970. Accuracy of throat cultures processed in physicians' offices. J. Pediatr., 76:606.

Rubinstein, E., Onderdonk, A. B., and Rahal, J. J. 1974. Peritonsillar infection and bacteremia caused by Fusobacterium gonidiaformans J. Pediatr., 85:673.

Siegel, A. C., Johnson, E. E., and Stollerman, G. H. 1961. Controlled studies of streptococcal pharyngitis in a pediatric population. I. Factors related to the attack rate of rheumatic fever. N. Engl. J. Med., 265:559.

Steigman, A. J., Lipton, M. M., and Braspenickx, H. 1962. Acute lymphonodular pharyngitis: A newly-described condition due to Coxsackie A virus. J. Pediatr., 61:331.

Steinhauer, P. F. 1967. Ludwig's angina: Report of case in a 12-day-old boy. J. Oral Surg., 25:251.

Tahernia, A. C. 1969. Electrocardiographic abnormalities and serum transaminase levels in diphtheritic myocarditis. J. Pediatr., 75:1008.

Tyson, H. K. 1976. Tularemia: An unappreciated cause of exudative pharyngitis. Pediatrics, 58:864.

van der Veen, J., and Dijkman, J. H. 1962. Association of type 21 adenovirus with acute respiratory illness in military recruits. Am. J. Hyg., 76:149.

Wannamaker, L. W. 1954. The epidemiology of streptococcal infections. In McCarty, M. (Ed.) Streptococcal Infections. New York, Columbia University Press, p. 157.

Wannamaker, L. W. 1972. Perplexity and precision in the diagnosis of streptococcal pharyngitis. Am. J. Dis. Child. 124:352.

Weathers, D. R., and Griffin, J. W. 1970. Intraoral ulcerations of recurrent herpes simplex and recurrent aphthae: Two distinct clinical entities. J. Am. Dent. Assoc., 81:81.

Weinstein, L., and Le Frock, J. 1971. Does antimicrobial therapy of streptococcal pharyngitis or pyoderma alter the risk of glomerulonephritis? J. Infect. Dis., 124:229.

Wiesner, P. J., Tronca, E., Bonin, P., et al. 1973. Clinical spectrum of pharyngeal gonococcal infections. N. Engl. J. Med., 288:181.

Zimmerman, R. A., Cross, W. M., Miller, D. R., et al. 1966. A streptococcal epidemic in an isolated civilian population with institution of mass prophylaxis. J. Pediatr., 69:40.

Chapter 48

TONSILLECTOMY AND ADENOIDECTOMY

Jack L. Paradise, M.D.

No practice involving health care for children has excited more heated controversy among health professionals than has surgical removal of the tonsils and adenoids. Long the most common major operation carried out on children, tonsillectomy-and-adenoidectomy (T&A) continues to draw professional, legislative, and lay attention as a treatment whose benefits in relation to costs and risks have never been adequately assessed and whose indications remain largely ill-defined. Nonetheless, the continuously high rate of performance of T&A, despite some decline in recent years, attests to its strong hold on the minds of many physicians and parents as a treatment of importance and value. Annual expenditures for tonsil and adenoid surgery in the United States probably exceed a half billion dollars.

While T&A is often thought of, and most often carried out, as a single, combined operation, it is obvious that in considering indications for operating, each of the two components — tonsillectomy and adenoidectomy — requires attention individually.

HISTORY

Tonsillectomy has been known as a surgical procedure for at least two millenia, a technique for the operation having been described by Celsus as early as 50 A.D. (Kaiser, 1932). Adenoidectomy, by contrast, was probably not undertaken until the latter half of the 19th century, when Wilhelm Meyer of Copenhagen indicated that adenoid vegetations are responsible for both nasal symptoms and impaired hearing (Meyer, 1870). The two operations began increasingly to be carried out together early in the 20th century, as the then-popular "focus of infection" theory attributed various systemic disorders, most notably "rheumatism," to diseased tonsils and adenoids, and as enthusiasts proceeded even further to recommend T&A as a treatment for such diverse conditions as anorexia, mental retardation, and enuresis, or simply as a general measure to promote good health (Kaiser, 1932; Hays, 1924). Perhaps the ultimate in enthusiasm for T&A was manifested in certain communities in wholesale surgery on entire populations of school children in public school buildings (Baker, 1978).

Skepticism regarding the propriety of subjecting such large numbers of children to T&A began to be voiced increasingly in the 1930s (Kaiser, 1932; American Child Health Association, 1934) and 1940s (Bakwin, 1945). This skepticism received powerful reinforcement as (1) epidemiologic studies pointed to a natural decline in the incidence of upper respiratory infections in children after the first few years in school (Townsend and Sydenstricker, 1927; Van Volkenburgh and Frost, 1933; Tucker et al., 1952; Badger et al., 1953; McCammon, 1971); (2) recognition spread, in the period preceding the development of an effective vaccine, that individuals who had recently undergone tonsillectomy were at greatly increased risk of developing poliomyelitis, particularly of the bulbar type (Eley and Flake, 1938; Francis et al, 1942; Lucchesi and LaBoccetta, 1944; Anderson and Rondeau, 1954; Fisher et al., 1963); (3) a succession of effective antimicrobial agents became available for treating bacterial respiratory infections; and (4) a number of studies were published that purposed to show that tonsil and adenoid surgery was, after all, ineffective (Paton, 1943; McCorkle et al., 1955; Chamovitz et al., 1960).

Antipathy toward T&A, particularly in pediatric circles, mounted, exacerbated by frequent instances in which operation had been undertaken for obviously insubstantial indications. Occasional newspaper accounts of family-wide tonsillectomy (Fig. 48–1) added to collective righteous indignation about unnecessary surgery on children. During the 1950s, a major health care program, the United Mine Workers Welfare and Retirement Fund, hoping to both improve quality of care and reduce costs, instituted as a requirement for paying for a tonsil or adenoid operation prior endorsement of the procedure by one of a select panel of pediatricians or internists. In the late 1960s an account in a standard pediatric textbook questioned the very existence of indications for tonsillectomy (Einhorn, 1968), while a critical review in a prestigious journal termed tonsillectomy "rit-

ualistic surgery" (Bolande, 1969). As recently as 1976, the suggestion was made that tonsil and adenoid surgery be suspended entirely until such time as its efficacy could be established in properly conducted trials (Shaikh et al., 1976).

Notwithstanding this climate ranging from skepticism to outright condemnation, support for T&A has continued throughout many segments of the medical community. This support derives variously from (1) attitudes acquired during training; (2) judgments drawn from personal clinical experience; (3) newer studies, embodying for the first time randomized, clinical trials, which despite their limitations suggested that the operations *were* in some degree efficacious (McKee, 1936a, 1963b; Mawson et al., 1967; Roydhouse, 1970); (4) contentions by orthodontists that sustained mouthbreathing due to large adenoids may cause abnormalities in the growth and development of the facial skeleton and dentition (Subtelny, 1954; Linder-Aronson, 1970, 1974); and (5) accumulating reports of instances of life-threatening airway obstruction attributable to

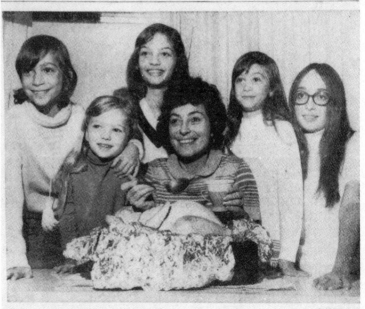

Figure 48–1 Newspaper photograph of five children in one family who underwent T&A on the same day. (Courtesy of the Pittsburgh Post-Gazette.)

enlarged tonsils and adenoids that was relieved by their removal (Menashe et al., 1965; Noonan, 1965; Luke et al., 1966; Levy et al., 1967; Macartney et al., 1969).

The net result of conflicting precepts, preconceptions, and polemics regarding tonsil and adenoid surgery, combined with the lack of conclusive evidence regarding its efficacy or inefficacy as generally undertaken, has been striking variation among both practitioners and academicians in their recommended indications for surgery (Modern Medicine Poll on Medical Practice, 1969; Sullivan, 1974).

PATTERNS OF PERFORMANCE

Current Trends

Table 48–1 shows data concerning the numbers of tonsil and adenoid operations carried out in the United States during the period from 1969 to 1977. Little change over the years has occurred in the frequency of tonsillectomy, whereas the frequency of adenoidectomy has increased steadily. By contrast, a striking decline has occurred in the frequency of the combined procedure (T&A), attributable to reductions more or less equally in the actual rate of operation and in the number of children in the "target" age groups.

Age

Age is an important factor in tonsil and adenoid surgical statistics. Three-quarters of all the operations are performed on children 15 years of age and under (Van DeMoortel, 1970).

In the age group under three years, tonsillectomy without adenoidectomy is performed rarely, while adenoidectomy and T&A are performed in about equal numbers. In children between three and 10 years of age, tonsillectomy alone continues to be performed infrequently, while T&As increase precipitously and outnumber adenoidectomies by about five to one. Between 10 and 20 years of age, adenoidectomy without tonsillectomy is performed relatively infrequently, and tonsillectomy alone and T&A are performed in about equal numbers (Bear, 1977).

Sex

Sex also influences surgical rates. The rate of adenoidectomy is about 1.5 times as high in males as in females, while the rate of tonsillectomy is about twice as high in females as in males. The rate of T&A — the procedure most commonly performed in both sexes — is slightly higher in males (National Center for Health Statistics, 1974).

Locale, Setting, and Surgeons

Striking variability in tonsil and adenoid surgery rates is noted between nations (Pearson, et al., 1968), regions (Nickerson and Colton, 1975; Lewis, 1969; Bunker, 1970), and even adjoining communities of similar population makeup (Glover, 1938; Massachusetts Dept. of Public Health, 1971; Gittlesohn and Wennberg, 1977; Bloor et al., 1978). Ultimately, of course, these variations must reflect underlying differences in attitude and practice among physicians. That the presence or absence of financial incentives

Table 48–1 FREQUENCY, IN THOUSANDS, OF TONSILLECTOMY, T&A, AND ADENOIDECTOMY (ALL U.S. SHORT-TERM NONFEDERAL GENERAL HOSPITALS)

Year	Tonsillectomy	Adenoidectomy	T&A	Total
1969	236	34	908	1178
1971	246	48	771	1065
1973	255	51	663	969
1975	234	70	482	786
1977	219	84	398	701
1979	209	83	342	634

Adapted from Bear, M. R. 1977. PAS Reporter, 15(5):1–8, and updated by personal communication, Commission on Professional and Hospital Activities, Ann Arbor, Mich.

may be one factor that influences physicians' decisions to perform these operations is suggested by the comparatively low frequency with which such surgery is performed in certain group practice, prepayment insurance programs in which the surgeon's income is not geared to the volume of surgery performed (Perrott, 1970; Klevit and Oleinick, 1971).

Currently it appears that although most tonsil and adenoid surgery in the United States is performed by physicians who report otolaryngology as their primary specialty, less than 40 per cent is performed by those who are Board-certified (American College of Surgeons, 1975). Substantial numbers of operations are performed also by general surgeons and general practitioners, the latter particularly in the Northwest (Nickerson et al., 1976, 1978).

CLINICAL INDICATIONS FOR SURGERY

Most indications used by those recommending or performing tonsil and adenoid surgery are encompassed by two categories of problems affecting the upper respiratory tract: *infection* that is recurrent or chronic, and *obstruction*. The infections involve variously the middle ears, mastoid air cells, nose, nasopharynx, adenoids, paranasal sinuses, oropharynx, tonsils, peritonsillar tissues, and cervical lymph nodes; the obstructions involve the nasopharyngeal 'and oropharyngeal airways and the oropharyngeal deglutitory pathway.

Certain variations on the themes of infection and obstruction are often cited in the case of the middle ear; adenoidectomy or T&A may be performed because of concern about *nonsuppurative* (secretory or serous) otitis media, a condition in which infection generally plays an initiating but not necessarily continuing role. Here the surgery is intended not only to eliminate presumed sources of infection in the adenoids or tonsils, or both, but also, in the case of adenoidectomy, to relieve presumed eustachian tube obstruction.

Wide differences of opinion prevail concerning how extensive, severe, and longstanding these various conditions should be in order to justify surgery. Opinions differ also as to whether, under various clinical circumstances, surgery should consist of tonsillectomy only, or adenoidectomy only, or the combined procedure (Modern Medicine Poll on Medical Practice, 1969; Sullivan, 1974). Tonsillectomy has generally been considered the component of tonsil and adenoid surgery that is efficacious with regard to recurrent throat infection (McKee, 1963a; Kaiser, 1930), and adenoidectomy the component efficacious with regard to middle ear disease (McKee, 1963b; Meyer, 1870; Crowe et al., 1917; Kaiser, 1930; Howard, 1972; Dealing, 1978). Nonetheless, when either operation alone appears indicated for a specific category of illness, the other operation often is added to the procedure to "take advantage" of the hospitalization and anesthesia and in the belief that more is to be gained than lost by performing the maximal removal of pharyngeal lymphoid tissue.

Other more general complaints, such as poor appetite or slow weight gain, that used to be widely accepted as indications for tonsil and adenoid surgery, may still occasionally be invoked as justifying surgery, but how often this occurs is impossible to determine.

The enormous variations in attitude and practice that exist in the medical community concerning tonsil and adenoid surgery are not surprising in light of the striking disparities that exist in the recommendations of current authorities. Contrast, for example, the American Academy of Pediatrics (1975) and AMA/PSRO (1976) criterion for tonsillectomy of "four or more episodes of tonsillitis with cervical adenitis within the preceding year," with this statement in a recent standard pediatric textbook: ". . . the presence or absence of tonsils does not affect the frequency, the course, or the complications of (acute pharyngitis) or susceptibility to it . . . so 'frequent sore throats' do not represent a valid indication for (tonsillectomy) . . ." (Eichenwald and McCracken, 1975).

WHY THE CONTROVERSY? PREVIOUS CLINICAL TRIALS OF TONSILLECTOMY AND ADENOIDECTOMY

One need not search far for an explanation of the continuing controversy concerning tonsil and adenoid surgery. It lies simply in the lack of convincing evidence that tonsillectomy and adenoidectomy, in the conditions for which they are usually undertaken, are superior in efficacy to conservative management. Such evidence can come only from properly designed and carefully conducted prospective clinical trials, and unfortunately, the trials reported have been not only few—six in all (McKee, 1963a, 1963b; Mawson et al., 1967; Roydhouse, 1970; Kaiser, 1930; Rynnel-Dagöö et al., 1978)—but also as a group, inadequate and inconclusive. Their methodological limitations and flaws in experimental design have received extensive discussion previously (Illingworth, 1950; Feinstein and Levitt, 1970; Paradise, 1972, 1976; Paradise and Bluestone, 1976) and will not be reviewed here in detail. Suffice it to say that the most important of the various shortcomings were the exclusion from most of the studies, on ethical grounds, of the very children most severely affected—particularly by middle ear disorders—along with admission to trial of children who were only mildly affected and in whom, therefore, benefits of surgery could at best be slight.

As for their findings, these reported studies agreed in general that T&A resulted in reductions in the incidence of throat infection that were significant statistically but not necessarily meaningful biologically. The studies were in disagreement over whether adenoidectomy, with or without tonsillectomy, resulted in a reduction in middle ear disease. It must be reemphasized that no study to date has provided data concerning the efficacy of tonsil or adenoid surgery in severely affected children. The unavoidable conclusions to be drawn from the current paucity of data have been stated previously: ". . . most judgments in favor of tonsillectomy, adenoidectomy, or both must be based either on unwarranted interpretations of the results of existing studies or on personal opinion or experience. Similarly, it seems . . . that some of the decisions against surgery also lack scientific support, or stem from prejudice against tonsillectomy and adenoidectomy engendered by its apparently excessive performance" (Paradise, 1976).

The current Children's Hospital of Pittsburgh study, to be discussed later, was designed to avoid the various shortcomings of earlier studies. In particular, by employing stringent surgical criteria, it focuses on children who are severely affected and who

therefore should stand the best chance of showing meaningful improvement if tonsil and adenoid surgery is indeed efficacious.

COST VS. BENEFITS OF TONSIL AND ADENOID SURGERY

The efficacy of an operation is a familiar concept for physicians, but the cost:benefit ratio of an operation, or of withholding an operation, may not be and deserves brief attention. The costs and potential benefits of tonsil and adenoid surgery are summarized in Table 48–2.

If surgery is resorted to, involved are not only financial costs, but also, and more importantly, risks of potentially lethal or damaging mishaps such as malignant hyperthermia (Snow et al., 1972) or cardiac arrhythmia, and of other adverse outcomes of varying nature include hemorrhage, airway obstruction, bronchopulmonary infection, transient or lasting velopharyngeal insufficiency, postoperative otitis media, and emotional upsets. There may also be other risks, such as immunologic ones (Ogra, 1971), that have yet to be elucidated fully.

Offsetting costs and risks, however, are potential benefits that could be substantial. Reduction in the frequency of episodes of ear, nose, and throat illness would involve corresponding reductions for children in discomfort, inconvenience, and school absence and for parents in anxiety, time missed from work, costs and inconvenience of physician office visits, and costs of medications. Reduction in nasal obstruction, if it were to occur, might conceivably result in improved respiratory function, lower incidence or lesser severity of upper respiratory infections, improved comfort, more restful sleep, more normal craniofacial growth and development, and more generally acceptable facial appearance. The remaining potential benefits shown in Table 48–2 — for children, reduction in hearing impairment and improvement in growth and overall well-being and for parents, reduction in overall anxiety — would, if they in fact resulted, obviously be important.

Most of the benefits listed in Table 48–2 might reasonably be grouped under the general heading of improved quality of life. Applying actual monetary values to such benefits constitutes an exercise termed by econ-

Table 48-2   COSTS AND POTENTIAL BENEFITS OF TONSILLECTOMY OR
ADENOIDECTOMY OR BOTH

Costs	Potential Benefits if Efficacious

Currently (March, 1980) $1500 at Children's Hospital of Pittsburgh	Reduction in frequency of ear, nose, or throat illness:
	  discomfort
	  inconvenience
	  school absence
	  parental anxiety
	  work missed by parents
	  costs of physician visits and drugs

Risk of anesthetic accidents:
  malignant hyperthermia
  cardiac arrhythmia
  vocal cord trauma
  aspiration with resulting bronchopulmonary
    obstruction or infection	

Risk of miscellaneous surgical or postoperative complications:
  hemorrhage
  airway obstruction due to edema of tongue,
    palate, or nasopharynx, or to retropharyngeal
    hematoma
  palatopharyngeal insufficiency
  otitis media
  emotional upset
	Reduction in nasal obstruction with improved
	  respiratory function
	  morbidity
	  comfort
	  sleep
	  craniofacial growth and development
	  appearance
	
	Reduction in hearing impairment

Unknown risks	Improved growth and overall well-being Reduction in long-term parental anxiety

omists as "shadow pricing" and is used by them in attempting to translate into economic terms value judgments that are biosocial in nature (Abt, 1977; Enthoven, 1978). This is an approach that merits the attention of physicians but is beyond the scope of the present discussion. Attempts at economic quantification aside, it is certain that physicians would be better able to judge whether the overall biosocial benefits of a tonsil or adenoid operation appear likely to outweigh its risks and costs if data were available regarding the degree of improvement the operation could be expected to bring about — that is to say, its efficacy.

To summarize what has been stated thus far, in order to arrive at rational indications for tonsil and adenoid surgery, groups of children must first be defined who have particular symptom complexes severe enough to justify particular operations; in those groups, the efficacy of the operations must then be tested by means of an integrated group of randomized, controlled trials; finally, if the operations prove efficacious, their overall impact must be assessed as critically as possible in relation to their risks and costs. It was with this frame of reference that the current Children's Hospital of Pittsburgh study was designed and undertaken.

THE CHILDREN'S HOSPITAL OF PITTSBURGH STUDY

Goals, Design, and Methodology

The Children's Hospital of Pittsburgh study, instituted on a pilot basis in 1971, supported since 1973 by the National Institute of Child Health and Human Development, and still in progress, addresses a number of questions involving both the natural history of presumably tonsil- and adenoid-related problems and the results of tonsil and adenoid surgery (Paradise, 1975, 1976; Paradise and Bluestone, 1976). In particular, the study focuses on three main questions: (1) the efficacy of tonsillectomy in reducing the frequency and severity of episodes of pharyngitis, (2) the efficacy of adenoidectomy in reducing the frequency and severity of episodes of otitis media, and (3) the effect of adenoidectomy on the course of nasal obstruction due to large adenoids.

Salient characteristics of the study include the following: (1) A team of individuals is employed specifically for the work of the study; virtually all historical accounts are obtained, and virtually all examinations are conducted by study personnel. (2) On entry, each subject receives independent evaluations by a

Table 48–3   CHILDREN'S HOSPITAL OF PITTSBURGH T&A STUDY: CRITERIA FOR ENTERING CONTROLLED, RANDOMIZED TRIAL OF TONSILLECTOMY

1. Recurrent throat infection
   a. at least three episodes in each of three years or
      five episodes in each of two years or
      seven episodes in one year, and

   b. each episode must have been characterized by one or more of
      the following:
         oral temperature 101°F (38.3°C) or higher
         enlarged (>2 cm) or tender anterior cervical lymph nodes
         tonsillar exudate
         positive culture for Group A β-hemolytic *Streptococcus*

   c. apparently adequate antibiotic therapy must have been administered for
      proven or suspected streptococcal episodes and

   d. each episode must have been confirmed by examination and its qualifying
      features described in a clinical record at the time of occurrence

or 2. Peritonsillar abscess

or 3. Chronic (minimum 6 months' duration) tonsillitis, persisting despite appropriate
      antimicrobial therapy

or 4. Nonurgent obstructive symptoms if tonsils very large, including
      a. stertorous breathing or mouthbreathing, with or without episodes of obstructive
         sleep apnea (Kravath et al., 1977)
      b. muffled "hot potato" voice if child is at least 6 years old

or 5. Chronic (minimum 6 months' duration) enlargement (>2 cm) or tenderness of
      anterior cervical lymph nodes, persisting despite appropriate antimicrobial therapy

pediatrician and an otolaryngologist. (3) Tonsillectomy and adenoidectomy are treated as separate procedures. (4) Criteria for entering the clinical trials of tonsillectomy and of adenoidectomy are specified (Tables 48–3 and 48–4). (5) Criteria are specified (Table 48–5) for exclusion from randomization (i.e., when indications for operation appear compelling). (6) Standardized systems are used for quantifying or rating relevant clinical findings and diagnoses. (7) A continuing process of testing the interobserver reliability of study staff members is maintained. (8) Assessment of middle ear status is based on combined otoscopic, tympanometric, and audiometric examinations. (9) Standardized cephalometric radiographs are used in assessing adenoid size. (10) Each subject receives a screening allergy/immunology evaluation that includes both skin tests and determina-

Table 48–4   CHILDREN'S HOSPITAL OF PITTSBURGH T&A STUDY: CRITERIA FOR ENTERING CONTROLLED, RANDOMIZED TRIAL OF ADENOIDECTOMY

1. Recurrent suppurative or nonsuppurative otitis media, if myringotomy and insertion of
   tympanostomy tube have been performed at least once previously

or 2. Persistent nasal obstruction
      a. manifested by stertorous breathing or mouthbreathing, with or without episodes
         of obstructive sleep apnea (Kravath et al., 1977), and by hyponasal speech, and
      b. accompanied by roentgenographic evidence of adenoid hypertrophy, and
      c. apparently not due to allergy

or 3. Chronic sinusitis or nasopharyngitis
      a. accompanied by both clinical and roentgenographic evidence of adenoid
         hypertrophy, and
      b. apparently not due to allergy, and
      c. persisting despite appropriate antimicrobial and other medical therapy

Table 48-5   CHILDREN'S HOSPITAL OF PITTSBURGH T&A STUDY: CRITERIA FOR
EXCLUSION FROM CONTROLLED, RANDOMIZED TRIAL AND FOR
PROMPT SURGICAL INTERVENTION

Indications	Treatment	
	Tonsillectomy	*Adenoidectomy*
Upper airway obstruction apparently due to large tonsils or adenoids or both, and accompanied by evidence of alveolar hypoventilation or cor pulmonale	x	x
Consistent interference with swallowing apparently due to tonsillar enlargement	x	
Severe nasal obstruction due to adenoid enlargement, resulting in apparent discomfort in breathing		x

tion of serum immunoglobulin levels. (11) Standardized dental and orthodontic observations concerning each subject are recorded by a pedodontist. (12) Follow-up of each subject is carried out by direct clinical examination at six-week intervals and also at the time of intercurrent respiratory illness and is supplemented by biweekly, standardized telephone inquiries.

Preliminary Findings

Limitations of Undocumented Histories of Recurrent Throat Infection.   Many of the children referred to in the study as potential candidates for the tonsillectomy trial have histories of recurrent throat infection episodes that appear to meet all the entry standards listed in Table 48-3 except for documentation. These children are admitted to the study and followed prospectively, and if at least two observed episodes of throat infection then develop with patterns of frequency and clinical features that match or exceed those described in their presenting histories, they become eligible for the tonsillectomy trial. To date, a large majority of such children have failed to develop frequent or severe episodes of throat infection (Paradise et al., 1978). From this experience, it may be reasonably concluded that histories of recurrent throat infection that are undocumented do not validly forecast subsequent experience and hence do not constitute an adequate basis for subjecting children to tonsillectomy.

The Clinical Trial of Tonsillectomy. Preliminary findings to date indicate that in children with recurrent episodes of throat infection that meet the entry criteria shown in Table 48-3, tonsillectomy is indeed effective in reducing throat infection morbidity over a period of at least two years. On the other hand, it is noteworthy that the absolute morbidity from throat infection experienced by control subjects has in general not been extreme; about half of the control subjects have thus far each experienced fewer than three episodes of throat infection per year, and almost two-thirds of these episodes have been rated clinically as mild.

With regard to the efficacy of tonsillectomy for, respectively, peritonsillar abscess, chronic (as distinct from recurrent acute) tonsillitis, and chronic isolated cervical lymphadenitis, the numbers of subjects with these conditions admitted to the study have been too few to warrant drawing conclusions.

Regarding those obstructive symptoms unequivocally attributable to large tonsils, tonsillectomy when carried out has consistently afforded complete relief; in children not operated on, data currently available are insufficient to indicate the extent to which such symptoms and the underlying tonsillar hypertrophy may subside spontaneously.

The Clinical Trial of Adenoidectomy for Otitis Media.   In order to define a population at high risk of developing otitis media, the protocol of the current study specifies that, as a prerequisite to entering the trial of adenoidectomy on the basis of recurrent otitis media, a child must have received myringotomy and tympanostomy tube insertion in the past and must subsequently have experienced at least one episode of either suppurative or nonsuppurative otitis media (Table 48-4).

Summarizing preliminary data, it is certain that in such children adenoidectomy by no means eliminates the problem of recurrent otitis media, but it remains uncertain whether adenoidectomy somewhat reduces the rate, severity, or duration of recurrent episodes. The question is particularly complex because of the large number of variables that may potentially influence outcome. A large number of study subjects will be required in order to reach firm conclusions concerning this question.

The Clinical Trial of Adenoidectomy for Nasal Obstruction. Children are admitted to the clinical trial of adenoidectomy for nasal obstruction only if the obstruction is appreciable (Table 48–4) and can be shown with reasonable certainty to be due wholly or mainly to large adenoids (Fig. 48–2.) At the time of this writing, such children who have received adenoidectomy appear to be experiencing almost uniformly excellent results persisting for at least two years. In the control group, spontaneous improvement of some degree has developed within the first year or two in some of the subjects, but complete resolution of nasal obstruction has developed in relatively few (Paradise et al., 1978a, 1978b). The children providing these data have been mainly five and six year olds, and information regarding children either younger or older is as yet inadequate for analysis.

It is important to consider whether the significantly greater relief of nasal obstruction achieved in the operated group resulted in benefits to the children that offset the cost and risks of the operation (Table 48–2). In an effort to test the development of one such benefit—improved nasal function—we have assessed olfaction in a group of study children using varying concentrations of phenylethyl alcohol, a rose-like odorant. We found that children rated as having no nasal obstruction showed almost uniformly good olfactory function, whereas most of those with severe obstruction showed poor function (Ghorbanian et al., 1978).

Other hoped-for outcomes of adenoidectomy remain to be evaluated. For example, certain orthodontists have attributed presumably abnormal growth patterns — long and narrow faces, low tongue placement, narrow upper jaws, steep mandibles, and open anterior bites — to large adenoids and have advocated surgery to prevent or ameliorate the so-called adenoid facies (Subtelny, 1954; Linder-Aronson, 1970, 1974). One study claimed improvement in dentofacial measurements following adenoidectomy but failed to include unoperated control subjects (Linder-Aronson, 1974). Comparative analysis of the standardized cephalometric roentgenographs obtained periodically from adenoidectomy and control subjects in the Pittsburgh study may help clarify this question. Certain other hoped-for outcomes of adenoidectomy, such as an increased sense of comfort in breathing and improved facial appearance, are essentially subjective and not readily measurable.

CURRENTLY ACCEPTABLE SURGICAL INDICATIONS AND SURGICAL DECISION-MAKING

Notwithstanding the large remaining areas of uncertainty about the efficacy of tonsillectomy and of adenoidectomy, it is obvious that decisions about surgery must be made currently on the basis of information now avail-

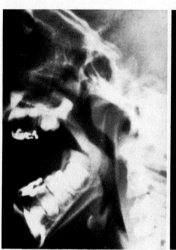 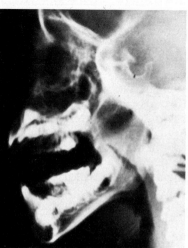

Figure 48–2 Lateral roentgenograms of children showing (left) normal adenoids and adequate airway and (right) adenoids encroaching on nasopharyngeal airway.

able. Operation is clearly indicated in a small number of severely affected children and clearly is not indicated in the great majority of children in whom the degree of tonsil- or adenoid-related illness or disability is insubstantial. Between these extremes lies an intermediate group concerning whom there is room for legitimate controversy. The uncertainty regarding these latter children is of two general categories: (1) the tonsil or adenoid surgery is of uncertain efficacy, as in the case of recurrent otitis media; or (2) efficacy appears to be reasonably well established, as in the case of adenoidectomy for nasal obstruction due to large adenoids, but in the patient at hand, the clinical severity, prognosis, or both may be in doubt. For example, it may not be possible to determine satisfactorily (a) whether a particular child is affected severely enough to justify an operation, (b) whether another child is so severely affected as to make surgery mandatory rather than optional, or (c) whether a third child is likely to soon "outgrow" the condition and thus to render operation of only short-term value.

Definite Surgical Indications

Operation is clearly indicated (Table 48–5) in those unusual circumstances in which massive hypertrophy of tonsils or adenoids or both results in unquestioned dysphagia, extreme discomfort in breathing, or even more extremely, in alveolar hypoventilation or cor pulmonale (Menashe et al., 1965; Noonan, 1965; Luke et al., 1966; Levy et al., 1967, Macartney et al., 1969).

Alveolar hypoventilation is a diagnosis difficult to be sure of, short of the development of clinical, roentgenographic, or electrocardiographic evidence of cor pulmonale. Required is the measurement of blood P_{O_2} and P_{CO_2} both when awake and during sleep (Mandel et al., 1980), a procedure which at present writing cannot be accomplished noninvasively. Extremely stertorous breathing when awake and frequently occurring episodes of obstructive apnea during sleep are signs that should lead to a high index of suspicion of the presence of alveolar hypoventilation. It appears likely that the condition, while admittedly unusual, may be more common than generally is appreciated.

On the other hand, even in children with symptoms or signs of appreciable obstruc-

tion, surgery should not immediately be resorted to automatically. Seemingly dramatic obstructive manifestations, even when long-standing, may sometimes be due to edema accompanying relatively inapparent infection rather than to fixed structural changes. Such obstructive symptoms may sometimes lessen considerably when vigorous antimicrobial treatment is applied. Accordingly, a trial of an appropriate antimicrobial agent is often advisable before deciding finally whether surgery is mandatory or even reasonably indicated.

Uncertain but Reasonable Indications for Surgery

At present writing, the conditions listed in Table 48–3 and 48–4, while still being tested, appear to constitute reasonable indications for tonsillectomy and adenoidectomy, respectively. For all these conditions, the common denominator is an arbitrarily arrived at minimum degree of severity, frequency, or duration. Equally reasonable, however, might be modifications that preserve intact the general principles of these minimum standards. For example, in the case of frequently recurring or persistent episodes of recurrent otitis media, it would appear acceptable, given the present limitations of our knowledge, (1) not to require prior tympanostomy tube placement before considering adenoidectomy or (2) to include tonsillectomy if adenoidectomy were being embarked upon as a treatment option.

However, the fact that a child indeed meets the outlined criteria should not necessarily lead to a decision in favor of surgery. Each decision should be individualized. For example, in the case of recurrent tonsillopharyngitis, additional factors that might properly tilt the decision one way or the other include accessibility of health care, school achievement and progress, potential tolerance of illness, other family stresses, and the relative out-of-pocket costs to the family of medical and surgical management, respectively. One study argues in favor of tonsillectomy for the patient with rheumatic heart disease who has large tonsils and in whom antistreptococcal prophylaxis cannot be maintained with confidence (Feinstein and Levitt, 1970).

Regarding the question of using surgical criteria less stringent than those listed in

Tables 48–3 and 48–4 (such as the criteria listed by a committee of the American Academy of Pediatrics in 1975), it should be kept in mind that the purpose of those criteria was to define a *minimally acceptable* standard of care rather than *optimal* care. Recognizing that the criteria in Tables 48–3 and 48–4 are arbitrary, it nonetheless appears that relaxing them would rarely bring about appreciable benefits but might, on the other hand, lead many children to undergo surgery needlessly. The Children's Hospital of Pittsburgh study should eventually provide information regarding the expected illness experience of the children who fall just short of meeting these criteria, since such children also are followed in the study prospectively. Should their prognosis prove in general benign, relaxing the criteria would hardly seem appropriate. If, on the other hand, these children are found in general to have experienced appreciable tonsil- or adenoid-related illness, further study of the efficacy of surgery in such children would be called for.

One distressing condition not heretofore considered — *halitosis* due to the accumulation of debris in tonsillar crypts — may justify tonsillectomy in those unusual circumstances in which more conservative measures, such as gargling or pharyngeal douche, prove ineffective.

Contraindications to Tonsil and Adenoid Surgery

Contraindications to surgery concern four general categories: velopharyngeal, hematologic, immunologic, and infectional.

A number of abnormal conditions that result in *velopharyngeal insufficiency* constitute contraindications to adenoidectomy. These include overt cleft of the palate; submucous (covert) cleft of the palate; neurologic or neuromuscular abnormalities leading to impaired palatal function; and the unusually capacious pharynx. In each of these conditions, the presenting complaint is likely to be *hyper*nasality, a symptom that the unwary observer may fail to distinguish from *hypo*nasality. If adenoidectomy is undertaken to improve the "nasal" speech of such children, the symptom may worsen markedly, since the adenoids had been serving to help fill the relative velopharyngeal void and thus facilitate normal speech production (Fig. 48–3).

Suspicion that a submucous cleft of the palate is present should be aroused when a bifid uvula is observed, or when widening and attenuation of the median raphe of the soft palate are present. The question may be clarified by palpating along the junction of the hard and soft palates, where a V-shaped midline notch, rather than the normal rounded curve, strongly suggests the presence of a submucous cleft (Fig. 48–4). This examination should be performed on all children, with or without hypernasality, for whom adenoidectomy is being considered. Irrespective of the findings, if hypernasality due to velopharyngeal insufficiency is suspected, it is advisable to refer the patient to an individual or a team skilled in cleft palate evaluation and management.

Hematologic contraindications to tonsil or adenoid surgery consist of (1) anemia and (2) disorders of hemostasis. Surgery should not be undertaken if the hemoglobin concentration is less than 10 gm per dl or if the hematocrit is less than 30 per cent. When surgery is being considered, careful inquiry should always be made about a family or past history of unusual bleeding or bruising, as certain rare hemostatic disorders may not be detectable with readily available tests. Routine preoperative studies should include measurements of the hemoglobin or hematocrit, prothrombin time and partial thromboplastin time and an estimate of the platelets, usually from a stained blood smear.

In the view of some clinicians, the existence of frank respiratory *allergy* that has not been treated for at least six months constitutes a contraindication to tonsil or adenoid surgery unless urgent, obstructive symptoms are present (Avery and Harris, 1976). The opinion that tonsil or adenoid surgery in allergic children may precipitate the development of asthma (Clein, 1952) has not been tested in clinical studies. Certainly in children with nonurgent obstructive symptoms who have both upper respiratory allergy and large tonsils or adenoids, a reasonable trial of antiallergic management as a precursor to considering surgery seems prudent.

Tonsillectomy or adenoidectomy should not be undertaken in the face of local infection unless urgent obstructive symptoms are present or unless appropriate, prolonged antimicrobial treatment has been maintained unsuccessfully, or, in the view of some (Brandow, 1973), unless a peritonsillar abscess is

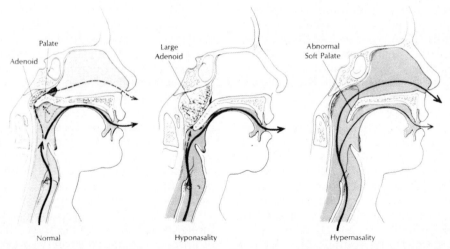

Figure 48–3 Functional and anatomic relationships in nasality are diagrammed. Normally, soft palate reaches posterior pharyngeal wall during production of sibilant and plosive sounds (solid arrow, left). With other sounds, passage is open enough for normal nasal resonance (dashed arrow, left). Large adenoids (center) interfere with air flow and produce hyponasality. Velopharyngeal insufficiency (as in submucous cleft) lets sound escape through nose and produces hypernasality (right). (Figure by C. Donner. *In* Paradise, J. L., and Bluestone, C. D. 1976. Toward rational indications for tonsil and adenoid surgery. Hosp. Pract., *11*[2]:79–87.)

present. Ordinarily, an interval of at least three weeks following an episode of acute infection will both allow for general recuperation and reduce the risk of operative hemorrhage.

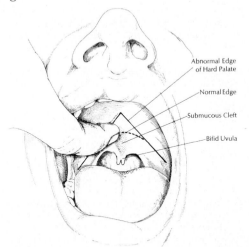

Figure 48–4 In patients with cleft palate, either overt or submucous, adenoidectomy is usually contraindicated since it would tend to worsen hypernasality. Palpation for diagnosis of submucous cleft palate — which may be easily overlooked — is diagrammed. Bifida uvula, widening and attenuation of the median raphe of the soft palate, and a V-shaped midline notch, rather than smooth curve, are diagnostic and should be looked for. (Figure by C. Donner. *In* Paradise, J. L., and Bluestone, C. D. 1976. Toward rational implications for tonsil and adenoid surgery. Hosp. Pract., *11*[2]:79–87.)

Adverse Effects of Tonsil and Adenoid Surgery: Real and Potential

Any physician who recommends tonsil or adenoid surgery must weigh the possibility of resulting harm. The possible adverse consequences range from death to nonfatal direct and indirect anesthetic and surgical complications, to hypothetical interference with immunologic defense mechanisms. Unfortunately, accurate statistics regarding mortality and morbidity in large patient populations are not available.

The death of a child as a consequence of tonsil or adenoid surgery is tragic in any circumstance, but particularly so if, as is usually the case, the operation was elective in nature. Case fatality rates have been variously reported during the past quarter century as ranging from 1 in 1000 to 1 in 27,000 (Avery and Harris, 1976; Bluestone et al., 1975), but the validity of these reports is open to question. Except for a probably irreducible minimum of anesthesia-related deaths (the anesthesia-related mortality rate unadjusted for age was recently reported at 1 in 14,000 [Avery and Harris, 1976]), death as a result of tonsil or adenoid surgery should be entirely preventable under present-day circumstances of care.

The possible nonfatal complications of tonsil or adenoid surgery are summarized in

Table 48–2, and two of them — *velopharyngeal insufficiency* and *emotional upsets* — are discussed in detail in this chapter. The risk of *hemorrhage* can be minimized by avoiding operation during or immediately following episodes of infection, by careful attention to surgical technique (DeWeese and Saunders, 1968), and by avoiding the use of aspirin for relief of postoperative pain. Nonetheless, hemorrhage, either primary or secondary, is bound to occur in some cases, and transfusion will occasionally be required. Data reported from a large number of hospitals surveyed during 1965 indicate a transfusion rate of 0.4 per cent (Avery and Harris, 1976). *Otitis media* has been reported as a not infrequent postoperative complication (McKee, 1963a and b), but it is not clear that the risk is higher than in comparable patients not operated upon.

Whether tonsil or adenoid surgery imposes *immunologic risks* of any practical consequence remains uncertain. The heightened risk of poliomyelitis that was an important deterrent to surgery before the advent of an effective vaccine and for which an immunologic basis has more recently been elucidated (Ogra, 1971; Surjan et al., 1972) is no longer of practical concern in this era of virtually universal immunization. Also, the concern that tonsillectomy might predispose to the development of Hodgkins disease (Vianna et al., 1971) has been apparently dispelled by more recent epidemiologic investigations (Johnson and Johnson, 1972; Guttensohn et al., 1975). It remains possible that removal of the immunologically active tonsils and adenoids will someday prove to undermine resistance to disease of some sort, but at present writing the likelihood seems small.

PREPARATION FOR HOSPITALIZATION AND SURGERY AND CARE IN THE HOSPITAL

Children who are to undergo surgery should be prepared specifically for the experience well in advance. Parents should describe the expected course of events in as much detail and as frankly as possible, commensurate with the child's ability to comprehend. Children should be told that a certain amount of discomfort will be entailed but that every effort will be made by hospital personnel to minimize it. Many hospitals permit advance visits so that children may see firsthand the facilities and equipment to be used and become acquainted with some of the personnel. Coloring or story books can also be helpful in the familiarization process. Once admitted to the hospital, children should have free and unlimited access to parents or parent surrogates, and parental rooming-in should be encouraged, especially for children of younger than school age. In any event, one or both parents should remain with the child during the period immediately preceding the trip to the operating room and should be at the bedside when the child returns. Careful preparation and kind, thoughtful management of the entire process of hospitalization and surgery should virtually eliminate the risk of untoward psychological consequences in previously well-adjusted children. For the child who is emotionally disturbed, the same general principles apply, but in addition, specialized professional advice may be appropriate to help minimize the risk of the child's neurotically misinterpreting the operative event (Jessner et al., 1952).

REFERENCES

Abt, C. C. 1977. The issue of social costs in cost-benefit analysis of surgery: *In* Bunker, J. P., Barnes, B. A., and Mosteller, F. (Eds.) Costs, Risks, and Benefits of Surgery. New York, Oxford University Press, pp. 40–55.

American Academy of Pediatrics, 1975–1976 Committee on Hospital Care. Pediatric Model Criteria Sets. Evanston, IL, American Academy of Pediatrics, p. 32.

American Child Health Association. 1934. Physical Defects: The Pathway to Correction. New York, American Child Health Association, Chap. 8, pp. 80–96.

American Medical Association. 1976. Sample criteria for short-stay hospital review: Screening criteria to assist PSROs in quality assurance. Chicago, American Medical Association, pp. 457–458.

Anderson, G. W., and Rondeau, J. L. 1954. Absence of tonsils as a factor in the development of bulbar poliomyelitis. J.A.M.A., *155*:1123–1130.

Avery, A. D., and Harris, L. J. 1976. Tonsillectomy, adenoidectomy, and tonsillectomy with adenoidectomy: Assessing the quality of care using short-term outcome measures. Quality of Medical Care Assessment Using Outcome Measures: Eight disease-specific applications. Santa Monica, California, Rand Corp., pp. 651–727.

Badger, G. F., Dingle, J. H., Feller, A. E., et al. 1953. A study of illness in a group of Cleveland families. II. Incidence of the common respiratory diseases. Am. J. Hyg., *58*:31–40.

Baker, S. J. 1939. Fighting for Life. New York, Macmillan Co., pp. 140–141. Cited in Pediatrics, *62*:559, 1978.

Bakwin, H. 1945. Pseudodoxia pediatrica. N. Engl. J. Med., *232*:691–697.

Bear, M. R. 1977. Downward trend in the incidence of tonsillectomy with adenoidectomy. PAS Reporter, *15*(5):1–8.

Bloor, M. J., Venters, G. A., and Samphier, M. L. 1978. Geographical variation in the incidence of operations on the tonsils and adenoids: An epidemiological and sociological investigation. Part I. J. Laryngol. Otol., *92*:791–801.

Bluestone, C. D., Paradise, J. L., Kass, E. H., et al. 1975. The workshop on tonsillectomy and adenoidectomy. Ann. Otol. Rhinol. Laryngol., *84* (Suppl. 19):1–79.

Bolande, R. P. 1969. Ritualistic surgery — circumcision and tonsillectomy. N. Engl. J. Med., *280*:591–596.

Brandow, E. C., Jr. 1973. Immediate tonsillectomy for peritonsillar abscess. Trans. Am. Acad. Ophthalmol. Otolaryngol., *77*:1412–1416.

Bunker, J. P. 1970. Surgical manpower: A comparison of operations and surgeons in the United States and in England and Wales. N. Engl. J. Med., *282*:135–144.

Chamovitz, R., Rammelkamp, C. H., Wannamaker, L. W., and Denny, F. W., Jr. 1960. The effect of tonsillectomy on the incidence of streptococcal respiratory disease and its complications. Pediatrics, *26*:355–367.

Clein, N. W. 1952. Influence of tonsillectomy and adenoidectomy on children with special reference to the allergic implications of respiratory symptoms. Ann. Allergy, *10*:568–573.

Crowe, S. J., Watkins, S. S., and Rothholz, A. S. 1917. Relation of tonsillar and nasopharyngeal infections to general systemic disorders. Bull. Johns Hopkins Hosp., *28*(311):2–3.

Dealing with fluid in the middle ear (editorial). 1978. Lancet, *1*:1297.

DeWeese, D. D., and Saunders, W. H. 1968. Textbook of Otolaryngology, 3rd ed. St. Louis, The C. V. Mosby Co., pp. 72–78.

Eichenwald, H. F., and McCracken, G. H., Jr. 1975. Tonsils and adenoids. In Vaughan, V. C., III, and McKay, R. J. (Eds.) Nelson Textbook of Pediatrics, 10th ed. Philadelphia, W. B. Saunders Co., pp. 947–950.

Einhorn, A. H. 1968. The nose, paranasal sinuses and pharynx. In Barnett, H. L. (Ed.) Pediatrics, 14th ed. New York, Appleton-Century-Crofts, pp. 1675–1677.

Eley, R. C., and Flake, C. G. 1938. Acute anterior poliomyelitis following tonsillectomy and adenoidectomy with special reference to the bulbar form. J. Pediatr., *13*:63–70.

Enthoven, A. C. 1978. Shattuck lecture. Cutting cost without cutting the quality of care. N. Engl. J. Med., *298*:1229–1238.

Feinstein, A. R., and Levitt, M. 1970. The role of tonsils in predisposing to streptococcal infections and recurrences of rheumatic fever. N. Engl. J. Med., *282*:285–291.

Fisher, A. E., Lucchesi, P. F., Marks, H. H., et al. 1963. Poliomyelitic paralysis and tonsillectomy. J.A.M.A., *186*:873.

Francis, T., Jr., Krill, C. E., Toomey, J. A., et al. 1942. Poliomyelitis following tonsillectomy in five members of a family. J.A.M.A., *119*:1392–1396.

Ghorbanian, S. N., Paradise, J. L., and Doty, R. L. 1978. Odor perception in children in relation to nasal obstruction (abstract). Pediatr. Res., *12*:371.

Gittelsohn, A. M., and Wennberg, J. E. 1977. On the incidence of tonsillectomy and other common surgical procedures. In Bunker, J. P., Barnes, B. A., and Mosteller, F. (Eds.) Costs, Risks, and Benefits of Surgery. New York, Oxford University Press, pp. 91–106.

Glover, J. A. 1938. The incidence of tonsillectomy in school children. Proc. R. Soc. Med., *31*:1219–1236.

Gutensohn, N., Li, F. P., Johnson, R. E., et al. 1975. Hodgkin's disease, tonsillectomy and family size. N. Engl. J. Med., *292*:22–25.

Hays, H. M. 1924. Diseases of pharynx, nasopharynx and hypopharynx. In Abt, I. A. (Ed.) Pediatrics, 3rd ed. Philadelphia, W. B. Saunders Co., pp. 217–218.

Howard, W. A. 1972. The tonsil and adenoid problem. In Ferguson, C. F., and Kendig, E. L., Jr. (Eds.) Pediatric Otolaryngology, 2nd ed. Philadelphia, W. B. Saunders Co., p. 1093.

Illingworth, R. S. 1950. Discussion on the tonsil and adenoid problem. Proc. R. Soc. Med., *43*:317–324.

Jessner, L., Blom, G. E., and Waldfogel, S. 1952. Emotional implications of tonsillectomy and adenoidectomy in children. Psychoanalyt. Stud. Child., *7*:126–169.

Johnson, S. K., and Johnson, R. E. 1972. Tonsillectomy history in Hodgkin's disease. N. Engl. J. Med., *287*:1122–1125.

Kaiser, A. D. 1930. Results of tonsillectomy: A comparative study of 2200 tonsillectomized children with an equal number of controls three and ten years after operation. J.A.M.A., *95*:837–842.

Kaiser, A. D. 1932. Children's Tonsils In or Out. Philadelphia, J. B. Lippincott, pp. vii, 2–3, 8–10.

Klevit, H. D., and Oleinick, A. 1971. The decline of tonsillectomy in a prepayment practice. Proceedings of the 13th International Congress of Pediatrics, Vienna, pp. 135–140.

Kravath, R. E., Pollak, C. P., and Borowiecki, B. 1977. Hypoventilation during sleep in children who have lymphoid airway obstruction treated by nasopharyngeal tube and T and A. Pediatrics, *59*:865–871.

Levy, A. M., Tabakin, B. S., Hanson, J. S., et al. 1967. Hypertrophied adenoids causing pulmonary hypertension and severe congestive heart failure. N. Engl. J. Med., *277*:506–511.

Lewis, C. E. 1969. Variations in the incidence of surgery. N. Engl. J. Med., *281*:880–884.

Linder-Aronson, S. 1970. Adenoids: Their effect on mode of breathing and nasal airflow and their relationship to characteristics of the facial skeleton and the dentition. Acta Otolaryngol. Suppl., *265*:1–32.

Linder-Aronson, S. 1974. Effects of adenoidectomy on dentition and nasopharynx. Am. J. Orthod., *65*:1–15.

Lucchesi, P. F., and LaBoccetta, A. C. 1944. Relationship of tonsils and adenoids to the type of poliomyelitis: An analysis of four hundred and thirty-two cases. Am. J. Dis. Child., *68*:1–4.

Luke, M. J., Mehrizi, A., Folger, G. M., Jr., et al. 1966. Chronic nasopharyngeal obstruction as a cause of cardiomegaly, cor pulmonale, and pulmonary edema. Pediatrics, *37*:762–768.

Mandel, E. M., Paradise, J. L., Bluestone, C. D., et al. 1980. Large tonsils without large adenoids as a cause of upper airway obstruction, alveolar hypoventilation, and cor pulmonale (abstract). Pediatr. Res., *14*:647.

Massachusetts Department of Public Health. 1971. Tonsillectomy and adenoidectomy in Massachusetts. N. Engl. J. Med., 285:1537.

Mawson, S. R., Adlington, P., and Evans, M. 1967. A controlled study evaluation of adeno-tonsillectomy in children. J. Laryngol. Otol., 81:777–790.

McCammon, R. W. 1971. Natural history of respiratory tract infection patterns in basically healthy individuals. Am. J. Dis. Child., 122:232–236.

Macartney, F. J., Panday, J., and Scott, O. 1969. Cor pulmonale as a result of chronic nasopharyngeal obstruction due to hypertrophied tonsils and adenoids. Arch. Dis. Child., 44:585–592.

McCorkle, L. P., Hodges, R. G., Badger, G. F., Dingle, J. H., and Jordans, W. S., Jr. 1955. A study of illness in a group of Cleveland families. VIII. Relation of tonsillectomy to incidence of common respiratory disease in children. N. Engl. J. Med., 252:1066–1069.

McKee, W. J. E. 1963a. A controlled study of the effects of tonsillectomy and adenoidectomy in children. Br. J. Prev. Soc. Med., 17:49–69.

McKee, W. J. E. 1963b. The part played by adenoidectomy in the combined operation of tonsillectomy with adenoidectomy: Second part of a controlled study in children. Br. J. Prev. Soc. Med., 17:133–140.

Menashe, V. D., Ferrehi, C., and Miller, M. 1965. Hypoventilation and cor pulmonale due to chronic upper airway obstruction. J. Pediatr., 67:198–203.

Meyer, M. 1870. On adenoid vegetations in the nasopharyngeal cavity: Their pathology, diagnosis, and treatment. Medico-chirugical Trans. (London), 53:191–215.

Modern Medicine. 1969. Poll on medical practice, 37:77–88, Feb. 10.

National Center for Health Statistics. 1974. Surgical Operations in Short-Stay Hospitals, United States, 1971. Rockville, MD, U.S. Dept. of Health, Education, and Welfare (DHEW Publication No. HRA 75–1769).

Nickerson, R. J., and Colton, T. 1975. Area studies: Surgery in the United States. In Zuidema, G. D. (Ed.) A Summary Report of the Study on Surgical Services for the United States. Baltimore, R. R. Donnelley & Sons, pp. 36–55.

Nickerson, R. J., Colton, T., Peterson, O. L., et al. 1976. Doctors who perform operations: A study on inhospital surgery in four diverse geographic areas. N. Engl. J. Med., 295:921–926, 982–989.

Nickerson, R. J., Hauck, W. W., Bloom, B. S., et al. 1978. Otolaryngologists and their surgical practice. Arch. Otolaryngol., 104:718–724.

Noonan, J. A. 1965. Reversible cor pulmonale due to hypertrophied tonsils and adenoids: Studies in two cases. Circulation, 32 (Suppl. 2):164.

Ogra, P. L. 1971. Effect of tonsillectomy and adenoidectomy on nasopharyngeal antibody response to poliovirus. N. Engl. J. Med., 284:59–64.

Paradise, J. L. 1972. Why T&A remains moot. Pediatrics, 49:648–651.

Paradise, J. L. 1975. Pittsburgh tonsillectomy and adenoidectomy study: Differences from earlier studies and problems of execution. Ann. Otol. Rhinol. Laryngol., 84 (Suppl. 19):15–19.

Paradise, J. L. 1976. Clinical trials of tonsillectomy and adenoidectomy: Limitations of existing studies and a current effort to evaluate efficacy. South. Med. J., 69:1049–1053.

Paradise, J. L., and Bluestone, C. D. 1976. Toward rational indications for tonsil and adenoid surgery. Hosp. Pract., 11(2):79–87.

Paradise, J. L., Bluestone, C. D., Bachman, Z., et al. 1978a. History of recurrent sore throat as an indication for tonsillectomy: Predictive limitations of histories that are undocumented. N. Engl. J. Med., 298:409–413.

Paradise, J. L., Bluestone, C. D., and Carrasco, M. M. 1978b. Nasal obstruction due to adenoid hypertrophy: Two-year course with and without adenoidectomy. Abstracts, 18th annual meeting of the Ambulatory Pediatric Association, New York City, April 25, p. 43.

Paton, J. H. P. 1943. Tonsil-adenoid operation in relation to health of group of school girls. Quart. J. Med., 12:119–128.

Pearson, R. J., Smedley, B., Berfenstam, R., et al. 1968. Hospital caseloads in Liverpool, New England, and Uppsala: An international comparison. Lancet, 2:559–566.

Perrott, G. S. 1970. The Federal Employees Health Benefits Program: Seventh term (1967) coverage and utilization. Selected data prepared for Group Health Association annual meeting, Washington, DC, March 21.

Roydhouse, N. 1970. A controlled study of adeno-tonsillectomy. Arch. Otolaryngol., 92:611–616.

Rynnel-Dagöö, B., Ahlbom, A., and Schiratzki, H. 1978. Effects of adenoidectomy: a controlled two-year follow-up. Ann. Otol. Rhinol. Laryngol., 87:272–278.

Shaikh, W., Vayda, E., and Feldman, W. 1976. A systematic review of the literature on evaluative studies of tonsillectomy and adenoidectomy. Pediatrics, 57:401–407.

Snow, J. C., Healy, G. B., Vaughan, C. W., et al. 1972. Malignant hyperthermia during anesthesia for adenoidectomy. Arch. Otolaryngol., 95:442–447.

Subtelny, J. D. 1954. The significance of adenoid tissue in orthodontia. Angle Orthod., 24:59–69.

Sullivan, M. A. 1974. Physician attitudes toward tonsillectomy and adenoidectomy: A critical analysis. Thesis, Johns Hopkins University School of Hygiene and Public Health, Baltimore.

Surjan, L., Surjan, L., Jr., and Surjan, M. 1972. Further investigation into the immunological role of the tonsils. Acta Otolaryngol., 73:222–226.

Townsend, J. G., and Sydenstricker, E. 1927. Epidemiological study of minor respiratory disease. Public Health Rep., 42:99–121.

Tucker, D., Coulter, J. E., and Downes, J. 1952. Incidence of acute respiratory illness among males and females at specific ages. Milbank Mem. Fund Q., 30:42–60.

Van De Moortel, V. A. 1970. T&A profile. The Record, 8:1–3.

Van Volkenburgh, V. A., and Frost, W. H. 1933. Acute minor respiratory diseases prevailing in a group of families residing in Baltimore, Maryland, 1928–1930: Prevalence, distribution, and clinical description of observed cases. Am. J. Hyg., 17:122–153.

Vianna, N. J., Greenwald, P., and Davies, J. N. P. 1971. Tonsillectomy and Hodgkin's disease: The lymphoid tissue barrier. Lancet, 1:431–432.

Chapter 49

OROPHARYNGEAL MANIFESTATIONS OF SYSTEMIC DISEASE

William Schwartz, M.D.

INTRODUCTION

The oropharynx is frequently involved in generalized diseases. Careful and systematic examination of the oropharynx will yield clues to the presence of systemic disorders. Because the oropharynx is easily examined and contains an abundant supply of blood vessels, nerves and exocrine glands, systemic disorders will be identifiable in the course of a complete physical examination. Oral lesions may be the presenting symptom or a sign of a more generalized disease or, conversely, oropharyngeal problems such as bleeding gingiva or difficulty swallowing may be independent problems and unrelated to a systemic disorder.

Dryness of the mouth may be an indicator of dehydration from loss of fluids, or it may be a sign of ingestion of an atropine-related drug. Masses in the oropharynx may represent localized abscesses or tumors, or may be manifestations of a systemic disease, such as neurofibromatosis, thus alerting the physician to organize a more complete evaluation of the other organ systems. Changes in color may also indicate serious conditions. Paleness of the mucosa occurs in various anemias and pigmentation of the gingiva is seen in prolonged exposure to lead. Certain congenital defects, such as cleft palate, may be isolated problems or part of a syndrome involving other organs, such as is seen in trisomy 13 or 18.

This chapter will describe pertinent organic diseases seen in pediatrics that have manifestations in the oropharynx (Table 49–1).

Some of the specific disorders are described also in Chapters 42, 43, 45, 47, 50, 51, and 52.

INFECTIONS

Candida albicans

Oral infections with *Candida albicans* may be a localized problem (thrush) or associated with a disease such as hypoparathyroidism,

Table 49–1 CLASSIFICATIONS OF OROPHARYNGEAL MANIFESTATIONS OF SYSTEMIC DISEASE

Infections
    Candida albicans
    DiGeorge syndrome
    Mucocutaneous candidiasis
    Common childhood infections
        Varicella (chickenpox)
        Rubella (measles)
        Infectious mononucleosis
Tumors
    Leukemia
    Neurofibromatosis or von Recklinghausen
      disease
Metabolic diseases
    Lesch-Nyhan syndrome
    Reticuloendotheliosis
Bleeding disorders
    Idiopathic thrombocytopenia
    Hemophilia
    Von Willebrand disease
Inflammatory diseases
    Lupus erythematosus
    Sjögren's syndrome

diabetes, adrenal insufficiency, hypothyroidism, leukemia, or immunodeficiency such as DiGeorge syndrome.

DiGeorge Syndrome

DiGeorge syndrome, or the third and fourth pharyngeal pouch syndrome, is an absence or hypoplasia of the thymus and parathyroid (Lischner, 1972). This syndrome is characterized clinically by neonatal tetany, relapsing hypocalcemia, oral and cutaneous moniliasis, increased susceptibility to infection, failure to thrive, malformation of the ear, micrognathia, blunted nose, neck anomalies, great vessel lesions such as a double aortic arch, and cardiac lesions such as endocardial cushion defects.

The etiology is unclear, but it is related to a defect in the third and fourth pharyngeal pouches from which the parathyroid and thymus normally evolve. The range of symptoms and laboratory findings is related to the amount of thymus and parathyroid tissue that is present. There is a potential DiGeorge syndrome in which a small amount of histologically normal thymus may be seen.

The laboratory findings in this disease are related to the amount of thymus tissue that is present. Usually the levels of immunoglobulins are normal, but the thymus-dependent functions are affected, leading to delayed skin reaction to antigens (*Candida*) and inability to reject a skin graft, depressed proliferative responsiveness of peripheral blood lymphocytes to phytohemagglutination, and depressed antibody response to specific immunization.

Children with this syndrome have difficulty with fungal and viral diseases and may succumb to live virus immunization. Fetal thymus transplantation may be helpful to therapy.

Mucocutaneous Candidiasis

This disease is characterized by persistent monilial infections of the oral mucosa and the nails, without systemic symptoms. In contrast to patients with DiGeorge syndrome, these patients have normal reactions to viral infections and vaccines. They may have a transient defect in response to the *Candida* antigen skin test. Many patients respond to mystatin or amphotericin therapy. There are reports of the use of transfer factor.

Common Childhood Infections

The widespread use of immunization and the improvement of living conditions have contributed to a decrease of some of the common infectious diseases in children. They are still present, however, and those infections that are seen in the oropharynx have systemic manifestations as well. Some infections, such as certain specific group A beta hemolytic streptococcal infections of the pharynx, will institute an immune complex disease that affects the collagen vascular system, with emphasis on the heart in rheumatic fever, or, on the kidney in acute poststreptococcal glomerulonephritis several weeks after the primary pharyngeal infection has abated. Several of the more common childhood infections such as varicella (chickenpox), rubeola (measles), and infectious mononucleosis are discussed in this section, to emphasize the systemic aspects of these infections.

Varicella.   Varicella is a highly contagious disease that is spread by droplets. It has an incubation period of 13 to 17 days. An infected individual is contagious from 24 hours before the rash to 6 to 7 days after the vesicular lesions appear. The lesions usually start on the trunk and spread to the head. The vesicles in the mouth rapidly become macerated and may form shallow ulcers. The larynx is rarely involved, but when it is, respiratory distress may develop. The most common complication of varicella is secondary bacterial infection, usually staphylococcal or beta streptococcal. Impetigo or osteomyelitis are also frequently seen. Varicella pneumonitis is a serious and, at times, fatal complication. It fortunately is rare in children, but it is seen in adults. Other complications include myocarditis, pericarditis, endocarditis, hepatitis, and glomerulonephritis. Ten per cent of Reye syndrome (encephalopathy with fatty degeneration of the liver) cases are associated with varicella. Other central nervous system involvement of varicella includes encephalitis, cerebellar ataxia, and ascending paralysis (Guillain-Barré syndrome).

In individuals at risk, such as those with malignancies and those on immunosuppressive drugs, Zooster immune globulin (ZIG) may be given within 72 hours of exposure to prevent development of varicella. Otherwise, treatment is symptomatic for relief of pruritus.

Measles (Rubeola).   Measles is characterized by a cough, coryza, conjunctivitis, a generalized maculopapular rash, and Koplik spots in the mouth. It is transmitted by air-borne spread of droplets. The incubation period is usually 10 to 12 days. Infected individuals are contagious from the fifth day of incubation to several days after the rash appears.

Typically the patient has a cough and fever similar to those of a common upper respiratory infection. Several days prior to the rash, the typical Koplik spots (red lesions with a bluish-white speck in the center) appear on the buccal mucosa. The cough becomes more brassy or harsh and will persist when the rash and conjunctivitis recede.

The major systemic reactions are in the respiratory tract and central nervous system. Otitis media, cervical lymphadenitis, laryngotracheobronchitis, and pneumonia may develop. The pneumonia is characterized by giant cell infiltration and may take several weeks to resolve.

Encephalitis develops in 0.1 per cent of measles cases. More than half of the cases of encephalitis result in permanent damage such as mental retardation, epilepsy, neuromuscular dysfunction, or deafness.

Infectious Mononucleosis. Infectious mononucleosis is characterized by fever, pharyngitis, cervical adenopathy, and splenomegaly (Fernbach and Starling, 1972). It is most likely caused by the Epstein-Barr (EB) virus. The incubation period is variable (average 50 days) and there are many EB virus infections in children without the complete clinical picture of infectious mononucleosis. The symptoms include a sore throat accompanied by a gray exudate and an edematous soft palate with petechiae. In one third of the cases, beta hemolytic streptococcus can be cultured from the throat.

Lymphadenopathy is a feature of the disease. The nodes in the cervical area may become so prominent that a "bull neck" appearance may result. Splenomegaly occurs in about 50 per cent of the cases and hepatitis in about 10 per cent of cases. Other systemic involvement includes pneumonia, aseptic meningitis, encephalitis, coma, and transverse myelitis.

The diagnosis is made by documenting lymphocytosis: 10 to 20 per cent atypical lymphocytes and a positive heterophil test. The heterophil antibody is also present in serum sickness as well as in infectious mononucleosis. The antibody is absorbed by beef red blood cells in infectious mononucleosis, but in serum sickness it is not. There are also commercial screening tests such as Monospot that are helpful in making the diagnosis.

The treatment is usually supportive, but in cases of severe adenitis and pharyngeal edema that compromise the airway and cause respiratory distress corticosteroids may be used.

TUMORS

Tumors limited to the oropharynx are rare and are discussed in Chapter 52. There are two generalized tumor conditions that deserve special mention — leukemia and neurofibromatosis.

Leukemia

Various forms of acute and chronic leukemia will cause bleeding of the gums and other soft tissues because of the decreased number of platelets or because of direct infiltration of leukemic cells. Additional physical findings of enlarged lymph nodes and splenomegaly are consistent with the diagnosis. A blood smear and bone marrow examination are necessary to make the diagnosis.

Neurofibromatosis (von Recklinghausen Disease)

This is an autosomal dominant disorder that consists of pigmentation of the skin plus neurofibromas of the cranial, spinal, and peripheral nerves (Fienman and Yakovac, 1970). Neurofibromas can cause large tongues or can present as postpharyngeal masses that press down on the soft palate and cause speech with a nasal escape sound. The auditory nerve is sometimes involved, and bilateral tumors of the acoustic nerve are seen in certain families. Other central nervous system tumors include meningiomagliomas, astrocytomas, and spinal cord ependymomas. For the uncomplicated neurofibroma, there is no special treatment. The tumor should be removed if it causes pressure symptoms.

METABOLIC DISEASES

Lesch-Nyhan Syndrome

This is a sex-linked recessive disorder of uric acid metabolism whose features are self-mutilation, choreoathetosis, spasticity, and mental retardation. Typically the lip is bitten off and the finger tips may be chewed off (Lesch and Nyhan, 1964). Other features include hyperuricemia, acute arthritis, hematuria, and renal calculi. The underlying defect is a deficiency of hypoxanthine-guanine phosphoribosyltransferase.

Treatment with allopurinol will interfere with uric acid production and decrease the incidence of gout, arthritis, or renal stones. It has no effect on the cerebral manifestations.

Reticuloendotheliosis

Reticuloendothelial cells are found in all tissues of the body. They have phagocytic functions that are involved in hematopoiesis; they form antibodies and have an important role in local and systemic reactions to infection. Reticuloendotheliosis includes a group of diseases in which there is a proliferation of cellular elements of the reticuloendothelial system, sometimes forming granulomatous lesions (Lahey, 1975). The clinical symptoms depend upon the involved organ system, so there may be only an isolated lesion of bone or soft tissue or there may be a total systemic malignant process. Formerly three separate syndromes were recognized — Hand-Schüller-Christian, Letterer-Siwe, and eosinophilic granuloma — but today they are considered a spectrum of the basic disease process of the reticuloendothelial cells and are labeled histiocytosis X.

In the acute disseminated form, many organs are involved, especially gingival mucosa, skin (eczematoid rash), spleen, liver, lungs, and lymph nodes. Bone marrow involvement will be manifested as hypoplastic anemia, thrombocytopenia, leukopenia, and bleeding tendencies. In the mouth there is gingival swelling, ulceration, bleeding, and infection. The teeth may be loose, and frequently unexplained loss of teeth will be an early complaint. This generalized involvement is usually found in young children and is associated with an early death.

A more chronic and milder form of this disease is seen in older children. The major organs involved are skin, bones, middle ear, spleen, liver, and lymph nodes. Dramatic symptoms include exophthalmos, loosening of teeth, and diabetes insipidus. Lytic lesions may be seen in all bones and lead to symptoms such as loose teeth, exophthalmic pituitary dysfunction, labyrinthine dysfunction,

or pseudotumor cerebri. The course is variable and is less favorable in young children.

Treatment by chemotherapy is most promising. Radiotherapy or surgical excision is effective in isolated lesions. Radiotherapy should be limited to cases in which surgical removal is not practicable.

BLEEDING DISORDERS

Bleeding gums or coagulation problems in the mouth may reflect (a) decreased platelets from generalized sepsis, lupus, leukemia, or idiopathic thrombocytopenia or (b) coagulation defects, such as hemophilia or plasma thromboplastin component (PTC) deficiency. As the mouth is subject to minor and major trauma, bleeding disorders are frequently first detected in the mouth.

Idiopathic Thrombocytopenia

Idiopathic thrombocytopenia (ITP) is a presumed immunologic disorder in which platelets are first sensitized and then destroyed by the spleen or liver (Shende and Lanzkowsky, 1974). Clinical symptoms include epistaxis, bleeding gums, sublingual hematoma, or postpharyngeal bleeding. The peripheral smear shows decreased or absent platelets. Prothrombin time and partial thromboplastin time are normal, and bone marrow examination shows an increased number of megakaryocytes. Most cases remit spontaneously and require no specific treatment, while 10 per cent may progress to chronic thrombocytopenia requiring corticosteroid therapy or at times splenectomy.

Hemophilia

Hemophilia is a sex-linked genetic disease that is a result of a deficiency of clotting factor VIII.

Bleeding may be spontaneous, cyclic, or the result of minor trauma to the mouth, joints, or soft tissue. Hemarthrosis is painful and may lead to destruction of the synovial membrane and joint contractions. The partial thromboplastin time (PTT) is prolonged while the bleeding and clotting times are normal. The diagnosis is confirmed with a specific factor VIII assay.

The treatment of hemophilia is by replacement of factor VIII with cryoprecipitate or fresh frozen plasma. For bleeding of oral mucosa, epsilon-aminocaproic acid, an inhibitor of the fibrinolytic system, is used with factor VIII concentrates (Abildgaard, 1975).

Von Willebrand Disease

Von Willebrand disease (pseudohemophilia) is an autosomal dominant disease that involves dysfunction of the platelets and lower levels of factor VIII. The clinical symptoms are epistaxis and mucous membrane and skin bleeding. Bleeding may also occur after dental procedures and mouth trauma. There is a reduction in plasma factor VII and a prolonged bleeding time and prolonged partial thromboplastin time (PTT). Platelet aggregation is abnormal. Treatment is mainly by localized pressure and rarely is supplementation of factor VIII necessary.

INFLAMMATORY DISEASES

The oropharynx is frequently involved in systemic inflammatory or collagen diseases. Frequently ulcerations secondary to vasculitis are the major problems, but there can be dryness if the salivary glands are involved and bleeding if the bone marrow is affected or platelet antibodies depress the platelet count.

Lupus Erythematosus

Oral lesions occur in about 25 per cent of patients. The lesions are found on the tongue, hard palate, and mucosa of the lips and cheeks. Systemic involvement includes photosensitivity and vasculitis, changes of the skin, and the classic butterfly rash over the malar area (although any area of skin can be involved). Alopecia is common. The other major symptom is arthritis. Vasculitic changes in the brain may produce seizures or personality changes, and cardiac symptoms include cardiomyopathy, tachycardia, pericardial effusion, and endocarditic vegetations. In children the type and severity of glomerulonephritis is a major determinant in the prognosis.

Diagnosis of lupus erythematosus is made by positive antinuclear antibody and DNA binding and positive LE preparations. The patients have anemia and decreased platelets and may have diseased complement and positive Coombs' test and serologic test for syphilis (STS).

The treatment depends on the severity of the problem. Rarely will salicylates control the symptoms in children, as they will in adults. More frequently, corticosteroids are required for children. If renal involvement is extensive, cyclophosphamide (Cytoxan) is added. The prognosis is variable and is dependent on the renal involvement and the susceptibility to infection.

Sjögren Syndrome

This syndrome involving the salivary glands and lacrimal glands presents with keratoconjunctivitis and dry mouth (xerostomia). In 50 per cent of the cases in children, rheumatoid arthritis is also present. There is also an associated decrease in secretions in the tracheobronchial tree, upper gastrointestinal tract, and pancreas.

The major symptoms include dry mouth and difficulty in chewing, swallowing, and speaking. Dental caries are common, and ulcers of the tongue, lips, and mucous membranes are present. In the eyes, there is photosensitivity, dryness, and keratoconjunctivitis.

The laboratory tests show nonspecific evidence of an inflammatory process. There is anemia, elevated sedimentation rate, positive antinuclear antibody (ANA), positive rheumatoid factor, and positive Coombs' test. Specific anti-salivary duct antibody can be demonstrated by immunofluorescent techniques.

Treatment is symptomatic. The eyes must be lubricated. Corticosteroids may be used to control the associated systemic involvement. The prognosis is related to the associated disease that occur with Sjögren syndrome, such as lupus, rheumatoid arthritis, and malignancy.

SELECTED REFERENCES

Krugman, S., and Ward, R. 1973. Infectious Diseases of Children and Adults, 5th ed. St. Louis, C. V. Mosby Co.
  This text outlines in detail the important infectious diseases that affect the head and neck as well as other organ systems. It has good illustrations, diagrams, and references.

Nathan, D. G., and Oski, F. A. 1974. Hematology of Infancy and Childhood. Philadelphia, W. B. Saunders Co.
  This text, well written and comprehensive, contains the pathophysiology and clinical aspects of children's blood problems.

Vaughan, V. C., III, McKay, R. J., and Behrman, R. E. (Eds.) 1979. Nelson Textbook of Pediatrics. 11th ed. Philadelphia, W. B. Saunders Co.

A complete pediatric textbook written by more than 100 contributors. This is an excellent general reference, with a listing of additional references.

REFERENCES

Abildgaard, C. F. 1975. Current concepts in the management of hemophilia. Semin. Hematol., *122*:223.

Fernbach, D. J., and Starling, K. A. 1972. Infectious mononucleosis. Pediatr. Clin. North Am., *19*:957.

Fienman, N. L., and Yakovac, W. C. 1970. Neurofibromatosis in childhood. J. Pediatr., *76*:339.

Lahey, M. E. 1975. Histiocytosis X—An analysis of prognostic factors. J. Pediatr., *87*:184.

Lesch, M. and Nyhan, W. L. 1964. A familial disorder of uric acid metabolisms and central nervous system findings. Am. J. Med., *36*:561.

Lischner, H. 1972. DiGeorge syndrome(s). J. Pediatr., *81*:1042–44.

Shende, A., and Lanzkowsky, P. 1974. Thrombocytopenia in childhood. Pediatr. Ann., *3*(54):71.

Chapter 50

IDIOPATHIC CONDITIONS OF THE MOUTH AND PHARYNX

George H. Conner, M.D.

Idiopathic conditions include a group of disorders that vary from those which are frequently seen to those which are very rare. For a classification of idiopathic oral and pharyngeal disease, see Table 50–1.

ULCERATIVE DISEASES

Ulcerative diseases of the mouth are common, being second only in frequency to gingivitis (Zagarelli, 1969). The patients characteristically describe an abrupt onset of

Table 50–1 IDIOPATHIC CONDITIONS OF THE MOUTH AND PHARYNX

I. Ulcerative diseases
  1. Acute necrotizing ulcerative gingivitis
  2. Recurrent ulcerative stomatitis
  3. Recurrent scarifying ulcerative stomatitis (Sutton disease)
  4. Behçet syndrome
  5. Angular stomatitis
  6. Noma
  7. Geographic tongue
  8. Cheilitis granulomatosa

II. Vesiculobullous diseases
  1. Erythema multiforme
  2. Epidermolysis bullosa

III. Keratotic diseases
  1. Lichen planus
  2. Hereditary keratosis
    a. Familial white folded dysplasia
    b. Keratosis follicularis (Darier disease)
  3. Chronic discoid lupus erythematosus

ulcerations with pain, which last from one to three weeks. Most oral ulcers may be diagnosed by their clinical appearance; however, in some instances a biopsy may be necessary.

Systemic diseases with oral manifestations, especially blood dyscrasias or nutritional deficiency states, should always be considered.

Acute Necrotizing Ulcerative Gingivitis (Vincent Infection, Vincent Stomatitis, Trench Mouth)

Natural History. Most cases of acute necrotizing ulcerative gingivitis are seen in teenagers or young adults, as the condition is less common in older persons. When it is found in younger children, a thorough investigation for debilitating systemic disease, particularly for blood dyscrasias, should be carried out. Systemic signs and symptoms such as fever, pallor, and fatigue may be prominent (Zagarelli, 1969).

Etiology. The exact etiology of this type of gingivitis is unknown, although poor oral hygiene, food impactions, malocclusion, and local dental diseases may contribute to this condition. Since many patients with acute necrotizing ulcerative gingivitis are high school or college students, unusual physical or emotional stress may play a role (Zagarelli, 1969). Similarly, dietary imbalances and fatigue may also be of significance. Underlying systemic disease such as nutritional deficiency states and blood dyscrasias seen with this

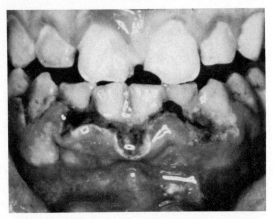

Figure 50-1 Acute necrotizing ulcerative gingivitis. Ulcerations at the base of the teeth are covered with a dirty, gray, necrotic membrane. There is associated local pain and bleeding with a foul mouth odor. (Bailliere's Medical Transparencies, London.)

condition may only represent lowered local tissue resistance to bacterial invasion.

There are no specific confirmatory laboratory tests. The presence of Vincent microorganisms is not definite proof of the existence of acute recurrent ulcerative stomatitis, since 80 per cent of healthy individuals have these organisms within their mouths. It is probably not possible to transmit this disease to a healthy mouth (Zagarelli, 1969).

Clinical Picture. Most patients present with a complaint of painful, bleeding gums, a bad taste in the mouth, or a foul mouth odor. Examination reveals the presence of gingivitis of variable severity. Ulcerations at the base of the teeth are covered by dirty, gray necrotic membranes that adhere loosely. Removal of this necrotic slough reveals a painful ulceration at the base of the tooth. Occasionally the buccal mucosa or other tissues of the mouth will become involved (Fig. 50-1).

Management. The treatment of acute necrotizing ulcerative gingivitis consists of (1) searching for and eliminating any local or systemic contributing disorder and (2) gentle mechanical cleansing of involved areas and improvement of oral hygiene. Water irrigating devices are useful.

Prognosis. Provided that there is no underlying systemic condition, local measures should result in gradual improvement. In rare instances, infection of a severe degree has been known to invade the underlying bone, leading to marked tissue destruction and necrosis that is sometimes severe enough to expose bone (Zagarelli, 1969). In the vast majority of cases, however, the prognosis is good.

Recurrent Ulcerative Stomatitis

Natural History. Recurrent ulcerative stomatitis is a frustrating disease characterized by painful oral ulcerations that tend to recur.

Etiology. Recurrent ulcerative stomatitis may be caused by a variety of etiologic factors, but no single specific cause can be found in the majority of cases. Hormonal disorders may play a role since the onset of ulcerations in females may occur simultaneously with menses or only during pregnancy (McCarthy, 1964). Nutritional disturbances are probably not of significance in that most patients with recurrent ulcerative stomatitis do not seem to have other signs of systemic nutritional deficiency states and rarely benefit from vitamin or nutritional regimens. Iron, folic acids, and Vitamin B_{12} deficiencies, however, have been described (Wray, 1975) so that a complete hematological screening should be carried out. Allergies have similarly been implicated since cures have been claimed by avoidance of such allergenic foods as fruits, chocolates, nuts, and shellfish. Local trauma (Lund, 1976), gastrointestinal upsets, emotional disturbances, and the like all have been implicated but never proven to be specific etiological agents (Zagarelli, 1969).

Clinical Picture. In most cases the general health of the individual is good. There are no accompanying signs of fever, malaise, or skin eruptions. The ulcerative episodes usually last from one to three weeks and are often followed by a remission of two weeks to two months or longer. Occasionally remissions may be virtually absent, with one crop of ulcerations being superimposed on those not yet fully healed from a previous episode. The overall duration of the disease is quite variable, lasting from weeks to intermittent occurrences of many months.

Prodromal signs and symptoms may include itching, burning, and a tingling sensation 24 to 48 hours prior to the onset of the development of mucosal ulcers. Occasionally the prodromal stage may consist of one or more reddish spots or macules or elevated papules or vesicles where the ulcerations eventually develop (Zagarelli, 1969).

The ulcers may vary in size from 1 to 10 mm in diameter, may be round or oval in shape, and usually have a yellow membrane surrounded by a narrow zone of inflammation. The buccal mucosa, lips, and tongue are most commonly involved, with associated local pain and tenderness.

Management. Therapy remains symptomatic with no regimen being successful in preventing recurrences. Local applications of silver nitrate, trichloroacetic acid, topical protectorants, and topical steroids offer variable degrees of palliation. Coexisting deficiency states should be corrected (Wray, 1975).

Prognosis. The overall prognosis of this disorder is good. There seems to be no relationship between this problem and the development of other, more serious disorders such as erythema multiforme, pemphigus, or mouth cancer. However, such lesions may represent the initial stages of Behçet disease.

Recurrent Scarifying Ulcerative Stomatitis (Sutton Disease)

Natural History. Recurrent scarifying ulcerative stomatitis is characterized by a pattern of intermittent oral ulcerations lasting two to four weeks. In contrast to recurrent ulcerative stomatitis, the ulcers are larger and more penetrating and have a much greater tendency to scarify upon healing (Lund, 1976). Remissions may occur which last for weeks or months, although occasional patients suffer ulcerations continuously (Zagarelli, 1969).

Etiology. There is no known cause for recurrent scarifying ulcerative stomatitis. The usual variety of factors have been implicated: allergy, viral infections, malnutrition, deficiency states, emotional disturbances, and the like. It may be that recurrent scarifying ulcerative stomatitis is only a more severe form of recurrent ulcerative stomatitis.

Clinical Picture. The ulcers of recurrent scarifying ulcerative stomatitis are usually multiple and distributed throughout the buccal mucosa and tongue. The ulcers are large, with considerable necrosis covering all or part of the ulcer, which has an elevated rim and which may have a malignant appearance. Scarring is of prime diagnostic importance and is often severe enough to cause distortion of the surrounding mucosa, leading to an impairment of mouth function. The scars are firm and are usually grayish or pale pink in color.

Pain and local discomfort are the main symptoms and may require analgesics or narcotics for control. Tender submaxillary adenopathy is commonly present.

Management. Presently there is no effective specific therapy for this condition. Biop-sies should be taken to rule out the possibility of malignancies. Topical steroids and analgesics are about all that can be offered for palliation.

Prognosis. The overall prognosis is good, although occasionally the scarring can be sufficient to distort surrounding tissues and interfere with oral or chewing functions (Zagarelli, 1969).

Behçet Disease

Natural History. Behçet disease is a rare condition characterized by a triad of symptoms involving ocular inflammation with oral mucosal and external genitalia aphthous ulceration. It is seen in young adults of either sex. Ulcerations involving the oral and genital areas are discrete and resemble the lesions of aphthous stomatitis. Such lesions may be recurrent for many years. Neurologic involvement may occur in as high as 25 per cent of cases (Wolf, 1965). Eye manifestations such as uveitis, iridocyclitis, and hypopyon, which eventually lead to blindness, may also occur (O'Duffy, 1976). Other systems with involvement include esophageal ulceration with chest pain (Kaplinsky, 1977; Lockhart, 1976), recurrent pneumonia with hemoptysis (Petty, 1977), as well as colitis, vasculitis, thrombophlebitis, large artery aneurysms, and encephalitis (O'Duffy, 1977).

Etiology. The etiology of Behçet disease is unknown, although the possibility of a specific virus or an immune response to an unknown substance has long been debated (O'Duffy, 1976).

Clinical Picture. The usual presenting complaint is that of a painful ulcer in the mouth. Such ulcers may resemble aphthous ulcerations or the lesions of recurrent ulcerative stomatitis. The ulcers may be multiple, small, and shallow and covered with a yellow serofibrous exudate. Larger ulcers may be somewhat depressed in the center with elevated rims. The mouth lesions per se are not specific and are not diagnostic (Zagarelli, 1969). In most cases mouth lesions will be accompanied by genital and/or eye lesions, and it is on the basis of these multiple-site lesions that the diagnosis is made. The genital lesions are similar in appearance to those of the mouth and affect the vulvar folds or vaginal canal in females and the scrotal sac or penis in males. The eye lesions may consist of purulent conjunctivitis and uveitis, iridocyclitis, or hypopyon. When the eye is involved, progression to blindness is almost the rule (Mamo, 1976).

Occasionally the skin will be involved with a cutaneous vasculitis. The joints may exhibit synovitis and the central nervous system involvement may be manifested by paresis, cerebellar ataxia, pseudobulbar palsy, or ocular palsies (O'Duffy, 1976).

Management. Remissions may occur with vigorous therapy, including systemic corticosteroids, azathioprine, and chlorambucil (Mamo, 1976) and, more recently, transfer factor (Wolf, 1977). Exacerbations may occur when steroid dosages are reduced (O'Duffy, 1976). Chlorambucil should be given for at least six months after complete remission has occurred (Mamo, 1976).

Prognosis. Behçet disease usually is a recurrent disease that lasts for years. The more benign forms may respond to early systemic steroids. Long-term combination therapy may be curative. Deaths have been reported when neurological involvement has occurred. The most significant complication is that of extensive scarring about the eye, with resultant diminished vision or blindness. This occurs on the average of 3.36 years after the onset of eye symptoms (Mamo, 1976).

Angular Stomatitis

Natural History. Angular stomatitis is the occurrence of an inflammatory lesion at the corner of the mouth. The usual lesion begins at the mucocutaneous junction and extends onto the skin (Fig. 50–2).

Etiology. Angular stomatitis is an easily recognized condition and in most cases has an underlying cause such as a riboflavin deficiency. It is referred to as "cheilosis" in such instances (McCarthy, 1964). However, occasionally no apparent etiology can be found.

"Pseudocheilosis" is a term used to describe a situation in which a decrease in the intermaxillary distance results in an accentuation of the transverse folds of the skin at the angle of the mouth with pooling of the saliva in the corners leading to drying and crusting that cause local inflammation. This is usually a result of loss of dentition and is therefore more common in the elderly (Zagarelli, 1969).

The lesions at the angle of the mouth may be complicated by secondary invasion of microorganisms of the oral flora, particularly streptococci, staphylococci, and monilia.

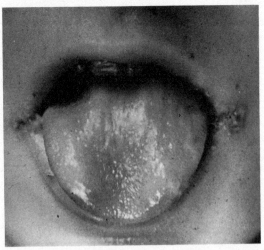

Figure 50–2 Angular stomatitis in a child with nutritional deficiency. Such areas can become secondarily invaded by normal oral flora or *Candida albicans*. (From Dreizen, S. The Mouth in Medicine. Multi Media Postgraduate Medicine, 1971.)

When *Candida albicans* is predominant, the condition is referred to as "perlèche" (McCarthy, 1964).

Angular stomatitis may also be due to an allergic or toxic reaction to such substances as cosmetics, lipsticks, or ointments.

Management. Every attempt should be made to determine the underlying cause of the inflammation. Nutritional deficiency states, mechanical problems, and allergic disorders should all be investigated. In cases in which there is a secondary invasion by local microorganisms, the topical application of antibiotic or antifungal ointments is often successful. In the occasional case in which there is no clear-cut etiology for the angular stomatitis, symptomatic improvement may be observed with topical corticosteroid medications (Zagarelli, 1969).

Prognosis. The prognosis is good, provided that there is no serious underlying disorder.

Noma (Gangrenous Stomatitis, Cancrum Oris)

Natural History. Noma is a gangrenous disease that involves the lips, cheek, face, maxilla, or mandible and occurs most commonly in children. Although rare in the western world, it is still a major health problem in many developing countries (Tempest, 1966).

Noma may be initiated by necrotic foci developing in areas of preexistent inflammation such as partially erupted teeth. The acute lesion develops into an indolent ulcer that rapidly increases in depth and size. Acute inflammation occurs in the overlying skin, followed by necrosis and sloughing. The gangrenous area may rapidly expand, with indistinct margins between the necrotic tissue and the surrounding inflammation. Perforation of the lips or cheeks occurs early and is often accompanied by a foul odor. There is a significant mortality rate if treatment is delayed or unsuccessful. In fetal cases there is a downhill course with development of aspiration pneumonia, septicemia, and death (Zagarelli, 1969).

Etiology. The specific etiology of noma is unknown, although it is seen in debilitative states, malnutrition, or following an acute infectious process or exanthem. Most cases are reported in areas of the world where malnutrition and avitaminosis are prevalent. Often measles will precede the onset of the disease (Tempest, 1964). No specific organisms are ordinarily found in the necrotic material.

Clinical Picture. The picture is usually that of a toxic child with an acute inflammation that often involves the buccal mucosa adjacent to a sharp, carious, or partially impacted tooth. An ulceration appears with pain, edema, and acute inflammation involving the overlying skin. This is followed by rapid necrosis with formation of a grayish or black purulent slough that expands rapidly. Perforation of the lips or cheeks is the forerunner of a steadily worsening course of pneumonia and septicemia, leading to death.

Management. Vigorous treatment with antibiotics and supportive measures, with extensive local debridement, may be successful. Severe disfigurement often with ankylosis of the jaw, requiring surgical correction at a later date, is typical in survivors (Oluwasanmi, 1976).

Geographic Tongue

Natural History. Geographic tongue is a common condition that is seen in all age groups. This condition may occur suddenly and last for many weeks or even years. Often there is an associated fissuring of the tongue.

Etiology. There is no known etiology for this condition.

Clinical Picture. The involved areas of the tongue are smooth and red and the

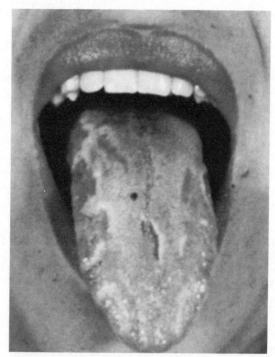

Figure 50–3 Geographic tongue. Patchy areas of loss of filiform papillae result in the appearance of smooth, red areas surrounded by zones of elevated, white exudate. Often there is an associated fissuring.

fungiform papillae are easily observable. This is due to a loss of filiform papillae in well-defined areas, which are surrounded by an elevated zone of white exudate. The symptoms are usually mild and accompanied by varying degrees of discomfort (Fig. 50–3).

Management. Therapy for geographic tongue is directed toward providing local comfort. Topical anesthetic agents and the avoidance of hot or spicy foods may be helpful. The prognosis is good (Zagarelli, 1969).

Cheilitis Granulomatosa

Natural History. Cheilitis granulomatosa begins as a diffuse swelling of the lips, more commonly involving the lower lip. It is a rare condition, which results in chronic and persistent enlargement of the lips.

Clinical Picture. The lower lip is usually involved. The swelling is firm and elastic to touch. Scaling and fissuring may be present. Microscopically, there is chronic, nonspecific inflammation with local granuloma formation. When the condition is associated with facial paralysis and a congenitally fissured tongue, it is known as Melkersson-Rosenthal syndrome (McCarthy, 1964).

Management. Since there is no known etiology, there is no reliable or specific therapy. However, the prognosis for resolution of the problem is good.

VESICULOBULLOUS DISORDERS

Erythema Multiforme

Natural History. Erythema multiforme is an acute inflammatory disease that may be accompanied by a variety of skin lesions, which are often self-limiting. Oral lesions are often present, involving the lips with bullae, which then form ulcers and are covered by hemorrhagic exudate (Haskell, 1976). The skin lesions begin as macules and papules that eventually become vesicles and bullae and break down to become erosions and ulcerations. An iris-like "target lesion" on the skin is diagnostic. The condition comes on acutely and may recur frequently. In the mild form it may heal spontaneously in about two weeks. There may be seasonal variations, with the disorder occurring more often in the winter and the early spring.

Etiology. The etiology of erythema multiforme is not known, although it frequently occurs following inflammatory disorders, especially herpes simplex, and after vaccinations. It may also be precipitated by a variety of agents such as penicillin, barbiturates, sulfonamides, and others (Safai, 1977; Baer, 1976). *Mycoplasma pneumoniae* has been cultured from the throat and bullae of some patients but it is not known what role, if any, it may play in the disease.

Clinical Picture. Erythema multiforme usually has an abrupt onset accompanied by fatigue, malaise, and fever. The latter, however, may be absent when the eruptions are restricted to the mouth (Fig. 50–4).

The oral mucosal lesions of erythema multiforme may be large and irregular with a raw base. Necrotic sloughs may occur that are firmly adherent. The lips are covered by a hemorrhagic exudate (Haskell, 1976). Iris-like "target lesions" may occur on the skin, especially on the palms of the hands and are diagnostic of the condition. In severe cases, when associated with purulent conjunctivitis, fever, leukopenia, macular erythematous necrotic skin lesions, and bullous stomatitis, the name Stevens-Johnson syndrome is given to this disorder.

Management. Treatment of erythema

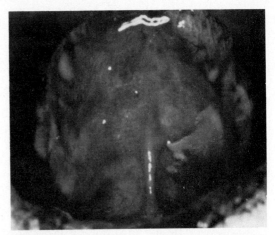

Figure 50–4 Erythema multiforme involving the tongue. Superficial necrotic sloughs may be multiple within the mouth. The lesions may be large and irregular with a raw base. (Bailliere's Medical Transparencies, London.)

multiforme is palliative in mild cases, with antihistamines (Bhargava, 1977) and local moist compresses for erosive lesions. Hydrogen peroxide (3 per cent) mouthwash and topical anesthetic agents are helpful for the oral lesions. Tetracycline or erythromycin may be used for suspected *M pneumoniae* infections (Haskell, 1976). Systemic corticosteroids are indicated when involvement is more severe.

In cases of Stevens-Johnson syndrome, treatment should include immediate hospitalization, intravenous fluids, and systemic corticosteroids in high doses given initially and tapered off over a two to three week period. Additionally, local care as outlined above for skin lesions should be instituted. This form of the disorder runs a one to four week course, usually with the recovery of the individual although fatalities may occur, particularly with severe pulmonary involvement (Zagarelli, 1969).

Complications. Blindness as a result of severe purulent conjunctivitis has been reported.

Epidermolysis Bullosa

Natural History. Epidermolysis bullosa is a rare connective tissue disorder in which there is a lack of adherence of the epidermis to the dermis, which results in a separation leading to bullous formations.

Oral lesions occur as a result of minor

trauma or even normal oral activity such as sucking. Any trauma to the skin will cause vesicles and bullae to develop.

Etiology. In most cases there is a family history of the disorder.

Clinical Picture. Epidermolysis bullosa is divided into two types: epidermolysis simplex and epidermolysis dystrophica.

Epidermolysis simplex is the milder form of the disorder, appearing at birth or shortly thereafter. Small bullae containing serous fluid appear on areas of trauma, especially over joints and on the hands and feet. These areas will heal without scarring unless secondary infection becomes a problem. Oral lesions frequently occur. The first evidence may be on the lips of an infant as a result of forceful or prolonged sucking. Later, any traumatic experience will result in lifting of the epidermis and subsequent erosion.

Epidermolysis bullosa dystrophica is the serious form of the disease; it appears in infancy and rapidly leads to death. Bullae appear following minor trauma. The area may then become hemorrhagic. Large sheets of epidermis may come loose, denuding much of the surface of the body and allowing for rapid fluid and protein loss and secondary infection. The oral lesions in such cases may be so severe as to prevent feeding, thus contributing to the rapid demise of the infant.

Management. Treatment is directed at protecting the individual from any form of traumatic experience. This is likely to be successful only in the milder or epidermolysis simplex cases. Administration of corticosteroids may bring improvement (McCarthy, 1964).

KERATOTIC DISEASES

Lichen Planus

Natural History. Lichen planus is a fairly common dermatologic disorder involving the mucous membranes and the skin. It occurs in older children and young adults as well as in older populations. It is seen with equal frequency in males and females. The lesions are usually discovered accidentally when the patient sees or feels them or when they are noted by a dentist or physician.

Etiology. The etiology of lichen planus is unknown although trauma, emotional disturbances, toxic reactions, and infections have been implicated. A relationship to lupus

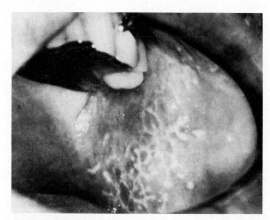

Figure 50–5 Lichen planus involving the buccal mucosa with a reticular pattern. Other lesions may consist of glistening white papules or plaques. (Bailliere's Medical Transparencies, London.)

erythematosus has been suggested (Davies, 1977; Romero, 1977).

Clinical Picture. The mouth is the most frequently affected site, with the buccal mucosa and tongue being most commonly involved. The lesions may vary in size from a papule a few millimeters in diameter to involvement of the entire buccal mucosa. Often the lesions will appear in a reticular pattern although papules, plaques, and ulcerative forms may occur (McCarthy, 1964). The reticular pattern is the most easily recognized and occurs most often on the buccal mucosa (Fig. 50–5). It is composed of narrow, slightly elevated graywhite lines that join each other at angles to form a network-like pattern. The papular pattern consists of pinhead-sized, slightly raised, glistening white spots that occur in groups or diffusely over the oral mucosa. Frequently it takes the form of a solid, raised, white plaque. Magnified examination of such plaques reveal them to be composed of large numbers of tiny papules.

The symptoms of lichen planus are variable. The patient may be symptom-free; however, if ulcerations are present, local discomfort and burning sensations will occur. The history is usually one of remission and exacerbation for years (Zagarelli, 1969).

The diagnosis is confirmed by a biopsy specimen that shows keratosis and parakeratosis with a moth-eaten pattern of destruction of the basal cells. A broad band of inflammatory cells, usually lymphocytes, is located directly beneath the basal epithelium.

Management. There is no known effective treatment. Reassurance that the condition is benign and not precancerous is important. When the condition is ulcerative, systemic corticosteroids are occasionally effective. Intralesional injection of steroids may also promote healing (Ferguson, 1977).

Prognosis. The prognosis is good although symptoms may persist indefinitely.

Hereditary Keratoses

By definition hereditary disorders cannot be considered idiopathic and are technically out of place in this chapter. However, for the purpose of differential diagnosis, two keratotic disorders of the mouth will be covered briefly: (1) familial, white folded dysplasia (white sponge nevus) and (2) keratosis follicularis (Darier disease).

White Folded Dysplasia

Natural History. This is probably a hereditary condition, which can be noted at birth. Lesions of gray-white spongy areas with fissures and folds may be noted on the tongue or buccal mucosa. Progressive involvement continues until adolescence when the extent of the disorder tends to stabilize. Lesions of a similar nature may also be found on the vaginal, rectal, or nasal mucosae.

Clinical Picture. The lesions are white, soft, and spongy in appearance and resemble diffuse leukoplakia. The entire oral mucosa tends to be involved, with the most obvious lesions in the buccal mucosa, floor of the mouth, and the ventral surface of the tongue. The lesions are entirely asymptomatic.

Diagnosis is dependent on the clinical appearance and the presence of a similar condition in a sibling, parent, or grandparent. The histologic findings are those of thickening of the epithelium with acanthosis with an intact basal cell layer. Intracellular edema and vacuolization of the prickle cell layer is present. There is little or no cornification.

Management. There is no specific therapy and since these patients are virtually symptom-free, generally no therapy is needed. Reassurance that this is not a malignant condition and that it will usually arrest itself during adolescence is given. There usually are no complications or sequelae (McCarthy, 1964).

Keratosis Follicularis (Darier Disease)

Natural History. This is a rare hereditary condition that involves the epidermis of the skin and mucous membranes. The disease is generally slowly progressive with periods of remission and exacerbation. The mucous membranes tend to be less frequently involved than the skin.

Clinical Picture. The skin lesions may appear as small, firm, red papules which may ulcerate, coalesce, and form crusts. The skin lesions are most commonly found on the face, neck, shoulders, and axillae. Secondary infections are common, especially during warm, humid weather. Remissions may occur, usually during the winter months. The oral lesions are firm nodules or papules, usually on the palate, although the tongue and buccal mucosa may be involved. The mouth lesions are usually asymptomatic.

Etiology. Nothing is known concerning the cause of Darier keratosis follicularis except for its familial tendency.

Management. There is no known effective treatment; however, some improvement with Vitamin A therapy has been reported (McCarthy, 1964).

Chronic Discoid Lupus Erythematosus

Natural History. This is a collagen disorder that involves the skin and the mucous membranes. It is rare in childhood. It is included in this section because the oral manifestations demonstrate areas of patchy hyperkeratosis.

The natural course of the disease is one of pronounced chronicity with periods of remission and exacerbation. There is a tendency for gradual remission, and eventually many cases seem to burn out over a period of years.

With chronic discoid lupus erythematosus there are very few associated signs or symptoms, and generally this does not progress to the acute or disseminated forms of the disease. Occasionally it will be seen with lichen planus (Davies, 1977).

Etiology. The cause of chronic discoid lupus erythematosis is unknown, although it is felt that it is in some way related to the autoimmune disorders.

Clinical Picture. Chronic discoid lupus erythematosus is a mucocutaneous disorder that affects either sex with a slight predilection for females. It is rare in childhood, being seen usually between the ages of 20 and 40. About 25 per cent of the patients will show lesions on the oral mucosa, with the buccal mucosa being the most common site. Photosensitivity may exist (Prystowsky, 1977).

The characteristic oral lesion is usually a well-defined area of irregular configuration with loss of epithelium mixed with patches of hyperkeratosis and exudates. A unique radial arrangement of capillaries at the periphery of the lesion extending into the surrounding tissues is present. Scarring will occur with older lesions along with irregular white patches.

Patients with oral lesions almost invariably have skin manifestations. Usually this takes the form of the characteristic butterfly configuration over the nose and cheeks.

Histologically, the oral lesions will demonstrate hyperkeratosis, parakeratosis, and degeneration of the stratum germinativum with hyaline-like degeneration of the connective tissue collagens and lymphocytic infiltration in clumps, usually in a perivascular pattern. The periodic acid–Schiff staining procedure for mucopolysaccharides reveals an intense reaction in the areas of collagen degeneration (McCarthy, 1964). Immunofluorescence techniques may be helpful in establishing a diagnosis (Davies, 1977).

Management. The treatment of chronic discoid lupus erythematosus consists of the use of antimalarial drugs, such as chloroquine, antipyrine, and primaquine, as well as topical and systemic steroids. The overall prognosis for this ailment is good.

SELECTED REFERENCES

Lund, W. S. 1976. Treatment of superficial lesions of the mouth and pharynx. J. Laryngol. Otol., 90(1): 101–104.

A brief, concise article that clearly describes virtually all the lesions that commonly occur in the mouth. Up-to-date treatment is also discussed.

O'Duffy, J. D., and Goldstein, N. P. 1976. Neurologic involvement in seven patients with Behçet's disease. Am. J. Med., 61:(2), 170–178.

This is an extremely readable and complete article on this subject. It is probably the most complete article on neurologic disorders of Behçet's disease, but, additionally, it has excellent covering of all manifestations and current treatments.

Tempest, M. N. 1966. Cancrum oris. Br. J. Surg., 53:949–969.

This is an excellent and very complete article about all the ravages of this severe disorder. It contains numerous illustrations and recommendations for immediate and rehabilitative therapy.

Two books are worthy of mention and deserve to be in the library of any physician interested in diseases of the mouth:

McCarthy, P. L., and Gerald, S. 1964. Diseases of the Oral Mucosa. New York, McGraw-Hill Book Co.

Zagarelli, E. V., Kutscher, A. H., and Hyman, G. A. 1969. Diseases of the Mouth and Jaws, Philadelphia, Lea & Febiger.

Together these two texts provide a complete reference source for virtually all diseases of the mouth.

REFERENCES

Ackerman, A. B., Penneys, N. S., and Clark, W. H. 1971. Erythema multiforme exudativum: Distinctive pathological process. Br. J. Dermatol., 84:554–566.

Baer, R. L. 1976. Perspective: Erythema multiforme — 1976. Am. J. Med. Sci., 271(1):119–120.

Bhargava, R. K., Singh, V., and Soni, V. 1977. Erythema multiforme resulting from insecticide spray. Arch. Dermatol., 113(5):686–687.

Bjornberg, A., and Hellgren, L. 1976. Treatment of chronic discoid lupus erythematosus with betamethasone-17,21-dipropionate. Curr. Ther. Res., 19(4):442–443.

Colvard, D. M., Robertson, D. M., and O'Duffy, J. D. 1977. The ocular manifestations of Behçet's disease. Arch. Ophthalmol., 95(10):1813–1817.

Davies, M. G., Gorkiewicz, A., Knight, A., et al. 1977. Is there a relationship between lupus erythematosus and lichen planus? Br. J. Dermatol. 96(2):145–154.

Ferguson, M. M. 1977. Treatment of erosive lichen planus of the oral mucosa with depot steroids. Lancet, 2(8041):771–772.

Haim, S. 1975. Behçet's disease: Etiology and treatment. Dermatologica, 150:163–168.

Haskell, R. 1976. Oral vesiculo-bullous lesions. J. Laryngol. Otol., 90(1):101–104.

Kaplinsky, N., Neumann, G., Harzahav, Y., et al. 1977. Esophageal ulceration in Behçet's syndrome. Gastrointest. Endosc., 23(3):160.

Limongelli, W. A., Clark, M. S., and Williams, A. C. 1976. Nomalike lesion in a patient with chronic lymphocytic leukemia. Oral Surg., 41(1):40–51.

Lockhart, J. M., McIntyre, W., and Caperton, E. M. Jr., 1976. Esophageal ulceration in Behçet's syndrome. Ann. Intern. Med., 84(5):572–573.

Lund, W. S. 1976. Treatment of superficial lesions of the mouth and pharynx. J. Laryngol. Otol., 90(1):105–112.

Mamo, J. G. 1976. Treatment of Behçet's disease with chlorambucil. Arch. Ophthalmol., 94(4):580–583.

Martin, S. 1977. Clarification of lichen planus actinicus. Arch. Dermatol., 113(11):1615.

McCarthy, P. L., and Gerald, S. 1964. Diseases of the Oral Mucosa. New York, McGraw-Hill Book Co.

O'Duffy, J. D., and Goldstein, N. P. 1976. Neurologic involvement in seven patients with Behçet's disease. Am. J. Med., 61(2):170–178.

Oluwasanmi, J. O., Lagundoye, S. B., and Akinyemi, O. O, 1976. Ankylosis of the mandible from cancrum oris. Plast. Reconstr. Surg., 57(3):342–350.

Prystowsky, S. D., and Gilliam, J. N. 1977. Antinuclear antibody studies in chronic cutaneous discoid lupus erythematosus. Arch. Dermatol., 113(2):183–186.

Prystowsky, S. D., Herndon, J. H. Jr., and Gilliam, J. N. 1976. Chronic cutaneous lupus erythematosus (DLE) — a clinical and laboratory investigation of 80 patients. Medicine, 55(2):183–191.

Rekant, S. I. 1976. Lichen planus and bullous pemphigoid. Arch. Dermatol., 112(11):1613.

Rogers, R. S., III, Movius, D. L., and Pierre, R. V. 1976.

Lymphocyte–epithelial cell interactions in oral mucosal inflammatory diseases. J. Invest. Dermatol., *67*(5):599–602.

Romero, R. W., Nesbitt, L. T., Jr., and Reed, R. J. 1977. Unusual variant of lupus erythematosus or lichen planus. Arch. Dermatol., *113*(6):741–748.

Safai, B., Good, R. A., and Day, N. K. 1977. Erythema multiforme: Report of two cases and speculation on immune mechanisms involved in the pathogenesis. Clin. Immunol. Immunopathol., *7*(3):379–385.

Tempest, M. N. 1966. Cancrum oris. Br. J. Surg., *53*:949–969.

Walker, D. M., and Dolby, A. E., 1976. Recurrent aphthous ulceration. Int. J. Dermatol., *15*(8):589–591.

Williams, B. D., and Lehner, T. 1977. Immune complexes in Behçet's syndrome and recurrent oral ulceration. Br. Med. J., *1*(6073):1387–1389.

Wolf, R. E., Fudenberg, H. H., Welch, T. M., et al. 1977. Treatment of Behçet's syndrome with transfer factor. J.A.M.A., *238*(8):869–871.

Wolf, S. M., Schotland, D. L. and Phillips, L. L. 1965. Involvement of nervous system in Behçet's syndrome. Arch. Neurol., *12*:315.

Wray, D., Ferguson, M. M., Mason, D. K., et al. 1975. Recurrent aphthae: Treatment with vitamin B_{12}, folic acid, and iron. Br. Med. J., *1*:490–493.

Zagarelli, E. V., Kutscher, A. H., and Hyman, G. A. 1969. Diseases of the Mouth and Jaws. Philadelphia, Lea and Febiger.

Chapter 51

DISEASES OF THE SALIVARY GLANDS

George A. Gates, M.D.

INTRODUCTION

Even though disorders originating in or involving the salivary glands comprise a minor part of the daily problems encountered by pediatricians and otolaryngologists, these disorders include a number of interesting and diverse pathologic states, the diagnosis of which is made difficult by the similarities of their clinical presentations and the management of which is hampered by the complex regional anatomy and the rather indolent but tenacious nature of many of these problems. With the exception of viral parotitis (mumps), all salivary gland disorders are more common in adults than in children; effective immunization against the mumps virus will probably remove this exception as well.

Most pediatric salivary gland problems are characterized by a painful swelling of a gland or, less commonly, a painless mass within a gland. These two clinical presentations encompass a large variety of causative agents. The differential diagnosis is often challenging, if difficult, yet the experienced clinician usually has little difficulty in defining the general nature of the problem by routine clinical methods, even though precise diagnosis may require the use of invasive techniques.

This chapter will describe the relevant clinical features and treatment of those salivary gland problems likely to be seen by the pediatrician. The description also includes basic information about the anatomy and physiology of the glands. This discussion is limited to the parotid and submandibular glands. Diseases of the minor salivary glands are covered in Chapter 52.

The objective of this chapter will be met if the reader acquires or improves diagnostic skills and knowledge of pediatric salivary gland disorders.

BASIC SCIENCE

Clinical Anatomy

The parotid gland fills the irregular space between the mandible and the ear canal and overlaps the mandible both medially and, to a greater extent, laterally where its duct crosses the masseter muscle and opens into the mouth opposite the second maxillary molar tooth. The external fascial envelope so tightly binds the gland to adjacent structures that in the normal subject the borders of the gland cannot be seen or felt. When swollen by a diffuse pathologic condition, the external contour of the gland can be seen in front of and below the external ear, often pushing the lobule up; the lower border frequently projects into the upper neck. Rarely, tumefactions will enlarge medially to displace the tonsil and soft palate toward the midline as the mass enlarges in the parapharyngeal space. Gland enlargements do not, as a rule, cause swelling of the cheek except in the immediate preauricular area. Swelling of the accessory lobe, which is located anterior to the main part of the gland, may occasionally produce an isolated midcheek mass. Fascial septa divide the gland into noncommunicating compartments; as a result, coalescence of abscesses seldom occurs.

The submandibular gland can be seen as a smooth bulge in the submandibular triangle. It can be felt externally in the upper neck as well as intraorally in both the normal and pathologic states. Enlargements or masses confined to the gland do not extend above the lower border of the ramus of the mandible owing to the fascial attachments there. The duct can be seen intraorally under the mucosa of the floor of the mouth, where it opens into a papilla located just lateral to the midline frenulum of the tongue. The duct has a right angle bend at the hilum and a long uphill course: these conditions predispose to calculi. There are several lymph nodes overlying the submandibular gland which, when enlarged, can simulate disease in the gland. Often these can be differentiated anatomically because the examiner's finger can displace them superiorly over the ramus of the mandible.

The neural relationships of the glands aid in diagnosis and therapy. Paralysis or even weakness of adjacent nerves is prima facie evidence of malignancy; this condition is more common in the parotid where the facial nerve is quite vulnerable as it passes through the substance of the gland. By contrast, the lingual and hypoglossal nerves lie outside the capsule of the submandibular gland and are less commonly involved. The location of the secretomotor fibers to the glands readily permits preganglionic denervation via the tympanic cavity: the chorda tympani nerve innervates the submandibular gland; the tympanic plexus innervates the parotid gland. Postganglionic denervation is more difficult, requiring near removal of the particular gland for surgical access.

Physiology

General. The sole function of the salivary glands is to produce saliva, a complex fluid of variable composition that has the following functions: (1) moistening the mouth for hygiene, protection, speech, and chewing; (2) lubricating food for mastication, taste sensation, and deglutition; and (3) initiating the preliminary phase of starch digestion by alpha amylase. The salivary glands indirectly participate in water regulation because dehydration leads to diminished salivary flow; the subsequent oral dryness stimulates the sensation of thirst.

Production. Saliva formation is the result of the separate activities of the acini and ducts. The former are the source of the water and various protein components of saliva; the latter are concerned largely with ion transport. The primary fluid has the composition of an isotonic ultrafiltrate of serum; it enters the lumen of the acinus via the intracellular transport mechanisms of pinocytosis and active ion pumping. With secretomotor stimulation, the acinar cells become electronegative because of the outward flow of potassium. The protein component of acinar secretion consists primarily of the salivary amylases plus other glycoproteins and mucopolysaccharides, including, in the submandibular gland, the blood group antigens. These materials enter the acinar lumen via disruption of secretory (zymogen) granules in the apical ends of the cells. The acinar fluid is carried distally by a pressure gradient and by contraction of the myoepithelial cells, which surround the acinus.

In the striated duct, hyperosmolar reabsorption of electrolytes leaves a fluid that is hypotonic and low in sodium, chloride, calcium, and bicarbonates and high in potassium. Electrolyte composition is dependent on the flow rate except for potassium; at low flow rates, contact time in the ducts allows greater reabsorption of electrolytes, whereas at high flow rates, rapid transit time prevents ductal reabsorption. In the unstimulated or resting gland, saliva flow rate approximates 0.05 ml per min and reaches rates of 0.5 ml per min under conditions of physiologic stimulation. Figure 51–1 shows the secretory unit of the salivary gland.

Regulation of Secretion. Continuous lubrication of the oral cavity results from the constant secretion of the minor salivary glands of the palate, cheeks, tongue, and lips. The major glands secrete only in response to reflex stimuli, primarily tactile and gustatory but olfactory as well. Psychic stimulation of saliva probably does not occur in humans (Enfors, 1962). Afferents reach the salivary nuclei in the brain stem by their respective pathways; efferents follow two different routes: those to the submandibular gland arise in the superior salivary nucleus, exit in the nervus intermedius of the seventh cranial nerve, pass in the chorda tympani nerve, and synapse in the small ganglion located on the gland; parotid secretomotor fibers begin more caudally (in the inferior salivary nucleus), exit in the ninth cranial nerve, cross the promontory of the middle ear in the tympanic plexus, and synapse in the otic ganglion located just external to the foramen ovale. Postganglionic fibers are carried in the auric-

SALIVARY GLAND UNIT

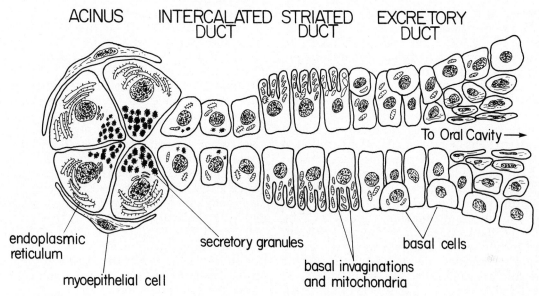

Figure 51–1 The secretory unit: several acinar cells are depicted around a central lumen, which empties into the intercalated duct and thence into the striated duct and, finally, into the excretory duct.

ulotemporal nerve. Although interruption of the preganglionic parasympathetic fibers in the middle ear abolishes reflex secretory activity, the gland continues to secrete because of its intact sympathetic innervation and because of the appearance, within three weeks, of denervation hypersensitivity. This is a paralytic secretion condition in which the gland responds excessively to circulating acetylcholine and catecholamines.

Gland secretion and saliva flow result from both parasympathetic and sympathetic stimuli: the former is watery, copious, and persists indefinitely, whereas sympathetic saliva is thick and viscid, small in volume, and gradually stops even with prolonged stimulation. It is generally felt that in humans reflex salivation occurs largely as the result of parasympathetic discharge and that sympathetic stimulation results in expulsion of preformed saliva. Beta adrenergic blocking agents, for example, prevent the release of amylase secretory granules and result in a net increase in gland content of amylase (Arglebe et al., 1976).

Many drugs inhibit secretion. Those possessing anticholinergic activity such as atropine are most notable, but postganglionic sympathetic blocking agents have a similar effect. Glandular stimulation results from acetylcholine and other parasympathomimetic agents, such as pilocarpine and methacholine. Undesirable side effects, such as increased bowel and bladder contractions, preclude the clinical use of these drugs for correction of hyposalivation. Adrenergic drugs induce salivation when administered intraductally, intraarterially, or in large intravenous dosages but are less effective than the parasympathomimetic drugs. Many of the sympathomimetic drugs used for nasal decongestion appear to decrease salivation slightly as well. Antidepressant agents, such as the dibenzazepine derivatives, imipramine and amitryptyline, exert an atropine-like side effect on the salivary glands, which occasionally may result in a secondary stomatitis.

Pathophysiology

Disturbances in gland function are uncommon but are generally severe. Hypofunction is more common than hypersalivation. True hypersalivation is rare and is usually associated with local irritation, which produces a reflex salivation. Apparent hypersalivation (ptyalism) is, however, a common complaint. Functional disturbances may result in alterations in the composition of saliva as well as alterations in volume.

Hyposalivation. Causes of decreased salivation are protean but may be divided into four categories: dehydration, gland disease, radiation damage, and drugs.

Cessation of salivation is one of the first sequelae of hypovolemia. This leads to dryness of the oral mucous membranes and the sensation of thirst which, in the normal individual, results in water intake. Dehydration in the debilitated or unconscious patient is an important predisposing cause for oral sepsis and acute suppurative sialadenitis, particularly of the parotid gland.

Virtually all inflammatory disorders of the salivary glands result in temporary cessation of function, which usually is recovered as the disorder subsides. The secretions in chronic parotitis are diminished but are also changed in character, becoming more viscid and opalescent. Sjögren syndrome is characterized by a moderate to severe decrease in saliva volume. Sodium and chloride concentrations are moderately increased in acute inflammation and even more so in Sjögren syndrome. Some systemic disorders are associated with a dry mouth: diabetes (Liu and Lin, 1969), hypertension (Wotman et al., 1967), and some hypogeusic conditions (Henkin et al., 1971). Anxiety and fear produce a severe dry mouth, presumably as the result of increased circulating catecholamines (Jenkins and Dawes, 1966). Dry mouth also occurs in some postmenopausal women (Kullander and Sonesson, 1965).

Severe xerostomia is an inevitable side effect of ionizing radiation to the salivary glands and oral cavity as, for example, that used in the treatment of head and neck cancer. In some cases the xerostomia is total. This has a devastating effect on teeth, often resulting in rampant caries. Similar but less profound changes follow the use of radioactive iodine as in the treatment of hyperthyroidism or metastatic thyroid cancer. The iodide salt is excreted into saliva by the ductal epithelium; it is at this anatomic site that the destructive effect of the iodine-131 occurs. Dry mouth is a common complaint of patients receiving tricyclic antidepressant medication. In some cases the drugs have to be discontinued because of secondary stomatitis; pilocarpine-containing lozenges to counter

this problem have not been very effective. Sympathomimetic agents used for nasal decongestion and ganglionic blocking agents used for hypertension also produce variable degrees of oral dryness.

Hypersalivation. True hypersalivation is rare and usually occurs as the result of painful or noxious stimuli from oral disease or from heavy metal poisoning in which oral irritation is a prominent factor. Hypersalivation and drooling are common in children during teething. Hypersalivation is also a part of the nausea syndrome, presumably for protection of the oral cavity should vomiting occur. Apparent hypersalivation (ptyalism) occurs in Parkinson disease, pregnancy, and in children with cerebral palsy. The problem is usually one of decreased ability to swallow and to clear the oral cavity. Drooling in palsied children can be corrected surgically. Salivary suppressant medication is inappropriate for long-term use because drying of the tracheobronchial mucosa and subsequent infection will result.

Altered Composition. Changes in the chemical or physical nature of saliva occur but are seldom a problem to patients except in cases of postradiation xerostomia where the secretions are very viscid and difficult to swallow. Children with cystic fibrosis have excessive amounts of salivary calcium and phosphorus, which predispose them to dental calculi but not to salivary calculi (Wotman et al., 1973). Salivary uric acid levels increase in gout and may be associated with uric acid calculi (Blatt et al., 1958).

Saliva is normally tasteless because of the low concentrations of sodium and glucose. Active secretion of drugs or other compounds into saliva may produce peculiar taste sensations as, for example, certain iodine-containing materials. Salivary potassium is elevated in aldosteronism and in digitalis toxicity. The potential usefulness of salivary analysis for diagnosis and monitoring is limited by the variable of the secretory rate influence on concentration and by the technical awkwardness of collection devices.

CLINICAL PATHOLOGY

This section classifies, defines, and briefly describes in clinical terms the major and the most common salivary gland problems seen in children. Limitations of space preclude the classic histologic descriptive approach to the study of salivary gland pathology — the reader is referred to the Selected References for greater detail. For purposes of discussion, salivary gland disorders may be divided into three groups: (1) systemic disorders that involve the salivary glands, (2) primary non-neoplastic disorders, and (3) primary neoplastic diseases.

Systemic Disorders

The salivary glands may be involved by viral infection (mumps), by generalized endocrine/metabolic dysfunctions such as obesity, starvation, or diabetes, by autoimmune disorders (Sjögren syndrome), by generalized exocrine gland dysfunction (mucoviscidosis), and by extension of local diseases into the gland from the surrounding tissues, particularly the lymph nodes. In some instances, allergy is thought to play a role. It is important to keep these possibilities in mind when evaluating a swollen gland or a mass involving the gland lest one overlook the possibility of nonregional etiology.

Viral Parotitis (Mumps). Mumps is an acute, contagious illness that usually causes fever and painful parotid enlargement; in many cases other organ system involvement occurs with meningoencephalitis, orchitis, pancreatitis, or deafness. The cause is usually the mumps virus; however, echovirus, coxsackie A virus, and lymphocytic choriomeningitis virus have also been implicated as occasional causes of epidemic parotitis (Zollar and Mufson, 1970).

There is an 18 to 21 day incubation period and a one to three day prodromal period of malaise prior to the parotitis. In some cases parotitis may be absent; in others all four major salivary glands may become acutely enlarged and, rarely, only one submandibular gland may be affected.

Meningoencephalitis, varying from mild headache and lassitude (common) to seizure, coma, and death (rare) occurs in about 25 of every 1000 cases of mumps; death occurs in only one to two per cent of these cases (Modlin, 1975). Pancreatitis is probably more common than has been suspected. The sensation of vertigo and nausea may be due to central nervous system involvement, to pancreatitis, or to the labyrinthitis that commonly results in unilateral deafness with or without detectable loss of vestibular function. Why the deafness is usually unilateral and total is not clear. Although immunization against mumps using the live attenuated Jeryl-Lynn strain has not been universally practiced (only 39 per cent of children had been vaccinated in 1974), a high seroconversion rate (greater than 95 per cent) is noted, and a 38 per cent reduction in the incidence of mumps and its complications was reported by the Center for Disease Control (Modlin, 1975).

Lymphadenitis. The parotid gland has many lymph nodes on its lateral surface or within its substance; these may be involved by lymphoma or granuloma (such as animal scratch fever and actinomycosis), as well as by suppurative infection originating in the scalp, face, or nasopharynx. Although the tissues over the submandibular gland contain fewer nodes than the parotid, these are more commonly involved by atypical mycobacterial infections. Sarcoid is a common cause of bilateral parotid enlargement in young black patients; when the uveal tract is involved the term uveoparotid fever (Heerfordt disease) is used.

The clinical distinction between a lymph node disorder and a salivary gland disorder is difficult and often can be made only by excisional biopsy.

Endocrine and Metabolic Disorders. Salivary gland enlargement occurs by infiltration of fat in some diabetics and in grossly obese people, by a functional hypertrophy in persons who consume a carbohydrate diet exclusively, or as a result of autoimmune processes in Sjögren syndrome. The latter disorder may begin in childhood and is typified clinically by progressive enlargement of the salivary glands, lacrimal glands, or both; by dryness of the oral and conjunctival membranes; and by evidence of a collagen vascular disorder, such as rheumatoid arthritis. Any of these classical clinical manifestations may be absent. Sialograms usually reveal sialectasis. Tests for antinuclear antibody and latex agglutination are often positive. Histologically the gland shows acinar atrophy and marked lymphocyte infiltration, often with germinal centers: the lymphocytes are of both T and B cell derivation. The disorder is progressive; steroid therapy is of little help in the amelioration of symptoms.

Mucoviscidosis. Alterations in salivary composition consist mainly of elevated calcium and phosphorus content. The elevation of sodium and chloride levels seen in other secretions is inconsistently manifested in saliva and varies appreciably with the flow rate;

measurements of salivary electrolytes are not recommended as a screening test for cystic fibrosis (Kaiser et al., 1974). The submandibular glands are enlarged in over 90 per cent of cases (Barbero and Sibinga, 1962), but there are no other symptoms. The mechanism is unknown.

Allergy. Some feel that hypersensitivity to certain foods, such as strawberries and seafoods, may precipitate a sudden, short-lived, often bilateral, painless parotid swelling that is frequently accompanied by other commonly accepted indications of allergy, such as hives and bronchospasm. The mechanism for such an event is not clear, but a rapid increase in the viscosity of the saliva may be responsible. Efforts to establish that acute, painless parotid swelling can be allergic in nature should include cytologic examination of saliva (looking for eosinophils and ruling out bacterial infection), a differential white blood cell count, a family history, and provocative testing.

Iodine-containing compounds may produce parotid enlargement when given systemically (as for angiography or pyelography), orally, or intraductally for sialography. Whether this is due to allergy or to local toxicity from the concentrated iodine in the saliva is not known.

Primary Nonneoplastic Diseases of the Salivary Glands

Most disorders that involve the gland parenchyma are either of systemic origin (see the preceding section) or are neoplastic. The vast majority of primary nonneoplastic disorders begin within the ductal system and are characterized by recurrent painful swelling; most have some degree of bacterial infection, either primarily or secondarily, in the presence of stones, a stricture, or sialectasis. In some cases, more than one pathophysiologic mechanism may be involved; i.e., a primary duct stricture can lead to stone formation because of salivary stasis and can be associated with secondary bacterial suppuration. Alternatively, a primary calculus can cause both suppuration and stricture at its point of lodgment.

Sialectasis. Saccular dilatation of the small, intercalated ducts that connect the acini with the striated ducts is one of the more common congenital abnormalities of the salivary glands. Since there is no obstruction to

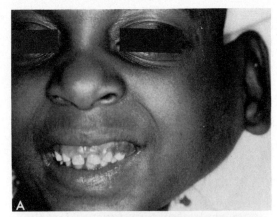

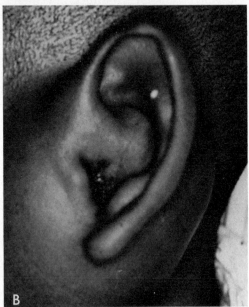

Figure 51–2 *A,* Anterior view of the left parotid hemangioma. Note normal facial motion. *B,* Lateral photograph of a left parotid hemangioma.

flow, the term nonobstructive sialectasis has been used to differentiate this condition from dilatation of the larger ducts that occurs with distal ductal obstruction (obstructive sialodochiectasis). Although both parotids usually display the typical radiographic findings (Fig. 51–2), the symptoms are most often confined to one gland and are due to recurrent bacterial infection rather than to the sialectasis per se. Submandibular involvement is rare. The clinical picture is one of painful gland enlargement associated with systemic inflammatory signs such as fever, leukocytosis, and elevated sedimentation rate. With repeated infection the gland becomes permanently enlarged and the ductal ectasia may worsen. Control of infection by medical means and manual emptying of the gland by massage can prevent progression of the disorder.

Other problems characterized by nonobstructive sialectasis are Sjögren syndrome and postinfectious sialectasis. The latter is very uncommon and may, in reality, be a clinical variant of congenital sialectasis. It is important to include the possibility of Sjögren syndrome because a small number of cases may develop overt lymphoma in the affected gland or elsewhere.

Stricture.   Narrowing of a major duct may result from faulty chewing habits (which traumatize the punctum) or from external trauma. Rarely, pneumococcal infection of the duct may occur; this results in multiple strictures. Strictures can also be secondary to calculi. Dilatation of the duct proximal to the stricture will be seen in long-standing cases (obstructive sialodochiectasis) as a result of weakening of the duct wall from secretory pressure and infection. Patients note recurrent acute parotid or submandibular swelling early in the course of a meal as the reflex secretory pressure and flow approach maximum. This is painful and may cause the patient to stop eating. Eventually reflex stimulation ceases, the gland slowly empties, and the swelling recedes; this usually takes two hours. Generally only one gland is affected.

Sialolithiasis.   Stones in the salivary gland ducts are due to local causes and are not associated with hyperparathyroidism as are renal stones. Calculous disease is quite different in the parotid and in the submandibular glands, and they should be considered separately in this respect.

The submandibular gland is more prone to stones than the parotid because of anatomic differences (a longer, uphill duct) and chemical differences (submandibular saliva is more alkaline, more viscous, and has a higher concentration of calcium and phosphorus compounds). Precipitation of these salts occurs as a result of stasis or increased concentration of salts. Most stones contain calcium apatite; 80 per cent of all submandibular stones are radiopaque. The intraductal calculi are smooth, elongated, and elliptical and may move within the duct to impinge on the punctum by the pressure of mealtime salivation. The stone may extrude through the punctum spontaneously, in which case the symptoms begin to subside immediately. If impacted into the punctum the gland will slowly decrease in size over a two hour period owing to cessation of salivation by pressure

and the slow escape of saliva around the stone. Strictures may form owing to ulceration and secondary infection. Secondary infection is common and may confuse the clinical picture. One should search for a stone in every case of submandibular suppuration; in a majority of cases one or more will be found. Intraglandular stones form at the hilum where the duct makes a 90 degree turn. These tend to be large, irregular, and fixed and may cause no symptoms until they are quite large when the symptoms are those of chronic enlargement and tenderness of the gland rather than intermittent painful swelling. Erosion into the soft tissues and even fistulization into the mouth may occur.

Parotid stones are far less common than are submandibular stones. This probably is a reflection of the differences in anatomy and secretion of the two glands. In addition, parotid stones are usually radiolucent because they tend to form around a bacterial nidus or may be due entirely to noncalcium materials, such as the uric acid calculi seen in gout. Calcified masses in the parotid are as likely to be phleboliths or calcified lymph nodes as they are to be intraductal calculi; sialography is essential for diagnosis in these cases.

Cysts.   Most cystic lesions occur in the parotid gland; they may be congenital, posttraumatic, retention cysts, or cystic degeneration of neoplasms. Approximately two per cent of all parotid masses are cystic.

The most common congenital cyst arises from the first branchial arch and contains epithelium only (Type I) or epithelium and adnexal structures (Type II) (Work, 1972). Both are duplication anomalies of the external auditory canal and regardless of their external position (Type I is intraparotid, Type II is infraparotid) the tract comes into deep relationship with the canal. The tract always passes near the facial nerve; in one case reported by Work (1972), the tract was surrounded by a split in the main trunk.

These and other congenital cysts (dermoid) become clinically evident because of infection within the cyst leading to abscess, rupture, and sinus tract formation.

Primary Neoplasms

The most common tumors of the salivary glands in children are of vascular origin — hemangioma and lymphangioma. If vascular lesions are excluded and only the solid or

Table 51–1 SALIVARY GLAND NEOPLASMS IN CHILDREN (TOTAL: 428)*

Benign		Malignant	
Hemangioma	111	Mucoepidermoid carcinoma	73
Mixed tumor	94	Acinous cell carcinoma	18
"Vascular proliferative"	40	Undifferentiated carcinoma	14
Lymphangioma	18	Undifferentiated sarcoma	9
Lymphoepithelial tumor	3	Carcinoma ex mixed tumor	9
Cystadenoma	3	Adenocarcinoma	11
Warthin tumor	3	Adenoid cystic carcinoma	6
Plexiform neurofibroma	2	Squamous cell carcinoma	3
Xanthoma	2	Mesenchymal sarcoma	2
Neurilemoma	1	Rhabdomyosarcoma	2
Adenoma	1	Malignant epithelial tumor	1
Lipoma	1	Ganglioneuroblastoma	1
TOTAL	279	TOTAL	149

*Adapted from Schuller, D. E., and McCabe, B. F. 1977. Salivary gland neoplasms in children. Otolaryngol. Clin. North Am., *10*(2):399–412.

firm masses are considered, only 3.2 per cent of all salivary gland neoplasms occur in persons less than 16 years old. Of these, 57.1 per cent are malignant (Schuller and McCabe, 1977). Neoplasms are far more common (10:1) than solid non-neoplastic tumefactions; most of the latter are due to localized chronic sialadenitis or lymph node hyperplasia. These statistics emphasize the fact that a solid mass in the parotid or submandibular gland of a child has a greater than 50 per cent chance of being malignant.

Clinically, salivary gland tumors fall into three groups: benign, low-grade malignancy, and high-grade malignancy. In adults the ratios of these three types are 70:20:10; in children they are 43:35:22. In children there is essentially only one benign epithelial tumor, the mixed tumor. All other benign lesions are rare and usually are of supporting tissue origin. The low-grade malignancies are the mucoepidermoid carcinoma and acinous cell carcinoma. The high-grade malignancy group consists of a variety of adenocarcinomas and sarcomas (Table 51–1).

Solid Tumors

Benign Tumors. Several neoplasms of epithelial origin occur in the adult that are universally considered to be benign: mixed tumor (pleomorphic adenoma), Warthin tumor, oncocytoma, a variety of adenomas, and the lymphoepithelial lesion. Only the mixed tumor occurs with any regularity in children; it accounts for 4.5 per cent of all mixed tumors (Schuller and McCabe, 1977),

and it is the single most common solid gland tumor seen in pediatric patients.

The mixed tumor is composed of two cellular elements that are derived from the intercalated duct reserve cell: the epithelial cell and the myoepithelial cell (Regezi and Batsakis, 1977). In addition there is usually a distinct stromal component. The cellular and stromal components can vary greatly in amount and composition; the characteristic pattern is one of stellate cells in a loose myxoid stroma. The capsule is thin, and the surface is often irregular and lobulated with microscopic bosses projecting through the capsule.

This type of tumor usually arises in the lateral portion of the gland, grows slowly, is painless, and has been present for 15 months prior to removal in most children. The average age of children undergoing an operation for this problem is 9.5 years. The mass averages 2.7 cm in diameter, is firm and freely mobile, and there is no evidence of facial nerve weakness associated with the tumor.

Obtaining a biopsy specimen by incision is contraindicated in these cases because of the danger of seeding, which causes recurrence of an otherwise curable lesion; the diagnosis is made by removal of that portion of the gland containing the tumor.

Other solid, benign tumors, such as adenoma and neurofibroma, occur too infrequently for any generalizations to be made about their clinical behaviors.

Low-grade Malignancy. Two low-grade malignant neoplasms appear occasionally in children: mucoepidermoid carcinoma and acinous cell carcinoma (acinic cell carcinoma). Both lesions have a generally benign course in the majority of cases, but because occasionally some exhibit malignant behavior, it is inappropriate to classify either one as completely benign or malignant. In addition, it is very difficult to predict the biologic behavior of either one of these tumors on histologic grounds alone; therefore, it is generally felt that they should be classified in a separate category.

The mucoepidermoid carcinoma is composed of epithelial cells derived from the excretory duct. These may be differentiated into squamous cells in the high-grade tumor, mucous cells in the low-grade tumor, and a cell intermediate in the formation of both; these cells are noted to be present in varying proportions in most cases. The presence of intracellular mucin as detected by Alcian blue or other stains is necessary to establish the diagnosis and to distinguish the high-grade tumor from a squamous cell carcinoma.

The acinous cell carcinoma may be recognized histologically by its uniform, large, round clear cells, which have abundant basophilic or clear cytoplasm. These cells are thought to arise from precursors of the acinar cell. The five year control rate of this tumor is excellent, but control falls to 50 per cent after 25 years (Eneroth and Hamberger, 1974).

Both lesions tend to be clinically similar to the mixed tumor: a solitary, firm, mobile, slow-growing, painless mass located in the parotid (most commonly) or submandibular gland. Clinical evidence of malignancy, such as rapid growth, pain, fixation, or facial paralysis, is uncommon and should alert the clinician to the probability that the lesion is *not* a mixed tumor.

High-grade Malignancy. A large number of cell types can be considered in this category (Table 51–1); a detailed discussion of the clinical pathology of each type sufficient to be meaningful would be unnecessarily lengthy and repetitive since most of these lesions have similar clinical manifestations and show aggressive biologic behavior. Individual tumor characteristics that are important for treatment will be discussed in the section on management. The reader is referred to the selected readings for greater detail.

High-grade malignancies tend to occur at a younger age (average 5.3 years) than do the low-grade and benign tumors (9.7 and 9.5 years average, respectively) (Schuller and McCabe, 1977). The rate of growth and the severity of local symptoms are generally more pronounced than in the benign and low-grade tumors. Facial paralysis and fixation are the classic physical findings of malignant parotid tumors; in the submandibular gland, fixation and involvement of the lingual, hypoglossal, or marginal mandibular branch of the facial nerve similarly indicate advanced disease. Metastases to the regional lymph nodes are not uncommon, and hematogenous spread to the lungs, liver, and bone may occur. Excisional biopsy, when technically feasible, or incisional biopsy when not, is essential for proper diagnosis. Even then, because of the undifferentiated nature of many of these lesions, a specific cell-type diagnosis may often only be inferred, and the treatment must be based on consultations among the otolaryngologist, pediatrician, pathologist, radiation therapist, and the pediatric chemotherapist.

Fluctuant Masses

Approximately 60 per cent of all pediatric salivary gland masses are soft, compressible lesions of vascular origin: hemangiomas or, less frequently, lymphangiomas. Most arise in the parotid gland. Congenital cysts also may be noticeably fluctuant, but they are generally firmer and more discrete. These masses usually appear in the first few months or weeks after birth; many enlarge rapidly and create great concern for the infant's welfare, even though malignant transformation of these lesions is unknown in this age group. Many regress spontaneously but not predictably.

The hemangioma is composed of solid masses of cells and of capillary-like vascular spaces that have replaced the secretory tissue of the gland, leaving only widely spaced ducts. The tumor usually infiltrates the entire gland, limited only by the fascial envelope of the gland, which results in a rather characteristic appearance (Fig. 51–2). The mass is warm, soft, compressible, does not transilluminate, and grows more tense with crying or straining. If large, it extends into the upper neck. There is no facial weakness. Regression of this cellular type of hemangioma begins after a variable period of growth; cavernous hemangiomas that appear later in childhood tend not to regress spontaneously. The exact percentage of tumors that disappears is not known because many are resected. The complications of parotidectomy for hemangioma that have been reported (Williams, 1975), such as facial paralysis, recurrent tumor, and postoperative deaths, are persuasive of the adoption of a wait-and-see approach. Taking a small biopsy specimen to confirm the diagnosis is recommended. If excision is contemplated after a period of observation, an experienced parotid surgeon should be consulted.

Lymphangioma occurs less commonly, is softer and more diffuse, and transilluminates more readily than a hemangioma. Approximately 50 per cent of lymphangiomas are present at birth. Grossly, the tumor extends beyond the anatomic borders of the gland and invades rather than replaces the gland. Microscopically lymphangiomas may be composed of small, capillary-sized spaces, cavernous dilated spaces, or both. When the lesion is large and composed more of loculated lymph cysts than channels, the term cystic hygroma is used. Spontaneous regression is uncommon.

Metastatic Neoplasm

The parotid gland is a common site for metastases of primary lesions of the scalp, face, cheek, orbit, and external nose. One should search for a primary lesion outside of the gland in all cases of suspected malignancy. The clinical behavior of metastatic tumors reflects the biology of the primary neoplasm.

Lymphoma

Primary lymphoma of the salivary glands is rare; Regezi and Batsakis (1977) reviewed six reported series composed of 2924 parotid neoplasms of which seven were lymphomas. Many of these were associated with Sjögren syndrome, in which case the outlook was poor. The others had favorable prognoses. The reported cases have all occurred in the parotid gland.

DIAGNOSIS

History

As in most areas of medicine, the time-related events surrounding a particular ill-ness involving the salivary glands are generally easy to establish by direct inquiry and provide important diagnostic perspective; i.e., was the particular episode of enlargement the first or merely one of a series of problems? Mumps, after all, only occurs once in each person. The time relationship of the enlargement to eating indicates a lesion obstructing salivary outflow; this is confirmed by subsidence of pain and swelling in the first two postprandial hours. Inflammatory lesions do not subside so promptly. Progressively enlarging masses usually are neoplastic in nature, although some granulomas can behave this way. An aggressive malignancy can grow so fast that one suspects inflammation as the cause.

Physical Examination

Three distinct observations need to be made: Is the entire gland enlarged, or just a part of it? If part, is the mass in or around the glands? If in the glands, is the mass solid, cystic, or inflammatory? In addition, one needs to note signs of tenderness, nerve or skin involvement, fixation, and, lastly, the character of the saliva or other fluid expressible from the duct. Facial paralysis associated with a parotid mass indicates neoplasm until proved otherwise; benign lesions do not, as a rule, disrupt neural function. A similar rule can be made for the submandibular gland, especially since the adjacent nerves (marginal mandibular branch of the seventh cranial nerve, lingual nerve, and hypoglossal nerve) are some distance away from the gland; here neural findings may indicate nonresectability as well.

The ductal orifice should be inspected, and the nature of the saliva should be noted. Saliva can be expressed by manual pressure on the gland exerted in a behind-to-forward stripping motion. Normal saliva is crystal clear. Redness of the punctum and clear saliva suggest viral infection. Purulent secretions are seen in cases of bacterial infection. Opalescent saliva is common in many types of chronic glandular dysfunction. Palpation of the duct may reveal a stone, but dilatation of the punctum and insertion of a probe into the lumen is often more helpful in this regard: the probe will encounter the stone and impart a feeling of resistance to the examiner's hand. A stricture of the duct or punctum is readily evident when attempting to dilate prior to probing.

Laboratory Examination of Saliva

Three examinations can be done on saliva: culture, cytology, and sialochemistry. The validity of culture data is greatest when the specimen is most carefully obtained. Ideally, needle aspiration (after careful skin preparation) or intraductal aspiration via a catheter should be attempted. Cultures made from specimens obtained by simple swabbing of the duct opening usually grow the usual mouth flora; this may be misleading.

Cytologic and chemical examinations of saliva are best done on fluid obtained from an intraductal catheter or a vacuum-held collection cup placed over the orifice. In this way fluid from abnormal glands will be obtained undiluted by saliva from the other glands. Fluid flow should be stimulated by applying 6 per cent citric acid or whole lemon juice to the tongue.

Cytologic examination will reveal tumor cells in over two thirds of cases and, if interpreted by an experienced cytopathologist, the results may provide a histologic diagnosis prior to biopsy. Chemical examination of the saliva is not useful for the diagnosis of salivary gland disorders but is used as a research tool in pharmacology and toxicology.

Examination of submaxillary saliva electrolytes as a screening test for disorders such as aldosteronism has been advocated (Wotman et al., 1970). The salivary electrolyte composition varies with the flow rate, however, and flow rate is difficult to standardize, so such tests are seldom used.

Radiographic Examination

Three different techniques are available: plain films, sialograms, and radionuclide scans. The techniques and normal findings are noted in Chapter 40.

Plain films are used to locate radiopaque calculi, to detect dystrophic calcification, and to assess the bony structures adjacent to a mass. Approximately 20 per cent of submandibular calculi and 80 per cent of parotid calculi are radiolucent, however, and some of the rest are too small or too hidden by overlying structures to be seen. The use of intraoral dental film, high resolution commercial-grade emulsions, and multiple views may help overcome problems locating occult calculi.

Contrast sialograms will display the radiolucent calculus as a filling defect (assuming there are no air bubbles in the contrast medium). Sialograms are essential in evaluating children with recurrent sialadenitis and should be done routinely to determine if there is an underlying anatomic abnormality, such as a duct stricture, calculus, or sialectasis. In small children sedation or general anesthesia may be required to do the examination, which is slightly painful and requires considerable patient cooperation. Sialograms are not much help in tumor diagnosis, however.

Radionuclide scans (radiosialography) made with the Anger camera can outline the vascular compartments of the gland, the lesion, or both immediately after injection. After 30 minutes the radioactivity is concentrated within the gland parenchyma and ducts, where an outline of the gland, tumor, or both is apparent. A third study can be made after the patient uses a sialagogue such as a fresh lemon to determine how much of the radioactive saliva can be expelled into the oral cavity; this provides a rough measure of the secretory function of the gland. Tumor imaging for size and detail is best done on the rectilinear scanner, even though the examination takes longer.

Although all these scan techniques have been used for adults, their applicability to the diagnosis of pediatric salivary gland problems is limited by considerations of radiation exposure, requirements for patient cooperation, and the general vagueness of the examination results. Certainly the scan cannot substitute for a tissue diagnosis where a tumor is suspected in children. (The Warthin tumor and the oncocytoma have a characteristic scan appearance, but these are almost exclusively adult tumors.)

Biopsy

Incisional biopsy is rarely indicated. If a histologic diagnosis is required when, for example, neoplasm is suspected, excisional biopsy is preferred for several reasons: (1) the pathologist usually needs to study the entire tumor to make an accurate diagnosis (this is why needle biopsy is of questionable value); (2) complete excision avoids cutting and spillage of the tumor (benign tumors seldom recur except when seeded; then recurrence is the rule); (3) for the majority of cases complete excision will be indicated; and, (4) formal operating room excisional biopsy avoids the hazards of accidental nerve injury from limited exposure approaches. Incisional biopsy may be helpful in the presence of an obvious, advanced malignancy to determine the cell type prior to radiation therapy or chemotherapy. If it is helpful to confirm a diagnosis of Sjögren syndrome, one can do an incisional biopsy of the minor salivary glands of the labial or buccal mucosa; these may show the same histologic abnormality as in the major glands.

MANAGEMENT

In this section the principles and some specific techniques of management of common childhood salivary disorders will be discussed. The term "management" rather than treatment is used because there is no specific therapy for some disorders and, in addition, the author wishes to stress the unique interrelationship between diagnosis and treatment of salivary gland tumors.

Functional Disturbances

Xerostomia. Drug therapy is generally of no help in xerostomia; it is better to remove the cause, where possible. Pilocarpine lozenges have been used with limited success. For intractable dry mouth, such as after radiation therapy, an artificial saliva preparation frequently instilled into the mouth will facilitate deglutition and help oral hygiene. One such formula is methylcellulose 4 per cent — 20 ml, glycerine — 10 ml, and lemon oil — 1 drop. Sialagogues, such as sour lemon drops, are also very helpful.

Drooling. For children with uncontrollable drooling, such as occurs in cerebral palsy, surgical rerouting of the parotid ducts into the fauces plus bilateral submandibular gland excision have been performed. Wilkie and Brody (1977) report getting 86 per cent good to excellent results in 123 patients; there was one death, and 20 patients required reoperation because of stenosis. Parotid denervation by tympanic neurectomy, however, substantially reduces sialorrhea to acceptable levels in 66 per cent of patients with none of the morbidity of the Wilkie procedure (Townsend et al., 1973). It is reasonable, therefore, to recommend the less morbid procedure, the bilateral transtympanic neurectomy, as the initial treatment for intractable drooling. (Chorda tympani neurec-

tomy will reduce the sialorrhea even more, but the taste sense from the anterior tongue is sacrificed.) For the one third of cases not controlled by this procedure, bilateral submandibular gland excision can be added to the treatment regimen. The Wilkie parotid duct rerouting procedure can be held in reserve for those patients not responding to the preceding two steps.

Management of the Acutely Swollen Salivary Gland

Mumps. An acutely swollen, tender parotid gland, clear saliva, a red punctum, fever, lymphocytosis, and no prior history of sialadenopathy typify mumps. No treatment exists; supportive care consists of recommendations for a bland liquid or very soft diet, analgesics, and antipyretics. The child should be isolated until the gland swelling and fever are gone.

Mumps immunization is available and is recommended as part of the routine immunization series.

Acute Submandibular Sialadenitis. Mumps seldom affects only one submandibular gland. One should look for another cause, in particular a calculus, by performing a radiologic examination of the area even if the physical examination is inconclusive. Many stones are too small to be felt in acutely edematous tissue. Dilatation, slitting the punctum, or both procedures will allow the small stone to pass. This is an office procedure for adults but requires general anesthesia for most children. A suture should be passed around the duct proximal to the stone before probing; otherwise the stone may be inadvertently pushed back into the gland. Larger stones or those within the hilum require excision of the gland for control; lesser procedures often result in recurrent stone formation and infection.

Management of the Recurrently Swollen Salivary Gland

Recurrent Parotitis. This common salivary gland problem is characterized by painful enlargement of the gland associated with low-grade fever, leukocytosis, and purulent exudate in the duct. Although individual episodes respond to proper antibiotic treatment, recurrence is common. Sialography usually reveals punctate sialectasis. Total gland excision is the only completely effective treatment, but the hazard of postoperative facial weakness usually persuades the parents to continue medical therapy for each episode. The percentage of cases that subside with time is not known; probably most do.

If sialography reveals duct stricture, calculi, or both, dilatation is recommended for primary management; most parotid stones are small and will pass through the dilated duct. Stones should be analyzed for their chemical composition.

Recurrent Submandibular Sialadenopathy. Here, stones, strictures, and local sepsis are all commonly identified as contributing factors. Excision of the gland is the most efficacious therapy.

Management of the Progressively Enlarging Gland

An important distinction must be made between the enlarging gland as discussed here and an enlarging mass within the gland as discussed in the next section. If in doubt, it is best to manage it as a mass and obtain a tissue diagnosis.

Parotid Gland. Bilaterally symmetrical enlargement of the entire gland that is soft and nonnodular usually requires no more than the history and physical examination for local evaluation, but this situation should prompt a search for an underlying metabolic problem, particularly diabetes. Weight reduction and limitation of carbohydrate intake are helpful in these cases.

Diffuse enlargement of a single parotid gland generally is of greater concern, and one should search for an underlying granuloma, such as tuberculosis or sarcoid, by appropriate skin tests, laboratory examinations, and biopsy.

Both parotids are usually involved in Sjögren syndrome. The diagnosis is suspected by history and physical examination and confirmed by sialogram, lip biopsy, and occasionally by parotid biopsy. Treatment is supportive: manual emptying of the gland after meals, meticulous oral hygiene, and sialogogues and artificial saliva. Steroid therapy is reserved for acute episodes of associated arthropathy.

Submandibular Gland. Progressive diffuse enlargement is seen in mucoviscidosis and as a side effect of drug therapy with adrenergic blocking agents. Less commonly, this gland may be involved along with the parotids in Sjögren syndrome.

Enlargement of a single gland is of concern, and neoplasm should be suspected in the majority of cases. Unlike the parotid where a discrete mass is easily discerned because the gland is attached to surrounding structures, the more mobile submandibular gland conforms to the pressure of the enlarging mass within it.

Management of an Enlarging Mass in the Salivary Gland

Parotid

Primary Epithelial Neoplasms. An enlarging mass in or about the parotid gland most frequently is a neoplasm. Occasionally, congenital cysts, benign lymphadenopathy, and granulomata are found. The safest rule to follow is to consider that all parotid masses are neoplastic until proved otherwise. After appropriate studies have been done, such as skin tests, plain radiographs, and routine hematologic tests, one must decide if the clinical picture is probably that of a benign neoplasm or not. If the usual criteria are met, i.e., slow, painless growth, no nerve involvement, and no fixation to surrounding structures, then an excisional biopsy should be performed. This is, in fact, the definitive treatment for the majority of cases because the specimen containing the tumor consists of the bulk of the gland; no further surgery is necessary for the benign tumor or for the small, low-grade malignancy.

This approach, wherein definitive treatment is carried out prior to a tissue diagnosis, has become standard practice for salivary neoplasms because incisional biopsy prior to therapy leads to seeding of the wound and tumor recurrence. A frozen section pathology report is obtained to confirm the diagnosis.

Occasionally the permanent section pathology report will differ from the frozen section. If the diagnosis is downgraded to a frank malignancy where none was clinically apparent, further surgery, postoperative radiotherapy, or both can be carried out as indicated. If the frozen section indicates malignancy in the absence of clinical verification, the operation is terminated after the excisional parotid biopsy. Further treatment should be delayed until the permanent sections have been thoroughly studied. In general, radical surgery, including nerve sacrifice, is not performed on the basis of frozen section interpretation because a suspicious report may be upgraded later.

For patients with clinically apparent malignancy, one of two treatment programs is used depending on the surgeon's estimate of the resectability of the mass: radical operation followed by postoperative radiotherapy and chemotherapy for probably resectable lesions; or incisional biopsy plus radiotherapy and chemotherapy for the nonresectable lesion followed by later excision, if warranted. Most salivary gland malignancies respond so poorly to radiation therapy or chemotherapy that surgical removal or debulking should be carried out first to increase the likelihood of a favorable response to radiation or drugs. The notable exception is the rhabdomyosarcoma, in the treatment of which radiation and therapy with vincristine, actinomycin D, and cyclophosphamide (Cytoxan) (VAC therapy) are so effective that deforming surgery should not be done until the results of this treatment are evident.

Hemangioma and Lymphangioma. The diagnosis of these masses is usually evident from the physical examination. Resection should be delayed as long as possible to allow for spontaneous regression of the hemangioma to occur and to let the child grow. Removal of the hemangioma is difficult because of bleeding, and it seems unreasonable to place the facial nerve at risk for a benign disease that has a high rate of spontaneous regression. The lymphangioma, on the other hand, generally continues to enlarge slowly and may press on the airway or foodway sufficiently to produce difficulty. Needle aspiration is contraindicated, first because it does no good (the fluid-filled spaces are noncommunicating) and, second, as it may result in infection with acute exacerbation of obstructive symptoms. Excision of the lymphangioma is always incomplete because of its diffuse and invasive growth pattern, but subtotal removal is usually sufficient to relieve the patient of the symptoms of the mass.

Submandibular Gland

The principles of management of neoplasms outlined for the parotid gland are equally applicable to those arising in the submandibular gland. Because tumors of the submandibular gland are so uncommon in children, they are generally misdiagnosed and adequate treatment is not planned for.

SUMMARY

In this chapter, the most common and the most important salivary gland disorders seen in children have been reviewed. The author hopes that the reader will find this review helpful in learning about and caring for patients with these interesting and perplexing problems.

SELECTED REFERENCES

Conley, J. J. 1975. Salivary Glands and the Facial Nerve. New York, Grune and Stratton.
    The extensive experience of this distinguished surgeon and teacher, along with contributions from other eminent authorities, is combined into a readable and very well illustrated volume which should be required reading for all serious students of salivary gland diseases.

Rankow, R. M., and Polayes, I. M. 1976. Diseases of the Salivary Glands. Philadelphia, W. B. Saunders Co.
    This is a well illustrated work that covers all aspects of salivary gland diseases from basic anatomy and physiology to diagnosis, treatment, and reconstruction. In Chapter 11, salivary gland disorders in infancy and childhood are discussed.

The Otolaryngologic Clinics of North America. 1977. Philadelphia, W. B. Saunders Co., *10*(2).
    This multiauthored series of articles succinctly summarized the current state of knowledge regarding salivary glands and their diseases. It is a good learning text as well as a handy reference source. It is recommended reading for all residents interested in these problems.

REFERENCES

Arglebe, C., Eysholdt, U., and Chilla, R. 1976. Pharmacological inhibition of salivary glands: a possible therapy for sialosis and sialoadenitis. Effect of experimentally induced beta-receptor block on the rat parotid gland. ORL, *38*(4):218–229.

Barbero, G., and Sibinga, M. 1962. Enlargement of the submaxillary salivary glands in cystic fibrosis. Pediatrics, *29*:788–793.

Blatt, I. M., Denning, R. M., Zumberge, J. H., et al. 1958. Studies in sialolithiasis. The structure and mineralogical composition of salivary gland calculi. Ann. Otol. Rhinol. Laryngol., *67*(3):595–617.

Eneroth, C. M., and Hamberger, C. A. 1974. Principles of treatment of different types of parotid tumors. Laryngoscope, Suppl, *84*:1732–1740.

Enfors, B. O. 1962. The parotid and submandibular secretion in man. Quantitative recordings of the normal and pathological activity. Acta Otolaryngol., Suppl., *172*:1–67.

Henkin, R. I., Schechter, P. J., Hoye, R., et al. 1971. Idiopathic hypogeusia with dysgeusia, hyposmia, and dysosmia. A new syndrome. J.A.M.A., *217*:434–440.

Jenkins, G. N., and Dawes, C.: 1966. The psychic flow of saliva in man. Arch. Oral. Biol., *11*:1203–1204.

Kaiser, D., Schoni, M., and Drack, E. 1974. Anionen- und Lationenausscheidung per Parotis in Abhängigkeit von der Fliessrate bei Mukoviszidosepatienten und Gesunden. Helv. Paediat. Acta., *29*:145–150.

Kullander, S., and Sonesson, B. 1965. Studies on saliva in menstruating, pregnant, and postmenopausal women. Acta. Endocrinol. (Copenh.), *48*:329–336.

Liu, F. T., and Lin, H. S., 1969. Role of insulin in body growth and in the growth of salivary and endocrine glands in rats. J. Dent. Res., *48*:559–567.

Modlin, J. F. 1975. Current status of mumps in the United States. Infection, *132*(1):106–109.

Rairkow, R. M., and Polayes, I. M. 1976. Diseases of the Salivary Glands. Philadelphia, W. B. Saunders Co.

Regezi, J. A., and Batsakis, J. G. 1977. Histogenesis of salivary gland neoplasms. Otolaryngol. Clin. North Am., *10*(2):297–307.

Schuller, D. E., and McCabe, B. F. 1977. Salivary gland neoplasms in children. Otolaryngol. Clin. North Am., *10*(2):399–412.

Townsend, G. L., Morimoto, A. M., and Kralemann, H. 1973. Management of sialorrhea in mentally retarded patients by transtympanic neurectomy. Mayo Clin. Proc., *48*:776–779.

Wilkie, T. F., and Brody, G. S. 1977. The surgical treatment of drooling. A ten year review. Plast. Reconstr. Surg., *59*(6):791–798.

Williams, H. B. 1975. Hemangiomas of the parotid gland in children. Plast. Reconstr. Surg., *56*(1):29–34.

Work, W. P. 1972. Newer concepts of first branchial cleft defects. Laryngoscope, *82*:1581–1593.

Wotman, S., Baer, L., Mandel, I. D., et al. 1970. Submaxillary potassium concentration in true and pseudo-primary aldosteronism. Arch. Intern. Med., *126*:248–251.

Wotman, S., Mandel, I. D., Thompson, R. H., et al. 1967. Salivary electrolytes, urea nitrogen, uric acid and salt taste thresholds in hypertension. J. Oral. Ther., *3*:239–250.

Wotman, S., Mercadente, J., Mandel, I. D., et al. 1973. The occurrence of calculus in normal children, children with cystic fibrosis, and children with asthma. J. Periodontol., *44*:278–280.

Zollar, L. M., and Mufson, M. A. 1970. Acute parotitis associated with parainfluenza 3 virus infection. Am. J. Dis. Child., *119*:147–148.

Chapter 52

TUMORS OF THE MOUTH AND PHARYNX

James M. Toomey, M.D., D.M.D.

Benign tumors are relatively common in the oral cavity of the child as compared to both the infrequent appearance of benign mass lesions in the oropharynx or hypopharynx and to the distinctly rare occurrence of malignancies in any of the sites in this age group (Table 52–1). However, Bhaskar (1963) has reported that only approximately 3 per cent of all tumors of the oral cavity, jaws, and salivary glands are seen in children. One may conclude, therefore, that tumors of any type are somewhat unusual in the young, and this fact, coupled with the wide variety of congenital and acquired oral and pharyngeal neoplasms encountered in the pediatric age group, underscores the need for the oto-laryngologist to have a systematized diagnostic approach to these lesions (Table 52–2).

The head and neck area, excluding the central nervous system, is the site of about 5 to 10 per cent of all childhood malignancies (Rush et al., 1963), while at the same time being the locus of 1 per cent or less of all head and neck cancers in all age groups (Ariel and Pack, 1960; Krolls and Hoffman, 1976). The few cancers arising in the oral cavity, oropharynx, or hypopharynx are more often of mesodermal than of ectodermal or endodermal origin, although this tendency is less marked than the 9:1 ratio of sarcomas to carcinomas described for all tumors in all sites in children might suggest (Jones and

Table 52–1 ESTIMATED RELATIVE FREQUENCY OF TUMORS OF THE MOUTH AND PHARYNX IN CHILDREN

Tumor Type	% of All Tumors	Tumor Subtypes	% of All Tumors	Comment
Benign	92%	Mesenchymal	78%	
		hemangioma	30%	Most common tumor
		epulis	27%	
		hamartoma	7%	
		Epithelial	14%	
		papilloma	8%	Most common epithelial tumor
Malignant	8%	Sarcoma		
		rhabdomyosarcoma	Sarcoma predominates;	Most common primary malignancy
		other sarcomas	number of reported	
		lymphoma/leukemia	cases too small to pro-	
		Carcinoma	duce meaningful figures	Least common single type

Table 52-2 CLASSIFICATION OF BENIGN AND MALIGNANT TUMORS OF THE MOUTH AND PHARYNX IN CHILDREN

I. *Oral Cavity*
   A. Benign tumors
      1. Labial, buccal, and palatal mucosa
         a. hemangioma
         b. lymphangioma
         c. fibrous tumors
         d. epithelial tumors
            1) white sponge nevus
            2) Heck disease
            3) papilloma
            4) dermoid cysts
            5) other cysts
         e. hamartomas and choristomas
         f. miscellaneous tumors
      2. Tongue and floor of the mouth
         a. hemangioma
         b. lymphangioma
         c. epithelial tumors—dermoid cysts
         d. other cystic lesions
            1) ranula
            2) branchial cysts
            3) thyroglossal duct cysts
         e. rests, hamartomas, and choristomas
         f. miscellaneous tumors
      3. The gingiva and jaws
         a. gingival tumors
            1) congenital epulis
            2) melanotic neuroectodermal tumor
            3) giant cell reparative granuloma
            4) hemangioma
            5) gingival hypertrophies
         b. odontogenic tumors
            1) cysts
            2) cementomas
            3) ameloblastomas
            4) myxomas
            5) central fibromas
         c. nonodontogenic tumors
            1) hemorrhagic cysts
            2) aneurysmal bone cysts
            3) solid tumors
               a) fibrous dysplasia
               b) cherubism
   B. Malignant tumors
      1. Oral soft tissues
         a. rhabdomyosarcomas
         b. other sarcomas
         c. epidermoid carcinomas
         d. miscellaneous malignancies
      2. Jaws
         a. Burkitt lymphoma
         b. fibrosarcoma
         c. osteogenic sarcoma
         d. Ewing sarcoma
         e. chondrosarcoma
II. *Pharynx*
   A. Benign tumors
      1. Primary tumors
      2. Tumors impinging upon the pharynx
   B. Malignant tumors
      1. Malignant lymphoma
      2. Rhabdomyosarcoma

Campbell, 1976). The fact that 40 of 48 reported cases of epidermoid carcinoma in children occurred in the mouth and pharynx again emphasizes the relative frequency of this tumor type in the mouth and pharynx (Moore, 1958).

The diagnostic identification of an oral or pharyngeal mass in a youthful patient can often be made with considerable accuracy if one combines a history of the age at which the mass appeared and its subsequent clinical evolution with careful inspection and palpation of the presenting lesion.

Details in the history should include information regarding the age of onset of the mass; the rapidity of its growth and extension; subsequent size increase, decrease, or stability; the relationship of tumor growth rate to growth rate of the child; random fluctuations in size; the presence or absence of inflammation, ulcerations, bleeding, or drainage; alterations in color, texture, or consistency; the presence of any local or referred pain; local or regional paresthesia or anesthesia; the presence of possibly associated, contiguous, or distant similar lesions or anomalies; family history of similar lesions; and the possible presence of any initiating events.

Physical examination should take note of the precise site, size, color, and texture of the tumor, whether it is sessile or pedunculated, fixed or mobile, tender or painless, mucosal or submucosal, ulcerated or infected, whether or not it blanches on pressure, transilluminates, is fluctuant, has a bruit, extends to or from neighboring structures, or tends to interfere in deglutition, speech, or respiration. The location and appearance of the mass should be related to known embryologic events in that locale.

In consequence, history and physical examination alone can identify a number of pediatric oral or pharyngeal tumors with considerable certainty (e.g., cavernous hemangiomas and torus palatinus) and others with probability (e.g., sublingual dermoid and lingual thyroid). Those lesions that continue to enlarge, interfere with function, cause persistent symptoms, or remain diagnostically obscure should be excised if accessible, or a biopsy should be taken to determine the need for additional therapy.

It is difficult in dealing with certain individual lesions of the oral and pharyngeal tissues in children to determine whether the mass is a true tumor or not, and, if so, what its subsequent biologic behavior will be. The fibromatous and fibroblastic tumors of the head and neck provide an example. An attempt will be made to identify these problem areas and to indicate where recent clarifying evidence is available.

ORAL CAVITY

Benign tumors of the labial, buccal, and palatal mucosae will be considered initially. Subsequently, nonmalignant lesions of the tongue and floor of the mouth and of the gingiva and jaws will be discussed. Finally, the malignant neoplasms of specific soft tissues and the jaws will be presented. This anatomic division of tumors in the mouth has the advantages of grouping certain particular varieties of tumors and of identifying similar or related structures, which may modify the clinical presentation or course of some of the tumors at certain sites.

Benign Tumors

In a study of 293 oral tumors in children, Bhaskar (1963) found that 91 per cent were benign and 9 per cent were malignant. Thirty-nine per cent of the tumors were found in the first four years of life, while the remaining 61 per cent appeared between ages 5 and 14. Males and females were about equally affected (47.5 and 52.5 per cent, respectively). Over two thirds of the lesions arose from oral soft tissues, with 27 per cent being derived from the jaws and 5 per cent from salivary glands. The four most common benign oral tumors were vascular and lymphatic (27 per cent), fibrous (15 per cent), odontogenic (15 per cent), and nonodontogenic (12 per cent). Further, in order of decreasing frequency, epithelial lesions, hamartomas or choristomas, salivary gland hemangiomas, miscellaneous soft tissue tumors, and a variety of other salivary gland masses were reported. The relatively large proportion of jaw lesions in this series may well reflect the dental origin of much of the patient material.

Benign Tumors of the Labial, Buccal, and Palatal Mucosa

Hemangiomas. Hemangioma is the single most common head and neck tumor of

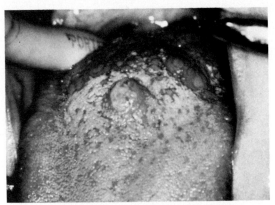

Figure 52–1 Pyogenic granuloma of the tongue. The sessile, fleshy, vascular appearance of the lesion is typical.

childhood (Batsakis, 1974; Bhaskar, 1963). In one large series the lip was most often involved, with the cheek and tongue being less common sites (Batsakis, 1974). In unusual instances other oral or pharyngeal structures may harbor a hemangioma.

Histologically an oral hemangioma may be cellular (juvenile), capillary, mixed, or cavernous. It has been proposed on the basis of transition areas in some such lesions that there may be a maturation of the cellular type to the capillary and thence to the cavernous variety (Batsakis, 1974). Clinical behavior can rarely be predicted on the basis of microscopic appearance alone.

Many oral hemangiomas are diagnosed in early infancy and may be malformations rather than true neoplasms. Others, which become evident later in childhood, may represent a local response to trauma, i.e., pyogenic granuloma (Fig. 52–1).

The oral lesions may be small and superficial, in which case they present as blue or purplish, sessile, compressible masses. More deeply seated hemangiomas are generally more extensive and are often recognized by age five. They are firm, less well defined, and may exhibit only irregular bluish discoloration through the overlying mucosa. Extensive replacement of the lip (macrocheilia) or of the tongue (macroglossia) has been described.

A number of syndromes may be recognized by associated vascular lesions. The angiomatous lesions of hereditary hemorrhagic telangiectasia appear frequently at the labial mucocutaneous junction or on the anterior tongue as friable, small, abnormal collections of vessels that may be spider-like, puncti-form, or nodular in type. Batsakis also mentions that the Sturge-Weber, Maffucci, or Von Hippel-Lindau syndromes can include oral vascular lesions (Batsakis, 1974). Juvenile nasopharyngeal angiofibroma has been described as having presented by eroding the palate.

The small, superficial, asymptomatic, nondeforming, clinically nonaggressive oral hemangioma can usually be observed for signs of spontaneous involution. More extensive, strategically located lesions, particularly if recurrent or bothersome to the patient, may later be treated by complete local excision. Cryosurgery offers an attractive alternative for treatment of large, partially accessible intraoral masses. There is no convincing evidence that benign hemangiomas give rise to malignant vascular tumors.

Lymphangiomas. Lymphangiomas are said to involve the oral cavity more often than any other area (Bhaskar, 1963). Some 50 to 60 per cent are recognized at birth and 80 to 90 per cent are evident by the end of the second year of life in relation to the period of greatest lymphatic growth (Bill and Summer, 1965).

According to the unified concept of lymphatic tumors proposed by Bill and Summer (1965), the histologic types of lymphangioma simplex (capillary type), cavernous lymphangioma, and cystic hygroma are variants of the same process, with histologic differences being dependent upon anatomic location. The typical appearance of a given variety in a particular site is related to that site in the sense that the larger, cystic lesions arise in the loose tissue planes of the neck, whereas the simple and cavernous types tend to occur in the more compact tissues of the lower face and mouth (Bill and Summer, 1965). The lips, cheek, and tongue are common locations for the latter lesions, the cavernous type predominating. Diffuse involvement of the lower lip may result in macrocheilia. Cystic hygroma may on occasion extend from the neck to involve the floor of the mouth, tongue, cheek, or parotid region.

Oral lymphangiomas generally appear as whitish or pink, fluctuant, superficial lesions that transilluminate. Larger and deeper tumors are usually ill-defined and woody with little mucosal color change.

Some of the smaller lesions may undergo spontaneous fibrous obliteration, whereas others may be excised locally if such a course

is clinically indicated. The larger, deeper, cavernous or cystic lesions are often difficult to eradicate surgically, largely because of their poorly defined interface with surrounding tissue.

Fibrous Tumors. Bhaskar (1963) noted that 15 per cent of his series of pediatric oral tumors were of fibrous tissue origin, but he did not elaborate further. The wide range of fibrous lesions that are found in the head and neck has been logically classified and described by Batsakis (1974) and need not be repeated here.

Dehner and Askin (1976) reported on 66 children with tumors of fibrous tissue origin, of which 33 per cent arose in the head and neck region. Five of the 22 head and neck lesions occurred in the oral cavity, three on the tongue, and one each on maxillary gingiva and retromolar trigone. The average age of the 22 patients was 5.7 years. Thirty-two per cent of the treated lesions recurred, and 4 per cent of the patients died of their disease. It was stated that adequate local surgery was generally successful.

True oral fibromas are probably unusual. It is at least very difficult to distinguish histologically between true benign fibrous neoplasms and induced hyperplasias.

Kaufman and Stout (1961) have reported upon two children with benign histiocytomas of the lip.

Extensive submucosal fibrosis of the oral cavity, which shows a marked predilection for natives of India, rarely occurs in children as young as 10 years. The palate, faucial pillars, buccal mucosa, and lower lip are especially affected. Severe late oral crippling, a lack of effective therapy, and an eventual association with oral carcinoma are typical sequelae.

Epithelial Tumors. White sponge nevus is a rare familial form of epithelial hyperplasia of the oral mucosa. The abnormality has been reported only in Caucasians, and males and females are equally affected. Fewer than 50 cases have been recorded (Kamalamma et al., 1970). The lesion appears at birth or later in childhood as a diffuse, whitish, thickened, folded-appearing, asymptomatic lesion, particularly involving the buccal mucosa, lips, floor of the mouth, and ventral surface of the tongue (Bhaskar, 1966a). Epithelial thickening and parakeratosis are seen microscopically. The lesions tend to progress but are felt to be entirely benign and to require no treatment.

Focal epithelial hyperplasia (Heck disease)

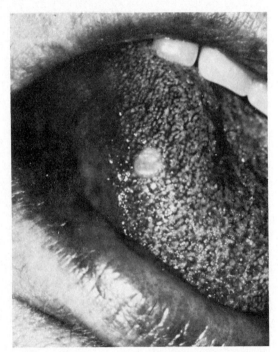

Figure 52–2 Squamous papilloma of the tongue. The tumor is white, firm, raised, and sharply demarcated.

is a familial form of epithelial hyperplasia found in children of American Indian parentage (Witkop and Niswander, 1965). Single cases have been reported in children of other races. Multiple soft, pale papules and confluent patches are evident on the oral mucosa, particularly on the lower lip. Acanthosis and parakeratosis are prominent histologically. No serious late sequelae have been identified.

Squamous papillomas of the oral mucosa are much less common in children than in adults (Fig. 52–2). Eversole and Sorensen (1974) recently reported the case of a 13 year old white male with Down syndrome who had florid confluent squamous papillomatosis of the lips, gingiva, buccal mucosa, tongue, palate, and oropharynx. Multiple papillomas of the lips, oral cavity, and oropharynx are also seen in association with multiple hamartomas of the skin, other mucosae, breast, GI tract, and thyroid in Cowden disease. Finally, Darier disease is an inherited abnormality in which crusted hyperkeratotic oral papular lesions exist in the absence of systemic findings (Greer et al., 1976).

A small number of dermoid cysts of the lip and palate have been presented in the literature. They usually occur at or near the midline as globular, submucosal masses of moderate size with a doughy feeling on palpation. Intraoral excision is generally indicated.

Among the occasional case reports of isolated epithelial cysts in the oral cavity of children has been that of Bhaskar (1966b) in which he noted the rare appearance of lymphoepithelial cysts in the mouth.

Hamartomas and Choristomas. These developmental abnormalities are relatively common in the tongue and will be described with benign lesions of that organ. However, the appearance of masses of unexpected tissue components in other oral locations should call this possibility to mind in the young child.

Miscellaneous Tumors. Mucoceles of the lip, cheek, or tongue appear as relatively common, small, pale, globular lesions in early life. Knapp (1970) has described single or multiple, 1 to 3 mm, smooth, pink, nodular masses of the oral cavity, which on the basis of histologic examination he termed oral tonsils. The soft palate is most often involved, and the floor of the mouth or tongue are involved less frequently. A small number of leiomyomas of the cheek have been recorded.

Multiple neuromas of the lip (bumpy lip syndrome), tongue, and larynx have been observed in association with pheochromocytomas, medullary carcinoma of the thyroid gland, and hyperparathyroidism (Sipple syndrome) (Bartley et al., 1976). Neurofibromas, either solitary or representing the oral manifestation of von Recklinghausen syndrome, are seen occasionally in pediatric patients. The plexiform type may be particularly difficult to control locally (Smith et al., 1977). Oral mucosal neurofibromas are also found in the neuropolyendocrine syndrome along with multiple endocrine adenomas and medullary carcinoma of the thyroid gland. Neurilemoma occurs rarely.

Fordyce disease (Fordyce granules) is a relatively common developmental abnormality in which ectopic sebaceous glands occur submucosally in the oral cavity, typically beneath the posterior buccal mucosa near the line of occlusion. The glands appear as 1 to 2 mm yellowish masses. They have no clinical significance.

Five teratomas of the face, attached to the host child in the region of the cheek, were reported by Gifford and MacCollum (1972). Neural elements predominated and early total excision was advised.

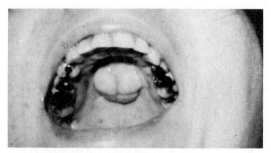

Figure 52–3 Torus palatinus. This bony, hard, midline palatal mass is lobulated and mucosa-covered.

Epignathi attached to the palate have been described by Jones and Campbell (1976) and by Mahour et al. (1974).

A torus is an exophytic, benign, bony overgrowth that most often arises in the oral cavity (in about 20 per cent of the general population), often at puberty, in the midline of the hard palate (Batsakis, 1974). There is, in addition, an 8 per cent incidence of tori on the lingual aspect of the mandible in the premolar region. The mass may be lobulated (Fig. 52–3). Although these are clearly not mucosal lesions, the overlying mucosa is ulcerated occasionally.

Benign Tumors of the Tongue and Floor of the Mouth

Hemangiomas. As mentioned previously, the tongue is the second or third most common intraoral site of hemangioma. On occasion, the floor of the mouth is the site of such a lesion. Extensive lesions may be successfully treated with one or several applications of cryosurgery (Figs. 52–4 and 52–5). Diffuse lingual hemangioma as a cause of macroglossia can almost always be distinguished easily from other forms of symmetrical enlargement of the tongue on the basis of its obvious vascular nature. Macroglossia may also represent an isolated congenital anomaly or may be due to lymphangiomatosis, plexiform neurofibromatosis, or mucopolysaccharidosis; or it may be part of Beckwith syndrome (visceromegaly, omphalocele, and hypoglycemia) (Beckwith, 1969).

Lymphangiomas. The tongue is a fairly frequent site of isolated capillary or cavernous lymphangioma, more often the latter. By contrast, the majority of lymphangiomas of the floor of the mouth contain a mixture of lymphangioma and cystic hygroma (Bill and Summer, 1965). In a few cases, cystic hy-

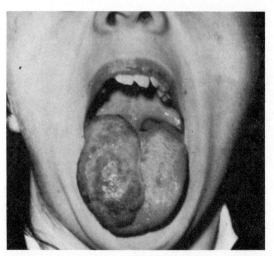

Figure 52–4 Extensive cavernous hemangioma of the tongue. The entire right half of the tongue is replaced by an irregularly nodular, purplish, compressible vascular mass.

groma may also extend into the tongue, although Batsakis (1974) points out that apparent lingual involvement may in fact represent an associated local lymphomatous malformation. Seven per cent of cystic hygroma patients are said to have this diffuse angiomatosis.

An isolated lymphangioma of the tongue or floor of the mouth often causes both some asymmetry and restriction of tongue movement. The lesion is somewhat rubbery on palpation. The surface mucosa may be pale and contain small translucent cysts.

Epithelial Tumors. Approximately 1.6 per cent of all dermoids and 20 per cent of head and neck dermoids occur in the oral cavity, and the vast majority of these are

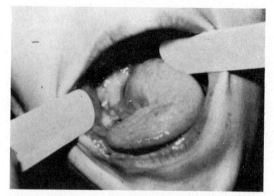

Figure 52–5 Cavernous hemangioma of the tongue. Same lesion as in Figure 52–4, 18 days following cryosurgery. The tumor has sloughed and healing is satisfactory.

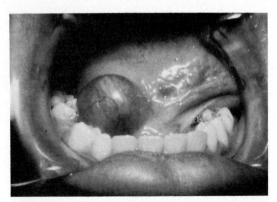

Figure 52–6 Ranula. The pale, cystic, translucent nature of this lesion of the floor of the mouth is evident.

located in the anterior part of the floor of the mouth. The tumor may be evident at birth or may not become manifest until the second or third decade of life (Resouly, 1976). The sexes are equally affected. Dermoids in the floor of the mouth may be located above the mylohyoid diaphragm and displace the tongue upward or they may appear below the mylohyoid where they produce a double chin effect. The lesions are found in or close to the midline. Seemingly aberrant dermoids are felt, in fact, to be choristomas in most, if not all, cases. Complete excision is the preferred treatment.

Cystic Lesions. A ranula is a large, lateralized, retention cyst of the floor of the mouth usually secondary to obstruction of the sublingual or another major salivary gland duct. A few may represent cervical sinus remnants (Batsakis, 1974). The lesion is mucosa-covered and typically has a translucent, bluish white, frog belly appearance (Fig. 52–6). Secondary salivary gland inflammation is rare. Treatment of the enlarging mass commonly takes the form of marsupialization, thus avoiding widespread dissection in the floor of the mouth.

Robins (1969) has discussed seven cases of sublingual branchial cleft cyst, all microscopically confirmed. His case was that of a four year old black female who had had a mass in the submental and submaxillary triangles since age one. Excision was performed through an external incision.

Thyroglossal duct cysts rarely may occur in the substance of the midline of the base of the tongue. It is important to distinguish this lesion from the more common lingual thyroid.

Rests, Hamartomas, and Choristomas. Lingual thyroid represents a rest of thyroid tissue that is found in the midline of the dorsum of the base of the tongue between the foramen cecum and the vallecula. The mass is globular, reddish, highly vascular, smooth or lobulated, firm or soft, and may have intact or superficially ulcerated mucosa covering it. The tumor may become clinically apparent at any time from birth through adulthood. Females are predominantly affected. Dysphagia is the most common presenting symptom, although a muffled voice, dyspnea, orthopnea, or hemorrhage are also seen. Normally functioning thyroid tissue is usually present in the mass. About 3 per cent of all lesions have malignant changes present. Uptake and scan studies are requisite to demonstrate the functional status of the mass and the presence or absence of functioning thyroid tissue elsewhere in the neck. Taking a biopsy specimen may induce necrosis and is not advised. Symptomatic masses may be handled by ablation and replacement therapy or by removal and autotransplantation of the tissue into a suitable skeletal muscle bed.

The tongue is the most common oral site for hamartomas. Tissues indigenous to the area comprise these tumor-like masses. Some authors consider granular cell myoblastoma to be a hamartoma. Choristomas of the region contain unexpected tissue such as glandular acini, glial tissue, cartilage, or bone (Krolls et al., 1971). Oral cysts containing gastric mucosa occur in the tongue or floor of the mouth of infants or young children and are felt to be choristomas (Gorlin and Jirasek, 1970). Choristomas, particularly if highly cellular, may be diagnostically confusing initially. Hamartomas and choristomas can generally be excised without difficulty.

Miscellaneous Tumors. Leiomyomas occur in the tongue as well as elsewhere in the oral cavity (Cherrick et al., 1973). Origin from undifferentiated mesenchyme, from smooth muscle of local blood vessels, or from both sources has been postulated.

Benign Tumors of the Gingiva and Jaws

A wide variety of mass lesions may arise in children from the gingival soft tissues or as odontogenic or nonodontogenic cysts or tumors of the mandible or maxilla. The precise incidence of these major types of lesion is difficult to ascertain largely because the smaller and more common lesions are either not treated or do not come to the attention of the pathologist. In general, however, it appears safe to say that gingival lesions are most common, odontogenic neoplasms next most frequent, and nonodontogenic tumors of the jaws least common.

Further confusion arises both from inaccurate classification of some lesions and from the continued use of ill-defined clinical terms such as epulis and epignathus. Epulis literally means "on the gum" and has been applied to (a) congenital epulis (granular cell tumor), (b) vascular epulis (hemangioma), (c) fibrous epulis (pyogenic granuloma), (d) epulis of pregnancy (granuloma graviderum), and (e) giant cell epulis (giant cell reparative granuloma). Thus, it is obvious that "epulis" is used to refer to any localized, fleshy, small-to-moderate-sized gingival mass regardless of its etiology or histology. Epignathus can indicate any mass present at birth and attached to the jaw(s), the hard palate, or both (Jones and Campbell, 1976). This latter term has been variously used to describe hamartomas, choristomas, or teratomas of the region present at birth and believed to be monozygotic in origin or examples of incomplete dizygotic twinning, whether these abnormalities arose in the jaws, palate, or nasopharynx.

Gingival Tumors. Localized benign tumors include congenital epulis, the melanotic neuroectodermal tumor of infancy, giant cell reparative granuloma, hemangioma, and pyogenic granuloma.

Congenital epulis is a rare, benign gingival tumor of the newborn that affects females 80 per cent of the time and occurs on the anterior maxillary gingiva in about 70 per cent of cases. Multiple lesions are seen occasionally. The mass is generally pink, spherical, lobulated, pedunculated, and mucosa-covered. It may range from 5 mm to 9 cm in greatest diameter (Custer and Fust, 1952). Microscopically the component cells resemble those of granular cell myoblastoma, although ultrastructural studies have suggested that the lesion may represent an abortive ameloblastoma (Kay et al., 1971). Local resection is indicated. Recurrences are unknown.

Melanotic neuroectodermal tumor of infancy has in the past been referred to by such terms as melanotic progonoma, retinal anlage tumor, or pigmented ameloblastoma. Fewer than 100 cases have been reported. In most instances the lesion becomes evident during the first six months of life as a 1 to 3 cm mass of the anterior maxilla near the junction of the globular and maxillary processes. The circumscribed mass is covered with mucosa through which grey, tan, brown, or black pigment is visible in some cases (Kaye et al., 1966). The mandible and remote sites are involved occasionally. Females are more commonly affected. The histopathology is said to be pathognomonic. A moderately vascular fibrous stroma divides the tumor cells into islands which in turn contain irregular, slit-like alveoli. The alveoli are lined with large cells, the abundant cytoplasm of which contains melanin. Smaller cells with dark nuclei and little cytoplasm fill the alveoli. Mitoses are absent (Batsakis, 1974). The mass displaces tooth buds. This fact coupled with microscopic observations tends to favor neuroectodermal derivation. Complete local excision is required. Recurrences are not uncommon (Jones and Campbell, 1976).

Giant cell reparative granuloma is a sessile, reddish mass of young vascular connective tissue containing multinucleated giant cells, which may present as a 4.5-cm or smaller lesion of the gingiva of either jaw in children or young adults. Boys and girls are equally affected (Dehner, 1973). The gingiva anterior to the premolars is most often involved. Central endosteal lesions are described below. It is felt that there is an underlying injury involved. Excision or curettage is usually curative, but the question of possible recurrence has not been settled.

Hemangioma has been described as a small, sessile, reddish lesion of the gingiva in a small number of cases. Pyogenic granuloma as a response to minor trauma is very likely a more common lesion of the gums and is often grossly and microscopically indistinguishable from hemangioma. A third similar gingival lesion, granuloma graviderum, is seen in the early part of pregnancy in some women.

Epstein pearls are small keratin cysts seen on the alveoli or palate of newborn infants. The lesions exfoliate within a few weeks.

In Caffey disease, bilateral firm soft tissue swellings occur over the mandible, along with local new bone formation, hyperirritability, and fever (Gorlin and Pindborg, 1964).

Diffuse enlargement of the gingiva may be either generalized or localized. Hereditary gingival fibromatosis is transmitted as an autosomal dominant and leads to generalized gingival hypertrophy, usually at the time of permanent tooth eruption, due to collagenous fibrous connective tissue accumulation. Hypertrichosis or cherubism are associated at times. Sporadic cases are termed idiopathic.

Acquired generalized gingival hypertrophy may be due to poor oral hygiene, diphenylhydantoin (Dilantin) ingestion, leukemia, the Sturge-Weber syndrome, cyclic neutropenia, or scurvy. Massive hyperplasia may be seen several months after beginning Dilantin therapy and regresses if the drug is discontinued. At least one third of childhood leukemics exhibit gingival enlargement that is spongy and friable and may be associated with other oral ulcerations or infiltrations. The Sturge-Weber syndrome can also lead to highly vascular gingival hypertrophy (Mostehy and Stallard, 1969).

Localized gingival enlargement takes the form of bilateral involvement in the region of the maxillary or mandibular tuberosities as a hereditary or idiopathic abnormality (Zagarelli et al., 1963) or may be found as a randomly located sporadic lesion in response to local irritation.

Persistent forms of gingival enlargement that do not respond to therapy in good-prognosis patients may require periodontal treatment and surgery.

Odontogenic Tumors. In a small percentage of cases any of a multitude of lesions of certain or probable odontogenic origin may expand intraorally to present as oral tumors. This possibility will be the major focus of this section. Among the lesions to be considered are odontogenic cysts, cementoma, dentinoma, odontoma, ameloblastoma, odontogenic myxoma, and odontogenic fibroma.

Odontogenic cysts may be periodontal, dentigerous, or primordial (Killey and Kay, 1966). Primordial cysts arise in the enamel organ before the formation of calcified structures, and they are more common in the mandible than the maxilla. The third molar region is a site of predilection. The tooth of origin is missing. The cyst may attain considerable size and extend through the cortex of the jaw. Dentigerous cysts arise in the enamel organ after amelogenesis is complete, and posterior mandible is again a frequent site. The formed associated teeth are unerupted or their eruption is delayed. These cystic lesions may also enlarge beyond the confines of the jaw of origin. Periodontal cysts that result from root canal infection are relatively

rare in children, and only a small percentage of that number enlarge to the point of producing external deformity of the bone.

In the basal cell nevus syndrome both jaws, particularly the mandible, often contain multiple keratocysts, which may reach several centimeters in size.

Cementoma, consisting of a mass of cementum around a tooth root apex; dentinoma, made up of a small paradental collection of dentin; or odontoma, a probably hamartomatous mixture of ameloblastic epithelium, dentine, cementum, and connective tissue, are all very unusual in childhood and rarely, if ever, become large enough to impinge upon the oral cavity.

Ameloblastoma is a benign odontogenic cystic neoplasm that is seen at times in children, particularly in tropical countries. Blacks are somewhat more commonly affected. The mandible is the area of usual involvement. The tumor is multicystic, osteolytic, and expansile, and the diagnosis may be made by the onset of a soft swelling in the mouth.

Most myxomas of the jaws are believed to be odontogenic in origin. One hundred and sixteen such cases had been reported by 1969 (Batsakis, 1974). Two thirds of myxomas of the jaws become apparent between 10 and 29 years of age, and the two jaws are equally affected, usually posteriorly. Not infrequently myxoma leads to loosening of the teeth locally and bulging of the contiguous bone. The tumor is locally aggressive and must be treated by rather wide excision if the reported 25 per cent recurrence rate is to be avoided.

Central fibroma of the jaws (usually the maxilla) has been reported in a small number of cases. It is not certain whether the lesion is of odontogenic derivation, nor can any certain statement be made regarding its incidence in children or its expansile capabilities.

Nonodontogenic Tumors of the Jaws. A considerable number of nonodontogenic cystic and solid tumors that may occur in the mandible or maxilla of the young patient can enlarge sufficiently to produce an intraoral mass. The bone cysts involved are the fissural, hemorrhagic, and aneurysmal types. Fissural cysts are presumed to arise from epithelial inclusions in embryonic lines of closure of from epithelial rests. These cysts are subclassified as nasopalatine, globulomaxillary, nasolabial, median mandibular, or median fissural according to their anatomic locations (Killey and Kay, 1966). In unusual cases in children any of these cysts is capable of enlarging sufficiently to produce a bulge within the mouth. Enucleation of the offending cyst is predictably curative.

Hemorrhagic cyst (solitary or traumatic bone cyst) is an idiopathic cavity most commonly found in the posterior portion of the mandible or the incisor region in males 10 to 20 years of age. In excess of 150 cases have been recorded (Huebner and Turlington, 1971). The etiology may be local trauma, and painless enlargement is the usual mode of presentation. Surgical obliteration may be required.

Aneurysmal bone cyst is rare and occurs most often as a honeycombed, enlarging mass in the body of the mandible in females. The cyst may be secondary to vascular changes initiated by a preexisting primary lesion of bone (Buraczewski and Dabska, 1971). The lesion is highly vascular and responds in most cases to curettage.

Solid, nonodontogenic jaw tumors, which have been reported to present or conceivably can present as intraoral swellings, include isolated osteoma, the multiple osteomas of Gardner syndrome, exostosis (torus mandibularis), hemangioma, lipoma, neurogenous tumors, the nonodontogenic varieties of fibroma and myxoma, fibrous histiocytoma, the fibrous gingival tumors associated with tuberous sclerosis, central giant cell reparative granuloma, bony involvement by histiocytosis X (particularly eosinophilic granuloma), the bone lesions of hyperparathyroidism, fibrous dysplasia, and cherubism. Space does not permit a detailed description of the clinical, radiologic, and pathologic features that help to differentiate among these tumors. However, if one encounters a youthful patient with an expansile lesion of the mandible or maxilla in whom there is no convincing clinical evidence for an odontogenic lesion, this nonodontogenic group of neoplasms should be considered. Fibrous dysplasia and cherubism as causes of major facial and oral deformity in childhood deserve mention.

Fibrous dysplasia of the jaw is usually monostotic and is not associated with the other stigmata of Albright syndrome. The process appears to be a hamartomatous replacement of bone with collagen, fibroblasts, and osteoid and exhibits its phase of rapid growth in the period from early childhood to adolescence. The lesion is generally unilateral and involves the maxilla more frequently than the mandible. Maxillary lesions tend to expand into the canine fossa and zygomatic areas and may, in addition, lead to proptosis. The mandibular angle is the common site of involvement of that bone, and painless swelling is the typical mode of clinical presentation. The dentition is usually not affected, and the lesion tends to stabilize with maturity. Deformity, pain, or interference with function are reasons for conservative subtotal resection. A late growth spurt, particularly following early radiotherapy, may herald sarcomatous change.

Cherubism is a developmental process of familial incidence in which bone is replaced by fibrous tissue with giant cells. The lesion is somewhat clinically similar but histologically different from fibrous dysplasia and may be microscopically similar but clinically unlike giant cell reparative granuloma. The process classically begins as a symmetrical fullness of both mandibular angle regions in the second or third year of life. Enlargement of the involved portions of the bones is greatest during the following one to two years and ceases at about 10 years of age with considerable regression of the lesion following puberty. Maxillary involvement is seen in approximately two thirds of cases. The deciduous teeth are shed prematurely, and the permanent teeth often fail to erupt into the mouth. The cherub-like appearance results from a combination of the rounded face and retraction of the lower eyelids, producing a "raised to heaven" effect (Batsakis, 1974). Pain or functional disability seldom occur, although reactive cervical lymph node hyperplasia is common. Surgical recontouring of cosmetically disturbing areas is the only therapy required in most patients. Occasional cases may be unilateral or otherwise atypical.

Malignant Tumors

Malignancies of the oral cavity are notably unusual in the pediatric age group. Approximately 5 to 10 per cent of all oral tumors in childhood fall into this category. The accumulated experience with many tumor types is so small that no meaningful generalizations can be made regarding relative incidence, biologic behavior, therapy, or prognosis. Three groups of lesions are sufficiently com-

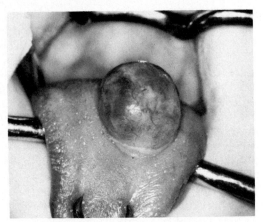

Figure 52–7   Rhabdomyosarcoma of the tongue in a 10 month old infant. The tumor appears innocent but had appeared recently and grown rapidly.

mon to permit the formulation of some useful conclusions. In descending order of frequency, these are rhabdomyosarcoma, other sarcomas, and epidermoid carcinoma. Again, however, absolute or relative incidence figures are difficult to ascertain.

Malignant Tumors of the Oral Soft Tissues

Rhabdomyosarcoma.   Rhabdomyosarcoma is an embryonic malignancy of skeletal muscle. It is the most common primary soft tissue head and neck cancer in children. A significant proportion of all rhabdomyosarcomas occur in the head and neck and, of these, about 30 per cent are found in the oral, pharyngeal, and nasopharyngeal cavities (Dito and Batsakis, 1963).

Li and Fraumeni (1969) studied the epidemiology of rhabdomyosarcoma and found five families among 698 patients in which a second child had a soft tissue sarcoma and in which other close relatives had a high incidence of early-onset breast and other cancers suggesting a familial syndrome of multiple primary neoplasms. They also noted that the tumor was not associated with congenital defects as are many other neoplasms of early inception and that there are no variations of incidence with time or place that might suggest environmental influences.

Within the oral cavity the tongue, palate, and cheek are relatively common sites of origin (Fig. 52–7). Among other structures reportedly involved have been gingiva, retromolar trigone, floor of the mouth, and the lip. Jones and Campbell (1976) state that

rhabdomyosarcoma is the commonest primary malignancy of the tongue in children.

In most instances the tumor appears during the first decade of life, and about 40 per cent are seen before age six. A small number of cases are congenital (less than 5 per cent) and a few occur in older age groups. Racial distribution is predominantly white.

Rhabdomyosarcoma nearly always presents as a mass which may or may not be symptomatic. Initially the mass may have an innocent polypoid appearance, but subsequent rapid growth, ulceration, and bleeding suggest the diagnosis. The bulk of the tongue tends to mask the tumor so that any asymmetric expanding mass of that organ in a young child must be considered as possible rhabdomyosarcoma. On the order of half the cases have until recently shown local recurrence, distant metastases or both; nodal metastases are not necessarily regional, and lung and bone spread is also common.

A microscopically embryonal tumor and a more differentiated pleomorphic type of tumor are recognized. Alveolar and botryoid varieties have also been described, but these may represent variants of the embryonal tumor. Most head and neck rhabdomyosarcomas are embryonal. However, the great majority of tongue lesions have pleomorphic characteristics.

Until recently survival rates in treated patients were discouragingly small. Of the 170 cases studied by Dito and Batsakis (1963), there was a 15.8 per cent three year survival rate and an 8.2 per cent five year survival rate. In 1973, Donaldson et al. reported that 74 per cent of 19 patients were alive two years after therapy consisting of local excision if possible, 6000 rads of radiotherapy, and chemotherapy with vincristine, actinomycin D, and cyclophosphamide. Similarly, Ghavimi et al. (1975) later recorded that 29 patients displayed no evidence of disease 4 to 42 months following surgical debulking, 4500 to 7000 rads of radiation, and long-term use of dactinomycin, Adriamycin, vincristine, and cyclophosphamide. The tumors in these two series were mostly not in the head and neck, but these short-term results are encouraging.

Other Oral Sarcomas.   The epidemiologic study of 696 childhood sarcomas by Chabalko et al. (1974) pointed out that the tumors were found primarily in the head and neck in younger children and in the lower extremities in adolescence. This, they felt, might be related to differences in the timing of rapid growth phases. Fifty-seven of 297 sarcomas studied in hospitalized patients were located in the head and neck. Among the specific sarcomas reported in pediatric patients have been fibrosarcoma (tongue, gingiva), leiomyosarcoma (palate, floor of the mouth, tongue, gingiva), angiosarcoma (lip, tongue), Kaposi sarcoma (unspecified secondary involvement), reticulum cell sarcoma (sites unspecified), and undifferentiated sarcoma (lip, cheek, palate, tongue). In general, therefore, almost any type of sarcoma can appear in the oral cavity of a child. The patient is usually in his earlier years and is found to have a bulky, infiltrating, often submucosal mass. The long-term results of combined surgical, radiotherapy and chemotherapy are usually fair to poor. Exceptions, as with well-differentiated fibrosarcoma, exist.

Epidermoid Carcinoma of the Mouth. The relative rarity of epidermoid carcinoma in this region is reflected in Conley's series (1970) of head and neck malignancies in children in which only 4 of 88 tumors were of this type. In a study of 9775 cases of oral squamous cell carcinoma, Krolls and Hoffman (1976) found that 0.05 per cent of the total occurred in patients up to 14 years of age and another 0.15 per cent in patients between 15 and 19 years of age. Further, in 1958, Moore found a total of 40 cases of squamous cancer of the mouth and pharynx in children in the literature, of which 8 were in the oral cavity (tongue — 4, lip — 2, gingiva — 1, unspecified site — 1). Fourteen years later Pichler et al. (1972), in their review, identified a total of 11 reported cases of tongue carcinoma.

Despite the restricted number of cases, Jones (1970) felt that certain generalizations could be made: tumor growth rate is rapid in the growing host, symptom duration is usually measured in weeks, regional metastases occur early, and no exogenous etiologic factors are obvious. Preexisting ectodermal defects may predispose a child to tumor formation (Lancaster and Fournet, 1969).

The tongue is the site of predilection, particularly at the junction of the anterior two thirds and the base. The lip, palate, and gingiva have also been reported sites.

Treatment is comparable to that in the adult, but salvage rates are certainly not as good.

Miscellaneous Oral Malignancies. Among other cancers found in the oral cavity of the child have been malignant mesenchymoma, neuroblastoma, neuroepithelioma, malignant paraganglioma, hemangiopericytoma, Hand-Schüller-Christian disease, lymphoma, mucoepidermoid carcinoma, adenoid cystic carcinoma, and melanoma. All are extremely rare. Finally, Li et al. (1975) found 19 second primary tumors in 414 long-term survivors of other childhood malignancies. Seventeen of these patients had received radiotherapy.

Malignant Tumors of the Jaws

Malignant jaw tumors tend to become clinically evident by causing some combination of expansion of the gingiva, loosening and displacement of teeth, soft tissue ulceration, toothache and local pain, paresthesia or anesthesia in the area, or trismus.

These tumors are very uncommon. For example, only 4 of the 189 head and neck childhood malignancies studied by Sutow and Matgue (1967) involved the jaws. It is, therefore, obvious that it is not possible to characterize the behavior of most specific tumor types. The lesions involved are essentially all mesodermal, and the ultimate prognosis is felt to be poor.

Sporadic reports have indicated that osteogenic sarcoma, fibrosarcoma, osteochondrosarcoma, chondrosarcoma, myxofibrosarcoma, Burkitt sarcoma, Ewing sarcoma, malignant fibrous histiocytoma, or carcinoma occur in the jaws of children. Wilms tumor metastatic to the mandible has also been documented.

Available information justifies some statements about the more common of these malignant tumors.

Burkitt lymphoma was originally described as a process in children of central Africa that often began as jaw tumors and later became generalized. It is now recognized that both the age and geographic distributions are much broader. Jaw involvement is not universal and attains its highest incidence at age three years. Males are more often afflicted, and the maxilla is involved twice as often as the mandible. A single posterior maxillary lesion is most often seen first, although multiple lesions of the maxilla or of both jaws may be present, especially if searched for roentgenographically. The tumor is osteolytic and is seen clinically as a whitish mass that expands the alveolus and loosens or displaces the teeth with minimal pain or paresthesia. Untreated patients die in four to six months. The process responds briskly to debulking of large lesions plus a number of cytotoxic agents. A 20 to 25 per cent long-term remission rate is induced, which may relate as much to the patient's immunologic response as to the therapy.

The majority of oral fibrosarcomas are periosteal in origin. More rarely a medullary-endosteal type occurs. The tumor is osteolytic and is associated with a high local recurrence and metastatic rate.

Osteogenic sarcoma appears to affect males and the mandible predominantly. It is usually a painful, osteolytic, multicystic malignancy with a poor prognosis.

Ewing sarcoma is more often found in the mandible. It probably originates in marrow and has a five year survival rate of about 15 per cent.

Chondrosarcoma tends to involve either the anterior maxilla or the posterior (angle) mandible.

PHARYNX

Neither the orpharynx nor the hypopharynx is at all a common site for tumor formation. As a result most of the available information consists of isolated case reports and anecdotal statements. Only a very few lesions, most notably malignant lymphoma of the oropharynx, have been reported often enough to justify any meaningful statements regarding their specific behavior in the rather large area extending from the level of the soft palate to the cricoid. Benign lesions are more frequently encountered than malignant lesions.

Benign Tumors

An impressive variety of benign lesions may exist in the pharynx of the child. These may represent developmental errors, acquired neoplasia, reaction to local irritation or inflammation, or impingement upon the pharyngeal cavity from masses in contiguous areas.

Tumors that have been reported include hamartoma, choristoma, hemangioma, rhab-

domyoma, melanotic neuroectodermal tumor plus brain heterotopia, granular cell myoblastoma, leiomyoma, lipoma, myxoma, fibrous histiocytoma, papilloma, teratoma, pleomorphic adenoma, neurofibroma, localized fibrous lesions, fibromatous polyp, or pyogenic granuloma. Fibromatous polyp is generally seen as a sessile mass of variable size projecting from the posterior hypopharyngeal wall. It probably represents herniation of adipose or fibrous tissue through a portion of the pharyngeal wall weakened by injury or inflammation. Pyogenic granuloma may appear anywhere in the pharynx as a reaction to minor trauma, but such lesions in the tonsillar region can specifically be caused by endotracheal intubation.

The wall of the pharynx can be impinged upon by branchial cleft cysts, neurofibromas, or other cervical or parapharyngeal space masses. In addition, any of a number of polypoid nasopharyngeal tumors may present in the mesopharynx. This latter group includes dermoids (hairy polyp), other teratomas, gliomas, and, on rare occasions, angiofibroma, antrochoanal polyp, or chordoma.

If any of the benign tumors primary in the oropharynx or hypopharynx are enlarging, symptomatic, or otherwise the source of concern, an excisional biopsy should be obtained.

Malignant Tumors

Malignant lymphoma and rhabdomyosarcoma are the two most frequently encountered mesopharyngeal or hypopharyngeal cancers. Sporadic reports of other lesions, such as fibrosarcoma of the oropharynx or epidermoid carcinoma of the hypopharynx or tonsil in childhood, have been made.

Malignant lymphoma is most frequently diagnosed as a tumor of the oropharynx in children of from 5 to 10 years of age. The tumor may be found in the structures of the Waldeyer ring (tonsil or base of tongue) or the pharyngeal wall proper. If the former is involved, cervical nodes are usually also positive. In either case no conclusion can be reached about possible infradiaphragmatic disease without a specific search for disseminated tumor. The diagnosis is suggested by a bulky, enlarging oropharyngeal mass, particularly if one tonsil is involved. There may be difficulty swallowing, snoring, a muffled voice, or stridor. If a tonsil is the site of the tumor its normal cryptitic appearance is often replaced by a cauliflower-like neoplasm, the surface of which may be ulcerated or hemorrhagic. Cervical nodes, especially the jugulodigastric, may well be palpable. An excisional biopsy of the affected tonsil is indicated. If the process is limited to the pharynx, radiotherapy may be effective. Chemotherapy is reserved for systemic disease.

Rhabdomyosarcoma of the pharynx is of the embryonal type in most cases. The region is one of the least often affected in the head and neck. In the oropharynx the tumor may arise beneath the tonsil and pharyngeal wall and thus initially may mimic peritonsillar, retropharyngeal, or lateral pharyngeal abscess. Treatment is the same as for the tumor in other sites.

SELECTED REFERENCES

Batsakis, J. G. 1974. Tumors of the Head and Neck. Baltimore, Williams and Wilkins.
Most of the head and neck tumors commonly encountered in infants and children are described in a concise and accurate way that reflects recent pathologic opinion. A number of controversial groups of lesions are covered effectively.

Bhaskar, S. N. 1963. Oral tumors of infancy and childhood. J. Pediatr., 63:195.
This is an excellent review of a series of 293 oral tumors in children. Appropriate statistics are provided. Clinical descriptions of the major lesions are supplemented with numerous illustrations.

Jones, P. G., and Campbell, P. E. (Eds.) 1976. Tumors of Infancy and Childhood. London, Blackwell Scientific Pub. Chapter 14, Tumors of the head and neck, pp. 295–396.
This is a well-organized, complete, and clearly presented overview of the spectrum of pediatric head and neck tumors. An extensive list of references is provided.

REFERENCES

Ariel, I. M., and Pack, G. T. (Eds.) 1960. Cancer and Allied Diseases of Infancy and Childhood. Boston, Little, Brown & Co., pp. 51–98.

Bartley, P. C., Lloyd, H. M., and Aitken, R. E. 1976. Medullary carcinoma of the thyroid, multiple pheochromocytoma, mucosal neuromas, Marfanoid habitus and other abnormalities (Sipple's syndrome). Med. J. Aust., 2:1973.

Batsakis, J. G. 1974. Tumors of the Head and Neck. Baltimore, Williams and Wilkins Co.

Beckwith, J. B. 1969. Macroglossia, omphalocele, adrenal cytomegaly, gigantism and hyperplastic viscceromegaly. Birth Defects, 5(2):188.

Bhaskar, S. N. 1963. Oral tumors of infancy and childhood. J. Pediatr., 63:195.

Bhaskar, S. N. 1966a. Oral lesions in infants and children. Dent. Clin. North Am., July, 421–435.

Bhaskar, S. N. 1966b. Lymphoepithelial cysts of the oral cavity. Oral Surg., 21:120.

Bill, A. H., Jr., and Summer, D. S. 1965. A unified concept of lymphangioma and cystic hygroma. Surg. Gynecol. Obstet., 120:79.

Buraczewski, J., and Dabska, M. 1971. Pathogenesis of aneurysmal bone cyst: relationship between the aneurysmal bone cyst and fibrous dysplasia of bone. Cancer, 28:597.

Chabalko, J. J., Creagan, E. T., and Fraumeni, J. F., Jr. 1974. Epidemiology of selected sarcomas in children. J. Natl. Cancer Inst., 53:675.

Cherrick, H. M., Dunlap, C. E. and King, O. H., Jr. 1973. Leiomyomas of the oral cavity. Oral Surg., 35:54.

Conley, J. 1970. Concepts in Head and Neck Surgery. New York, Grune and Stratton, p. 187.

Custer, R. P., and Fust, J. A. 1952. Congenital epulis. Am. J. Clin. Pathol., 22:1044.

Dehner, L. P. 1973. Tumors of the mandible and maxilla in children. I. Clinicopathological study of 46 histologically benign lesions. Cancer, 31:364.

Dehner, L. P., and Askin, F. B. 1976. Tumors of fibrous tissue origin in childhood. Cancer, 38:888.

Dito, W. R., and Batsakis, J. G. 1963. Intra-oral, pharyngeal and nasopharyngeal rhabdomyosarcomas. Arch. Otolaryngol., 77:123.

Donaldson, S. S., Castro, J. R., Wilbur J. R., et al. 1973. Rhabdomyosarcoma of head and neck in children. Cancer, 31:26.

Eversole, L. R., and Sorenson, H. W. 1974. Oral florid papillomatosis in Down's syndrome. Oral Surg., 37:202.

Ghavimi, F., et al. 1975. Multidisciplinary treatment of embryonal rhabdomyosarcoma in children. Cancer, 35:677.

Gifford, G. H., and MacCollum, D. W. 1972. Facial teratomas in the newborn. J. Plast. Reconst Surg., 49:616.

Gorlin, R. J., and Pindborg, J. J. 1964. Syndromes of the Head and Neck. New York, McGraw-Hill Book Co. pp. 325–330.

Gorlin, R. J., and Jirasek, J. E. 1970. Oral cysts containing gastric or intestinal mucosa. Arch. Otolaryngol., 91:594.

Greer, R. O., Jr., Pooper, H. A., and DeMento, F. J. 1976. Cowden's disease (multiple hamartoma syndrome). Report of a limited mucocutaneous form. J. Periodontol., 47:531.

Huebner, G. R., and Turlington, E. G. 1971. So-called traumatic (hemorrhagic) bone cysts of the jaws. Oral Surg., 31:354.

Jones, J. H. 1970. Oral carcinoma in the young patient with a report of two cases. Brit. J. Oral Surg., 8:159.

Jones, P. G., and Campbell, P. E. (Eds.) 1976. Tumors of the head and neck. *In* Tumors of Infancy and Childhood. London, Blackwell Scientific Pub. pp. 295–396.

Kamalamma, M. K., et al. 1970. The white sponge nevus. Oral Surg., 30:51.

Kaufman, S. L., and Stout, A. P. 1961. Histiocytic tumors (fibrous xanthoma and histiocytoma) in children. Cancer, 14:469.

Kay, S., Elzay, R., and Willson, M. 1971. Ultrastructural

observations on a gingival cell tumor (congenital epulis). Cancer, *27*:674.

Kaye, B. L., Robinson, D. W., Masters, F. W., et al. 1966. Tumors of the premaxilla in children: report of two unusual cases and a review. Plast. Reconstr. Surg., *37*:131.

Killey, H. C., and Kay, L. W. 1966. Benign Cystic Lesions of the Jaws. Edinburgh and London, E. & S. Livingstone, Ltd.

Knapp, M. J. 1970. Oral tonsils: location, distribution and histology. Oral Surg., *29*:155.

Krolls, S. O., Jacoway, J. R., and Alexander, W. N. 1971. Osseous choristomas (osteomas) of intraoral soft tissues. Oral Surg., *32*:588.

Krolls, S. O., and Hoffman, S. 1976. Squamous cell carcinoma of the oral soft tissues: a statistical analysis of 14,253 cases by age, sex and race of patients. J. Am. Dent. Assoc., *92*:571.

Lancaster, L., and Fournet, L. F. 1969. Carcinoma of the tongue in a child. J. Oral Surg., *27*:269.

Li, F. P., and Fraumeni, J. F. 1969. Rhabdomyosarcoma in children: epidemiologic study and identification of a familial cancer syndrome. J. Natl. Cancer Inst., *43*:1365.

Li, F. P., Cassady, J. R., and Jaffe, N. 1975. Risk of second tumors in survivors of childhood cancer. Cancer, *35*:1230.

Mahour, G. H., Woolley, M. M., Trivedi, S. N., et al. 1974. Teratomas in infancy and childhood: experience with 81 cases. Surgery, *76*:309.

Moore, C. 1958. Visceral squamous cancer in childhood. Pediatrics, *21*:573.

Mostehy, M. R., and Stallard, R. E. 1969. The Sturge-Weber syndrome: its periodontal significance. J. Periodontol., *40*:243.

Pichler, A. G., Williams, J. R., and Moore, J. A. 1972. Carcinoma of the tongue in childhood and adolescence: report of a case and review of the literature. Arch. Otolaryngol., *95*:178.

Resouly, A. 1976. Sublingual dermoids. J. Laryngol. Otol., *90*:487.

Robins, R. B. 1969. Sublingual branchial cleft cyst: a case report. Laryngoscope, *79*:288.

Rush, B. F. Jr., Chambers, R. G., and Ravitch, M. M. 1963. Cancer of the head and neck in children. Surgery, *53*:210.

Smith, R. F., Toomey, J. M., and Snyder, G. G., III. 1977. Facial plexiform neurofibroma. Laryngoscope, *87*:2101.

Sutow, W. W., and Montague, E. D. 1967. Pediatric tumors. *In* MacComb W. S., and Fletcher, G. H. (Eds.) Cancer of the Head and Neck, Baltimore, Williams and Wilkins, pp. 428–446.

Witkop, C. J., and Niswander, J. D. 1965. Focal epithelial hyperplasia in Central and South American Indians and Latinos. Oral Surg., *20*:213.

Zagarelli, E. V., Kutscher, A. H., and Lichtenthal, R. 1963. Idiopathic gingival fibromatosis: report of 20 cases. Am. J. Dig. Dis., *8*:782.

Chapter 53

CONGENITAL MALFORMATIONS OF THE ESOPHAGUS

John C. Adkins, M.D.
William B. Kiesewetter, M.D.

Most congenital esophageal malformations manifest themselves early by rendering feeding difficult or impossible or by causing respiratory difficulty. Yet diagnosis of some of these abnormalities eludes all but the most tenacious investigative approaches. Although it is incumbent upon the physician to diagnose these disorders correctly before their complications jeopardize the life or development of the patient, overzealous use of diagnostic tests can pose as much of a threat to the child as the malformation itself. The following outline of outstanding features of important lesions affecting the esophagus and our discussion of the diagnosis and management of these disorders should guide the physician along the thin line between diagnosis and overstudy for these congenital problems.

ESOPHAGEAL ATRESIA AND TRACHEOESOPHAGEAL FISTULA

Thomas Gibson, in 1696, was the first to mention tracheoesophageal fistula and esophageal atresia. More than a century passed before other reports of cases began to trickle into the literature. The disorder was uniformly fatal, although surgical attempts at repair or palliation were made at the turn of this century (Hoffman, 1899; Brennemann, 1913). In 1939, Ladd and Leven, within 24 hours of each other, performed gastrostomy as the initial step in the first successful surgical approaches to complete reconstruction of the esophagus as treatment for this disorder (Ladd, 1944; Leven, 1940–41). They ulti-

mately fashioned antethoracic skin tubes to connect the upper esophagus with the stomach. Cameron Haight, in 1941, performed the first successful primary end-to-end repair of the esophagus in a 13 day old girl (Haight and Towsley, 1943). After a half century of frustration in trying to find a treatment for children with esophageal atresia or tracheoesophageal fistula, surgeons not only developed a technique that allowed their survival but within 16 months had also developed a standard surgical technique that is still viable.

Embryology

Between 21 and 23 days of gestation the primitive trachea, bronchi, and lung buds appear as a ventral pouch on the foregut. During the next seven to nine days in normal development the tracheoesophageal septum proliferates and elongates, pinching off the trachea from the esophagus. Smith (1957) gives the most convincing explanation for the teratology of anomalies that occur during this last step. At about 26 days, paired lateral esophageal grooves indent the lateral walls of the esophagus from the trachea obliquely in a dorsocaudal direction. He postulates that these grooves for some reason may meet within the lumen and coalesce, obliterating the esophageal lumen. Tracheoesophageal fistulae result from incomplete development of the tracheoesophageal septum. A variety of forms of coalescence of the lateral esophageal grooves and the septum may occur; the particular anomaly that develops would depend on the type of coalescence which occurred.

Classification and Incidence

Numerous schemata for classifying these anomalies have been proposed in the past, giving rise to considerable confusion. We shall avoid this by using the anatomic description of the particular anomaly being considered. The most useful categorization to date is that by Kluth (1976).

The anomaly appears once in every 3000 to 5000 live births. Figure 53–1 shows the more frequently encountered variations of the anomaly, and the frequency of each is among 1058 infants reported upon by Holder et al. (1964) for the Surgical Section of the American Academy of Pediatrics.

The cause of tracheoesophageal fistula with esophageal atresia is unknown, but there are several reports of its repeated occurrence

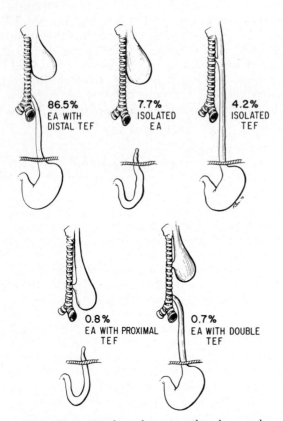

Figure 53–1 Esophageal atresia and tracheoesophageal fistula. A schematic representation of the more common anomalies within the complex. The rarer varieties are not depicted. EA, esophageal atresia; TEF, tracheoesophageal fistula.

in families (Hausmann et al., 1957) (see Fig. 53–4).

Presentation and Diagnosis

Eighty-five per cent of children with esophageal atresia alone and 32 per cent of those with atresia with fistula (Waterston et al., 1963) have a gestational history of hydramnios. Conversely, 7 per cent of children with such a history will have esophageal atresia (Scott and Wilson, 1957). Any child with such a history must be suspected of having this lesion.

We favor the routine passage of a soft No. 8 or No. 10 French catheter through the mouth and into the stomach, with aspiration of gastric contents, as part of the initial examination of the newborn. Inability to pass the catheter or the presence of more than 30 ml of gastric fluid is abnormal and warrants further investigation. Inability to pass the catheter indicates esophageal obstruction; the presence of excess gastric fluid indicates gastric or upper intestinal obstruction (Quinn, 1971). Although complications such as bleeding and pharyngeal perforation (Girdany et al., 1969; Heller et al., 1977) have rarely occurred with this procedure, the early diagnosis of children with esophageal atresia or upper gastrointestinal obstructive anomalies supports the use of this technique. Figure 53–2 presents a radiograph of an infant with the catheter curled in the obstructed upper pouch, a sign pathognomonic of esophageal atresia. If the catheter seems to pass but gastric contents cannot be aspirated, anteroposterior and lateral radiographs will demonstrate whether the catheter has passed posteriorly down the esophagus or anteriorly into the trachea.

Contrast studies, if necessary, should not be performed except at the hospital where definitive surgery is to be performed, and then only with the responsible surgeon in attendance. We have rarely needed such studies to make a diagnosis, but when performed they are best done using 0.5 ml injections of sterile, finely dispersed barium. A water-soluble contrast medium such as meglucamine diatrizoate (Gastrografin), if aspirated, will spark a fulminant pneumonitis. Figure 53–3 shows the roentgenogram of a child into whom the proper amount of barium was instilled. More than one infant has been referred to us after an unnecessary

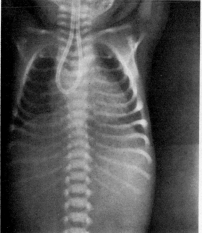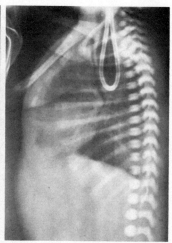

Figure 53–2 Esophageal atresia demonstrated by curled catheter in the upper esophageal pouch. This technique is the recommended one for establishing the diagnosis. Absence of gas within the abdomen strongly suggests the absence of a fistula.

and improperly performed barium swallow has resulted in massive aspiration. The aspiration invariably has caused a most stormy bout of pneumonia in an infant whose condition is already precarious.

Absence of air in the abdomen ordinarily indicates that there is no distal fistula (Fig. 53–2).In cases of esophageal atresia without fistula, the distal portion of the esophagus is short, extending only a centimeter or two above the diaphragm; for this reason, the possibility of primary esophageal anastomosis is remote in these cases.

The child whose anomaly is not discovered at the time of the neonatal examination will usually be described as having excessive salivation or mucus, choking, and, except in

cases of isolated tracheoesophageal fistula without esophageal atresia, an absolute inability to take feedings. These symptoms mandate that the physician use the catheter technique described to verify the presence of the anomaly.

The *isolated tracheoesophageal fistula* may be subtle in its presentation and elusive in its diagnosis. It is often missed in the neonatal period, and its presence is suggested later by recurrent bouts of pneumonia, coughing episodes when fed, or unexplained periods of abdominal distention. The diagnosis may be made by careful cineradiography (Fig. 53–4); positioning the child in the prone, head-down position during the study will enhance the likelihood that a small fistula will be

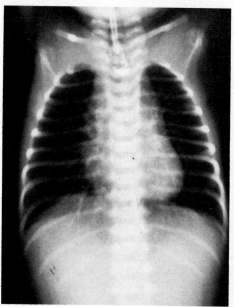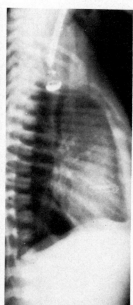

Figure 53–3 Esophageal atresia demonstrated by barium instillation. When necessary, this method of contrast illumination will outline the pouch and simultaneously minimize aspiration by overflow or via a proximal fistula.

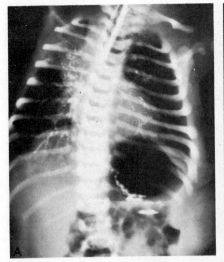
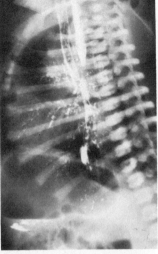
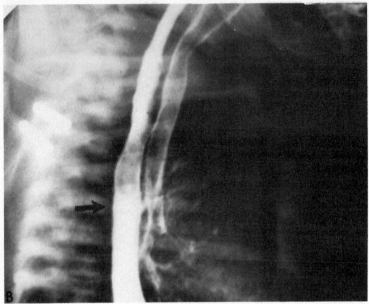

Figure 53–4 The father of this 6 week old baby had been operated upon 21 years previously for esophageal atresia with tracheoesophageal fistula. Since birth, she had had several episodes of apparent aspiration when feeding, as well as multiple bouts of abdominal distention with crying. A barium swallow did not demonstrate any fistula. Suddenly on this examination, the fistula opened, outlining the trachea generously and causing some aspiration. Only a mild pneumonia occurred. *A,* Anteroposterior and lateral films do not definitely demonstrate the fistula. *B,* From the cineradiographic study, this frame nicely demonstrates the fistula to be located considerably lower than usual (arrow)

detected (Keats and Smith, 1973). When the presence of this fistula is strongly suggested by the persistence of symptoms but it cannot be confirmed radiologically, endoscopic procedures may show the fistula as a dimple in the membranous trachea. Methylene blue instilled into the esophagus will occasionally bubble through the fistula into the trachea when the fistula could not otherwise be seen. We agree with the recommendation that exploration for an isolated tracheosophageal fistula is *never* indicated unless the fistula has been demonstrated.

The evaluation of children with esophageal anomalies must include a careful search for other abnormalities that may have a strong bearing upon the care of the child. Table 53–1 lists the common, associated anomalies encountered in the Surgical Section survey (Holder et al., 1964). The presence of many of these anomalies or of prematurity will have a substantial impact on the management and mortality of these children (Holder et al., 1964). Many authors have elaborated upon the diagnosis and management of these associated anomalies (Weigel and Kaufmann, 1976; Quan and Smith, 1973; Bachiller et al., 1976; Landing, 1975).

Treatment

Preparation. Once the diagnosis of esophageal atresia, tracheoesophageal fistula, or both has been established, the usual care of the newborn (including temperature control and proper hydration) must be continued. A Replogle sump tube (Replogle, 1963) is positioned in the upper esophageal pouch and connected to low suction in order to avoid aspiration of saliva. Antibiotics are administered routinely because of the possibility of aspiration; the infant who presents with pneumonia requires even more strenuous efforts to avoid worsening of this potentially lethal complication.

Although some surgeons practice a less aggressive approach, we strongly recommend that these anomalies be handled as surgical emergencies. Even with a perfectly functioning Replogle sump tube, the distal esophageal fistula can reflux gastric secretions into the trachea, initiating one of the most virulent forms of pneumonitis. In addition, breathing and crying insufflate much air into the stomach. Such abdominal distention will further compromise ventilation as well as result in reflex vomiting up through the fistula.

In preparation for operation, the chest radiograph must be carefully studied to determine the level of the upper pouch, to detect evidence of congenital heart disease, and to rule out the presence of a right aortic arch. (If the arch lies on the right, cardiac anomalies are more likely to be present, and, of more immediate importance, any esophageal anastomosis will be made much more difficult or impossible to perform through the standard right thoracotomy incision.)

Operation. At the time of surgery the child initially undergoes a routine Stamm gastrostomy; care must be taken to anchor the stomach securely to the anterior abdominal wall; we prefer to use Malecot catheters, No. 20 or larger, for this procedure. The baby is then positioned for a right lateral thoracotomy through the bed of the fourth rib (unless the presence of a right aortic arch necessitates a left-sided approach). An extrapleural approach is preferred because of the better survival rate in case of an anastomotic leak. The fistula is identified and divided at the level of the trachea. The trachea is closed with a continuous interlocking 5-0 silk suture *during division* to minimize the air leak. Care is taken neither to narrow the trachea nor to leave a posterior tracheal pouch. The upper esophageal pouch is then identified and dissected. The anesthetist can facilitate this identification by passage of a stiff No. 10 French catheter into the pouch. Dissection of the pouch is carried as high as possible, taking care not to injure the trachea anteriorly or the vagi laterally. The anterior dissection should be careful and complete as, rarely, a proximal fistula may be present and may only be discovered in this manner.

Figure 53–5 depicts the anastomotic techniques currently practiced. At present, we feel the Haight anastomosis is the safest, although each anastomosis has its own drawbacks. These are discussed in the figure legend.

Table 53–1　ASSOCIATED ANOMALIES IN 1058 PATIENTS WITH ESOPHAGEAL ATRESIA AND/OR TRACHEOESOPHAGEAL FISTULA

Anomalies	Number		Per Cent	
None	553		52	
Associated anomalies (849 anomalies)	505		48	
Congenital heart disease	201		19	
Gastrointestinal	134		13	
Intestinal atresia		38		3.6
Malrotation		21		2.0
Genitourinary	109		10	
Imperforate anus	99		9.4	
Musculoskeletal	91		8.6	
Arm and hand		45		4.3
Hemivertebrae		19		1.8
Face	53		5.0	
Cleft lip and/or palate		28		2.6
Central nervous system	35		3.3	
Down syndrome	28		2.6	
Larynx, trachea, and lung	19		1.8	
Diaphragm	17		1.6	
Vascular	11		1.0	
Liver and spleen	8		0.8	
Miscellaneous	43		4.1	

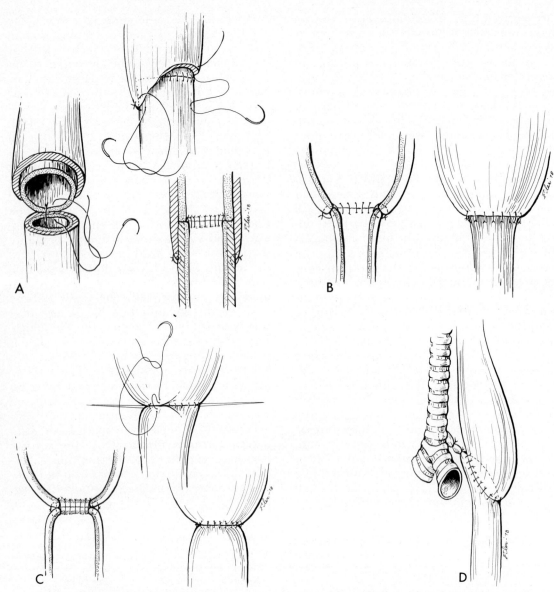

Figure 53-5 *A*, Haight anastomosis. Advantage: low incidence of leakage. Disadvantages: (1) increased tension on anastomosis, (2) high (36 per cent) incidence of anastomotic stricture. *B*, Single-layer anastomosis. Advantages: (1) rapidly performed, (2) reduced tension on anastomosis, (3) low (19 per cent) incidence of anastomotic stricture. Disadvantage: somewhat higher incidence of leakage. *C*, Two-layer anastomosis. Advantage: moderate incidence of leakage. Disadvantages: (1) technically difficult, (2) increased tension on anastomosis, (3) high incidence of stricture. *D*, Duhamel anastomosis. Advantages: (1) reduced tension, (2) widely patent anastomosis. Disadvantage: increased incidence of recurrent fistula.

The esophagus at the level of the fistula is dissected as little as possible because of its precarious blood supply, derived from the intercostal vessels. After completion of the esophageal anastomosis, a judgment can be made regarding the tension on it. If this tension is excessive, it is prudent to oversew the distal esophagus at the level of the fistula, perform a cervical esophagostomy on the left,

and plan a colon interposition at a later date. Staged repair, with upper pouch bougienage and stretching preparatory to a second attempt at end-to-end anastomosis, has not been satisfactory in our experience. Hendren has reported the successful use of intermittent electromagnetic bougienage in these cases (Hendren and Hale, 1976).

The isolated tracheoesophageal fistula can

usually be approached satisfactorily through a cervical incision, since most of these fistulas occur in the neck. The placement of a ureteral catheter across the fistula preoperatively greatly facilitates its identification at the time of surgery. Care must be exercised to avoid injuring the laryngeal nerves during such a procedure.

Care of the infant after repair of an esophageal atresia or tracheoesophageal fistula requires the facilities and expertise of a neonatal intensive care unit. Frequent suctioning of the infant's pharynx is necessary to prevent aspiration before the anastomosis functions. A barium swallow is done after seven days, and if no leak is present, oral feedings are initiated. The gastrostomy tube is left in place until the surgeon is reasonably certain that there is no anastomotic stricture.

The child who requires gastrostomy and esophagostomy can be started on gastrostomy feedings after three days. It is important to give simulated oral feedings simultaneously in order to maintain the infant's ability to swallow and to associate oral feeding with relief of hunger. Otherwise, after colon interposition, the child will have to learn to swallow and this may be difficult.

Complications

An acute, massive, postoperative pneumothorax almost always signals dehiscence of the anastomosis. Prompt reoperation and the performance of an esophagostomy are necessary if the baby is to survive. Smaller anastomotic disruptions may be heralded by the presence of saliva in the chest tube, and these can be treated conservatively with antibiotics. They almost always close spontaneously, but it may be necessary to reoperate if the child becomes septic and remains so. Tiny leaks may show up only at the time of the postoperative esophagogram, and they are usually self-limited. Fortunately, the use of the extrapleural approach mitigates the effect of an anastomotic leak, avoiding the devastating effects of empyema.

The sudden postoperative appearance of choking or the abrupt development of pneumonia may herald recurrence of the tracheoesophageal fistula. This may occur at any time up to a month or more following the operation. When the recurrence has been clearly demonstrated it is necessary to reoperate, but the results of this second surgery are generally good. The Duhamel type of anastomosis is particularly subject to recanalization of the fistula.

Fixed narrowing of the anastomosis as noted by fluoroscopic esophagography indicates the presence of a stricture. Enlargement of the upper esophageal pouch may persist despite an adequate anastomosis. Esophageal strictures are by far the most common postoperative complications. In a study of 127 patients at the Children's Hospital of Pittsburgh who underwent repair of the common upper pouch–lower fistula anomaly, 40 (31 per cent) developed strictures that required dilatations more than four times. Haight and two-layer anastomoses were particularly subject to this complication. If an anastomotic leak occurs, the patient is at high risk of developing a stricture. The gastrostomy tube should be left in place in a patient who has a leak or who has a narrowing of the esophagus demonstrated by esophagography. Early "calibration" of the anastomosis by passing a bougie or by direct esophagoscopy may abort the development of a stricture. Esophagoscopy may also allow removal of an intraluminal suture that is serving as the nidus for inflammation.

The gastrostomy simplifies esophageal dilatations by permitting Tucker dilators to be used in a retrograde fashion. Most esophageal strictures will eventually respond to continued dilatations and will not need to be handled surgically. Persistence of a stricture may be due to continued inflammation from gastroesophageal reflux (Pieretti et al., 1974; Ashcraft et al., 1977) (Fig. 53–6) which, if present, may require gastric fundoplication (see Hiatal Hernia) to eliminate. Rarely a patient may require resection of an esophageal stricture.

Obstruction of the esophagus by a foreign body occurred on 60 occasions in 35 of our 127 patients. Patients both with and without strictures may become so obstructed. These foreign bodies can occasionally be pushed through the anastomosis by using a nasogastric tube, but often they require removal by esophagoscopy. Foreign body obstruction with concomitant choking is a perennial lethal possibility in these children. For this reason, blenderized food and ground meats are given at least until the child is of school age, when he or she can understand the need for, and practice, the necessary chewing of food. Hot dogs and hard candy are probably best avoided until the teens.

Certain patients will have postoperative re-

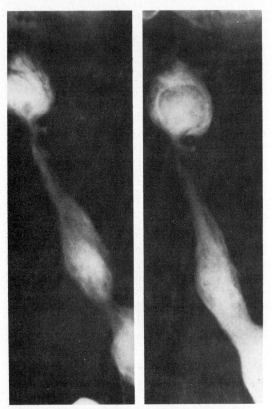

Figure 53–6 Esophageal anastomotic stricture and ulcer secondary to reflux. This child underwent repair of esophageal atresia and tracheoesophageal fistula. A persistent anastomotic narrowing was noted to recur repeatedly, and an ulcer developed at the anastomosis. Gastrointestinal series demonstrated reflux on several occasions. Gastric fundoplication resulted in prompt resolution of the stricture.

spiratory problems. The barking cough and hoarse cry, which are characteristic of these patients, are not causes for concern. Some patients, however, have anoxic spells or pneumonia seemingly unassociated with aspiration or tracheal narrowing. Filler et al. (1976) suggest that tracheal compression between the aorta or innominate artery and the esophagus causes this potentially lethal complication. They recommend anterior suspension of the offending vessel.

Functional swallowing disorders are very common in these patients, and these are discussed in Chapter 54.

Esophageal Replacement

Patients in whom a primary esophageal repair is impossible or unsuccessful will require colon interposition for esophageal reconstruction (Gross and Firestone, 1967;

German and Waterston, 1976). Although White (1976) has reported satisfactory results with performing this procedure on children as young as five weeks of age, we prefer to wait until the child is 9 to 11 months old to perform this extensive procedure. We use the left colon, mobilized on the left colic artery, and placed in a left posterior retropleural position. The lower anastomosis is made to the esophagus, preserving the gastroesophageal junction and its antireflux function. Further details of the operation will not be given here.

Early complications of this procedure are related to anastomotic leaks, particularly at the upper anastomosis. These usually respond after a few days to conservative treatment and observation. Leaks from the lower anastomosis may result in extrapleural collections, which require prolonged drainage, but these, too, can be expected eventually to close.

Twisting, kinking, compression, or spasm of the blood supply to the interposed colon may result in catastrophic early sloughing of the intestine. Removal of the infarcted colon, drainage, and, if the patient survives, a second interposition, will be necessary in these cases.

The segment of colon used for esophageal replacement has no peristaltic function: it acts as a passive conduit for swallowed food. For this reason, redundancy or kinking will give rise to varying degrees of dysphagia. Either anastomosis may be the site of foreign body obstruction, and endoscopy using the rigid scope may not be possible, although flexible esophagocologastroscopy may simplify management of some of these children. Dysphagia may also occur during bouts of intestinal viral infection owing to secretion of mucus by the colon segment. This is easily managed by encouraging increased intake of liquids.

The high position of the upper esophageal pouch requires a long vascular pedicle for interposed bowel segments. For this reason, jejunal segments are not satisfactory for esophageal replacement because of the relatively short mesentery to the small intestine.

Reversed gastric tubes, utilizing the left gastroepiploic artery, have been successfully used for esophageal replacement both for lye strictures and esophageal atresia (Anderson and Randolph, 1973). We see little to recommend this procedure over colon interposition, although it may be of value if the latter is impossible or has previously failed.

Holder and Ashcraft (1966) and Myers and Aberdeen (1979) offer excellent and extensive discussions of the subject of tracheoesophageal fistula and esophageal atresia.

CONGENITAL ESOPHAGEAL STENOSIS

Stenosis of the esophagus may be due to webs, fibromuscular or hamartomatous rings, or fibrous strictures. Depending upon the degree of narrowing, they may present during infancy or later, even into adulthood.

These lesions will be discussed more fully in Chapter 54.

DUPLICATIONS OF THE ESOPHAGUS

Esophageal duplications are theorized to occur as a result of incomplete twinning or because of disturbed recanalization following the solid stage of embryologic development. Others, usually of the cystic variety, probably represent foregut rests. Most esophageal duplications occur in or along the lower third of the esophagus. The lumen of the duplication may or may not communicate with the normal esophagus, although a common muscular wall is often shared. Foregut cysts may occur anywhere in the superior or posterior mediastinum, and there may be a connection with the subdiaphragmatic gut. Bower et al. (1978) found that 20 per cent of alimentary tract duplications were located within the thorax. The lining epithelium of these structures may be squamous, respiratory, intestinal, or mixed. Those with secretory epithelium undergo gradual progressive enlargement, and this often accounts for their symptomatic presentation. Often, gastric acid-secreting mucosa is found to line the structures; ulceration with bleeding is a complication with this type of duplication. Certain pulmonary sequestrations, often referred to in the literature as esophageal lungs, demonstrate a communication between the sequestration bronchus and the esophagus (Heithoff et al., 1976).

Presentation and Diagnosis

Unlike most other esophageal lesions, duplications and cysts usually do not include swallowing difficulties among the presenting symptoms. Respiratory complaints such as stridor, pneumonia, and cough predominate, and Haller et al. (1975) emphasized that in cases of neonatal respiratory obstruction these lesions must be considered. Many such lesions remain asymptomatic until adolescence or later and are often found incidentally on chest radiographs, although some come to medical attention because of failure to thrive in infancy, vomiting, or esophageal obstruction.

As with other foregut anomalies, there is a high incidence of associated vertebral abnormalities. Cervical or thoracic myeloceles occasionally occur concomitantly with these lesions and may lead to confusion or error in their diagnosis. Communications between the neural tube and the lumen of the cyst or duplication occur rarely but are of obvious importance.

Radiographic studies, including plane films and fluoroscopic evaluation of the esophagus, are virtually always of value. Studies of the thoracic and cervical spine are performed as indicated. Routine or computed tomography may assist in the detection of spinal defects or communications, although myelography may ultimately be required to define the problem. Ultrasound studies may occasionally be of help in distinguishing mediastinal cysts from solid masses. The use of sonography to detect intrathoracic lesions is difficult, however, even in experienced hands.

Endoscopic studies, although frequently performed, rarely demonstrate more than external compression.

Treatment

Surgical removal of these duplications is virtually always recommended. The cystic lesions are relatively easily removed, although inflammation may make dissection from adjacent structures difficult. Any communication with the subdiaphragmatic gut should be dissected to the entry point and closed. Laparotomy may or may not be required for this to be accomplished completely and safely.

Most esophageal duplications offer no difficulty in complete removal, although an occasional one of great length, sharing a common wall with the main esophagus, will present difficulties. Construction of a reentry portal at the most distal point of the duplication without resection may be the safest procedure.

Neurenteric communications must be assiduously dissected and closed. Cooperation with neurosurgeons in these cases is generally wise.

Most complications in the treatment of these lesions arise from unrecognized injury to an adjacent viscus or failure to recognize a communication with the gut or neural tube. The best way to avoid complications is careful and meticulous dissection.

HIATAL HERNIA

Esophageal hiatal hernias were first described by Richard Bright in an autopsy series. Almost a century passed before Findlay and Kelly first reported its occurrence in infants and children in 1931. There has been an increasing incidence in the diagnosis of

the disorder since that time. For many years, European clinics have reported more cases and a higher incidence of operation for this disorder than have clinics in the United States (Jewett and Waterston, 1975). Recently, certain North American children's hospitals have been reporting large numbers of cases, more closely reflecting the European experience (Randolph et al., 1974). True congenital esophageal hiatal hernias are relatively rare; they usually occur in association with connective tissue disorders such as cutis laxa. Figure 53–7 illustrates such an example. Unfortunately, these infants ordinarily have a poor prognosis because of the seriousness of pulmonary involvement and other complications of their generalized disease. The recurrence rate following operation in these children is rather high.

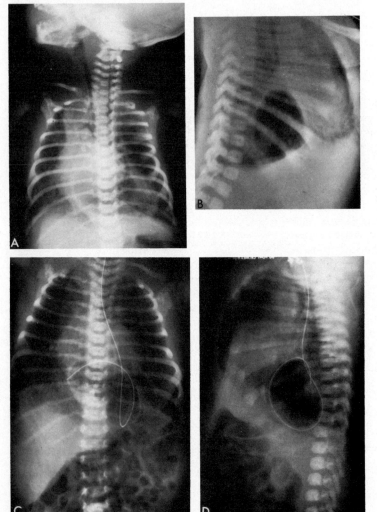

Figure 53–7   Congenital, massive, esophageal hiatal hernia. This baby, noted at birth to have cutis laxa, developed respiratory difficulty. A and B illustrate the posterior mediastinal radiolucency which proved to be the stomach upon insertion of a nasogastric tube (C and D). The infant required repair of the hernia in the newborn period because of gastric obstruction, but he died at 6 weeks of age owing to progressive respiratory failure.

Of more clinical importance are those cases that appear in infants and children after the perinatal period. Hiatal hernias in infancy may be difficult to distinguish from chalasia (Chap. 54), and, indeed, they may result from inadequate treatment of chalasia. Pediatric surgeons recognize that infants operated upon for esophageal atresias often develop symptoms of reflux, and occasionally a hiatal hernia may be demonstrated in such a child.

Hiatal hernias occur in two forms: sliding (the more common type) and paraesophageal. The sliding type is characterized by displacement of the esophagogastric junction from its normal intraabdominal position into the chest. As with other sliding hernias, visceral peritoneum comprises one wall of the hernia sac. Paraesophageal hernias are described as herniation of abdominal organs (usually the stomach) into the chest through the esophageal hiatus and alongside the esophagus, with the esophagogastric junction lying in its normal position. Combined hernias do occur rarely, usually as a result of trauma.

The esophageal hiatus lies anterior to and to the left of the aortic hiatus. It is generally slightly constricting to the esophagus. The stomach is held in its abdominal position by the tough posterior layer of the phrenoesophageal ligament, which passes behind and above the gastroesophageal junction; by the somewhat flimsy anterior leaf of this ligament, which passes anterior to the esophagus; as well as by the constricting nature of the diaphragmatic crura and the bulk of the stomach.

Pressure tracings of the normal esophagus demonstrate an area of higher tonic contraction pressure located in the esophagus 5 cm or so below the esophageal hiatus. This esophageal high-pressure zone, which relaxes only with swallowing, is largely responsible for prevention of gastroesophageal reflux.

Presentation and Diagnosis

Uncomplicated paraesophageal hernias are usually asymptomatic, but complications such as incarceration, strangulation, gangrene, ulceration, bleeding, and perforation of the herniated viscus can develop. The diagnosis may be suggested before complications develop by vague complaints of epigastric discomfort in the older child. These hernias are uncommon, but because of the possibility of complications, most authors recommend prompt surgical treatment.

Sliding hiatal hernias, unless quite large, are ordinarily no problem if unaccompanied by gastroesophageal reflux. Reflux is very often associated with these hernias, but this is not always so. This attests to the fact that the lower esophageal sphincter — the high-pressure zone — can remain functional even if displaced into the thorax. However, since young infants seem to have an imperfectly functioning sphincter, a hiatal hernia will usually accentuate reflux in these children. The diagnosis of a sliding hernia may be suggested in an infant by recurrent bouts of pneumonitis, iron deficiency anemia, or dysphagia, with any of these symptoms being accompanied or unaccompanied by vomiting. Certain patients who are brought to medical attention because of a failure to thrive have poor feeding patterns because of the presence of a hiatal hernia.

Complaints of frequent vomiting — occasionally projectile enough to suggest pyloric stenosis — may require full investigation, including an upper gastrointestinal series. This study may also be performed because of symptoms and signs of complications of reflux, such as complaints of heartburn in an older child or fussiness of an infant when he or she is laid down after feeding. Difficulty taking feedings suggests an esophageal stricture. Hematemesis occasionally occurs as a manifestation of a more severe esophagitis. Indeed, such a child may be evaluated for anemia or melena. Evaluation of recurrent respiratory infections should include an esophagram.

When a clinically important hiatal hernia is present, a barium swallow will usually demonstrate major gastroesophageal reflux. The radiographic significance of the size of the hiatal hernia is debatable, but the importance of reflux is unquestioned. *Clinically significant reflux can occur in the absence of any radiographically demonstrable hiatal herniation.* Indeed, operation may be indicated in some cases in which the hernia cannot be visualized radiographically. It is also important to examine such a child for the presence of esophageal ulceration or stricturing.

Esophagoscopy is usually indicated in the child who has significant reflux, and it is always indicated in the child who has any suggestion of esophagitis with stricture, ulceration, or bleeding. We prefer rigid endoscopy, but fiberoptic instruments have also been used with success (Forget and Meradji, 1976).

Treatment

Once the diagnosis is established, a simple yet rigid approach is taken to avoid reflux. The regimen consists of keeping the child in the sitting position and giving frequent feedings of thickened formula. The importance of strict adherence to this regimen cannot be overstressed to the parents. Close follow-up is mandatory, and, if complications develop, prompt operative treatment is imperative to prevent progression of strictures or aspiration pneumonitis.

The patient who has an isolated stricture secondary to reflux can sometimes be treated by esophageal dilatation. This may be initiated at the time of esophagoscopy and followed up by dilatations from above. It is often more desirable to perform retrograde dilatations following placement of a gastrostomy tube. Either of these approaches *must* be accompanied by the routine nonoperative regimen outlined above. This approach will occasionally avoid a more extensive operation, but care must be taken not to procrastinate in the face of worsening symptoms. Periodic esophagography and esophagoscopy are helpful in assessing the effectiveness of this approach.

With the development of any complications or in a static situation, a more definitive operation is mandatory. At the present time, virtually all pediatric centers utilize the Nissen gastric fundoplication operation, or a modification of it, for the treatment of esophageal reflux. Less importance is placed upon actual closure of the esophageal hiatus, although we have found that it is important to close the hiatus somewhat in order to avoid postoperative paraesophageal herniation of the gastric fundus. During the procedure, a large esophageal bougie should be placed through the gastroesophageal junction to prevent excessive narrowing. A gastrostomy is recommended if there is an esophageal stricture for which postoperative retrograde dilatations are planned.

It is extremely unusual for a child not to respond to the above regimen. Even a prolonged course of dilatations would be preferable to any esophageal resection or replacement procedure. Perseverance is the key to satisfactory treatment of these difficult cases.

Complications

The fundoplication procedure is, fortunately, relatively free of complications. An excessively tight fundoplication can result in the "gas-bloat" phenomenon of inability to vomit or eructate. For this reason, the fundoplication is performed rather loosely. Severe symptoms of gastric distention are simply treated by passage of an orogastric or nasogastric tube.

On rare occasions, the fundoplication can slip down over the stomach, creating severe gastric obstruction. This is diagnosed by an upper gastrointestinal radiograph series and requires an immediate operation to secure the fundoplication at the level of the esophagogastric junction. Cephalad slipping of the fundoplication can also occur and results in an immediate failure of the operation to prevent reflux. This complication is also diagnosed by an upper gastrointestinal series, and reoperation is necessary if reflux is significant.

Rarely a child will develop postoperative symptoms due to herniation of the stomach through the esophageal hiatus if it is not closed sufficiently. This is unusual. Most authors feel that one of the special benefits of the fundoplication is that it continues to function even when the stomach is partially displaced into the chest.

A special category of hiatal hernia may be seen in the patient who has undergone repair of esophageal atresia and tracheoesophageal fistula. Occasionally one of these patients develops an anastomotic stricture that does not respond to dilatation. Esophagoscopy will demonstrate a continuing, active, inflammatory process at the level of the anastomosis. Some degree of esophageal reflux may be demonstrated on an upper gastrointestinal radiographic series. These patients represent a problem in that there is sufficient esophageal reflux to prevent complete healing of the anastomosis because of continued inflammation, but the reflux is unassociated with distal esophageal inflammation. We agree with Fonkalsrud (1979) that persistence with the esophageal dilatations usually fails, and we recommend early operation and fundoplication. The anastomosis heals following elimination of reflux, but anastomotic dilatation may be required during and for a few weeks after this healing phase.

SELECTED REFERENCES

Holder, T. M., and Ashcraft, K. W. 1966. Esophageal atresia and tracheoesophageal fistula. Curr. Prob. Surg., Aug.
  This monograph represents one of the most extensive discussions on the entire subject.
Myers, N. A., and Aberdeen, E. 1979. Congenital esophageal atresia and tracheoesophageal fistula. *In* Pediatric Surgery, 3rd ed. Chicago Year Book Medical Pub. p. 446.
  This extensive chapter covers the subject in detail and is directed primarily toward the pediatric surgeon.

REFERENCES

Anderson, K. D., and Randolph, J. G. 1973. The gastric tube for esophageal replacement in children, J. Thorac. Cardiovasc. Surg., 66:333.

Ashcraft, K. W., Goodwin, C., Amoury, R. A., et al. 1977. Early recognition and aggressive treatment of gastroesophageal reflux following repair of esophageal atresia. J. Pediatr. Surg., 12:317.

Bachiller, M. C., Juareguizar, E., and Martinez, A. 1976. Malformaciones digestivas asociadas a la atresia de esofago. Estudio de 125 casos. Ann. Esp. Pediatr. (Madrid), 9:11.

Bower, R. J., Sieber, W. K., and Kiesewetter, W. B. 1978. Alimentary tract duplications in children, Ann. Surg., 188:669.

Brennemann, J. 1913. Congenital atresia of the esophagus with report of three cases. Am. J. Dis. Child., 5:143.

Bright, R. 1836. Tabular view of the morbid appearances in 100 cases connected with albuminous urine and observations. Guy Hosp. Rep., 1:398.

Filler, R. M., Rossello, P. J., and Lebowitz, R. L. 1976. Life-threatening anoxic spells caused by tracheal compression after repair of esophageal atresia: correction by surgery, J. Pediatr. Surg., 11:739.

Findlay, L., and Kelly, A. B. 1931. Congenital shortening of the esophagus and the thoracic stomach resulting therefrom. J. Laryngol., 46:797.

Fonkalsrud, E. W. 1979. Gastroesophageal fundoplication for reflux following repair of esophageal atresia. Arch. Surg., 114:48.

Forget, P. P., and Meradji, M. 1976. Contribution of fiberoptic endoscopy to diagnosis and management of children with gastroesophageal reflux. Arch. Dis. Child., 51:60.

German, J. C., and Waterston, D. J. 1976. Colon interposition for the replacement of the esophagus in children, J. Pediatr. Surg., 11:227.

Gibson, T. 1696. The anatomy of humane bodies epitomized, 5th ed. London, Awnsham and Churchill, p. 240.

Girdany, B. R., Sieber, W. K., and Osman, M. F. 1969. Traumatic pseudodiverticula of the pharynx in newborn infants. N. Engl. J. Med., 280:237.

Gross, R. E., and Firestone, F. N. 1967. Colonic reconstruction of the esophagus in infants and children. Surgery, 61:955.

Haight, C., and Towsley, H. A. 1943. Congenital atresia of the esophagus with tracheoesophageal fistula; extrapleural ligation of fistula and end-to-end anastomosis of esophageal segments. Surg. Gynecol. Obstet., 76:672.

Haller, J. A., Jr., Shermeta, D. W., Donahoo, J. S., et al. 1975. Life-threatening respiratory distress from mediastinal masses in infants. Ann. Thorac. Surg., 19:364.

Hausmann, P. F., Close, A. S., and Williams, L. P. 1957. Occurrence of tracheoesophageal fistula in three consecutive siblings. Surgery, 41:542.

Heithoff, K. B., Sane, S. M., Williams, H. J., et al. 1976. Bronchopulmonary foregut malformation: a unifying etiological concept. Am. J. Roentgenol., 126:46.

Heller, R. M., Kirchner, G., and O'Neill, J. A. 1977. Perforation of the pharynx in the newborn: a near look-alike for esophageal atresia, Am. J. Roentgenol., 129:335.

Hendren, W. H., and Hale, J. P. 1976. Esophageal atresia treated by electromagnetic bougienage and subsequent repair. J. Pediatr. Surg., 11:713.

Hoffman, W. 1899. Atresia oesophagi et communicato inter-oesophagum et tracheam, Inaugural dissertation (Griefswald, Druk Von Julius Abel).

Holder, T. M., and Ashcraft, K. W. 1966. Esophageal atresia and tracheoesophageal fistula. Curr. Prob. Surg., Aug.

Holder, T. M., Cloud, D. T., Lewis, J. E., et al. 1964. Esophageal atresia and tracheoesophageal fistula, a survey of its members by the Surgical Section of the American Academy of Pediatrics. Pediatrics, 34:542.

Jewett, T. C., and Waterston, D. J. 1975. Surgical management of hiatal hernia in children. J. Pediatr. Surg., 10:757.

Keats, T. E., and Smith, T. H. 1973. An improved positioning technique for radiological demonstration of infantile tracheoesophageal fistulae: a technical note. Radiology, 109:727.

Kluth, D. 1976. Atlas of esophageal atresia. J. Pediatr. Surg., 11:901.

Ladd, W. E. 1944. The surgical treatment of esophageal atresia and tracheoesophageal fistula. N. Engl. J. Med., 230:625.

Landing, B. H. 1975. Syndromes of congenital heart disease with tracheobronchial anomalies. Am. J. Roentgenol. Rad. Ther. Nucl. Med., 123:679.

Leven, N. L. 1940–41. Congenital atresia of the esophagus with tracheoesophageal fistula: report of successful extrapleural ligation of fistulous communication and cervical esophagostomy. J. Thorac. Surg., 10:648.

Myers, N. A., and Aberdeen, E. 1979. Congenital esophageal atresia and tracheoesophageal fistula. *In* Pediatric Surgery, 3rd ed. Chicago, Year Book Medical Pub., p. 446.

Pieretti, R., Shandling, B., and Stephens, C. A. 1974. Resistant esophageal stenosis associated with reflux after repair of esophageal atresia: a therapeutic approach. J. Pediatr. Surg., 9:355.

Quan, L., and Smith, D. W. 1973. The Vater association. Vertebral defects, anal atresia, T-E fistula with esophageal atresia, radial and renal dysplasia: a spectrum of associated defects, J. Pediatr., 82:104.

Quinn, N. J., Jr. 1971. Diagnostic catheter examinations of the newborn, should these be done routinely? Clin. Pediatr., 10:251.

Randolph, J. G., Lilly, J. R., and Anderson, K. D. 1974. Surgical treatment of gastroesophageal reflux in infants. Ann. Surg., *180*:479.

Replogle, R. L. 1963. Esophageal atresia: plastic sump catheter for drainage of the proximal pouch. Surgery, *54*:296.

Scott, J. S., and Wilson, J. K. 1957. Hydramnios as an early sign of esophageal atresia. Lancet, *2*:569.

Smith, E. I. 1957. The early development of the trachea and esophagus in relation to atresia of the esophagus and tracheoesophageal fistula. Contrib. Embryol. Carnegie Inst., Wash., 245–36–41.

Waterston, D. J., Bonham-Carter, R. E., and Aberdeen, E. 1963. Congenital tracheoesophageal fistula in association with oesophageal atresia. Lancet, *2*:55.

Weigel, W., and Kaufmann, H. J. 1976. The frequency and types of other congenital anomalies in association with tracheoesophageal malformations, radiologic studies of 83 such infants. Clin. Pediatr., *15*:819.

White, J. J. 1976. Early short segment left colon interposition for esophageal atresia. J. Pediatr. Surg., *11*:735.

Chapter 54

FUNCTIONAL ABNORMALITIES OF THE ESOPHAGUS

William K. Sieber, M.D.

DEFINITION

Functional abnormalities of the esophagus in infants and children are associated with symptoms of dysphagia, partial obstruction with regurgitation and vomiting, and respiratory symptoms due to aspiration. Dysphagia indicates difficulty in swallowing and usually means sticking of food somewhere between the mouth and the stomach or pain during swallowing. Infants may respond by refusing feedings or choking on feedings. The clinical course may suggest the diagnosis, but definitive recognition rests upon the results of appropriate radiologic studies, endoscopy, and manometry. Esophagoscopy, although it usually discloses no pathologic condition, may be therapeutic in some instances, such as in achalasia. Newer radiologic equipment, which visualizes the esophagus by cine studies and videotaping, often allows good visualization of esophageal motor activity. Manometry documents the actual motor activity of the esophagus and finds its greatest value in the diagnosis and management of these functional disorders.

ESOPHAGEAL MANOMETRY

Study Methods

The normal muscular movements of the esophagus can be documented accurately and objectively by manometry (Goyal, 1976). The method introduced by Hightower and Code (1949) is generally used for these studies. The equipment necessary for manometry includes three water-filled polyethylene catheters connected to transducers, the outputs of which activate a four-channel recorder. Each catheter has an opening on the side as well as at the end; the side opening is 2, 3, or 5 cm from the tip, depending on the size catheter used, which in turn depends on the size of the patient and the intent of the study. Respiratory movement pressures are recorded on the fourth channel of the recorder.

To study children by this method it is necessary that the patient be sedated. (We recommend secobarbital, 5.0 mg per kg body weight, meperidine, 1.0 mg per kg body weight, or both.) After sedation of the patient, the catheter unit is introduced into the stomach. The gastric-fundal pressure is recorded, and the tube is withdrawn 0.5 to 1 cm at a time, recording the resting pressure at each level with a dry swallow and with a swallow of water at each level. Pressures are recorded in either millimeters of mercury or centimeters of water. Infinite patience and diligent attention to detail are essential for the completion of a single, acceptable, reproducible study in an infant, as crying, movement, sobbing, and coughing alter the record. A quiet, cooperative, but conscious child willing to swallow is necessary for a successful study.

Gastric fundic pressure is the zero reference point. The inferior esophageal sphincter is identified as the lower 1 to 3 cm of the esophagus where a resting expiratory phase pressure 0.3 to 5 mm of Hg above the gastric fundic pressure is recorded. The wave of relaxation preceding the passage of a primary peristaltic wave further identifies this in-

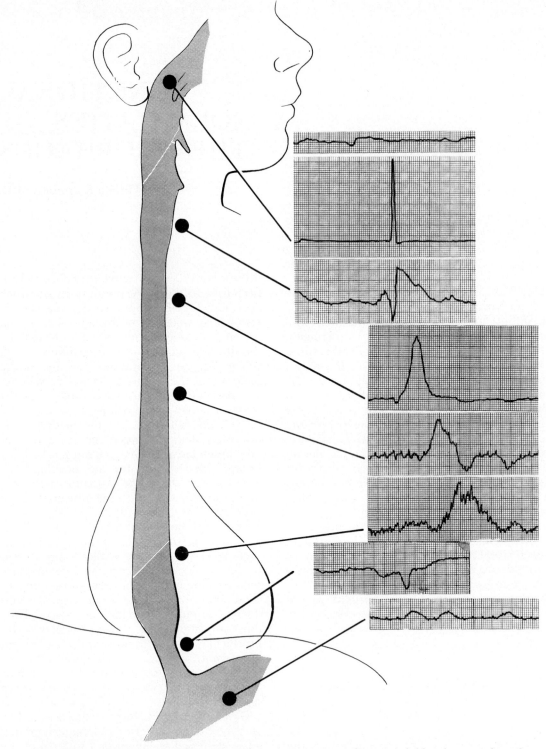

Figure 54–1 Manometric intraluminal esophageal pressure recordings in a child without esophageal abnormality. The character, duration, pressure generated, and time relationship at various levels are illustrated. Relaxation of the superior and inferior sphincters precedes the pressure wave. The top tracing records respirations; the bottom records gastric fundal pressure.

ferior esophageal sphincter. Respiratory phase reversal occurs where positive inspiratory pressure changes to negative inspiratory pressure; this is assumed to occur at the level of the diaphragm, and in most infants and children the inferior sphincter is below or coincides with this point. A primary peristaltic wave is a wave of pressure initiated by swallowing which passes sequentially to the stomach, preceded by relaxation of the superior and inferior sphincters. Such a wave normally follows 80 to 100 per cent of swallows. A secondary peristaltic wave is one not initiated by a swallow; such waves of pressure occur as artifacts during movements of tubes, from irrigation of tubes, and at times from intrinsic esophageal pathology. They normally occur in limited numbers in the smooth muscle part of the esophagus. Tertiary waves are nonperistaltic and are noted when there is deficient or absent peristalsis.

The superior esophageal sphincter is a zone of higher pressure in the upper esophagus, which may be recognized by identical pressure profiles at all three levels of the esophagus monitored and indicates simultaneous, identical pressures occurring at these points.

Variations in the technique of manometry include the use of tiny balloons rather than openings in the catheters, the recording of end rather than side pressures, constant slow infusion of the catheters, and, most recently, the use of tiny transducers embedded in the tube to be swallowed. Balloons and constant infusion techniques tend to exaggerate pressure waves in an area of stenosis and in the sphincters since they record not only the resting pressure but also the resistance to distention by the balloon or the infusing fluid. Figure 54–1 illustrates manometric intraluminal esophageal pressure recordings in a child with no esophageal abnormalities.

Manometric studies identify esophageal motility abnormalities by detecting (1) failure to contract (owing to weakness or paralysis); (2) failure to relax (as in achalasia); (3) lack of coordination (simultaneous contractions); and (4) excessive contractions (identified as a spasm). Harris (1966), reviewing the status of esophageal manometry, suggests that the technique of recording intraluminal pressures of the esophagus may be relatively simple, but the interpretation of these recordings may be difficult, too readily accepted, and at times misleading.

FUNCTIONAL ABNORMALITIES OF SWALLOWING AND ESOPHAGEAL FUNCTION

Functional disorders of the pharynx and esophagus result from impaired neurologic control, abnormalities of the muscle, or replacement of the esophageal muscle fibers by fibrous tissue.

Illingworth (1969) reviewed the world literature about dysphagia in infancy and concluded that the causes could be classified into two general categories: those associated with gross anatomic abnormalities and those associated with neuromuscular problems. To these two general headings should be added those abnormalities of esophageal function associated with systemic illness and those due to local trauma (Table 54–1). The gross anatomic congenital defects causing functional abnormalities of the esophagus are described in Chapter 53.

Delayed maturation in the premature infant is often associated with transient pharyngeal incoordination, which when treated by the use of feeding tubes, should lead to complete recovery in weeks to months. Swallowing improves as compensatory movements of the tongue are acquired. It is notable that extraluminal pressure or aberrant position of the esophagus are rarely causes of motility disturbances. Systemic disorders associated with esophageal motor dysfunction include connective tissue disorders, metabolic and endocrine diseases, disorders of the nervous system, and a group of miscellaneous disorders. Such disordered motility is often transitory and overlooked because of the primary disorder. In scleroderma and other connective tissue diseases, progressive replacement of the esophageal connective tissue by fibrosis causes aperistalsis, dysphagia, and inability to swallow. The full-thickness fibrosis occurring with lye burns results in the same findings, and the first indication of tetanus neonatorum is commonly dysphagia, due to stiffness of the jaws, which makes swallowing impossible.

Suprabulbar paresis (pseudobulbar palsy) denotes a lesion in the nerve pathways above the medulla, which carry motor fibers from the cortical motor areas for the tongue, palate, and lips to the motor nuclei in the medulla; the symptoms of this lesion include weakness and spasticity of the lips, tongue, palate, pharynx, and laryngeal muscles with resul-

Table 54–1 CAUSES OF FUNCTIONAL ABNORMALITIES OF THE PHARYNX AND ESOPHAGUS IN INFANTS AND CHILDREN

I. Gross Anatomic Congenital Defects
1. Palate — cleft palate
2. Tongue — macroglossia
    cysts, tumors
    lymphangioma
    ankyloglossia superior
3. Nasopharynx — choanal atresia
4. Mandible — micrognathia
    Pierre-Robin syndrome
    temporomandibular joint ankylosis and/or hypoplasia
5. Pharynx — cyst, diverticulum, tumor
6. Larynx — cleft, cyst, defect
7. Esophagus — atresia, stenosis, duplication, tracheoesophageal fistula, hiatal hernia, pseudodiverticulum, foregut cyst
8. Thorax — dysphagia lusorum, mediastinal cysts or tumors

II. Neuromuscular Causes
1. Delayed maturation (prematurity)
2. Cerebral palsy
3. Bulbar and suprabulbar palsy
4. Cricopharyngeal achalasia
5. Achalasia of the esophagus
6. Chalasia of the esophagus
7. Muscular diseases
    a. Muscular dystrophy
    b. Myotonic dystrophy
    c. Myasthenia gravis
    d. Amyotonia, hypotonia
8. Syndromes
    a. Möbius
    b. Cornelia DeLange
    c. Riley-Day
    d. Prader-Willi
9. Systemic infections
    a. Tetanus
    b. Diphtheria
    c. Poliomyelitis

III. Systemic Illnesses
1. Infections — local and systemic
2. Connective tissue diseases
    Scleroderma — mixed connective tissue disease
3. Endocrine problems (diabetes mellitus)

IV. Local Trauma
1. Ingestion of corrosive substances (lye burns)
2. Reflux esophagitis

tant dysphagia. With this ailment the jaw jerk is exaggerated, but there is no tongue fasciculation or atrophy. Suprabulbar paresis is often associated with other manifestations of cerebral (upper motor neuron) palsy, whereas true bulbar palsy implies lower motor neuron injury and is associated with muscle hypotonia, atrophy, and often facial paralysis. Tube feedings and frequent pharyngeal and tracheal aspiration are necessary in infants suffering from pseudobulbar paresis, but remarkable return of function may occur after weeks, months, and even years.

Amyotonia congenita may appear at birth as swallowing and perhaps sucking difficulties associated with general weakness, hypotonicity, and respiratory as well as swallowing weakness. The response to appropriate drug therapy is usually prompt, and the condition is rarely progressive.

Practically all patients with familial dysautonomia (Riley-Day syndrome) have feeding problems from birth, often requiring tube feeding for the first few months owing to disruption of swallowing reflexes. This inheritable disease seems to be limited to persons of Jewish extraction. Its most striking features are disturbances of autonomic function, manifested by reduced or absent tear production during crying, postural hypotension, coldness of hands and feet, excessive perspiration, poor motor coordination with speech difficulty, difficulty in swallowing and eating, and emotional instability. Delayed cricopharyngeal opening in response to swallowing has been documented as a cause of aspiration in these patients (Kilman, 1976), and vomiting attacks often cause aspiration and pneumonitis. The treatment is symptomatic and the prognosis for life is poor, although performance of a gastrostomy has not usually been necessary.

Another syndrome associated with esophageal abnormality is the Prader-Willi syndrome. Patients with the Prader-Willi syndrome may require tube feeding because of weak or absent swallowing reflexes that result in dysphagia. These feeding difficulties tend to disappear after a few months, but hyperphagia and, later, obesity become evident.

The treatment of buccopharyngeal dysphagia in infants and young children is dependent upon the etiology. Since the functional disturbance is often transient, nasogastric tube feeding may suffice. Gastrostomy is rarely indicated, but when it is proposed contrast studies are a necessary part of the preoperative evaluation to detect associated gastroesophageal reflux. Should this be present, an antireflux (Nissen) procedure or cross-stapling with double gastrostomies will avoid troublesome regurgitation and aspiration of gastrostomy feedings.

Persistent functional abnormalities of the esophagus in infants and children occur with achalasia of the superior or inferior esophageal sphincters, following repair of esophageal atresia, associated with congenital esophageal stenosis, and in some children with unremitting gastroesophageal reflux. These problems merit consideration in more detail.

ESOPHAGEAL FUNCTION IN REPAIRED ESOPHAGEAL ATRESIA WITH AND WITHOUT TRACHEOESOPHAGEAL FISTULA

Despite successful surgical repair of esophageal atresia, some infants continue to have swallowing difficulties manifested by dysphagia, episodes of aspiration with pneumonitis, and foreign' body impaction (Chap. 53). These symptoms may occur in the absence of stenosis or a recurring tracheoesophageal fistula and are due to motility abnormalities of the repaired esophagus. Whether these motility disturbances are an associated part of the original anomaly or the result of the surgery necessary for its correction is difficult to ascertain. It is known that similar abnormalities have been identified in patients with tracheoesophageal fistula prior to surgery and that these changes have persisted postoperatively (Orringer et al., 1977).

The symptoms in these children consist of episodes of aspiration, pneumonia, paroxysms of coughing that are associated with aspiration, and, as the children become older, painful swallowing and dysphagia (Crispen et al., 1966).

Deficient motor activity of the distal esophagus in patients with repaired esophageal atresia and tracheoesophageal fistula has been recognized clinically and radiographically (Duranceau et al., 1977). Intraluminal manometric recording of pressures generated during swallowing provides objective evaluation of esophageal motor activity.

Radiographic studies may reveal several abnormalities (Crispen et al., 1966), including absence of the normal effective stripping wave, which therefore leaves a residue in the esophagus and never clears the barium from the esophagus. In some patients, this esophageal residue undergoes a "yo-yo" type of movement as intermittent spontaneous contractions of the lower part of the esophagus force the residue superiorly, expelling it into the upper esophagus with each contraction. Contractions from above then push the material again into the lower esophagus. This so-called "yo-yo" movement can result in reflux as high as the pharynx, but the vestibule appears to act as a stopgap. Associated hiatal hernias are seen in as many as 10 per cent of the patients with repaired esophageal atresia and tracheoesophageal fistula (Orringer et al., 1977). Inefficient esophageal contractility adds to the problem, and repetitious swallowing occurs. There is often retrograde esophageal flow in addition to the reflux movement, and tracheal aspiration is commonly noted at the time of barium esophagram studies. Radiographically these findings can be seen as inefficient primary stripping peristaltic waves that leave an esophageal residue after deglutition and that are associated with reflux action and often with sliding hernias as described by Kirkpatrick et al. (1961).

Motor abnormalities yield consistently abnormal or bizarre manometric results (Shepard et al., 1966; Duranceau et al., 1977; Orringer et al., 1977). Manometry is the most sensitive method of demonstrating the motility abnormalities present to some extent in all patients with repaired esophageal atresia. These abnormalities may involve the greater part of the esophagus or may involve only small parts of the midesophagus at the area distal to the anastomosis after repair of the atresia. The superior esophageal sphincteric mechanism is generally intact, the resting pressure being normal with reference to control patients. The inferior esophageal sphincter, however, is often not identifiable as a high-pressure zone. While relaxation is readily identified, as is the following wave, in most instances the pressure generated in the distal sphincteric area is less than it is in normal control patients. The upper esophagus corresponding to the area above the anastomosis responds to swallowing with the primary wave of pressure, which at times is followed with some delay through the area of the anastomosis to the distal esophagus. The area of the anastomosis is generally identified by the absence or by greatly diminished amplitude of the pressure wave. The segment of the esophagus that is aperistaltic may represent as little as 10 per cent to as much as 60 per cent of the entire length of the esophagus. Below this level, the esophagus responds to the primary wave by spasm without pre-

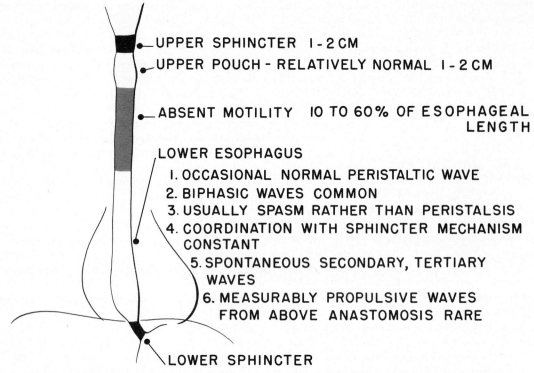

UPPER SPHINCTER 1-2CM

UPPER POUCH - RELATIVELY NORMAL 1-2CM

ABSENT MOTILITY 10 TO 60% OF ESOPHAGEAL LENGTH

LOWER ESOPHAGUS

1. OCCASIONAL NORMAL PERISTALTIC WAVE
2. BIPHASIC WAVES COMMON
3. USUALLY SPASM RATHER THAN PERISTALSIS
4. COORDINATION WITH SPHINCTER MECHANISM CONSTANT
5. SPONTANEOUS SECONDARY, TERTIARY WAVES
6. MEASURABLY PROPULSIVE WAVES FROM ABOVE ANASTOMOSIS RARE

LOWER SPHINCTER

Figure 54–2 Summary of esophageal manometric findings in children with repaired esophageal atresia with tracheoesophageal fistula.

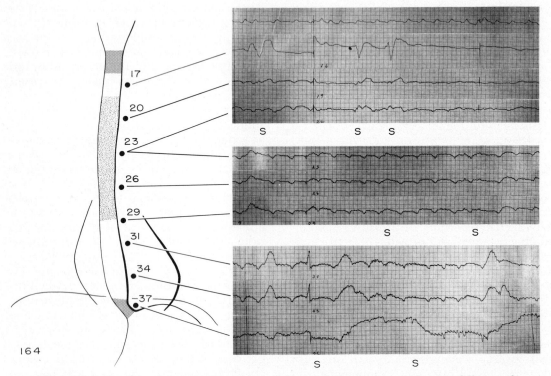

Figure 54–3 Esophageal manometric study in a patient with poor esophageal function following the successful repair of his esophageal atresia with tracheoesophageal fistula. Note the inadequate upper esophageal waves and the short length of the functioning upper segment.

76-2

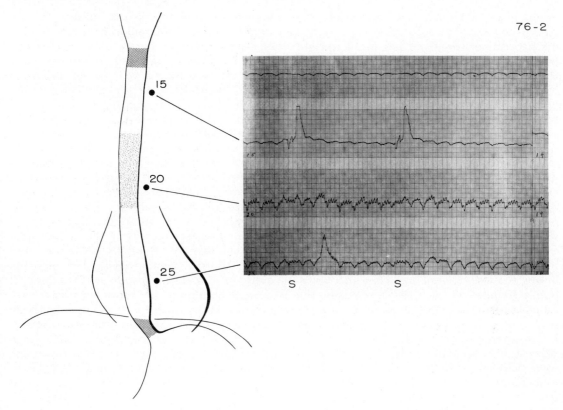

Figure 54-4 Esophageal manometric study in a patient with good esophageal function following successful repair of esophageal atresia with tracheoesophageal fistula. Note the large effective primary wave reappearing in the distal esophagus. In the second swallow the primary wave does not appear distally.

ceding relaxation. Often the activity of this lower segment of the esophagus occurs as a secondary wave unrelated to the upper pouch wave. Biphasic, tertiary, and retrograde waves are commonly identified in this distal third of the esophagus. Although the inferior esophageal sphincter is usually at or below the diaphragm, as determined by the respiratory reversal of the pressure pattern, it has been noted to be above the diaphragm and associated with a hiatal hernia in approx-imately 10 per cent of surgically treated patients. The characteristic pressure profile pattern of infants and children with repaired esophageal atresias is summarized in Figure 54-2.

The clinical status of the child's swallowing correlates well with variations in this general pattern. Long segments of aperistalsis, low amplitude of upper esophageal segment pressure waves, repeat secondary and tertiary waves, and retrograde peristalsis are common in those infants and children who show the poorest function (Fig. 54-3). Where the amplitude of the waves is high, the contour and

duration normal, and the aperistaltic segment short, the function is excellent (Fig. 54-4). Changes identified manometrically and radiographically in an infant are still present as the body matures: the relative length of the aperistaltic segment with relation to other segments of the esophagus is static. However, the length of the upper esophageal sphincter and the pressure generated by the upper esophagus, especially by the cricopharyngeus, during deglutition increases as the infant gets older. Correlation of manometry findings with cine-esophagrams and clinical observation has been excellent. The aperistaltic section of the esophagus is probably the area of the anastomosis and may be the result of fibrosis secondary to the surgical procedure. Vagal injury or a congenital abnormality could account for the distal motility changes and spasm. Congenital deficiencies of vagal innervation are difficult to diagnose with certainty since preoperative manometry is rarely possible.

The treatment of these functional abnormalities depends upon the severity of the symptoms. Generally, education of the parents to the child's need for being propped up at bedtime, for being fed in an upright position, and for being kept propped up for a reasonable period of time after feeding, will relieve the symptoms. The symptoms can also be relieved by training the child to sleep in a semi-sitting position. When choking and very severe symptoms of dysphagia and "dying spells" with feeding occur, a temporary gastrostomy may be life-saving. In such patients it is essential that hiatal hernia and gastroesophageal reflux be eliminated as a cause of the symptoms since they should be treated by performance of an antireflux procedure (Nissen fundoplication procedure).

The progressive clinical improvement of these patients who are having difficulty swallowing is a well-documented clinical observation (Orringer et al., 1977). Initially the esophagus still has poor function postoperatively, but as the infant grows there is dramatic improvement, especially during the first year of life. Sometimes, however, there is some initial improvement, which we attribute to increasing activity of the superior esophageal sphincter and upper esophagus as the infant grows. In addition, the high closure pressure of the superior esophageal sphincter provides a backstop for the generation of very high upper pouch pressures to propel the bolus through the aperistaltic segment. Improvement in function of the esophagus after surgical repair may also be due to the acquisition by children of eating habits such as drinking more water with meals, eating more slowly, and chewing food more thoroughly. Thus, these children to a certain extent treat themselves. As the esophagus is studied over periods of time, no evidence of change in the motility pattern is apparent.

Studies of infants who underwent end-to-side esophageal anastomosis with fistula ligation as advocated by Beardmore (Ty et al., 1967) demonstrate the same motility pattern and problems as those repaired in the conventional fashion.

ACHALASIA OF THE ESOPHAGUS (MEGAESOPHAGUS), CARDIOSPASM

Achalasia of the esophagus is a neuromuscular disorder of the esophagus characterized by abnormal motility of the esophagus and failure of relaxation of the distal esophageal sphincter with swallowing. This entity, well known in adolescents and adults, is seen rarely in infants and children. It has, however, been seen in newborns, and surgical treatment by cardiomyotomy has been necessary in infants less than a year of age (Moazam and Rodgers, 1976; Asch et al., 1974).

The incidence of achalasia in newborns is only 3 to 5 per cent of all collected series of patients with this disorder and is equal in boys and girls. The etiology of the abnormality is obscure, although histologic studies of biopsies of the musculature of the lower esophagus in patients with achalasia indicate that approximately half the patients are without ganglion cells. In some there is hypoganglionosis, but in general the lack of ganglion cells cannot be implicated as the cause of the disorder. Along with the lack of relaxation of the distal esophagus is a lack of normal motility in the esophagus itself. Abnormal extraesophageal innervation has been suggested as a cause (Ellis and Olsen, 1969).

In young children and in infants huge propulsive waves convey material down the esophagus to the cardiac sphincter. Occasionally reverse peristalsis occurs, but in general there is fairly normal motility associated with this reversing peristalsis. However, in older patients this motility changes to spasm and finally to aperistalsis, changes that can often be coordinated with the changes in the radiologic picture seen as the disease advances. There is initially ballooning out of the distal esophagus followed by aperistalsis and enlarging of the entire esophagus; finally the esophagus becomes a huge, sigmoid-like sac projecting into the right hemithorax. The response of the child to treatment for this problem will depend upon the stage at which treatment is instituted.

Diagnosis of achalasia in children usually depends upon the child's showing symptoms of regurgitation. Respiratory symptoms are much more common in children than in adults, and often the children are seen because of repeated episodes of pneumonitis and aspiration pneumonia. Such infants are noisy breathers, especially at night, although a sitting position for sleeping may prevent noisy breathing and aspiration. The vomiting that may occur with this disorder is associated with regurgitation rather than being projectile. The vomitus is undigested material with a fetid odor since it may have remained in the esophagus for a long period of time before being ejected (Singh et al., 1969).

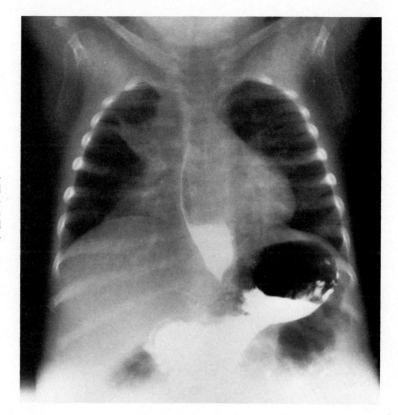

Figure 54–5 Contrast roentgenogram of the chest in a 4 month old girl (J.G.) with esophageal achalasia. There is aspiration pneumonitis with atelectasis, and the enlarged esophagus and beaklike cardioesophageal narrowing are apparent.

The diagnosis of achalasia is established radiographically by plain films of the chest, which show a fluid level in the visibly enlarged esophagus, either in the anterior–posterior or in the lateral view; the esophagus may be air-filled or partially fluid-filled. In addition, there may frequently be evidence of aspiration pneumonitis (Fig. 54–5). The size and extent of the esophagus should be identified on an esophagram, and the beak-like narrowing of the distal esophagus, tapering down to a point, may be seen. The stomach may be small and contain relatively small amounts of air; emptying into the stomach from the esophagus may be prolonged and incomplete. Children with this disorder rarely demonstrate other abnormalities.

The results of manometric studies vary considerably in patients with achalasia. In young children it may be quite difficult to introduce the recording catheters through the cardia and into the stomach, but the studies are misleading unless this is done. With balloon-tip recording tubes the pressure may be quite high, whereas with lateral recording orifices and with the perfused recording tubes the diagnosis may be obtained most readily. In most manometric studies the inferior cardiac sphincter fails to relax (Fig. 54–6). The pressure does not elevate in some studies, although in occasional cases it does: either a spasm or lack of motility in the body of the esophagus leads to inefficient contractions that fail to move material through the narrowed area so that drainage is primarily by gravity. Huge peristaltic waves are often noted in the distal esophagus in children, although the upper sphincter is usually quite normal. The Mecholyl test is rarely done to verify the diagnosis in children.

When esophagoscopy is performed on patients with achalasia, the esophagus is usually seen to be dilated with retained particulate matter. The superior sphincter is usually normal, and although the distal sphincter is usually closed, it will open promptly to allow the esophagoscope to enter the stomach, so few abnormalities other than transient closure of the distal esophageal lumen are usually noted.

The initial treatment for achalasia in infants and children is dilatation of the esophagus. This is most effective when done forcefully with a hydrostatic or pneumatic bag, but such procedures are dangerous, and equipment and experience for treating infants are

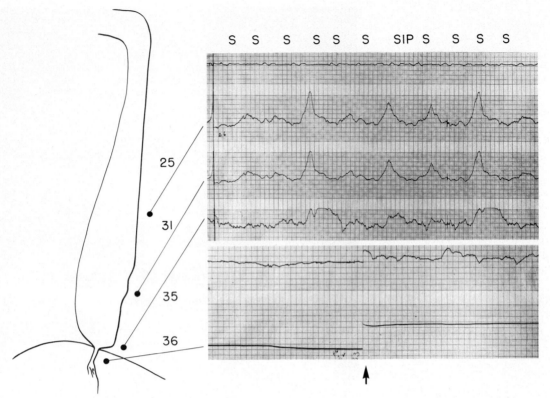

S   S   S   S   S   S   SIP S   S   S   S

25

31

35

36

Figure 54–6 Esophageal motility study in an 11 year old girl with achalasia of the esophagus. The top three tracings at three levels indicate identical pressures (spasm) at the first two levels. There is no evidence of relaxation of the inferior esophageal sphincter at the 35-cm level. There is, however, spontaneous sphincter muscular activity and a pressure wave coinciding with those above but no preceding relaxation. The lower two tracings indicate pressure at the inferior sphincter and intraluminal pH. Note the abrupt elevation as the probe passes above the sphincter. This study was done using water-filled tubes without perfusion.

rarely available. Also, since esophageal rupture from forceful dilatation is a catastrophic complication, conventional dilatation methods are usually used to provide temporary improvement but rarely a cure.

The definitive treatment of esophageal achalasia in children, as in adults, is a cardiomyotomy or Heller procedure performed either abdominally or transthoracically. The operative procedure is a straightforward one, and the complication most commonly encountered postoperatively is cardioesophageal reflux. Should this occur, later esophagitis, peptic ulceration, and stricture formation may nullify the initially good results of surgery. It is for this reason that the patients undergoing a Heller procedure for cardiospasm should be followed by periodic checkups, and it is now common practice to include an antireflux procedure (fundoplication, full or incomplete) as an essential part of the operative procedure. Most series in children

are small, and those that are presented rarely give long-term follow-up information.

In our experience a cardiomyotomy consistently relieves the obstruction initially (Fig. 54–7), but many years later problems may occur. In these children, dilatations and even esophageal replacement procedures may be necessary.

Other pathologic conditions may produce symptoms and roentgenographic findings similar to those of achalasia of the esophagus. There may be a stricture at the cardiac end of the stomach, which will yield to initial dilatations. This is most commonly seen in newborns or very young children. In occasional children with neurologic abnormalities, there are abnormalities including the whole esophagus associated with cardiospasm. These children, just as those with cricopharyngeal achalasia, often improve as they get older, and in them no surgical treatment is indicated. The indication for surgery should be continuing

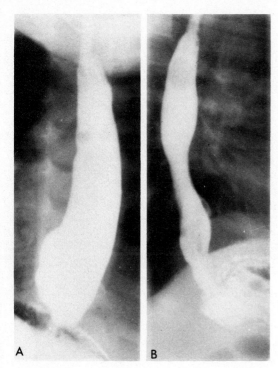

Figure 54–7 (J.G.) Preoperative (A) and post-Heller procedure (B) esophagrams. Note the enlarged cardioesophageal lumen and the return of the esophagus to normal caliber.

esophageal dysfunction after esophageal dilatation has failed to provide relief.

ESOPHAGEAL SPASM

This is a motility disorder involving the entire esophagus, and while it has been recognized in adults, it is rarely seen in infants and children. Irregular, uncoordinated contractions beginning as secondary waves below the arch of the aorta cause intermittent dysphagia and severe substernal pain in this abnormality of hypermotility. Radiologic examination identifies areas of localized esophageal constriction — the so-called "corkscrew esophagus" — and the nature of the motility disturbance is further documented by a characteristic manometric pattern of spasm and tertiary waves. The treatment consists of atropine sulfate 1:1000 sol before each feeding; warm liquids often help also. Dilatation of the esophagus may be necessary when these measures fail. Extensive submucosal myotomies, such as those that are performed on adults, have not been reported in infants or children.

CRICOPHARYNGEAL DYSFUNCTION

Just as spasm or lack of relaxation of the distal esophageal sphincter can produce dysphagia and swallowing difficulties, so may the superior esophageal sphincter cause similar but more apparent symptoms. The lack of relaxation of the superior sphincter may be difficult to identify manometrically or radiologically. Whether true spasm exists or whether this is actually the lack of ability to relax with the initiation of swallowing is difficult to prove (Palmer, 1976). Delayed cricopharyngeal opening, premature closing (as in the Riley-Day syndrome), incomplete relaxation, and loss of resting tone have all been implicated as the mechanism of cricopharyngeal dysfunction.

Cricopharyngeal achalasia, an entity not uncommon in debilitated elderly individuals, has only recently been identified in infants and young children (Reichert et al., 1977). The etiology is usually obscure, but brain damage, bulbar poliomyelitis, cerebrovascular accidents, and other neuromuscular deficiencies are commonly associated with this entity.

When noted, the predominant symptom in infants and children is dysphagia while eating. Two or three conscious swallowing efforts may be necessary; however, once the food is swallowed, there does not appear to be regurgitation from the esophagus or from the stomach. Aspiration is commonly seen as a part of attempted swallowing; however, except in severely brain-damaged children coughing will rapidly clear the trachea. Aspiration during sleep is unlikely. Commonly, this disorder is seen in neonates as a transitory phenomenon in mildly neurologically damaged children. It has been identified occasionally in children with brain tumors, and in some instances it has been identified in the absence of any neurologic abnormality.

Identification depends upon the radiologic demonstration of a shelf-like spasm of a cricopharyngeal muscle in the lateral view. This narrowing of the upper esophagus in the area of the superior sphincter is apparent only with barium swallows. There is no proximal dilatation, and the only identifying symptom is this shelf-like narrowing. The association with aspiration is a constant one in neonates, right upper lobe aspiration pneumonitis being common in this group of patients.

Manometric studies may be disappointing

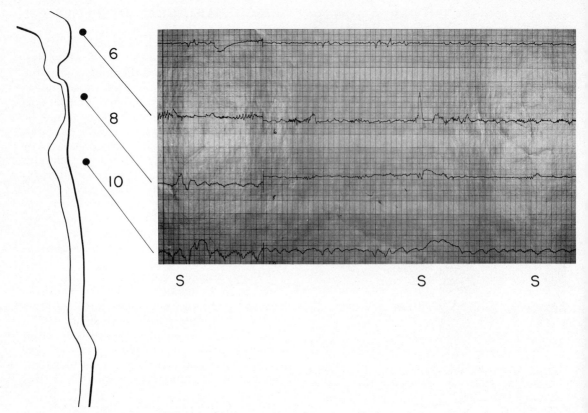

Figure 54–8 (G.E.) A 1 month old infant with cricopharyngeal achalasia. The superior sphincter at the 8-cm level fails to relax adequately with swallowing.

and unrewarding when performed in infants with cricopharyngeal achalasia. Although balloon probes or constant infusion monitoring of the pressure are preferable, the continuous infusion technique may be dangerous. Open tip catheters with a side vent tend to record lower pressures and tend to be obliterated with swallowing. In our experience, conclusive, helpful manometric studies have been difficult to obtain in infants with suspected cricopharyngeal achalasia (Fig. 54–8).

The treatment for cricopharyngeal achalasia in the past has depended upon the age of the patient and the degree of involvement of the cricopharyngeus. In those children with severe neurologic abnormalities, if nasogastric feeding must be prolonged, a gastrostomy is done. There are often distal functional abnormalities of the esophagus as determined by manometry; occasionally there is associated gastroesophageal reflux. Radiologic studies are necessary to identify such reflux prior to gastrostomy so that an antireflux procedure, such as fundoplication

or gastric division and double gastrostomies, can be done to prevent reflux and aspiration pneumonitis.

Many infants suffering initially from cricopharyngeal spasm will improve in the first month or six weeks of life. Others tend to remain the same or become worse. Cricopharyngeal myotomy, an operative procedure, may be indicated in some of these children. Bishop (1974) reports a dramatic, sustained improvement in swallowing following cricopharyngeal myotomy in a 4½ year old boy, but it is unlikely that any large number of children with cricopharyngeal achalasia will experience a dramatic improvement with this procedure.

CONGENITAL ESOPHAGEAL STENOSIS

Congenital esophageal stenosis may be suggested in the newborn period by the presence of excessive oral mucus, regurgitation with feedings, choking with feedings, and respiratory distress from aspiration pneumonitis. In older children, foreign body and food impactions may call attention to the stenosis. The esophageal stricture may be at the area of the junction of the upper third and middle third of the esophagus or at the junction of the middle and distal thirds. More commonly it is in the latter. When more proximally located, the lesion may be interpreted as abortive esophageal atresia, and when the lesion is in the distal area, stricture secondary to peptic esophagitis must be eliminated as the cause. However, when no reflux exists and the narrowing appears to be located in one of these two areas, true congenital stenosis may be diagnosed. Esophagrams demonstrate the stenotic area and show that in the absence of a foreign body impaction there is no proximal dilatation and the distal esophagus is often of normal caliber. The narrow segment can be overlooked easily unless it is sought for. Esophagoscopy discloses a remarkably normal mucosa with stenosis, which is usually ring-like in character. After dilatation, a repeated esophagoscopy rarely identifies any abnormality. Manometric studies in these patients identify an aperistaltic zone that coincides with the narrowed area of the esophagus identified radiologically. The lack of pressure changes with respirations reflects the decreased pliability of the esophageal wall in the area of the stenosis. These abnormalities do not change as the child is followed into later life.

The great majority of such congenital stenotic lesions respond to simple dilatation to relieve the anatomic stricture (Bluestone et al., 1969). However, the function remains abnormal, and such patients who have been followed for as long as 25 years continue upon occasion to suffer obstruction from foreign bodies requiring esophagoscopy for removal. In these patients, the esophagram and esophagoscopy results show a normal esophagus, and the only explanation for the continuing problem is the motor function abnormality (Figs. 54–9 and 54–10).

Surgical excision may be indicated in those instances in which the anatomic narrowing is persistent or unimproved by repeated dilatations. However, in most instances congenital stenosis of the esophagus is a truly functional abnormality and will not respond to any surgical treatment other than dilatation. High-grade stenosis in infancy may require a temporary gastrostomy for feeding and for retrograde esophageal dilatation.

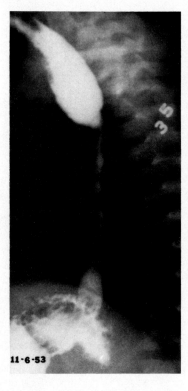
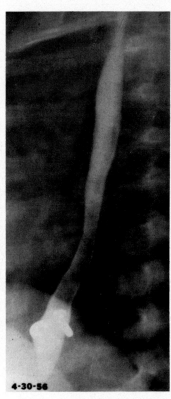

Figure 54–9 Congenital stenosis of the junction of the upper third and the middle third of the esophagus in a 3 week old infant with follow-up 2½ years later demonstrating an anatomically normal esophagus following dilatation.

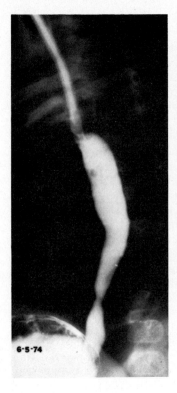

6-5-74

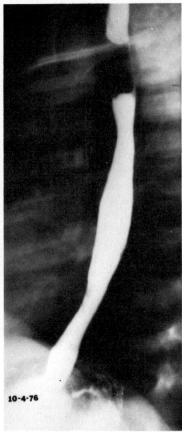

10-4-76

Figure 54–10 Congenital stenosis of the junction of the distal and the middle thirds of the esophagus in a 3 year old girl with an essentially normal esophagram two years later following dilatations.

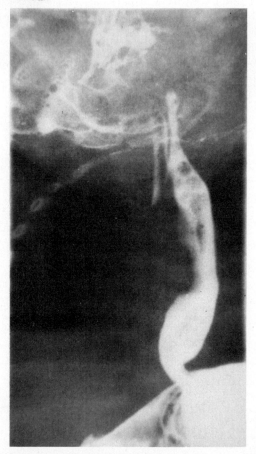

Figure 54–11 Chalasia in a 1 month old infant with regurgitant vomiting. Note the radiopaque material in the trachea. This infant was gaining weight, was able to clear the trachea promptly, and improved with positioning in a "burp" chair. At 10 months of age all vomiting had ceased.

GASTROESOPHAGEAL REFLUX (CHALASIA)

Chalasia is massive gastroesophageal reflux in infancy in the absence of a detectable hiatal hernia (Berenberg and Neuhauser, 1950). True chalasia is rare, and chalasia usually disappears as infants become older. Gryboski et al. (1963) has documented the fact that the cardiac sphincter in the newborn is inactive and unpredictable until a month to six weeks of life and that the sphincter becomes more receptive to ingestion of food as the infant gets older. Asymptomatic and minimal gastroesophageal reflux in the first few weeks of life is commonplace, perhaps universally present, and of no pathologic significance. Infants with chalasia have a continuation of this infantile abnormality. In such infants, nonprojectile vomiting begins in the first few days to weeks of life, is persistent, most apparent when the infant is recumbent, and is often confused with pyloric stenosis. The infant, however, gains weight normally, positioning usually diminishes the vomiting, and complete recovery may be expected by about one year of age. When chalasia persists beyond the usual 10 to 12 month duration, investigation to identify possible peptic ulceration and anatomic as well as functional abnormalities is indicated. Aspiration and pulmonary infection are complications of persistent regurgitant vomiting. The diagnosis is established by an esophagram, which demonstrates reproducible free reflux from the barium-filled stomach into the esophagus in the absence of a hiatal hernia (Fig. 54–11). The treatment consists of positioning in the upright position. Persistence of symptoms is an indication of other pathologic conditions.

The benign nature of persistent reflux is questioned by Lilly et al. (1969) and Leape et al. (1977) who advise a more aggressive diagnostic and therapeutic approach (Chap. 53).

SELECTED REFERENCES

Ellis, H. H., Jr., and Olsen, A. M. 1969. Achalasia of the Esophagus. Philadelphia, W. B. Saunders Co.
A classic monograph on esophageal achalasia.

Goyal, R. K. (Ed.). 1976. Symposium on esophageal motility. Arch. Intern. Med., *136*:511–601.
This current symposium is an excellent comprehensive review of esophageal manometry and disorders of esophageal motility.

Gryboski, J. 1975. Gastrointestinal Problems in the Infant. Philadelphia, W. B. Saunders Co., pp. 87–97.

A superb review of functional esophageal abnormalities in infants and children.

Illingworth, R. S. 1969. Sucking and swallowing difficulties in infancy: Diagnostic problem of dysphagia. Arch. Dis. Child., *44*:655–665.
A complete review with extensive personal experience. Information is consolidated from many sources and is not easily available elsewhere.

REFERENCES

Asch, M. J., Liebnian, W., Lochman, R. S., et al. 1974. Esophageal achalasia: Diagnosis and cardiomyotomy in a newborn infant. J. Pediatr. Surg., *9*:911.

Berenberg, W., and Neuhauser, E. B. D. 1950. Cardioesophageal relaxation (chalasia) as a cause of vomiting in infants. Pediatrics, *5*:414.

Bishop, H. C. 1974. Cricopharyngeal achalasia in childhood. J. Pediatr. Surg., *9*:775.

Bluestone, C. D., Kerry, R., and Sieber, W. K. 1969. Congenital esophageal stenosis. Laryngoscope, *54*:1095–1104.

Crispen, A. R., Friedland, G. W., and Waterston, D. J. 1966. Aspiration pneumonia and dysphagia after technically successful repair of aesophageal atresia. Thorax, *21*:104.

Duranceau, A., Fisher, S. R., Flye, M. W., et al. 1977. Motor function of the esophagus after repair of esophageal atresia and tracheoesophageal fistula. Surgery, *82*:116–123.

Ellis, H. H., Jr., and Olsen, A. M. 1969. Achalasia of the Esophagus. Philadelphia, W. B. Saunders Co.

Goyal, R. K., 1976. Symposium on esophageal motility. Arch. Intern. Med., *136*:511–601.

Gryboski, J. D., Thayer, N. R., Jr., and Spiro, H. M. 1963. Esophageal motility in infants and children. Pediatrics, *31*:382.

Harris, L. D. 1966. Editorial: The present status of esophageal manometry. Gastroenterology, *50*:708–710.

Hightower, N. C., Jr., Code, C. F., and Maher, F. T. 1949. A method for the study of gastrointestinal motor activity in human beings. Proc. Staff Meet., Mayo Clin., *24*:453–462, Aug. 31.

Illingworth, R. S. 1969. Sucking and swallowing difficulties in infancy: Diagnostic problem of dysphagia. Arch. Dis. Child., *44*:655–665.

Kilman, W. J. 1976. Disorders of pharyngeal and upper esophageal sphincter motor function. Arch. Intern. Med., *136*:592.

Kirkpatrick, J. H., Cresson, S. L., and Pilling, G. P., IV. 1961. The motor activity of the esophagus in association with esophageal atresia and tracheoesophageal fistula. Am. J. Roentgenol., *86*:884–887.

Leape, L. L., Holder, T. M., Franklin, J. D., et al. 1977. Respiratory arrest in infants secondary to gastroesophageal reflux. Pediatrics, *60*:924.

Lilly, J. R., and Randolph, J. G. 1969. Hiatal hernia and gastroesophageal reflux in infants and children. J. Thorac. Cardiovasc. Surg., *65*:42.

Moazam, F., and Rodgers, B. M. 1976. Infantile achalasia. J. Thorac. Cardiovasc. Surg., *72*:809–811.

Orringer, M. B., Kirsh, M. M., and Sloan, H. 1977. Long term esophageal function following repair of esophageal atresia. Ann. Surg., *186*:436.

Palmer, E. D. 1976. Disorders of the cricopharyngeus muscle: A review. Gastroenterology, *71*:510–519.

Reichert, T. J., Bluestone, C. D., Stool, S. E., et al. 1977. Congenital cricopharyngeal achalasia. Ann. Otol. Rhinol. Laryngol. *86*:603–610.

Shepard, R., Fenn, S., and Sieber, W. K. 1966. Evaluation of esophageal function in postoperative esophageal atresia and tracheoesophageal fistula. Surgery, *59*:608–617.

Singh, H., Gupta, H. L., Sethi, R. S. et al. 1969. Cardiac achalasia in childhood. Postgrad. Med. J., *45*:327–335.

Ty, T. C., Brunet, C., and Beardmore, H. C. 1967. A variation in the operative technique for the treatment of esophageal atresia with tracheoesophageal fistula. J. Pediatr. Surg., *2*:118–126.

Chapter **55**

BURNS AND ACQUIRED STRICTURES OF THE ESOPHAGUS

Keith H. Riding, M.D.
Charles D. Bluestone, M.D.

INTRODUCTION

History. Toward the end of the 19th century and the beginning of the 20th century, lye products became commercially available for domestic use, primarily as drain cleaners (Jackson, 1931). Coincident with the rising availability of these products in the home was the increasing number of children with esophageal burns due to accidental ingestion. Chevalier Jackson saw the need for publicity campaigns warning mothers of the dangers of lye products and for labeling such products as poisonous. After several years of effort and against a certain amount of opposition, he was able to initiate a law that required lye products to be labeled as poisonous and to have antidote advice on the label. This law was the Federal Caustic Act of 1927, enacted by President Coolidge on March 2nd of that year.

Laws. Since 1927 further regulations have come into being, namely the Poison Prevention Packaging Act, 1970, and the Federal Hazardous Substances Act, 1972; both are administered by the U.S. Consumer Product Safety Commission. These require child-resistant packaging for sodium hydroxide or potassium hydroxide in the dry form or in solutions greater than 2 per cent. As well as containing the manufacturer's name, the chemical name, and the words "Keep out of the reach of children," labels for solutions of sodium or potassium hydroxide of between 2 and 5 per cent concentration should contain the word "danger" and possibly "fatal if swallowed." For solutions of over 10 per cent, the label should have the word "poison" instead of "danger." On every label, suitable handling and antidote procedures are required to be listed. Acids and other caustic substances are to be treated similarly.

The Food and Drug Administration has authority over lye products that are not commercially available by the Federal Food, Drug, and Cosmetic Act. These would include such products as Clinitest tablets, which contain sodium hydroxide.

Incidence. It has been estimated that there are as many as 5000 accidental lye ingestions per year by children under five years of age in the United States (Sobel, 1970; Leape et al., 1971).

Children in the first decade of life constitute the largest group affected, with an especially high incidence in the first three years. Mentally defective children or adults attempting suicide form another group, and in this group females tend to outnumber males. Laboratory accidents may account for a few cases each year.

An example of the frequency of caustic esophageal burns can be seen in Figure 55–1. These figures are taken from the Children's Hospital of Pittsburgh. A sharp rise in frequency in 1968 and 1969 may be accounted

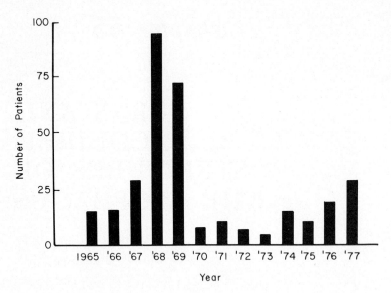

Figure 55–1 Incidence of caustic burns of the esophagus at Children's Hospital of Pittsburgh.

for by the introduction and widespread advertising of liquid drain cleaners (containing approximately 30.5 per cent NaOH) to the market.

In all reported series, the substances causing burns most frequently were the alkalis (60 to 80 per cent). The remainder were caused by such substances as Lysol (phenol), Clorox, and acids (Alford et al., 1959, Bikhazi et al., 1969; Daly and Cardona, 1961; Yarington et al., 1964; Holinger and Johnston, 1950; Owens, 1954).

Action on Drains. In 1970, a consumer organization investigated drain cleaners (Consumer Reports, 1970). The action of sodium or potassium hydroxide on a blocked U-shaped trap under the sink is first to generate intense heat when it comes in contact with water and then to attack fat and other chemicals by reacting with them. The intense reaction causes spattering of the chemical into the air around the sink, and it was recommended that most lye products were only acceptable if the user wore rubber or plastic gloves, rubber or plastic aprons, and goggles or face masks. Most products were inefficient at removing the obstruction. Complete banning of most household drain cleaners was recommended.

TYPES OF CORROSIVES

Alkalis are bases that dissolve in water. They contain a positive radical and a hydroxyl group. The common alkalis are sodium, potassium, and ammonium hydroxides (NaOH, KOH, NH₄OH).

Acids are compounds that contain hydrogen and one or more nonmetals. Most are soluble in water. Common acids are hydrochloric, sulfuric, and nitric (HCl, H₂SO₄, HNO₃).

Other corrosive substances commonly encountered are:

Phenol or hydroxybenzene (C_6H_5OH). It is a crystalline, acidic compound that is very caustic. When a little water or alcohol is added to it, it is sold as carbolic acid or Lysol in drugstores.

Bleach — The active ingredient in bleach is hypochlorous acid (HClO). Usually it is sold as a salt (e.g., Clorox) which is 5.25 per cent sodium hypochlorite. When it gives up its oxygen, hydrochloric acid is formed.

Other substances, such as kerosene, creosote, potassium permanganate, and sodium dichromate, may also be corrosive.

Common household products that may contain caustic substances are listed in Table 55–1.

PATHOLOGY

Effects of Corrosives on the Esophagus. Krey (1952) reviewed the literature and experimented on rabbits with lye. From this excellent article, the natural history of the burned esophagus can be followed. The extent of corrosive ulcers and the degree of penetration into the esophageal wall depend on the *type, concentration, amount,* and *time of contact* of the corrosive agent.

Types of Corrosive. Acids cause a *coagulation* necrosis from which an eschar forms. This tends to keep the corrosive from penetrating to deeper layers of tissues. Alkalis, on the other hand, produce *liquefaction* necrosis with an edematous loosening of the tissue and with diffusion of the corrosive into the deeper layers. Lesions caused by acids are thus more superficial and have a more favorable prognosis than the deeper alkali lesions.

Concentrations of Corrosive. The concentration of sodium hydroxide required to produce a lesion is somewhere between 0.5 and 1 per cent. If a solution is stronger than this it is likely to cause a lesion. For example, 3.8 per cent sodium hydroxide (1N) causes necrosis of the mucosa and submucosa with some involvement of the inner longitudinal fibers; 10.7 per cent sodium hydroxide (3N) causes necrosis extending into the circular muscle layer; 16.9 per cent (5N) causes necrosis extending into the outer longitudinal muscle; and solutions greater than 22.5 per cent cause necrosis through the whole esophageal wall and also affect the periesophageal connective tissue.

Weeks and Ravitch (1969) reported an experiment in which cats were exposed to liquid chlorine bleach (sodium hypochlorite 0.05 per cent, sodium hydroxide 5.25 per cent). This solution resulted in burns of the stomach and esophagus with late stricture formation in some animals. It was suggested that the damage was done by oxidation rather than by chlorination.

Ashcroft and Padula (1974) used sulfuric acid, less than 10 per cent, in cats and produced severe esophageal damage after a 30 second exposure.

Amount. Leape and his associates (1971) reported that 1 cc of highly concentrated liquid lye solution produced esophageal lesions in cats.

Ashcroft and Padula (1974) reported that even small amounts of concentrated sodium hydroxide caused lesions in children; in one case, a patient placed a discarded cap from a bottle of drain cleaner in her mouth and suffered esophageal burns.

The Time of Contact. Krey (1952) showed that areas of physiologic narrowing of the esophagus — the cricopharyngeal opening, the crossing of the aorta and left mainstem bronchus, and also the fundus where the esophagus passes through the dia-

Table 55–1   COMPOSITION OF SOME OF THE MORE COMMONLY
USED DRAIN CLEANERS

Name of Product	Manufacturer	Active Ingredient	Concentration (%)
Granular			
Plumite	Simoniz Co., Chicago	Sodium hydroxide	92%
Rooto Heavy-Duty Drain Cleaner	Roota Corp., Farmington, Michigan	Potassium hydroxide	71%
Mitee	DAP Inc., Dayton, Ohio	Sodium hydroxide	<10%
Drano	Drackett Prod. Co., Cincinnati	Sodium hydroxide	54%
Liquid			
Liquid Drano	Drackett Prod. Co., Cincinnati	Sodium hydroxide	9.5%
Glamorene Drain Powder	Glamorene Prod. Corp. Clifton, N.J.	Potassium hydroxide	35%
Mister Plumber	National Solvent Corp., Cleveland	Conc. sulfuric acid	99.5%
Plunge	Drackett Prod. Co.	Sodium hydroxide	9.5%
Down the Drain	Lehn & Fink Prop., Montvale, N.J.	Potassium hydroxide	36.5%
Liquid Plumr	Clorox Corp., Oakland, California	Sodium hydroxide	12%

phragm — were often more severely affected because of the longer amount of time spent by the corrosive at these sites. Leape et al. (1971) showed that highly concentrated liquid lye caused ulceration and eventual stricture of the esophagus in cats even after one second of exposure.

Pathologic Stages of the Burn. Krey (1952) was able to observe by the naked eye and by microscopic examination the progress of discrete burns in the esophagus caused by varying concentrations of sodium hydroxide. On the first day the edge of the lesion is poorly defined, but after a few days a distinct ulcer is seen that is covered by a crust and has discrete edges. Between 15 and 20 days, the necrotic area is shed, leaving granulation tissue in the ulcer with patches of irregular epithelialization. Thirty to 40 days later, the ulcer is still not covered by epithelium, but the wall around the ulcer is thickened. Microscopically, no epithelial remnants can be found after 24 hours, and the connective tissue of the submucosa remains as a few degenerated connective tissue fibrils. The muscle fibers are slightly swollen and held apart by a leukocyte-rich inflammatory exudate. The inflammatory process is not limited to the immediate vicinity of the necrotic area but extends for some distance into the surrounding esophageal wall and into the periesophageal connective tissue. After two to four days, granulation tissue consisting of newly formed blood vessels and young connective tissue develops between the necrotic area and the intact tissue. By five to eight days, a well-marked necrotic area can be seen as a result of the increase in granulation tissue. By 10 days, the greater part of the ulcer is filled with granulation tissue, which forces the necrotic area into the esophageal lumen. By 15 days, the whole ulcer is filled with granulation tissue, and the necrotic area is shed. Small remnants of this necrotic tissue can remain adherent to the surface of the ulcer for up to 30 to 40 days. The esophageal wall at the site of the lesion is greatly thickened into the rich development of granulation tissue, which is transformed into connective tissue in the deeper layers. After 20 to 25 days, the surface of the ulcer is covered with a purulent, fibrinous exudate in which necrotic particles can be seen. The fibrous conversion of the granulation tissue in the deeper layers of the wound begins to predominate over the cellular components. After 30 to 40 days,

complete epithelialization of the ulcer is still not present. The underlying connective tissue becomes richer in collagen, and this, eventually, forms the scar, which contracts and leads to constriction of the lumen.

From the pathology, it can be seen that there are three stages: acute, intermediate, and late, which correspond clinically to immediate pain, discomfort and difficulty in swallowing, gradually easing over the first two weeks, followed by a relatively asymptomatic period lasting for a week or more; then a period of increasing difficulty swallowing leading in some cases to a complete inability to swallow as strictures develop.

CLINICAL PICTURE

Cardona and Daly (1971) classified patients into five categories, depending upon the severity of their burns, for the purpose of comparing results and evaluating the effect of treatment. These were based on both clinical observation and esophagoscopy.

Mild, Nonulcerative Esophagitis. These patients have very little discomfort on swallowing. Esophagoscopy shows hyperemia of the esophageal mucosa without ulceration.

Mild, Ulcerative Esophagitis. These patients usually have discomfort and difficulty swallowing. They have shallow ulcers in the esophagus that seem to involve the mucosa only. These may form strictures, and the patient will go through the three clinical stages of esophageal burns.

Moderate to Severe Ulcerative Esophagitis. These patients have lesions that produce deep craters. The muscle layers of the esophagus and sometimes even the entire wall are involved. There may be a single ulceration, or there may be multiple ulcers with viable mucosa in between. These patients, untreated, will inevitably develop strictures.

Severe Ulcerative, Uncomplicated Esophagitis. Most of the esophageal mucosa is involved with very few areas of intact mucosa remaining. Sloughing and necrosis are deep, involving most of the layers.

Severe Ulcerative Esophagitis with Complications. In these cases perforation occurs, resulting in mediastinitis or localized mediastinal abscesses. Perforation of the stomach or duodenum may also occur, leading to peritonitis. The larynx may also be burned, leading to upper airway obstruction, and there may be acid–base metabolic disturbances.

DIAGNOSIS

In the emergency room, it is important to find out the type of substance that was ingested or suspected to have been ingested. Most often the parents or the people accompanying the patient can provide only the name of the substance. In this case, the information as to the constitution and concentration of the substance can be obtained from the nearest poison center. An attempt should be made to estimate how much of the substance was ingested. In children, this is usually very difficult. It should be emphasized that even small amounts of caustic products can cause severe damage to the esophagus and that once a substance has touched a child's tongue, the natural reflex leads to swallowing. *Thus, parents should not be reassured that no damage has been done until the child has been fully examined.* It is important to know whether the patient vomited after ingestion or was made to vomit, since this would increase the length of time the esophagus was exposed to the agent.

Examination of the patient, especially a child, may reveal that there are burns on the lips, chin, hands, or chest due to manipulation of the substance and possible regurgitation. The patient may be in severe pain and unable to swallow even his own saliva. There may be burns in the mouth. The presence of burns in the mouth has been shown to correlate very poorly with burns in the esophagus; so it should not be assumed that because of the absence of burns in the mouth, esophageal burns are unlikely and vice versa.

The complications of acute laryngitis that lead to airway obstruction should be searched for. Mediastinitis, which may cause severe chest pains, especially on respiration, should be looked for. The abdomen should also be examined for signs of peritonitis.

From the history and examination it may be possible to place the patient into one of three categories. The first category would be the mild, ulcerative esophagitis in which the patient is relatively asymptomatic. The second category would include mild, moderate to severe, and uncomplicated severe ulcerative esophagitis in which the patient would show definite evidence of ingestion with burns of the mouth, surrounding skin, or both, and pain in swallowing. In the third category would be the patients with severe ulcerative esophagitis with complications.

MANAGEMENT

Aim. The aim of management is to prevent stricture formation. Any management modality that reduces the amount of granulation tissue, the number and activity of fibroblasts, or both will contribute to this end.

Acute Management of Uncomplicated Esophagitis

Analgesics. Having once established that there is no airway obstruction, mediastinitis, or peritonitis present, intramuscular or intravenous narcotics may be administered.

Alimentation and Fluid Balance. The patient, if able to swallow, should be allowed only clear liquids. Krey (1952) showed that particles of food become caught up in necrotic tissue and produce more granulation tissue. If the patient is unable to swallow, fluids are given intravenously. At the same time as the intravenous line is being established it is possible to take blood for electrolyte estimation.

Chest Radiograph. Posteroanterior and lateral views should be obtained in all cases as a baseline and also to detect evidence of mediastinitis or aspiration pneumonia.

Antibiotics. Krey (1952) also showed that epithelialization occurred more quickly when his animals were treated with antibiotics. By reducing the number of bacteria present in the burn tissue, granulation tissue can be reduced. It is usual to use ampicillin, 50 to 100 mg per kg per day, either intravenously or, if the patient can swallow, by mouth where it has a local effect as well as a systemic effect.

Steroids. Spain and others (1950) showed that cortisone given to a group of mice with wounds on their backs showed an almost complete lack of exudate and fibrin in the wounds, together with marked diminution of cellular elements as compared with a group of controlled mice. However, if the steroids were given more than 48 hours after wounding, there was no significant difference between the group receiving the drug and the control group. Johnson (1963) experimented on dogs and showed that steroid therapy, if started early, definitely inhibited inflammatory response and granulation tissue formation with subsequent decrease in stricture formation. Since that time, many patients with caustic burns of the esophagus have been treated with steroids combined with antibiotics. Haller and Bachman (1964), Middelkamp and others (1969), Ray (1956), Ritter and others (1968), Rosenberg and others (1951, 1953), Yarington and Heatley (1963), Yarington and others (1964), and Weisskopf (1952) all treated patients with a combination of antibiotics and steroids, finding the incidence of stricture formation much lower than previously. The usual dose is methylprednisolone sodium succinate, 20 mg every 8 hours for patients under the age of two years, or 40 mg every 8 hours or its equivalent for older patients.

Esophagoscopy. Cardona and Daly (1971) have emphasized the poor correlation between oral or pharyngeal ulcerations and esophageal ulcerations. The presence of burns in the esophagus can be definitely established only by direct visualization. For this reason, esophagoscopy should be carried out within 48 to 72 hours after ingestion. If esophagoscopy is performed within the first 24 hours, a lesion may be overlooked, since in nearly all animal experiments it took at least 24 hours for lesions to become visible to the naked eye. Esophagoscopy performed later than 72 hours may cause the patient to have had unnecessary medical treatment and hospitalization if no burns of the esophagus are found. The esophagoscope should not be advanced beyond the first area of a severe burn, since the danger of perforation is greater in these cases than normally. However, advancement of an esophagoscope with a telescope or fiberoptic flexible esophagoscope may be performed when a mild burn is visualized in the proximal esophagus, since a severe burn may be present in the distal esophagus.

Later Management

No Burn. If no burn is seen on esophagoscopy, medication is discontinued, and an esophagogram is performed before the patient is discharged from the hospital, both as a baseline and as a precaution in case of an overlooked lesion. The patient is discharged from the hospital but seen again in six to eight weeks when a second esophagogram is performed. If the patient is still asymptomatic and the esophagogram is normal, there is no follow-up necessary.

Burn. If, on the basis of the esophagoscopic results, the patient is considered to have either a mild or moderate ulcerative esophagitis, the combination of antibiotic and steroid therapy should be continued for three to six weeks. The child should be maintained on clear liquids or intravenous fluids for most of this time, but towards the end of this time the patient may begin a soft diet. After about three weeks an esophagogram should be performed. If the child is asymptomatic and the esophagogram is normal, the medication can be discontinued, and the patient may be discharged from the hospital. The esophagogram should be repeated in six to eight weeks, and the patient is seen every three months for one year. If the child has difficulty swallowing or the esophagogram shows evidence of early stricture formation, or both, the cortisone should be discontinued and prograde bougienage should be begun. Initially this should be performed under general anesthesia through an esophagoscope using filiform dilators.

Hurst Mercury Bougies. Dilatation may be carried out without general anesthetic using the Hurst mercury bougies. This may be done in very young children who must, however, usually be wrapped in a blanket and held upright on the lap of an assistant (Fig. 55–2). A bougie of suitable size may be selected at the time of esophagoscopy. The tip of the dilator should be inserted into the patient's mouth and held high above his head so that the weight of the mercury encourages the passage of the tube down the esophagus. Unfortunately, in some of the smaller-sized bougies, the weight of the mercury is not great enough to carry the bougie down the esophagus, so that gentle insertion of the bougie by the operator may be necessary. The size of the dilator is then increased until one size is found that will not pass down the esophagus. The intervals between dilatations are governed by how well the patient can swallow food. He will probably need dilatation for the rest of his life, but the length of time between dilatations should increase as the patient grows. Periodically throughout this time, esophagograms and esophagoscopy should be performed in order to follow the extent of the disease. If prograde dilatation

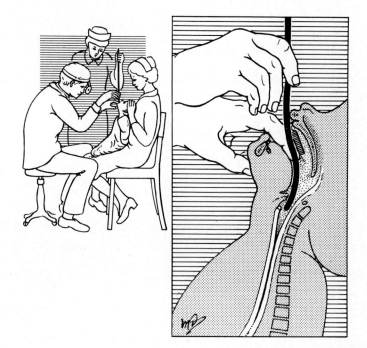

Figure 55–2 Prograde esophageal dilatation.

fails, it may be necessary to resort to gastrostomy and retrograde dilatation.

Psychiatric Consultation. Sobel, in 1970, studied 367 families whose children had been involved in accidental poisonings. In this study he found that the frequency of poisoning was unrelated to the accessibility of toxic substances which, he pointed out, was contrary to common sense. There was also found to be no relation between the level of motor development, intelligence of the child, birth complications, or parental accident-proneness. There was, however, significant association between accidental poisoning and measures of maternal psychopathology, such as the mother's marital dissatisfaction, mental illness, poor ego strength, and sexual dissatisfaction. His data suggested the hypothesis that a net role performance on the mother's part generates a power struggle with the child, which may eventually result in the ingestion of forbidden substances by the child as an act of defiance and rebellion. Accidental poisoning, therefore, should always be treated as a symptom of family disturbance. It is felt that psychiatric consultation is essential for giving emotional support to the mothers who are unable to cope with the stress placed upon them by their maternal and marital roles.

The mental trauma, both for the child and the family, in a severe case of poisoning would also warrant psychiatric support. The prolonged treatment necessary if a stricture develops, with frequent and, to the young child often unpleasant, visits to the hospital will also necessitate psychiatric support. In cases where suicide has been attempted by the older child, psychiatric consultation is mandatory.

Severe Uncomplicated Esophagitis. Initially these patients are treated the same as less severely burned patients, but as soon as the extent of the burn is realized by esophagoscopy, the steroids are discontinued. This should be done because when the whole wall of the esophagus is necrotic, the danger of perforation occurring when the patient is taking steroids is very great. In these cases the best method of treatment is to rest the esophagus, which is best done by performing a gastrostomy.

Gastrostomy. Krey (1952) found that the best results were obtained in reducing stricture formation by resting the esophagus, which may be accomplished by performing a gastrostomy and using antibiotics. A string should be passed through the esophagus and brought out through the gastrostomy. The upper end of the string is brought out through the nose and tied to the lower end so that there is a continuous loop of string through the esophagus. The patient may facilitate placement of the string by swallowing it first before esophagoscopy. After two or three weeks, retrograde bougienage may commence.

Retrograde Bougienage (Fig. 55–3). This may be done while the patient is awake, even in a very young child (Fig. 55–3A). The technique, described by Tucker (1924), should be such that the string is always present in the esphagus (Fig. 55–3B). The loop is first cut, and two pieces of string are tied to the lower end (Fig. 55–3C). By pulling on the upper end, two new pieces of string are pulled out through the nose (Fig.

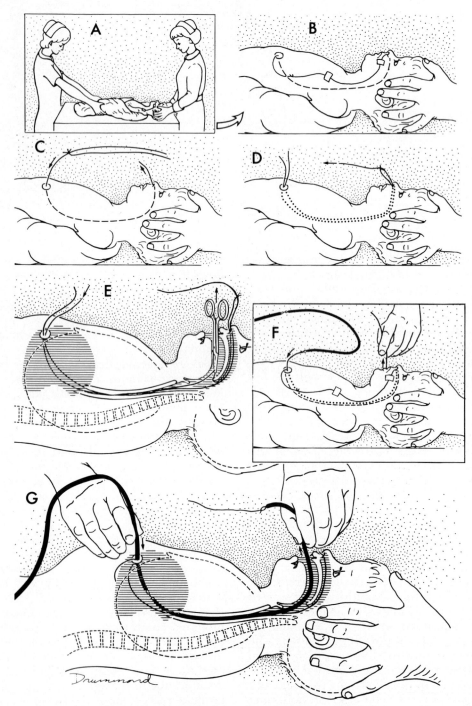

Figure 55–3   Retrograde esophageal dilatation (see text).

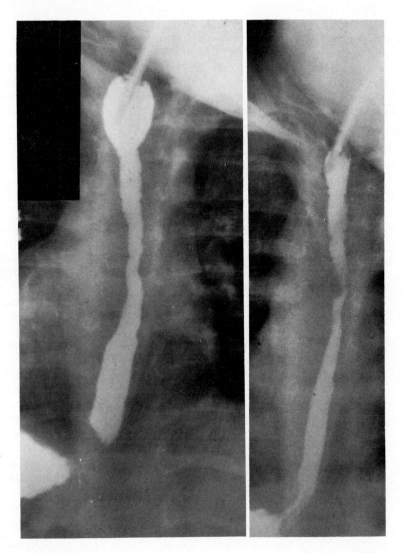

Figure 55–4 Example of esophageal stricture due to caustic burn.

55–3*D*). The upper end of one of these pieces of string is tied to the lower end of the same string. This will be the loop that remains in the esophagus after dilatation. The second loop is brought out through the mouth using forceps (Fig. 55–3*E*). A Tucker dilator is tied to the lower end of the string, and by a combination of pulling on the upper string and pushing the dilator, it can be passed up the esophagus and into the mouth (Fig. 55–3*F*). Dilators of increasing size can be tied end to end like a string of sausages, and the whole string can be pulled right out through the mouth (Fig. 55–3*G*). Alternatively, the first dilator can be pulled through the gastrostomy, and the string should be reattached to the second dilator. This procedure can be undertaken daily at first, and after a while it may be possible to progress to prograde dilatation. Prograde dilatation may continue for

the rest of the patient's life at varying intervals. Periodic esophagoscopy and esophagograms (Fig. 55–4) will be necessary to follow the course of the disease. If retrograde bougienage fails, then colon interposition may be the only alternative. However, a functioning esophagus is better than a colon interposition; so every effort should be made to maintain the esophageal function as long as possible.

Management of Acute, Complicated Esophagitis

The mortality of patients in this group is very high.

Shock and Metabolic Acid–Base Disturbance. This is treated along basic surgical principles with intravenous replacement therapy and correction of acid–base balance.

Upper Airway Obstruction. The larynx may have been burned to a varying degree. Edema and inflammation may cause an upper airway obstruction, which is relieved by tracheostomy. The larynx may be affected in the same way as the esophagus with a good deal of tissue destruction leading to stricture formation later on. This may require laryngeal surgery at a later date.

Mediastinitis. This occurs owing to perforation of the esophagus. It may lead to the development of small, localized abscesses around the esophagus or to full-blown mediastinitis. In the case of small, localized abscesses, the help of a thoracic surgeon may be necessary to place a drain in the chest. Severe mediastinitis may require immediate esophagectomy. Ritter (1971) recommended radical treatment for these cases since the mortality is so high. An immediate esophagectomy is sometimes recommended, leaving the patient with a cervical esophagostomy and gastrostomy. This means a colon interposition would be required at a later date. However, the radical surgery is reserved for the most severely perforated esophagus.

Peritonitis. A burn of sufficient severity to cause mediastinitis may also cause perforation of the stomach or duodenum, or both, leading to peritonitis. In these cases, again, immediate esophagogastrectomy is recommended to remove dead and necrotic tissue in order to reduce the morbidity and mortality rates.

Summary

The severity of burns of the esophagus caused by a caustic agent depends on the type, concentration, amount of agent, and time of contact. The aim of therapy is to reduce the amount of granulation tissue and, hence, the likelihood of stricture formation, by resting the esophagus and administering antibiotics and steroids. For the more severe burns, more drastic measures are necessary. Once a stricture has formed, periodic dilatations, either prograde or retrograde, are undertaken, every effort being made to maintain some sort of functioning esophagus in preference to performing a colon interposition.

ACQUIRED STRICTURES

Repaired Congenital Atresia of the Esophagus. One of the major problems following repair of congenital esophageal atresia is stenosis at the site of anastomosis. Holinger and Johnston (1963) and Morrison (1959) believe that stenosis may occur at the anastomotic site of a direct end-to-end anastomosis of the two segments of the esophagus; at the esophagogastric, esophagoduodenal, or esophagocolic anastomosis; and also at the colic-gastric anastomosis. The management following the repair of esophageal atresia seems to be the most significant factor in preventing stenoses. Morrison (1959) found that the most satisfactory management plan was to perform a gastrostomy a day or two following surgery. Gastrostomy provides the means for nutrition and also an avenue for a nasogastric string, which maintains a lumen in the esophagus and permits esophageal dilatation. It is felt that early dilatation is more likely to maintain the esophageal lumen than waiting for a tight, well-established stricture to develop and then trying to dilate it. Dilatation is carried out, therefore, at the end of the second or third postoperative week, starting with retrograde Tucker bougies, size 12 French. The size of bougie is increased very slowly, and by six months a size 18 French or 26 French can be achieved. Gastrostomy is maintained for 12 to 18 months, and dilatations are carried out periodically. Sometimes no dilatations are done for months at a time. After the gastrostomy is closed, a Hurst mercury bougie is used, at least once or twice every year, to measure the size of the esophagus and to help maintain the lumen. Size 30 to 34 French was used for this. Holinger and Johnston (1963) stressed the importance of the suture technique used for the anastomosis. They point out that the approach to the repair is somewhat controversial. The transpleural approach permits better exposure and greater ease in freeing the segments to permit anastomosis with lower morbidity and mortality rates but is accompanied by the serious complication of fistula formation. Their regime involves the performance of a fluoroscopic esophageal examination with barium 10 days following surgery. This is repeated in one month and then in three months if no narrowing is noted. If narrowing is demonstrated, bougienage is begun daily or once, twice, or three times a week. The dilatations may be accomplished with dilators of increasing diameter up to 22, 24, or 26 French, depending on the age and size of the patient.

Strictures Induced by Foreign Bodies or

Caustic Burns.   It is rather uncommon for a foreign body to lead to stricture, and there is very little information in the literature with regard to the incidence of this type of stricture. However, sharp foreign bodies may damage the esophageal wall, and this damage is increased when the foreign body is removed. A web-like stricture is most likely to develop following this sort of trauma.

The first evidence of the presence of a stricture may be the presentation of a patient in whose esophagus a foreign body is lodged. This may have been from caustic ingestion in early childhood and may occur many years later. Similarly, the foreign body lodgment occurs quite frequently in patients who have had congenital esophageal atresia repairs. The principles of treatment have already been discussed. Prograde dilatation is begun using increasing sizes of Hurst mercury bougies at increasing intervals until a satisfactory lumen is maintained. The follow-up treatment in these patients must be lifelong. It is only if prograde dilatation fails to maintain a lumen that retrograde dilatation is considered with gastrostomy. Mendelsohn and Maloney (1970) suggested injection of steroids into the stricture at esophagoscopy. They found that this was useful if the stricture was resistant and if progress towards increasing the lumen was slow by prograde dilatation. They used 1.5 to 2 cc of hydrocortisone acetate or triamcinolone acetonide (40 mg per cc) injected through the esophagoscope with a long needle. One cc of hyaluronidase is mixed with this steroid to act as a spreading agent. This is followed by immediate dilatation, using dilators two or four French sizes greater than in previous dilatations. Bleeding is a warning sign to stop the dilatation. They had no problems with infection, abscess, or perimediastinitis and felt that the stricture was softened and dilatation was able to be carried out more rapidly.

Stenosis at the Esophagocolic Junction Following Colon Interposition.   This may occur after replacement of all or part of the esophagus following caustic ingestion and is treated by early dilatation as outlined in the preceding section.

SELECTED REFERENCES

Jackson, C. 1931. The Life of Chevalier Jackson (An Autobiography). New York, The MacMillan Co.
  An interesting perspective on the historical background of caustic burns.

Johnson, E. 1963. A study of corrosive esophagitis. Laryngoscope, *73*:1651–1696.
  Another excellent article describing experimental studies on dogs using controlled, immediate antibiotic therapy, immediate steroid therapy, immediate steroid-antibiotic therapy, delayed antibiotic-steroid therapy, etc. It provides the basis of our clinical management today.

Krey, H. 1952. On the treatment of corrosive lesions in the oesophagus; an experimental study. Acta Oto-Laryngol., Suppl. 102.
  This is an excellent article that reviews the literature up to 1952. It includes a series of experiments on rabbits by which the natural history of esophageal burns can be followed, together with various treatment modalities in a controlled series. From this stems the procedure of antibiotic therapy and resting the esophagus.

Spain, D. M., Molomut, N., and Haber, A. 1950. The effect of cortisone on the formation of granulation tissue in mice. Am. J. Pathol., *261*:710.
  Based on the findings of this study, steroids were used in the treatment of caustic burns of the esophagus. This is a very short article.

REFERENCES

Alford, B. R., and Harris, H. H. 1959. Chemical burns of the mouth, pharynx, and esophagus. Ann. Otol., Rhinol., Laryngol., *68*:122–128.

Ashcroft, K. W., and Padula, R. T. 1974. The effect of dilute corrosives on the esophagus. Pediatrics, *53*:226–232.

Bikhazi, H. B., Thompson, E. R., and Shumrick, D. A. 1969. Caustic ingestion: Current status, a report of 105 cases. Arch. Otolaryngol., *89*:112–115.

Cardona, J. C., and Daly, J. F. 1971. Current management of corrosive esophagitis. Ann. Otol., Rhinol., Laryngol., *80*:521–527.

Consumer Reports. 1970. Drain cleaners. *35*:481–484.

Daly, J. F., and Cardona, J. C. 1961. Acute corrosive esophagitis. Arch. Otolaryngol., *74*:41–46.

Haller, J. A., and Bachman, K. 1964. The comparative effect of current therapy on experimental caustic burns of the esophagus. Pediatrics, *34*:236–245.

Holinger, P. H. 1960. Endoscopic aspects of esophagitis and esophageal hiatal hernia. J.A.M.A., *172*:313–324.

Holinger, P. H., and Johnston, K. C. 1950. Caustic strictures of the esophagus. IMJ, *98*:246–250.

Holinger, P. H., and Johnston, K. C. 1963. Postsurgical endoscopic problems of congenital esophageal atresia. Ann. Otol., Rhinol., Laryngol., *72*:1035–1049.

Jackson, C. 1931. The Life of Chevalier Jackson (An Autobiography). New York, The MacMillian Co., pp. 208–211.

Johnson E. E. 1963. A study of corrosive esophagitis. Laryngoscope, *73*:1651–1696.

Krey, H. 1952. On the treatment of corrosive lesions in the oesophagus, an experiment study. Acta Oto-laryngol., Suppl. 102.

Leape, L. L., Ashcraft, K. W., Scarpelli, D. G., and Holder, T. M. 1971. Hazard to health, liquid lye. N. Engl. J. Med., *284*:578–581.

Mendelsohn, H. J., and Maloney, W. H. 1970. The treatment of benign strictures of the esophagus with cortisone injection. Ann. Otol., Rhinol., Laryngol., *79*:900–906.

Middelkamp, J. N. , Ferguson, T. B., Roper, C. L. et al.

1969. The management of problems of caustic burns in children. J. Thorac. Cardiovasc. Surg., 57:341–347.

Morrison, L. E. 1959. Experiences with dilatation of the esophagus following surgery for esophageal atresia. Ann. Otol., Rhinol., Laryngol., 68:581–594.

Owens, H. 1954. Chemical burns of the esophagus; the importance of various chemicals as etiologic agents in stricture formation. Arch. Otolaryngol., 60:482–486.

Ray, E. S., and Morgan, D. L. 1956. Cortisone therapy of lye burns of the esophagus. J. Pediatr., 49:394–397.

Ritter, F. N., Gago, O., Kirsh, M., et al. 1971. The rationale of emergency esophagogastrectomy in the treatment of liquid caustic burns of the esophagus and stomach. Arch. Otolaryngol., 80:513–520.

Ritter, F. N., Newman, M. H., and Newman, D. E. 1968. A clinical and experimental study of corrosive burns of the stomach. Ann. Otol., Rhinol., Laryngol., 67:830–842.

Rosenberg, N., Kunderman, P. J., Vroman, L., et al. 1951. Prevention of experimental lye strictures of the esophagus by cortisone. Arch. Surg., 63:147–151.

Rosenberg, N., Kunderman, P. J., Vroman, L. et al.

1953. Prevention of experimental esophageal stricture by cortisone. Arch. Surg., 66:593–598.

Sobel, R. 1970. The psychiatric implications of accidental poisoning in childhood. Pediatr. Clin. North Am., 17:653–685.

Spain, D. M., Molomut, N., and Haber, A. 1950. The effect of cortisone on the formation of granulation tissue in mice. Am. J. Pathol., 261:710–711.

Tucker, G. 1924. Cicatricial stenosis of the esophagus with particular reference to treatment by continuous string, retrograde bouginage with the author's bougie. Ann. Otol., Rhinol., Laryngol., 69:1180–1214.

Weeks, R., and Ravitch, M. M. 1969. Esophageal injury by liquid chlorine bleach: Experimental study. J. Pediatr., 74:911–916.

Weisskopf, A. 1952. Effects of cortisone on experimental lye burn of the esophagus. Ann. Otol., Rhinol., Laryngol., 61:681–691.

Yarington, C. T., Jr., and Heatley, C. A. 1963. Steroids, antibiotics, and early esophagoscopy in caustic esophageal trauma. N. Y. State J. Med., 63:2960–2963.

Yarington, C. T., Jr., Bales, G. A., and Frazer, J. P. 1964. A study of the management of caustic esophageal trauma. Ann. Otol., Rhinol., Laryngol., 73:1130–1135.

Chapter 56

FOREIGN BODIES OF THE PHARYNX AND ESOPHAGUS

Myles G. Turtz, M.D.
Sylvan E. Stool, M.D.

"Bid the patient attend to you and say 'Bone (or whatever it is) come forth, like as Christ brought Lazarus from the tomb and Jonah from the whale,' then take him by the throat and say, 'Blasius, Martyr and servant of Christ, saith, "either come up or go down."'" Aetius (ca. A.D. 500–550).

INCIDENCE OF FOREIGN BODIES

Foreign body removal is the reason for performing approximately 5 per cent of all pediatric peroral endoscopic procedures; more than half of these foreign bodies occur in the esophagus (Turtz and Tucker, 1972). The children most at risk are those between the ages of 14 months (the inquisitive, orally oriented toddler) and six years (when the back molars appear). Coins in the esophagus are the most common pediatric foreign body in the United States, whereas in a series of cases from Hong Kong, fish bones were seen with equal frequency (Nandi and Ong, 1978).

CLINICAL HISTORY

Less than 50 per cent of children who present with foreign bodies of the pharynx or esophagus have histories of ingestion. Therefore, the physician must be suspicious of the possibility of foreign body ingestion when dealing with the pediatric population, even when there is no behavioral evidence of in-

gestion. Frequently, even when the family gives a history of presumed ingestion, few have actually observed the act. In such cases the burden of proof is on the physician, and the necessary studies must be done in order to discover the truth of the assumption.

SIGNS AND SYMPTOMS

Most foreign bodies, whether ingested or aspirated, will initially cause laryngeal irritation, coughing, or choking. Subsequent signs or symptoms will be a function of the nature of the foreign body, the preexisting status of the esophagus, the length of time the foreign body has been in the esophagus, the place of the arrest of the foreign body, and complications inherent in the nature of the foreign body itself. The order of frequency of symptoms reported by Nandi and Ong (1978) was: (1) refusal to take feedings, (2) increased salivation, (3) pain or discomfort on swallowing, and (4) vomiting.

THE NATURE OF THE FOREIGN BODY

Most ingested foreign bodies will pass through the esophagus (Tucker, 1964). The symptoms at the time of presentation depend on the size and shape of the foreign body relative to the patient's size; the characteristics of the object also affect the level at which the object lodges and the difficulty of extract-

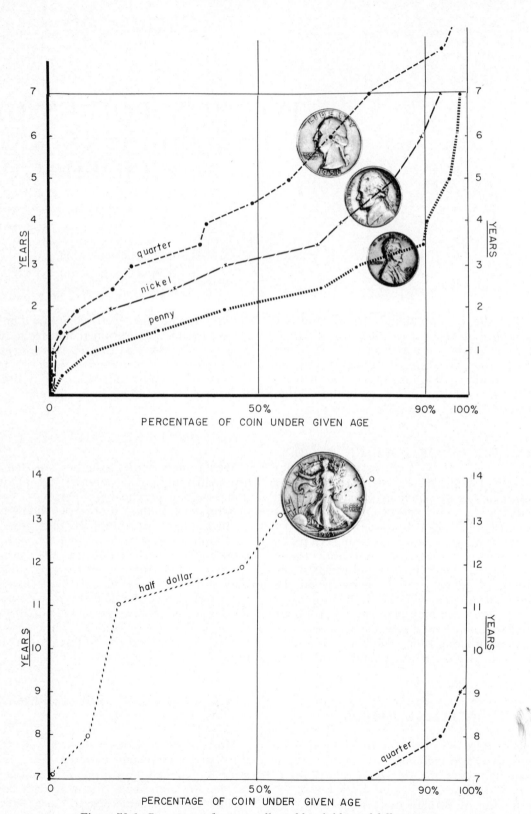

Figure 56–1 Percentage of coins swallowed by children of different ages.

ing the foreign body (Fig. 56–1). Smooth, slippery, plastic objects without burrs tend to traverse the swallowing passage without incident. However, if these plastic objects lodge in the esophagus, their very slipperiness can make it difficult to grasp them with forceps to remove them. Occasionally an irregularly shaped plastic object (Fig. 56–2) can also present problems. The type of toy varies with the area of the world (the toy in Figure 56–3 is common in Australia), but children around the globe seem to have equal propensities for swallowing their playthings.

The number of products fabricated from plastic and aluminum, which are not easily visualized radiographically, is increasing every year. For instance, there have been numerous cases of ingestion of beverage pull tabs, which are difficult to detect radiographically (Burrington, 1976). The use of special methods, such as contrast studies and xerography, thus becomes more valuable in making a diagnosis and identifying the foreign object (Thompson, 1978). Most emergency situations involving foreign bodies develop because of the sharpness of the object and its potential for perforation; the open safety pin is a classic example (and a perennial one) of this situation (Fig. 56–4). When a common safety pin has been swallowed, it should spontaneously pass through the gastrointestinal tract of a two year old child without the need for endoscopic or surgical intervention if it is less than two inches long and closed. In other instances, special treatments are necessary. Food, a common esophageal foreign body in adults, is uncommon in children *when the esophagus is otherwise normal.* Obviously, if the child has some other abnormality of the esophagus, feeding may present problems,

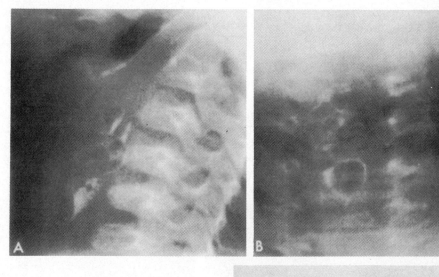

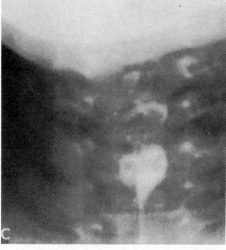

Figure 56–2 Lateral (A) and anteroposterior (B and C) views of a barium coated toy in the esophagus.

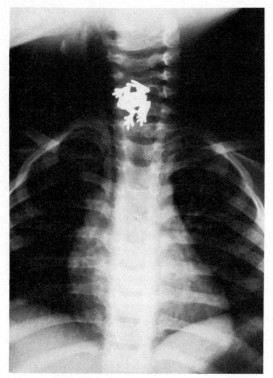

Figure 56-3 A toy in the esophagus of a child from Australia.

attended to quickly because of their potential to endanger the airway and also because their descent may create more severe problems.

PREEXISTING STATUS OF THE ESOPHAGUS

The three physiologic areas of narrowing in the healthy esophagus are the cricopharyngeus, the area of the aortic crossing, and the cardioesophageal sphincter. The most common site of foreign body arrest is at the cricopharyngeus; the most dangerous is at the crossing of the aorta, especially when the foreign body is sharp. Abnormalities of the esophagus can cause ingested material that would normally pass through the esophagus to act as a foreign body. For instance, congenital stenosis of the esophagus, vascular compressions of the esophagus (notably double aortic arches, almost never aberrant subclavian arteries), or any trauma to the esophagus (for instance, after repair of esophageal atresia or esophageal duplications, interpositions, or strictures), and ectopic gastric mucosa with stricture of the mediastinal mass can all lead to problems with swallowing and thus to foreign body obstruction with passage of "normal" boluses of food. In these cases, the actual site of arrest of the foreign body is a function not only of the foreign body itself but also of the specific esophageal pathology (Fig. 56-5).

and food may thus act as a foreign body in the esophagus. Large, sharp, or irregularly shaped foreign bodies may lodge in the hypopharynx and present as airway emergencies. Hypopharyngeal foreign bodies should be

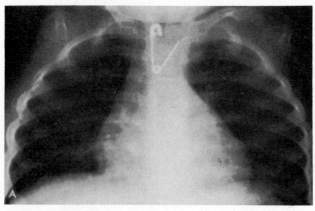

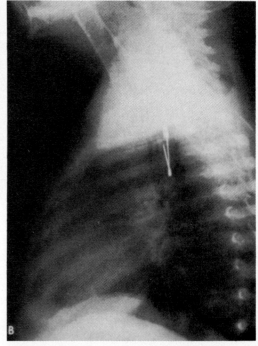

Figure 56-4 Anteroposterior (A) and lateral (B) views of an open safety pin.

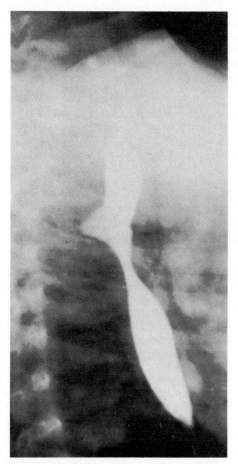

Figure 56–5 Esophageal abnormalities years after repair of esophageal atresia with fistula. Foreign bodies were repeatedly impacted proximal to the stenosis.

DURATION OF FOREIGN BODY OBSTRUCTION

In general, the longer the foreign body has been in the swallowing passages the greater will be the tissue reaction. Likewise, the foreign body will be more difficult to extract and complications will arise more frequently when the object has remained in the esophagus for some period of time. Duration of the obstruction is more significant when the object is sharp or metallic, but it can also be significant when the object is smooth.

DISTURBANCES IN DEGLUTITION

Occasionally, the foreign body will completely obstruct the swallowing passage, and the child will be unable to clear secretions. Other patients present with difficulty in swallowing that varies in degree with the nature of the object, duration of obstruction, and other previously mentioned factors. It is not uncommon for the child to have no early symptoms or signs of foreign body ingestion. It should be kept in mind that all children who have had esophageal surgery will have disturbances in the normal synchrony of swallowing, probably secondary to some interruption of the nervous supply to the esophageal wall (Kirkpatrick et al., 1961; Laks et al., 1972). In general, however, when any child without a history of such disturbances presents with swallowing difficulty, ingestion of a foreign body should be suspected.

RADIOGRAPHIC STUDIES

Neck and chest radiographs will usually identify radiopaque foreign bodies. The films should be made in both the lateral and anteroposterior planes. If the radiographs show evidence of a foreign body in the esophagus, a radiograph should be taken in the plane of the largest diameter of the presumed foreign body. A radiograph taken in such a plane will help to identify the object (especially flat bones and plates of metal, which are best seen on end). It will also help the endoscopist to formulate a three-dimensional concept of the foreign body, and it will allow the physician to determine the possibility of the presence of multiple coins or discs (Fig. 56–6). If there is a lack of plane radiographic evidence for presence of a foreign body but the clinical evidence for an esophageal foreign body is compelling, if the esophagus or mediastinum is widened, or if there is air in the upper esophagus, then a barium esophagogram is done. The danger that the child will aspirate the barium is real, but the test is justified in these instances. Performing a barium esophagogram with devices such as cotton pledgets has not been useful to us because such "aids" frequently confuse the endoscopic picture and occasionally complicate the clinical status of the patient. As previously stated, xerography is becoming a valuable technique in managing such cases (Thompson, 1978).

THE ENDOSCOPIC PROCEDURE

General Considerations

Few foreign bodies present such dire emergencies that some basic preliminaries cannot be performed before the removal is attempted. Discussion with the parents, total medical evaluation of the patient, practicing

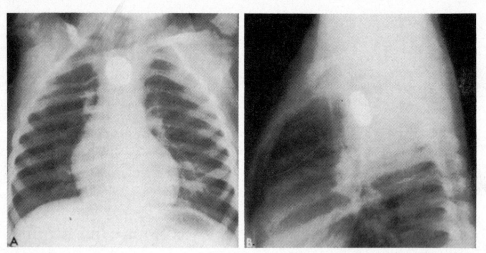

Figure 56–6 Esophageal coins (rouleaux) shown in anteroposterior (A) and lateral (B) views.

foreign body removal with a duplicate foreign body, and careful planning of the procedure by the endoscopic team should all precede the actual removal of the foreign body.

Discussion with the Parents

The family must be made aware of the possible complications of endoscopy. Since virtually all children who swallowed or could have swallowed a foreign body have been seen first by another physician before being referred to the otolaryngologist, it may be assumed that the parents have discussed the situation with another physician. Thus it is surprising that, except when the child has swallowed a sharp foreign body, many families are unaware of the potential complications that can arise from the removal of any foreign body. Unfortunately, families who are most aware of the problems incident upon foreign body extraction are those in whose child previous attempts at extraction of the object have failed. As a rule, it should *never* be suggested that the foreign body will be removed at the first attempt. The parents should be asked to agree to an examination of the child to determine if an extraction should be attempted at that time. Occasionally, an otherwise straightforward foreign body will not be extractable during the first procedure for any one of a myriad of reasons, and thus another course of action may be planned and discussed with the parents without having

failed to perform a promised extraction and without having lost their faith in your abilities.

Medical Evaluation of the Patient

Although the focus of the family and endoscopist is on the foreign body problem, a careful general history must be taken and a physical performed on each child who presents with this complaint. Special attention should be given to underlying illnesses, medications, and the states of hydration and nutrition of the child. Consultation with a pediatrician is routine in many institutions.

Practice on a Duplicate

Except for common esophageal foreign bodies, e.g., coins, it is highly desirable to practice extraction on a duplicate foreign body. Many unexpected problems of forceps purchase, changes in foreign body rotation and position, and insecure fit can become obvious, and the solutions to these problems can be developed in a practice session.

Planning with the Endoscopic Team

Whenever possible, the anesthesiologist is considered as part of the endoscopic team for foreign body removal. The history, physical findings, laboratory results, and radiographs

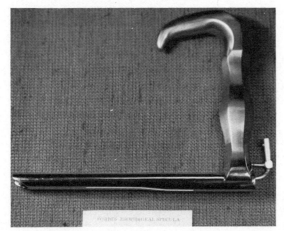

Figure 56-7 Forbes esophageal speculum – a useful instrument for removal of foreign bodies in the region of the cricopharyngeus.

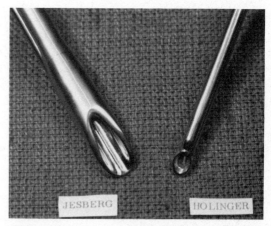

Figure 56-8 Distal end of the Holinger and Jesburg esophagoscopes. Lighting is provided with distal illumination.

should be reviewed by the team as a whole preoperatively.

SELECTION OF INSTRUMENTS

Esophagoscopes

The majority of esophageal foreign bodies lodge at the cricopharyngeus. A useful esophagoscope for these foreign bodies is the Forbes esophageal speculum (Fig. 56–7). The Forbes speculum gives direct access to the area, opens the sphincter, and allows for the use of laryngeal forceps. Foreign bodies in the esophagus require the use of longer esophagoscopes for their removal. The largest possible esophagoscope should be used in each case. The choice is usually between the

Holinger and Jesburg esophagoscopes (Fig. 56–8), although some pediatric endoscopists prefer the Storz esophagoscope (Fig. 56–9), with which the Hopkins rod lens telescope may be used to provide superb visualization of the object. However, the Storz endoscope does not have a suction channel. The Jesburg esophagoscope allows for a larger working area but has two disadvantages: there is no slide channel for continuous suctioning, and the Jesburg esophagoscope should be kept in the plane of intubation throughout the procedure, thus somewhat limiting the ability of the operator to use the Jesburg esophagoscope itself as a foreign body manipulator and rotator. Flexible esophagoscopes thus far have had limited application in foreign body removal, but as techniques and instruments improve they will surely be utilized more

Figure 56–9 Storz esophagoscopes and bronchoscopes: A, Child-size bronchoscope. B, Hopkins rod lens telescope with air sheath. C, Child-size esophagoscope. D, Infant-size bronchoscope. E, Infant-size esophagoscope. F, Prismatic deflector for proximal lighting. A 16 mm film – *Pediatric Bronchoscopy*, Order No. C6011–R16–is available which demonstrates the assembly and application of this instrument; the film may be obtained through the Karl Storz Co., 658 S. San Vicente Blvd., Los Angeles, CA 90048.

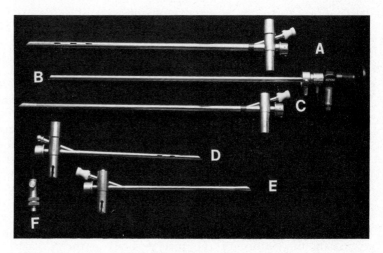

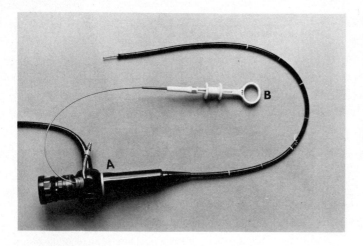

Figure 56–10 The flexible esophagoscope has been utilized for gastric and some esophageal foreign body removals. *A,* Esophagoscope. *B,* Biopsy forceps. Other types of foreign body forceps are available.

often (Fig. 56–10) (De Luca et al., 1976; Kline, 1974).

Forceps and Foreign Bodies

The endoscopist should have available a wide selection of forceps; the problem of the technique of removal should be a function *only* of the foreign body itself and not due to an incomplete armamentarium. Attempting to force the foreign body to accommodate to an inappropriate set of instruments can be dangerous. The classic reference work in the field of foreign bodies of the air and food passages is that by Jackson and Jackson (1936), which presents a distillate of hundreds of experiences in the removal of foreign bodies by skilled hands. Some of the forceps designed to be used with the Storz instrument are illustrated in Figures 56–11, 56–12, and 56–13. The Domia basket has also been used with the Storz esophagoscope, as well as has the conventional esophagoscope, for removal of a spherical foreign body (Schiratzki, 1976).

In recent years there have been tremendous advances in the development of flexible fiberoptic instrumentation. These instruments have been used for gastroscopy for removal of foreign bodies (Christie and Ament, 1976). There are also several case reports that describe the removal of foreign bodies without endoscopy, using a Foley catheter guided by a fluoroscope (Brown et al., 1972). This method may have some merit in very specific circumstances, such as in isolated medical facilities and when there is no doubt regarding the nature of the foreign body

(Stool and Dietch, 1973), but it does present some hazards.

The problem of the open safety pin in the esophagus serves as a model for many of the considerations and problems inherent in the removal of any foreign body. The patients are usually small. The history may be positive, or the discovery of the foreign body may occur during a study of associated signs or symptoms, such as stridor, feeding problems, fever, pneumonias, pneumothorax, failure to thrive, hematemesis, hemoptysis, subcutaneous emphysema, a neck mass, irritability, or pain. The child may appear to be healthy or in the throes of a catastrophic illness. The open safety pin may be in the patient's mouth (Fig. 56–14), allowing for office removal (given the ready availability of the appropriate assistance and equipment). More commonly the open safety pin is in the esophagus itself, necessitating peroral endoscopy (Fig. 56–4). In any event, a sense of urgency exists. The "anatomy" of the safety pin is reviewed: point, point shaft, spring, keeper shaft, and keeper. The point is invariably "up" (cephalad); the keeper is usually the presenting part.

Although there are several methods of esophageal safety pin removal (straightening, endogastric version, point-sheathing, and closing), all are based on the dictum "advancing points perforate; trailing points do not" (Jackson and Jackson, 1936). Various techniques for removal should all be practiced before being attempted *in vivo,* and a judgment must be made as to whether or not fluoroscopic guidance is indicated (Fig. 56–15). If biplane fluoroscopy is not available, the "C" arm is portable and may be used in

Figure 56–11 Optical fenestrated forward grasping forceps.

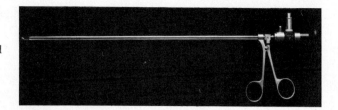

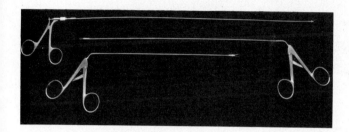

Figure 56–12 Alligator forceps for use with the open tube esophagoscope.

Figure 56–13 *A*, Fenestrated forward grasping forceps for use with the open tube Storz esophagoscope. *B*, Alligator forceps to be used through the instrument channel with the Storz Hopkins telescope. *C*, Cup forceps for use through the instrument channel of the Storz Hopkins esophagoscope.

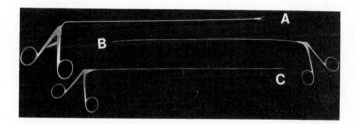

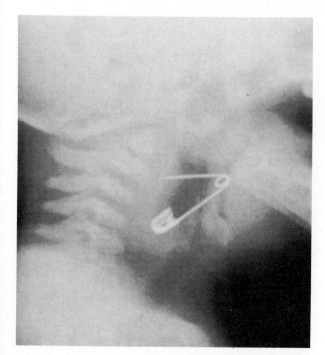

Figure 56–14 Hypopharyngeal presentation of open safety pin.

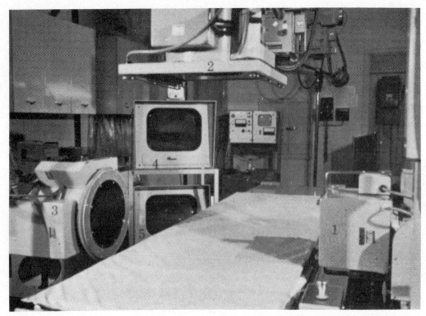

Figure 56–15   Biplane fluoroscope. (1) Tube for horizontal beam, (2) and (3) dual field 6 to 9 inch image intensifiers for vertical and horizontal beam projections, (4) and (5) television monitors for horizontal and vertical beam projections. (From Norris et al., 1971. Bronchoesophagologic application of recent advance of fluoroscopy. Ann. Otol., *80*:528.

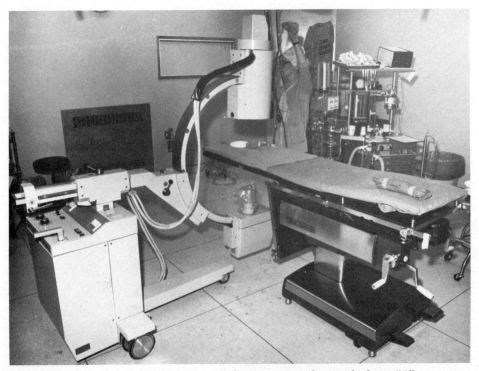

Figure 56–16   Portable fluoroscope with image intensifier attached to a "C" arm.

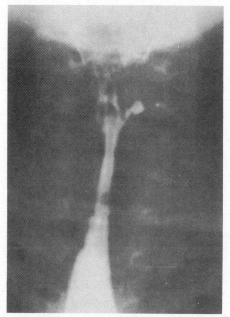

Figure 56–17 Sinus following removal of jackstone.

the operating room (Fig. 56–16). All forceps and esophagoscopes that may possibly be used are tested for fit and function. Anesthesia is effected by the techniques described in the next section. The mechanical approach to the foreign body, as well as the manipulation of it, is done with a conscious effort by the endoscopist to be *slow and deliberate*. Postoperatively, the patient is observed for signs of perforation (Fig. 56–17). Because of possible masking of symptoms of perforation, many endoscopists avoid the use of either adrenocorticosteroids or antibiotics after removal of the foreign body. If no signs or symptoms of perforation appear within 24 hours, clear liquids may be begun by mouth and the diet subsequently advanced. An esophagogram is usually obtained postoperatively.

TECHNIQUE FOR THE REMOVAL OF ESOPHAGEAL FOREIGN BODIES

General Considerations

With few exceptions, the discussion of technique here will be confined to nonemergency situations. All foreign body removals are considered to be major surgical procedures. The special considerations here include location of the foreign body, plan of extraction by the endoscopist, rating of the physical status of the patient, need for inhalation anesthesia, indications or contraindications for endotracheal intubation, need for tissue paralysis, contents of the stomach, contraindications to the use of nasogastric tubes in the presence of esophageal foreign bodies, and the possibility that creation of cricoid pressure in order to prevent regurgitation in "crash anesthesia" may be contraindicated (it frequently is).

Gastric Preparation of Children for Endoscopy

Children should not be given food or liquid by mouth according to the following guidelines: (1) no solids or milk for 12 hours prior to endoscopy for all ages; (2) for children 0 to 6 months, no clear liquids for 4 hours; (3) for children ages 6 to 36 months, no clear liquids for 6 hours; and (4) for children over the age of 36 months, no clear liquids for 8 hours.

Preoperative Medications

For sedation preoperatively, we use pentobarbital, 1 to 2 mg per kg; hydroxyzine, 0.25 mg per kg; and atropine, 0.02 mg per kg (minimum 0.15 mg).

For children under one year of age we use atropine alone.

We recommend succinylcholine, 1 mg per kg intravenously, as a muscle relaxant preoperatively.

MONITORING

All patients are continuously monitored with a precordial stethoscope, electrocardiogram equipment, sphygmomanometer, and thermometer. All patients should have an intravenous line securely placed.

Intubation Technique

Hypopharyngeal Foreign Bodies without Intubation

Induction. A nitrous oxide-halothane mixture is given by mask until the eyelid reflex is lost. The nitrous oxide is then discontinued, and the patient is allowed to spontaneously breathe a 2 per cent halothane/98 per cent oxygen mixture. After six to 10 minutes, the patient is given to the endoscopist.

Special Problems. Airway obstruction and laryngeal spasm, accidental dislodgment of the foreign body with an oral airway, possible regurgitation, and aspiration can occur. Because of these special problems in their removal, hypopharyngeal foreign bodies are frequently removed while the patient is awake.

Esophageal Foreign Bodies

Induction. Nitrous oxide/halothane is administered by mask, and when the patient is breathing regularly and quietly the nitrous oxide is discontinued and a mixture of halothane (2 per cent) and oxygen (98 per cent) is delivered by mask with positive pressure. Succinylcholine 1 mg per kg, is administered intravenously, and after fasciculation the trachea is intubated. After intubation the nitrous oxide is reintroduced to the halothane/oxygen mixture. An alternative induction technique is to administer ketamine (0.5 mg per kg intravenously) or pentobarbital (4 mg per kg intravenously), followed by the 2 per cent halothane/98 per cent oxygen mixture.

Special Problems. Contraindications to the use of nasogastric tubes include possible involvement of the posterior or subglottic larynx by edema, dislodgment of the endotracheal tube during manipulation or extraction of the object, the possibility of perforation (leading to pneumothorax or other complications), postoperative croup, excessive secretions in those patients who are totally obstructed, and compression of the endotracheal tube by the esophagoscope.

COMPLICATIONS OF ESOPHAGOSCOPY

Complications from peroral endoscopy in infants and children should be uncommon (Figs. 56–17 and 56–18). The complications resulting from endoscopic removal of foreign bodies, therefore, are largely a result of the foreign body itself, the peculiarities of its presentation, and the length of time that has elapsed from ingestion to removal (Yee et al., 1975). Most complications occur before re-

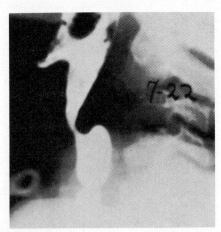

Figure 56–18 Granulations and stenosis following toy extraction.

moval is attempted. The most common complications are pneumothorax, pneumomediastinitis, mediastinitis, croup, pneumonia, airway obstruction, dysphagia, or odynophagia. Death is a rarity. In general, complications occur in less than 2 per cent of procedures.

ILLUSTRATIVE CASES

As with all pediatric bronchoesophagologic operations, selection of the proper size of endoscope is critical. Too large an instrument will unnecessarily traumatize tissues; one that is too small will limit the operator's ability to manipulate the foreign body. Rigid rules regarding the appropriate size for an endoscope should be avoided, but Table 56–1 may serve as a general guide.

Coin

Figure 56–6 shows a two year old girl who swallowed two coins. The presenting complaint was that the parents saw the child "swallow a nickel." The child was asymptomatic. The radiographs showed a coin. No anesthesia was used in the retraction of this foreign body, and a Forbes esophageal speculum was used in order to insert laryngeal grasping forceps, which were able to gain purchase on the presenting part: the edges of two nickels in rouleaux. There were no complications. After removal of both nickels, the child recalled swallowing the other coin two

Table 56–1 SELECTION OF ENDOSCOPE SIZE

	Laryngoscope*	Bronchoscope†	Esophagoscope†
Newborn	7, 9	2½, 3	3
10–20 lbs.	9	3, 3½	4
20–30 lbs.	9, 10½	3½, 3¾, 4	4, 5
30–40 lbs.	10½	4	5
50–70 lbs.	10½, 11, 12	4, 5	5

*Numbers refer to working length in centimeters.
†Numbers refer to internal diameter in millimeters.

weeks prior to the one her parents saw her swallow.

Jackstone

Figure 56–19 shows a jackstone in the esophagus of a four year old boy. The presenting complaint was dysphagia, and the child's history was negative for ingestion. General anesthesia was used, and the Forbes esophageal speculum was used to pass ball forceps, which grasped the ball of the jackstone. The child required tracheotomy 10 hours after esophagoscopy. Jackstones are a fairly common pediatric foreign body, although even when they are demonstrated on

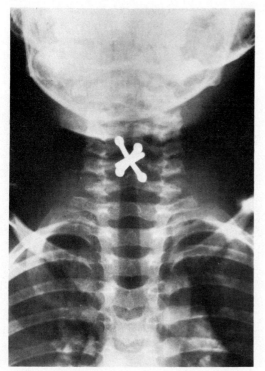

Figure 56–19 Jackstone present in esophagus.

radiographs children frequently deny ingestion of the objects. Because of their irregular shape, large size, rigidity, and usually high level of presentation, some airway distress occurs in approximately a third of cases.

Wire-spring

Figure 56–20 shows a wire-spring in the esophagus of a 14 year old male. The presenting complaint was recurrent croup, bronchitis, and a cough for six months. The history was negative for foreign body ingestion, but the radiograph showed a spring in the midthoracic esophagus. A barium swallow showed a narrowing of the barium column, but it did not contact the coil of the spring. Anesthesia was general, and the esophagoscope used was a 6 by 20 inch Holinger. The presenting part of the wire-spring was the granulations, which were grasped with laryngeal grasping forceps. Manipulation of the spring dislodged the endotracheal tube, and a bronchoscope was required to establish the airway. In this case of a long-standing esophageal foreign body presenting with respiratory distress, the foreign body was found to be so completely embedded as to be invisible endoscopically, and biplane fluoroscopic guidance was required to extract the object.

Plastic Wheels and Axle

Figure 56–2 shows the barium swallow of a three year old girl with a plastic toy in the esophagus. The presenting complaint was that the parents saw the child swallow and gag on the foreign body 10 months prior to admission. On admission the child was cachectic and could swallow only liquids. A radiograph confirmed the presence of the

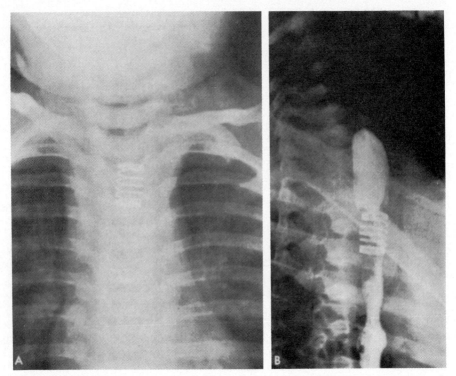

Figure 56–20   *A*, Spring in esophagus. *B*, Spring seen during barium study.

foreign body with a barium coating. Anesthesia was general, and the Forbes esophageal speculum was used to pass laryngeal rotation forceps, which grasped an upper wheel. Complications of this case included the need to perform a tracheotomy and a gastrostomy for retrograde dilatations of esophageal stenosis. The parents of this child saw many physicians over the 10 month period before admission to our service. Plain radiographs of the neck and chest were done repeatedly for this radiolucent foreign body. One week prior to referral, an otolaryngologist saw the foreign body during a mirror laryngoscopy, and a barium swallow confirmed the presence of the foreign body.

Open Safety Pin

Figure 56–4 shows a 16 month old male who swallowed an open safety pin. The presenting complaint was that the child "wouldn't eat and was irritable." The radiograph showed the open safety pin, which was removed under general anesthesia. A No. 4 Holinger esophagoscope was used to pass ring rotation forceps, which grasped the spring of the safety pin. The safety pin's presenting part was the keeper, and it was

then extracted by version. There were no complications.

Gastric Coin

Figure 56–21 is the radiograph of a coin lodged in the abdomen of an infant. The

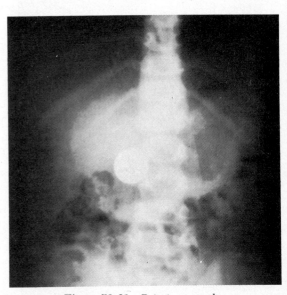

Figure 56–21   Coin in stomach.

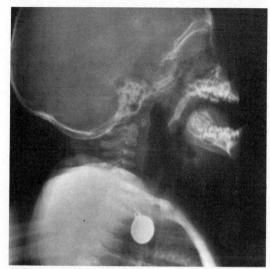

Figure 56–22 Medallion in esophagus causing respiratory obstruction and stridor.

presenting complaint in this case was that the child had "swallowed a quarter." The radiograph showed the coin to be located in the stomach. It was removed under general anesthesia with a No. 5 Jackson esophagoscope being used to pass forward-grasping forceps. The forceps were passed with fluoroscopic guidance and grasped the presenting part, the edge of the coin in the stomach. There were no complications of extraction, but the coin had been in the stomach for at least nine weeks, and the child had required a repair of a pyloric stenosis, which left scars.

Medallion

Figure 56–22 shows a one year old child who presented with stridor of two months duration. General anesthesia was used to pass a Storz 5 mm esophagoscope, through which Storz alligator forceps were able to grasp the edge of the coin the child had swallowed. There were no complications of removal of this foreign body. There have been a number of reports of cases similar to this one (Tauscher, 1978; Peroff, 1972; Pasquariello, 1975).

SELECTED REFERENCES

Jackson, C., and Jackson, C. L. 1936. Diseases of the Air and Food Passages of Foreign Body Origin. Philadelphia, W. B. Saunders Co.

This text is the definitive foreign body reference for

endoscopists. It is detailed and full of techniques, problems, and solutions.

Kirkpatrick, J. V., Cresson, S. L., and Pilling, G. P., IV. 1961. The motor activity of the esophagus in association with esophageal atresia and tracheal esophageal fistula. Am. J. Roentgenol., *86*:884.

This is one of the first studies to explain swallowing problems universal in children with repaired esophageal atresias with fistula.

Laks, H., Wilkinson, R. H., and Schuster, S. R. 1972. Long term results following correction of esophageal atresia with tracheoesophageal fistula: A clinical and cinefluorographic study. J. Pediatr. Surg., 7:7591.

This article updates and discusses that by Kirkpatrick et al. (1961).

Norris, C. M., Tucker, G. F., Jr., and Woloshin, H. J. 1971. Bronchoesophagologic application of recent advances of fluoroscopy. Ann. Otol. Rhinol. Laryngol., *80*:528.

These authors present good guidelines for the use of biplane fluoroscopy.

Tucker, G. F., Jr. 1964. The age incidence of lodgement of single coins in the esophagus. Trans. Am. Bronchoesophagol. Assoc., *44*:145.

The graph from this article in this chapter allows the reader to predict which coins will pass spontaneously and makes the point that not everything ingested will arrest in the food passages.

Turtz, M. G., and Tucker, G. F., Jr. 1972. The present day spectrum of pediatric bronchoesophagology. Laryngoscope, *82*:945.

This article reviews 906 bronchoesophagologic procedures in a pediatric hospital.

REFERENCES

Brown, E., Hughes, P., and Koenig, H. 1972. Removal of foreign bodies lodged in esophagus by a Foley catheter without endoscopy. Clin. Pediatr., *11*(8):468–471.

Burrington, J. D. 1976. Aluminum "pop tops." J.A.M.A. *235*:2614–2617.

Christie, D. L., and Ament, M. E. 1976. Removal of foreign bodies from esophagus and stomach with flexible fiberoptic panendoscopes. Pediatrics, *57*:931–934.

DeLuca, R., Ferrer, J., and Wortzel, E. 1976. Polypectomy snare extraction of foreign bodies from the esophagus. Am. J. Gastroenterol., *66*:374–376.

Ferguson, C. F., and Kendig, E. L. 1972. Pediatric Otolaryngology. Philadelphia, W. B. Saunders Co.

Jackson, C., and Jackson, C. L. 1936. Diseases of the Air and Food Passages of Foreign Body Origin. Philadelphia, W. B. Saunders Co.

Kirkpatrick, J. V., Cresson, S. L., and Pilling, G. P., IV. 1961. The motor activity of the esophagus in association with esophageal atresia and tracheal esophageal fistula. Am. J. Roentgenol., *86*:884.

Kline, M. 1974. Endoscopic snare in removal of an esophageal foreign body. Gastrointest. Endosc., *20*:165–166.

Laks, H., Wilkinson, R. H., and Schuster, S. R. 1972. Long term results following correction of esophageal atresia with tracheoesophageal fistula: A clinical and cinefluorographic study. J. Pediatr. Surg., 7:7591.

Nandi, P., and Ong, G. B. 1978. Foreign body in the oesophagus: Review of 2394 cases. Brit. J. Surg., 65:5–9.

Norris, C. M., Tucker, G. F., Jr., and Woloshin, H. J. 1971. Bronchoesophagologic application of recent advances in fluoroscopy. Ann. Otol., Rhinol. Laryngol., 80:528.

Pasquariello, P. S., Jr. 1975. Cyanosis from a foreign body in the esophagus. Clin. Pediatr., 14:223–225.

Peroff, R. P. 1972. Esophageal foreign body presenting with respiratory symptoms and signs. Can. J. Otolaryngol., 1(2):141–145.

Schiratzki, H. 1976. Removal of foreign bodies in the esophagus. Arch. Otolaryngol., 102:238–240.

Stool, S., and Dietch, M. 1973. Potential danger of catheter removal of foreign body. Pediatrics, 51:313–314.

Tauscher, J. W. 1978. Esophageal foreign body: An uncommon cause of stridor. Pediatrics, 61:657–658.

Thompson, D. H. 1978. Xerographic detection of foreign bodies. Laryngoscope, 82:254–259.

Tucker, G. F., Jr. 1964. The age incidence of lodgement of single coins in the esophagus. Trans. Am. Bronchoesophagol. Assoc., 44:145.

Turtz, M. G., and Tucker, G. F., Jr. 1972. The present day spectrum of pediatric bronchoesophagology. Laryngoscope, 82:945.

Yee, K. F., Schild, J. A., and Holinger, P. H. 1975. Extraluminal foreign bodies (coins) in the food and air passages. Ann. Otol. Rhinol. Laryngol., 84:619–623.

Chapter 57

INJURIES OF THE MOUTH, PHARYNX, AND ESOPHAGUS

Robert H. Maisel, M.D.
Robert H. Mathog, M.D.

Injuries to the mouth, pharynx, and esophagus need careful and complete evaluation in order to prevent later problems in speech and eating. Early and precise diagnosis of the location and extent of tissue damage is essential and often requires contrast radiography and general anesthesia with peroral endoscopy. Tracheostomy may be necessary to assist in the evaluation and to prevent airway obstruction.

The early wound care, debridement, and repair of soft tissue depend on the location and cause of the injury. Burns will require observation for a period of time to determine the extent of tissue destruction. Generalized debilitation from malnutrition will require correction prior to definitive reconstruction. The aim in all treatment is rapid rehabilitation, a short period of hospitalization, and preservation of normal psychosocial development.

INJURIES FROM ACCIDENTS

Accidents are the major causes of death and injury in children, and include animal bites, intraoral penetration by foreign bodies, automobile accidents, and injuries from knives, guns, and endoscopic instruments. These injuries usually spare the upper digestive and respiratory tracts, but the lip and cheek are frequently involved. Curiosity, belligerence, and carelessness frequently lead to accidents of this type. In many cases parental neglect and abuse have also been factors.

Intraoral Foreign Bodies

Probably the most common injuries to the upper aerodigestive tract are those that occur from foreign objects placed in the mouth. Toys, sticks, pencils, and similar objects cause lacerations and puncture wounds of the oral and pharyngeal mucosae. Occasionally the foreign body penetrates a vulnerable structure, but more often the injuries are minor. Major problems may occur if the object breaks and becomes imbedded in the tissue, leading to a foreign body reaction.

In general, minor wounds require no specific therapy except antibiotics to prevent infection. The patient should be watched closely in case the injury causes swelling and respiratory embarrassment. The physician must be certain that all foreign material is removed from the wound. If a neck abscess should develop, the wound may require drainage through the neck and healing through secondary intention.

Vehicle Accidents

Automobile and bicycle accidents often result in injuries of the head and neck, causing facial fractures as well as soft tissue damage. Proper use of seat belt restraints has reduced the incidence and seriousness of adult trauma, but in the child the effects of these preventive measures are less certain. Seatbelts are often too loose, and the shoulder strap may strangle a child. Infant seats are

1111

not always adequate to prevent the release and propulsion of the child.

In vehicle-caused accidents involving the head and neck, the location and extent of damage to the child must be evaluated. The primary concern should be possible swelling of the oropharyngeal airway and subsequent respiratory distress. With fracture of the lower jaw, support of the tongue is absent, and the tongue may fall back into the pharynx, causing an obstruction. Swelling at the base of the tongue or in the pharyngeal walls may present similar difficulties. In cases where the larynx is injured directly, the airway may be compromised. Secretions and blood in the pharynx of the obtunded individual will compound the respiratory difficulties.

The airway, if compromised, should be secured by suction, an endotracheal tube, or both. The chest should be evaluated for possible hemothorax and pneumothorax, and

cervical spine films should be taken if indicated.

The evaluation and repair of facial fractures are discussed in Chapter 35. In cases of soft tissue injury (lacerations, avulsions, or a combination), the site should be cleaned with copious amounts of normal saline. Obviously, dead tissue should be debrided, whereas viable tissue should be retained. All landmarks should be marked with Bonney's Blue or similar marking solution before infiltration with local anesthetics.

Lip Injury. Lip lacerations and small avulsions (up to one third of the lip) should be repaired by direct approximation (Fig. 57–1). Frequently, a shieldlike extension of the wound or a W incision made inferiorly to the defect is useful to close the wound. Absorbable sutures should be placed to bring the lacerated orbicularis oris muscle together. It is only when this layer is satisfactorily approximated that further closure is possible.

AVULSION OF LIP

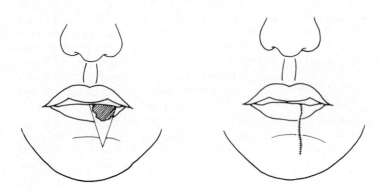

Wedge Excision

Figure 57–1 "Lip Switch" procedure.

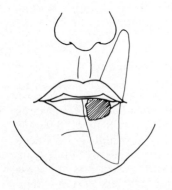
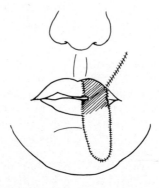

"Lip Switch" Procedure

Nonabsorbable sutures are used to bring the skin edges together exactly at the vermilion border.

When avulsions extend beyond one third of the lip, local flaps must be used for repair. The preferred flaps are the Abbe flap, which is a staged, cross-lip flap, and the Estlander flap, which is similar but involves the commissure of the mouth (Fig. 57–1, bottom). These flaps are designed so that the bulk of mobilized tissue is equal to approximately 50 per cent of the defect. When the Abbe flap is used, the pedicle is left in place for 10 to 14 days, after which the base is cut and returned to the opposite lip. When the Estlander flap is used, the procedure can be performed in one stage, although a secondary commissuroplasty may be necessary in some cases. Often the appearance of the commissure improves with time, so revision surgery should be delayed for several months in children.

For mobilization of large volumes of soft tissue, the Gillies fan flap is useful. In these cases, tissue from the nasolabial fold is transposed to repair large median defects of the upper or lower lip. The cosmetic results are not as desirable as with the "lip switch" procedures just described, and often a "fishmouth" deformity will require a later revision.

Regional flaps are also very useful in correction of large defects of the lip. Flaps from the forehead and neck are necessary when there are large areas in and around the mouth and when bone is exposed. Temporal artery-based forehead flaps may be used for replacement of the entire upper and lower lips. Similar flaps may be developed in the neck area.

Tongue Injury. Reconstruction of the tongue is not usually important, as primary healing often occurs rapidly because of the rich blood supply to the tongue. In addition, it is difficult to immobilize the tongue for suturing using local anesthesia in children. Only with large lacerations (longer than 2 cm) is it necessary to attempt closure, and in the child this usually must be done under general anesthesia or heavy sedation. Loss of the tongue tip from extensive injury usually produces no permanent deficit since the tongue hypertrophies to rebulk itself over a period of six months.

Many times a laceration in which a flap of muscle is elevated may be ignored, and this results in some distortion of the tongue, which is of concern to the parent and later to the child. Another special group of injuries to the tongue are those that occur in children with coagulation defects. These tend to heal very slowly, and although they may heal primarily the process may take weeks in a child who has hemophilia. It is important that healing take place rapidly since it is necessary to maintain the child on coagulation factors. Therefore, suture of a relatively small injury might be advisable in these cases. In addition, a dentist should be asked to provide a smooth splint for the upper teeth to prevent the child from irritating the injury.

For effective function following the proper repair of the lip and tongue, early motion is advisable. Within several days after removal of the sutures, the patient should be executing stretching exercises. Contracture of the lips, commissure, and buccal areas can be prevented by passive opening of the mouth with tongue blades or a clothespin. These exercises should be continued until the tissues soften and the period of wound contracture has passed.

Palate Injuries. The hard palate, because of its firm, bony support, is rarely penetrated by sharp objects, but it may be fractured in the midline with a severe injury that involves a maxillary fracture. The soft palate, composed of muscle and mucosa, is occasionally penetrated when a child holding a straight object in his mouth trips and falls. Frequent offenders in these cases are pens, pencils, and popsicle sticks. The injury may produce acute oral bleeding, but an examination usually shows only a small tear in the mucosa with only occasionally complete penetration to the nasopharynx. These injuries are usually not sutured if the bleeding stops expeditiously. The only severe complication of this type of injury is penetration through the posterior wall to the venous plexus surrounding the carotid artery. This is obviously very rare, and tamponade of the artery would be required to allow it to heal. Lacerations of the mucous membrane will heal spontaneously if kept clean, and the only repair should be secondary in cases of persistent fistula.

Pharynx and Larynx Injury. Lacerations and avulsions of the pharynx and supraglottis require careful evaluation of the extent and location of the injury and, when necessary, an airway bypass. Injuries to the supraglottic larynx are evaluated radiologically and by indirect and direct endoscopy.

When the epiglottis occludes the airway, it

has usually been avulsed at its petiole. If left unattended, the avulsed tissue will heal in a position of partial obstruction and will impair speech, swallowing, and also evaluation of the underlying tissue. To prevent these problems, a large chromic suture is placed around the hyoid bone and used to fix the epiglottis anteriorly. In cases where there is more extensive injury, a supraglottic laryngectomy is performed. The tracheostomy tube is not removed until the patient is able to breathe satisfactorily with a small tube plugged for at least 48 hours. Deglutition must also be satisfactory before extubation. In children, partial (horizontal) resection of the larynx will result in a nearly normal voice and excellent deglutition.

Laryngeal lacerations that expose cartilage require open exploration and approximation of cartilage and mucosa. Fractures of the hyoid bone usually are not repaired unless the airway is compromised. Fragments of the thyroid cartilage may be sutured with a small wire, but if the fragments are markedly displaced and difficult to position, an intralaryngeal stent is used.

If the vocal cords are paralyzed or scarred, resulting in glottic incompetence characterized by either a weak voice or aspiration, polytetrafluoroethylene can later be injected into the vocal cords to improve their function.

Occasionally, following the treatment of laryngeal injuries, scarring causes a contracture of the glottis and fixation of the cords. Dilatation, steroid injection, and excision of the scar tissue with replacement of mucosa with skin grafts may be necessary. In cases where the recurrent nerve is damaged and the airway is inadequate, the surgeon may attempt to transplant the ansa hypoglossi nerves to the intrinsic muscles of the larynx. Excellent success has been reported, and little morbidity occurs with this procedure.

Guns and Knives

Damage from guns and knives used irresponsibly or with provocation is commonly observed. Most civilian gunshot wounds are caused by low-velocity projectiles, which cause moderate soft tissue destruction and bone injury in their path. Often these bullets pass around arteries and nerves without injury and penetrate fixed structures such as the pharynx and esophagus. In contrast, the

shotgun wound causes extensive destruction, frequently shattering the mandible and maxilla with significant loss of bone. Knife wounds are extremely dangerous, and although the entry wound may not be large, these sharp instruments may easily lacerate nerves and other vital structures.

In cases of neck wounds penetrating beyond the platysma, the patient should be admitted to the hospital and should be evaluated systematically. Although many physicians prefer to explore all patients with neck injuries, the procedure for selecting appropriate cases for exploration proposed by May (1976) may be advisable.

The care of soft tissue lacerations and avulsions and of injuries to the larynx is discussed in the section on vehicle accidents in this chapter. For information on injuries to the major vessels and nerves, the reader is referred to May's original article (1975).

An esophageal injury must be evaluated immediately. The extent and location of esophageal lacerations and avulsions can be evaluated only by endoscopy with a nonflexible endoscope and radiologic fluoroscopic studies. If a torn viscus is suspected, use of the locally toxic Hypaque contrast material should be avoided. Should the physician suspect a tracheoesophageal fistula or aspiration, Dionosil is the indicated contrast agent. Barium should be avoided where there is a risk of chemical pneumonitis (May, 1975).

With all tears and lacerations of the digestive system, antibiotic treatment is necessary. Exploration through the neck or through a combined neck-chest incision is desirable to drain any abscesses. Should there be mediastinitis, chest tubes may be placed and irrigated with antibiotics. Ordinarily, uncomplicated pharyngeal tears are allowed to heal by secondary intention while esophageal injuries should be explored surgically (McInnis et al., 1975).

Instrument Injuries

Instruments are a common cause of injury to the esophagus. These injuries can occur during the removal of foreign bodies, biopsies, or diagnostic evaluations. Although the flexible endoscope has reduced the likelihood of such complications, the rigid endoscope is often necessary to carry out many of the procedures.

The most common site of injury to the

esophagus during endoscopy is at the cricopharyngeus. It is not clear whether the use of local or general anesthesia affects the incidence of such a complication. Occasionally, the injury goes unnoticed until the patient complains of chest pain. A widening of the mediastinum on radiographs, and fever, tachycardia, and elevation of the white blood count are symptoms of the injury and indicate the possibility of mediastinitis.

The treatment of esophageal tears consists of immediate prescription of antibiotics and evaluation of the extent of the tear with Dionosil or Gastrografin. If the injury appears to be significant (extravasation is noted), early drainage of the mediastinum may be indicated. In cases in which the infection progresses to an abscess, drainage is essential to treat this life-threatening complication (Paparella and Shumrick, 1980).

Animal Bites

Animal bites may also be a cause of injuries to the upper digestive and respiratory tracts. Approximately 8 per cent of animal bites occur in the head and neck and primarily affect the middle and lower face. Most of the bites are ascribed to family dogs or at least a dog known in the neighborhood who is provoked by removal of food or a litter. In some cases, kissing and playing with the animal have accounted for the injuries. In contrast to automobile accidents, animal bites frequently involve soft tissues and spare bony structures.

The mild, acute swelling that may occur with these mucosal injuries may be treated with cold compresses and steroids to reduce the inflammation. Antibiotics are administered to reduce the likelihood of infection.

Tetanus prophylaxis is prescribed when there are entry wounds on the face or lips. As recommended by the World Health Organization, bites from animals suspected to be rabid require rabies prophylaxis. In such instances, patients should be started on a course of antiserum while the animal is observed; then, if the animal develops rabies the vaccine should be given. Recommended doses are 40 IU per kg of antirabies serum intramuscularly or half of the dose given intramuscularly and the other half of the dose injected into the wound. If necessary, the vaccine should be given for 21 days subcutaneously, followed by two booster doses. Human rabies immunoglobulin, 15 to 40 IU per kg, can be substituted in individuals sensitive to the serum.

The types of injuries observed with animal bites usually are puncture wounds, lacerations, and avulsions. All areas of injury should be irrigated with benzalkonium chloride (Mathog, 1978).

INJURY FROM HEAT

Electrical Burns

Electrical burns of the head and neck, and especially those of the mouth, account for a significant number of childhood injuries. Perioral damage from electricity accounts for 4000 outpatient visits per year and 4 per cent of burn patient admissions (Crikelair and Dhalival, 1976).

Usually, electrical burns occur in children who are less than two years of age. Over 50 per cent of the injuries are due to sucking on the end of a live extension cord, while another 40 per cent of the injuries occur when the child places the connection between two cords into his mouth. Rarely does the child ever bite through the cover of a live wire, although injury from sucking on an exposed wire has been reported.

The location of tissue injury is determined by the current (amperage) of the line. The current (I) is calculated from the voltage (V) and resistance (R) according to Ohm's law ($I=V/R$). Since most household voltage is 110 volts, current flow and current intensity will vary according to the local and distant resistance. Electric current can be fatal if it flows throughout the body and disrupts cardiac rhythm (Fig. 57–2). Local damage will occur primarily if the current flows only through one area of reduced resistance (Thomson et al. 1965).

The degree of injury from electricity is related to the thermal energy expended, which varies with resistance and the square of the current ($H=I^2R$). Current, which is the most important factor, depends on the local tissue electrical resistance. Dry skin has a high resistance of 40,000 to 100,000 ohms per cm^2 and allows minimal current flow, but mucous membrane resistance may be as low as 100 ohms per cm^2 allowing high current flow. Thus, the low resistance of mucosa may lead to intense oral burns (Fig. 57–3). The high resistance distally explains the low incidence

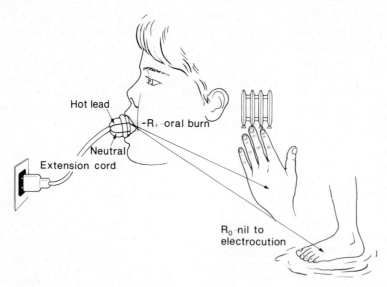

Figure 57–2 Mechanism of oral burn. When regional resistance is low and peripheral resistance is high $(R+)$, then oral burn results. When regional resistance is low and peripheral resistance is low (Ro), then tingling or electrocution results. (From Small, A. 1976. Early surgery for electrical mouth burns. AORN J., 23:128. Reproduced with permission from the American Association of Operating Room Nurses and Allen Small, M.D.)

of death or cardiac arrhythmia in these children.

The lower lip is usually more severely burned than the upper lip, and most damage of the lip occurs at the vermilion border. Approximately 25 per cent of all electrical lip burn injuries occur to the middle of the lip, while the remainder involve the commissure. Extensive burns may involve the labial and lingual mucosa and extend into the alveolar process. In such cases, the burn can devitalize deciduous teeth and cause mucous membrane and periosteal necrosis. Alveolar bone exposure and sequestration can occur, often with significant pain. Curiously, the unerupted permanent dentition is never destroyed in these children.

The tongue is often involved by the burn, and its destruction may later cause loss of mobility with poor speech and difficulty with deglutition. Deeper structures in the oral cavity usually show minimal damage except when they are the site of exit of the electrical current.

The early appearance of an oral burn wound is similar to that of any third-degree burn, with a gray central depression or ulcer surrounded by a pale elevation of the skin. Hyperemia haloes the immediately adjacent skin. The lesions are usually avascular, cold, and relatively painless owing to cauterization of the sensory nerves. Histologically, coagulation necrosis extends beyond the gross margins of the wound. The media of blood vessel walls is often destroyed and may cause late, brisk bleeding. An exposed eroded labial artery can bleed extensively, either soon after the injury (within 10 days) or later with the sloughing of the eschar over the burn site.

In the acute care phase, to encourage development of a "clean" eschar, the burn injury is treated with antibiotic ointment and frequent hydrogen peroxide swabbings. Tetanus prophylaxis is administered, and fluids

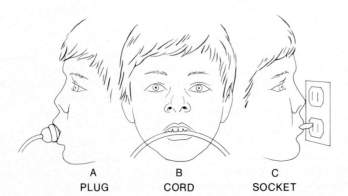

Figure 57–3 Thirst and dryness may be factors causing children to chew or suck on electrical cords. (From Small, A. 1976. Early surgery for electrical mouth burns. AORN J., 23:128. Reproduced with permission from the American Association of Operating Room Nurses and Allen Small, M.D.)

| A | B | C |
| PLUG | CORD | SOCKET |

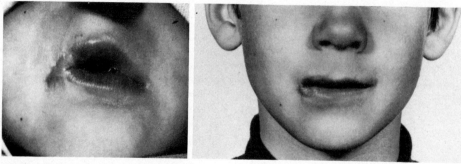

Figure 57–4   Electrical burn of the lip demonstrating severe contracture and correction by excision and advancement of local mucosal flaps.

are permitted if swallowing is satisfactory. Supplemental intravenous infusions are used if needed.

The timing of surgical repair and débridement of these wounds is a topic of debate (Small, 1976). Classicists advocate local conservative care so that the burn will demarcate prior to excision. Approximately one to two weeks are needed for the coagulation necrosis to become obvious. Advocates of the conservative school note that early surgery may cause removal of otherwise viable and vital tissues, which are needed for the repair. The proponents of acute surgical débridement and excision claim that a 20 per cent incidence of labial artery bleeding can be prevented by early surgery. Moreover, these surgeons believe that when the wound is excised and approximated, healing from secondary intention is avoided, contracture is minimized, and ultimately less scarring will occur.

The method of repair will depend upon the degree of destruction and availability of local tissues. Minimal burns of the lip heal satisfactorily per primum (Fig. 57–4). In more extensive injuries, lip repair requires restoration of muscle activity, mucosal covering and reconstitution of a vermilion border with labial eversion (Fig. 57–5).

In all lip lesions, the scar or destroyed tissues must be removed completely. In pure, midlip lesions that do not involve the corner of the mouth, the surface should be repaired with intraoral mucosa, which is undermined and advanced to replace the destroyed tissue. Pedicled grafts of buccal or labial gingival mucosa are also useful for this purpose. In lesions that are deeper, requiring bulk replacement, wedge excision and direct repair are appropriate techniques. In lesions involving half of the lip, Abbe-Estlander flaps and cross-lip flaps of the Abbe-Stein-Estlander type may be necessary. The choice of methods will often depend on the extent of loss of tissue and the status of possible donor tissue.

In burns involving the corner of the mouth, the injury destroys the commissure as well as the mucosa of the adjacent upper and lower lips. Treatment should be directed to the prevention of contractures and fusion of the upper and lower lips, which could result in relative microstomia. In a small superficial burn of the commissure, debridement of the eschar and advancement of mucous membrane from the adjacent lip will restore the angle of the mouth. For more significant defects where deep scarring has occurred, the lesions will require excision of the contracted commissure and advancement of buccal and labial mucosa to the lip. This injury is shown in Figure 57–5.

Extensive burns that involve more than half of the lip with destruction of the alveolar ridge may require local full-thickness flaps. A cheek flap can be designed for this purpose.

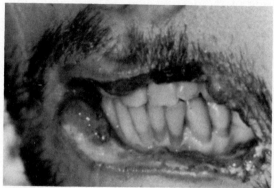

Figure 57–5   Severe lip burn which required cheek flap for repair.

The prevention of lip burns is extremely important. Easy access to electrical sources is probably the most significant problem with children. Fortunately, new plug designs make it difficult for children to put them into their mouths, but parental education is also important in keeping the child off the floor and in keeping him from tampering with electrical systems.

Smoke and Fire

Injuries from fire burns are usually limited to the lips, pharynx, tongue, and supraglottic airway. Below the level of the glottis, burn damage to the airway and digestive tract is unusual. Hot air and other gases carry little thermal energy, and thus with increasing distance from the source damage is minimal to the cool, moist, surface epithelium. Hot liquids and steam can transfer large quantities of heat and can cause respiratory tract and esophageal burns, but fortunately these burns are rare. Also in these cases, the exposure of the glottic aperture to heat causes reflex vocal cord closure and protection of the trachea, while similar spasm prevents thermal damage to the esophagus.

The burn injury can become complicated beyond just surface damage. In a confined area, the patient exposed to thermal sources may be forced to inhale smoke and toxic gases. These substances irritate and inflame the bronchial mucosa and cause protein, which can obstruct alveoli and bronchioles, to be exuded from lung epithelium. Casts of the bronchi or trachea may be formed, and respiratory death can occur owing to pulmonary edema, lower airway obstruction, or both.

Extensive surface burns of the face and neck can also cause thermal injury and swelling of the deep tissues of the pharynx and oral cavity. The inflamed area usually responds quickly to treatment, but airway control is needed during the early phases.

The mechanism of injury from burns has been studied extensively. Following the initial injury, cell membranes become abnormally permeable and molecules up to 125,000 mol wt escape to the extravascular space. Plasma, protein, and fibrinogen enter the extravascular and extracellular spaces. Fluids shift into these spaces with the protein, and although these shifts are significant for burns over more than 10 per cent of the body, burns confined to the head and neck do not cover this great an area. Plasma and extracellular fluid losses occur mostly during the first 12 hours after injury and continue for only 6 to 12 hours beyond that time. The shifts in fluid may cause soft tissue edema, obstruction of the airway, and difficulty in swallowing (Beal, 1970).

During the acute phase following smoke inhalation, the main problems are bronchospasm and airway edema. Intubation or tracheostomy must be performed in the burn patient who has a compromised upper airway. Some studies have shown that pulmonary sepsis in burn patients is six times more common in patients with tracheostomy than in those who did not require such a procedure. Bacteria identical to those in the burn wound can be cultured from the endotracheal aspirate. To avoid infection, nasal or oral intubation is usually preferred, and tracheostomy is even more carefully considered than in the usual airway obstruction before the operation is undertaken.

Some of the indications for early intubation in the burn patient include charring, edema of the posterior pharynx with the threat of upper airway obstruction, full-thickness burns of the entire face, severe hoarseness or stridor, and obvious smoke inhalation with signs of pulmonary contamination from carbon. Severe orofacial burns and coma at the time of admission similarly suggest the need for airway control. In patients with smoke inhalation without a severe burn, the main indication for intubation is evidence of central nervous system depression. Delay in intubation makes the procedure difficult because of upper airway edema, and tracheostomy may then be necessary. Patients can be intubated for several days, although in the presence of an upper airway burn the possibility of eventual scarring of the larynx and subglottis must be considered.

The effectiveness of steroids in the treatment of smoke inhalation is still a matter of debate. It appears that very early in the course of the disease, steroids with high glucocorticoid activity, such as methylprednisolone and dexamethasone, are helpful. Mineralocorticoid drugs, such as cortisone or hydrocortisone, have been found to be ineffective in animal studies and may cause sodium retention and possible fluid overload.

Significant burns of the lip with tissue destruction are reconstructed by the techniques described for repair following electrical injury. Pharyngeal contractures usually need no late treatment, but when they are significant in extent, they are treated best by split-thickness skin graft repair and rotation mucosal flaps. Esophageal injuries due to thermal energy and smoke inhalation are very rare, and these stenoses are best managed by dilatation. Small vocal cord webs may be lysed endoscopically, whereas large ones should be treated with thyrotomy and insertion of a McNaught keel. Extensive stenosis may require excision of scar tissue and insertion of stents to prevent reformation of the adhesions.

Stenosis of the supraglottic larynx is treated by dilatation or by subtotal supraglottic laryngectomy with removal of the false vocal cords and epiglottis. The usual closure of the base of the tongue to the larynx is satisfactory and permits an adequate airway.

CHEMICAL INJURIES

Although the evaluation and treatment of caustic burns are discussed in Chapter 55, it should be noted that acid and alkali are common causes of injury to the mouth and oral cavity.

Injury from chemicals is initially evaluated by direct inspection for extent and depth. After 24 to 48 hours, necrosis may become more apparent. As with more distal esophageal injuries, the patient with a pharyngeal burn is immediately started on a broad-spectrum antibiotic. A nasogastric tube is inserted to maintain a feeding schedule. Steroids may be administered to patients with more significant injury to prevent excessive stenoses. Treatment for pharyngeal stenoses following the healing phases would require skin grafts, flaps, Z-plasty, or a combination of these procedures.

Steroids are rarely used in patients with oral burns. They are frequently used in pharyngeal burns and are the usual treatment in esophageal burns that show erosion deeper than the mucosa.

SELECTED REFERENCES

May, M., Chadaratana, P., West, J. W., 1975. Penetrating neck wounds: Selective exploration. Laryngoscope, 85:57.

This review of the authors' experiences with trauma is well organized and concise, and his treatment concurs with current otolaryngologic recommendations for handling this injury.

Moncrief, J. A. 1973. Burns. N. Engl. J. Med., 288:444.

Military and university centers headed by this author are unparalleled in treatment of burns, and his recommendations are logical and universally respected.

Thomson, H., Juckes, A. W., and Farmer, A. W. 1965. Electric burns to the mouth in children. Plast. Reconstr. Surg., 35:466.

This article summarizes the authors' extensive experiences with this problem and describes the etiology of this type of injury.

REFERENCES

Beal, D. D. 1970. Respiratory tract injury: A guide to management following smoke and thermal injury. Laryngoscope, 80:25.

Crikelair, G. F., and Dhaliwal, A. S. 1976. The cause and prevention of electrical burns of the mouth in children. Plast. Reconstr. Surg., 58:206.

Mathog, R. H., Wurman, L., and Pollak, D. 1977. Animal bites to the head and neck. *In* Sisson, G. A., and Tardy, M. E. Plastic and Reconstructive Surgery of the Face and Neck, Vol. 2, Rehabilitative Surgery. Proceedings of the second international symposium, New York, Grune & Stratton.

May, M., Chadaratana, P., West, J. W., et al. 1975. Penetrating neck wounds: Selective exploration. Laryngoscope, 85:57.

May, M., Tucker, H. M., and Dillard, B. M. 1976. Penetrating wounds in the neck in civilians. Otolaryngol. Clin. North Am., 9:361.

McInnis, W. B., Cruz, A. B., and Aust, J. B. 1975. Penetrating injuries to the neck: Pitfalls in management. Am. J. Surg., 130:416.

Moncrief, J. A. 1959. Tracheotomy in burns. Arch. Surg., 79:45.

Moncrief, J. A. 1973. Burns. N. Engl. J. Med., 288:444.

Paparella, M. M., and Shumrick, D. A. 1980. Otolaryngology, 2nd ed. Philadelphia, W. B. Saunders Co.

Small, A. 1976. Early surgery for electrical mouth burns. AORN J., 23:126.

Thomson, H., Juckes, A. W., and Farmer, A. W. 1965. Electric burns to the mouth in children. Plast. Reconstr. Surg., 35:466.

Chapter 58

NEUROLOGIC DISORDERS OF THE MOUTH, PHARYNX, AND ESOPHAGUS

Michael J. Painter, M.D.

INTRODUCTION

Many significant neurologic disorders have oral, pharyngeal, or esophageal manifestations. A knowledge of these manifestations is often important in making a differential diagnosis and in planning patient care. The physician examining the oropharynx should consider lesions of neurologic significance when encountering clefts of the hard or soft palate, for example. These clefts are occasionally associated with midline anomalies of the brain, with encephaloceles, or with anomalies of the cervical spine. Failure to discover these abnormalities would result in failure to consider lesions of chromosomal and genetic importance or lesions that would eventually cause cervical spinal cord compression. Failure to recognize an encephalocele would result in improper surgical approaches to correction of the cleft, with disastrous consequences. The realization that both teeth and brain originate from neuroectodermal tissue is of value in recognizing disorders that may have neurologic implications when examining a patient with malformed or hypoplastic teeth. Nails and skin are also of ectodermal origin, and those of patients with dental malformations should be examined for the same reason. It is of paramount importance for the physician confronted with a patient who takes an abnormally long time to feed, who has impaired swallowing, or who drools excessively to realize that these are problems not uncommonly seen in bilateral cerebral hemisphere disease,

brain stem lesions, or neuromuscular lesions. The neurologist also must realize the important implications of impaired swallowing; difficulty swallowing secondary to any neurologic lesions indicates a significant risk of aspiration, but it is of most concern when encountered in neuromuscular disorders, such as myasthenia gravis and dermatomyositis.

THE MOUTH

The structures of the mouth that are often affected in disorders involving the nervous system include the lingual, gingival, and buccal mucosae, the teeth and tongue, and the hard and soft palates, as well as the salivary glands.

Lingual, Gingival, Glossal, and Buccal Mucosae

Ulcerative, Nodular, and Inflammatory Lesions

Inflammatory lesions of the mouth are occasionally associated with inflammatory, vascular, or progressive disorders of the central nervous system. Recurrent ulcerative lesions involving any surface of the mouth are seen with ataxia telangiectasia (Louis-Bar syndrome) and with Chédiak-Higashi syndrome (Hamilton et al., 1974) owing to immunosuppression. Ataxia telangiectasia is a familial autosomal recessive disorder characterized by

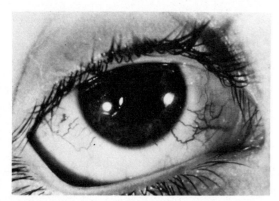

Figure 58–1 Ocular telangiectasia in ataxia telangiectasia.

progressive ataxia, choreoathetosis, oculocutaneous telangiectasis (Fig. 58–1), recurrent sinopulmonary infections, and susceptibility to lymphoreticular malignancies (McForlin, 1972). Ataxia is often noted in very early childhood as the infant first begins to ambulate. This abnormality initially involves truncal musculature and then spreads to involve the extremities. Speech, when it develops, is dysarthric. Subsequently choreoathetosis, myoclonus, and intention tremors are noted. Usually, recurrent, discrete episodes of infection develop between three and eight years of age. Chronic otitis, sinusitis, bronchitis, and eventually bronchiectases are most often noted, and it is at that time that recurrent oral inflammatory lesions may be observed. A clue to the presence of an immune defect is the absence of lymphadenopathy and small tonsillar mass during these infectious episodes. At about the same time that infections become prevalent, telangiectasis of the conjunctivae and exposed areas of the skin are usually noted. The bridge of the nose, the flexor surfaces of the neck and extremities, and the supraclavicular fossae are typical sites of occurrence. The telangiectases are not seen on mucosal surfaces, but depigmented lesions may be noticeable on skin surfaces. Approximately 30 to 50 per cent of children with ataxia telangiectasia are mentally retarded. The vast majority die as a result of chronic infection in late childhood to early adulthood.

Chédiak-Higashi disease is a rare autosomal recessive disorder characterized by dramatic deficiencies in pigmentation of the skin, hair, and irides. In addition, these patients manifest weakness, peripheral neurop-

athy, pancytopenia, atopia, and nystagmus. Decreased resistance to infection, due to impaired granulocyte function, results in recurrent oral inflammatory lesions, and increased susceptibility to lymphoreticular malignancies has also been noted in these patients. Chédiak-Higashi disease becomes evident in the first two years of life. Some findings in patients with this syndrome resemble those seen in the familial spinocerebellar degenerations.

Behçet syndrome is characterized by recurrent oral and genital ulcers associated with uveitis, meningitis, a confusional state, and increased intracranial pressure (Kalbian and Challis, 1970). The oral ulcers seen in virtually all cases are often the first manifestation of the disorder, and the patient may be seen for months or years for this problem before eye or central nervous system abnormalities become manifest. The oral lesions are painful and not uncommonly associated with fever, malaise, and an elevated sedimentation rate (Johnson, 1972). Esophageal ulcerations identical in all respects to those seen in the mouth have also been described in Behcet syndrome (Lockhart et al., 1976). Systemic and topical steroids have no effect on the course of the oral ulcers and may aggravate or precipitate the genital lesions. Neurologic manifestations occur in 10 to 25 per cent of patients with Behçet syndrome (Kozen et al., 1977). The neurologic manifestations, in order of decreasing frequency, consist of hemiparesis or quadriparesis, cranial nerve palsies, cerebellar signs, dementia, organic brain syndrome, meningoencephalitis, focal or generalized seizures, pseudobulbar palsy, pseudotumor cerebri, extrapyramidal tract signs, spinal cord lesions, and cauda equina syndrome. Pleocytosis and elevated cerebrospinal fluid protein are often but not invariably found when the cerebrospinal fluid is examined. Neuropathologic findings include demyelinization and encephalomalacia adjacent to arterioles and venules with a perivascular inflammatory response. These findings are felt to be compatible with diffuse vasculitis. Neuroradiologic procedures, including angiography and computerized tomography (CT) scanning have demonstrated lesions most compatible with infarction. Topical and systemic steroids have been said to improve the course of the uveitis and on occasion have been felt to be beneficial in management of the central nervous system manifestations of the disease, but there is no established efficacious treatment for Behçet syndrome. Recent data, however, show promise that transfer factor may be of value (Wolf et al., 1975). Although the etiology of the disease is unknown, several investigators have postulated a viral connection, whereas other investigators have demonstrated the dissimilarity between Behçet syndrome and known viral diseases (Dudgeon, 1961). Recent work has focused on an allergic etiology (Kalbian and Challis, 1970). Further clinical characteristics of and therapy for this difficult disease are discussed in Chapter 50.

Acute oral ulceration may occur in association with known infectious central nervous system illnesses. Herpes, coxsackie A, ECHO virus, histoplasmosis, and blastomycosis all produce CNS and oral lesions. Herpes encephalitis is most often a primary herpetic infection and as such may be associated with vesiculobullous eruptions of the lingual, gingival, buccal, or pharyngeal mucous membranes. The oral lesions are most often vesicular, multiple, and widespread and progress through ulcerative, hemorrhagic, crusted, and confluent stages (Muller, 1971). High fever, lymphadenopathy, and prominent gastrointestinal symptoms accompany the oral ulceration. Central nervous system manifestations include disorientation, meningismus, and seizures (Meyers et al., 1970). The brain lesions of herpes simplex are hemorrhagic and may be diffuse but tend to have an orbital frontal and temporal lobe preponderance. This localization is reflected in a high incidence of psychomotor seizures. Approximately 50 per cent of the patients with central nervous system herpes will have hemorrhagic cerebrospinal fluid associated more commonly with pleocytosis. The mortality of patients with herpes encephalitis is 20 to 30 per cent, and although uridine derivatives and cytosine arabinoside have been advocated by some, there is no proven therapy. Coxsackie A infections are accompanied by well-circumscribed, small ulcers of the anterior tonsillar pillars. This finding may be a clue as to the responsible agent in a patient with meningoencephalitis.

This same agent is also responsible for acute bulbar and spinal cord lesions, which result in flaccid paralysis difficult to distinguish from, but significantly less severe than, poliomyelitis. The ulcerative lesions seen with ECHO virus infections are less specific. Both coxsackie and ECHO meningoencephalitis tend to occur in the spring and fall.

Histoplasmosis, blastomycosis, and actinomycosis will produce nodular lesions of the tongue, palate, or lips. These lesions ulcerate and are painful (Bell and McCormick, 1975). Regional nodes enlarge and, in the case of blastomycosis, ulcerate. In disseminated histoplasmosis the CNS is involved about 25 per cent of the time, resulting in disseminated meningoencephalitis or localized granulomas (Nelson, 1961). In disseminated blastomycosis the CNS is involved in up to a third of the cases, with leptomeningitis, multiple microscopic abscesses, or large confluent abscesses being noted (London and Lawson, 1961). Actinomycosis causes fulminant meningitis with markedly purulent cerebrospinal fluid (CSF) when the CNS is involved (Edwards et al., 1951). In all these fungal processes the results of examining a biopsy specimen of the oral lesions, if they are present, are of value in establishing the diagnosis.

Vesicular lesions of the buccal mucosa, including the anterior tonsillar pillars, may be seen in association with paralysis of the fifth, eighth, and tenth cranial nerves. Although the classic Ramsey-Hunt syndrome is described as facial paralysis associated with vesicles in the external ear canal secondary to varicella zoster infection of the geniculate ganglion, the trigeminal and other brain stem ganglia may be involved; when this occurs, vesicular, ulcerative lesions may be observed in the distribution of the trigeminal nerve. Awareness of this fact will result in a more specific diagnosis when the physician evaluates a patient with idiopathic "Bell's palsy."

Oral ulcerative lesions, particularly glossitis, are seen in vitamin deficiency states. This occurs especially in patients suffering from deficiencies of thiamine (B_1), nicotinamide (B_2), pyridoxine (B_6), and riboflavin (Barness, 1977). The tongue and buccal mucosae are red, swollen, and fissured with these conditions, and the concomitant CNS manifestations of these deficiency states include psychic disturbances, dementia, cranial nerve abnormalities, and peripheral neuropathy. Although uncommon in the well child, these deficiency states may be observed in the child receiving antimetabolite therapy for malignancy, as poor oral intake associated with the ingestion or injection of vitamin antagonists may produce these deficiency states. Wernicke encephalopathy has been reported in a child with acute leukemia (Shah and Wolff, 1973).

A number of heavy metal intoxications that involve the mouth and the CNS have been described. Mercury, bismuth, lead, thallium, and arsenic poisoning all produce inflammation or discoloration of the mucosa of the mouth. Arsenic is a constituent of a variety of insect sprays and may contaminate unwashed fruits and vegetables (Arena, 1974). Occasionally arsenic is found in rural asthma remedies. This metal will result in acute hemorrhagic encephalopathy, polyneuropathy, or both when taken in sufficient quantity. Lead encephalopathy is well known and in a small percentage of cases is associated with a blueblack line on the gingivae; this line is due to the precipitation of lead sulfide.

Thallium poisoning is uncommon, but this metal is present in a variety of depilatory agents and in a rodent and ant poison known as Zelipaste or Zelio. Occasional ingestion of these agents by the young child still occurs. Thallium intoxication often produces a green-black discoloration of the tongue with CNS manifestations, including irritability, lethargy, convulsions, choreiform movements, and neuropathy. Alopecia often develops in the course of thallium poisoning (Cohen and Flora, 1976).

Mercury is present in local antiseptics and fungicides and in a variety of industrial products, including industrial waste. This metal also volatilizes at room temperature and thus may enter the body through respiration (Cohen and Flora, 1976). In acute mercury intoxication, inflammation of the mucous membranes of the mouth is a constant feature. Neurologically a wide variety of symptoms are evident, ranging from encephalopathy with or without movement disorders to syndromes mimicking Guillain-Barré.

Pigmentary and Vascular Lesions

Adrenoleukodystrophy is an X-linked recessive disorder that is first seen in children between the ages of 5 and 15 years. Most patients are males, and the disorder has both addisonian and progressive CNS degenerative features. Increased pigmentation of nonexposed body surfaces, including the buccal, gingival, and lingual mucosae, is an early feature of this disease (Schamburg, 1975). Mild infections are tolerated poorly owing to lack of corticosteroid response secondary to adrenal atrophy. Neurologically these patients develop progressive deterioration of gait associated with extensor plantar responses and spasticity. Focal signs, such as hemiparesis or visual field defects, may be noted. Occasionally the disorder may be acute and associated with increased intracranial pressure. Psychiatric manifestations, including psychosis and personality disorders, may be prominent; dementia may become evident after the long tract abnormalities are noted, but seizures are not usually prominent.

The vascular nevus of Sturge-Weber disease often extends to involve the mouth when the mandibular or maxillary distribution of the trigeminal nerve is involved. This disorder is due to the presence of capillary venous angiomas in the meninges resulting in impaired cerebral blood flow. There is loss of cortical neurons with extensive gliosis and calcification of superficial and deep cortical layers. The occipital and temporal lobes ipsilateral to the nevus are involved in the vast majority of cases. In those patients with the CNS lesion, the facial angioma is always in the ophthalmic distribution of the trigeminal nerve. The maxillary and mandibular divisions may also exhibit the nevus, but only in association with an ophthalmic division component (Alexander and Norman, 1960). Retinal angiomas and glaucoma are commonly seen on the affected side. Refractory seizures, behavioral disturbances, and contralateral progressive hemiparesis characterize Sturge-Weber disease.

Hereditary hemorrhagic telangiectasia (Rendu-Osler-Weber disease) characteristically produces small angiomas over the buccal and lingual mucosae. This familial disorder is transmitted as an autosomal dominant trait of high penetrance. The classic manifestations of this disease are recurrent epistaxis and gastrointestinal hemorrhages, but subarachnoid hemorrhages and neurologic manifestations have been reported. Hydrocephalus with unruptured intracranial angiomas has been seen (Boynton and Morgan, 1973). Recurrent syncope, diplopia, vertigo, visual and auditory disturbances, and brain abscesses have been seen secondary to pulmonary arteriovenous fistulae, which occur with this disorder (Roman et al., 1978).

Angiokeratoma corporis diffusum (Fabry disease) is an X-linked recessive condition caused by absence of the enzyme ceramide trihexosidase and subsequent accumulation of ceramide-trihexoside in the corneas, peripheral nerves, kidneys, brain, and spinal cord. Characteristically, red-purple angiomas known as angiokeratoma corporis diffusum are present over the scrotum, penis, or umbilical area. Small angiomas may be present over the lingual or buccal mucosae. The skin and mucous membrane lesions are usually present in the first decade. In the pediatric age range, spontaneous, lightning-like pains and dysesthesia are seen secondary to the neuropathy. Phenytoin has been successful in relieving the neuritis pain (Lockman et al., 1973). Renal failure is a common cause of disability in early adulthood.

Hypoalphalipoproteinemia (Tangier disease) is a rare autosomal recessive disorder, the pathognomonic finding of which is yellowish-orange enlargement of the tonsils. The absence of alpha lipoproteins results in elevated triglyceride levels with low cholesterol. Triglyceride is stored in the organs of the reticuloendothelial system, resulting in splenomegaly and enlarged lymph nodes. The palatine tonsils are thus enlarged and orange in color. Patients may develop symptomatic polyneuropathy in childhood (Kocen et al., 1967); this neuropathy is asymmetric and manifest by relapsing weakness and sensory loss.

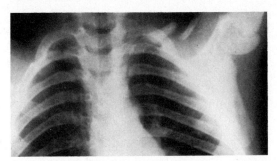

Figure 58–2   Cleidocranial dysostosis: partial clavicular agenesis.

tumors involving the hypothalamus (the most common of which is craniopharyngioma) and in cleidocranial dysostosis (Dixon and Stewart, 1976). Not only is eruption delayed, but, once erupted, the deciduous teeth fail to shed, resulting in crowding of primary and secondary teeth and the development of bizarre malocclusions. These dental abnormalities may precede the more common tumor manifestations of increased intracranial pressure and gait abnormalities.

Cleidocranial dysostosis is recognized by partial or complete absence of the clavicles (Fig. 58–2), by abnormalities of the wormian bones of the skull (Fig. 58–3), and by relative macrocephaly. Spastic paraparesis, syringo-

Abnormalities of the Teeth and Gingivae Associated with Neurologic Disorders

Early in human development, cells destined to form teeth migrate from the neural crest into the developing oral and face regions. The association, therefore, of developmental disorders of the CNS with cutaneous abnormalities and disordered formation of the teeth has its origin in early embryogenesis. (The reader is referred to Chapter 45 for a discussion of normal dental development.) Certain endocrinologic disorders may have both dental and neurologic implications. These abnormalities of teeth include disordered morphodifferentiation, impaired eruption, and early or delayed shedding of deciduous teeth. Therapeutic agents used in neurology, particularly phenytoin, which is often used in the control of seizures, will cause gingival changes that may mask underlying gingival abnormalities.

Delayed eruption of teeth is seen with

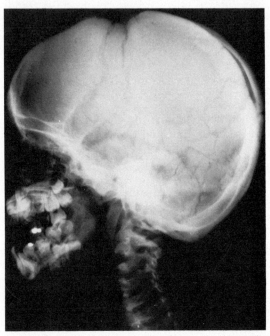

Figure 58–3   Cleidocranial dysostosis: wormian bones of the skull.

myelia, basilar impression, and hydrocephalus have also been described in cleidocranial dysostosis.

Conical defects of the teeth are seen in incontinentia pigmenti, Rieger syndrome, and Williams syndrome. Incontinentia pigmenti (Morgan, 1971) presents with a papular or bullous eruption following a dermatomal distribution in the newborn period (Fig. 58–4). These lesions resolve to a pigmented, whorled, spidery pattern in the same distribution. Dystrophic fingernails and toenails are often noted, and a significant number of the patients demonstrate mental deficiency, microcephaly, and seizures. Microgyria has been noted in the few autopsied cases. Approximately a third of these patients have hypodontia, delayed eruption, or malformation of the teeth (Fig. 58–5).

Rieger syndrome consists of dysplasia of the iris, hypodontia, and partial adontia. A variable number of these patients also have

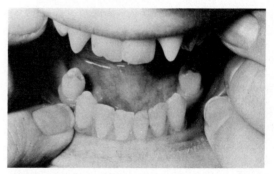

Figure 58–5 Incontinentia pigmenti. Note conical bicuspid defects and partial adontia.

myotonic dystrophy. Craniosynostosis has also been described with this entity (Pearce and Kerr, 1965).

Williams syndrome consists of variable infantile hypercalcemia, a fish-shaped mouth, supravalvular aortic stenosis, and mental retardation. Partial adontia and malformed teeth are seen in a significant number of these patients (Kelly and Barr, 1975).

Three relatively common but often subtle neurologic disorders that may be quite difficult to diagnose also involve abnormalities of the teeth, gingivae, or both. These entities are tuberous sclerosis, neurofibromatosis, and Lesch-Nyhan syndrome. All three may involve hypoplasia and hypocalcification of the teeth. In addition, the angiomas of tuberous sclerosis and the neurofibromas of neurofibromatosis are not infrequently found in the mouth (Fig. 58–6). The classic case of tuberous sclerosis, consisting of seizures, mental retardation, adenoma sebaceum, shagreen patches, and intracranial calcifications, is not difficult to recognize, but the disorder is often much more subtle. In the patient with only seizures and scattered depigmented le-

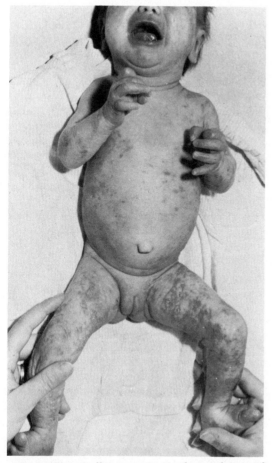

Figure 58–4 Bullous eruption in the newborn with incontinentia pigmenti.

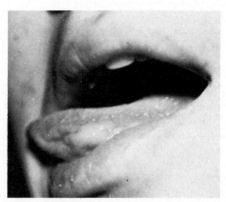

Figure 58–6 Neurofibroma of the tongue.

sions on the skin, recognition of the associated oral and dental defects is of value in diagnosing the disease. It is said that 11 per cent of patients with tuberous sclerosis have associated oral abnormalities; enamel pits appear to be quite common and have a distribution that is characteristic of this disorder (Hoff, 1975).

The Lesch-Nyhan syndrome also is not difficult to diagnose when choreoathetosis, mental retardation, seizures, and self-mutilation, often consisting of chewing of the lips and buccal mucosa, are present. However, self-mutilation is not a constant feature of this disease. The disorder is due to absence of the enzyme hypoxanthine-guanine-phosphoribosyl transferase, resulting in increased uric acid accumulation that may be reflected in hyperuricemia and hyperuricosuria. In the patient with isolated choreoathetosis, mental retardation, and seizures, further clues to the diagnosis may be found in associated dental abnormalities: Nyhan has described a child with tooth dysplasia, hyperuricemia, mental retardation, and absence of tears. The metabolic changes appear to be secondary to an increased rate of purine synthesis and are distinct from those in the classic Lesch-Nyhan syndrome. It is not uncommon for patients with any of the three previously mentioned disorders to be diagnosed as suffering from an idiopathic seizure disorder and to be given anticonvulsants on this basis. The physician evaluating a child for phenytoin-induced gingival hyperplasia would be wise to consider the possibility of these underlying disabilities.

In both pseudohypoparathyroidism and hypoparathyroidism, the associated hypocalcemia leads to tetany, convulsions, and muscle cramps. Both disorders are commonly mistaken for epilepsy and have been diagnosed by dentists examining the mouth for phenytoin-induced gingival hyperplasia. Pseudohypoparathyroidism is inherited as an X-linked trait in which dental as well as biochemical manifestations vary according to the sex of the patient. Males are more severely affected than females, but female patients are more commonly encountered. These patients are short, stout, and have round facies; also the fourth metacarpal is usually short. Central nervous system calcifications are seen. Defective teeth have been found in up to 50 per cent of patients with pseudohypoparathyroidism; they occur more frequently and with greater severity in males and appear in the order of tooth development: if the first permanent molars are hypoplastic, teeth that develop thereafter, including the bicuspids, cuspids, and the second and third molars, are also hypoplastic. In addition, pitting enamel defects have also been noted in these patients.

The mucopolysaccharidoses and the mucolipidoses comprise a group of 20 or more heterogenous, rare, but phenotypically similar and genetically distinct inborn errors of metabolism. Clinically these disorders are characterized by coarse features not initially present at birth but becoming evident in later infancy. A variety of ocular and bony abnormalities and variable mental retardation characterize these syndromes (Tegum et al., 1976). Although oral manifestations are obvious in a number of these disorders, such as Hurler syndrome (widely spaced teeth and alveolar hypoplasia), a careful systematic evaluation of the oral manifestations in these disorders is not available. The hypoplastic, malformed teeth noted in a variety of these disorders may be due to an enamel defect but may also be due to the effects of bruxism. Gingival biopsy has demonstrated metachromatic material and characteristic Hurler cells in Hurler syndrome. This material most likely takes time to accumulate, and the technique is probably not of value in the diagnosis of the young child (Gardner, 1971). Obliteration of the pulp chambers has been described in dental radiographs of patients with Sanfilippo syndrome (Webman, 1977). Electron microscopic evaluation of conjunctival biopsy specimens appears to be promising in the diagnosis of mucolipidosis (Kenyon and Sensenbrenner, 1971), and enzyme determinations on fibroblasts are available for studying different types of saccharidosis.

The Tongue

As the tongue is basically a structure composed of muscle covered by mucous membrane, clinical involvement of this organ is seen very early in denervation processes. The patient may note and complain of impaired deglutition and articulation. In intrinsic brain stem disease involving the hypoglossal nucleus, such as syringobulbia, pontine telangiectasis, or brain stem glioma, atrophy and fasciculations of the tongue are early findings. In disorders involving the hypoglossal nerve distal to the nucleus, fasciculations are usually not seen, but atrophy and weakness are prominent. Involvement of the hypoglossal nerve occurs in traumatic lesions involving the base of the skull, exudative meningitis, and various extramedullary tumors. Prominent furrowing of the tongue (lingua plicata) may be seen in association with recurrent edema of the lips or face and unilateral or bilateral facial palsy (Zecho et al., 1976). This clinical complex is known as Melkersson syndrome and occurs occasionally in the pediatric age group. When present, the tongue furrowing is a constant feature, whereas the edema and facial paralysis may or may not occur. There is no proven therapy for this problem, and the edema and facial paralysis usually resolve over days to weeks.

Familial dysautonomia (Riley-Day syndrome) is a neurologic disorder characterized by alacrimation, areflexia, autonomic disturbances, multiple sensory deficits, and poor growth (Pearson, 1974). The tongue shows absence of fungiform papillae resulting in a smooth, gray appearance of the mucous membrane. Normally the fungiform papillae, because of their high vascularity, comprise the red projections amongst the more numerous gray filiform papillae. The vallate papillae are intact in familial dysautonomia, but taste abnormalities in this disease are pathognomonic: inability to discriminate between acid and sweet solutions. Familial dysautonomia is virtually limited to the Ashkenazi-Jewish population and is an autosomal recessive disorder without sex predilection. The infant is hypotonic as a newborn, and episodes of flushing, cyanosis, and aspiration are common. Mental retardation, areflexia, and growth failure become evident as the child grows older. Swallowing disorders, primarily due to impaired pharyngeal and esophageal motility, are prominent in the Riley-Day syndrome. The prognosis is poor, and few children reach adolescence or early adulthood. Neuropathologic examination reveals loss of autonomic neurons, which may account for the impaired vasomotor reflexes.

The Palate

The mucosa covering the bony palate is subject to those disorders that have been

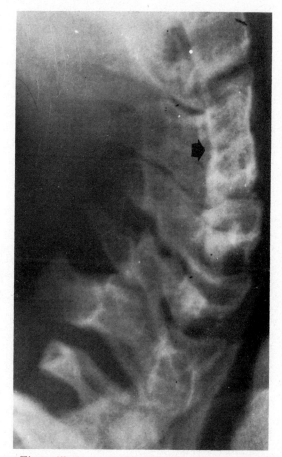

Figure 58–7 Cervical spine radiograph of a patient with Klippel-Feil syndrome. Note bony fusion (arrow).

discussed as affecting the buccal and lingual mucosae.

The vast majority of patients with cleft palate do not have associated neurologic disorders. A small but significant percentage, however, may have associated abnormalities with neurologic implications, and it is good to be aware of this association (Gorlin, 1971). It is estimated that 2 per cent of patients with cleft palate have Klippel-Feil abnormalities. This syndrome is characterized by defects of segmentation of the cervical vertebrae resulting in reduction in the number of and abnormal fusion of vertebrae (Fig. 58–7). The infant appears to have no neck, and the head rests directly on the shoulders. Anteroposterior and rotatory movements of the cervical spine may be limited, and scoliosis, platybasia, and hydrocephalus have been reported to accompany this syndrome. Narrowing of the cervical spinal canal, when present, renders the patient susceptible to myelopathy following episodes of minor trauma. Decompressive laminectomy may be beneficial in selected cases.

Occasionally Duane syndrome may be associated with cleft palate. This disorder is due to developmental fibrosis of the lateral rectus muscle unilaterally or bilaterally. There is paralysis of abduction of the affected eye, and on adduction there is retraction and elevation of the affected side. Duane syndrome is not uncommonly confused with abducens nerve paralysis.

Approximately 5 per cent of encephaloceles are frontal in location and may be associated with cleft palate. The encephalocele mass may extend through defects in the sphenoid bone, ethmoidal bone, or both bones into the nasal cavity and occasionally to the oral cavity. In one series, two of eight transphenoidal and transethmoidal encephaloceles had associated cleft palates. In this situation, it is important that the lesions not be mistaken for a nasal polyp or adenoidal mass; death following an operative approach based on mistaking these lesions for an adenoidal mass has been reported (Pollock et al., 1968). Variable amounts of brain tissue, including the hypothalamus, corpus callosum, and optic chiasm may be present in the encephalocele (Fig. 58–8).

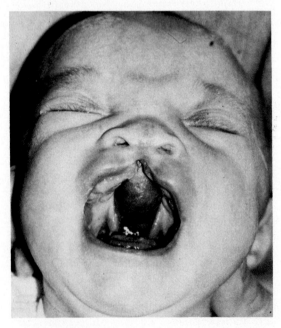

Figure 58–8   Child with a cleft palate and a nasofrontal encephalocele.

Table 58–1   GROSS CHROMOSOMAL CLEFT SYNDROMES

4p-
5p-
Trisomy C mosaicism
Trisomy 13
Dp-
14q-
Trisomy 18
18p-
18q-
Trisomy 21
XXXXY syndrome
Various translocations
Supernumerary G-sized fragment
Monosomy G
Triploidy

A variety of chromosomal abnormalities has been associated with cleft palate. In the vast majority of these cases, the children demonstrated profound mental retardation (Webman et al., 1977) (Table 58–1).

PHARYNX AND ESOPHAGUS

Inflammatory, congenital, neuromuscular, and vascular CNS disorders may have significant pharyngeal and esophageal components.

The most common complaint and physical finding in infectious mononucleosis is sore throat. Exudate over the palatine tonsils is present approximately half the time. Neurologic complications occur in a variable number of patients. In one study approximately a quarter of patients with infectious mononucleosis had cerebrospinal fluid pleocytosis, and a third had EEG abnormalities (Karzon, 1976). Clinical neurologic presentations have run the gamut of Guillain-Barré syndrome, myelitis, encephalitis, facial nerve paresis, and aseptic meningitis. In addition, associated cases of Reye syndrome have been found to have typical hematologic and pathologic features of infectious mononucleosis.

A variety of CNS and neuromuscular disorders results in impairment of the swallowing mechanism. Assessment of swallowing function is important in neurologic disorders because dysfunction is not uncommon and predisposes to aspiration. As a rule, neuromuscular disorders result in impaired motility, whereas CNS disorders impair motility and cricopharyngeal relaxation. Disorders producing brain stem distortion not uncommonly involve the lower cranial nerves. In childhood this is seen to be associated with myelomeningocele and the Arnold-Chiari malformation (Jehon, 1975). Paralysis of the palate may occur, or there also may be associated cricopharyngeal achalasia (Jehon, 1975). As noted by Kelman and Goyal (1976), the specific type of swallowing dysfunction encountered depends on the muscle involved.

Weakness of the buccal and glossal muscles results in drooling, dribbling, hesitation in the initiation of the swallowing reflex, and defective bolus formation. Weakness of the superior pharyngeal constrictor, palatopharyngeus, and levator palati muscles results in velopharyngeal incompetence and nasal regurgitation. Impaired pharyngeal and esophageal motility results in slow propulsion, asymmetry of the food column, and pooling in the recesses of the pharynx. Subsequently regurgitation to the oral pharynx will occur. If pooling persists beyond the period when respiratory effort must occur, laryngeal aspiration results (Kelman and Goyal, 1976). A detailed discussion of the swallowing mechanism is given in Chapter 42.

Impaired pharyngeal and esophageal motility are commonly encountered in myotonic dystrophy. In one series of adults approximately half of the patients complained of dysphagia, but all had radiologically abnormal esophageal motility. Laryngeal aspiration is a clinical problem in this disorder. When myotonic dystrophy presents in the newborn period, impaired swallowing necessitating prolonged nasogastric tube feeding is present in the majority of infants. These infants often have a tented upper lip (Fig. 58–9), but myotonia, elicited either electrically or by percussion, is usually absent. The diagnosis is best confirmed by examining the mother, who will most likely have easily demonstrable myotonia. This is an autosomal dominant syndrome that also manifests mental retardation, cataracts, testicular atrophy, premature baldness, pulmonary dysfunction, and a high incidence of infertility.

Oculopharyngeal dystrophy is a rare disorder, encountered primarily in the elderly and only very rarely appearing in the teenage years. Bilateral progressive ptosis is the initial symptom in 60 to 70 per cent of the cases, but dysphagia may be the initial manifestation in 20 per cent (Kelman and Goyal, 1976). The

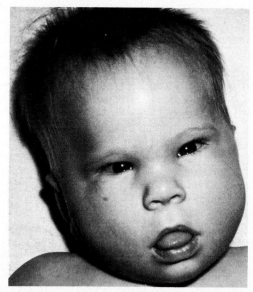

Figure 58–9   Myotonic dystrophy in a neonate. Note tented upper lip.

disease is slowly progressive. Usually the dysphagia is mild, but pooling in the pyriform recesses and valleculae may occur. In more severe cases troublesome aspiration has been seen. Unlike myotonic dystrophy, the esophagus is not involved in this disorder. Motility studies reveal weakness of the pharyngeal constrictors, low cricopharyngeal basal pressure, and normal relaxation.

In the pediatric age group, myasthenia gravis presents in two distinct fashions, and both have important implications regarding swallowing. Transient, neonatal myasthenia gravis occurs in 17 per cent of infants born to mothers with myasthenia (Namba et al., 1970). These infants do not have chronic myasthenia but manifest moderate to severe weakness for a variable period, up to weeks, beyond delivery. Although as of yet unidentified, it is presumed that a transplacentally acquired agent is responsible for their weakness. If symptomatic they always present in the first 10 days after delivery. Extraocular muscle abnormalities and ptosis are characteristically absent. Respiratory and feeding difficulties are the rule and have resulted in death. These infants will respond to anticholinesterase medication.

In juvenile myasthenia gravis the majority of cases are ocular and confined to the extraocular muscles. The pupils are not involved. In the smaller percentage who develop generalized myasthenia dysarthria, choking and aspiration are significant problems. In the classical case the patient notes progressive swallowing difficulty from the beginning to the end of a meal. Tongue weakness will result in impaired bolus formation, and velopalatal weakness leads to nasal regurgitation. Radiologic investigation reveals pooling of barium in the pharyngeal recesses. Cricopharyngeal dysfunction almost never occurs in this condition. The pharyngeal, lingual, and esophageal abnormalities will respond to anticholinesterase medication. Steroids and thymectomy are the most frequently used current treatment modalities (Mann, 1976).

Childhood dermatomyositis may also involve the muscles concerned with swallowing. In one series of 18 cases, two patients were also noted to have dysphagia (Sullivan et al., 1972), while in one other series the incidence has been as high as 50 per cent (Bitnum et al, 1964). Petechial and plaque lesions of the buccal mucosa are also common and may undergo leukoplastic changes. Characteristically progressive muscle weakness is the predominant complaint. Proximal leg muscle weakness is seen earliest. Intermittent fever is present in most instances, and approximately two thirds of patients will have the characteristic violaceous heliotrope discoloration of the upper eyelids and scaly erythematous eruptions over the malar areas (Sullivan, 1972). Bitnum and others (1964) noted that palatal respiratory involvement in this disorder is a common cause of death in the pediatric age group. High-dose steroid therapy appears to be beneficial in this disorder, and cricopharyngeal myotomy has been performed with improved swallowing function in an adult (Kelman and Goyal, 1976; Porubsky et al., 1973).

The innervation of the cricopharyngeus muscle is imperfectly understood, but it is definitely different from innervation of the other pharyngeal muscles. Detailed neurologic studies have been carried out in dogs, but the prominent vagal branch seen in the dog has no counterpart in the human. The sympathetic innervation is controversial if present at all. The parasympathetic nerve supply is vagal, but the course of the fibers is not clear. Most experiments accept that the visceral afferents reach the nucleus solitarius and relay to the nucleus ambiguus. The vagal fibers then run in the pharyngeal plexus. It is unlikely that innervation of this muscle is via the recurrent nerves, as dysfunction of this muscle is not seen in recurrent nerve injury. Resection of cervical sympathetic fibers produces no swallowing difficulties. Cricopharyngeal malfunction is, however, seen in a variety of neurologic disorders common to children. Cricopharyngeal muscle disturbance is said to be rare in childhood, but we agree with Bishop that this is because it is not looked for (Bishop, 1974). Reichert (Reichert et al., 1977) has reported on a series of 15 cases of childhood cricopharyngeal muscle disturbance in which 11 patients had associated CNS abnormalities. We have seen this disorder in children with cerebral palsy, brain stem abnormalities, and metabolic disorders affecting the central nervous system. Dysfunction has been encountered in bulbar poliomyelitis, amyotrophic lateral sclerosis, posteroinferior cerebellar and basilar artery thrombosis, transient neonatal pharyngeal paralysis, brain stem tumor, and myotonic dystrophy (Palmer, 1976). Dystrophies other than myotonic characteristically spare the swallowing mechanism. Bilateral cerebral hemispheric diseases most commonly encountered in the pediatric age group, and loosely defined as cerebral palsy, result in disturbances of the muscles of mastication, the tongue, and the pharyngeal musculature. The associated difficulties with swallowing may lead to chronic, recurrent aspiration. These abnormalities include disorders of pharyngeal and esophageal motility associated with abnormalities of cricopharyngeus muscle function. About 10 per cent of patients with cerebral palsy have severe difficulties with chronic drooling (Friedman et al., 1975). The difficulties with swallowing involve impaired coordination between tongue movements and the pharyngeal and esophageal phases of swallowing. Drooling is due to impaired removal of saliva by dysfunctional swallowing mechanisms. Tympanic neurectomy and recessing of the salivary ducts has been of value in treating severe, incapacitating drooling (Palmer, 1976; Friedman et al., 1975).

REFERENCES

Alexander, G. C., and Norman, R. M. 1960. The Sturge-Weber syndrome. Baltimore, Williams and Wilkins Co.

Arena, J. 1974. Poisoning. Springfield, IL, Charles C Thomas.

Bell, W., and McCormick, W. 1975. Neurologic Infections in Children. Philadelphia, W. B. Saunders Co.

Bishop, H. 1974. Cricopharyngeal achalasia in childhood. J. Pediatr. Surg., 9:775.

Bitnum, S., Daeschner, C. W., Jr., Travis, L. B., et al. 1964. Dermatomyositis. J. Pediatr., 64:101.

Barness, L. A. 1977. Vitamins in nutrition. In Kelley, V. (Ed.), Practice of Pediatrics. New York, Harper & Row.

Boynton, R. C., and Morgan, B. C. 1973. Cerebral arteriovenous fistula with possible hereditary telangiectasis. Am. J. Dis. Child., 125:99.

Cohen, M., and Flora, G. 1976. Cerebral intoxication. In Baker, A. B. (Ed.) Clinical Neurology. Hagerstown, MD, Harper & Row.

Dixon, G., and Stewart, R. 1976. Genetic aspects of anomalous tooth development in oral facial genetics. St. Louis, C. V. Mosby Co.

Dudgeon, J. A. 1961. Virological aspects of Behçet's disease. Proc. Roy. Soc. Med., 54:104.

Edwards, C., Elliott, W. A., and Randall, K. J. 1951. Spinal meningitis due to Actinomyces bovis treated with penicillin and streptomycin. J. Neurol. Neurosurg. Psychiatr., 14:134.

Friedman, W. H., and Kaplan, B. 1975. Tympanic neurectomy. Correction of drooling in cerebral palsy. N. Y. State J. Med., 75:2419.

Gardner, D. G. 1971. The oral manifestations of Hurler's syndrome. Oral Surg., 32:46.

Gorlin, R. J. 1971. Facial clefting and its syndrome. Birth Defects, 7:35.

Hamilton, R. E., Jr., and Giansanti, J. S. 1974. The Chediak-Higashi syndrome. Report of a case and review of the literature. Oral Surg., 37:754.

Haymaker, W., and Kuhlenbeck, H. 1976. Disorders of the brain stem and its cranial nerves. In Baker, A. B. (Ed.) Clinical Neurology. Hagerstown, MD, Harper & Row.

Hoff, M. 1975. Enamel defects associated with tuberous sclerosis. Oral Surg., 40:261.

Jehon, P. 1975. Laryngo-pharyngeal paralysis. Complications during the course of myelomeningocele. Arch. Fr. Pediatr., 32:49.

Johnson, R. L. 1972. Ulcerative lesions of the oral cavity. Otolaryngol. Clin. North Am., 5:213.

Kalbian, V., and Challis, M. 1970. Behçet's disease. Am. J. Med., 48:823.

Karzon, D. 1976. Infectious mononucleosis. Adv. Pediatr., 22:231.

Kelly, J. R., and Barr, E. J. 1975. The elfin facies syndrome. Oral Surg., 40:205.

Kelman, W. J., and Goyal, R. K. 1976. Disorders of the pharyngeal and upper esophageal motor function. Arch. Intern. Med., 136:592.

Kenyon, K., and Sensenbrenner, J. 1971. Mucolipidosis II (I-cell disease): ultrastructural observations of conjunctiva and skin. Invest. Ophthalmol., 10:555.

Kocen, R. S., Lloyd, J. K., Lascelles, P. T., et al. 1967. Familial and lipoprotein deficiency (Tangier disease) with neurological abnormalities. Lancet, 1:1341.

Kozin, F., Haughton, V., and Bernhard, G. C. 1977. Neuro-Behçet disease: Two cases and neuroradiologic findings. Neurology, 27:1148.

Legum, C. P., Schorr, S., and Berman, E. R. 1976. The genetic mucopolysaccharidosis and mucolipidoses: Review and comment. Adv. Pediatr., 22:305.

Lockhart, J. M., McIntyre, W., and Caperton, E. M., Jr. 1976. Esophageal ulceration in Behçet's syndrome. Ann. Intern. Med., 84:572.

Lockman, L. A., Hunninghake, D. B., Krivitt, W., et al. 1973. Relief of pain in Fabry's disease by diphenylhydantoin. Neurology, 23:871.

London, R. G., and Lawson, R. A., Jr. 1961. Systemic blastomycosis. Recurrent neurological relapse in a case treated with amphotericin. Br. Ann. Intern. Med., 55:139.

Mann, J. D. 1976. Long term prednisone followed by thymectomy in myasthenia gravis. Ann. N. Y. Acad. Sci., 274:608.

McForlin, D. E. 1972. Ataxia telangiectasis. Medicine, 51:281.

Meyer, J. S., Bauer, R. B., Rivera-Olmos, V. M., et al. 1970. Herpes encephalitis. Arch. Neurol., 23:438.

Morgan, J. D. 1971. Incontinentia pigmenti. Am. J. Dis. Child., 122:294.

Muller, J. 1971. Viral infections of the skin and mouth. Oral Surg., 32:752.

Namba, T., Brown, J., and Grub, D. 1970. Neonatal myasthenia gravis. Report of two cases and review of the literature. Pediatrics, 45:488.

Nelson, J. D. 1961. Histoplasma meningitis. Recovery following Amphotericin B therapy. Am. J. Dis. Child., 102:218.

Palmer, E. 1976. Disorders of the cricopharyngeus muscle. Gastroenterology, 71:510.

Pearce, W. G., and Kerr, C. B. 1965. Inherited variation in Rieger's malformation. Brit. J. Ophthalmol., 49:530.

Pearson, J. 1974. Current concepts of dysautonomia: neuropathological defects. Ann. N. Y. Acad. Sci., 228:288.

Pollock, J. A., Newton, T. H., and Hoyt, W. F. 1968. Transsphenoidal and transethmoidal encephaloceles. A review of clinical and roentgen features in eight cases. Radiology, 90:442.

Porubsky, E. S., Murray, J. P., and Pratt, L. L. 1973. Cricopharyngeal achalasia in dermatomyositis. Arch. Otolaryngol., 98:428.

Reichert, T., Bluestone, C., Stool, S., et al. 1977. Congenital cricopharyngeal achalasia. Ann. Otol. Rhinol. Laryngol., 86:603.

Roman, G., Fisher, M., Perl, D. et al. 1978. Neurological manifestations of hereditary hemorrhagic telangiectasia (Rendu-Osler-Weber disease): Report of two cases and review of the literature. Ann. Neurol., 4:130.

Schaumburg, H. H., Powers, J. M., Raine, C. S., et al., 1975. Adrenoleukodystrophy: A clinical and pathological study of 17 cases. Arch. Neurol., 32:577.

Shah, N., and Wolff, J. 1973. Thiamine deficiency. Probably Wernicke's encephalopathy successfully treated in a child with acute lymphocytic leukemia. Pediatrics, 51:750.

Sullivan, D. B., Cassidy, J. T., Petty, R. E., et al. 1972. Prognosis in childhood dermatomyositis. J. Pediatr., 80:555.

Webman, M. S., Hirsch, S. A., Webman, H., et al. 1977. Obliterated pulp cavities in the Sanfilippo syndrome (mucopolysaccharidosis III). Oral Surg., 43:734.

Wolf, R. E., Fundenberg, H. H., Spitler, L. E., et al. 1975. Treatment of Behçet's syndrome with transfer factor. (Abstr) Arthritis Rheum., 18:432.

Zecha, J. J., Van Dijk, L., and Hadders, H. N. 1976. Cheilitis granulomatosa (Melkersson-Rosenthal syndrome). Oral Surg., 42:254.

Section V

THE LARYNX, TRACHEA, BRONCHI, AND LUNGS

Chapter 59

EMBRYOLOGY AND ANATOMY

J. Thomas Love, Jr., M.D.

INTRODUCTION

This chapter reviews the developmental embryology and anatomy of the larynx and lower respiratory tract, with an emphasis on their clinical significance and relevance.

Phylogenetically, the lungs and larynx developed when air-breathing vertebrates evolved from lower vertebrates that lived in the water. The lungs provide the surface area for the exchange of gases between living tissues and ambient air; the trachea and bronchi are the passages for air to and from the lungs; and the larynx is the sphincteric protective mechanism for the lower airways. Only after complete development of the protective role of the larynx does vocalization evolve as a major, although secondary, function of that structure.

The face, larynx, trachea, bronchi, and lungs, as well as other related structures, are all partially derived from the fifth and sixth branchial arches and from the third, fourth, fifth, and sixth visceral arches (Arey, 1965; Moore, 1973).

The ectodermal derivatives of these arches form the cranial and spinal nerves; the entodermal layer develops into the epithelium of the tongue, the alimentary tract, the pharynx, larynx, trachea, parathyroids, thyroid gland, and the alveoli; the mesoderm forms the connective tissue elements of voluntary and involuntary muscles, blood vessels, lymphatics, and skeletal elements of the head and neck (Davies, 1973).

Although the connective tissue elements may migrate from the skeletal elements of the primordial arch from which they develop, the neural components remain attached to the site of origin. Hence, misaligned muscle elements may be identified as to their origin by their nerve supplies (Moore, 1973).

LARYNX

Embryology

One of the earliest life forms demonstrating a sphincteric mechanism for protecting the lower respiratory system is the African lungfish. In this primitive larynx model, the glottis is constricted by a single abductor muscle, the constrictor pharyngis. A higher life form of air-breathing animal, the salamander, has arytenoid-like cartilages, whereas the alligator has cartilage forms representative of the cricoid and thyroid cartilages. A mammalian prototype larynx model may be seen very clearly in the cat, which has a well-defined larynx with true thyroarytenoid muscle and an epiglottis (Arey, 1965).

More refined laryngeal development may be seen in the monkey larynx, which develops vestibular folds, ventricles, sacculi, and aryepiglottic muscles. The human larynx shows complete, sequential ontogenesis of this phylogenetic pattern (Arey, 1965).

The Carnegie system of classification can be used for the most accurate staging of embryonic development of the human larynx (Tucker et al., 1978; Tucker and O'Rahilly, 1972). The larynx, trachea, bronchi, and lungs arise from a tracheobronchial groove located in the ventromedial aspect of the foregut, caudal to the pharyngeal pouches. (Tucker et al., 1978; Tucker and O'Rahilly, 1972). This ridge or groove forms the respiratory diverticulum, which is present in

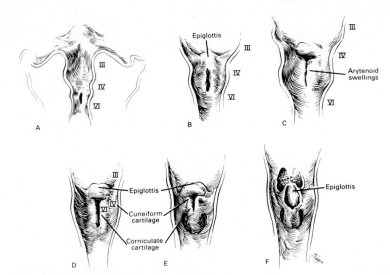

Figure 59–1 Development of the human larynx. *A,* four weeks; *B,* five weeks; *C,* six weeks; *D,* seven weeks; *E,* ten weeks; *F,* infant larynx at birth. Roman numerals refer to visceral arch derivatives.

the ninth Carnegie stage (approximately 20 day old embryo). Furrows along the lateral aspect of the tracheobronchial groove gradually deepen and eventually unite, effectively separating the laryngotracheal tube from the esophagus. The anterior portion of the cranial end of this tube forms the laryngeal slit, or aditus, in the tenth Carnegie embryonic stage, or about the 22nd day of development. Caudally, the laryngotracheal tube progresses to form lung buds in Carnegie stage 11 on or about the 24th day of development (Arey, 1965; Moore, 1973) (Fig. 59–1).

The recurrent laryngeal nerve can be identified by Carnegie stage 13, 37 days of gestational age. In Carnegie stage 14 (the 5 to 7 mm embryo) at approximately 30 to 32 days of gestation, the epiglottis begins to form from the hypobranchial eminence of the third and fourth arches and the anlage of the arytenoid cartilages on both aspects of the laryngeal slit. These anatomic anlages grow during the fifth week (6 to 9 mm embryo, Carnegie stage 15) (Tucker et al., 1978; Tucker and O'Rahilly, 1972), approximating each other medially and toward the base of the tongue. Growth and movement of these masses alter the aditus or laryngeal slit, producing the "I" or "Y" shape of the future glottis. By this stage, the superior laryngeal nerve can be identified (Tucker et al., 1978; O'Rahilly and Tucker, 1973), and the tracheoesophageal septum is complete to the level of the as yet posteriorly unfused cricoid cartilage (sixth arch) (Arey, 1965; Moore, 1973). Incomplete development at this stage may produce variable degrees of persistent laryngeal cleft (Ferguson, 1970). The eventual ventral and dorsal fusion of two lateral mesenchymal masses will form the complete cricoid cartilage. A definite larynx may be seen by Carnegie stage 17 (41 days of gestation). Fusion of the cricoid cartilage usually occurs by Carnegie stage 18, 42 to 44 days of development (Arey, 1965; Moore, 1973).

Differentiation of the laryngeal musculature is dependent upon the cartilaginous development with which each muscle is associated. Some authors consider the inferior pharyngeal constrictor to be a laryngeal muscle with its attachments to the thyroid (fourth arch) and cricoid (sixth arch) cartilages (Arey, 1965). The internal laryngeal constrictors begin as primitive cell masses lying medial to the thyroid cartilage, lateral and dorsal to the arytenoid areas, and lateral to the cricoid cartilage. As the cricoid develops (sixth arch), the muscles of the internal larynx also begin differentiating; the first distinct muscle of this group is the interarytenoid (which appears at five to six weeks of gestation). The cricothyroid muscle may also be distinguished at about this same stage of development as it arises from the anlage of the inferior pharyngeal constrictor (Arey, 1965). Soon thereafter, the lateral cricoarytenoid cartilage becomes visible (Carnegie stage 18, 44 days of gestation) (Tucker et al., 1978; Tucker and O'Rahilly, 1972), while the arytenoids themselves have not yet separated completely from the cricoid anlage.

The cricothyroid muscle develops during the fifth and sixth weeks of gestation, after the development of the anlage of the inferior pharyngeal constrictor. As the thyroid cartilage develops, the inferior cornu separates the tissue of the inferior constrictor into two bundles; the superior bundle develops into the inferior pharyngeal constrictor muscle, and the inferior forms the cricothyroid muscle. Developing independently of the remaining intrinsic laryngeal muscles, the cricothyroid is the only laryngeal muscle derived from the fourth arch and is, therefore, the only muscle innervated by the nerve of the fourth arch, the superior laryngeal nerve (Arey, 1965; Moore, 1973).

The cricoid and thyroid cartilages begin to develop prior to the arytenoids and begin chondrification at about seven weeks of gestation. Arytenoid chondrification is accordingly later, beginning at about 12 weeks of gestation. The corniculates also chondrify at about the 12th week, and the vocal processes are the last of the cartilaginous structures to undergo this development.

The epiglottis begins to develop during the eighth week of gestation, chondrifying during the fifth fetal month. Cuneiform cartilages develop within the aryepiglottic folds late in the seventh fetal month. The anlage of the thyroarytenoid muscle may be seen in the five to six week old embryo, but this muscle and true cords are not well differentiated until the formation of the glottis. As the thyroid cartilages develop, the glottis deepens and the true cords are aligned within the thyroid lamina. Failure of the true cords to split at ten weeks of gestation to form the primitive glottis results in congenital atresia of the larynx or, more often, a complete or partial congenital laryngeal web (Ferguson, 1970). Although these webs may be supraglottic (at the level of the false cord) or subglottic, most webs occur at the level of the glottis.

The laryngeal ventricle appears during the development of the true cords. It begins as an evagination in the laryngeal cavity during the eighth week (22 to 24 mm embryo). This outpouching of the endolarynx separates the true and false cords during the middle of the third month. The false cords have no muscle component, and the fibrous stroma that comprises them develops from condensed mesenchyme.

Aryepiglottic folds develop from the lateral boundaries of the fourth arch along a line from the hypobranchial eminence (epiglottis) to the arytenoid eminence of the sixth arch. Congenital cysts of the supraglottic region are possibly remnants of the third branchial pouch and lie superior to the derivations of the fourth arch (Ferguson, 1970).

By the tenth to eleventh weeks of gestation, the major structures of the larynx have developed and the cartilages are chondrifying. Refining and definition of structural features then begins and occurs more slowly than initial development. By the end of the second trimester of pregnancy the larynx has assumed a more completely developed, cone-shaped form, with the narrow subglottic lumen of the human fetus. In addition, laryngeal epithelium has changed from primitive mesenchyme into cuboidal and stratified squamous epithelium.

Fetal Anatomy of the Larynx

The fetal larynx forms an obtuse angle with the mandible, with the anterior portion of the hyoid overlapping the superior aspect of the thyroid cartilage. This relationship persists until after the first postnatal year. In addition, the fetal larynx is positioned high in the neck, between cervical vertebrae one and four (usually at the level of the second or third vertebra) and is about 2 cm long at birth (Fig. 59–1). The maximum width of the larynx at the level of the upper thyroid cartilage is also approximately 2 cm. The internal dimensions of the larynx at birth are approximately one third those of the adult (Crelin, 1973), but the larynx of the infant has a greater internal area proportional to total body size than does the adult larynx. The thyroid cartilage lies closer to the hyoid in the infant, and the laryngeal prominence and notch are insignificantly developed in the infant compared to these structures in the adult. Whereas the thyroid cartilage of infants is relatively shorter and broader than an adult's, the cricoid cartilage remains in essentially the same shape throughout life. The infant's vocal cords are 4.0 to 4.5 mm long, relatively shorter than those of the child or adult (Crelin, 1973). Internally, the infantile larynx is shorter and more funnel-shaped than that of an adult, with the ventricle being relatively small, although the laryngeal saccule is variable in size and often large. The infantile subglottic larynx makes an angle with the supraglottic portion, descending downward and dorsally rather than forming the vertical column present in older children and adults. This is important to remember when selecting laryngeal tube size and shape should intubation of the infant be necessary, since mucosal irritation with a straight, rigid

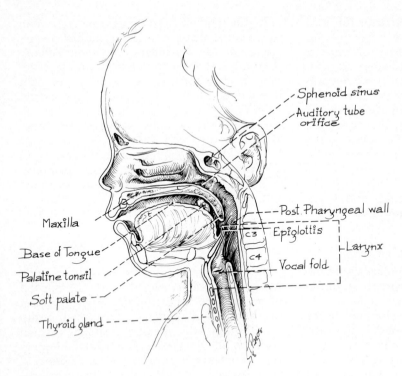

Maxilla

Base of Tongue

Palatine tonsil

Soft palate

Thyroid gland

Sphenoid sinus

Auditory tube orifice

Post. Pharyngeal wall

Epiglottis

C3

C4

Vocal fold

Larynx

Figure 59–2 Development of the lower airway through the eighth week of gestation.

tube may lead to submucosal edema and consequent occlusion of the airway (Fig. 59–2).

By about the third year of life some difference according to sex may be seen in the pediatric larynx. Boys develop a longer and larger internal larynx, whereas the angle of the thyroid laminae becomes greater in girls. At puberty, these changes are accentuated as the size of the male larynx increases more rapidly. The angle of the thyroid laminae develops to about 90 degrees in males and to about 120 degrees in females, the difference being responsible for the laryngeal prominence in males. In addition, boys at puberty develop thicker and longer vocal cords, producing the characteristic change in voice quality at puberty (Crelin, 1973).

TRACHEA AND BRONCHI

Embryology

Within the 4 mm embryo (Carnegie stage 11, approximately 24 days of gestation), the tracheobronchial groove has completely developed and the primitive "lung bud" has bifurcated, forming two primary bronchi. These primitive trachea and bronchi are in the shape of an inverted "Y." The right bronchus forms a more obtuse angle with the trachea than does the left, a feature that

remains constant even into adulthood. This accounts for the more frequent aspiration of foreign bodies into the right bronchus (Arey, 1965; Crelin, 1973; Moore, 1973). The primary bronchi curve dorsally to lie next to the esophagus in Carnegie stage 14 (O'Rahilly and Tucker, 1973). Secondary proliferations at the site of future secondary bronchi may also be seen. By Carnegie stage 15, lobar bronchial buds may be seen, and capillary plexes cover the developing pulmonary tree (O'Rahilly and Tucker, 1973).

Lung buds develop at the caudal end of the laryngotracheal tube. These buds differentiate into the bronchi and eventually lead to the developing lung. The left lung bud, in addition to forming a more acute angle with the trachea, is slightly smaller than the right. During the fefth fetal week, these buds extend laterally into the pericardioperitoneal canals, which are the primitive pleural spaces.

At the same time, the right bud forms two secondary buds, while the left forms only one. Hence, the right adult lung has three primary bronchi and the left has two (see Fig. 59–3). Each of the secondary bronchi forms two branches until there are approximately 24 orders or branches present by the 16th week of fetal development (Arey, 1965; Moore, 1973).

The developing lungs acquire a layer of

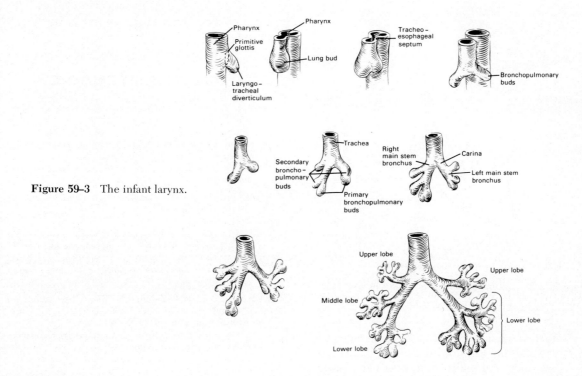

Figure 59–3 The infant larynx.

visceral pleura from the splanchnic meso-derm, which expands with the lungs during growth. With continued growth, the lungs extend caudally into the body wall mesen-chyme. Thus, the thoracic body wall becomes lined with parietal pleura derived from the somatic mesenchyme.

Most authors divide the developmental process of the lungs into three or four stages (Arey, 1965; Moore, 1973); these stages are as follows.

Stage 1 (5 to 17 weeks of gestation). The air conduction system of bronchi and bron-chioles is developed. Because the developing lung at this stage has the microscopic appear-ance of a gland, this stage has been termed the "glandular" or "pseudoglandular" stage. The bronchi and bronchioles are lined with cuboidal epithelium.

Stage 2 (13 to 25 weeks of gestation). During this stage the respiratory bronchioles are developed. Lung tissues become very vascular, and at about 24 weeks of gestation each terminal bronchiole gives rise to two or more respiratory bronchioles, which fur-ther divide into three to six sacculations, or alveolar ducts. The cuboidal lining of these alveolar ducts becomes smaller; later in devel-opment this shrinking permits close approx-imation of the blood capillaries to the air spaces.

Stage 3 (24 weeks of gestation to birth). Alveolar ducts continue to develop and give rise to clusters of primitive pulmonary alveoli. Capillary growth increases within the sur-rounding mesenchyme, as does concurrent lymphatic proliferation. By the 26th to 28th week of gestation the fetus should weigh about 1000 gm, and the terminal alveoli should be sufficiently developed to permit survival of a premature infant. Prior to this critical time the vascular development about the alveoli is insufficient for adequate gas exchange.

Stage 4 (birth to approximately eight years). The epithelium of the alveoli contin-ues to thin, and the number of alveoli in-creases. In fact, about one sixth to one eighth of the total number of alveoli of an adult are present at birth. Respiratory movement is present prior to birth, and the lungs are about half full of liquid that has been swal-lowed from the amnionic cavity. This fluid is believed to be removed during birth by com-pression of the chest and by absorption into the pulmonary blood vessels and the lym-phatics. The newborn lungs are shown in Figure 59–4.

Surfactant lowers the surface tension of the air–alveoli interface, maintaining the patency of the alveoli and preventing atelectasis. The absence of or a decrease in the amount of

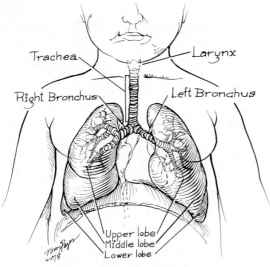

Figure 59–4 The infant lungs.

surfactant is believed to be a major cause of hyaline membrane disease (Crelin, 1973).

Congenital malformations of the lower respiratory tract include tracheoesophageal fistula, which occurs in about one in 2500 births. It is believed that this malformation results from incomplete division of the foregut into the separate precursors of the esophagus and trachea (Crelin, 1973). The incomplete fission of the tracheoesophageal folds produces incomplete tracheal and esophageal separation. Four main variations of this defect exist, but the most common is a condition in which the upper esophagus ends blindly while the lower esophagus enters the trachea near the bifurcation of the trachea.

Tracheal stenosis, or atresia, is a rare defect and usually occurs with a tracheoesophageal fistula. These abnormalities are usually due to unequal partitioning of the foregut during the development of the esophagus and trachea.

Tracheal diverticula are rare. They are blind branches of a bronchus and are significant only in instances of foreign body aspiration. Bronchial cysts may form from ab-

normal saccular enlargements during development.

SELECTED REFERENCES

Arey, L. B. 1965. Developmental Anatomy: A Textbook and Laboratory Manual of Embrology, 7th ed. Philadelphia, W. B. Saunders Co., pp 263–271.
> *This book presents a good overview of the embryology of the larynx and lower airway. The author is an anatomist rather than a physician, and presents his material from that standpoint.*

Fergusion, C. F. 1970. Congenital abnormalities of the infant larynx. Otolaryngol. Clin. North Am., 3(6):185–200.
> *This article presents a general discussion of development of the normal infant larynx and of congenital abnormalities of the larynx. It offers good suggestions for clinical application of information available on problems of development of the larynx.*

Tucker, J. A., and O'Rahilly, R. 1972. Observations on the embryology of the human larynx. Ann. Otol., Rhinol. Laryngol., 81:520–523.
> *This article presents the Carnegie system for staging embryonic laryngeal development.*

REFERENCES

Arey, L. B. 1965. Developmental Anatomy: A Textbook and Laboratory Manual of Embryology, 7th ed. Philadelphia, W. B. Saunders Co., pp 263–271.

Crelin, E. S. 1973. Functional Anatomy of the Newborn. New Haven, Yale University Press, pp 16–51.

Davies, J. 1973. Embryology and anatomy of the head and neck. In Paparella, M. M., and Shumrick, D. A. (Eds.) Otolaryngology, Vol. 1. Philadelphia, W. B. Saunders Co., pp 111–149.

Ferguson, C. F. 1970. Congenital abnormalities of the infant larynx. Otolaryngol. Clin. North Am., 3(6):185–200.

Moore, K. L. 1973. The Developing Human: Clinically Oriented Embryology. Philadelphia, W. B. Saunders Co., pp 168–174.

O'Rahilly, R., and Tucker, J. 1973. The early development of the larynx in staged human embryos. Ann. Otol., Rhinol. Laryngol., Suppl 7, 82.

Tucker, J. A., Tucker, G., and Vidic, B. 1978. Clinical correlation of anomalies of the supraglottic larynx with the stage sequences of normal human development. Ann. Otol., Rhinol. Laryngol., 87:636–644.

Tucker, J. A., and O'Rahilly, R. 1972. Observations on the embryology of the human larynx. Ann. Otol., Rhinol. Laryngol., 81:520–523.

Chapter 60

PHYSIOLOGY OF THE LARYNX, AIRWAYS, AND LUNGS

Robert E. Wood, Ph.D., M.D.

THE LARYNX

Structure

The larynx is composed of the cricoid, thyroid, and arytenoid cartilages, the epiglottis, the vocal cords, and associated muscles and ligaments. The details of laryngeal structure may be found in any standard anatomy text and in Chapter 59 of this book.

Innervation

Innervation of the larynx, both motor and sensory, is from the tenth cranial nerve via the superior and inferior laryngeal nerves. Since there is bilateral cortical representation to each side, motor paralysis of the larynx is almost always due to a peripheral lesion. Innervation to all the intrinsic muscles of the larynx is by the recurrent laryngeal nerves except for the cricothyroid muscle, which is innervated by the external branch of the superior laryngeal nerve. The sensory supply of the epiglottis, aryepiglottic folds, and the laryngeal mucosa (including the subglottic space) comes from the internal branch of the superior laryngeal nerve.

There are many laryngeal reflexes, some of which are poorly defined and understood. Reflexes arising in the larynx may alter the function of the cardiovascular system, as well as that of the lower airways and the respiratory center in the brain. Bradycardia, apnea, laryngospasm, and bronchoconstriction are among the effects produced by these reflexes. In addition, systemic alterations, such as hypoxemia or hypercapnia, may reflexly alter laryngeal muscle tone. Many of the laryngeal reflexes may be abolished or modified by topical anesthetics or vagolytic drugs.

Intrinsic Laryngeal Musculature

There are four important functions of the intrinsic laryngeal muscles: (1) The *glottis is opened* by rotation of the arytenoid cartilages, which are moved by the posterior cricoarytenoid muscles. (2) The *glottis is closed* by the action of the lateral cricoarytenoid muscles, which rotate the arytenoids in a direction opposite to that which opens the glottis. This action is supplemented by that of the arytenoideus muscle, which approximates the arytenoids and shortens the posterior commissure. In addition, the cricothyroid muscle tenses the vocal cords and thus also may participate in glottic closure. (3) *Vocal cord tension* is regulated by two sets of muscles. The cricothyroid muscle tilts the cricoid cartilage backwards, tensing and lengthening the vocal cords. This is important in phonation as well as in glottic closure. The thyroarytenoid muscle relaxes the cords and shortens them. The vocalis muscle, a part of the thyroarytenoid, "fine tunes" vocal cord tension and is thus very important in phonation. (4) The fourth muscle function of the larynx is that of *lowering and raising the epiglottis*. The aryepiglotticus lowers the epiglottis to cover the glottic chink, while the thyroepiglotticus,

1141

extending from the anterior portion of the epiglottis to the thyroid cartilage, raises the epiglottis, thus exposing the glottis.

Laryngeal Functions

The larynx serves three important functions: it acts as an airway, it serves as an instrument of phonation, and it protects the lower airways. The larynx is the narrowest portion of the entire airway system and as such is particularly vulnerable to obstruction. The subglottic space is entirely surrounded by the cricoid cartilage, which serves a protective function but which also may be a contributing factor to airway obstruction should mucosal edema occur, since the only direction in which the mucosa may swell is into the airway lumen. Complete or partial closure of the glottis during expiration results in increased intrathoracic pressure. This is essential for coughing or for forceful expulsion of abdominal contents (Valsalva maneuver) and may improve airway dynamics or gas exchange in pathologic conditions, as discussed later in this chapter.

The vocal function of the larynx is a complex subject that will not be addressed here.

The larynx protects the airway in several ways. Most importantly, it effects complete and automatic closure of the glottis during swallowing; contrary to popular belief, the epiglottis is not necessary for glottic closure nor for prevention of aspiration. During swallowing the vocal cords are completely closed, and the epiglottis is brought down over the glottis, thus deflecting the bolus of swallowed material to either side and posteriorly into the esophageal orifice. The other major protective function of the larynx is its role in the cough reflex, which is triggered by sensitive receptors in the larynx and the subglottic space. Stimulation of these receptors results in immediate closure of the glottis, which is followed by an explosive cough. The importance of this reflex mechanism in homeostasis cannot be overemphasized.

Important Physiologic Derangements in Laryngeal Function

Cord Paralysis

Paralysis of the vocal cords may result from injury to the recurrent laryngeal nerves. Because of the longer course of the left recurrent laryngeal nerve (which passes around the aortic arch), it is more susceptible to injury than the right recurrent nerve, and it may also be involved by mediastinal lesions. Birth trauma is a relatively common cause of transient cord paralysis. *Abductor paralysis* (paralysis of the posterior cricoarytenoid muscles) results in midline paralysis with airway obstruction. In this circumstance, phonation or cry is often fairly normal, although infants may be stridorous and adults may experience dyspnea. *Adductor paralysis* (paralysis of the lateral cricoarytenoid and arytenoideus muscles) results in the inability to close the glottis, thus leading to aspiration and an ineffective cough. Unilateral adductor paralysis may lead to aspiration, whereas unilateral abductor paralysis is often relatively asymptomatic.

Obstruction

Laryngeal obstruction may result from abductor paralysis as noted previously or, more commonly, from infection or trauma leading to edema. Laryngeal edema may be generalized, as with thermal burns, or it may be localized to either the subglottic or supraglottic regions. Supraglottic edema is most often associated with acute infectious epiglottitis and is discussed elsewhere in this text. Subglottic edema may result from viral infections (croup) or may be the result of mechanical trauma (such as intubation or bronchoscopy). Other causes of laryngeal obstruction include foreign bodies and congenital lesions, such as laryngeal webs, cysts, or subglottic stenosis, which are discussed in other chapters of this text.

An important laryngeal obstructive lesion in infancy is the result of immaturity of the laryngeal cartilage, called *laryngomalacia*. This condition is usually benign and self-limited but may be severe enough to require tracheostomy to achieve an adequate airway. The most common findings associated with laryngomalacia are a very floppy epiglottis (which may fall into the glottic chink during inspiration), large redundant aryepiglottic folds, which may also occlude the glottis during inspiration, and large or redundant arytenoid processes. In severe cases the cricoid and thyroid cartilages themselves may be so soft that the entire larynx tends to collapse during inspiration. Stridor associated with laryngomalacia is predominantly inspiratory, and there is usually little obstruction during expiration. However, stridor is always more apparent when the rate and depth of respiration are increased, as in crying or with exercise. Two factors contribute to this phenomenon: (1) because of the Bernoulli effect (lateral pressure in a flowing stream decreases as the velocity of flow increases), the laryngeal structures tend to collapse, producing more obstruction as the airflow velocity increases; (2) higher flow velocity increases the turbulence of the flow and therefore the noise of respiration. Laryngomalacia is discussed in more detail elsewhere in this text.

Severe laryngeal obstruction leads to alveolar hypoxia. This, in turn, leads to pulmonary arteriolar constriction and elevation of pulmonary arterial pressure. Eventually, permanent changes may occur in the pulmonary arterial tree that lead to irreversible pulmonary hypertension, cor pulmonale, and death.

THE AIRWAYS

Structure

One of the most important features of the structure of the airways is their ability to remain patent despite relatively large shifts in intrathoracic pressure during respiration. This characteristic is due to the fact that airways as small as 1 to 2 mm in diameter have enough cartilage to maintain their shape in the face of moderate pressure changes. In the trachea and major bronchi the cartilage is in the form of rough, C-shaped rings, but in more peripheral airways the cartilage becomes more irregular and less prominent. Only in the subglottic space does the cartilage (cricoid) completely encircle the airway. Small airways (less than 1 mm in diameter) are supported entirely by the elastic properties of the pulmonary parenchyma, and surfactant may play an important role in maintaining patency of these airways. Larger airways are surrounded by strands of smooth muscle fiber, particularly between the ends of the cartilaginous rings, contraction of which results in decreased diameter of the airways and increased resistance to airflow. However, in the trachea and largest bronchi, smooth muscle contraction may actually stabilize the airway.

An important microscopic feature of the airway mucosa is the presence of mixed seromucous glands, which are numerous in the larger airways (approximately one gland per square millimeter) but which become quite sparse after the first several generations of airways. Goblet cells are numerous in the upper airways and extend further into the respiratory tree than do the glands, but under normal circumstances they are not present in the smaller airways. The epithelium of the respiratory mucosa from the posterior laryngeal commissure to the smaller airways is pseudostratified and ciliated. At the bronchiolar level the epithelium becomes more cuboidal in nature, and the number of cilia are decreased. No cilia are found in the respiratory bronchioles or smaller airways.

The airways are lined with a thin (perhaps discontinuous) layer of mucus that overlies the tips of the cilia on the epithelial cells. Secretion of mucus and fluid by the mucosal glands is under parasympathetic nervous control; goblet cells discharge their contents (mucus) primarily in response to irritative phenomena. Surrounding the cilia is a fluid whose precise composition is unknown, but which for hydrodynamic reasons must be assumed to have a low viscosity; the origin and control of secretion of this periciliary fluid is unknown.

Innervation

Sensory innervation of the trachea and airways is entirely via the vagus nerve. The receptors are primarily irritant receptors, stimulation of which results in effects very similar to those that are seen with stimulation of the larynx. Motor innervation is both vagal and sympathetic, as is the nerve supply of the mucosal glands.

Function

The major function of the airways is air conduction. The velocity of airflow at any point depends on respiratory frequency, tidal volume, and airway diameter. In normal adults tracheal flow velocity is approximately 1.5 meters per second during quiet breathing. With an effective cough, the tracheal flow velocity may approach two thirds the speed of sound. The total cross-sectional area of the airways increases dramatically with increasing distal branching, and thus the linear flow velocity decreases the further out it is measured in the respiratory tree. In the large aiways (except the trachea), airflow patterns are turbulent or nearly so, and it is this turbulent flow that produces normal breath sounds. In smaller airways airflow becomes

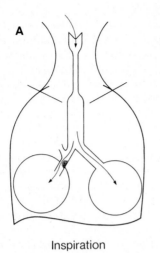
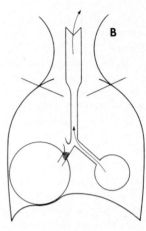

Inspiration   Expiration

Figure 60–1 During exhalation (A) intrathoracic pressure is less than atmospheric, thus leading to distention of the intrathoracic airways. The extrathoracic portion of the trachea is surrounded by atmospheric pressure and may become narrower. During expiration (B) intrathoracic pressure is higher than atmospheric and intrathoracic airways narrow, while the extrathoracic trachea may distend or remain at normal caliber. The dimensions on this diagram are exaggerated to approximate those of a patient with significant tracheomalacia.

The lower airways are not as well supported as is the trachea, and their change in size with respiration may be more pronounced. This diagram illustrates that in the presence of partial bronchial obstruction (as by a foreign body), air may be able to enter the lung distal to the obstruction during inspiration but may not exit during exhalation, thus leading to air trapping and overinflation of that part of the lung (obstructive emphysema).

laminar, and at the level of the alveolar ducts and alveoli, linear flow velocity is so low that molecular diffusion may account for a significant proportion of gas movement.

Inspiration occurs when intrathoracic pressure is lower than atmospheric, and expiration occurs when intrathoracic pressure becomes greater than atmospheric. The airways have some degree of compliance, increasing in diameter during inspiration and decreasing in diameter during expiration (Fig. 60–1). Because of this, the shear force exerted by the air on the secretions on the airway walls is greater during expiration than during inspiration — a fact that may play some role in keeping the airways clear of secretions. This phenomenon is exaggerated during hyperventilation, which perhaps helps to explain the effectiveness of exercise in stimulating a productive cough. Narrowing of the lumen of the larger airways during coughing (by active muscle contraction as well as by increased intrathoracic pressure) increases the linear flow velocity and thus leads to a more effective cough.

The ventilatory function of the lung may be described in terms of volumes, flow rates, and airway resistance (the most common parameters of pulmonary function measured in the laboratory). Total lung capacity is divided into several components (Fig. 60–2). The reference point for all volume measurements is functional residual capacity, which is defined as the volume of gas contained in the

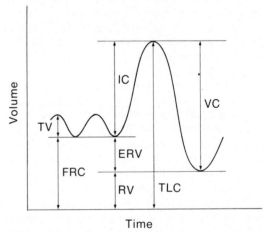

Figure 60–2 This spirogram indicates the subdivisions of lung volume. TV (tidal volume), VC (vital capacity), ERV (expiratory reserve volume), and IC (inspiratory capacity) are relative volumes and may be measured with a simple spirometer. The absolute lung volumes, TLC (total lung capacity), FRC (functional residual capacity), and RV (residual volume) cannot be determined by use of a simple spirometer but must be measured by gas dilution plethysmographic techniques.

lung when all forces acting on the lung are in equilibrium. In practice, this occurs at the end of a quiet, relaxed, normal exhalation. Residual volume is the volume of gas remaining in the lung at the end of a maximal exhalation. Vital capacity (total lung capacity minus residual volume) and its subdivisions (inspiratory capacity and expiratory reserve volume) are usually measured with a simple spirometer. Measurements of absolute lung volumes (functional residual capacity, residual volume, and total lung capacity) require more sophisticated methodology. The simplest technique for measurement of functional residual capacity (from which all other absolute lung volumes are calculated) is to have the subject rebreathe from a closed container of known volume that at the start has a known concentration of helium. After rebreathing and equilibration (usually for seven minutes), the volume of gas contained in the lungs can be calculated from the ratio of the initial and final helium concentrations and the initial volume of the container. Measurement of functional residual capacity with a body plethysmograph, although requiring more complex and expensive equipment, has the advantage of rapid measurement and is more accurate in subjects with poor gas mixing in the lung (as with significant airway obstruction).

Flow rates are affected by both the neuromuscular and mechanical components of ventilation. The most common measurement

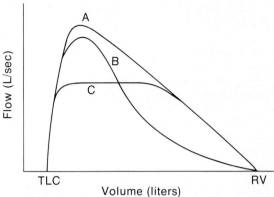

Figure 60–4   The expiratory flow–volume curve presents the same data as are shown in a conventional spirogram but in a more easily interpreted form. Curve A is a normal tracing in which the peak flow is achieved after 10 to 15 per cent of the vital capacity has been exhaled; the remainder of the curve has a nearly constant slope. The tail of the curve is relatively effort-independent. Curve B is a tracing obtained from a subject with lower airway obstruction. Flow rates at low lung volumes are markedly decreased, while the peak flow is maintained at a nearly normal level. Curve C is a tracing obtained in a subject with high airway obstruction (tracheal or laryngeal) in which the expiratory flow is limited at high lung volumes but not at lower lung volumes. TLC, total lung capacity; RV, residual volume.

of flow is the forced expiratory volume in the first second ($FEV_{1.0}$), which is measured with a spirometer (Fig. 60–3). Normally the $FEV_{1.0}$ is at least 80 per cent of the vital capacity. Decreased $FEV_{1.0}$ may be due to poor effort or muscle weakness but is usually a manifestation of airway obstruction. The $FEV_{1.0}$ may not reflect significant increases in airflow resistance in airways less than about 2 mm in diameter.

A spirometric tracing shows expired volume versus time. Plotting the first derivative of the spirometric tracing (i.e., volume per unit time) against expired volume yields the so-called "flow–volume curve" (Fig. 60–4). From this graphic presentation of the expiratory flow maneuver, inferences may be made about the state of the small airways. The slope of the flow–volume curve below approximately 50 per cent of vital capacity is relatively independent of effort. In contrast, the $FEV_{1.0}$ is highly effort-dependent. Small airway obstruction will be manifest primarily by lower flow rates at low lung volumes, thus giving a concave flow–volume curve. High airway obstruction (at the larynx or in the trachea) will yield a curve with a truncated peak˙(Fig. 60–4). Flow–volume curves are ordinarily generated with an electronic pneu-

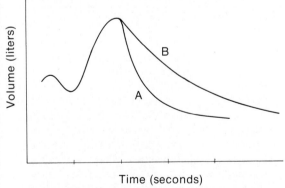

Figure 60–3   This spirogram shows forced expiratory maneuvers. Curve A represents a normal tracing, in which approximately 86 per cent of the vital capacity is expelled in the first second ($FEV_{1.0}/VC$ = .86). Curve *B* is an abnormal tracing recorded from a patient with airway obstruction ($FEV_{1.0}/VC$ = .49). The administration of a bronchodilator will usually result in an increase in the expiratory flow rate ($FEV_{1.0}$) in a subject with physiologic airway obstruction.

motachometer in which flow rate is measured directly and integrated against time to yield volume.

Airway resistance is defined as the pressure required to produce a given flow rate and is expressed in units of centimeters of water pressure per liter per second of airflow. Airway resistance is measured in a body plethysmograph and varies inversely with the volume at which the measurement is taken. Airway resistance measured at low lung volumes will be higher than that measured at high lung volumes owing to the increase in the size of the airways during inspiration. This may be taken into account by multiplying the airway resistance by the lung volume at which the measurements were taken; the resulting measurement is called the specific airway resistance. Airway resistance increases inversely as the fourth power of the radius of the airway. Thus, although there are a very large number of small airways, their total cross-sectional area is large, and they contribute approximately one fourth or less of the total pulmonary resistance. This means that measurements of airway resistance primarily reflect changes in the *larger* airways.

Another important function of the airways is *humidification* of inspired air. At 37°C air saturated with water vapor contains 44 mg water per liter, while at room temperature air contains 10 to 15 mg water per liter, depending on the relative humidity. Thus, a large amount of water must be added to the inspired air. During normal nasal breathing a major portion of the humidification occurs in the upper airway (above the glottis), but further warming and humidification take place in the trachea and mainstem bronchi. When the nose is bypassed, either by mouth breathing or by an artificial airway, the lower airways must assume a much greater role in humidification and warming.

Important Derangements in Airway Function

Mechanical obstruction of the airways may be the result of extrinsic compression (as by mass lesions or enlarged great vessels) but more commonly is due to an intrinsic airway lesion. There are many causes of intrinsic airway obstruction, including endobronchial masses, airway stenosis (congenital or acquired). an aspirated foreign body, mucosal edema, and increased tracheobronchial se-

cretions. Increased secretions with decreased airway clearance is the single most common cause of chronic obstruction (as in chronic bronchitis or cystic fibrosis).

Physiologic obstruction is most often the result of increased bronchomotor tone (bronchospasm). This is usually transient and reversible but may be intractable and life-threatening (status asthmaticus). In an asthma attack, several mechanisms operate to produce obstruction, including increased bronchomotor tone, increased secretions, increased viscosity of secretions, mucosal edema, and impaired mucociliary transport. Bronchomotor tone is increased by parasympathetic effectors and may be decreased by beta-adrenergic stimulating agents or by parasympatholytic agents such as atropine. Physiologic airway obstruction may be the result not only of increased bronchomotor tone but also of *decreased* bronchomotor tone, which may result in increased compliance of the airway walls. If the airways are *too* compliant, as in bronchiectasis, collapse may occur during exhalation, and air will be trapped in the lung. Diffuse distal airway obstruction, as occurs with asthma or bronchiolitis, may lead to proximal airway collapse with air trapping because of the increased intrathoracic pressure generated in the effort to overcome the expiratory resistance. This may to some extent be overcome by partial glottic closure during exhalation ("grunting" or pursed-lip breathing) so that the major pressure drop occurs at the glottis. In much the same way and for the same reasons, an infant with surfactant deficiency will grunt to maintain a higher intrathoracic pressure during exhalation.

The dynamics of the trachea are different from those of other airways, since part of the trachea lies outside the thorax. The extrathoracic trachea is in effect surrounded by atmospheric pressure, which remains constant, in contrast to the intrathoracic trachea, which is surrounded by the varying pressures of the intrathoracic space. During inspiration the *extra*thoracic trachea tends to collapse, whereas the *intra*thoracic trachea tends to collapse during expiration (Fig. 60–1). Thus a patient with tracheomalacia may have both inspiratory and expiratory stridor. Contraction of the smooth muscle of the tracheal wall may reduce the compliance of the membranous portion of the wall, which normally tends to invaginate when intrathoracic pressure is increased. Because of this, some patients may develop increased expiratory obstruction after administration of a bronchodilator owing to loss of tracheal and large airway muscle tone.

THE PULMONARY PARENCHYMA

The pulmonary parenchyma can be considered to consist of the terminal airways, alveoli, pulmonary capillary bed, and their supporting tissues. The functional unit of the lung is the alveolar–capillary interface, across which gas exchange takes place.

Structure

Alveoli appear as outpouchings in the walls of respiratory bronchioles; they are more numerous in the alveolar ducts, which terminate in a cluster of alveolar sacs. Each alveolus is a rough hexagon, with one side open to the alveolar duct. The alveolar walls or septae are composed of two types of epithelial cells, reticular and elastic fibers, a thin basement membrane, and the capillary endothelium. Capillaries make up the majority of the septae. Small holes in the septae between adjacent alveoli provide an alternate route for movement of gases. Type I alveolar epithelial cells have a very thin cytoplasm through which gases diffuse readily. Type II alveolar epithelial cells are rich in mitochondria and endoplasmic reticulum and actively synthesize and secrete surfactant. The number of alveoli increases about tenfold from birth to adulthood, when it averages 300 to 400 million with a total surface area of 40 to 100 square meters.

The patency of the smallest airways is dependent upon the elastic properties of the lung parenchyma since these airways have no cartilaginous support. When lung elasticity is reduced, as in old age or emphysema, collapse of the smaller airways during exhalation may result in air trapping and impaired ventilation.

Compliance

Compliance is defined as the change in volume per unit change in transpulmonary pressure. In practice, compliance is more useful as a concept than as data, since its accurate measurement is relatively complex.

Compliance is decreased by the normal elastic forces in the lung and by surface tension in the alveoli, as well as by pathologic processes such as pneumonia, pulmonary edema, and interstitial fibrosis. Surfactant reduces surface tension, thus increasing pulmonary compliance.

Surfactant

Because the alveoli are so small, (the average diameter is approximately 0.25 mm) they have a significant amount of surface tension, which tends to make them collapse. This is countered by the presence of surfactant, which markedly reduces surface tension, especially during deflation of the lung. Surfactant is composed mostly of dipalmityl lecithin and is synthesized in Type II alveolar cells from choline and alpha-beta-diglycerides. This metabolic pathway matures at approximately 32 to 33 weeks in the human fetus, and infants born prior to that time usually have surfactant deficiency with the clinical syndrome of hyaline membrane disease (respiratory distress syndrome). The stress of birth or prolonged labor will result in the induction of the enzymes of this pathway in the immature newborn, as will exogenous administration of corticosteroids. Approximately 24 to 48 hours are required for full induction of the pathway and synthesis of sufficient surfactant to prevent hyaline membrane disease. Hypoxia and metabolic acidosis interfere with both enzyme induction and surfactant production and may contribute to the development of surfactant deficiency in a mature infant.

Surfactant deficiency increases alveolar surface tension and reduces pulmonary compliance so that more inspiratory effort is required to achieve adequate tidal volume. The functional residual capacity is decreased, and many alveoli may become completely atelectatic during expiration. Atelectasis and low functional residual capacity result in intrapulmonary shunting of blood and reduced arterial oxygen tension despite increased inspired oxygen concentrations. Alveolar collapse may be prevented by applying a constant positive distending pressure to the alveoli (CPAP — continuous positive airway pressure or CNP — continuous negative pressure applied to the thorax). This will increase pulmonary compliance and reduce the work of breathing. In patients whose ventilation is being assisted mechanically, positive end-expiratory pressure accomplishes the same end. The maintenance of a constant distending pressure, regardless of the mechanism by which it is produced, has greatly reduced mortality due to neonatal respiratory distress. Constant distending pressure is also used effectively in patients beyond the neonatal period who for some reason have lost surfactant (shock lung, etc.).

Gas Exchange

The major function of the lungs and respiratory system is gas exchange, for which there are three major requirements: pulmonary capillary blood flow, alveolar ventilation, and diffusion of gases across the alveolar capillary membrane.

Perfusion

Under normal circumstances the entire right ventricular output passes through the pulmonary arteries before returning to the left atrium. The regional distribution of pulmonary blood flow is regulated by the pulmonary arterioles, which are in turn controlled by the partial pressure of oxygen in the adjacent alveoli. Alveolar hypoxia results in pulmonary arteriolar constriction, which helps to maintain a uniform ratio of perfusion to ventilation. Gravitational effects are also important, as blood flow to dependent portions of the lung is increased.

Ventilation

The diaphragm and accessory muscles of respiration interact with the rigid chest wall to produce the negative intrathoracic pressure that is necessary for flow of air into the lungs. Relaxation of the muscles combined with elastic recoil of the lung parenchyma increases intrathoracic pressure and results in exhalation. Forced exhalation is accomplished by contraction of the abdominal muscles and the internal intercostal muscles.

The regional *distribution of ventilation* depends on several factors: (1) the distribution of intrathoracic pressure (in unilateral diaphragmatic paralysis, intrathoracic pressure on the paralyzed side will be less negative and therefore ventilation will be impaired on that side); (2) the distribution of airway resistance and lung compliance (areas with high airway resistance or low compliance will be relatively poorly ventilated); (3) respiratory frequency (at very low respiratory frequencies, the distribution of ventilation will be relatively even regardless of the distribution of airway resistance; however, as respiratory frequency increases, ventilation will be shunted preferentially to those areas of the lung having the lowest airway resistance); (4) depth of inspiration (tidal volume).

A factor of major importance in gas exchange is *matching of perfusion and ventilation.* "Wasted" ventilation occurs when areas of lung are ventilated but not perfused, but will not contribute to arterial desaturation. Wasted perfusion (areas of the lung perfused but not ventilated) will result in arterial hypoxemia by mixing the unoxygenated pulmonary arterial blood with the pulmonary venous return. Pulmonary arteriolar constriction in response to low alveolar oxygen tension is the most important mechanism for maintaining even distribution of perfusion and ventilation. Ventilation–perfusion mismatching due to uneven distribution of ventilation is the most common cause of hypoxemia.

The ratio of anatomic or physiologic dead space to tidal volume is another major factor involved in gas exchange. Physiologic dead space is the volume of air contained in the conducting airways that does not reach the alveoli and in those areas of the lung that are ventilated but not perfused. Normally the dead space accounts for approximately 30 per cent of the tidal volume. With disease that decreases the tidal volume or results in "wasted" ventilation, this ratio increases, and minute volume must be increased to maintain the same effective alveolar ventilation. Examples of conditions that may produce an increased ratio of dead space to tidal volume would include restrictive lung disease, severe obstructive lung disease, chest trauma, pneumothorax, and hypoventilation due to depressant drugs.

The *regulation of respiration* may be considered to have three major components (Berger et al., 1977): sensors (chemoreceptors and mechanical receptors), effectors (lungs and respiratory muscles), and the controller (the central nervous system).

Arterial chemoreceptors in the carotid bodies and the aortic bodies respond to changes in the arterial oxygen tension by increasing their output when the arterial oxygen tension decreases. Likewise, acidosis or an increase in arterial carbon dioxide tension will result in increased chemoreceptor activity. Central chemoreceptors in the medulla respond to changes in cerebrospinal fluid pH. Since the cerebrospinal fluid bicarbonate concentration equilibrates very slowly with that in the blood, the medullary chemoreceptor is essentially a carbon dioxide sensor. With long-standing hypercapnia and metabolic compensation (increased bicarbonate) the response of this chemoreceptor may be blunted, leaving the oxygen receptors as the primary functioning sensor. Since the activity of the peripheral arterial oxygen sensor begins to fall off rapidly as the arterial oxygen tension rises above 100 torr, it is evident that administering oxygen to a chronically hypercapnic patient may deprive him of much of his respiratory drive.

Pulmonary stretch receptors located within the airway smooth muscle are activated by inflation of the lungs and reflexly inhibit inspiration (the Hering-Breuer reflex).

Central control of respiration may be a voluntary, cortical function, but automatic respiration is a brain stem function. A number of different nuclei and tracts are involved in the generation of respiratory rhythm, the integration of efferent and afferent signals, and the responses to various respiratory stimuli.

Under normal circumstances, arterial carbon dioxide tension is the most important factor controlling overall ventilatory function: as it rises, so does minute ventilation. In most healthy subjects, minute ventilation increases by at least 1 liter per minute per torr of carbon dioxide, and the "sensitivity" to carbon dioxide is greater in younger subjects. The hypoxic respiratory drive is a nearly linear function of the desaturation of arterial hemoglobin, even though the chemoreceptors respond directly to changes in arterial oxygen tension. The individual response to hypoxia is quite variable and may be diminished in patients with chronic hypoxia.

Diffusion

Both oxygen and carbon dioxide must diffuse across the alveolar capillary membrane in order to achieve effective gas exchange. The rate of diffusion of carbon dioxide is much greater than that of oxygen, and carbon dioxide is usually not limited by diffusion. On the other hand, diffusion of oxygen may be impaired when the alveolar capillary membrane is thickened by disease (such as interstitial pneumonitis or fibrosis, or pulmonary edema), and arterial hypoxemia may result. The diffusing capacity of the lung for oxygen (D_{LO_2}) is estimated by measuring the diffusing capacity for carbon monoxide (D_{LCO}).

PULMONARY DEFENSE MECHANISMS

Pulmonary defense mechanisms may be divided into four different categories: mechanical, neurologic, humoral, and cellular.

Mechanical Defense Mechanisms

Mechanical defense mechanisms begin at the nares, where the nasal hairs provide an important *filtration* function. Turbulent airflow over the turbinates results in the deposition of many particles on the nasal mucosa. Those particles that survive in the airstream beyond the nose then are trapped in the mucous layer lining the airways, either by impaction or (in peripheral airways) by sedimentation. The depth to which particles penetrate the lung is a function of the size and density of the particles. Those particles trapped in the mucous layer are removed from the lung by mucociliary transport, by coughing, or both. Particulates that reach the alveolar spaces are removed by phagocytic cells. Another vitally important mechanical defense is cough, which may remove aspirated fluid as well as particulates and secretions.

Mucociliary transport serves to remove not only inhaled particulate matter but also secretions and cellular debris from the airways. The importance of mucociliary transport in maintaining pulmonary homeostasis is emphasized by the recent description of patients with immotile cilia, who develop chronic bronchitis and bronchiectasis at an early age (Eliasson et al., 1977).

Effective mucociliary transport requires the concurrent function of a number of elements. These include the number and distribution of cilia (or ciliated cells). Areas of squamous metaplasia may occur with various forms of insult and will result in diminished mucus transport. Ciliary beat frequency (normally 15 to 20 beats per second) and the direction of coordinated ciliary beat are important aspects of effective mucociliary function. The mucous layer (sometimes referred to as the "gel" layer) floats on the periciliary fluid and is propelled along by the tips of the cilia. High viscosity and effective intermolecular cross-bridging between the adjacent mucous glycoprotein molecules are necessary for effective mucociliary transport. This is a factor of clinical relevance, since the administration of mucolytic agents such as N-acetylcysteine may liquefy mucus and result in pooling of secretions in the airways rather than normal clearance. The periciliary fluid must have appropriate viscoelastic properties and must be of the correct depth. If this layer is relatively dehydrated, the tips of the cilia may be crushed by the overlying mucus, and if this layer is too deep, the mucus may float above the tips of the cilia. In either case, mucociliary transport will be impaired.

Many extrinsic factors may affect mucociliary transport. Trauma to the mucosa, as may occur with intubation or bronchoscopy, may impair transport until the mucosal damage has been repaired. Some viral infections, particularly influenza, produce a marked sloughing of ciliated cells, and many weeks may be required to achieve normal function again (which may explain the high incidence of bacterial superinfections associated with influenzal pneumonia). Bacterial infection or nonspecific inflammation may also interfere with mucus transport.

Dehydration of the tracheobronchial secretions will reduce mucociliary transport. Thus it is important to provide additional humidification of inspired air when normal humidification is impaired (as during intubation). Cigarette smoking and many disease states also interfere with effective mucociliary function. These include chronic bronchitis, cystic fibrosis, asthma, and Kartagener syndrome (now known to be associated with immotile cilia).

Mucociliary function may be improved by the administration of beta-adrenergic stimulating agents, by restoring normal humidification, by correcting nutritional or metabolic abnormalities, such as vitamin A deficiency, and by eliminating extrinsic factors, such as cigarette smoking.

Neurologic Defense Mechanisms

Neurologic pulmonary defense mechanisms primarily involve avoidance reflexes. A noxious odor will stimulate bronchospasm or even apnea so as to reduce the penetration of the material into the lung. On a more integrated basis, an organism will attempt to remove itself from a noxious environment.

Cough is also a neurologic defense mechanism in that it is a reflex involving the participation of the larynx, airways, and respiratory musculature and may be impaired by blocking the sensory pathways. A cough results when the chest is compressed against a closed glottis and then quickly released, resulting in a very high rate of expiratory airflow through the major airways.

Humoral Defense Mechanisms

Humoral defense mechanisms in the lung involve both local and systemic immune responses. Secretory IgA is produced locally in the upper airways. This immunoglobulin does not fix complement, nor does it have much opsonizing activity, but it is important in neutralization of viruses and toxins. In addition, it may agglutinate bacteria and reduce bacterial attachment to tissue.

Large amounts of lysozyme are secreted in the epithelium of the upper airways and may be important in antibacterial defenses, particularly against *Staphylococcus aureus* and other bacteria.

In the lower airways, IgG is the predominant immunoglobulin. There is both local production (mediated by the bronchial-associated lymphoid tissue) and transudation from the vascular bed. Other proteins, such as IgM and complement, are found in very small quantities in the pulmonary secretions, but all proteins enter the secretions more readily in the presence of inflammation.

Cellular Defense Mechanisms

The cellular defense mechanisms of the lung include alveolar macrophages, lymphocytes, and polymorphonuclear leukocytes. The alveolar macrophage is derived from blood monocytes, which are in turn derived from the bone marrow. The alveolar macrophage is a highly specialized cell and, in contrast to macrophages elsewhere in the body, is critically dependent on oxidative metabolism, becoming essentially nonfunctional at oxygen concentrations less than about 25 torr. Alveolar macrophages are primarily responsible for removal of particulate debris, including dead or damaged cells, from the alveoli and terminal airways.

Alveolar macrophages depend to a great extent on factors produced by lymphocytes, such as chemotactic factors and migration-inhibition factor (MIF), which invite macrophages into the lung and then make them feel at home. Mechanical factors may also result in mobilization of macrophages — particulate loads (such as are produced with cigarette smoking) lead to a great increase in the number of macrophages recoverable from the lung by saline lavage. "Activation" of macrophages by lymphocyte factors (possibly by migration-inhibition factor results in increased production of lysosomal enzymes, enhanced phagocytosis, and other phenomena. Alveolar macrophages may in turn stimulate lymphocytes by initial processing of antigens to which the lymphocytes then respond specifically. Macrophages are very important in killing intracellular organisms (such as mycobacteria and toxoplasma) as well as fungi, bacteria, and viruses. Activated macrophages are capable of recognizing and killing tumor cells.

Infections or other inflammatory reactions in the lung attract large numbers of polymorphonuclear leukocytes. These cells may be more important in dealing with established infection than are alveolar macrophages, since they are less dependent on oxygen and thus can operate within masses of secretions or hypoxic tissue.

REFERENCES

Bates, D. V., Macklem, P. T., and Christie, R. V. 1971. Respiratory Function in Disease, 2nd ed. Philadelphia, W. B. Saunders Co.

Berger, A. J., Mitchell, R. A., and Severinghaus, J. W. 1977. Regulation of respiration (three parts). N. Engl. J. Med., 297:194.

Breeze, R. G., and Wheeldon, E. B. 1977. The cells of the pulmonary airways. Am. Rev. Resp. Dis., 116:705.

Derene, J. P. H., Macklem, P. T., and Roussos, C. H. 1978. The respiratory muscles: mechanics, control, and pathophysiology (two parts). Am. Rev. Resp. Dis., 118:119, 373.

Eliasson, R. E., Mossberg, B., Camner, P., et al. 1977. The immotile cilia syndrome: A congenital ciliary abnormality as an etiologic factor in chronic airway infections and male sterility. N. Engl. J. Med., 297:1.

Farrell, P. M., and Avery, M. A. 1975. Hyaline membrane disease. Am. Rev. Resp. Dis., 111:657.

Green, G. M., Jakab, G. J., Low, R. B., et al. 1977. Defense mechanisms of the respiratory membrane. Am. Rev. Resp. Dis., 115:479–514.

Kaltreider, B. H. 1976. State of the art: Expression of immune mechanisms in the lung. Am. Rev. Resp. Dis., 113:347.

Proctor, D. F. 1977a. The upper airways. I. Nasal physiology and defense of the lungs. Am. Rev. Resp. Dis. 115:97.

Proctor, D. F. 1977b. The upper airways. II. The larynx and trachea. Am. Rev. Resp. Dis., 115:315.

Thurlbeck, W. M. 1975. Postnatal growth and development of the lung. Am. Rev. Resp. Dis., 111:803.

Wanner, A. 1977. Clinical aspects of mucociliary transport. Am. Rev. Resp. Dis., 116:73.

West, J. B. 1977. Ventilation-perfusion relationships. Am. Rev. Resp. Dis., 116:919.

Chapter 61

METHODS OF EXAMINATION

Byron J. Bailey, M.D.
John K. Jones, M.D.

INTRODUCTION

Several aspects of the history, physical examination, radiographic examination, and laboratory evaluation of the pediatric patient differ greatly from those of the adult patient. It is the purpose of this chapter to bring together information from our experience and a variety of other sources and to organize it into a framework that the otolaryngologist may use to facilitate his or her evaluation of the status of the pediatric patient's airway.

Any examination of the airway should answer three questions: Is the airway normal? If the airway is abnormal, is the pathologic condition in the upper or lower airway? If the airway is abnormal, what is the nature of the pathologic condition?

In order to answer the first question, the physician must evaluate the airway in terms of air movement (respiratory quality), ventilation (the intake of oxygen and the exhalation of carbon dioxide), the quality of the vocal output (including the cry and cough), and the ease of swallowing (freedom from drooling or evidence of aspiration).

If the airway is abnormal, it becomes extremely important for the physician to locate the pathologic state in the upper or lower airway and then establish a differential diagnosis. This chapter seeks to help the physician acquire a technique of examination of the airway of each patient that will provide the answers to the three key questions in such a manner that a diagnosis of the problem may be formed.

HISTORY

The general difficulty in obtaining a careful and precise history from the pediatric patient is widely appreciated. Thus, the necessary historical information must be obtained from the child's parents, from other physicians who have seen the child, and from all other appropriate sources.

The pediatric patient's history begins with the nature of the mother's pregnancy and the delivery of the patient. In dealing with a newborn infant, it is important to recognize the significance of medications the mother may have taken or infections she may have had during pregnancy. Length of the pregnancy (whether or not the baby was premature) is an important factor in establishing a diagnosis of respiratory distress syndrome in the neonate. A traumatic delivery is known to be a factor in some cases of vocal cord paralysis or nasal trauma, either of which may result in airway obstruction in the neonate.

Respiratory obstruction that presents between one and three weeks after delivery suggests laryngomalacia or congenital subglottic stenosis. If the respiratory distress has its onset between one and three months after delivery, one might suspect a subglottic hemangioma and should look carefully for cutaneous manifestations of this disorder, which will be found in approximately half of these neonates.

If the onset of respiratory distress has occurred immediately after a surgical procedure with intubation, one may suspect that

1152

inspissated subglottic mucus is the cause of the problem. However, if several hours pass following intubation before distress develops, the obstruction is more likely to be related to traumatic edema of the glottic and subglottic region. Development of distress within two to three weeks following intubation may indicate an early subglottic stenosis. Respiratory distress or hoarseness two to three months after intubation raises the possibility of vocal cord granuloma formation in the child.

Stridor that occurs following an apparently simple cold and cough that have lasted a few days is indicative of laryngotracheitis. The onset of supraglottitis (epiglottitis) is usually more rapid and can occur within a few hours. The child with epiglottitis will usually be in an older age group (three to six years) than the child with laryngotracheitis (six months to three years). Episodic coughing associated with wheezing and dyspnea should lead the physician to evaluate the patient for asthma.

A history of respiratory distress with feeding during the neonatal period suggests the possibility of a congenital anomaly, such as a tracheoesophageal fistula or a congenital posterior cleft of the larynx (Chaps. 53 & 66).

PHYSICAL EXAMINATION

General Pediatric Examination

In some instances, the child will be observed to have respiratory distress not associated with laryngotracheal pathology. For example, several supralaryngeal conditions can produce respiratory distress. Bilateral complete choanal atresia usually produces severe respiratory distress in the newborn who is an obligatory nose breather. The micrognathia and macroglossia of the Pierre-Robin syndrome also produce respiratory distress secondary to upper airway obstruction. Hypertrophy of the tonsils and adenoids has been shown to obstruct the airway and in more severe cases can result in cor pulmonale. Retropharyngeal and other pharyngeal abscesses, as well as abscess formation in the floor of the mouth, may compromise the oropharyngeal airway and result in respiratory distress.

Neck masses, such as a large lymphangioma or hemangioma, may compress the laryngeal and cervical tracheal airway. A large thyroglossal duct cyst, lingual thyroid gland, or branchial cleft cyst may also produce compression of the airway. Extrinsic pressure from a foreign body in the cervical segment of the esophagus can result in respiratory distress from airway compression.

Anomalous vascular rings can be extra-airway causes for respiratory distress. Congenital anomalies involving the central nervous system (CNS), such as the Arnold-Chiari syndrome, as well as inflammatory and neoplastic diseases involving the CNS, can cause respiratory distress. Certain systemic disorders, including high fever and anemia, severe biochemical alterations such as the metabolic acidosis occurring with diarrhea or diabetes, and respiratory alkalosis (e.g., salicylate toxicity) will produce tachypnea. Metabolic alkalosis, from pyloric stenosis and other causes of intractable vomiting, and respiratory acidosis, from the ingestion of opiates or tranquilizers, can produce a marked slowing of the respiratory rate (bradypnea).

Airway and Respiration in General

Inspection

This element of the examination begins with observations of the respiratory rate, which is most accurately measured when the child is asleep or completely relaxed. The normal respiratory rate varies with the age of the child, being rapid in the neonate and much slower in the adolescent (Fig. 61–1). Tachypnea refers to an increase in the rate of respiration. This is seen normally after exertion or when the child is anxious, but is also seen with a high fever, severe anemia, metabolic acidosis, or respiratory alkalosis. In addition, it is observed in the presence of bronchiolitis, pneumonia, pleural effusion, and pulmonary edema. Bradypnea is an abnormally slow respiratory rate and is seen in children with metabolic alkalosis, respiratory acidosis, and certain disorders of the CNS.

After measuring the rate, the examiner should observe and document the respiratory rhythm. Abnormalities of the respiratory rhythm include periodic breathing, in which the patient breathes normally for about 15 seconds and then stops breathing for a period of 5 to 10 seconds, and apneic spells, in which the nonbreathing interval is greater than 20 seconds. Cheyne-Stokes breathing refers to a waxing and waning of the depth of respiration followed by periods of apnea. This is

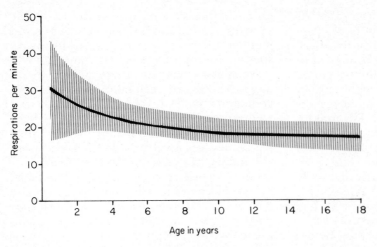

Figure 61–1 The effect of age on resting respiratory rate. (From Iliff, A., and Lee, V. 1952. Child Dev., 23(4).

observed in children with congestive heart failure, cerebral injury, and increased intracranial pressure. Biot breathing is a condition in which the child takes one or two breaths followed by long periods of apnea; it is associated with severe brain damage from trauma or encephalitis.

Next, one should note the depth of respiration. Variations from normal include hyperpnea (generally seen with tachypnea) and hypopnea (generally seen with bradypnea). Trepopnea refers to the condition in which a child finds it much easier to breathe when lying on one side. The child will lie with the better side upward.

Finally, one should note the ease of respiration. The normal child has relatively effortless respiration, known as eupnea. With some respiratory disorders, the child finds it much easier to breathe while sitting in the upright position (orthopnea), whereas in other disorders, breathing is difficult in all positions (dyspnea).

Observation of these features of the general respiratory pattern is followed by careful inspection of the child for other signs of respiratory distress. Specific features that may be seen in respiratory distress are head movement with respiration (head bobbing), flaring of the nasal alae with inspiration, circumoral pallor, and suprasternal and intercostal retraction. Intercostal retraction is a primary sign of respiratory obstruction and results from the unusually high negative pressure associated with labored inspiration.

The shape of the thorax varies with age. In the newborn and infant, the thorax is round when viewed from above, but with increasing age it becomes more oval and appears flatter anteriorly and posteriorly. Asymmetry of thoracic expansion may be observed with unilateral obstruction of one mainstem bronchus. The side with diminished motion may appear to be underinflated in the presence of a complete obstruction or overinflated in the presence of a ball valve obstruction. Paradoxical movement of half of the thorax occurs when one side of the thorax moves out of phase with the other. This may result from obstruction of a mainstem bronchus or may be seen in association with pneumothorax. It arises when there is a negative intrathoracic pressure on inspiration without subsequent inflation of the lung.

Palpation of the Neck

The infant larynx and trachea are soft and compressible. With increasing age, the cartilaginous framework of these structures becomes more firm, and landmarks such as the superior notch of the thyroid cartilage and the cricoid cartilage become easier to identify.

The trachea may normally be located very slightly to the right of the midline at the root of the neck. Deviation of the trachea from the midline can occur as a result of pathologic processes in the neck or inside the thorax. The first step is to determine whether the deviation is dynamic or fixed. In the case of a dynamic deviation there is a perceptible movement in the trachea with respiration (like a pendulum) as the mediastinum shifts owing to overinflation or underinflation of one lung. The trachea may be deviated from the midline in a fixed or static manner by pathologic processes that push or pull it to one side. Examples of the latter condition include tracheal displacement secondary to a large branchial cyst, cervical or mediastinal lymphadenopathy, or neoplasms of the thyroid or thymus.

Fracture of the larynx is unusual in the pediatric age group because of the elasticity of the airway cartilages and the great mobility of these structures in the child. Laryngeal fracture or laryngotracheal separation may result from a very forceful impact, such as striking the dashboard of an automobile during an accident, particularly with the head extended ("padded dashboard syndrome"). There are also numerous accounts of laryngotracheal separation associated with motorbike and snowmobile accidents. Palpation of the larynx will reveal areas of localized tenderness and may disclose palpable abnormalities of the laryngeal cartilage together with subcutaneous crepitus. It should be remembered that such severe trauma may also cause esophageal and cervical spine injuries.

Neck masses involving the larynx and cervical trachea are uncommon, but when they occur they may be of any consistency to the touch, from totally compressible to hard. A compressible mass adjacent to the larynx suggests the possibility of a laryngocele (rare in children), while a soft mass adjacent to the larynx may represent a congenital cyst or a laryngomucopyocele. A firm mass adjacent to the larynx or cervical trachea might be a chondroma or chondrosarcoma.

Subcutaneous emphysema is characterized by a distinctive crepitant sensation on palpation of the neck in a child with apparent neck swelling. It indicates a break in the integrity of the airway at some point between the pharynx and the terminal bronchioles, which may have resulted from trauma, instrumentation, or spontaneous rupture of the pulmonary alveoli (as may occur in emphysema). Radiographic and endoscopic evaluation are necessary in most instances to localize the area of airway injury. Clostridial infection may result in gas accumulation in the neck, but this is extremely rare.

Auscultation

Voice, Cry, and Cough. Important diagnostic information can sometimes be obtained by listening carefully to the child's voice, cry, or cough. Variations from the normal voice should be characterized precisely as coarse (gruff), muffled, aspirate (breathy), or high-pitched.

A coarse or gruff voice suggests either excessive vocal cord bulk from swelling of the cords or a tumor that is interfering with the normal vibratory pattern of the true cord. Examples of this type of problem are acute and chronic laryngitis, subglottic hemangioma, and certain endocrine disorders.

A muffled quality to the voice suggests the presence of a supraglottic obstructive process that is altering the normal modulation of the sound produced at the glottic level. A muffled voice will be noted in patients with acute epiglottitis, a large supraglottic laryngeal cyst, or a retropharyngeal abscess.

An aspirate (breathy) vocal quality is produced by the presence of a lesion that interferes with normal vocal fold approximation. This can be caused by any of the following: juvenile laryngeal papillomatosis, postintubation granuloma, vocal nodules, or a foreign body.

A high-pitched voice suggests excessive vocal cord tension or anatomically shortened vocal folds. A high-pitched voice is heard in children with a congenital web at the anterior commissure, underdevelopment of the larynx, and certain endocrine disorders.

Aphonia (inability to vocalize) is extremely rare. It may be produced by the presence of a foreign body lodged between the vocal folds, or it may be a manifestation of a psychogenic disorder.

The cri-du-chat syndrome is a chromosomal disorder in which the newborn infant cry is quite similar to the mewing sound of a cat.

Upper Airway. The respiratory sounds heard when the stethoscope is placed over the larynx and cervical trachea are described as "tubular" sounds. These are high-pitched and harsh in quality.

Stridor is a harsh, high-pitched, loud sound produced by high-velocity airflow through a small passage. It may occur predominantly during the inspiratory phase of respiration or during exhalation. Since the upper airway effectively decreases during inspiration, most obstructive lesions of the larynx and cervical trachea are associated with inspiratory stridor. Although stridor is audible without the aid of a stethoscope, this instrument may be used to localize the area of maximum obstruction.

Laryngomalacia (congenital laryngeal stridor) is the most commonly seen obstructive disorder in the newborn but is rarely severe enough to require tracheotomy. Most of these children are better by 12 to 18 months of age.

Croup (infectious laryngotracheobronchitis) and acute epiglottitis are characterized by the relatively sudden onset of inspiratory stridor and respiratory distress. Subglottic hemangioma is characterized by the slow onset of inspiratory stridor (most commonly between the ages of one and three months). Juvenile papillomatosis of the larynx presents the same slow onset of inspiratory stridor, usually between the ages of one and three years. A congenital web or cyst of the larynx may be suspected when there is noisy inspiration at birth.

Lungs. Auscultation of the lungs is best accomplished in the child with an adult stethoscope. This is not only more convenient but also will provide more auditory information than is usually obtained with a pediatric stethoscope.

Breath sounds are noted to change as one moves from the tracheal airway to the periphery of the lungs. Tracheal sounds are high-pitched, harsh, and tubular, whereas bronchial, bronchovesicular, and vesicular breath sounds are lower-pitched and soft on inspiration and are usually absent on expiration. The latter are actually vibrations produced by the movement of air through the tubular tracheobronchial tree; they vary with the size of the tubular passage and the intensity or velocity of the airflow.

Suppressed breath sounds (softer than normal) indicate underventilation, a condition that occurs in atelectasis of the newborn with respiratory insufficiency and which may or may not be associated with dullness to percussion.

Foreign bodies may be localized in some patients by careful attention to the process of auscultation. There may be a wheezing sound that is maximal over the foreign body as a reflection of diminished airway diameter and associated airflow turbulence. There may also be diminished breath sounds peripheral to the foreign body, and, on occasion, one may hear a slapping sound with respiration caused by the foreign body moving.

Rales, or crackles, are produced by small amounts of air bubbling through liquid. They are classified as fine (usually in the larger bronchioles) or coarse and are audible as a discontinuous crackling sound. It should be remembered that rales are not significant if they clear with coughing.

Rhonchi, or wheezes, are produced by air flowing past an obstruction at a high velocity and usually in association with some air turbulence. Rhonchi are classified as sibilant (high-pitched) or sonorous (low-pitched). They are persistent and musical in quality and are usually heard during the expiratory phase in the lower airway, as opposed to the stridor heard in the upper airway. This is because lower airway structures are larger during the inspiratory phase than during the expiratory phase.

A friction rub is a high-pitched squeaking sound that is produced by movement of the inflamed pulmonary and thoracic pleural layers against each other. This condition is occasionally heard in children with pneumonia.

Percussion is useful in the detection of areas of decreased aeration. Dullness to percussion in a localized area suggests the presence of atelectasis, and hyper-resonance indicates overinflation of the underlying tissue and may be found in children with a foreign body that is functioning as a ball valve or in children with pneumothorax. It is also useful in the detection of a mediastinal shift.

Visualization

The epiglottis can be visualized in most children by having the child open his or her mouth, protrude the tongue, and say "ah." Further depression of the tongue with a wooden blade may improve the view. Visualizing a swollen, red epiglottis in this matter is occasionally all that is needed to make the diagnosis of acute epiglottitis. However, this procedure can provoke acute, total respiratory obstruction, which is to be avoided; the presence of drooling and increased quantities of saliva in the pharynx should restrain the examiner from this procedure.

Indirect Examination. Indirect examination of the larynx can be accomplished in most children beyond the age of four years if the child's confidence is obtained by careful explanation and reassurance. If the child has been properly prepared, it will usually be unnecessary to spray the pharynx with a topical anesthetic. The patient should be positioned sitting upright in a chair with a light source behind it, while the examiner should position himself or herself so that the light reflected from the head mirror can be fo-

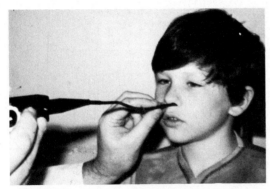

Figure 61–2 The flexible nasopharyngolaryngoscope in use. (Courtesy of Dr. Sylvan Stool, Children's Hospital of Pittsburgh, Pittsburgh, PA.)

cused onto the patient's mouth. The laryngeal mirror should be warmed and the temperature of the instrument tested on the skin of the physician. The child puts out his or her tongue, which is then held in a piece of gauze between the thumb and the index finger of the doctor. The patient is asked to breathe in as relaxed a fashion as possible while the mirror is inserted into the patient's mouth to rest on the soft palate. The back of the tongue should not be touched by the mirror. The examiner, by focusing the light onto the mirror, is able to see the hypopharynx and larynx, which should be examined systematically. The movement of the larynx and vocal cords can be seen when the patient vocalizes the sounds "aah" and "eee."

Office Endoscopy. Endoscopic examination in the office or in the hospital ward can be accomplished with some of the newer instruments that have been marketed in recent years. These include fiberoptic laryngoscopes and optical lens/mirror systems, which provide an excellent view of the larynx in a cooperative child.

The flexible fiberoptic nasopharyngolaryngoscope has been found to be valuable in examining the larynx and supralaryngeal area of the upper respiratory tract (Silberman, 1978).

In addition to affording a good view of the nasal passages, nasopharynx, and action of the palate, this endoscope enables the examiner to assess the larynx in its natural, dynamic state. General anesthesia is not required, although some children will require sedation. Figure 61–2 illustrates the nasopharyngolaryngoscope.

Before endoscopy, one of the nasal passages is anesthetized. The instrument is then passed along the nose into the nasopharynx under direct vision. It is helpful at this stage if the patient can breathe through the nose to allow the palate to drop down, thereby exposing the epiglottis. The instrument is further advanced to reveal the larynx, which can now be examined with particular reference to appearance and mobility. Swallowing by the patient usually eliminates any saliva, which may impair the view. The mobility of the larynx during this procedure makes instrumentation an imprecise and unwise maneuver that may induce laryngospasm.

The fiberoptic laryngopharyngoscope using the Hopkins rod lens system may be used in the older child (Ward et al., 1974). This method, like the mirror examination, demands cooperation from the patient. It has the advantage of uniform bright illumination and a wide angle field. The patient is positioned as for mirror examination, sitting upright in a chair with the tongue held forward (Fig. 61–3), and the instrument is passed through the mouth to rest on the palate. This provides an excellent view of the larynx and hypopharynx.

Both the flexible fiberoptic nasopharyngolaryngoscope and the Hopkins system permit documentation of the appearance of the

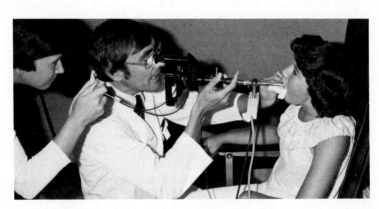

Figure 61–3 The indirect laryngopharyngoscope (Hopkins optical system) in use, showing camera attachment.

Table 61–1 NORMAL VALUES FOR PULMONARY STUDIES
(RANGES INCLUDE APPROXIMATELY 95% OF NORMAL VALUES:
VOLUMES IN LITERS, BTPS)*

Age (yrs) Length (cm)	Newborn 51	6 115	10 138	14 160	18 Men 175	Women 163
Vital capacity (L)	0.100	1.0–1.8	1.7–2.9	2.6–4.5	3.4–6.3	2.7–4.8
Peak expiratory flow rate (L/min)	7.1–10.1	130–236	217–391	294–534	390–770	295–535

*Table 61–1 is reproduced through the courtesy of Vaughan, V. C., McKay, R. J., and Nelson, W. E. (Eds.) 1975. Nelson Textbook of Pediatrics, 10th ed. Philadelphia, W. B. Saunders Co., p. 926.

larynx by photography. The examiner, however, must be sure that a significant pathologic state is not missed by an incomplete examination.

PULMONARY FUNCTION TESTS

This section will cover concisely the three primary tests employed in the evaluation of respiratory function in children. These tests are useful in quantifying the degree of disordered ventilation that is present.

The vital capacity test can provide information with regard to the quantity of air that is moved in and out with a single respiration. Results of this test are often observed to correlate directly with the degree of decreased compliance (stiffening) of the lung tissue and correlate inversely with the respiratory rate. They will be significantly altered in the presence of a complete obstruction of a major segment of the lung or will reflect the presence of an interstitial stiffening process, such as pneumonia or pulmonary edema. The McKesson Vitalor is an inexpensive and readily available item of equipment that can provide this information. Tables 61–1 and 61–2

Table 61–2 PULMONARY FUNCTION
TESTS IN OBSTRUCTIVE AIRWAY
DISEASE AND RESTRICTIVE LUNG
DISEASE

Test	Obstructive	Restrictive
Vital capacity (VC)	N*	↓
Peak expiratory flow rate	↓	N
Arterial oxygen tension (P_aO_2)	↓	↓
Arterial CO_2 tension (P_aCO_2)	N or ↑	↓

*N = Normal

give normal and abnormal pulmonary function test results for different age groups.

The peak expiratory flow rate can be determined using the Wright Peak Flowmeter. This measurement provides a good indication of the degree of severity in the case of obstructive airway disease and often correlates with the degree of effectiveness of the patient's cough. The peak expiratory flow rate is diminished in the presence of both localized obstructive lesions (foreign body, tracheal stenosis) and generalized airway narrowing (croup, asthmatic bronchitis).

Arterial blood gas analysis provides an indication of the effectiveness of the child's ventilatory effort in terms of oxygen intake and the exhalation of carbon dioxide. The radial artery is usually the source for the blood sample, which is obtained under anaerobic conditions. If the child is struggling and hyperventilating when the blood is taken, the sample obtained will not truly reflect the clinical state of the patient. Decreased ventilation is quantified in terms of the degrees of hypoxia (decreased oxygen in arterial blood) and of hypercarbia (increased carbon dioxide in the arterial blood sample) present. The physician must be particularly alert for the vicious cycle of prolonged hypoxia due to underventilation, which results in an increased respiratory effort that produces an exaggeration of the physiologic inward collapse of the tracheobronchial wall. This causes increased obstruction and hypoxia, which are exaggerated by the element of general fatigue. The end result in severe cases may be respiratory failure and death.

RADIOGRAPHIC EVALUATION

Roentgenographic studies of the larynx and tracheobronchial tree can be extremely valuable in supplementing the information obtained from the history and physical examination.

Plain films of the upper and lower airway can provide valuable information with regard to deviations from normal in the contour of the airway passages. A lateral, soft-tissue film of the neck is useful in the diagnosis of retropharyngeal abscess or acute epiglottitis. These views are taken with the head in the extended position, as flexion will produce a marked widening of the normal retropharyngeal soft tissue shadow.

The posterior–anterior view of the larynx and trachea can provide useful information in this area. The normal, slight deviation of the trachea to the right may be exaggerated during expiration. When films are obtained during phonation and deep respiration, they may be useful in documenting a vocal cord paralysis. Asymmetry of the subglottic region will be noted in the case of a unilateral subglottic hemangioma. Other irregularities in the contour of the airway can indicate external compression, inflammatory narrowing of the airway (croup), tracheal stenosis, or a foreign body. It has been observed that the "flip tops" from aluminum cans, even though they are metallic, may not be visualized easily on roentgenograms, unless they are viewed end-on.

Plain films of the lower airway are useful in the detection of three types of atelectasis, that which is (1) of the newborn, (2) due to a foreign body, and (3) postoperative. Interstitial disease, such as pneumonia or an abscess, can also be seen on plain radiography of the chest. Other diseases are characterized by the presence of hyperaeration, visible on the chest radiograph. This usually results from partial obstruction of the airway, which may be produced by asthma, cystic fibrosis, bronchiolitis, or the presence of a foreign body with trapping of air.

Polytomography and laminography may be useful in the clarification of indistinct areas of suspected pathologic conditions in the lung. They can differentiate between solid and cystic masses and in some cases are extremely important.

Xeroradiography can provide a very crisp image of the airway wall by virtue of its ability to enhance the contrast between air and soft tissue. One advantage of this technique is that it exposes the child to less irradiation than standard polytomography.

Contrast studies are sometimes necessary to evaluate the nature and extent of certain pulmonary diseases. These studies are rarely indicated and should be done only when the results are important in deciding on major aspects of therapy. Bronchography is usually performed under general anesthesia with a small endotracheal tube. A small catheter is placed into the trachea, and 1 cc of aqueous propyliodone (Dionosil) per year of age up to 8 cc is instilled into the airway. This is sufficient to provide a fine coat of contrast material on the walls of the tracheobronchial tree. Bronchography is felt to be indicated for the following conditions: (1) chronic, productive, purulent cough in a child who does not have cystic fibrosis; (2) recurrent unifocal pneumonia; (3) recurrent or severe hemoptysis; and (4) bronchiectasis that does not improve with medical management.

Contrast studies of the esophagus (esophagograms) are sometimes indicated in the case of children with respiratory problems. They are useful in the detection of a tracheoesophageal fistula, which is best shown in the left oblique position, and in some cases of persistent aspiration.

Cinefluoroscopy is helpful in evaluating the dynamics of respiration and may be particularly helpful in the evaluation and localization of a foreign body.

Angiography is indicated when there appears to be airway compression from a vascular anomaly, such as a right aortic arch, vascular duplication, or an anomalous vascular ring.

ENDOSCOPIC EXAMINATION

The indications for endoscopy are both diagnostic and therapeutic. The diagnostic uses are to inspect structural or functional abnormalities, to obtain cultures and biopsy specimens, and to assist in contrast radiograph studies. The therapeutic uses include removal of foreign bodies, removal of thickened secretions and bronchial lavage, removal of tumors (e.g., papillomata), dilatation of strictures, and to provide an airway in the obstructed child.

Any lesion should be documented by freehand drawings in the horizontal and vertical planes together with a written description of the lesion. Photographic documentation is useful if the equipment is available. Thus, any physician following the patient will have an accurate record of the original problem.

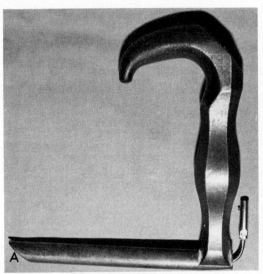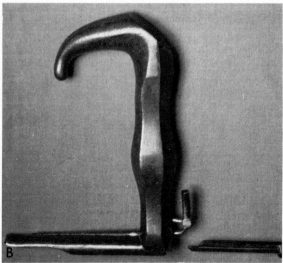

Figure 61–4   Infant laryngoscope: *A*, anterior commissure. *B*, Jackson with slide removed.

Direct Laryngoscopy

Direct laryngoscopy in the operating room is the primary technique for definitive diagnosis and management of laryngeal disease. There is still some argument as to whether or not general anesthesia is required to do direct laryngoscopy in infants. It is easier to view the larynx without the presence of an endotracheal tube, and, in the infant, the endoscopist can usually obtain an adequate assessment of the structures and mobility of the larynx without the use of anesthesia. Also, it is alleged that there is an increased likelihood of apnea in the obstructed child when general anesthesia is used. However, we feel that with modern anesthetic techniques this problem can be managed successfully.

When general anesthesia is used, it is important that both the endoscopist and the anesthesiologist are cognizant of the aims and technical details of the procedure. The individual role of each physician must be understood by the other. This facilitates the team approach that is necessary to achieve a controlled, safe airway. Because the patient under general anesthesia does not move, the endoscopist should feel less inclined to hurry and thus should be able to perform a careful assessment of the airway. Any endoscopic biopsy or surgery can therefore be carried out more precisely. It is the practice in our institution to perform most direct laryngoscopies and bronchoscopies in a well-equipped endoscopy room under general anesthesia. The cardiovascular and respiratory functions

of the child are monitored, as for any other operative procedure. Halothane is the most commonly used anesthetic agent, but it often has to be augmented by a 4 per cent lidocaine (Xylocaine) spray to provide local anesthesia in order to decrease the possibility of cardiac irregularities. In the infant, mask ventilation alone can be used if the procedure is short. Most laryngoscopies, however, are performed using endotracheal intubation, which provides a secure airway. The venturi apparatus can be used in situations in which the tube intrudes on the surgeon's view of the larynx and interferes with any surgery being performed. It is important to obtain paralysis of the vocal cords when using the venturi so that a glottic chink is always available for the passage of air.

There are three main types of laryngoscopes, each of which has a fiberoptic light carrier attached to a xenon light source. The anterior commissure laryngoscope permits a good assessment of the glottic area and anterior commissure with the advantage that it can be passed between the cords to inspect the subglottic area. The Jackson infant laryngoscope allows a wider view, and the presence of the slide enables the endoscopist to introduce a bronchoscope through the lumen. The modified anterior commissure endoscope with the widened lumen allows binocular vision to be utilized with the otomicroscope, and microsurgical procedures to be performed with greater ease. Figure 61–4 illustrates several types of laryngoscopes.

Before beginning the procedure, the laryngoscope and instruments to be used should be checked. It is important to remember that the entire procedure should be carried out with extreme gentleness. The patient is positioned with the head extended on the flexed neck. The upper teeth or gingivae are protected by a guard or gauze and should not be used as a fulcrum; the doctor's forefinger and thumb are used to support the endoscope. The distal end of the laryngoscope should be lubricated and inserted into the mouth; if the patient is not anesthetized it is usually advisable to introduce the instrument along the side of the tongue to reach the vallecula; otherwise the midline approach may be used. The larynx can be viewed initially by elevating the beak of the laryngoscope in the vallecula. It is important to use this approach when assessing the mobility of the cords as there is, at this stage, no restraining pressure from the laryngoscope.

Each area of the hypopharynx and larynx should be methodically and carefully examined. The appearance of the supraglottic structures should be noted, keeping in mind the possibility that an omega epiglottis (as in laryngomalacia), a cyst, or a web might be present. Subglottic stenosis can be viewed through the cords as an annular constriction. Hemangiomata are usually in the subglottic region and will appear as bluish swellings protruding from the laryngeal wall. As they partially empty under general anesthesia, their size will shrink and the mucosa will acquire a more normal color. This makes the smaller hemangiomata more difficult to diagnose.

The Zeiss microscope enables any surgical procedure to be performed more precisely. When doing examinations with this instrument, the laryngoscope is held in place with the suspension unit, and the larynx is viewed

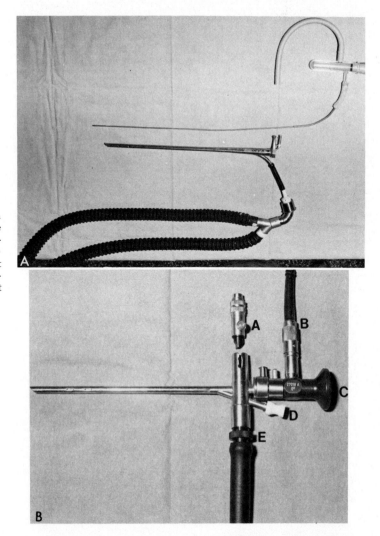

Figure 61–5 A, Bronchoscope with ventilating apparatus and Lukens tube attached to suction. B, 3.5 mm bronchoscope with Hopkins optical system: (A) prism attached to light source; (B) light source attached to telescope; (C) telescope; (D) aspiration and instrument channel; (E) ventilating tube.

Table 61–3 INDICATION FOR SIZE OF BRONCHOSCOPE AT DIFFERENT AGES

Bronchoscope Size	Indication for Use
3 mm	under 5 pounds
3.5 mm	up to 6 months
4 mm	up to 3 years
5 mm	up to 12 years
6 mm	over 12 years

through the microscope using a 400 mm objective lens.

Bronchoscopy

The question of whether bronchoscopy should be performed under general or local anesthesia can be answered with the arguments used in the section on direct laryngoscopy. We do the majority of our bronchoscopies under general anesthesia using the bronchoscope to ventilate the patient, since we feel that with modern anesthetic techniques being as safe as they are, there is very little place for bronchoscopy under local anesthesia in the child. If local anesthesia is used, it is imperative that the child be wrapped firmly and the head held to prevent any movement.

The rigid bronchoscope is used most commonly in children. The Jackson and Hollinger endoscopes (Fig. 61–5*A*) provide excellent views of the trachea and bronchi and allow the passage of instruments for aspiration, tissue biopsy, and removal of foreign bodies. Both endoscopes have a ventilating system that can be attached to the anesthetic equipment and, owing to their rigidity, can be used to dilate stenoses. Recently, Storz has

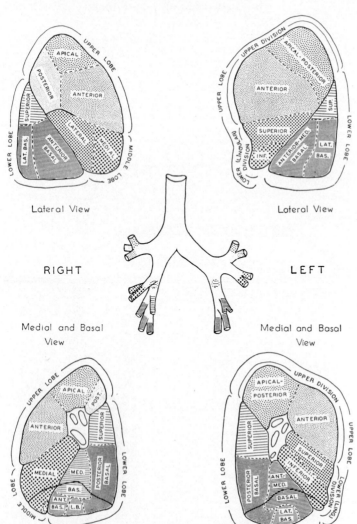

Lateral View   Lateral View

RIGHT   LEFT

Medial and Basal View   Medial and Basal View

Jackson Huber Nomenclature

Figure 61–6 Bronchopulmonary segments shown on both lateral (above) and mediastinal (below) aspects. (From Jackson, C., and Jackson, C. L., 1950. Bronchoesophagology. Philadelphia, W. B. Saunders Co., p. 1240, Fig. 6.)

developed a bronchoscope (Fig. 61–5*B*) using the Hopkins optical system that, in addition to the qualities of the Jackson and Hollinger bronchoscopes, has much improved illumination and magnification. All the above endoscopes can be used with straight forward, oblique, and lateral telescopes, which enable closer inspection of areas that cannot be seen with the bronchoscope tube. Specifically, they are useful to view the right and left upper bronchial orifices, the right middle bronchial orifices, and the basal bronchi.

The place of flexible bronchoscopy in children is limited to the older child because the instrument obstructs a considerable part of the airway and thus interferes with ventilation. It is useful for inspection of the peripheral bronchi and also allows a view of the trachea and inferior portion of the larynx via a tracheotomy.

As with direct laryngoscopy, successful and safe bronchoscopy can be attributed to good preparation and gentleness during the procedure. The time taken to carry out the bronchoscopy should be as short as possible, especially in the infant, as during prolonged examinations the subglottic area may be traumatized, resulting in obstructive edema. The bronchoscope should be the size that affords the physician the best possible view while causing the least trauma at the glottic and subglottic regions (Table 61–3).

Before the procedure, the instruments to be used should be checked to insure proper function. Radiographic evidence of a lesion should be translated into the anatomy of the bronchial tree as viewed through the bronchoscope (Fig. 61–6).

The child should be positioned with the head extended on the flexed neck. It is usual-

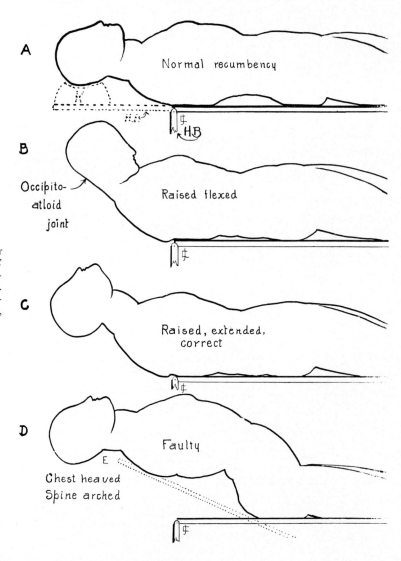

Figure 61–7 Positions for laryngoscopy or bronchoscopy (*C* is the best position). (From Jackson, C., and Jackson, C. L. 1950. Bronchoesophagology. Philadelphia, W. B. Saunders Co., p. 1236, Fig. 2.)

ly not necessary to have a person to hold the head in the young child, but a vertically moving headrest is often utilized. The same care should be taken of the teeth and gingivae as in direct laryngoscopy. The forefinger and the thumb of the doctor's left hand are used to support the instrument. Figure 61–7 shows the patient positioned for bronchoscopy or laryngoscopy, and Figure 61–8 illustrates the technique used to introduce the bronchoscope through the laryngoscope. It is considerably easier to use the Jackson laryngoscope with its slide to introduce the bronchoscope in the child. The laryngoscope is introduced, as previously described, until the glottis is in sight. The selected bronchoscope

is then passed through the lumen of the laryngoscope to the level of the true vocal cords. Next, the bronchoscope is turned at a right angle with its tip pointing to the right. The left vocal cord is centered in the field of vision by directing the bronchoscope to the left. This positions the tip of the bronchoscope in the glottis. A gentle twisting motion while advancing the tube allows entry into the subglottic area. Figure 61–9 illustrates the technique used to introduce the bronchoscope through the glottis.

If the laryngoscope is not used, it is easier for the physician to lose his or her way. However, in the older child the bronchoscope is often introduced on its own. The instru-

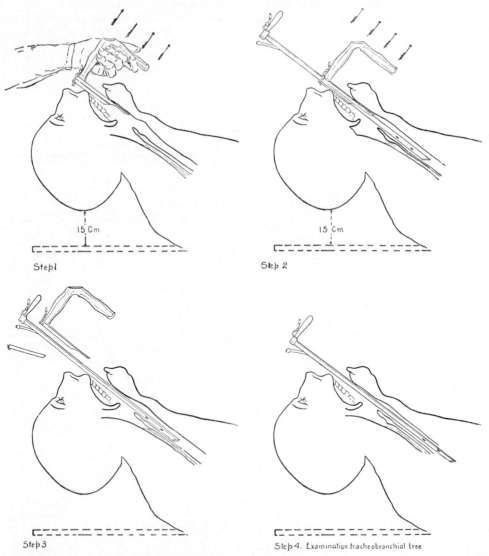

Figure 61–8 Technique of introduction of the bronchoscope through the laryngoscope; the head is lifted in the direction of the arrows. (From Jackson, C., and Jackson, C. L. 1950. Bronchoesophagology. Philadelphia, W. B. Saunders Co., p. 1237, Fig. 3.)

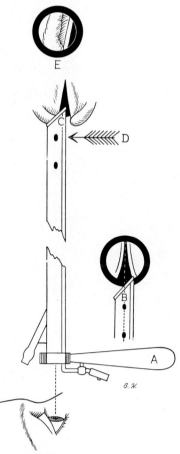

Figure 61–9 Introduction of bronchoscope through the glottis. *A*, Make sure the handle is on the right. *B*, Locate scope centrally. *C*, Insert the tip of the scope between the cords during inspiration by moving it slightly to the left. *D*, Obtain a glottic view. *E*, The glottic view. (From Jackson, C., and Jackson, C. L., 1950. Bronchoesophagology. Philadelphia, W. B. Saunders Co., p. 1238, Fig. 4.)

ment is passed to the back of the mouth where the vallecula and epiglottis are seen. The epiglottis is lifted forward on the beak of the bronchoscope, and, taking care to remain in the midline, the glottis is approached and entered as described previously.

The subglottic area and trachea are inspected. Attention should be paid to the lumen, mucosa, and secretions. Features such as narrowing, tumors, differences in mucosal coloration, pulsation, and collapsibility of the trachea should be noted and investigated appropriately. Abnormal secretions are collected for culture using a Lukens tube. The suction apparatus should be washed through with nonbacteriocidal saline so that all the secretions are collected in the Lukens tube. These are sent for cytologic inspection and

culture for bacteria, including tuberculi and fungi.

The bronchoscope is further advanced to the carina. This movement should be easy, but if there is any resistance, the physician should check that the head and neck are correctly positioned, that the lips are not caught on the bronchoscope, and that the jaw is freely open. The physician should also insure that the correct size of bronchoscope is being used. The carina should appear as a sharp, vertical spur dividing the entry into the two mainstem bronchi. Its appearance changes with respiration, becoming more blunt on expiration. Widening or decreased movement may be caused by pathologically enlarged hilar nodes. Figure 61–10 is a schematic drawing of the subdivision of the lobes into bronchopulmonary segments.

The right mainstem bronchus is the easier to enter as it meets the trachea at an angle of about 25 degrees, whereas the left mainstem bronchus is at a 75 degree angle to the trachea. Both sides of the lower respiratory tree should be inspected. Any abnormality in secretions or mucosal color and any tumors or narrowing of the lumen should be noted. It is advisable to complete the total bronchoscopic evaluation of both lung fields before performing any biopsy, as any resultant bleeding will make the subsequent examination more difficult. Secretions are aspirated from both mainstem bronchi, and, occasionally, bronchial washings are obtained by instilling nonbacteriocidal saline into the endoscope and suctioning it back into the sterile Lukens tube.

The right mainstem bronchus is entered by turning the lip of the bronchoscope in the direction of the bronchus and turning the head of the patient slightly to the left. A better view is always obtained if the axes of the bronchus to be viewed and the bronchoscope are coincident. The right upper lobe bronchus exits from the lateral wall of the mainstem bronchus. As in other parts of the bronchial tree, it is not uncommon to see variations in its anatomy, but the normal tripartite division into anterior, apical, and posterosuperior lobe bronchi can be seen with a lateral telescope. Just below, the superior bronchus of the lower lobe can be seen in the posterior wall. The bronchial divisions to the basal segments of the posterior lobe can then be identified and more carefully inspected using the straight forward telescope.

The left bronchial tree should then be examined. Because of the angle that the left

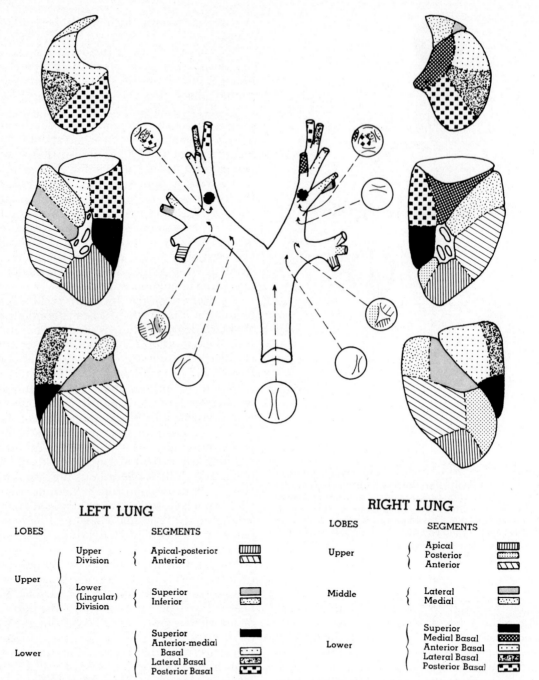

Figure 61–10   Schematic drawing of subdivision of lobes into bronchopulmonary segments. (From Jackson, C., and Jackson, C. L. 1950. Bronchoesophagology. Philadelphia, W. B. Saunders Co., p. 1239, Fig. 5.)

mainstem bronchus makes with the trachea, the head of the patient has to be turned towards the right shoulder to give easy access to this area. The obliquely lying carina, dividing the left upper lobe bronchus from the lower lobe bronchus, is seen running from a position of 12 o'clock to 8 o'clock on an imaginary clock face. It is sometimes possible to enter the left upper brochus with the bronchoscope, but on other occasions the lateral viewing telescope has to be used. The upper lobe bronchus quickly divides into its upper and lingular divisions. The bronchus leading to the lingular lobe then divides into its superior and inferior segments.

The left lower bronchus is longer than the

right, with a relatively higher origin for the posteriorly placed left superior lower bronchus. The basal branches are a mirror image of the right except that the medial basal branch arises from the anterior basal branch.

It is sometimes difficult to position the lateral viewing telescope to afford a view of the bronchus to be inspected. It is essential to first position the bronchoscope tube precisely and keep it correctly placed while the telescope is introduced (Fig. 61–11). The tube is inserted to the proximal lip of the bronchial orifice that is to be viewed and kept strictly aligned along the long axis of the bronchus. In this way the telescope can always be inserted to the same length, and any exaggerated movement will not injure the bronchial mucosa. The lateral viewing telescope is then passed through the tube facing the direction in which the bronchial orifice is located. Immediately after bronchial mucosa is seen, the opening of the bronchus can be found by moving the telescope, using a combination of rotary and piston-like actions.

At the completion of the examination, under direct vision in order to avoid any

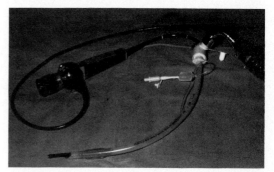

Figure 61–12 Flexible fiberoptic bronchoscope passing through the endotracheal tube.

unnecessary trauma, the bronchoscope should be removed with as much care as was used in its insertion.

The flexible fiberoptic bronchoscope can be used in the older child whose airway has reached a sufficient size to allow adequate ventilation around the instrument (Berci, 1978). Most flexible bronchoscopes have an optical channel and a channel for aspiration, biopsy, and brushings for cytology. The tip can be moved only in one plane by remote control. The bronchoscope is directed by adjusting the tip and rotating the whole instrument. It should be remembered that these are delicate instruments, the fibers of which can easily be broken by excessive bending or torque when rotating the bronchoscope.

The physician may introduce the flexible bronchoscope either through the nose or through a special-purpose endotracheal tube. In the former approach, the bronchoscope is manipulated through the nose and pharynx to enter the larynx, which can be inspected. The approach through the endotracheal tube permits easy access directly into the trachea but does not give a view of the larynx. The bronchoscope is passed systematically through the lower respiratory tract using a combination of pushing, pulling, and rotary movements on the instrument and adjusting the tip by the remote control. Attention is paid to the same details of anatomy as when the rigid bronchoscope is used. Specimens for cytologic examination can be obtained by aspirating secretions and collecting the results of brushings of the bronchial wall. Biopsy specimens can also be taken and small foreign bodies removed through the flexible bronchoscope.

The otolaryngologist should attempt to acquire familiarity with the use of both rigid

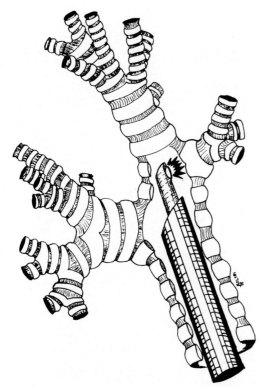

Figure 61–11 Relative position of telescope and bronchoscope to view the right upper lobe bronchus.

and flexible bronchoscopes, as each has a part to play in the examination and treatment of the lower respiratory tract.

The complications of endoscopic examination are laryngospasm, bronchospasm, trauma to the subglottic area resulting in edema and obstruction, and bleeding. These can best be avoided by as gentle and methodical an examination as possible.

REFERENCES

Berci, G. 1978. Analysis of new optical systems in bronchoesophagology: Chevalier Jackson lecture. Ann. Otol. Rhinol. Laryngol., *87*:451.

This article describes the use of the flexible and rigid fiberoptic endoscopes. Their use and limitations are described together with a comparison of different types of flexible bronchoscopes.

Silberman, H. D. 1978. The use of the flexible fiberoptic nasopharyngolaryngoscope in the pediatric upper airway. Otolaryngol. Clin. North Am., *11*:2.

This chapter describes the pediatric flexible fiberoptic nasopharyngolaryngoscope. A detailed account of the technique of introduction of the instrument and its application is given.

Ward, P. H., Berci, G., and Calcaterra, T. C. 1974. Advances in endoscopic examination of the respiratory system. Ann. Otol. Rhinol. Laryngol., *83*:754.

Dr. Ward documents the development of fiberoptic endoscopes and describes the Hopkins lens system. The advantages of these instruments are discussed, and reference is made to the relative quality of photographs obtained using these systems.

Chapter 62A

COUGH

Edward M. Sewell, M.D.

A cough is the most prominent symptom of respiratory disease and occurs more frequently than wheezing and dyspnea. It is embarrassing to the patient as well as annoying to the patient and others. It produces discomfort, is difficult to control, and is a source of considerable anxiety to parents.

To the parent, coughing is a sign of illness in the child. It is evidence of abnormality in the breathing apparatus and signals a malady in essential life-sustaining organs. Parents recognize it as an indicator of distress, from the cough itself and from the illness that causes the cough. The insistent, repeated sound of the cough is a spur to action. The parent feels obliged to take corrective measures and feels a need for explanation of the source of the cough and a determination of its prognosis.

Older patients recognize that coughing is a symptom of disease, but patients of any age are made uncomfortable by or at least annoyed by this symptom regardless of its diagnostic implications. It interrupts breathing, talking, and eating and may make it impossible even to sit quietly for any extended period of time. When coughing is frequent or prolonged it becomes painful. The force of the column of air impinging on the larynx, upper airway, and pharynx produces irritation, tenderness, and pain in these regions. The repeated forceful contracting of the diaphragm and intercostal muscles renders them sore and aching. Coughing is most troublesome because it interferes with sleep. All coughs seem to get worse after the sun goes down, and many coughs are noticeably more difficult to control when the patient is recumbent. Therefore, the relief that sleep brings to other symptoms is denied to the patient with a cough, who may find it impossible to fall asleep or who may soon awaken, if he does get a few minutes of relief.

COUGH AS A DEFENSE

Since coughing is such an anxiety-producing nuisance, many patients and parents forget that it is an essential component of the body's defense system. It is the primary guardian of the respiratory tract. The expulsive efforts of coughing are responsible for keeping the trachea and bronchi and their epithelial surfaces clear of the secretions that would otherwise prevent adequate respiration. This is especially necessary in disease states that increase either the quantity or the viscosity of mucous secretions. In addition, inhaled bacteria and fine particles are harmful to the lungs and must be expelled by coughing. Aspirated food and liquids, including blood and vomitus, can lead to serious lung damage if not promptly evacuated. Larger foreign bodies, when aspirated as they frequently are by children, can cause atelectasis, infection, and even bronchiectasis. The active cough reflex is our primitive, persistent, and usually most reliable defense mechanism against all these noxious agents.

CLASSIFICATION

Coughing is a symptom, not a disease. This makes classifying types of cough difficult. Logically a classification of types of cough should be based on etiology or reflect physiologic considerations, but there are many different causes for a cough of the same character. A cough represents a physiologic response to a variety of conditions. The stimulus to cough can come from any point along the respiratory tract, but the character of the response to the stimulus may not vary to any significant degree.

One useful approach is to use the common description of cough employed by parents and families as well as the medical community. They have characterized coughs as acute and self-limited or chronic and persistent. In addition, coughs may be described on the basis of the sound they produce. The amount of secretion moved by the cough is an important determinant of its sound, so that people talk of a dry cough or a loose cough. For example, in the early stages of an upper respiratory infection, children have an acute, self-limited, dry cough. On the other hand, the constant cough of the patient with cystic fibrosis is characterized by the sound of rattling sputum and is therefore of the chronic, loose variety. Unfortunately for purposes of consistent classification, one cannot always relate a single disease to one kind of cough because the nature of the cough changes from one stage of the disease process to another; what begins as an acute upper respiratory infection with a dry cough may evolve into a chronic cough when sinusitis develops as a complication.

PHYSIOLOGY OF COUGH

The production of a cough requires an intact neurosensory apparatus. Cough receptors located in the small airways, large airways, and nasopharynx carry stimuli along efferent pathways to respiratory centers in the medulla, and from these centers efferent pathways carry motor impulses to the expiratory musculature.

Mechanically a cough begins with a deep inspiration through a wide open larynx. The glottis then closes, and the effort of the expiratory muscles produces an increase in pressure behind this obstruction. The sudden opening of the glottis combined with continued expiratory effort generates a rapid flow of air through the air passages that is able to move both solid material and mucus.

The physiology and mechanics of coughing have been reviewed by Irwin and colleagues (1977). Inspiration leads to an increase in lung volume with a concomitant increase in the diameter of the airways, providing lowered airway resistance, which favors maximal expiratory flow rates. The bronchi appear on bronchography to lengthen by unrolling of their spiral arrangement with inspiration. Closure of the glottis, accompanied by the beginning of the contraction of the thoracic muscles of respiration and a fixed diaphragm, builds up considerable pressure against the closed cords of the larynx. (Although cough can occur without glottic closure, it is less effective.) With the opening of the glottis, pressure is released, and the rapid flow of air through the passages begins. The vibration of laryngeal structures aids in dislodging secretions. The action of the diaphragm and other muscles continues throughout the cough. Thoracic volume and airway diameter constantly decrease in order to maintain high pressures and increased rates of airflow. The compression of the tracheobronchial structures, which is so important in achieving this increased flow, probably does not extend below the third generation of bronchi. It is therefore in these larger airways that coughing is most effective. However, as bronchial structures decrease in diameter, compression may involve the next smaller passages. This helps to move secretions toward the larger airways, where they can be expelled with subsequent coughing.

We tend to think of coughing as symptomatic of problems in the lower respiratory tract. However, a cough may be stimulated from several other areas. For instance, many patients will cough in response to manipulation of the external auditory canal, and nerve endings in the nasopharynx respond to stimuli of touch, pain, and stretching and frequently initiate the cough reflex. Indeed, it is our belief that much of the coughing that accompanies an upper respiratory infection represents this latter kind of stimulation rather than indicating progress of the inflammatory process below the larynx. This is the most frequent type of cough in the pediatric age group. It may occur acutely with viral infections or more chronically as a result of allergic rhinitis with or without accompanying bacterial infection, which involves the sinuses and leads to postnasal drip (Irwin and Pratter, 1980).

COUGH AS A DIAGNOSTIC AID

Cough is an important diagnostic aid for the physician. Because a characteristic cough is regularly associated with certain disease states, it is important for the diagnostician to recognize the special character of the patient's cough. It is often helpful to describe the cough as carefully as possible. Characteristics of a cough that are useful to note include onset, frequency, time of day, force, pitch, and the presence of secretions. Moreover, some coughs may be associated with pain, an important symptom to note.

The onset of the cough may be significant. Mothers will frequently describe a cough as having been present since birth. Further questioning usually will reveal that this is somewhat of an exaggeration. However, for those few infants whose cough was apparent on or about the first day of life, this may indicate the presence of an important congenital anomaly (Chaps. 65 & 66A,B).

The frequency of the cough may shed light on the seriousness of the problem as well as give some indication of the cause. Children who live in an urban environment may cough on rare occasions, widely separated in time, without the presence of any abnormality. Failure to appreciate this fact causes a surprising number of parents to seek medical advice. Such parents need reassurance. It is often useful to inquire "Does the child cough every day?" A positive answer to this question usually indicates that further investigation is necessary.

The time of day at which the cough occurs can be important. The child who always has an episode of coughing on arising in the morning may have bronchiectatic lesions in which mucopurulent material collects at night. The increased activity and deeper breathing associated with waking move this material into proximal portions of the tracheobronchial tree, where it initiates a cough. If the coughing is associated with meal times or with drinking, aspiration may be the cause.

Congenital anomalies, such as a laryngeal cleft or a tracheoesophageal fistula, disorders of swallowing function secondary to neurologic problems, and gastroesophageal regurgitation can all lead to aspiration (Mellis, 1979) (Chaps. 66A,B). Coughing associated with postnasal drip is worse at night, and the nocturnal character of whooping cough is well known (Krugman et al., 1977) (Chaps. 67 & 69).

The force of the cough may vary greatly, from the almost inaudible "clearing of the throat" to the loud explosive sounds associated with aspiration of a foreign body (Chap. 71).

The pitch of the cough may give some indication of the offending lesion and its location. In general, a high-pitched sound is associated with lesions above the larynx, whereas deeper sounding coughs indicate problems below the larynx. However, this is not invariably true, since many respiratory problems cause difficulty throughout the respiratory tract.

The presence or absence of a liquid component in the cough is important in determining its sound. The cough may be dry and obviously nonproductive, or its rattling discontinuous nature can denote the presence of liquid. The fluid content of the cough associated with some conditions is characteristic, as in the bronchiectatic cough, which produces a significant amount of sputum at all times and is always loose and liquid in quality, or the amount of liquid may vary, leading to a change in the quality of the cough with time. For instance, the course of an acute upper respiratory tract infection of viral origin is marked by considerable change in the character of the cough as the infection evolves. It usually begins with a short, dry, hacking, and relatively infrequent cough, which rapidly increases in frequency and severity as the symptoms become full-blown. A few days into the course of the infection, a clear, relatively thin mucoid secretion is raised with each cough. This expectorated material gradually increases in amount, becomes more viscous, changes in color from clear to white, and may finally develop a yellowish, purulent character before the self-limited condition resolves itself.

Persistent, thick, purulent sputum, of course, suggests the presence of a chronic bronchial infection. Patients with cystic fibrosis will almost always have productive coughs. It is sometimes possible to guess at the predominating organism from the color of the sputum: *Staphylococcus* will cause the sputum to appear lemon-yellow or golden in color. When *Pseudomonas* becomes more prominent, the color will be brown or green.

The most frightening color that can appear in the sputum is the red color of blood. In this regard it is important to remember that true pulmonary bleeding, producing hemoptysis, is very rare in children, while blood from the nose, throat, teeth, or gastrointestinal tract may at times become mixed with respiratory mucus or sputum and lead to diagnostic difficulties. True hemoptysis in young children could be due to the presence of a foreign body, a congenital anomaly, or pulmonary hemosiderosis. In the older child, bronchiectasis and cystic fibrosis must be considered (Chap. 68).

The pain associated with a cough needs to be carefully described. Is the discomfort directly related to the inflammatory process giving rise to the cough? This may be true in laryngitis and tracheitis, in which a vicious cycle is set up: Inflammation produces a cough, which produces further inflammation. Is the patient's complaint of pain a reflection of the muscular effort that has gone into the coughing, or does the sharp, severe nature of the pain, its association with the respiratory movement required in coughing, and its sharp localization mark it as pleural in origin?

The response of the cough to therapy may be an important indicator of the severity of the problem. Coughs that respond to simple measures, such as increased humidification or non–codeine-containing cough medicines, are seldom associated with any serious difficulty. When more potent remedies, such as a cough sedative, are required to provide relief, a more serious problem may be present. Some coughing will not yield to any symptomatic therapy. The disappearance of the cough may have to await accurate diagnosis and specific treatment of the underlying problem.

COUGHING AS THERAPY

The cough is an important therapeutic tool for the physician. With the parents of children who have chronic pulmonary disease, one cannot emphasize too much the need to encourage purposeful, helpful coughing. While coughs should never be allowed to exhaust these children or any other patients, the therapeutic regimen must include the use of coughing to clear the respiratory tract. Many of the maneuvers of respiratory physical therapy are best thought of as adjuvants to the coughing mechanism. The position of the patient helps to direct the cough along lines of gravitational force. The force of percussion is added to the impulse generated by the cough and should help to move greater quantities of secretion. The use of breathing exercises may help to mobilize sputum for expectoration and is intended to increase the strength and efficiency of muscular contraction during coughing. It becomes the responsibility of the physicians who treat patients with coughs to instruct these patients and their parents in the positive aspects of coughing. One must resist pressures to eliminate a useful cough by sedation. It is better to teach techniques that effectively augment the cleansing action of coughing so that it can be used for therapeutic purposes.

An intact cough mechanism is very important in the prevention of pulmonary atelectasis and infection. Patients who have been deprived of coughing by coma or paralysis of the diaphragm or the intercostal muscles or in whom loss of laryngeal function makes it impossible to close the glottis may have their clinical course so seriously complicated by the loss of an effective cough that this absence becomes the most important factor in their survival. Such patients frequently require intubation, which eliminates natural coughing or reduces its effectiveness. It then becomes necessary to substitute for the cough by the mechanical removal of secretions by suction. At times an artificial cough may also be effective: The respiratory therapist provides positive pressure via the endotracheal tube and releases it suddenly while simultaneously applying expulsive force against the thoracic cage.

COUGHS OF SPECIAL SIGNIFICANCE

Some coughs are so characteristic of the condition with which they are associated that the physician may hazard a diagnosis on the basis of the cough alone. Patients with croup produce a singular cough. It is dry, relatively high-pitched, short, and resonant. It has been described as similar to the bark of a dog; however, it more nearly resembles the bark of a seal.

The cough of measles may be diagnostic. Its character is difficult to describe but is typical enough so that it carries, for the experienced clinician, a significance almost as reliable as that of Koplik's spots. It is short, nonproductive, hacking, frequent in occurrence, disturbing, and uncomfortable for the patient.

One of the most dramatic and most characteristic of coughs is associated with pertussis. A patient with this disease produces a series of short, sharp, staccato coughs rapidly getting closer and closer together in time and increasing in pitch and force. The expulsive efforts of coughing follow so quickly upon one another that the patient is unable to inspire between coughs. The face becomes plethoric, first red and then blue, and those observing the patient involuntarily hold their breath as the intensity and the frequency of the coughing mount until the paroxysm abruptly ends and the sudden, prolonged indrawing of air produces the high-pitched sound of the whoop. Such coughing may be followed by syncope or even convulsions. Sometimes the patient will retch or vomit after a paroxysm of such coughing.

In small infants, pneumonia caused by *Chlamydia trachomatis* may be confused with pertussis (Beem and Saxon, 1977). Both conditions produce episodes of short staccato coughing. These episodes may be accompanied by apnea and cyanosis. Pertussis in infants seldom produces the characteristic whoop. Chlamydial pneumonia usually has its onset around six weeks of age and is accompanied by conjunctivitis in 50 per cent of the cases (Chap. 67).

External compression of the trachea from enlarged lymph nodes or a vascular ring produces a cough that Schick (1910) has described as bitonal in character and expiratory without any audible inspiratory component. It consists of a short, nonproductive, high-pitched sound followed immediately by a lower-pitched, more resonant note.

It is now well established that coughing may be the only symptom of allergic bronchitis or asthma. Some patients present with a persistent, short, hacking nonproductive cough. The usual episodes of dyspnea and wheezing may be less frequent or absent altogether. In such cases, careful auscultation of the chest will detect wheezing at the end of full expiration. Children old enough to cooperate for pulmonary function testing will show evidence of obstructive lung disease with prolongation of expiration, which is reversible with bronchodilators (Chap. 61).

The cough that does not originate in any organic pathologic condition and that is caused by psychogenic factors may also reveal its nature by its character. Sometimes it is a short, hacking cough that is nonproductive and tends to increase at times of greater stress. Less frequently one encounters a more dramatic symptom in a great, booming, resonant, bellowing cough produced one cough at a time, seeming to come from the depths of the chest. The patient may complain about the cough but gives no visible evidence of distress. In our experience these patients have most frequently been adolescent females, and the cough is extremely resistant to all forms of therapy.

TREATMENT OF COUGHING

At times the disturbing and troublesome effects of a cough may be so severe that they outweigh the beneficial effects. This is true when the cough itself is contributing to the inflammation and irritation, when the cough produces exhaustion or interferes with sleep, or when the repeated paroxysmal nature of the cough leads to retching and vomiting. In such situations, modification of the cough with therapy is necessary. This therapy may employ physical means such as humidification or postural drainage, or it may involve the use of a pharmacologic agent such as a sedative or narcotic. Attempts to decrease the viscosity of sputum by orally administered expectorants are generally unsuccessful (Mellis, 1979) and, in our opinion, are not worth the effort.

REFERENCES

Beem, M. O., and Sazon, E. M. 1977. Respiratory tract colonization and a distinctive pneumonia syndrome in infants infected with *Chlamydia trachomatis*. N. Engl. J. Med., *296*:306.

Irwin, R. S., and Pratter, M. E. 1980. Postnasal drip and
    cough. Clin. Notes Resp. Dis., *18*:11–12.
Irwin, R. S., Rosen, M. J., and Braman, S. S. 1977.
    Cough. A comprehensive review. Arch. Intern.
    Med., *137*:1186–1191.
Krugman, S., Ward, R., and Katz, S. L. 1977. Infectious
    Diseases of Children, 6th ed. St. Louis, C. V. Mosby
    Co.

Mellis, C. M. 1979. Evaluation and treatment of chronic
    cough in children. Pediatr. Clin. North Am.,
    26:553–564.
Schick, B. 1910. Expiratorisches Keuchen als Symptoma-
    tologie im Ersten Lebensjahre, Wien. Klin.
    Wchnschr., *23*:153.

ASPIRATION

Arlen D. Meyers, M.D.

INTRODUCTION

Human survival depends on eating, and the ability of humans to swallow food without aspirating it represents a very advanced evolutionary event. The fact that the respiratory and digestive systems share a common conduit demands the use of unique physiologic adaptations.

In children, any important dysfunction of the swallowing mechanism will result in the impairment of the function of the respiratory tract (Cohen, 1955). To understand the causes and treatment of chronic aspiration, therefore, the physician must be acquainted with the anatomy and physiology of the swallowing mechanism and with those morbid and pathophysiologic events that alter it.

By definition, a child who chronically aspirates has an anatomic or physiologic abnormality that compromises the integrity of the respiratory tract. Congenital anomalies and neurologic diseases of the mouth, laryngopharynx, and esophagus are the most common causes of aspiration. The treatment of patients with recurrent aspiration pneumonia can begin only after a thorough history, physical examination, acquisition of laboratory data, and radiographic studies are performed.

ANATOMY AND PHYSIOLOGY

The anatomy and physiology of the mouth, pharynx, and esophagus have been discussed in detail in Chapters 38 and 39. Certain points should be stressed, however, with regard to disorders of swallowing and aspiration in children.

The swallowing mechanism can be divided into three phases — the oral phase, the buccopharyngeal phase, and the esophageal phase (Culley and Creamer, 1958; Ellingworth and Lister, 1964; Sessle and Hannam, 1976). In the oral phase food is deposited into the oral cavity. The tongue, lips, cheeks, and jaws process the food for swallowing. The physiology of sucking and swallowing in normal and abnormal infants has been discussed by several authors (Andross et al., 1958; Benson, 1962; Bishop, 1974; Bosma, 1957; Culley and Creamer, 1958; Frank and Baghdassrian-Gatewood, 1966; Grahamm, 1964; Margulies et al., 1968; Mistretta et al., 1975; Moosa, 1974; Utiam and Thomas, 1969). Squeezing the liquid from the nipple often seems to be part of the infant oral phase. Indeed, it appears that sucking is only half as effective as squeezing liquid from a nipple (Andross et al., 1958).

While food is being chewed, it is prevented from passing into the pharynx by apposition of the base of the tongue with the soft palate. The buccopharyngeal phase begins when the mylohyoid muscles elevate the base of the tongue and push the bolus into the pharynx. At this point, there is elevation of the pharyngeal tube, followed by peristalsis within it. Immediately prior to swallowing, the food is brought to a preparatory position. A conduit, the "palatopharyngeal partition" (Del Monico and Hoar, 1972), is formed by the apposing pharyngeal constrictors, palate, and palatopharyngeus and directs the food into the hypopharynx. Once the bolus passes through the partition, the mylohyoid rises from its intermediate position to a position of maximum elevation. The pharynx continues to elevate and engulfs the prepared food.

The buccopharyngeal phase and the third phase, the esophageal phase, are reflex actions. Sensory and proprioceptive impulses from the glossopharyngeal, trigeminal, and superior laryngeal nerves transmit impulses to the "swallowing center" in the floor of the fourth ventricle, the reticular substance of the medulla (Doty et al., 1967), which then relays signals to the muscles involved in swallowing.

While the bolus passes the oropharynx, several events occur. The upper esophageal sphincter relaxes, respiration stops, the larynx rises superiorly, the glottis closes, the nasopharynx is occluded by the velum, and peristalsis begins (Sessle and Hannam, 1976).

The swallowing mechanism of children varies in several ways from that of adults (Andross et al., 1958; Del Monico and Hoar, 1972). Since the hard palate is relatively closer to the base of the skull in children, angulation of the soft palate during nasopharyngeal closure is not a prominent feature, and the adenoid pad contributes to the closure. In addition, the tonsils act as directors of small quantities of food into the oropharynx and help to keep the airway open until the child is ready to swallow. Finally, since the larynx is relatively closer to the base of the skull in children, the upper and posterior movement of the hyoid and larynx is less.

Opening of the cricopharyngeus muscle initiates the third phase of swallowing, the esophageal phase. The sphincter opens for 200 msec and is followed 60 msec later by esophageal peristalsis (Andross et al., 1958; Hendrix, 1974). The above discussion displays the tremendously complex arrangement to keep the airway and digestive passages separate. Anatomic or physiologic variation in any of these mechanisms contributes to problems in deglutition and resultant aspiration.

In addition, the larynx is primarily a sphincter that guards the respiratory tract from particulate invasion. When the vocal cords are unable to protect the integrity of the airway, aspiration results. Although neurologic damage frequently results in dysfunction of both the pharyngeal and laryngeal musculature, isolated recurrent laryngeal nerve injury does occur with some regularity and can be responsible for recurrent aspiration (see Chapter 69).

HISTORY

The approach to a patient with recurrent aspiration begins with a thorough history, designed to uncover those symptoms suggestive of anatomic or physiologic abnormalities of the mouth, laryngopharynx, esophagus, or respiratory tract (Ekdahl et al., 1974).

One should seek a history of neurologic disease in the family. In addition, hydramnios should alert the physician to the possibility of an esophageal abnormality in the newborn. Although hydramnios is associated with defects of the esophagus, it appears to be, in addition, a defect in regulation of the production of amnionic fluid in the third trimester (Weathers et al., 1974). Poor sucking habits, as evidenced by the need for an enlarged nipple hole, inability to breathe and suck at the same time, and frequent choking and gagging may suggest a defect. Recurrent aspiration with dysphagia frequently leads to failure to thrive and possibly a developmental lag. It is important to note methods of improving a feeding problem. If an infant aspirates only liquids, attention should be directed to the extent of glottic competence as the basic problem.

Although seemingly benign, suction tubes and endotracheal tubes have resulted in damage to the infant hypopharynx (Meyers et al., 1978). Careful documentation of instrumentation during attempts at neonatal resuscitation will alert the physician to the possibility of laryngeal or hypopharyngeal damage resulting in aspiration. The following case illustrates this point.

A 3 kg girl was delivered after an uneventful pregnancy. At birth the patient's airway was obstructed with meconium, and resuscitative efforts included aspiration of the nasopharynx, oropharynx, and hypopharynx with a soft, Silastic suction catheter. After several unsuccessful attempts at nasotracheal intubation, an orotracheal tube was finally placed and removed a short time afterward.

Four hours after birth the child was noted to have copious pharyngeal secretions, labored respiration, and cyanosis on oral feeding. Subsequently, crepitus of the neck and upper thorax were noted. A chest film revealed a 50 per cent pneumothorax and aspiration pneumonia, and a subsequent barium swallow showed extravasation of dye into the posterior mediastinum from the hypopharynx (see Fig. 62B–1). Direct laryngos-

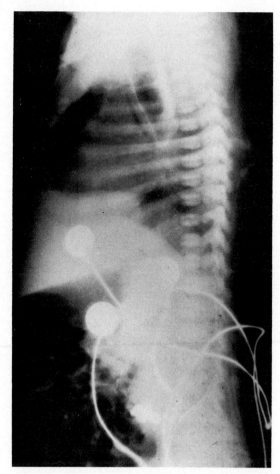

Figure 62B–1 Pseudodiverticulum of the hypopharynx. Lateral view of barium swallow shows extravasation of dye into the posterior mediastinum.

copy in the nursery showed no visible tears in the posterior hypopharyngeal mucosa. Conservative treatment with antibiotics and intravenous hyperalimentation was begun. Although the clinical course of the next 48 hours was complicated by intermittent apnea and bradycardia, the child remained afebrile. She continued to do well, and on the 17th hospital day a repeat barium swallow showed closure of the pseudodiverticulum. She was discharged three days later and continued to gain weight.

PHYSICAL EXAMINATION

Methods of examining the mouth, pharynx, and esophagus have been discussed in Chapter 40. Inspection and palpation of all mucous membranes of the nose, oral cavity, and oropharynx is essential in dealing with children who aspirate chronically. Specific information about feeding and feeding reflexes can be gained by the physician bottle feeding the patient (Ekdahl et al., 1974). Signs such as unusual feeding movements, difficulty in breathing, and drooling should be noted. Some feel that auscultation of the pharynx yields valuable information (Ekdahl et al., 1974). Several anatomic abnormalities can result in aspiration and should be noted (Table 62B–1). In addition, a general physical examination with attention to the neurologic system is basic to evaluation of children with feeding problems, since several syn-

Table 62B–1 ABNORMALITIES ASSOCIATED WITH CHRONIC ASPIRATION

Congenital Abnormalities
Partial or complete mandibular agenesis
First and second branchial arch syndromes
Cleft palate
Short palate
Macroglossia (Combs et al., 1965)
Microglossia
Ankyloglossia superior (Wilson et al., 1963)
Choanal atresia
Laryngeal cleft (Berkoritz et al., 1974; Delahunty and Cherry, 1969; Del Monico and Hoar, 1972)
Laryngeal ptosis
Esophageal absence
Esophageal stenosis, webs, atresia
Esophageal duplication
Tracheoesophageal fistula
Cardiovascular anomalies (Holinger et al., 1948)
Pharyngeal diverticulum or pouch (Britnall and Kridelbaugh, 1950; Clay, 1972)

Traumatic
Pseudodiverticulum of the pharynx (Meyers et al., 1978)
Foreign body
Laryngeal endotracheal tube damage or other trauma (Krajina et al., 1976)

Neoplasm

Infection

Neuromuscular
Central — tumor, degenerative disorders of the CNS (Cohen, 1955; Grahamm, 1964), immaturity of the newborn (Benson, 1962; Frank and Baghdassrian-Gatewood, 1966), cerebral palsy (Ekdahl et al., 1974), agenesis of nucleus ambiguous
Cricopharyngeal achalasia (Reichert et al., 1977)
Bulbar paralysis (Cohen, 1955)
Myotonic dystrophy (Delahunty and Cherry, 1969; Moosa, 1974)
Tetanus (Atharale and Pai, 1964)
Myasthenia gravis
Superior or recurrent laryngeal nerve paralysis

dromes of neurologic dysfunction are commonly associated with dysphagia and subsequent aspiration.

RADIOGRAPHY

Should the history and physical examination leave the physician in doubt as to the etiology of the aspiration, then a lateral neck film and cineradiography of the swallowing mechanism should be performed.

Several techniques for performing cineradiography in children have been described (Andross et al., 1958; O'Connor et al., 1976; Rossato, 1977; Weathers et al., 1974). Characteristic abnormalities of pharyngeal motion are readily visualized (Donner, 1974; Ekdahl et al., 1974; Moosa, 1974; Penchaszadeh, 1971).

Generally, aspiration occurs in one of two ways (Ekdahl et al., 1974): (1) directly, at the time of swallowing, or (2) later, with inspiration or expiration of barium running into the pharynx after the preceding swallow.

Abnormalities of swallowing and aspiration involve three pathologic mechanisms (Kilman et al., 1976). In the first, abnormal transport of barium through the pharynx can be seen. Repeated attempts at swallowing, sluggish or prolonged propulsion of the bolus, asymmetry or deviation of the food column, pharyngeal stasis, dilatation in the absence of distal obstruction, or pulling of dye into the valleculae or pyriform sinuses is abnormal.

A second abnormal sign is regurgitation of food into the mouth, nasopharynx, nasal cavity, or through the vocal cords.

Finally, abnormalities of the cricopharyngeus muscle prevent the proper passage of food into the esophagus with, in some instances, aspiration. Resting hypotension or hypertension of the cricopharyngeus muscle has been documented in some cases (Kilman et al., 1976). Most abnormalities of the cricopharyngeus muscle involve either delayed, premature, or incomplete relaxation with subsequent dysphagia and intermittent aspiration (Andross et al., 1958; Ekdahl et al., 1974; Seamen, 1976).

ENDOSCOPY

Endoscopy in children has been discussed in Chapter 61. If the history, physical exami-

nation, and results of radiography fail to reveal the etiology of chronic aspiration, then direct laryngoscopy, esophagoscopy, and bronchoscopy are indicated. Although some abnormalities, such as laryngotracheoesophageal cleft, are difficult to document endoscopically (Berkoritz et al., 1974; Delahunty and Cherry, 1969), most abnormalities are readily visible.

TREATMENT

The treatment of recurrent aspiration is primarily directed toward reestablishing the integrity of the respiratory tract. Life-threatening situations, such as tracheoesophageal fistula, bifid larynx, or laryngotracheoesophageal cleft, require repair as soon as possible. Iatrogenic causes should be recognized and remedied immediately (Meyers et al., 1978). Aspiration associated with other anatomic defects, however, is not usually quite so severe, and temporizing methods, such as nasogastric intubation, gastrostomy, esophagotomy, parenteral feeding, or tracheostomy may be of benefit until the abnormality is corrected.

Patients with neurologic or neuromuscular abnormalities frequently benefit from a program of physical therapy directed toward reeducating damaged pharyngeal or oral muscles. Several techniques for feeding and teaching patients with swallowing disabilities have been described and should be used before surgical intervention is entertained (Buckley et al., 1976; Bullock, 1975; Gaffney et al., 1975; Griffin, 1974; Holser-Beuhler, 1966; Larsen, 1972).

Surgery is of use when alternative methods of therapy have failed or when the patient's condition progressively deteriorates. Sometimes aspiration can be remedied by surgical procedures designed to manage specific diseases — for example, repositioning the parotid ducts and submaxillary gland excision in children with excessive drooling (Ekdahl et al., 1974), or cricopharyngeal myotomy in patients with cricopharyngeal spasticity, or removal of masses. If recurrent aspiration defies definition or if the pathophysiologic mechanism is defined but is not easily remedied by these procedures, closing the glottis and diverting the food stream (Habal and Murray, 1972; Lindeman, 1975; Montgomery, 1975) may be indicated.

SUMMARY

Children with chronic aspiration most commonly have associated anatomic or physiologic abnormalities that interfere with the three phases of swallowing. A thorough history and physical examination and complete radiographic and endoscopic evaluations are frequently necessary to define the etiology precisely. Although some patients have transient dysfunction (Benson, 1962; Bishop, 1974; Frank and Baghdassrian-Gatewood, 1966), most have permanent abnormalities that require treatment. Nutritional support and pulmonary toilet are of paramount importance. Although physical therapy is beneficial, many patients will continue to aspirate and may require appropriate surgical intervention.

SELECTED REFERENCES

Bosma, J. F. 1957. Deglutition, pharyngeal stage. Physiol. Rev., 37:275–300.

 Although somewhat dated, this article presents a comprehensive review of the physiology of the oral and pharyngeal stages of swallowing. It presents a nice framework of the neurologic pathways of deglutition, abnormalities of which are frequently found in newborns with aspiration.

Logan, W. J., and Bosma, J. F. 1967. Oral and pharyngeal dysphagia in infancy. Pediatr. Clin. North Am. 14:47.

 A complete review of swallowing problems in children is presented. Often, dysphagia is accompanied by aspiration, and identification of those factors responsible is the initial step in management.

Reichert, T. J., Bluestone, C. D., Stool, S. E., et al. 1977. Congenital cricopharyngeal achalasia. Ann. Otol. Rhinol, Laryngol., 76:603.

 The authors present in this article 13 cases of cricopharyngeal achalasia in children with comments on their management. The physiology and anatomy of the cricopharyngeal muscle are reviewed.

REFERENCES

Andross, G. M., Kemp, F. H., and Lind, J. 1958. A cineradiographic study of bottle feeding. Br. J. Radiol., 31:11.

Atharale, V. B., and Pai, P. N. 1964. Tetanus — clinical manifestations in children. J. Pediatr., 65:590.

Benson, P. F. 1962. Transient dysphagia due to muscular incoordination. Proc. R. Soc. Med., 55:237–240.

Berkoritz, R. N. P., Bos, C. E., and Struben, W. H. 1974. Congenital laryngotracheoesophageal cleft. Arch. Otolaryngol., 100:442–443.

Bishop, H. C. 1974. Cricopharyngeal achalasia and childhood. J. Pediatr. Surg., 9:775–778.

Bosma, J. F. 1957. Deglutition, pharyngeal stage. Physiol. Rev., 37:275–300.

Bosma, J. F. 1954. Hoarseness: infant oral function. *In* Symposium on oral sensation and perception. National Institute of Dental Research, Bethesda, MD.

Britnall, E. S., and Kridelbaugh, W. W. 1950. Congenital diverticulum of the posterior hypopharynx simulating atresia of the esophagus. Am. Surg., 131:564–574.

Buckley, J. E., Addicka, C. L., and Maniglia, J. 1976. Feeding patient with dysphagia. Nurs. Forum, 15(1):69–85.

Bullock, J. 1975. Dysphagia. Nurs. Time, 71(49):1928–30.

Clay, B. 1972. Congenital lateral pharyngeal diverticulum. Br. J. Radiol., 45:863–865.

Cohen, S. R. 1955. Congenital dysphagia. Neurogenic considerations. Laryngoscope, 65:515.

Combs, J. T., Grunt, J. A,. and Brandt, I. K. 1965. A new syndrome of neonatal hypoglycemia. Association with visceromegaly, macroglossia, microcephaly, and abnormal umbilicus. N. Engl. J. Med., 275:236–243.

Culley, J. R. T., and Creamer, B. 1958. Sucking and swallowing in infants. Br. Med. J., 2:422.

Delahunty, J. E., and Cherry, L. 1969. Congenital laryngeal cleft. Ann. Otol. Rhinol. Laryngol., 78:96–106.

Del Monico, M. L., and Hoar, J. G. 1972. Bifid epiglottis. Arch. Otolaryngol., 96:178–181.

Donner, M. W. 1974. Swallowing mechanism and neuromuscular disorders. Semin. Roentgenol., 9:273–283.

Doty, R. W., Richmond, W. H., and Storey, A. T. 1967. Effect of medullary lesions on coordination of deglutition. Exp. Neurol., 17:91.

Ekdahl, C., Mansson, I., and Sandberg, N. 1974. Swallowing dysfunction in the brain-damaged with drooling. Acta Otolaryngol., 78(1):141–149.

Ellingworth, R., and Lister, J. 1964. The critical or sensitive period with special reference to certain feeding problems in infants and children. J. Pediatr., 65:839.

Frank, M. M., and Baghdassrian-Gatewood, O. M. 1966. Transient pharyngeal incoordination in the newborn. Am. J. Dis. Child, 111:178–181.

Gaffney, T. W., and Campbell, R. P. 1974. Feeding techniques for dysphagic patients. Am. J. Nurs., 74(12):2194–2195.

Graham, P. J. 1964. Congenital flaccid bulbar palsy. Br. Med. J., 5400:26.

Griffin, K. M. 1974. Swallowing training for dysphagic patients. Arch. Phys. Med. Rehab., 55:467–470.

Habal, M. A., and Murray, J. E. 1972. Surgical treatment of life-endangering chronic aspiration pneumonia. J. Plast. Reconstr. Surg., 49:305–311.

Hendrix, T. R. 1974. The motility of the alimentary canal. *In* Mountcastle, U. B. (Ed.) Medical Physiology, St. Louis, The C. V. Mosby Co.

Holinger, P. H., Johnston, K. C., and Koss, A. R. 1948. Tracheal and bronchial obstruction due to congenital cardiovascular anomalies. Ann. Otol. Rhinol. Laryngol., 57:808.

Holinger, P. H., Johnston, K. C., and Patts, W. J. 1947. Congenital anomalies of the esophagus. Ann. Otol. Rhinol. Laryngol., 56:1007.

Holser-Beuhler, P. 1966. The Blanchard method of feeding the cerebral palsied. Am. J. Occup. Ther., 20:31–34.

Kaplan, S. 1951. Paralysis of deglutition, a post-poliomyelitis complication treated by section of the cricopharyngeus muscle. Am. Surg., *133*:572.

Kilman, W. J., and Rajk, G. 1976. Disorders of the pharyngeal and upper-esophageal sphincter motor function. Arch. Intern. Med., *136*(5):592–601.

Krajina, Z., and Vecerina, S. 1976. Act of swallowing in the fixed larynx. Acta Otolaryngol., *81*(3):323–329.

Larsen, G. L. 1972. Rehabilitation for dysphagia paralytica. J. Speech Hear. Disord., *37*:187–194.

Lindeman, R. C. 1975. Diverting the paralyzed larynx: a reversible procedure for intractable aspiration. Laryngoscope, *85*:157–180.

Logan, W. J., and Bosma, J. F. 1967. Oral and pharyngeal dysphagia in infancy. Pediatr. Clin. North Am., *14*:47.

Margulies, S. E., Brunt, P. W., Donner, M. W., et al. 1968. Familial dysautonomia. Radiology, *90*:107–112.

Meyers, A., Lillydahl, P., and Brown, G. 1978. Hypopharyngeal perforations in neonates. Arch. Otolaryngol., *104*:51.

Mistretta, C. M., and Bradley, R. M. 1975. Taste and swallowing in utero. Br. Med. Bull., *31*(1):80–84.

Montgomery, W. 1975. Surgery to prevent aspiration. Arch. Otolaryngol., *101*:679–682.

Moosa, A. 1974. The feeding difficulty in infantile myo-

tonic dystrophy. Dev. Med. Child Neurol., *16*(6):824–825.

O'Connor, A. F., and Ardran, G. M. 1976. Cineradiography in the diagnosis of pharyngeal palsies. J. Laryngol. Otol., *90*(11):1015–1019.

Penchaszadeh, V. 1971. Oculopharyngeal muscular dystrophy. Birth Defects, *7*(2):118.

Reichert, T. J., Bluestone, C. D., Stool, S. E., et al. 1977. Congenital cricopharyngeal achalasia. Ann. Otol. Rhinol. Laryngol., *76*:603.

Rossato, R. G. 1977. Dionosil swallow: a test of laryngeal protection. Surg. Neurol., *7*(1):24.

Seamen, W. B. 1976. Pharyngeal and upper esopharyngeal dysphagia. J.A.M.A., *235*(24):2643–2646.

Sessle, B. J., and Hannam, A. G. (Ed.) 1976. Mastication and Swallowing. Toronto, Univ. of Toronto Press.

Utiam, H. L., and Thomas, R. G. 1969. Cricopharyngeal incoordination in infancy. Pediatrics, *43*:402–406.

Weathers, R. M., Becker, M. H., and Genieser, N. B. 1974. Improved technique for study of swallowing function in infants. Radiol. Technol., *46*(2):98–100.

Wilson, R. A., Klimen, M. R., and Hardyment, A. F. 1963. Ankyloglossia superior (palatoglossal adhesion in the newborn infant). Pediatrics, *31*:1051.

Chapter 63

HOARSENESS

Jacob Friedberg, M.D.

Hoarseness is a common clinical complaint. The abnormal qualities of the hoarse voice may be described as breathy and harsh, husky or rough, strident or coarse. The term "hoarse" may also describe the quality of a conversational voice, the simple cry of a newborn infant, or any vocalization. Not all phonatory sounds are laryngeal in origin; they may result from constriction of any part of

the airway. If severe enough, the constriction may give rise to stridor in all phases of respiration. In the infant one may not be able to separate such sounds from an abnormal voice or cry, and indeed such a distinction is often meaningless from a diagnostic and therapeutic point of view. The same lesion that produces hoarseness in one patient may produce stridor and obstruction in another,

Table 63–1 DIFFERENTIAL DIAGNOSIS OF HOARSENESS IN CHILDREN

Congenital
1. Laryngeal Anomalies
   a. laryngomalacia
   b. glottic webs
   c. subglottic stenosis
   d. vocal cord sulcus
   e. laryngotracheoesophageal cleft
2. Cystic Lesions
   a. laryngocele
   b. mucus retention cyst
   c. thyroglossal duct cyst
   d. branchial cleft cyst
3. Aspirational Disorders
   a. tracheoesophageal fistula
   b. pharyngoesophageal dyskinesia
4. Angiomas
   a. lymphangioma (cystic hygroma)
   b. Hemangioma
5. Cri du Chat Syndrome

Neurogenic (Congenital and Acquired)
1. Supranuclear
   e.g., hydrocephalus, subdural hematoma, pseudo-bulbar palsy, meningocele
2. Nuclear
   e.g., brain stem compression (due to Arnold-Chiari malformation, Dandy Walker cyst, meningocele, etc.), bulbar poliomyelitis, Guillain-Barré syndrome
3. Peripheral
   e.g., cardiovascular anomalies, mediastinal cysts and tumors, neuropathies (lead, arsenic, diphtheria, postinfectious), myasthenia gravis, recurrent laryngeal nerve trauma, or invasion by tumor

Vocal Abuse
Vocal cord polyps, nodules

Neoplasia
1. Papilloma
2. Squamous cell carcinoma
3. Others

Physical Voice Change of Puberty

Inflammatory
1. Infectious
   a. simple laryngitis
   b. diphtheria
   c. laryngotracheitis
   d. supraglottitis (epiglottitis)
2. Noninfectious
   a. chronic laryngitis
   b. allergic laryngitis
   c. angioneurotic edema
   d. rheumatoid arthritis

Traumatic
1. Hematoma
2. Laryngeal cartilage fracture
3. Arytenoid dislocation
4. Impacted foreign body
5. Postoperative
   a. postintubation granuloma
   b. thyroidectomy
   c. tracheoesophageal fistula repair
   d. cardiac surgery
   e. tracheotomy

1181

depending upon the size and location of the lesion. Hoarseness always indicates some abnormality of structure or function. Because of the precision of laryngeal mechanics, hoarseness may result from a remarkably small lesion and thus may be a very early sign in the course of a disease process. Conversely, if the lesion's origin is remote from the vocal cords, hoarseness may obviously be a very late sign.

The present study of hoarseness will be approached in terms of its character, its associated symptoms and signs, and the age and mode of onset of the hoarseness. Indications for extended investigation will be discussed as well as those aspects of diagnosis pertinent to the evaluation of these lesions.

PATHOGENESIS

Although many lesions produce hoarseness, they can do so only in a limited number of ways. In most general terms, the intensity of the voice varies with the subglottic air pressure maintained against glottic resistance. Vocal pitch and timbre are affected by the length and tension of the vibrating segment of the vocal cords and by their mass, posture, and strength of movement. The shape of the free vocal cord margins also plays a role in determining voice quality. Thus a failure or aberration in any of these vocal components may result in hoarseness.

CLINICAL EVALUATION

Establishing a differential diagnosis (Holinger, 1961; Holinger et al., 1970; Lore, 1950; Murphy, 1967; Senturia and Wilson, 1968) of the causes of hoarseness is a lengthy process, and statistically the majority of these lesions are innocuous and self-limiting. Thus, because of the potential hazards of some of the diagnostic techniques, before proceeding beyond the clinical examination one must first decide how important it really is to establish a firm diagnosis of the cause of hoarseness.

The quality of the hoarseness (Holinger et al., 1952) will give limited but valuable clues to its etiology, while its other characteristics, such as age of onset, rate of progression, associated infection, history of trauma or surgery, and the presence of respiratory or cardiac distress, may be of much greater significance. A low-pitched, coarse, fluttering voice suggests a supraglottic or even hypopharyngeal lesion, while a more high-pitched, cracking voice or an aphonic or breathy voice suggests a cordal problem. An associated high-pitched stridor also suggests the presence of a glottic or a subglottic lesion. Hoarseness that is altered by a position change suggests a mobile lesion, such as a vallecular or aryepiglottic cyst or pedunculated polyp.

General examination is often helpful. Head and neck hemangiomas or lymphangiomas strongly suggest the possibility of a similar laryngeal lesion as the source of hoarseness. Central nervous system depression, as in birth trauma or other head injury, diminished level of consciousness, abnormal muscle tone or coordination, increased intracranial pressure, or the presence of a meningocele should alert the clinician to the possibility of laryngeal nerve palsy. Associated dysphagia, regurgitation, aspiration, and pooling of pharyngeal secretions in the absence of esophageal obstruction or fistula should also suggest the possibility of neurologic lesion, usually bulbar, as a cause of hoarseness. Neck masses, tracheal shift, and abnormal heart sounds and murmurs indicate that the examiner should look for peripheral laryngeal nerve involvement. Palpation of the neck and larynx may define some of the preceding problems, but one should not overlook a brief but careful digital examination of the mouth and hypopharynx, which may reveal a lingual thyroid, vallecular cyst, or a parapharyngeal mass. No such manipulation should be done in the presence of potential airway obstruction unless one is fully prepared to establish an airway.

Indirect laryngoscopy may provide all the necessary diagnostic information required. With patience and gentleness, children from four years of age, or occasionally younger, may be examined. The alcohol flame for mirror warming is frightening and should be avoided. As defogging solutions are often foul tasting and local anesthetic spray may be quite startling, these should also be avoided. Warm water is quite adequate for demisting mirrors, and if topical anesthesia is required, it can generally be applied with cotton-tipped applicators. Because of the relatively high position of the child's larynx and the narrow epiglottis, a small web or papilloma at the anterior commissure may be missed, but a very adequate view of the remaining structures can readily be obtained (Chap. 61).

The Neonate

There are a number of congenital anomalies that may affect voice, airway, or both (Fearon, 1968; Ferguson, 1970), each in varying degrees, depending on the precise location and extent of the lesion. If the airway is significantly occluded, the resultant stridor, both inspiratory and expiratory, may be sufficiently noisy to obscure clinically any vocal sounds. This stridor may disappear at rest, but so will any active voice sounds in the small infant. The distinction is less than academic, and the primary problem in such cases is airway management, where indicated.

Congenital laryngeal stridor or laryngomalacia is characterized by a coarse, inspiratory stridor, but usually with a normal voice. With redundancy of the arytenoid and aryepiglottic mucosa, the infant's cry may have a noisy component to it, which is relieved in the prone position. Similarly, the infant with subglottic stenosis usually has a good voice that may be obscured by stridor. With sufficient stenosis, the air exchange is so poor that the cry is weak, if not truly hoarse. A posterior stenosis may be rigid enough to fix the cords partially, giving the cry a breathy as well as a stridorous quality.

A variety of cysts occur in or about the larynx (Desanto et al., 1969; Holinger and Brown, 1967). All are capable of affecting the voice or airway. Most of these are simple retention cysts of seromucinous glands, commonly occurring in the valleculae and aryepiglottic folds. Occasionally these may be subglottic and clinically indistinguishable from a fibrous subglottic stenosis. Still less common is the laryngocele (Holinger and Brown, 1967), which results from a functional occlusion of the neck of the saccule with subsequent dilatation with air or fluid. Hoarseness is an early sign of the presence of a laryngocele, but with enlargement and particularly with infection of the sac an acute airway problem may be precipitated. Once recognized, most of these can be managed by simple aspiration and marsupialization of the cyst, with dramatic relief of symptoms.

Laryngeal webs (Holinger and Brown, 1967), commonly glottic, vary in extent from a simple mucosal fold at the anterior commissure to a complete fibrous obliteration of the glottis. The latter is obviously incompatible with life unless breeched immediately after birth. The remainder may cause varying degrees of impairment, from mild hoarseness to aphonia, and respiratory signs, from minimal stridor and croupy cough to gross obstruction and severe distress. Diagnosis is by endoscopic examination findings. The smaller, thinner webs often respond well to dilatation. The more extensive lesions will require a tracheotomy for airway control and more definitive surgery, including incision and repeated dilatation, resection and use of the McNaught keel, and, more recently, CO_2 laser excision.

Complete failure of the thyroid gland to descend from the foramen cecum of the tongue to its usual pretracheal location will result in a so-called lingual thyroid in the base of the tongue. This is usually an asymptomatic structure unless it becomes enlarged owing to inflammation or endocrine disturbance, in which case both voice and airway may be disturbed. Symptomatic relief can be obtained by thyroid hormone suppression or by surgical transposition of the gland (Skolnik et al., 1976). Surgical ablation is not recommended, as this may be the only functional thyroid tissue in the body which may be demonstrated on a thyroid scan).

Any of the previously mentioned lesions in the base of the tongue or supraglottis may be readily missed by the examiner who looks only at the vocal cords for a source of hoarseness, particularly when the laryngoscope blade is just a little too large for the size of the child being examined.

Secretions spilling into or pooling on the larynx are a common cause of hoarseness in a neonate and may be aggravated by feeding or sleeping. Tracheoesophageal fistula, with or without atresia, may be considered, and it is usually readily diagnosed clinically, radiologically, and endoscopically. The much less common posterior-laryngotracheal cleft is less easy to recognize. The cry is weak, and aspiration is a constant problem. On direct examination, the endoscopist may miss the cleft unless the larynx is observed during vocal cord abduction or if one gently but deliberately applies pressure to the posterior commissure, thus opening the cleft. Once diagnosed, these should be repaired at the earliest possible date, either via a lateral pharyngotomy or endoscopically, to avoid the chronic lung problems of aspiration.

The "cri-du-chat" syndrome (Le Jeune, 1966) is a rare but interesting cause of an abnormal cry in that it is the result of a proven genetic defect. The cry is weak and high-pitched, characteristically like the mewing of a cat. The larynx is seen to be narrow with a diamond-shaped glottis during inspiration and a persistent posterior glottic chink on expiration, resulting in constant air leakage. Many anomalies, including gross retardation, microcephaly, and hypotonia, are also present.

Dysphonia in a neonate may be a clue to far-reaching damage to the vagus nerve system (Rontal and Rontal, 1977) from supranuclear to peripheral lesions with associated difficulty with deglutition and aspiration of secretions. Vocal cord movement is the simplest of the vagus nerve functions to recognize clinically and as such is a useful guide to the diagnosis of more extensive neurologic lesions. Diagnosis is best made endoscopically with care taken not to restrict cord movement with the laryngoscope. Unilateral cord palsy usually results in a hoarse cry only. This may improve in time, if not by recovery of function then by compensatory movement of the opposite cord. Airway obstruction is seldom a problem unless precipitated by minor swelling from an endotracheal intubation or a respiratory tract infection. The patient with a bilateral palsy, on the other hand, will have a clear but weak cry; however, dyspnea and stridor may be marked, and evidence of extensive central neuropathy is usually apparent. Again airway management takes priority, and is usually in the form of a tracheotomy; if recovery is not forthcoming, some form of cord lateralization will be indicated.

Neonatal myasthenia gravis may be seen in the infant of a patient with myasthenia. The larynx is commonly affected, resulting in a weak cry, which, however, may be overshadowed by widespread signs of neuromuscular weakness. Fortunately, this tends to regress in a few weeks (Chaps. 65, 66A, B & 69).

THE PROGRESSIVE LESION

Hoarseness in children tends to be overlooked or at least accepted until it reaches a certain level of severity. An accurate history of progression is often lacking but should be sought. The most common lesion (Arnold, 1962; Yairi et al., 1974) in this group is the simple laryngeal nodule, polyp, or keratosis of the vocal cord due to vocal abuse. As well

as progression of the hoarseness, there is a fluctuation in the severity of symptoms, which are aggravated by respiratory tract infections and relieved by periods of rest. Thus hoarseness may be worse at the end of the day, but the voice will be near normal in the morning. Dramatic deterioration may occur owing to sudden swelling of a polyp with infection or hemorrhage. This is seen in the vocally aggressive child who may share the disease with other members of the immediate family. The diagnosis of a vocal polyp is usually readily confirmed by mirror examination. For this self-limiting and self-correcting lesion, treatment should be conservative unless the voice is quite unacceptable. Speech therapy may be both corrective and reassuring (Wilson, 1968), but it is often more time-consuming than the symptom merits. Surgery also is unnecessary except, perhaps, for social reasons. In any event, unless underlying speech habits are corrected, the nodules are likely to recur. If there is any possibility that the lesion is anything other than a nodule, the taking of an excisional biopsy specimen is mandatory.

Relentlessly progressive hoarseness should suggest neoplasia, of which the juvenile laryngeal papilloma is by far the most common lesion as a cause. It is, however, not restricted to juveniles, but is seen in patients from birth well into adulthood. The treatments are legion and will not be dealt with here, except to recommend that representative biopsy specimens always be taken. Although the clinical appearance is usually typical, it may be indistinguishable from the rare but much more ominous laryngeal squamous cell carcinoma of childhood. Conversely, the rare but benign granular cell myoblastoma may present on the larynx. Inadequate biopsy specimens may be interpreted as being malignant because of the pseudoepitheliomatous hyperplasia overlying these lesions. Progressive hoarseness due to recurrent nerve invasion by malignancy is occasionally seen in the pediatric age group, particularly from thyroid carcinoma.

Laryngeal hemangiomas and lymphangiomas are not usually problematic at birth, but during the early months of life they may enlarge dramatically. As elsewhere, these tumors will tend to regress spontaneously in the first few years of life. The diagnosis is confirmed by the presence of similar lesions elsewhere in the body, by a positive isotope scan, and by direct visualization. A biopsy specimen is usually not necessary and should be avoided because of potential bleeding. In practice, however, bleeding is seldom a problem, as laryngeal hemangiomas tend to be rather fibrotic. These lesions are not resectable, and although they are radiosensitive, the hazards of using even a few hundred rads to this area in an infant must be fully appreciated. Hemangiomas may respond dramatically to a high dosage of corticosteroids, and this is certainly warranted. If no response is obtained, one must remember that spontaneous regression is the rule, and heroic measures can be avoided. Treatment should consist of control of the airway by tracheotomy, if necessary, and the maintenance of adequate nutrition by gastrostomy or gavage if feeding becomes a problem (Chap. 72).

Physiologic voice change at puberty should not be forgotten. The rapidly developing adolescent may require many months to gain control of his new larynx. However, such individuals are not immune to neoplasia and palsies, and a thorough clinical examination is still warranted.

Recurrent laryngeal nerve involvement, and thus hoarseness or breathiness, may be seen as part of a host of peripheral neuropathies (Chap. 69), including heavy metal poisonings, deficiency states, diabetes, postinfectious polyneuropathy, and infections, such as diphtheria, leprosy, and infectious mononucleosis. Hoarseness is often the least dramatic sign in such conditions but should alert the clinician to possible airway or aspirational problems.

Idiopathic unilateral and bilateral vocal cord palsies are seen in childhood and are often diagnosed as tracheitis or simple laryngitis. When these conditions fail to resolve as expected, a cord palsy must be ruled out.

INFLAMMATORY LESIONS

Hoarseness due to various laryngeal inflammations, including simple infective laryngitis, laryngotracheitis, supraglottitis, and associated exanthemata, is seldom a diagnostic or therapeutic problem. The concern is with the airway, and the voice change is viewed as incidental. Occasionally the systemic manifestations of the disease may be very mild, with voice change an early sign and airway obstruction comparatively late, catching the clinician unawares. Even epiglottitis may run a course of two or three days with

mild dysphagia and a "hot potato" voice as the only symptoms initially (Chap. 67).

Diphtheria, although admittedly very rare as a cause of acute laryngitis nowadays, is nevertheless still with us, and, with the growing degree of laxity by our population regarding primary immunization, may once again become a serious consideration.

The noninfectious cricoarytenoid joint inflammation of rheumatoid arthritis is seldom recognized in children. It is potentially reversible before permanent fixation with voice and airway changes occurs. Hoarseness, local discomfort, and dysphagia should suggest the diagnosis in the young rheumatoid arthritis patient; inflammatory changes of the arytenoid mucosa may also be apparent on mirror examination.

The presence of chronic rhinosinusitis or chest infection from any cause is commonly reflected in the laryngeal mucosa and associated voice changes. In the presence of chronic laryngeal irritation, as seen on mirror examination, a history of smoking should always be sought, regardless of the child's age.

Idiopathic atrophic changes of the respiratory tree may occur in the pediatric age group and may affect not only the nose in classical atrophic rhinitis but also the larynx and trachea. Loss of normal cilia, squamous cell metaplasia, secondary chronic infection, and retained secretions result in persistent hoarseness and may be readily assessed by indirect laryngoscopy (Chap. 67).

POST-TRAUMATIC HOARSENESS

Laryngeal trauma may begin in the newborn nursery. Common causes of laryngeal problems include frequent, overly aggressive pharyngeal aspiration in the newborn and repeated passage of a feeding tube. A weak cry should be a warning for the nursing personnel to be more gentle in their management (Chap. 70).

Blunt laryngeal trauma (Fitz-Hugh and Powell, 1970) is not common in children but is sometimes the result of a play injury in the preadolescent. A backhand from a bat or racquet, a fall on bicycle handlebars, or a blow from a swing seat are typical mischances that may result in laryngeal trauma. Gross signs of injury may be obvious, but even a minor change in voice quality should lead the physician to suspect a possible thyroid or cricoid fracture or arytenoid dislocation. Fortunately, children of this age group are usually readily examined, and when there is a good airway, normal laryngeal mobility, and apparent laryngeal symmetry, they can usually be managed conservatively. Hoarseness resulting from surgical emphysema, however, should warn the examiner of a more serious situation: the mucosa has obviously been breeched, and the progression of emphysema may result in local airway obstruction, pneumothorax, or both. Careful observation is therefore mandatory in these cases (Chap. 70).

POSTOPERATIVE HOARSENESS

Considering the frequency with which direct laryngoscopy and intubation are performed, often without the advantage of anesthesia, it is gratifying that injury occurs so rarely. However, of course it does occur, even when the procedures are performed carefully, so the physician should be aware of this possible cause of hoarseness (Chap. 68).

The newborn who becomes dysphonic or totally aphonic following intubation for assisted ventilation may have suffered an arytenoid dislocation. If recognized, this can be reduced by manipulation with an anterior commissure laryngoscope. During a transfer from the obstetrics to the anesthesia to the neonatology departments, however, such a sign may go unrecognized. In these cases direct laryngoscopy would be both diagnostic and therapeutic.

Prolonged orotracheal intubation or the use of an overly large tube may lead to varying degrees of ulceration of the larynx, damage to soft tissue and cartilage, granuloma formation and subsequent stenosis, webbing or airway obstruction, and even vocal cord palsy. Immediate postextubation vocal huskiness and croupy cough are common in these cases and indicate an impending complication. If all is proceeding well, this hoarseness should resolve in a few days; if not, direct visualization of the larynx should be considered.

With the increasing sophistication of ventilatory and resuscitative techniques, the performance of tracheostomies has become less common in recent years; consequently the expertise gained in this technique over the last few decades will likely be lost. Injury to the recurrent laryngeal nerves or the cricoid

and subglottic areas, although rare, will not be recognized until extubation is attempted, at which time irreversible damage may have been sustained. Coincidental with this trend is the increasing use of percutaneous needles or trocars into the larynx for topical anesthesia or for the establishment of an emergency airway. Here, too, the injury may go unrecognized until long after the acute episode is over, but damage to the voice should be minimal. Although the risk of local damage from these techniques may be small, adjacent structures are vulnerable; indeed, even the cervical spinal cord has been injured.

Thyroid surgery, except for malignancy, has largely become a thing of the past, but in cases where it is performed, postoperative hoarseness may be the result of intubation or recurrent laryngeal nerve injury, making routine preoperative and postoperative visualization of the larynx of value. Late onset of hoarseness — months or even a year after thyroid surgery — should suggest the development of a delayed palsy, presumably from fibrosis or ischemia or, in the case of malignancy, from recurrent disease. Bilateral recurrent nerve injury with the cords in a paramedian position retains a remarkably good voice; however, the examiner may recognize the presence of a problem since, if not hoarse, the voice is at least weak and slightly breathy, depending on the precise vocal cord position.

The vulnerability of the recurrent laryngeal nerves in the surgical repair of tracheoesophageal fistula (Bedard et al., 1974; Robertson, 1977), with or without atresia, by direct anastomosis or by segmental replacement by a gastric tube or colon, is obvious. The apparently low incidence of such injury may simply reflect our lack of follow-up investigations. Many of the infants who undergo repair of a tracheoesophageal fistula will have an endotracheal or nasogastric tube in place for a long time, so that any transient voice problems may go unnoticed. Compensation with a unilateral palsy is usually excellent, and no treatment is indicated. Persistent hoarseness or breathiness, however, requires a direct examination. Bilateral palsy usually demands that a tracheostomy be performed.

Vocal changes following cardiac surgery, particularly for the repair of a patent ductus, double aortic arch, or pulmonary artery anomalies, should not automatically be attributed to intubation. The left recurrent laryngeal nerve is very much at risk, as it passes around the arch of the aorta, and should be examined for normal function in these cases.

The Older Child

Many congenital lesions may, of course, manifest themselves at any age, as may the results of trauma and infection. The older child is subject to essentially the very same causes of hoarseness as is the adult (Schwartz et al., 1966) (Chaps. 66 & 70).

INDICATIONS FOR INVESTIGATION

Certainly not every child with a hoarse voice or cry merits investigation beyond an assessment of the symptom. In the presence of hoarseness with respiratory distress, tachypnea, decreased air entry, tachycardia or cyanosis, however, the larynx must be visualized, and a firm diagnosis of the cause of hoarseness must be made. A laryngeal examination should also be carried out when hoarseness is associated with recognized cardiac, esophageal, or nervous system disease. Such an examination may well precipitate an acute airway obstruction, necessitating intubation; this should be done preferably with a bronchoscope and subsequent tracheostomy. As much as one may wish to avoid this possibility, it should at least occur at the time and place chosen by the examiner under a controlled situation with minimal risk to life, rather than on an emergency basis.

Progressive hoarseness also merits investigation, and one need not wait until total aphonia or airway problems occur. Progression usually indicates a developmental lesion, such as a laryngeal or hypopharyngeal cyst; a neoplasm, such as papilloma or hemangioma; or, indeed, the occasional malignancy. Hoarseness in the presence of lesions such as cutaneous hemangiomata or head and neck lymphangioma should lead the examiner to exclude the presence of a similar lesion in or about the larynx. Hoarseness in the newborn with recognized cardiac or central nervous system anomalies or swallowing difficulties similarly merits a direct examination to rule out the various palsies and fistulae that may be present.

Social embarrassment or poor intelligibility of speech, particularly in the school-age child, does merit thorough assessment and, whenever possible, correction (Putney, 1965).

Hoarseness following external trauma or an otherwise uneventful intubation should also not go unchecked. Many granulomata will resolve in time if untreated, but a dislocated arytenoid, once fixed out of position, will never be made normally functional.

The hoarseness that has been, according to the history, "present since birth" is very difficult to evaluate in regard to infant and childhood vocal quality. So often one discovers the offending lesions to be simple vocal nodules, likely due to vocal abuse, and hardly congenital. Thus, such a history should prompt an investigation to rule out laryngeal web, cyst, palsy, or angioma, all of which may be treated readily but which have the potential to obstruct the airway. In these cases a diagnosis should be made (Chap. 61).

RADIOLOGIC EXAMINATION

As many of the lesions causing hoarseness in infants and children have the potential for airway obstruction, particularly with endoscopic manipulation, a variety of noninvasive techniques have been developed for investigation of the larynx and adjacent airway. Simple soft tissue lateral radiographs are easily obtained, even in the very small infant, and may give good demonstration of a hypopharyngeal lesion, such as a vallecular cyst, lingual thyroid, or lymphangioma, or a retropharyngeal mass with secondary vocal and airway symptoms. The epiglottis itself may be noted to be enlarged in epiglottitis or with angioneurotic swelling in this view. The overlying bony density of the cervical spine, however, makes the corresponding anteroposterior view a poor one. High kilovoltage magnification techniques (Slovis, 1977) minimize x-ray absorption by bone and result in good visualization of the airway with delineation of papillomatous masses, granulomata, or cord palsy, as indicated by a failure of effacement of the cord and lack of obliteration of the ventricle on inspiration.

Xeroradiographs (Holinger et al., 1972; Noyek et al., 1976) with their properties of edge enhancement, are particularly helpful in visualizing any lesion encroaching on the airway. The lateral view shows good detail of valleculae, epiglottis, aryepiglottic folds, cords, ventricles, and the subglottic region. When combined with tomographic techniques, the cervical spine density may be eliminated. The radiation dosage in this technique is about four times that of conventional radiographs, and its use should therefore be limited.

Although contrast studies of the larynx may give good laryngeal detail, they are usually not warranted because of limited patient cooperation in the pediatric age group and the risk of compromising an already limited airway. Contrast studies of the esophagus are, however, often done as part of the assessment of lesions that affect the airway and voice as well as swallowing. Evidence of aspiration and leakage through a fistula should be sought and may result in an unanticipated but nevertheless helpful laryngogram.

Tomography, similarly, may provide good views of the larynx, but the technique is not very satisfactory in uncooperative children. Radioisotope scans are of particular help in demonstrating laryngeal angiomata, particularly in the presence of a known lesion in the adjacent neck or pharyngeal structures. An isolated hemangioma of less than 1 cm diameter may, however, go unrecognized. Lingual thyroid can be nicely confirmed by iodine 131 or pertechnetate scanning. Ultrasound techniques are at present of little value in pediatric laryngology but, with refinement, will likely be useful in demonstrating cartilage defects or displacements as well as cystic lesions.

A plain chest film may demonstrate any one of a number of mediastinal lesions, including inflammatory or neoplastic lymph nodes, neurogenic tumors, bronchial or esophageal cysts or duplications, as well as a number of cardiac and vascular anomalies that may affect the recurrent laryngeal nerves.

Computerized tomography of the neck and chest region has been of limited usefulness in children because of the need for immobility during the scan. Newer units with shorter exposure times may be most helpful.

FLEXIBLE FIBEROPTIC NASOPHARYNGOLARYNGOSCOPE

Until recently, flexible fiberoptic and endoscopic equipment (Silberman et al., 1976) has been too large for widespread use in children; however, instruments of 3.9 mm diameter have become available, which, except for the smallest newborn, can usually be passed nasally for visualization of the hypopharynx

and larynx. In the infant this is done without anesthesia, while for the older child, topical anesthesia to the nasal mucosa is adequate. It allows observation of the larynx without the shortcomings of general anesthesia or the fixation artifacts of the rigid endoscopes. These instruments are, however, expensive and delicate but will probably play an ever-increasing role in laryngeal assessment.

DIRECT LARYNGOSCOPY

The diagnostic information provided by a properly conducted laryngoscopic examination is still without equal. More important is the control that the examiner has over the possibly compromised airway and his or her ability to relieve or correct immediately a significant number of the lesions that may be encountered. It is generally a safe procedure; however, it is not without some risk to maxillofacial and pharyngeal structures, as well as to the cervical spine, the larynx, and the airway and should not be undertaken merely out of curiosity. With few exceptions, if there is significant airway obstruction, a general anesthetic must not be used.

Even with a compromised airway, the maintenance of normal oropharyngeal muscle tone and spontaneous respiration provides a great safety factor. In the neonate or small infant, anesthesia is not necessary. Structural lesions, such as webs, cysts, and polyps, are readily appreciated; however, functional disorders, such as cordal spasm or paresis, may be difficult to appreciate, particularly if obscured by struggling, swallowing movements, coughing, irregular respiration, and secretions. Once physical obstruction has been ruled out and the examiner is confident of his or her ability to establish and maintain an airway, anesthesia may be induced with the patient breathing spontaneously. Topical anesthesia will eliminate any tendency to laryngospasm. Quiet respiration facilitates the use of the otomicroscope, which may reveal lesions not apparent to the naked eye, such as small capillary malformations of the cord, which are indicative of a more extensive underlying hemangioma. Similarly, a pinpoint nodule on the free margin of the cord, which may result in an extraordinary degree of hoarseness for its size, can be seen readily. Palpation of the cords for passive mobility may be carried out at this time.

As the patient is awakened, the cords may

be examined at leisure for mobility, with care being taken, however, not to inadvertently fix one or both cords with an improperly placed laryngoscope. Passive movement with increasing depth of respiration may be mistaken for active cord movement by the inexperienced examiner, who should learn to coordinate visualization of cord movement with chest movement. Passive abduction is in the expiratory phase, whereas active abduction is inspiratory. Similarly, the marked abduction with coughing should not be mistaken for active movement on awakening. It bears repeating that at all times during the course of this examination one should be prepared to establish an airway by orotracheal intubation or bronchoscopy and to institute appropriate resuscitative measures.

CONCLUSION

The list of lesions capable of causing hoarseness in childhood has not been exhausted here. In the majority of instances, the problem is innocuous, self-limiting, and usually reversible. However, some causes of hoarseness are progressive, potentially life-threatening, or symptomatic of extensive disease, and a precise diagnosis of the cause is thus required.

SELECTED REFERENCES

Ferguson, C. F. 1970. Congenital abnormalities of the infant larynx. Otolaryngol. Clin. North Am., *3*(2): 185–200.

Holinger, P. H. 1961. Clinical aspects of congenital anomalies of the larynx, trachea, bronchi and esophagus. J. Laryngol., *75*:1–44.

These two articles, based on the authors' best personal clinical experiences, provide a most comprehensive view of many of the lesions responsible for hoarseness in the infant.

Rontal, M., and Rontal, E. 1977. Lesions of the vagus nerve: Diagnosis, treatment and rehabilitation. Laryngoscope, *87*(1):72–86.

The multiplicity of neurogenic vocal problems has been dealt with in a very convenient and useful fashion, providing the clinician with an orderly approach to this sometimes confusing subject.

REFERENCES

Arnold, G. E. 1962. Vocal nodules and polyps: Laryngeal tissue reaction to habitual hyperkinetic dysphonia, J. Speech Hear. Disord. *27*:205–217.

Bedard, T., Girvan, D. P., and Shandling, B. 1974. Congenital H-type tracheoesophageal fistula, J. Pediatr. Surg., *9*(5):63–68.

Desanto, L., Devine, K., and Weiland, L. 1969. Cysts of the larynx, classification. Laryngoscope, *79*(1): 145–176.

Fearon, B. 1968. Respiratory distress in the newborn. Otolaryngol. Clin. North Am., *1*(1):147–169.

Ferguson, C. F. 1970. Congenital abnormalities of the infant larynx. Otolaryngol. Clin. North Am., *3*(2): 185–200.

Fitz-Hugh, G. S., and Powell, J. B. 1970. Acute traumatic injuries of the oropharynx and laryngopharynx and cervical trachea in children. Otol. Clin. North Am., *3*(2):375–393.

Holinger, P. H. 1961. Clinical aspects of congenital anomalies of the larynx, trachea, bronchi and esophagus. J. Laryngol., *75*:1–44.

Holinger, P. H., and Brown, W. T. 1967. Congenital webs, cysts, laryngoceles and other anomalies of the larynx. Ann. Otol. Rhinol. Laryngol., *76*:744–752.

Holinger, P. H., et al. 1972. Xeroradiography of the larynx. Ann. Otol. Rhinol. Laryngol., *81*:806–808.

Holinger, P. H., Johnson, K. C., and McMahon, R. J. 1952. Hoarseness in infants and children. Eye, Ear, Nose Throat Monthly, *31*(5):247–251.

Holinger, P. H., Schild, J. A., and Weprin, L. 1970. Pediatric laryngology. Otolaryngol. Clin. North Am., *3*(3):625–637.

LeJeune, J. 1966. Cri du chat syndrome, chromosome deletion causes severe retardation. J.A.M.A., *197*:40.

Lore, J. M., Jr. 1950. Hoarseness in children. Arch. Otolaryngol., *51*:814–825.

Murphy, R. S. 1967. Hoarseness. Nova Scotia Med. Bull., *46*(8):177–179.

Noyek, A. M., Friedberg, J., Steinhardt, M. I., et al. 1976. Xeroradiography in the assessment of the paediatric larynx and trachea, J. Otolaryngol., *5*(6):468–474.

Putney, F. J. 1965. Hoarseness: Management of common causes. Med. Clin. North Am.: *49*(5):1295–1308.

Robertson, J. R., and Birck, H. G. 1977. Laryngeal problems following infant esophageal surgery. Laryngoscope, *86*(7):72–86.

Rontal, M., and Rontal, E. 1977. Lesions of the vagus nerve, diagnosis, treatment and rehabilitation. Laryngoscope, *87*(1):72–86.

Schwartz, L., Noyek, A. M., and Naiberg, D. 1966. Persistent hoarseness, N.Y. State J. Med., *66*(20):2658–2662.

Senturia, B. H., and Wilson, F. E. 1968. Otolaryngologic findings in children with voice deviation. Ann. Otol. Rhinol. Laryngol., *77*:1027–1041.

Skolnik, E. M., Yee, K. F., and Golden, T. A. 1976. Transposition of the lingual thyroid. Laryngoscope, *86*(6):785–791.

Slovis, T. L. 1977. Non-invasive evaluation of the pediatric airway. A recent advance. Pediatrics, *59*(6):877–880.

Silberman, H. D., Wilf, H., and Tucker, J. A. 1976. Flexible fiberoptic nasopharyngolaryngoscope. Ann. Otol. Rhinol. Laryngol., *85*(5):640–645.

Wilson, D. K. 1968. Voice therapy for children with laryngeal dysfunction. Southern Med. J., *61*:956–962.

Yairi, E., Currin, L. H., and Bulian, N. 1974. Incidence of hoarseness in school children over a one year period. J. Communication Disorders, *7*:321–328.

Chapter 64

STRIDOR AND AIRWAY OBSTRUCTION

Robin Cotton, M.D.
James S. Reilly, M.D.

Stridor is a physical sign that is characterized by a harsh sound produced by turbulence of airflow through a partial obstruction, creating a composite of vibrations of the surrounding tissues. This sign merits immediate investigation, for its presence heralds a pathologic narrowing of the airway, potential respiratory obstruction, and even death. The precise underlying cause must be sought in every case. The time allotted to make the diagnosis may be only a matter of minutes if the onset of stridor is both sudden and associated with severe airway obstruction. In the absence of respiratory distress, a prompt but more thorough investigation can be made before making a diagnosis and deciding upon medical or surgical therapy. With rare exception, there is only one correct diagnosis.

The site of the obstruction causing the stridor must be in the airway, but the lesion may, on occasion, be extrinsic and may compress the softer, flaccid airway of the child (Tables 64–1 and 64–2). Because of the child's absolute small airway dimensions, even if the obstruction is very slight, stridor will be accompanied by signs indicative of respiratory obstruction, such as movement of alae nasi, suprasternal, sternal, and intercostal retractions, dyspnea, and cyanosis. The purpose of this chapter is to assist the physician in an orderly approach to the diagnosis of stridor (Chaps. 65–72).

PATHOPHYSIOLOGY

A review of physics is appropriate in order to understand the mechanisms involved in the production of a pathologic adventitious respiratory sound such as stridor. The movement of any gas through a partially closed tube is subject to certain principles of physics. The pressure exerted by a gas is equal in all directions, except when there is linear movement. Linear movement of a gas creates additional pressure in the forward vector, and because of the principle of conservation of energy, there is a corresponding fall in the lateral pressure, which is at a vector of 90 degrees. When a gas passes through a tube like the trachea that is narrowed, the lateral pressure (centrifugal) that has held the lumen open can drop precipitously and cause the tube to close. We call this phenomenon the Venturi principle (Forgacs, 1978).

The forces exerted by the Venturi principle cause the narrowed, flexible airway of the child to be momentarily forced closed during either inspiration or expiration. This closure obstructs airflow, and the pressure is released; the lumen then springs open. A pattern of intermittent flow creates a pattern of vibrations of the lumen wall that are often strong enough to result in audible sounds. The skilled clinician's ear is trained to recognize both normal respiratory sounds and pathologic adventitious sounds. The common pathologic sounds are well known and include, along with stridor, wheezes, rhonchi, and rales. Acoustic analysis of these pathologic sounds can differentiate them into two basic groups: musical and nonmusical. Most stridorous sounds are musical and are composed of an harmonious frequency and pitch. Stridor is acoustically similar to a wheeze. Rales, on the other hand, are popping, nonmusical sounds.

The narrow diseased portion of the child's

Table 64-1   CAUSES OF STRIDOR AND RESPIRATORY DISTRESS IN CHILDREN
ORIGINATING WITHIN THE UPPER RESPIRATORY TRACT

A. Supralaryngeal

Congenital
Nasal obstruction, e.g., choanal atresia, encephalocele
Macroglossia, e.g., cretinism, lymphangioma, hemangioma
Facial skeletal anomalies — Pierre Robin anomalad
                         cleft palate
                         Treacher-Collins syndrome
                         micrognathia
Facial edema (face presentation)
Congenital cysts — thyroglossal duct
                   dermoid of base of tongue
                   ranula
Lingual thyroid
Pharyngeal tumors, e.g., dermoid (Loeb and Smith, 1967)

Inflammatory
Retropharyngeal abscess
Infectious mononucleosis
Adenotonsillar hypertrophy
Ludwig angina
Severe maxillofacial trauma

Neoplasms
e.g., rhabdomyosarcoma

Neurologic Disease
Subacute sclerosing panencephalitis (Dawson disease)

Postoperative
Tongue obstruction

B. Supraglottic

Congenital Anomalies
Atresia
Web
Laryngomalacia
Cleft larynx — cleft arytenoid
              extensive cleft
Interarytenoid fixation (Cox and Simmons, 1974)
Ventricular band hypertrophy (Cavanaugh, 1965; Bowman and Jackson, 1939)
Bifid epiglottis (Healy et al., 1976)
Internal thyroglossal duct cyst
Cri-du-chat syndrome (Ward et al., 1968)
Cyst of epiglottis (Park and Israel, 1925; Altmeyer and Fechner, 1978)
Saccular cysts — anterior (DeSanto et al., 1970)
              lateral

Inflammatory
Epiglottitis — primary infection
             secondary to trauma
Abscess (Wilson, 1952)

Traumatic
Dislocated arytenoid
Edema — suctioning trauma
        allergic
        inhalation burns
        caustic ingestion
Fracture

Neoplasms
Hemangioma
Lymphangioma
Cystic hygroma
Recurrent respiratory papillomatosis
Chondroma

Table continued on the following page

Table 64–1 CAUSES OF STRIDOR AND RESPIRATORY DISTRESS IN CHILDREN
ORIGINATING WITHIN THE UPPER RESPIRATORY TRACT (*Continued*)

C. Glottic and Subglottic

Congenital
Atresia
Web
Stenosis — soft tissue
Vocal cord paralysis — unilateral
                          bilateral (Arnold-Chiari syndrome)
Cyst — thyroid cartilage foraminal cyst (DeSanto et al., 1970)

Inflammatory
Viral croup
Bacterial laryngotracheitis, including diphtheria
Tuberculosis (Wilson, 1962)
Fungal, e.g., coccidioidomycosis (Ward et al., 1977)
Allergic edema
Epidermolysis bullosa (Cohen et al., 1978e; Ramadass and Thangavelu, 1978)
Exanthemata, e.g., measles, whooping cough (Wilson, 1962)

Neoplasms
Benign — hemangioma
          granular cell myoblastoma (Kenefick, 1978)
          neurofibroma (Cohen et al., 1978f)
          hamartoma
          recurrent respiratory papilloma
Malignant — rhabdomyosarcoma
          lymphomatoid granulomatosis (Cohen et al., 1978b)
          plasmacytoma (Cohen et al., 1978c)
          Wegener granulomatosis (Cohen et al., 1978d)
          lymphosarcoma (Cohen et al., 1978b)
          fibrosarcoma (Rigby and Holinger, 1943)

Neurogenic
Vocal cord paralysis, e.g., syringobulbia (Duffy and Ziter, 1964; Alcala and Dodson, 1975)
Unilateral, e.g., post ductus ligation
                  postintubation (Salem et al., 1971)
Bilateral, e.g., meningomyelocele, hydrocephalus, ventriculoperitoneal
          shunt failure
          arthrogryphosis multiplex congenita (Cohen and Isaacs, 1976)
          hereditary abductor vocal cord paralysis (Gacek, 1976)

Trauma
Foreign body
Intubation — eventration of ventricle
          granulation tissue
          stenosis
          edema
Fracture
Postendoscopy

Miscellaneous
Tetanus
Tetany secondary to hypocalcemia

Table continued on opposite page

Table 64–1 CAUSES OF STRIDOR AND RESPIRATORY DISTRESS IN CHILDREN
ORIGINATING WITHIN THE UPPER RESPIRATORY TRACT *(Continued)*

D. Trachea

Congenital
Agenesis or atresia
Stenosis
    Fibrous strictures—webs (Miller and Morrison, 1978)
               fibrous stenosis of tracheal segments
               stenosis associated with tracheoesophageal fistula
    Absence or deformity of tracheal cartilage (Landing and Wells, 1973)
               tracheomalacia
               cartilage ring abnormalities (segmental malacia)
               calcification of tracheal cartilages (Goldbloom and Dunbar, 1960)
Tracheogenic cysts

Inflammatory
Membranous laryngotracheitis

Neoplastic
Fibrous histiocytoma

Traumatic
Foreign body
Intubation—granulation tissue
            ciliary ring (Lu et al., 1961)
            stenosis
Post-tracheotomy—granuloma, stenosis
Postsurgical—tracheoesophageal fistula repair

Table 64–2 CAUSES OF STRIDOR AND RESPIRATORY DISTRESS IN CHILDREN
ORIGINATING OUTSIDE THE UPPER RESPIRATORY TRACT

Outside Head and Neck

Extrathoracic—acute intra-abdominal catastrophe
             large abdominal mass
Intrathoracic
    Surgical—diaphragmatic hernia, paralysis, or eventration
             congenital lobar emphysema
    Medical—hyaline membrane disease
             aspiration pneumonia
             cardiac abnormality

Inside Head and Neck

Congenital
Vascular compression
Esophageal atresia
Tracheoesophageal fistula
Aberrant thyroid tissue
Congenital goiter
Esophageal reduplication cyst
Cystic hygroma

Inflammatory
Retropharyngeal abscess
Retroesophageal abscess
Retrotracheal lymphadenopathy (Johnson and Groff, 1972)

Trauma
Foreign body in esophagus

Tumors
Benign—plexiform neurofibroma
Malignant—neuroblastoma
             thyroid (Grünebaum, 1973)

airway commences to vibrate and produces a musical sound. The mechanism is analogous to the reed in the mouthpiece of a clarinet. The reed initiates a musical sound of well-defined pitch by means of an oscillating blade. The initial sound produced is then transmitted by the vibrations of the surrounding tissues of the neck or chest. These vibrations can often be easily heard as well as sometimes felt. A parent will often tell you that the child's chest "rattles" when held or touched.

The examining physician must monitor the pitch, duration, and timing of the stridorous sound, just as the conductor of a symphony orchestra must locate a musical note that is off key. Every adventitious sound will have a characteristic pitch, with varying complexity, duration, and location in the respiratory cycle. Clinical observations have shown that the characteristic pitch is primarily dependent on the thickness of the vibrating wall more than its absolute anatomic site (Forgacs, 1967). Virtually all detectable lung sounds are created by the major bronchioles and larger air passages where airflow is great enough to initiate air turbulence with vibrations. The duration of lung sound is a function of respiratory effort to move air along the passage. Anatomically fixed lesions will cause a reproducible sound, but foreign bodies can occasionally migrate and produce evanescent lung sounds that often result in delayed detection.

A symphony conductor divides an orchestra into sections — woodwinds, strings, and brasses — in order to help him or her in the orderly production of a muscial sound. The physician is helped by viewing the respiratory tree as a musical instrument and dividing it into three zones. These include (1) a supraglottic zone (including the pharynx), (2) an extrathoracic tracheal zone (including both glottis and subglottis), and (3) an intrathoracic tracheal zone (including primary and secondary bronchi). Certain zones tend to "play" and cause stridor more often during inspiration and others during expiration. Supraglottic lesions often cause stridor during inspiration, whereas lesions of the intrathoracic trachea or bronchi are aggravated during expiration.

The first zone, which is composed of the supraglottis, tongue, and pharynx, is relatively loosely supported and often falls or is drawn into the airway during inspiration. Inspiration is initiated by the expansion of the thorax, lung tissue, and intrathoracic bronchi. Vigorous inspiratory efforts, particularly when associated with "air hunger" requiring accessory muscle use, create a relative increase in pharyngeal pressure. As air passes through the narrowed diseased supraglottis, there is a combined effect of the Venturi principle and pharyngeal pressures to constrict the airway. Stridor for this zone is generally inspiratory. Expiration has the opposite effect on the supraglottic regions, forcing the airway open.

The second, or extrathoracic trachea, is a neutral zone, affected equally by both inspiration and expiration. The vocal ligament tightly supports the vocal cords between the thyroid and arytenoid cartilages and, in the absence of neural stimulation, is rigid. Similarly, the subglottic region is unyielding because of the cricoid ring. Both the vocal ligament and the subglottis are independent of fluid dynamics such as the Venturi principle. Airflow depends on absolute lumen size, since the airway cannot contract or expand dynamically. When stridor develops in this zone, the glottic and subglottic lumen has reached a critically small size. Stridor produced in this region is often "biphasic," being heard during both inspiration and expiration. Breathing requires tremendous effort to move air through a pinpoint opening, and biphasic stridor often heralds respiratory collapse. Biphasic stridor is a medical emergency that will often require intubation or tracheotomy.

In the third or intrathoracic bronchial zone, expiration commences by the contraction of the thorax. The relative positive pressures of expiratory forces within the chest wall will narrow the bronchial lumen in normal children. As air moves during expiration, the Venturi principle again adds a constricting force. Both forces act jointly to close the lumen against a foreign body or other lesion. The resultant sound is expiratory in phase and less harsh than stridor but retains a musical quality and is often called a wheeze. The term "wheeze" is derived from an old Norse word meaning "to hiss" and by common usage has come to be associated with, but is not restricted to, the hard breathing of asthma.

As a consequence of chronically increased negative pleural pressures during inspiration, retraction of the costal cartilages, sternum, and suprasternal tissues occurs. The degree of retraction is determined by the relative size of negative pleural pressure and the compliance of the rib cage. Young chil-

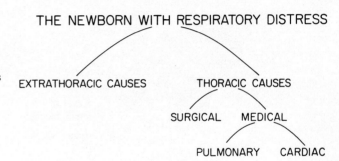

THE NEWBORN WITH RESPIRATORY DISTRESS

Figure 64–1 Causes of respiratory distress in the neonate.

dren have a highly compliant rib cage, and so sternal retraction is particularly marked. If an obstruction is long-standing, as may occur in laryngomalacia, a permanent pectus excavatum may result (Cavanaugh, 1965).

INITIAL HISTORY

Parents, grandparents, nurses in the neonatal unit, or other physicians may be the first to note "noisy respirations." Infants cannot yet verbalize, but their cry is a universal language and should be recognized when it is abnormal. Two points that must be promptly established by the responsible physician are the duration of the stridor and the presence of any respiratory distress. Both points of the initial history must not be confused. Stridor requires a lesion in a region of airflow. Respiratory distress can occur with or without airway obstruction (Chap. 61).

Over two score of nonairway lesions alone can cause respiratory distress in the neonate (Hanley, Braude, and Sweyer, 1963) (Fig. 64–1). Extrathoracic causes of respiratory distress without airway obstruction are intracranial hemorrhage, large abdominal mass, or neuromuscular disease, while intrathoracic examples include diaphragmatic abnormalities, pulmonary cysts, pneumomediastinum and pneumothorax, respiratory distress syndrome, transient tachypnea of the newborn, meconium aspiration, and cardiac abnormalities.

In the absence of severe respiratory distress, a careful history should be obtained. Information regarding time of onset, possible trauma, and characteristics of the cry are obviously important. The relationship of stridor to feeding and possibility of aspiration, reflux, and rumination may indicate that an investigation of the gastrointestinal tract is in order. In the presence of a normal birth history, hereditary congenital anomalies must

be considered. These can be expressed by external deformities, such as craniofacial anomalies, or internal changes, such as webs, cysts, fistulas, atresia, or duplications, all resulting from misdirected embryogenesis. Malformed neural or visceral structures, particularly cardiovascular, can occur in infants with normal external features.

If stridor has been present since birth, then the most likely causes are congenital laryngomalacia, subglottic stenosis, vocal cord paralysis, or a vascular ring. Bilateral vocal cord paralysis is most often seen in children with neurologic abnormalities, including Arnold-Chiari malformation and hydrocephalus, and may not develop until the first month or two of life. As increased intracranial pressure develops, the brain stem is forced through the foramen magnum, stretching the vagus nerves over the jugular foramen (Fig. 64–2).

Questioning is next directed to associated symptoms. Are there feeding difficulties that result in aspiration, cyanosis, regurgitation, or rumination and suggest that the sphincteric mechanism of the laryngeal muscles is malfunctioning or being flooded? This may be due to an incompetent or neurologically impaired cricopharyngeus or esophagus.

In contrast, children with congenital laryngomalacia have less feeding difficulty in the early days of life and make more noise when they are excited and crying. Infants with vascular rings, too, often have feeding problems, and some exhibit reflex apnea; in these episodes, the infant stops breathing for two to three minutes, leading to cyanosis and unconsciousness.

From a clinical point of view, infants with unilateral vocal cord paralysis often show some problems such as coughing and choking on feeding. Three possible causes for this are spasm or dysfunction of the cricopharyngeus muscle, allowing aspiration of fluids through the partially paralyzed larynx; loss of sensation to the superior half of the paralyzed

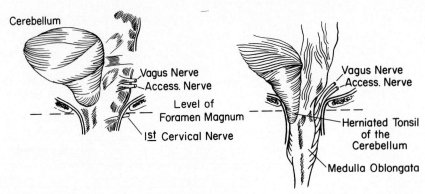

Figure 64–2 Dorsal view of the posterior fossa, foramen magnum, and upper cervical spine: left, normal; right, Arnold-Chiari malformation, showing the upward course of the lower cranial nerves and the pinching effect of the foramen magnum upon the upward coursing nerves.

larynx by superior laryngeal nerve injury; or esophageal atresia, constriction, or fistula. All of these possibilities must be considered.

The stridor of vocal cord paralysis is louder when awake than asleep and may be positional. These infants tend to sleep peacefully on the side of the paralyzed cord when gravity allows the cord to drop away from the midline of the larynx, thus opening the glottis, but they may become noisy and have respiratory distress when placed on the other side. Infants with a congenital saccular cyst (laryngocele) behave similarly.

A history of previous intubation should be carefully sought. Certainly, subglottic stenosis after prolonged intubation of the premature infant may not be apparent for many months after successful extubation. This is due to a combination of the failure of the damaged subglottic area to grow in pace with the child's respiratory needs and a worsening of the cicatricial process as granulation tissue matures into collagen. Minor degrees of obstruction may be quiescent for years and only be expressed by tachypnea and dyspnea when a child participates in strenuous play activities or experiences an upper respiratory infection.

If the onset of stridor is gradual and progressive over weeks or months, neoplastic growth compromising the airway must be considered and investigated. Tumors such as subglottic hemangiomas (Fig. 64–3) appear between one and three months of age, and 85 per cent may appear prior to six months of age. Fifty per cent will have associated skin hemangiomas (Calcaterra, 1968; Leikensohn et al., 1976). Papillomas of the larynx (Fig.

64–4) usually do not become symptomatic before six months of age. A history of maternal venereal condylomata should always be considered in a child gradually developing airway obstruction and voice change in this group. A gradual onset of stridor over weeks or even months can result by compression from a tumor, such as circumtracheal goiter (Fig. 64–5).

No history for stridor would be complete without careful, repeated questioning and a high degree of suspicion for an aspirated foreign body. The time relationship of the stridor may indicate the underlying pathology. Immediate onset of stridor, often accompanied by a choking spell, is strongly suggestive of a foreign body. It is important to realize that severe apnea and aphonia in the infant or child are not only symptoms of a laryngeal foreign body but also of an upper esophageal foreign body. The laryngeal cartilages and trachea are so compressible that airway problems develop rapidly after esophageal obstruction. Figure 64–6 is an anteroposterior view of a child three years of age in whom food has lodged at the site of a previous esophageal repair for tracheoesophageal fistula. On the lateral view (Fig. 64–7), compression of the tracheal air column is clearly evident. Compression of the trachea in both the anteroposterior and lateral views is noticeable in the radiograph of a two year old with a jingle bell in the esophagus (Fig. 64–8). Neonates, for instance, can receive and ingest bells or coins inadvertently fed to them by an older innocent sibling, and this can be undetected for months or years (Banks and Potsic, 1978).

Text continued on page 1200

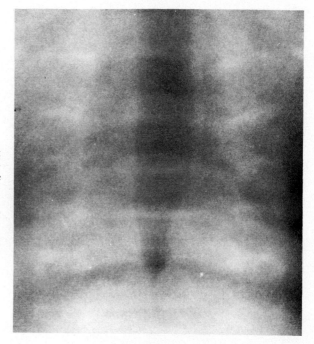

Figure 64–3 Anteroposterior radiograph of neck demonstrating an asymmetric appearance of the subglottic walls, a pathognomonic finding of subglottic hemangioma in an infant.

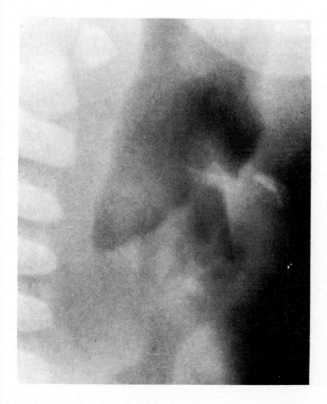

Figure 64–4 Lateral radiograph of neck in recurrent respiratory papillomatosis, demonstrating irregular soft tissue masses in the supraglottic and glottic areas.

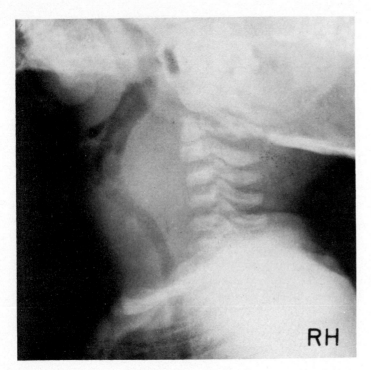

Figure 64–5 Lateral radiograph of neck demonstrating marked forward displacement of the larynx and upper trachea secondary to a circumtracheal goiter.

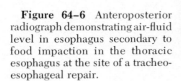

Figure 64–6 Anteroposterior radiograph demonstrating air-fluid level in esophagus secondary to food impaction in the thoracic esophagus at the site of a tracheo-esophageal repair.

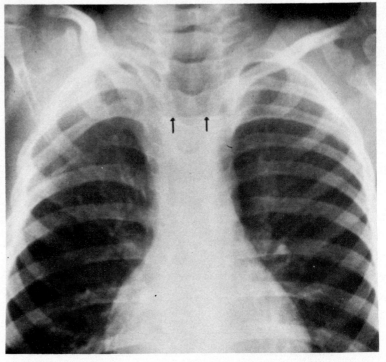

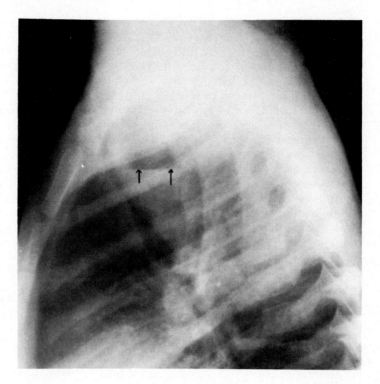

Figure 64–7 Lateral radiograph of the same case described in Figure 64–6. The tracheal lumen is considerably narrowed just below the air-fluid level secondary to the pressure of the esophageal contents.

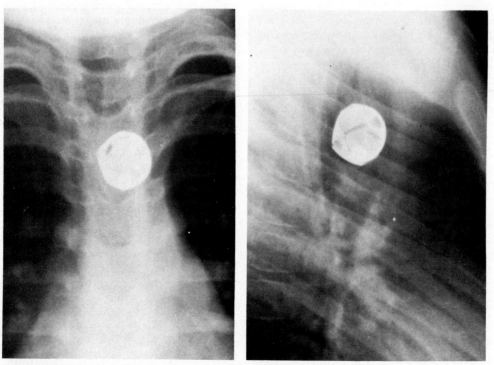

Figure 64–8 Jingle bell in esophagus causing stridor secondary to tracheal compression that is demonstrated in both the anteroposterior and lateral radiographs.

PHYSICAL EXAMINATION

The physical examination must be prompt, thorough, and organized. Careful inspection of the patient is the first priority. The child can remain in the parent's arms, and the physician can judge the respiratory rate and degree of distress. The physician should look for tachypnea or the onset of fatigue that may portend respiratory collapse. The presence of flaring of the nasal alae and the use of accessory neck or chest muscles demonstrates the degree of respiratory effort needed to maintain an oxygenated state. Increasing cyanosis and air hunger, particularly from supraglottic infection or a foreign body, will cause the patient to sit with the neck hyperextended in an attempt to improve airflow. The patient should be permitted to maintain such posture.

In a gravely ill child, additional examination should not be undertaken lest it precipitate respiratory arrest. The child requires prompt transport to an appropriate hospital via an emergency vehicle, accompanied by a physician who is capable of airway management. The hospital can provide two settings for additional examination and care: the emergency room and the operating suite. Resuscitation equipment for intubation of the airway, endoscopic evaluation, and possible tracheotomy must be immediately available, and a team of pediatricians, anesthesiologists, and otolaryngologists capable of airway management should be assembled.

In a well-oxygenated, stable child, additional examination can then proceed. Palpation can be performed gently. The texture of the skin can be noted for swelling or fever. Crepitations in the soft tissues of the face, neck, or chest can suggest subcutaneous emphysema and a tear of the air passage. The laryngeal and tracheal cartilages are noted to be midline and to have proper excursions during deglutition. Cysts and other tumors can often be palpated and any transmitted pulsations or thrills noted. Great caution must be exercised when deciding to palpate into the oral cavity or pharyngeal region, since sudden dislodgement of a foreign body or rupture of an abscessed cavity can aggravate an already compromised airway.

In cases of stridor, the most important part of the examination is auscultation, which is performed both with the ear and with the aid of a stethoscope. The pathologic respiratory condition is manifested through an acoustic signal that must be decoded by the physician. Sequential listening over the nose, open mouth, neck, and chest should be performed to localize its probable site of production by its heightened intensity. The presence or absence of normal breath sounds, in addition to the adventitious sounds, must be analyzed.

Attention is next directed to the respiratory cycle, which normally is composed of a shorter inspiratory phase and a longer expiratory phase. Is the phase prolonged or shortened by an obstruction, and are stridorous sounds present during that phase? Are the sounds monophonic or polyphonic, early or late? The same sound will be heard differently through the neck than through the chest because lung tissue serves as a high-frequency filter (Forgacs, 1978). Thus, in the region of the lower trachea, the pitch of a sound may change, but the musical quality, if present, will prevail and help identify its origin.

The infant should be placed in various positions to determine the effect of this upon the stridor. The stridors of laryngomalacia, micrognathia, macroglossia, and innominate artery compression diminish when the baby lies prone with the neck extended.

However, an aberrant great vessel can compress the airway, depending upon its course around the trachea. In older children, the ability to cough forcefully, as well as the presence or absence of a well-modulated voice, gives an indication of the dynamic state of the larynx.

The art of auscultation has been enhanced by tape recording respiratory sounds, and this has permitted acoustic analysis of children's cries and sounds (Hirschberg, 1980). Sonographic techniques permit classification of stridor into four basic categories based upon acoustic patterns. Distinct patterns of stridor include (1) pharyngeal, (2) laryngeal (the most musical), (3) subglottic, and (4) bronchial. When following chronic respiratory conditions, such data could be used for monitoring possible improvement or regression. It is hoped that with the help of computers, data could be stored and compared to assist physicians in accurate clinical impressions and as an adjunct to endoscopic evaluation.

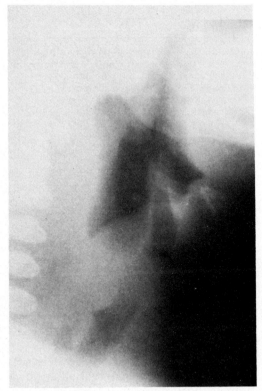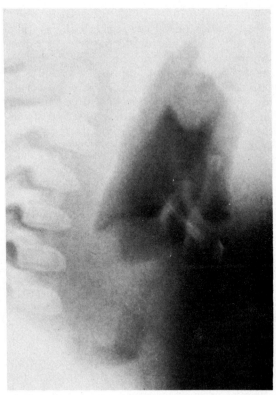

Figure 64–9 Views of neck showing mid-cervical tracheal buckling, a variant of normal. This may occur in normal studies or in association with croup, as in this case.

ROENTGENOGRAPHIC EVALUATION

After a careful history and physical examination, appropriate roentgenographic evaluation of the upper aerodigestive tract is indicated for patients without airway distress. The physician should request plain views of the soft tissues of the neck and chest in the anteroposterior and lateral planes. Fluoroscopy should often be performed to ascertain respiratory effort and segmental ventilation.

The physician should insist on high-quality roentgenograms (Dunbar, 1970). The lateral roentgenograms are particularly important in evaluating the upper respiratory tract in infants and children. A few degrees of rotation about either the coronal or sagittal axes can impair visualization by superimposing normal structures on the air column. Roentgenograms during both inspiration and expiration are particularly important in the infant, since mobile pharyngeal tissues bulge during expiration, mimicking a retropharyngeal abscess or mass. Even cartilaginous structures can buckle, as is seen in the normal trachea of a neonate (Fig. 64–9). If unable to obtain a roentgenogram in true expiration or inspiration, then fluoroscopy is indicated.

In the anteroposterior view, using a high-kilovolt technique, the tracheal air column is enhanced and should reveal a normal right lateral deviation just below the thoracic inlet caused by the presence of the aortic arch. Distortion of the air column to the left or into the midline suggests a right side aortic arch or mediastinal mass.

Examination of the pharynx, esophagus, and stomach with contrast media enables the physician to evaluate motility and rule out encroachment by an anomaly of the great vessels. Proper technique is especially important. Each study must include the oral, pharyngeal, and upper and lower esophageal views. In some departments, there is a tendency to use a catheter to instill the contrast medium into the esophagus; however, this may result in an incomplete study.

If indicated, additional special tests can be obtained. Xeroradiographs give improved visualization of soft tissues and can often demonstrate post-tracheotomy granulomas or subglottic stenosis but result in a higher radiation exposure, and, therefore, they should only be used sparingly. Tomography and angiography are both particularly helpful in evaluating the mediastinum for masses or aberrant vessels. Computerized tomography (CT) with enhancement has improved the art of radiographic evaluation, permitting analysis of both hard and soft tissue structures to within millimeters of size and location.

CLINICAL PHYSIOLOGIC TECHNIQUES

Pulmonary function testing, combined with arterial blood gases, can give an accurate, dynamic analysis of the respiratory state of both the neonate and the older child. Measurement of both inspiratory and expiratory airflow in relation to lung volume by means of a flow-volume loop can assist the physician in localizing obstructions or restrictions of the airway (Frenkiel et al., 1980). Sequential recordings and analysis will be helpful in monitoring functional state in children with chronic airway problems, such as laryngeal papillomatosis, subglottic stenosis, or tracheomalacia.

ENDOSCOPIC EVALUATION

Prior to endoscopy, there is no diagnosis, only impressions. Careful sequential inspection of the pharynx, larynx, trachea, and bronchi provides critical information of lumen size, vocal cord mobility, and the presence of dynamic compression or infection. In no surgical endeavor is cooperation and teamwork between surgeon and anesthesiologist so imperative as in the examination of the upper airway in children. With good teamwork, the responsibility is halved and the safety doubled (Pracy, 1965).

In the neonate in whom stridor is present, laryngoscopy should be performed without general anesthesia. Resuscitation equipment, including a tracheotomy tray, must always be at hand. The operating room is the safest place to perform the examination. Other upper airway endoscopy is usually performed in the operating room under general anesthesia. Atropine (0.02 mg per kg with minimum 0.1 mg) is given prior to induction. This drug suppresses the salivary secretions and

Table 64–3 EXPECTED SUBGLOTTIC SIZE

Age	Diameter—Minimum Internal
0–3 months	3.5 mm
3–9 months	4.0 mm
9–24 months	4.5 mm
2–4 years	5.0 mm
4–6 years	5.5 mm
6–8 years	6.0 mm
8–9 years	6.5 mm
10–12 years	7.0 mm
12–13 years	7.5 mm

(Adapted from Mustafa, S. M. 1976. Variations in subglottic size in children. Proc. R. Soc. Med., 69: 793.)

also the vagal reflexes, minimizing the risk of bradycardia. Slow induction is necessary to saturate the tissues with oxygen, so the surgeon must exhibit patience and vigilance. Lidocaine may be applied topically to the larynx for children over six months of age.

Prior to induction, the surgeon and operating room team must select the proper size bronchoscope and ascertain that all ancillary equipment, including lenses, side arm ventilation, suction tips, and forceps, are functioning properly. Subglottic size must be estimated (Table 64–3).

Laryngoscopy is performed using a straight blade and an open lumen scope. This examination should proceed carefully but promptly. The ventilating bronchoscope is then passed through the glottis under direct vision. The essential observations can then be made. These are (1) measurement of the size of the air passage, especially the subglottis; (2) inspection of anatomic and mucosal contour; and (3) maintenance of a channel to the lungs both to ventilate and for instrumentation to obtain a biopsy specimen, aspirate, and/or remove an obstruction. Based upon the lesion noted and its location, subsequent decisions on the ability and safety to intubate or perform a tracheotomy can be determined.

If the child can be bronchoscoped (critical size is 3.5 mm), then intubation is possible; laryngeal surgery can be performed using a suspension apparatus and microscope. Following intubation, a safe esophagoscopy or nasopharyngoscopy can be performed to rule out masses, foreign bodies, or fistulas. After endoscopic examination is completed, anesthesia is discontinued, and as the level becomes lighter, the laryngoscope can be reintroduced into the vallecula prior to extubation to permit inspection of vocal cord mobility during emergence. This is the last essential step. Active, bilateral movement must be observed. Passive movement and fluttering do not give information on the status of the laryngeal nerves.

With good teamwork between surgeon and anesthesiologist and with gentle instrumentation, edema of the larynx should rarely occur. If this is observed, postendoscopy treatment should include a cool mist tent and vaporized administration of racemic epinephrine for immediate relief. Cortisone can be administered to prevent delayed swelling, and the child should be observed closely for possible reintubation or tracheotomy. The child should remain hospitalized until the airway is stable.

The diagnosis, care, and protection of the child's airway should always be the cardinal concern of the responsible physician. A thorough understanding of respiratory dynamics, airflow, and the presence of abnormal lung sounds such as stridor remains as critical today as in the day of Laennec.

REFERENCES

Alcala, H., and Dodson, W. E. 1975. Syringobulbia as a cause of laryngeal stridor in childhood. Neurology, 25:875.

Altmeyer, V. L., and Fechner, R. E. 1978. Multiple epiglottic cysts. Arch. Otolaryngol., 104:673.

Banks, W., and Potsic, W. 1978. Unsuspected foreign bodies of the aerodigestive tract. Ann. Otol. Rhinol. Laryngol., 87:515–518.

Bowman, J. F., and Jackson, C. L. 1939. Chronic stridor in infancy. J. Pediatr., 15:476.

Calcaterra, T. C. 1968. An evaluation of the treatment of subglottic hemangioma. Laryngoscope, 78:1956.

Cavanaugh, F. 1965. Stridor in children. Proc. R. Soc. Med., 58:272.

Cohen, S. R., and Isaacs, H. 1976. Otolaryngological manifestations of arthrogryposis multiplex congenita. Ann. Otol. Rhinol. Laryngol., 85:484.

Cohen, S. R., Landing, B. H., and Isaacs, H. 1978a. Fibrous histiocytoma of the trachea. Ann. Otol. Rhinol. Laryngol., 87(52):2, 1978a.

Cohen, S. R., Landing, B. H., Siegel, S., et al. 1978b. Lymphatoid granulomatosis in a child with acute lymphatic leukemia in remission. Ann. Otol. Rhinol. Laryngol., 87(52):5.

Cohen, S. R., Landing, B., Isaacs, H., et al. 1978c. Solitary plasmacytoma of the larynx and upper trachea associated with systemic lupus erythematosus. Ann. Otol. Rhinol. Laryngol., 87(52):11.

Cohen, S. R., Landing, B. H., King, K. K., and Isaacs, H. 1978d. Wegener's granulomatosis causing laryngeal

and tracheobronchial obstruction in an adolescent girl. Ann. Otol. Rhinol. Laryngol., 87(52):15.

Cohen, S. R., Landing, B. H., and Isaacs, H. 1978e. Epidermolysis bullosa associated with laryngeal stenosis. Ann. Otol. Rhinol. Laryngol., 87(52):25.

Cohen, S. R., Landing, B. H., and Isaacs, H. 1978f. Neurofibroma of the larynx in a child. Ann. Otol. Rhinol. Laryngol., 87(52):29.

Cox, D. J., and Simmons, B. F. 1974. Midline vocal cord fixation in the newborn child. Arch. Otolaryngol., 100:219.

DeSanto, L. W., Devine, K. D., and Weiland, L. H. 1970. Cysts of the larynx: Classification. Laryngoscope, 80:145.

Duffy, P. E., and Ziter, F. A. 1964. Infantile syringobulbia. Neurology, 14:500.

Dunbar, J. S. 1970. Upper respiratory tract obstruction in infants and children. Am. J. Roentgenol., 109:227.

Forgacs, P. 1967. "Crackles and wheezes." Lancet, 2:203.

Forgacs, P. 1978. Lung Sounds. London, Balliere Tindall, pp. 12, 21–22.

Frenkiel, S., Desmond, K., Coates, A., et al. 1980. Upper airway obstruction in children. J. Otolaryngol., 9(1):7–11.

Gacek, R. R. 1976. Hereditary abductor vocal cord paralysis. Ann. Otol. Rhinol. Laryngol., 85:90.

Goldbloom, R. B., and Dunbar, J. S. 1960. Calcification of cartilage in the trachea and larynx in infancy associated with congenital stridor. Pediatrics, 23:669.

Grünebaum, M. 1973. Respiratory stridor — a challenge for the paediatric radiologist. Clin. Radiol., 24:485.

Hanley, W., Braude, M., and Sweyer, M. 1963. Neonatal respiratory distress. Can. Med. Assoc. J., 89:375–381.

Healy, G. B., Holt, G. P., and Tucker, J. A. 1976. Bifid epiglottis: A rare laryngeal anomaly. Laryngoscope, 86:1459.

Hirschberg, J. 1980. Acoustical analysis of pathological cries, stridor, and coughing sounds in infancy. Int. J. Pediatr. Otorhinolaryngol., 2:287–300.

Johnson, R. G., and Groff, D. B. 1972. Tracheal obstruction by a solitary lymph node. J. Pediatr. Surg., 7:440.

Kenefick, C. 1978. Granular cell myoblastoma of the larynx. J. Laryngol. Otol., 92:521.

Landing, B. H., and Wells, T. R. 1973. Tracheobronchial anomalies in children. Perspect. Pediatr. Pathol., 1:1.

Leikensohn, J. R., Benton, C., and Cotton, R. 1976. Subglottic hemangioma. J. Otolaryngol., 5(6):487.

Loeb, W. J., and Smith, E. E. Airway obstruction in a newborn by pedunculated pharyngeal dermoid. Pediatrics, 40:20.

Lu, A. T., Tamura, Y., and Koobs, D. H. 1961. The pathology of laryngotracheal complications. Arch. Otolaryngol., 74:323.

Miller, B. J., and Morrison, M. D. 1978. Congenital tracheal web — a case report. J. Otolaryngol., 7:218.

Mustafa, S. M. 1976. Variation in subglottic size in children. Proc. R. Soc. Med., 69:793.

Park, J. H., and Israel, S. 1925. Epiglottic cysts in infancy. South. Med. J., 18:128.

Pracy, R. 1965. Stridor in children. Proc. R. Soc. Med., 58:267.

Ramadass, T., and Thangavelu, T. A. 1978. Epidermolysis bullosa and its E.N.T. manifestations. J. Laryngol. Otol., *92*:441.

Rigby, R. G., and Holinger, P. H. 1943. Fibrosarcoma of the larynx. Arch. Otolaryngol., *37*:425.

Salem, M. R., Wong, A. Y., Barangan, V. C., et al. 1971. Vocal cord paralysis after intubation. Br. J. Anaesth., *43*:696.

Schroter, R. C., and Sudlow, M. F. 1969. Flow patterns in models of the human bronchial airways. Resp. Physiol., *7*:341.

Ward, P. H., Engel, E., and Nance, W. E. 1968. The larynx in the cri du chat syndrome. Laryngoscope, *78*:1716.

Ward, P. H., Berci, G., Morledge, D., and Schwartz, H. 1977. Coccidioidomycosis of the larynx in infants and adults. Ann. Otol. Rhinol. Laryngol., *86*:655.

Wilson, T. G. 1952. Discussion on stridor in infants. Proc. R. Soc. Med., *45*:355.

Wilson, T. G. 1962. Diseases of the Ear, Nose and Throat in Children. London, Heinemann, p. 259.

Chapter 65

RESPIRATORY DISORDERS OF THE NEWBORN

I. David Todres, M.D.

INTRODUCTION

Recently great advances have been made in the recognition and treatment of respiratory disorders in the newborn (Avery and Fletcher, 1974). Pediatric otolaryngologists have become active participants in the management of such children when endoscopy or tracheostomy becomes necessary or in dealing with the complications of respiratory therapy, such as laryngeal and tracheal granulations due to prolonged endotracheal intubation. A number of infants who present to the otolaryngologist with severe and recurrent otitis media have underlying chronic pulmonary disease that has its origin in the newborn period. Thus, a concise review of the current management of respiratory disorders in newborns should be useful background information for physicians confronted by children with these problems. We will begin our discussion with a review of the physiology of fetal and neonatal lungs as a first step toward understanding the pathologic conditions with which these structures may present.

PATHOPHYSIOLOGY

In fetal life the airways and terminal air spaces of the lung are filled with a liquid produced by the lung and containing surface-active lipoproteins. Gaseous exchange (uptake of oxygen and elimination of carbon dioxide) is carried out via the placenta. A small fraction (4 to 7 per cent) of the cardiac output perfuses the lungs. At birth, pulmonary vascular resistance decreases, the ductus arteriosus and foramen ovale close, and the total cardiac output perfuses the lungs, making independent extrauterine life possible.

At birth, pressures as high as 70 cm of H_2O may be necessary to initiate the introduction of air into the airless lung. After the first few breaths, inflation pressures are considerably less. The fluid in the lung is rapidly cleared during the process of delivery and by the pulmonary circulation and lymphatics. When terminal air spaces have been completely filled with air, they maintain their state through the presence of a phospholipid surface-active material known as surfactant. Only very small amounts of this material are produced before 35 weeks gestation, and production may be inhibited at any time by hypothermia, hypoxia, and acidosis.

ACUTE DISORDERS

Hyaline Membrane Disease

The most common form of respiratory distress in the newborn is hyaline membrane disease (HMD), also referred to as respiratory distress syndrome (RDS). The condition is more common in premature infants and is a significant cause of mortality and morbidity — 10,000 deaths per year occur in the United States (Wood and Farrell, 1974).

Pathophysiology

Hyaline membrane disease is the result of surfactant deficiency (Farrell and Avery,

1205

1975). Surfactant prevents the collapse of the alveoli at the end of expiration, and when surfactant is absent alveolar collapse results in intrapulmonary shunting and hypoxemia, which may progress in severe cases to death. In addition, pulmonary vasoconstriction occurs as a result of the hypoxemia, hypercarbia, and acidosis and leads to an increase in pulmonary vascular resistance, which in turn allows increased shunting of blood from right to left via the ductus arteriosus and foramen ovale. Hypoxemia increases and acidosis produces myocardial depression.

Clinical Presentation

The infant with hyaline membrane disease is usually premature and is distressed at birth or shortly thereafter with rapid respirations, retractions, and an audible grunt. The infant is also cyanotic when breathing room air. The grunt is a partial Valsalva maneuver and helps to maintain a positive end expiratory pressure of ± 3 cm of H_2O at the alveoli to prevent their collapse. The condition may rapidly worsen and commonly peaks at 48 hours of life. Hypovolemia frequently complicates the clinical condition.

Radiographic Findings

Air bronchograms show a characteristic diffuse reticulogranular pattern in both lung fields (Fig. 65–1).

Treatment

The primary goal of therapy is to relieve the hypoxemia. Oxygen is given to maintain an arterial Po_2 of 55 to 75 mm Hg. Oxygen is usually provided initially via an oxygen hood, but with worsening of the disease and increasing hypoxemia, adequate blood oxygen levels may be maintained only through the use of continuous positive airway pressure (CPAP) via nasal prongs (catheters) or an endotracheal tube (Gregory et al., 1971). Should the infant's ventilatory efforts decrease in effectiveness to the point where carbon dioxide accumulation occurs (Pco_2 >60 mm Hg), then mechanical ventilation is necessary. An endotracheal tube must be passed to permit mechanical ventilation; it may be placed either nasally or orally, although it is frequently passed orally because it is relatively easier to insert through the mouth. The tube should be securely taped in

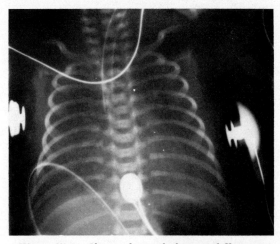

Figure 65–1 Chest radiograph showing diffuse granular opacification throughout both lung fields with air bronchograms bilaterally (hyaline membrane disease).

position, and movements of the infant's head should be limited to prevent displacement of the distal end of the tube, either into a mainstem bronchus (with head flexion) or possible extubation (with head extension) (Fig. 65–2). In most premature infants a 3.0 mm internal diameter tube may be passed, but for very low birth weight (less than 1000 to 1250 gm) infants a 2.5 mm endotracheal tube may be necessary. Full-term infants usually require a 3.5 mm tube. Suctioning for secretions must be carried out expeditiously to avoid increasing the hypoxemia, and the caretakers must be constantly on the alert for possible blockage of the endotracheal tube, a potentially lethal complication. Adequate humidification of air and suctioning of secretions should prevent tube obstruction. New models of mechanical respirators can provide the necessary amount of artificial ventilation while allowing the infant's spontaneous ventilations to continue unimpeded. In the severe forms of hyaline membrane disease in which the lungs have extremely low compliance, it is best to block out the inadequate spontaneous ventilatory efforts altogether with neuromuscular blocking agents, such as curare and pancuronium, and to rely totally upon mechanical ventilation.

Besides respiratory support of the infant with hyaline membrane disease, the physician must pay attention to the patient's hemodynamic status. Hypovolemia is frequently associated with respiratory distress and should be corrected with blood or colloid infusions. Other supportive measures are also essential:

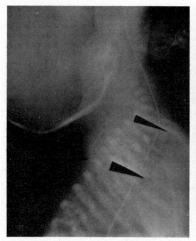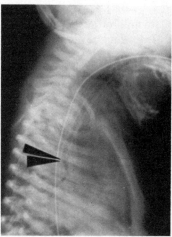

Figure 65–2 Relationship of the distal end of the endotracheal tube (upper arrow) to the carina (lower arrow) when the head is extended (left) and flexed (right).

maintenance of normal body temperature and of electrolyte balance, maintaining normal blood sugar, calcium ion concentration, total proteins, and optimal nutritional support.

Complications

Air Leaks and Pneumothorax. Leakage of air into the interstitium (emphysema) (Fig. 65–3) and pneumothorax occur predominantly when the infant is ventilated mechanically, and any sudden worsening in the infant's condition should suggest the possibility that this complication has occurred. The condition may occasionally be associated with a pneumopericardium. A tension pneumothorax is an emergency and must be diagnosed

rapidly and treated by insertion of a chest tube connected to an underwater seal (Fig. 65–4).

Persistent Patent Ductus Arteriosus (PDA). A persistent PDA frequently complicates the condition of the premature infant with hyaline membrane disease. It may cause congestive heart failure and delay the infant's weaning from the respirator. Many infants respond to medical therapy with digitalis, diuretics, and fluid restriction, but should this fail after an adequate trial, surgical ligation is necessary. Recently the use of indomethacin, a prostaglandin inhibitor that allows closure of the ductus, has proved to be successful in a significant number of infants, thus averting

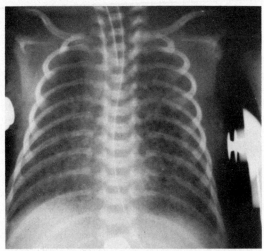

Figure 65–3 Chest radiograph of an infant with hyaline membrane disease showing multiple rounded lucencies, representing interstitial air, throughout both lung fields.

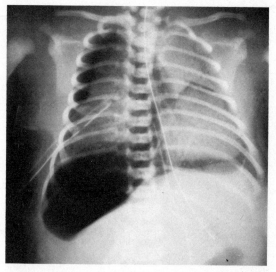

Figure 65–4 Infant with severe hyaline membrane disease who developed a massive tension pneumothorax on the right, shifting the heart to the left and depressing the right hemidiaphragm.

the need for surgical closure of the defect (Heyman et al., 1976).

Intraventricular Hemorrhage. Hemorrhage into the ventricles is frequently a lethal complication, particularly with very low birth weight infants. In fact, it is probably the most significant cause of morbidity and mortality in infants with hyaline membrane disease. Such a hemorrhage usually occurs on the third or fourth day of life and is heralded by apnea, bradycardia, cardiovascular collapse, or seizures. Computerized axial tomography (CAT scan) helps to define the extent of the hemorrhage and its possible long-term effects.

Bronchopulmonary Dysplasia (BPD). While most infants now recover fully from hyaline membrane disease, some later develop chronic lung changes termed bronchopulmonary dysplasia (Northway et al., 1967). Usually BPD occurs in infants who have required respiratory support for prolonged periods and especially when the oxygen concentration provided was high (more than 60 per cent oxygen). Pneumothorax has been correlated with an increased incidence of bronchopulmonary dysplasia, and a reduction in the incidence of BPD has been reported when inspiratory pressures delivered to the infant have been reduced. Bronchopulmonary dysplasia may progress to the point where the infant develops right heart failure (cor pulmonale) (Fig. 65–5).

Endotracheal Tube Complications. Endotracheal intubation in some infants produces significant trauma to the glottis and subglottic areas. When trauma is prolonged, granulomas may occur on or at the level of the vocal cords. In the subglottic area, ischemia and necrosis from compression may result in scarring with resultant subglottic stenosis, which may be minimized by the use of endotracheal tubes that are specially tested (I.T. and Z79 standards). Rubber endotracheal tubes are particularly notorious for causing damage to the mucosa, so that the tube material should be chosen with care. In addition, and most importantly, tubes should not fit too tightly; a slight leak is optimal. Nasotracheal intubation may be associated with ischemia and necrosis of the nares and in some cases the nasal septum with subsequent loss of the septal cartilage.

Prevention

Recent developments in the prevention of hyaline membrane disease include the use of biochemical tests (lecithin/sphingomyelin ratios) and foam stability tests on amnionic fluid to assess the degree of maturity of the fetus's lungs and thus the likelihood of hyaline membrane disease developing should the infant be delivered. The use of glucocorticoids in the pregnant mother for a period of 24 hours prior to delivery has been shown to reduce significantly the incidence of hyaline membrane disease in infants under 32 weeks gestation.

Transient Tachypnea of the Newborn

Newborns who show signs of transient tachypnea are usually full-term and begin to evidence tachypnea shortly after birth. Retractions are minimal, and although the infant may show some hypoxemia, alveolar ventilation is adequate as reflected by a normal P_{CO_2}. The course of this disorder is benign, with recovery occurring in 36 to 48 hours. Transient tachypnea is thought to be due to a delay in resorption of fetal lung fluid. Chest radiographs of these infants show ill-defined vascular markings and the presence of interstitial fluid. The lungs clear rapidly, however, and radiographs taken a few days to a week later show that the lungs have returned to normal. This condition must be differentiated from milder cases of hyaline membrane disease.

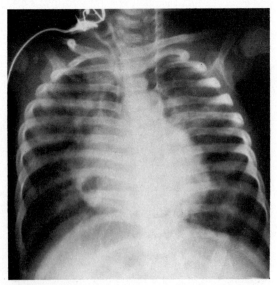

Figure 65–5 Chest radiograph showing alternating areas of collapse and hyperaeration within overall increased lung volumes.

Persistent Fetal Circulation

Increasingly, newborns with respiratory distress and cyanosis have been shown to have persistent fetal circulation. When infants undergo cardiac catheterization because of the possibility of underlying cyanotic heart disease, elevated pulmonary artery pressures and persistence of the fetal circulation (in the form of a patent ductus arteriosus and patent foramen ovale) are found. The condition may rapidly worsen with increasing hypoxemia and acidosis and may be fatal, or it may spontaneously correct itself within a few days. Recently, infusion of tolazoline (Priscoline), an alpha-adrenergic blocking agent that causes dilatation of the pulmonary vascular bed and promotes perfusion of the lungs and thus correction of the hypoxemia, has been found to be life-saving in some infants.

Aspiration Syndromes: Meconium Aspiration

Aspiration is a common cause of respiratory distress in the newborn. Postnatal aspiration of regurgitated feedings of dextrose water or milk is a potentially lethal complication, especially in the premature infant. Meconium aspiration is a significant cause of morbidity and mortality and will be described in more detail.

Aspiration of meconium *in utero* may result when a period of fetal asphyxia leads to the passage of meconium. Fetal overmaturity is frequently associated with aspiration. Along with the meconium, keratinized squamous cells and vernix may be aspirated into the terminal airways, resulting not only in intrapulmonary shunting but also in right-to-left shunting via the ductus arteriosus and foramen ovale, which leads to hypoxemia. The aspirated, inspissated plugs act like ball valves, allowing air to enter some alveoli and trapping it there. Air leaks and pneumothorax are thus common complications of this syndrome.

Clinical Presentation

The infant who has aspirated meconium is often in acute distress with tachypnea, retractions, and cyanosis evident, although the physical signs depend on the extent of the aspiration. The chest may appear to be hyperinflated, and rales and rhonchi are usually heard. Pneumothorax and pneumomediastinum may complicate the clinical picture.

Radiographic Findings

Coarse, irregular densities may be seen throughout both lung fields on chest radiographs, as may areas of hyperinflation or a flattened diaphragm. Clinical recovery usually occurs before resolution of the radiographic abnormalities, although air trapping may persist for months.

Treatment

Pharyngeal suctioning as the infant is delivered and before the first breath is taken significantly reduces the incidence of severe meconium aspiration. When particulate meconium is present at delivery the infant should be intubated and suctioned to prevent the possibly disastrous sequelae of aspiration. Oxygen, often high in concentration, is required to correct hypoxemia, and if respiratory distress is severe, as judged by clinical examination and arterial blood gas values, mechanical ventilation may be necessary.

Prognosis

The majority of infants suffering from aspiration syndromes recover in a few days. However, some infants may suffer severe cerebral hypoxemia with resulting morbidity and possibly death. In addition, complications of pneumomediastinum and pneumothorax are common; pneumonitis and septicemia may occur and require vigorous antibiotic therapy.

Pneumonia

Pneumonia is a significant cause of perinatal death. It may be acquired *in utero,* during labor or delivery, or after birth. Pneumonia is likely with infection of fetal membranes as a result of their prolonged rupture prior to delivery, usually more than 24 hours. Infection may also be blood-borne across the placenta.

Group B Streptococcal Infection

Infection with Group B streptococcus is becoming increasingly recognized as an important cause of mortality in the newborn. The disease may be clinically indistinguishable from hyaline membrane disease, and the physician must be alert for the possibility of infection to identify it early. Cultures from the mother's genital tract may reveal the organism and indicate the need for aggressive antibiotic therapy in the infant. Group B streptococci are susceptible to penicillin.

The infant with pneumonia is often depressed at birth. Respirations, once established, are rapid and associated with retractions. Fever may be absent. The classical physical chest signs of the adult are often absent, and the white blood cell count may be abnormally low, although in the majority of infants it is within the normal range. Blood cultures may be positive for infectious organisms. In severe cases, the infant may go into heart failure. Pneumonia is frequently associated with septicemia and should be suspected when the amnionic fluid is purulent or foul-smelling. A history of fever in the mother around the time of delivery, possibly due to amnionitis, should lead one to suspect that the infant may have pneumonia and septicemia. The organisms involved are most frequently *Pseudomonas aeruginosa, Aerobacter, Klebsiella, Streptococci,* and *Escherichia coli.*

Nursery-Acquired Pneumonias

The organisms that are usually found to cause nursery-acquired pneumonia include coagulase-positive staphylococci and Group A streptococci, although *E. coli* may also be responsible. The umbilical cord stump is often the primary site of infection. Staphylococcal infection is becoming more prevalent since soaps containing hexachlorophene used in the past to control staphylococcal outbreaks have been largely discontinued because of their potential neurotoxic properties. Staphylococcal pneumonia in the newborn may cause consolidation of a lobe or may involve both lungs diffusely. Pleural effusions and empyema may complicate the disease, and characteristically pneumatoceles appear, which may rupture to produce pneumothorax. The pneumonia may be associated with other staphylococcal infections that cause concomitant meningitis, osteomyelitis, or pericarditis. Oxacillin is the drug of choice for treating staphylococcal pneumonia, and it must be administered for at least 14 days to be effective. In addition, any abscesses present must be drained surgically in order to effect complete recovery.

The use of humidifiers and mechanical ventilators has been responsible for an increasing number of infections due to gram-negative organisms, *P. aeruginosa* and *Klebsiella.* In a compromised host they may cause acute and fulminating pneumonia but are often associated with chronic, low-grade infections. Other less common organisms that cause pneumonia in the newborn include the viruses, for example, the parainfluenza group. Rarely, pneumonia may be due to cytomegalic inclusion disease, toxoplasma, or congenital syphilis.

Atelectasis

Atelectasis is incomplete expansion of a lung or a portion of the lung and may be the result either of failure of the lung to expand or of collapse of a lung or a portion thereof that was previously expanded. Inadequate respiratory efforts in the newborn as a result of central nervous system depression or infection may be associated with incomplete lung expansion. Atelectasis may result from the inhalation of particulate amnionic fluid or mucous plugs that block the airways and prevent further air entry; when the distal air is absorbed the lung collapses. An entire lung, or a lobe, or multiple small areas of both lungs may collapse. Malpositioning of endotracheal tubes may cause collapse — not infrequently, the distal end of the tube may enter the right mainstem bronchus, resulting in collapse of the left lung and possibly of the right upper lobe. Deficiency of surfactant associated with hyaline membrane disease leads to atelectasis.

Diagnosis

The degree of clinical respiratory distress will depend upon the extent of the atelectasis. In addition, the collapse may be secondary to the existence of other pathologic conditions that are significant, such as pneumothorax. Clinically, atelectasis should be suspected in any distressed infant when inadequate chest excursion occurs with the heart shifted towards the side of the collapse. A chest radiograph will confirm the diagnosis. Atelectasis may be difficult to differentiate at times from pneumonia, but sequential chest films will often help to distinguish the two.

Treatment

Treatment of atelectasis is aimed at removing the cause of the problem, such as mucous plugs, by vigorous suctioning and physiotherapy or by correcting a malpositioned endotracheal tube.

Pulmonary Hemorrhage

Pulmonary hemorrhage is mostly seen as a complication of a generalized process, such as sepsis, pneumonia, hemolytic disease of the newborn, intracranial hemorrhage, or congenital heart disease. Rarely it appears as an isolated event. It may be associated with a generalized bleeding disorder or with disseminated intravascular coagulation. The infant may present with the sudden onset of severe respiratory distress associated with severe hypoxemia, and fresh blood may be suctioned from the trachea. Mechanical ventilation is often necessary, and the trachea may require frequent suctioning. The prognosis is usually grave. Underlying coagulation disorders should be sought for and actively treated, as should possible sepsis.

Lobar Emphysema

Lobar emphysema is characterized by emphysematous expansion of one lobe of the lung. The disease usually involves the upper lobes. Pathologically, the lobe may be overinflated with normal development of airways and alveoli. In some infants the numbers of alveoli and airways are diminished. Deficient cartilage has been found in some instances.

Clinical Presentation

Dyspnea and cyanosis associated with lobar emphysema appear most frequently between one week and one month of age. However, symptoms may occur at birth. On examination the infant is distressed, with chest retractions and the heart and mediastinum displaced away from the hyper-resonant side. A chest radiograph will show a hyperinflated lobe, usually the upper or right middle one (Fig. 65–6), with adjacent lobes collapsed.

Treatment

If the infant is in severe respiratory distress, surgical resection of the lung lobe is

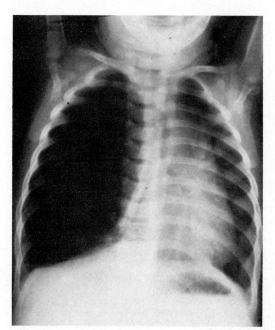

Figure 65–6 Infant with massive hyperinflation of the right upper lobe (lobar emphysema) compressing the right middle and lower lobes. Note shift of the mediastinum into the left chest.

necessary. Infants who are not in such distress should be carefully observed in an intensive care unit, as the lobar emphysema may spontaneously resolve.

Pulmonary Cysts

Pulmonary cysts may be congenital or acquired. They may exist singly or in groups and are significant in that they may become infected or enlarged with air or fluid to produce tension and compromise cardiac and pulmonary functions. The infant may be tachypneic from birth, and dyspnea may progress rapidly with tension.

On the chest radiograph the appearance of a pulmonary cyst under tension may simulate a pneumothorax. Multiple cysts may be congenital or may represent acquired emphysematous bullae. They may simulate a diaphragmatic hernia, in which case a barium swallow may be helpful in differentiating the two. Often pulmonary cysts are asymptomatic and are discovered only on a routine chest radiograph.

Most lung cysts will regress spontaneously, but if tension develops in the cyst, surgical exploration and excision are necessary.

With repeated infections that are unresponsive to antibiotic therapy, a lobectomy or pneumonectomy may be indicated.

Pneumothorax

A pneumothorax in the newborn is not uncommon. Its importance lies in its potential for becoming rapidly life-threatening. This condition is frequently the result of face mask and bag resuscitation or of mechanical ventilation associated with excessive pressures, but is also seen in infants whose ventilation has never been assisted. It is particularly common when particulate meconium has been aspirated, plugging the terminal airways and trapping air.

Clinical Presentation

The symptoms of pneumothorax may vary from none at all to severe distress with tachypnea, retractions, and cyanosis. The chest on the affected side may be seen to move less and on auscultation may be heard to have diminished breath sounds. However, it is important to appreciate that breath sounds are easily transmitted in the newborn so that auscultation may be misleading. The point of maximal cardiac impulse is shifted to the opposite side.

Diagnosis and Treatment

If the infant is seriously distressed with increasing hypoxemia and cardiovascular collapse, bradycardia, and hypotension, then *urgent* aspiration of the pneumothorax is essential. This diagnosis must always be suspected in any newborn with respiratory distress, and the pneumothorax should be relieved by aspiration with a needle placed at the level of the third interspace–anterior axillary line *before* confirmation by chest radiograph is obtained if the condition of the infant is critical. Although a chest radiograph is confirmatory of the diagnosis, one cannot always be obtained at a moment's notice; a newly developed technique of fiberoptic illumination of the chest may prove helpful as an aid to diagnosis in these situations. Although aspiration may be adequate to relieve the infant in an emergency situation, the air may reaccumulate, particularly if the infant requires mechanical ventilation. In this situation a chest tube should be placed to an underwater seal. Sometimes high concentra-

tions of oxygen may be administered to accelerate the resolution of a pneumothorax, on the theory that the oxygen replaces nitrogen that accumulated in the pleural space. However, this approach should be used only when the pneumothorax does not compromise the infant's condition.

Congenital Diaphragmatic Hernia

In a diaphragmatic hernia, the abdominal viscera herniate into the thoracic cavity above one or both diaphragms. The incidence of this disorder is about one in 3000 live births. It is a significant cause of respiratory distress in the newborn and one of the most urgent emergency problems encountered in the neonate. Most commonly, the diaphragmatic hernia arises as a result of incomplete closure of the foramen of Bochdalek situated posterolaterally in the diaphragm. The disorder has high morbidity and mortality rates.

Diagnosis

Most commonly the infant with a diaphragmatic hernia is in severe respiratory distress from birth. The degree of distress depends upon the volume of the abdominal viscera that have herniated into the chest. On occasion, respiratory distress may not appear until some hours or even days after birth.

Physical Examination

The infant may be cyanosed and in severe distress. The abdomen is scaphoid. The heart is significantly displaced to the opposite side, and the adjacent lung is severely atelectatic and usually hypoplastic.

A chest radiograph will confirm the diagnosis (Fig. 65–7).

Treatment

A diaphragmatic hernia should be suspected in any infant in respiratory distress. Once the condition is diagnosed, a nasogastric tube should be inserted to decompress the stomach and prevent further distress. The hernia is then corrected by emergency surgery.

Prognosis

Those infants presenting in significant distress in the first 24 hours after birth have a

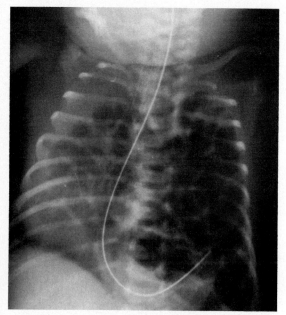

Figure 65–7 Multiple rounded lucencies within the left hemithorax with shift of the mediastinum into the right chest are notable.

high mortality rate: approximately 50 per cent. In those presenting after the first 24 hours, the prognosis is considerably better, with more than 90 per cent surviving. Survival also depends on other factors, such as early diagnosis, operative repair, degree of lung hypoplasia, associated congenital abnormalities, and postoperative intensive care management. Pneumothorax is a frequent occurrence postoperatively and is often unsuspected when it occurs on the contralateral side. A significant number of infants are hypoxemic postoperatively and develop high pulmonary-vascular resistance with right-to-left shunting through the foramen ovale and ductus arteriosus. Recently, the use of tolazoline (Priscoline) to dilate the pulmonary vascular bed and improve oxygenation has been life-saving.

Diaphragmatic Paralysis

A paralyzed diaphragm may be asymptomatic, or the infant may present with tachypnea and possibly cyanosis. The paralysis is most frequently right-sided and mostly associated with Erb palsy following a difficult breech extraction.

A chest radiograph may show an elevated diaphragm with basal atelectasis, which may become infected. Fluoroscopy will confirm the diagnosis, showing paradoxical movement of the affected diaphragm — elevation on inspiration and descent on expiration. A large number of infants recover spontaneously over a period of weeks to months, but the chances for complete recovery depend on the extent of the injury. Where symptoms persist with no evidence of improvement over a period of months, surgical plication is indicated.

Apnea

Apnea is frequently seen in the premature infant and is of significance when the cessation of respiration lasts more than 20 seconds or when there is a pause of any duration associated with cyanosis, bradycardia (heart rate less than 100 beats per minute), or both. Periodic breathing consists of regular clusters of 4 to 10 breaths followed by an apneic interval of up to 12 seconds in duration and not associated with cyanosis or bradycardia.

Etiology

The causes of apnea are multiple and include prematurity with or without hyaline membrane disease, infection, hypoxemia, hypothermia and hyperthermia, intracranial hemorrhage, and obstruction of the upper airway.

Management

The underlying cause of the apnea should be sought and treated. The infant is placed on an apnea monitoring device, and initially tactile stimulation is applied when the infant becomes apneic. If the episodes of apnea are frequent and do not readily respond to tactile stimulation, theophylline is administered (Shannon et al., 1975). Occasionally, mechanical ventilation is required.

CHRONIC RESPIRATORY DISORDERS

Bronchopulmonary Dysplasia (BPD)

Bronchopulmonary dysplasia may develop in low birth weight infants with a history of hyaline membrane disease who required high concentrations of oxygen and mechanical ventilatory support for prolonged periods. The infants are chronically ill and dependent on oxygen and intermittent ventilatory support. A radiograph of such a child's chest shows lung marking with areas of radiolucency or areas of atelectasis alternating with areas of hyperinflation. The etiology of BPD is not fully understood, although prolonged periods of breathing high concentrations of oxygen and the use of mechanical ventilation seen to be underlying factors. Reduction in inspiratory pressures associated with mechanical ventilation has been shown to reduce the incidence of BPD. Right heart failure may develop in severe cases.

Infants with this disorder require supplemental oxygen. Administration of diuretics and fluid restriction are necessary to control interstitial pulmonary edema. Under these conditions it is extremely difficult to provide sufficient caloric intake.

Mikity-Wilson Syndrome

The Mikity-Wilson syndrome occurs more frequently in very low birth weight infants. Often the infants have no respiratory distress at birth or during the first weeks of life but then insidiously develop tachypnea and possibly cyanosis in room air. These symptoms increase over a period of weeks and persist for several months. Striking oxygen dependence is noted. Occasionally, rales and wheezing are present. Lung compliance is reduced, and airway resistance is high. Hypoxemia and CO_2 retention occur. Cor pulmonale may develop later in the course of this disease.

When a child with Mikity-Wilson syndrome is examined radiographically, a bilateral, coarse, streaky infiltrate may be seen, which initially develops into cystic lesions. These lesions then enlarge and coalesce. Resolution of the lesions lags behind clinical improvement and may take years.

SELECTED REFERENCE

Avery, M. E., and Fletcher, B. D. 1974. The Lung and Its Disorders in the Newborn Infant, 3rd ed. Philadelphia, W. B. Saunders Co.
   Excellent general outline with good illustrations written by authorities on the subject.

REFERENCES

Avery, M. E., and Fletcher, B. D. 1974. The Lung and Its Disorders in the Newborn Infant, 3rd ed. Philadelphia, W. B. Saunders Co.

Farrel, P. M., and Avery, M. E. 1975. Hyaline membrane disease. Am. Rev. Respir. Dis., *111*:657.

Gregory, G. S., Kitterman, J. A., Phibbs, R. H., et al. 1971. Treatment of the idiopathic respiratory distress syndrome with continuous positive airway pressure. N. Engl. J. Med., *284*:1333.

Heyman, M. A., Rudolph, A. M., and Silverman, N. H. 1976. Closure of the ductus arteriosus in premature infants by inhibition of prostaglandin synthesis. N. Engl. J. Med., *294*:530.

Northway, W. H., Rosen, R. C., and Porter, D. Y. 1967. Pulmonary disease following respiratory therapy of hyaline membrane disease — bronchopulmonary dysplasia. N. Engl. J. Med., *276*:357.

Shannon, D. C., Gotay, F., Stein, I. M., et al. 1975. Prevention of apnea and bradycardia in low-birthweight infants. Pediatr., *55*:589.

Wood, R. E., and Farrell, P. M. 1974. Epidemiology of respiratory distress syndrome (RDS). Pediatr. Res., *8*:452.

Chapter **66A**

CONGENITAL MALFORMATIONS OF THE LARYNX

Robin Cotton, M.D.
James S. Reilly, M.D.

The larynx is a complex, evolutionary structure that permits the trachea and bronchi to be joined to the pharynx as a common aerodigestive pathway. The larynx serves the essential functions of (1) ventilation of the lungs, (2) protection of the lungs during deglutition by its sphincteric mechanism, (3) clearance of secretion by a vigorous cough, and (4) production of sound, i.e., vocalization. The survival of the infant is predicated upon the larynx being structurally and neurologically intact, or else prompt medical intervention for airway management is required.

The larynx is arbitrarily divided into three regions: supraglottis, glottis, and subglottis. The supraglottic larynx is composed of the epiglottis, aryepiglottic folds, arytenoid cartilage, ventricular folds, and sinus. The glottis comprises the vocal cords, also called vocal folds. The subglottic area extends from the undersurface of the vocal cords to the base of the cricoid cartilage. The size, location, configuration, and consistency of the laryngeal structures are all unique in the neonate, however. The purpose of this chapter will be to review both pertinent anatomy of the infant larynx and to discuss anomalies of structure or function that occur in each of these three regions (Table 66A–1).

ANATOMY

At birth the infant larynx is approximately one third the size of the adult larynx. The glottis of the neonate measures approximately 7 mm in the sagittal plane and 4 mm in the coronal plane. The vocal cords are 6 to 8 mm in length, with the posterior aspect composed

Table 66A–1 ANOMALIES OF THE PHARYNX

Supraglottic	Glottic	Subglottic
Congenital flaccid larynx	Vocal cord paralysis	Subglottic hemangioma
Supraglottic atresia	Laryngeal web	Subglottic web
Supraglottic hemangioma	Cri-du-chat syndrome	Subglottic atresia
Laryngocele	Laryngeal atresia	Subglottic stenosis
Bifid epiglottis	Anterior laryngeal cleft	Posterior laryngeal cleft
Anomalous cuneiform cartilage	Duplication of vocal folds	G syndrome
Absent epiglottis	Neurofibroma of larynx	
Supraglottic web	Plott syndrome	
Lymphangioma of vallecula	Arthrogryposis multiplex	
	Laryngoptosis	

of the cartilaginous process of the arytenoid. Subglottic diameter measures approximately 4.5 mm by 7 mm. A diameter of less than 3.5 mm suggests a marginal subglottic airway and is consistent with subglottic stenosis (Fearon and Cotton, 1972).

The superior border of the larynx is located as high as the first cervical vertebra. The inferior border of the infant larynx is determined by the cricoid cartilage, which is located at approximately the fourth cervical vertebra during infancy (Sasaki et al., 1977). The thyrohyoid membrane is foreshortened, and this results in the lingual hypopharyngeal laryngeal complex sitting more superiorly within the oral pharynx. Indeed, the hyoid cartilage can be located anterior to the thyroid cartilage (Tucker and Tucker, 1979). The severe superior condition of the larynx elevates the epiglottis approximately to the level of the palate and helps to explain the necessity of obligate nasal breathers over the first nine months of life (Negus, 1949). This position is further enhanced in nursing as forward thrust of the tongue causes increased elevation of the larynx. Gradually through childhood, the larynx descends to the sixth cervical vertebra and will approach adult size and configuration (Sasaki et al., 1977).

The configuration of the epiglottis is proportionally narrower than the adult and assumes either a tubular form or the shape of the Greek letter omega (Ω). The overall configuration of the air passage into the larynx has been a point of contention; in the child the epiglottis has a more vertical position and the larynx is at an angle from behind forward and downward. The cricoid cartilage is tilted posteriorly in the infant, creating more of a funnel-shaped lumen than in the adult. This funnel continues into the trachea. The lumen of the larynx in infants is relatively greater than that of the trachea. In later life the cricoid assumes a ring shape. The midline angle of the junction of the thyroid cartilage is obtuse in the child, approximately 110 to 120 degrees. At puberty, the angle narrows to 90 degrees. In the female this angulation remains about the same as it was in childhood (Stool and Tucker, 1970). Circumferential mucosal edema of 1 mm will create a glottis space to narrow by over 60 per cent (Tucker and Tucker, 1979).

The clinical manifestations associated with congenital anomalies of the larynx include (1) respiratory obstruction, (2) stridor, (3) a weakened or abnormal cry, (4) dyspnea, (5) tachypnea, (6) aspiration, and (7) sudden death. Congenital lesions that occur in the supraglottis, glottis, or subglottis will be discussed by region. Diagnosis can only be confirmed by endoscopic examination.

SUPRAGLOTTIS

Congenital Flaccid Larynx (Laryngomalacia)

Congenital flaccid larynx is a clinical entity that accounts for about 60 per cent of laryngeal problems in the newborn (Holinger, 1980). The diagnosis can be made only by clinical observation of the larynx during respiration. The abnormality appears to be a flaccidity or incoordination of the supralaryngeal cartilages, especially the arytenoids, that is expressed when the infant is stressed by excitation with an increased respiratory rate. Stridor is typically noted in the first few weeks of life and is characterized by fluttering inspiratory sounds. The supraglottic structures, unilaterally or bilaterally, are pulled into the lumen around a vertical axis with inspiration. Placing the child in the prone position with the neck hyperextended often will relieve the stridor. Eating difficulties and respiratory distress are rare (Holinger and Brown, 1967). Sternal retractions are seen frequently, with labored respiratory effort. It remains speculative as to whether the pectus excavatum that is often observed is a direct or indirect result of this condition.

Roentgenographic assessment can sometimes be a helpful adjunct to diagnosis if it captures the characteristic medial and inferior displacement of the arytenoid cartilage or epiglottis (Fig. 66A–1). Diagnosis in the neonate can be confirmed only by direct observation of movement of the supraglottis during respiration. The blade of the laryngoscope must be carefully placed to support the larynx without impeding normal mobility. The arytenoids will often appear more prominent than usual, and a deep interarytenoid cleft is seen. During inspiration the supraglottic structures collapse into the lumen, narrowing the air passage and creating an arrhythmic flutter. The diagnosis can also be confirmed by advancing the laryngoscope into the endolarynx and causing disappearance of the stridor. Careful sequential inspection of the respiratory tract is necessary to rule out associated secondary lesions, such as

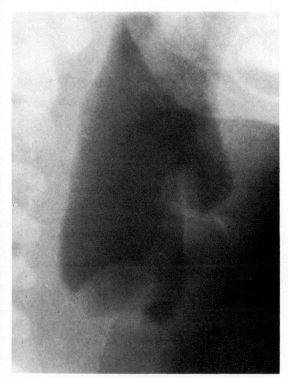

Figure 66A–1 Lateral radiograph of neck in laryngomalacia demonstrating forward bowing of aryepiglottic folds, ballooning of the hypopharynx, and dilation of the laryngeal ventricle.

innominate subglottic stenosis (Fearon and Ellis, 1971). Flexible, fiberoptic laryngoscopy can often be used to confirm an abnormality of the supraglottis but should be combined with rigid bronchoscopy to include subglottic evaluation.

The etiology remains enigmatic. Keleman (1953) reviewed histologic specimens of congenital laryngeal stridor and was impressed by the edematous nature of the aryepiglottic folds, particularly in the region of the ventricular bands. The suspension of the epiglottis is loose. The aryepiglottic fold can be devoid of musculature.

Holinger and Brown (1967) have proposed an explanation based upon an embryologic model. The epiglottis is formed by the third and fourth arches. More rapid growth by the third arch will elongate the arch and cause it to curl upon itself.

Martin (1963) noted the arytenoids to be brought into close apposition, foretilting inward. This is often noted to occur very early in respiration, prior to rapid airflow. Arytenoid movement is also arrhythmic and appears to be caused by muscle contraction. Martin postulates that neurologic immaturity

of the brain stem causes the infolding of the arytenoids.

Therapy consists of reassurance to the parents of a favorable prognosis for the child, as well as continued vigilance by the physician to be certain that the child continues to grow, feed, and breathe well. Surgical intervention via tracheotomy has rarely been reported as necessary for feeding difficulties (Holinger and Brown, 1967).

Supraglottic Atresia

Atresia represents one of the more severe forms of laryngeal anomalies, in contrast to webs or stenosis. Accordingly, there is a high frequency of associated anomalies, which can include esophageal atresia, tracheoesophageal fistula, urinary tract anomalies, and limb defects, particularly involving the radius. Survival time for affected children is usually short-lived, and limited ventilation occasionally occurs through a tracheoesophageal fistula (Smith and Bain, 1965). Tracheotomy is essential if the child is salvageable. Many children are not properly diagnosed antemortem.

Supraglottic Hemangioma

Hemangioma is a type of hamartoma that results in anomalous development of blood vessels in a particular region. Hemangiomas are most often located in the skin, and generally they have a secondary or tertiary location that could include the larynx (Liekensohn et al., 1976). Hemangiomas of the supraglottic structures are very rare and much less common than those of the subglottic area (Birch, 1961). Dyspnea, stridor, or feeding difficulties are frequent presenting symptoms. Treatment should be centered around an airway that is protected by a tracheotomy. Spontaneous regression generally occurs.

Laryngocele

The laryngocele is a sac-like structure with an internal lumen that is dilated and filled with air. It represents a dilatation of the ventricular sinus of Morgagni beyond the limits of the laryngeal cartilage (Canalis et al., 1976). Laryngoceles have been classified as internal if they are completely within the laryngeal cartilage or external if they pierce the thyrohyoid membrane. A third type is combined and extends both internally and externally (Holinger et al., 1978). Laryngoceles are extremely rare and, if present, cause intermittent hoarseness and dyspnea that increases with crying. Diagnosis is difficult since they can quickly contract when not filled with air and thus often cannot be observed when examined endoscopically under general anesthesia. A roentgenogram can sometimes be valuable in detecting such abnormalities.

By contrast, a saccular cyst is both a fluid-filled structure and lacks communication with the airway and should be distinguished from a laryngocele (DeSanto et al., 1968). Both the clinical and roentgenographic appearances of these two lesions can be identical. At endoscopy, a large, bluish, filled cyst can be seen occupying the area of the epiglottic fold. Attempts either to aspirate via a large-bore needle or to uncap the dome of the cyst will permit drainage of thick fluid. This procedure often has to be repeated multiple times because the cyst is quiescent. If postoperative edema is expected, the child should be kept intubated for several days to serve as a stent (Booth and Birck, 1981).

Bifid Epiglottis

Bifid epiglottis is a rare laryngeal anomaly resulting from a congenital absence of fusion of the epiglottis in the midline (Montrueil, 1949). The cleavage extends to just above the tubercle. There are fewer than 10 cases reported in the world literature. The patient's history frequently includes episodes of cyanosis associated with feeding and occasional airway obstruction. The presence of the midline split sometimes renders the epiglottis incompetent of its protective function of the airway (Delmonico and Harr, 1972). The epiglottis is also often unsupported and is drawn in with inspiration. There has been an association with the presence of polydactyly in about 40 per cent of cases. This is interesting because both the fingers and the epiglottis are at the same stage of human embryologic development and correlate with the emergence from the hypobranchial eminence of the epiglottis in the embryo (Healy et al., 1976).

When respiratory distress is present, a tracheotomy is often required for long-term management. Surgical removal of the epiglottis often improves airway function, but aspiration remains a minor problem (Montrueil, 1949).

Anomalous Cuneiform Cartilages

Templer et al. (1981) report a case of enlarged cuneiform cartilages associated with a small, floppy epiglottis that resulted in airway distress and stridor. The patient had chronic airway obstruction since birth and marked dyspnea on exertion. Indirect laryngoscopy confirmed that with strong respiratory effort, the accessory cartilages were drawn into the airway, resulting in temporary obstruction of the airway. Associated anomalies that have been reported included both ankyloglossia and macroglossia.

This embryologic abnormality is the result of a malformation of the lateral masses, which are derived from a portion of the sixth branchial arch.

Treatment included a tracheotomy followed by a supraglottic laryngectomy. This resulted in a marked improvement of the airway, and feeding has not been a major difficulty. A brief cough at the end of deglutition will clear endolaryngeal secretions.

Absence of Epiglottis

The failure of the epiglottis to develop requires that there be an embryologic abnormality that affects both the third and fourth branchial arches. Such an occurrence would invariably dramatically affect the formation of the larynx. Holinger and Brown (1967) encountered only two such lesions, and both were associated with severe stenosis of the glottis. Tracheotomy would be required in order to survive.

Supraglottic Web

Congenital webs are diaphragmatic growths of varying thickness that partially occlude the lumen. Supraglottic webs represent less than 2 per cent of a large series of congenital laryngeal webs (McHugh and Loch, 1942). Webs vary both in size and thickness. A web generally arises anteriorly, and, if partial, the air passage opens posteriorly. The web is generally thinner posteriorly and thickened anteriorly. The symptoms produced in each case depend on the size and position of the web. Symptoms can include dyspnea and voice change. Ten per cent of children with webs have associated anomalies.

Treatment consists of surgical lysis of the web followed by dilatation. Tracheotomy should be performed if the web is large or if manipulation will result in edema or airway compromise.

Supraglottic Lymphangioma (Vallecula)

Lymphangiomas are cystic malformations that result from abnormal development of lymphatic vessels (Morgenstern and LaSalla, 1953). When a lymphangioma is located close to a vital structure, it can compromise the function of that organ. Lymphangioma located in the vallecula can compress the epiglottis into the airway and cause airway distress. Symptoms include dyspnea and dysphagia. Treatment includes careful endoscopic confirmation, with the child intubated, followed by aspiration and marsupialization via cup forceps. The child must be carefully monitored postoperatively for any respiratory distress, and a tracheotomy should be performed if it becomes necessary. Recurrence of lymphangiomas is not uncommon and has been reported (Ruben et al., 1975).

GLOTTIS

Vocal Cord Paralysis

Absence of proper vocal cord mobility can occur unilaterally or bilaterally. Laryngeal paralysis may be present at birth or may become manifest in the first month or two of life. The neurologic impairment reflects an injury to the vagus nerve. The lesion can occur anywhere along its course from the brain through the neck, chest, and into the larynx. All these regions must be carefully investigated to attempt to locate a lesion. Many paralyses are idiopathic and an exact cause cannot be located (Ferguson, 1970). Stridor in the neonate in about 10 to 15 per cent of cases is the result of vocal paralysis (Holinger, 1980). This is perhaps lower than its actual occurrence since diagnosis can

occur and can be overlooked. The diagnosis is difficult, for improper positioning of the laryngoscopic blade or deep anesthesia can inhibit proper evaluation.

Unilateral paralysis generally results in a weakened cry but with an adequate airway unless stressed. The airway is stressed with vigorous activity, infections, or trauma. Roentgenographic examination remains important in the work-up of laryngeal paralysis. Unilateral paralysis is often associated with cardiac and great vessel anomalies, which chest films can confirm. Barium swallows and arteriograms are occasionally performed to confirm anomalies of the great vessels. Tracheotomy is rarely required in unilateral paralysis that may stretch the vagus.

Bilateral vocal cord paralysis results in the vocal cords being in the paramedian position, unable to abduct for inspiration. The airway is compromised markedly, causing stridor and cyanosis. The absence of a vigorous cough makes aspiration common and feeding hazardous. Tracheotomy to secure the airway is essential before additional testing is undertaken. In the presence of bilateral paralysis, the evaluation should include skull films with base views and tomograms of the base of the skull, including computerized tomography scans. Hydrocephalus and Arnold-Chiari malformation can result in herniation of the brain stem with stretching of the vagus nerves over the lip of the jugular foramen, causing paralysis.

A helpful aphorism to keep in mind is that unilateral vocal paralysis is often peripheral; bilateral paralysis often has a central cause.

Laryngeal Web

A web is formed during embryogenesis of the laryngotracheal groove, and if it persists at birth, it will cause respiratory distress. A web is a membrane of varying thickness that partially occludes a lumen. The degree of respiratory distress depends on the size of the tracheal lumen. Over 75 per cent of laryngeal webs are located at the level of the glottis. The web is generally located anteriorly with the concave posterior glottic opening. Most webs are thick and fibrous with subglottic extension and are difficult to lyse or remove (McHugh and Loch, 1942). A web that is thin enough to transilluminate easily can be transected with either knife or laser and followed up with repeated endoscopies, including dilatation of the larynx. A thick membranous web will require a tracheotomy, subsequent thyrotomy, lysis of the web, and implantation with a keel.

Laryngeal Atresia

Laryngeal atresia represents a complete failure of the embryo to recanalize the lumen of the larynx during the first trimester. Only a handful of cases have been properly diagnosed and treated in the delivery room with a tracheotomy. Many cases go undiagnosed and are simply recorded as stillbirths. Most data come from autopsy specimens that show complete occlusion of the laryngeal lumen.

On rare occasion there is a concomitant tracheoesophageal fistula that is large enough to sustain respiration. This has been reported in children with laryngeal atresia. For the child with laryngeal atresia to survive, a tracheotomy is essential.

Larynx and Cri-du-Chat Syndrome

This genetic syndrome is the result of a partial deletion of the short arm of chromosome No. 5 (B-group), as associated with peculiar congenital laryngeal stridor. When karyotypically confirmed, there is a characteristic high-pitched stridor that is similar to the "mew" of a cat. The endolarynx has been observed to be elongated and curved with a floppy epiglottis. During inspiration, the vocal cords are seen to be narrow and have a diamond-shaped appearance. This results from anterior approximation of the vocal cords with an abnormally large air status in the posterior commissure area. There is generally no associated respiratory distress with it, and tracheotomy is not required (Ward et al., 1968a, 1968b).

Anterior Laryngeal Cleft

Anterior nonfusions of the laminae of the thyroid cartilage creating an anterior midline defect have been reported by Montgomery and Smith (1976). There were no associated problems with either feeding or breathing. The only symptom was an increased pitch in the voice, and the diagnosis was not made until adulthood.

Duplication of Vocal Cord

Cited by Holinger and Brown (1967) but not demonstrated either clinically or histologically, an accessory vocal cord has been reported to exist immediately below the true vocal cord. The only associated symptom is hoarseness.

Neurofibromatosis of the Larynx

Von Recklinghausen's neurofibromatosis, an autosomal-dominant disorder with high penetrance, can produce clinical abnormalities as early as four years of age. These perineural fibromas produce symptoms of dyspnea or stridor and can be glottic or supraglottic (Zobell, 1964).

Congenital Neuromuscular Laryngeal Dysfunction

The Plott syndrome is a hereditary disorder that has congenital laryngeal adductor paralysis as a feature. The disorder is X-linked and associated with mental retardation. Symptoms include stridor and respiratory distress. Patients with this condition have a shortened life span (Plott, 1964).

Arthrogryposis Multiplex Congenita

This disorder is characterized by congenital joint deformities due to an intrauterine muscle weakness. Many children have dysfunction of the pharynx, palate, tongue, or larynx. About 20 per cent die, generally of respiratory problems.

Laryngoptosis

Laryngoptosis means that the larynx is positioned abnormally low into the neck, with the entire trachea being intrathoracic (Stewart et al., 1973). The larynx is structurally normal except for an "infantile epiglottis," which may cause some stridor. The voice is characteristically low-pitched and monotonic. The cause of laryngoptosis is debated. Some authors postulate that the cause is an abnormal, short trachea, while others have shown a fibrotic and contracted sternohyoid muscle, pulling the larynx inferiorly.

Surgery is best avoided, and attempts at tracheotomy are both hazardous and often unsuccessful.

SUBGLOTTIS

Subglottic Cleft

G Syndrome

G syndrome, which also includes abnormal facies, hypertelorism, wide anterior fontanel, low-set ears, hypospadias, and a hoarse cry, is secondary to a laryngeal cleft. This cleft can sometimes extend to the esophagus and can be associated with esophageal atresia (Opitz et al., 1969).

Subglottic Web

A membrane can form a web in the subglottic region. These lesions can often mimic a deformity of the cricoid cartilage or subglottic stenosis. About 7 per cent of laryngeal webs are in the subglottic region. They are generally anteriorly based with a small opening sometimes the size of a pinpoint posteriorly. The superior surface is covered with squamous epithelium and the inferior surface with mucous membrane. There is a slight female predominance (McHugh and Loch, 1942).

If there is respiratory distress, surgical intervention is indicated. An initial tracheotomy is placed to control the airway. Following this, various surgical approaches are available. Thin membranes respond to lysis and dilatation. Thicker webs, which are more common, require a cricothyrotomy with insertion of a keel.

Congenital Subglottic Stenosis

Subglottic stenosis occurs when the airway lumen in the region of the cricoid measures less than 3.5 mm in diameter in the newborn. Lesions in this area are congenital if they are the result of the abnormal development of the cricoid. An abnormality of the cartilage or the subglottic tissues that occurs in the absence of the history of trauma is generally congenital. This is important to distinguish from acquired subglottic stenosis, which can occur from intubation or other forms of laryngeal trauma. Histologic examination of the larynges most often reveals a soft tissue thickening of the subglottic area with additional thickening of the true vocal cords.

Mild cases of subglottic stenosis that result in a marginal airway are sometimes present in the first six months of life with a history of either recurrent infections or increasing respiratory distress precipitated by upper respiratory infection. Minimal laryngeal swelling precipitates airway obstruction since the cricoid cartilage prevents outward expansion, forcing edema internally, thus closing the airway. The greatest obstruction is generally 2 to 3 mm below the true cords.

Roentgenograms of the neck will frequently show a narrowing of the subglottic space and are helpful in the child who does not have associated respiratory distress. Diagnosis is confirmed by endoscopy. Over 40 per cent of a large series (Holinger et al., 1976) required tracheotomy, and it is our belief that if the airway does not permit easy passage of a 3.5 mm external diameter scope, then tracheotomy is essential (Marshak and Grundfast, 1981).

Congenital subglottic stenosis is often associated with other congenital lesions and syndromes. Children with trisomy 21 (Down syndrome) have a congenitally small larynx. Small larynges are very susceptible to injury by an endotracheal tube placed for surgery and can receive a secondary acquired stenosis. Once the airway is secured with the tracheotomy, additional intervention is only rarely required. This is because most congenital subglottic stenoses will improve as laryngeal growth occurs and do not require surgical intervention. Most children can be decannulated by approximately 24 to 36 months of age (Holinger et al., 1976).

Subglottic Hemangioma

A hemangioma is a hamartoma of blood vessel development and can be present in any organ system. These abnormalities are commonly seen on the skin and are frequently associated with internal hemangioma (Garfinkel and Handler, 1980). If a hemangioma is present in the subglottic region, there is frequently respiratory distress. Stridor that is exacerbated by crying or upper respiratory tract inflammation are common presenting symptoms. Associated symptoms include a harsh cry and dyspnea. Initially, difficulty with respiration can often be misdiagnosed as croup. However, the patient is afebrile and cough is not present. There is a large female preponderance, and most children present in the first six months of life (Liekensohn et al., 1976).

Roentgenographic examination will sometimes demonstrate an asymmetric narrowing of the subglottic airway. Endoscopic examination will reveal a soft compressible lesion of the subglottis, often arising posteriorly. The venous cysts within the hemangioma give them the characteristic blue color. Confirmation by biopsy is contraindicated because of fear of hemorrhage.

The natural course of hemangioma is one of growth over the first 6 to 18 months, followed by gradual regression. These lesions should be followed endoscopically to see if they conform to this pattern. Surgical laser therapy with adjunctive steroids has been advocated but has not been proved efficacious (Healy et al., 1980). Radiation therapy is contraindicated. The rarely encountered child who has a hemangioma and fails to regress can be considered a surgical candidate after three years of age.

Posterior Laryngeal Cleft

The laryngeal cleft arises at approximately 35 days of gestation for failure of rostral development of the tracheoesophageal septum. The absence of the septum prevents the proper formation of the cricoid cartilage ring (Lim et al., 1979). Respiratory distress is usually precipitated by feeding and associated with cyanosis. Infants with laryngeal clefts have recurrent aspiration leading to pneumonia and death. There is an associated 30 per cent history of maternal polyhydramnios, as well as a 20 per cent history of tracheoesophageal fistula. Multiple other congenital anomalies have been associated with this entity.

A chest film will frequently show aspiration pneumonitis that is severe. The esophagogram is the most important diagnostic tool for showing spillover of contrast material into the trachea. The diagnosis again is confirmed at endoscopy. Following direct laryngoscopy and bronchoscopy to confirm a patent airway, the child should be intubated (Pillsbury and Fischer, 1977). The endotracheal tube will hold open the edges of the cleft, which then can be easily seen when performing an esoph-

agoscopy. The length of the cleft should be noted in order to classify it. Most common is a partial laryngotracheal esophageal cleft. In an extensive cleft, initial airway maintenance should be maintained by either placement of the endotracheal tube or tracheotomy. In an extensive cleft, a tracheotomy tube often fails to be secure in the tracheal lumen and can frequently become displaced posteriorly. This can result in distress and respiratory arrest.

Prior to definitive repair, a feeding gastrostomy should be performed to prevent reflux and aspiration. Repair of the laryngeal cleft is best done via the lateral pharyngotomy. The multilayer closure is preferred up to the glottic area. The supraglottic area is not closed to prevent stenosis. If the cleft is mild, the child can be observed and surgery performed electively.

REFERENCES

Atkins, J. P. 1962. Laryngeal problems of infancy and childhood. Pediatr. Clin. North Am., 9:1125–1135.

Baker, D. C., and Savetsky, L. 1966. Congenital partial atresia of the larynx. Laryngoscope, 76:616–620.

Birch, D. A. 1961. Laryngeal stridor in infants and children — A study of 200 cases. J. Laryngol., 75:833–840.

Blumberg, J. B., Stevenson, J. K., Lemire, R. J., and Boyden, E. A. 1965. Laryngotracheoesophageal cleft — the embryological implication and review of the literature. Surgery, 57:559–566.

Booth, J. B., and Birck, H. B. 1981. Operative treatment and post-operative management of saccular cyst and laryngocele. Arch. Otolaryngol. 107:500–502.

Canalis, R. F., Maxwell, D. S., and Hemenway, M. G. 1977. The laryngocele — An updated review. J. Laryngol., 6(3):191–199.

Cavanaugh, F., 1965. Congenital laryngeal web. Proc. R. Soc. Med., 58:272–277.

Chamberlain, D. 1970. Congenital subglottic cyst of the larynx. Laryngoscope, 80:254–259.

Cohen, S. R., and Isacs, H. J. 1976. Otolaryngologic manifestations of arthrogryposis multiplex congenita. Ann. Otol. Rhinol. Laryngol., 85:484–490.

Cotton, R. F., and Richardson, M. 1981. Congenital laryngeal anomalies. Otol. Clin. North Am., 14:203–218.

Dayal, D., and Singh, A. P. 1971. Congenital laryngoptosis: A case report. Ann. Otol. Rhinol. Laryngol., 80:244–245.

Delahant, J. E., and Cherry, J. 1969. Congenital laryngeal cleft. Ann. Otol. Rhinol. Laryngol., 78:96–106.

DelMonico, M. L., and Harr, J. G. 1972. Bifid epiglottis — A case report. Arch. Otolaryngol., 96:178–181.

DeSanto, L. W., Devine, K. D., and Weiland, L. H. 1968. Cysts of the larynx — a classification. Laryngoscope, 78:145–176.

Donegan, J. O., Strife, J. L., Seid, A. B., et al. 1980. Internal laryngocele and saccular cysts in children. Ann. Otol. Rhinol. Laryngol., *89*:409–413.

Donahue, P. K., and Hendren, W. H. 1972. The surgical management of laryngotracheoesophageal cleft with tracheoesophageal fistula, and esophageal atresia. Surgery, *71*:363–368.

Fearon, B., and Ellis, D. 1971. The management of long term airway problems in infants and children. Ann. Otol. Rhinol. Laryngol., *80*:669–677.

Fearon, B., and Whalen, J. S. 1967. Tracheal dimensions in the living infant. Ann. Otol. Rhinol. Laryngol., *76*:964–974.

Fearon, B. 1968. Respiratory distress in the newborn. Otol. Clin. North Am., *1*:147–169.

Fearon, B., and Cotton, R. B. 1972. Subglottic stenosis in infants and children. The clinical problem and experimental surgical correction. Can. J. Otol., *1*:281–289.

Ferguson, C. G. 1970. Congenital anomalies of the infant larynx. Otolaryngol. Clin. North Am., *3*:185–200.

Ferguson, C. F., and Flake, C. G. 1961. Subglottic hemangioma as a cause of respiratory distress in infants. Ann. Otol. Rhinol. Laryngol., *70*:1095–1112.

Fuerstein, S. S. 1973. Subglottic hemangioma in infants. Laryngoscope, *83*:466–475.

Garfinkel, T. J., and Handler, S. D. 1980. Hemangioma of the head and neck. J. Otolaryngol., *9(5)*:435–450.

Gaskill, J. R., and Bailey, B. J. 1964. Congenital posterior clefts of the trachea and larynx. Trans. Pac. Coast Otoophthalmol. Soc., *51*:259–264.

Gilbert, E. F., and Opitz, J. M. 1976. The pathology of some malformations and hereditary diseases of the respiratory tract. Birth Defects, *12(6)*:239–270.

Hanallah, R., and Rosales, J. K. 1975. Laryngeal web in infant with tracheoesophageal fistula. Anesthesia, *42*:96–97.

Hast, M. 1970. The developmental anatomy of the larynx. Otol. Clin. North Am., 7:413–438.

Healy, G. B., Holt, G. P., and Tucker, J. A. 1976. Bifid epiglottis — A rare laryngeal anomaly. Laryngoscope, *86*:1459–1467.

Healy, G. B., Fearon, B., French, B., et al. 1980. Treatment of subglottic hemangioma. Laryngoscope, *90*:809–813.

Hoefer, P. A., and Ohman, J. 1974. Laryngeal lesions in Urbach Wilthe disease (lipoglycoproteinosis, lipoid proteinosis, hyalinosis cutis and mucosae). Acta Pathol. Microbiol. Scand. (A), *82*:547–558.

Holinger, L. D., Barnes, D. R., Sneid, L. J., and Holinger, P. H. 1978. Laryngocele and saccular cysts. Ann. Otol. Rhinol. Laryngol., *87*:675–685.

Holinger, L. D. 1980. Etiology of stridor in the neonate, infant and child. Ann. Otol. Rhinol. Laryngol., *89*:397–400.

Holinger, P. H., Johnson, K. C., and Schiller, F. 1954. Congenital anomalies of the larynx. Ann. Otol. Rhinol. Laryngol., *24*:581–606.

Holinger, P. H. 1964. Congenital anomalies of the tracheo bronchial tree. Postgrad. Med., *36*:454–469.

Holinger, P. H., and Brown, W. T. 1967. Congenital webs, cysts, laryngoceles, and other anomalies of the larynx. Ann. Otol. Rhinol. Laryngol., *76*:744–752.

Holinger, P. H., Kutnick, S., Schild, J. A., et al. 1976. Subglottic stenosis in infants and children. Ann. Otol. Rhinol. Laryngol., *85*:591–599.

Imbrie, J. D., and Doyle, P. J. 1969. Laryngotracheoesophageal cleft: Report of a case and review of the literature. Laryngoscope, *79*:1252–1574.

Keleman, G. 1953. Congenital laryngeal stridor. Arch. Otolaryngol., *58*:245–268.

Kahn, A., Baran, D., Spehl, M., et al. 1977. Congenital stridor in infancy. Clin. Pediatr. *16*:19–26.

Lacassie, Y., and McKusick, V. A. 1975. The G syndrome. Analysis of 2 cases. Birth Defects, *11*:334.

Landing, B. H. 1979. Congenital malformations and genetic disorders of the respiratory tract. Am. Rev. Respir. Dis. *120*:151–185.

Liekensohn, G. V., Benton, C., and Cotton, R. 1976. Subglottic hemangioma. J. Otolaryngol., *5(6)*:487–492.

Lin, J. A., Spanier, S. S., and Kohut, P. T. 1979. Laryngeal clefts: A histopathological review study. Ann. Otol. Rhinol. Laryngol., *88*:1837–1845.

Marshak, G., and Grundfast, K. 1981. Subglottic stenosis. Pediatr. Clin. North Ann., *28*:941–948.

Martin, J. A. 1963. Congenital laryngeal stridor. J. Laryngol., *77*:290–298.

Mastafa, S. M. 1976. Variation in subglottic size in children. Proc. R. Soc. Med., *69*:793–795.

McHugh, H. E., and Loch, W. E. 1942. Congenital webs of the larynx. Laryngoscope, *52*:43–65.

McMillan, W. G., and Duvall, A. J. 1968. Congenital subglottic stenosis. Arch. Otolaryngol., *87*:70–76.

Montgomery, W. W., and Smith, S. A. 1976. Congenital laryngeal defect in the adult. Ann. Otol. Rhinol. Laryngol., *85*:491–497.

Montrueil, F. 1948. Bifid epiglottis — A case report. Laryngoscope, *59*:194–199.

Morganstern, D. J., and LaSalla, A. M. 1953. Cysts of the larynx. Arch. Otolaryngol., *58*:179–182.

Negus, V. 1949. The Comparative Anatomy and Physiology of the Larynx. New York, Harper and Row.

Opitz, J. M., Frias, J. L., Gutenberger, J. E., et al. 1969. The G syndrome of multiple congenital anomalies. In Bergsma, D. (ed.): Malformation Syndromes, Birth Defects: Orig. Art. Ser., Vol. V, No. 2. Part II. White Plains: The National Foundation — March of Dimes, 1969, pp. 95–101.

Opitz, J. M., Kaveggia, E. G., Durkin-Stamm, M.V., et al. 1978. Diagnostic/genetic studies in severe mental retardation. Birth Defects, *14*:1–38.

Parkin, J. L., Steven, M. H., and Jung, A. L. 1976. Acquired and congenital subglottic stenosis in the infant. Ann. Otol. Rhinol. Laryngol., *85*:573–581.

Phelan, P. D., Stocks, J. G., Williams, H. E., and Donks, D. N. 1973. Familial occurrence of congenital laryngeal clefts. Arch. Dis. Child., *48*:275–278.

Pillsbury, H. C., and Fischer, N. D. 1977. Laryngotracheoesophageal cleft. Arch. Otolaryngol., *103*: 735–737.

Pracy, R. 1965. Stridor in children. Proc. R. Soc. Med., *58*:267–270.

Pracy, R. 1970. Children's laryngology. J. Laryngol. Otol., *84*:37–40.

Pracy, R., and Steel, P. M. 1974. Laryngeal cleft: Diagnosis and management. J. Laryngol. Otol., *88*:483–486.

Plott, D. 1964. Congenital laryngeal abductor paralysis due to nucleus ambiguus dysgenesis in three brothers. J.A.M.A., *27*:593–594.

Puveendran, A. 1972. Congenital subglottic atresia: A case report. J. Laryngol. Otol., *86*:847–852.

Ruben, R. J., Kucinski, S. A., and Greenstein, N. 1975. Cystic lymphangioma of the vallecula. Can. J. Otol., *4(1)*:180–184.

Sasaki, C. T., Levin, P. A., Lautman, M. P., et al. 1977. Postnatal descent of the epiglottis in man. Arch. Otolaryngol., *103*:169–171.

Seuhs, O. W., and Powell, D. B. 1967. Congenital cysts of larynx in infants. Laryngoscope, 77:654–662.

Shearer, W. T., Biller, H. F., Ogura, J. H., et al. 1972. Congenital laryngeal web and interventricular septal defect. Am. J. Dis. Child., 123:605–607.

Smith, H., and Bain, A. D. 1965. Congenital atresia of the larynx: A report of nine cases. Ann. Otol. Rhinol. Laryngol., 74:338–349.

Smoler, J., Viran, G., and Levey, P. S. 1966. Multiple neurofibromatosis with laryngeal involvement. Ann. Otol Rhinol. Laryngol., 75:968–974.

Stewart, K., Smith, R., and Tohme, S. M. 1973. Laryngoptosis. Arch Otolaryngol., 98:356–357.

Stool, S. E., and Tucker, J. A. 1970. Larynx, trachea, and endoscopy. In Kelley, V. C.: Brenneman's Practice of Pediatrics, Vol. IV, Chap. 48, pp. 1–11. Hagerstown, MD, Harper & Row.

Templer, J., Hast, M., Thomas, J. R., et al. 1981. Congenital laryngeal stridor secondary to flaccid epiglottis, anomalous accessory cartilages, and redundant aryepiglottic folds. Laryngoscope, 91:394–397.

Too-Chung, M. A., and Green, J. R. 1974. The rate of growth of the cricoid cartilage. J. Laryngol., 86:65–70.

Tucker, G. F., Osoff, R. R., and Holinger, L. D. 1979. Histopathology of subglottic stenosis. Laryngoscope, 89;866–877.

Tucker, G. F. 1979. Congenital anomalies of the infant larynx. In Healy, G. B., and McGill, J. (eds.): Laryngotracheal Problems in the Pediatric Patient, Chap. 7. Springfield, IL, Charles C Thomas, 1979, pp. 63–71.

Tucker, G. F., Tucker, J. A., and Vidic, B. 1977. Anatomy and development of the cricoid. Ann. Otol. Rhinol. Laryngol., 86:766–769.

Tucker, J. A., Tucker, G. F., and Vidic, B. 1978. Clinical correlation of anomalies of the supraglottic larynx with the staged sequence of normal human laryngeal development. Ann. Otol. Rhinol. Laryngol., 87:636–644.

Tucker, J. A., and Tucker, G. F. 1979. A clinical perspective on the development and anatomical aspects of the infant larynx and trachea. In Healy, G. B., and McGill, T. J. (eds.): Laryngotracheal Problems in the Pediatric Patient, Springfield, IL, Charles C Thomas.

Tucker, J. A., and Tucker, G. F. 1975. Some aspects of fetal laryngeal development. Ann. Otol. Rhinol. Laryngol., 84:49–55.

Tucker, J. A., Vidic, B., Tucker, G. F., et al. 1976. Survey of the development of the laryngeal epithelium. Ann. Otol. Rhinol. Laryngol., 85 (Suppl. 30):1–16.

Tucker, G. 1937. Laryngoptosis. Arch Otolaryngol., 25:389–392.

Vanden Brock, P., and Brinkman, W. F. B. 1979. Congenital laryngeal defects. Int. J. Pediatr. Otolaryngol., 1:71–78.

Ward, P. H., Engel, E., and Nance, W. E. 1968. The larynx in the cri du chat syndrome. Trans. Am. Acad. Ophthalmol. Otolaryngol., 72:90–102.

Ward, P. H., Engel, E., and Nance, W. E. 1968. The larynx in the cri du chat syndrome. Laryngoscope, 78:1716–1733.

Watters, G. V., and Fitch, N. 1973. Familial laryngeal abductor paralysis and psychomotoretardation. Clin. Genet., 4:429.

Yee, R. D., and Helper, R. S. 1973. Congenital hemangioma of the skin with orbital and subglottic involvement. Am. J. Ophthalmol., 75:876–879.

Zobell, D. H., 1964. Massive neurofibroma of the larynx: A case report. Laryngoscope, 74:233–240.

CONGENITAL MALFORMATIONS OF THE TRACHEA AND BRONCHI

Joyce A. Schild, M.D.

As may be seen from a scanning of previous chapters in this book, there are many pitfalls on the path to normal embryologic development of the tracheobronchial tree. The abnormally formed tracheobronchial tree may be so severely deranged that the infant dies shortly after delivery, or at the other end of the scale, the anomalies may be so minor as to be totally asymptomatic throughout the individual's life. A working classification modified from Holinger et al., (1972) of anomalies ranging from agenesis of the tracheobronchial structures to supernumerary formation of these structures is given in Table 66B–1 (Avery and Fletcher, 1974).

ANOMALIES OF THE TRACHEA

Agenesis or Atresia

Tracheal agenesis is a rare developmental defect which at present is not correctable. Probably as the result of defective differentiation in the third to fourth week of embryonic life (Smith, 1957), the trachea may be completely or only partially absent, and there is no continuity of the larynx and subglottic space with the bronchi. These infants may make respiratory efforts but cannot inflate the lungs.

Short-term survival of these infants is possible if there is a connection between the esophagus and the bronchi for passage of air (Peison et al., 1970). Surgical attempts at utilizing the esophagus as an air conduit have been only temporarily successful, however. The frequently associated severe anomalies of other body systems have made survival of these infants impossible (Joshi, 1969).

Constrictions of the Trachea

Fibrous Strictures

Webs. Webs are localized narrowings of the trachea that occur as films of fibrous tissue across the lumen and are not associated with gross deformity of the underlying cartilage. They can be of different thicknesses; the aperture remaining is of variable diameter, which results in variation in severity of respiratory obstruction. Treatment will depend on the firmness and thickness of the web, although usually simple rupture with dilatation is sufficient. However, in the more stubborn webs, repeated dilatation may be necessary (Holinger and Johnston, 1957).

Stenosis of Tracheal Segments. Fibrous strictures may occur in any portion of the trachea. The involved area is more lengthy than the simple membrane web and appears to involve a greater depth of tissue as well (Holinger et al., 1950). Because of this, the treatment may be more difficult, requiring multiple careful dilatations with either solid metal tracheal dilators or with direct visualization through bronchoscopes of increasing diameters. If the stenosis occurs in the cervi-

Table 66B–1   CLASSIFICATION OF
CONGENITAL ANOMALIES OF THE
TRACHEOBRONCHIAL TREE

I. Anomalies of the trachea
    A. Agenesis or atresia
    B. Constriction
        1. Fibrous strictures
            a. Webs
            b. Fibrous stenosis of tracheal segments
            c. Stenosis associated with tracheo-
               esophageal fistula
        2. Absence or deformity of tracheal cartilages
            a. Tracheomalacia
            b. Deformity due to vascular anomalies
            c. Individual cartilage deformity
    C. Tracheal enlargement (congenital trachiectasis)
    D. Tracheal evaginations or outgrowths
        1. Tracheoceles, cysts
        2. Fistulas
    E. Abnormal bifurcation
        1. Tracheal bronchus
        2. Other anomalies of gross morphology
II. Anomalies of bronchi and lungs
    A. Agenesis or atresia
    B. Constriction
        1. Fibrous strictures
            a. Webs
            b. Fibrous stenosis of bronchial segments
        2. Absence or deformity of bronchial cartilages
            a. Bronchomalacia
            b. Bronchial hypoplasia
    C. Bronchial enlargements
        1. Congenital bronchiectasis
        2. Kartagener syndrome
    D. Bronchial evaginations
        1. Bronchoceles, cysts
        2. Fistulas
    E. Abnormal bifurcation
    F. Anomalous attachments
        1. Sequestered lung
        2. Lung tissue attached to the
           gastrointestinal tract

·Adapted from Holinger, P. H., Zimmerman, A. A.,
and Schild, J. A. 1972. Tracheobronchial tree malformations. *In* Ferguson, C. F., and Kendig, E. L., Jr. (Eds.)
Pediatric Otolaryngology, Vol. 2, 2nd ed. Philadelphia,
W. B. Saunders Co., p. 1286.

cal trachea and is particularly severe and the
trauma of the dilatation results in edema, a
tracheostomy may be required for maintenance of the patient's airway and may need to
remain until the stenosis is relieved. Treatment of a low tracheal stenosis requires extremely careful manipulations to avoid the
airway obstruction that any edema produces.
Tracheal stenting has been found to be of use
by Leape (1973), while Cantrell and Guild
(1964) have successfully repaired localized
defects by resection and reanastomosis of the
trachea (Fig. 66B–1).

Stenosis with Tracheoesophageal Fistula.
Narrowing of the trachea has been seen in
patients with tracheoesophageal fistula; however, the problem is usually not recognized
until postoperatively. It is, therefore, impossible to define it as a true congenital
malformation, as it is most probably related
to the surgical correction of the primary
defect (Holinger et al., 1950).

Absence or Deformity of Tracheal Cartilages

Tracheomalacia.   Tracheomalacia occurs
independently of laryngomalacia (but may be
associated with it) and results in an expiratory
stridor (Baxter and Dunbar, 1963). In the
absence of other disease, the normal mobility
of the trachea and bronchi with respiration is
markedly exaggerated so that the posterior
membranous wall of the tracheobronchial
tree is seen nearly to approximate the anterior cartilaginous wall and, indeed, with
forced expiration (as in crying or coughing)
the walls may actually touch. The resultant
air turbulence causes an audible stridor that
is sometimes quite high-pitched and reminis-
cent of asthmatic wheezing. The onset may be
at birth, but this stridor is usually more noticeable in the older, more active infant and is
particularly noisy with respiratory infections.
When excess secretions are present, the infant may have difficulty expelling them because of the diminished lumen available. The
condition improves gradually with growth as
the tracheobronchial tree enlarges, and
usually disappears by 12 to 18 months of age.
To avoid respiratory distress or even atelectasis, secretions must be controlled by mucolytic
medications and careful control of environmental humidity, especially in the winter (Fig.
66B–2).

Deformity Due to Vascular Anomalies.
Complete vascular rings are the result of
faulty embryonic development, leaving vessels surrounding the trachea and esophagus.
The structure may have a large anterior or
posterior component, may be associated with
a right-descending aorta, or may have a
ligamentum arteriosum rather than ductus
communication (Lincoln et al., 1969). The
result is compression of both the trachea and
esophagus with symptoms referable to both:
dysphagia, dyspnea, cough, and stridor. Esophageal films show circumferential compression of the barium column. Endoscopy will

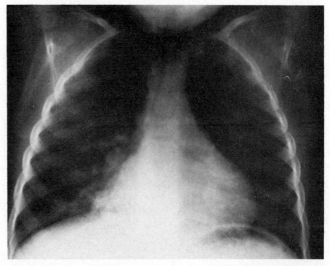

Figure 66B–1 Tracheal stenosis visible in the lower third of the trachea of a three year old child with noisy breathing since infancy. (Courtesy of Children's Memorial Hospital, Chicago.)

show narrowing of the trachea and esophagus of varying degrees, and compression of involved vessels by the advancing endoscope may result in disappearance of radial or carotid artery pulsations while the instrument is in place. The treatment is surgical division if the ring is tight. Swallowing is usually immediately improved by this treatment; however, symptoms of airway obstruction may take some time to improve because of the tracheal cartilage deformity present in association with the vascular problem (Fig. 66B–3).

Vascular anomalies other than complete rings also can cause compression of the trachea. The innominate artery having an anomalous origin from the aorta more distal than usual will necessarily cross the trachea posteroanteriorly and obliquely from left to right. Unless the vessel length is generous, there will be compression of the anterior wall

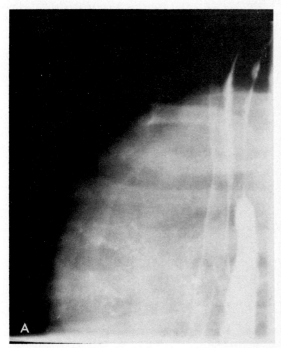

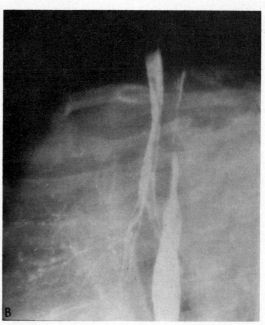

Figure 66B–2 Tracheogram of a three month old with tracheomalacia showing the marked reduction in lumen size from inspiration (A) to expiration (B). (Courtesy of Children's Memorial Hospital, Chicago.)

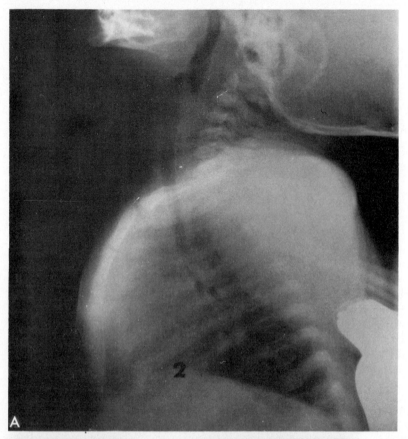

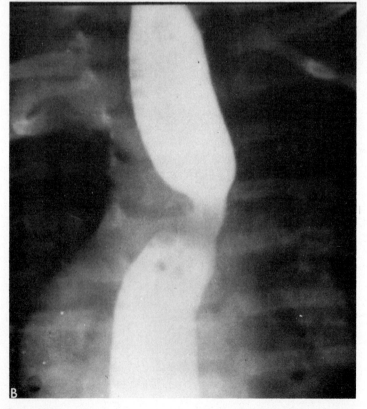

Figure 66B-3 Compression from a vascular ring seen in the lateral view (A) as a narrowing above the tracheal bifurcation and in the esophagograms (B) as a circumferential indentation especially notable on the right. (Courtesy of Children's Memorial Hospital, Chicago.)

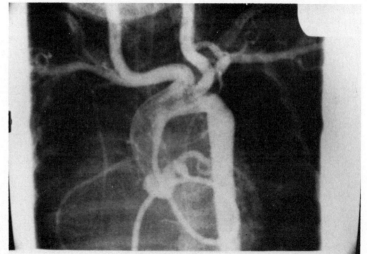

Figure 66B–4 Arteriogram showing the anomalous course of the innominate artery as it crosses the trachea, which is indicated by the endotracheal tube. (Courtesy of Children's Memorial Hospital, Chicago.)

of the trachea, which can be visualized bronchoscopically above the carina as described by Fearon and Shortreed (1963) and Moes and colleagues (1975). Associated symptoms in these children are stridor, dyspnea, reflex apnea, and recurrent respiratory infections. Radiographs of the chest show anterior compression of the trachea but no esophageal deformity. Surgical correction involves suspending the artery anteriorly from the sternum, which will relieve the arterial pressure against the trachea (Fig. 66B–4).

Pulmonary artery anomalies will also cause compression of the trachea and right bronchus. Dilatations of the pulmonary artery in association with cardiac defects result in com-

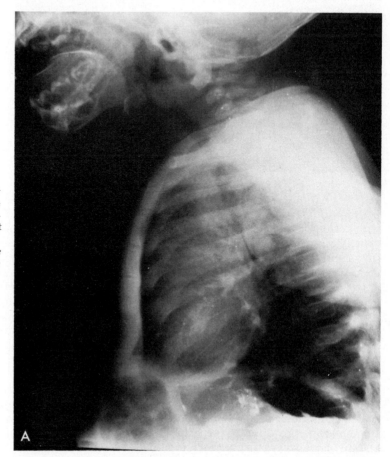

Figure 66B–5 *A*, "Pulmonary artery sling" effects seen in a five month old as lower tracheal compression visible on lateral chest film.

Illustration continued on the following page

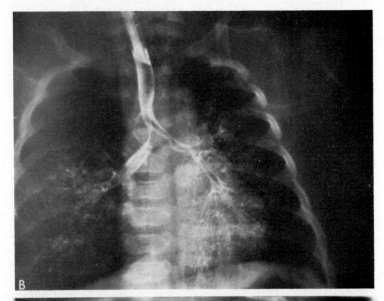

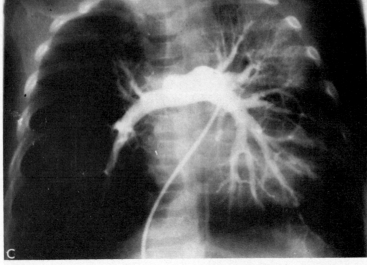

Figure 66B–5 *Continued* Right bronchial narrowing and lung hyperaeration seen with bronchogram (*B*) and the aberrant left pulmonary take-off as indicated by angiography (*C*). (Courtesy of Children's Memorial Hospital, Chicago.)

pression of the distal trachea and bifurcation with resultant respiratory distress. The aberrant left pulmonary artery ("pulmonary artery sling") likewise causes compression of the distal trachea as well as the right bronchus (Potts et al., 1954), since the left pulmonary artery arises on the right and passes between the trachea and esophagus, putting pressure on both. Narrowing of the posterior wall of the trachea can be seen on lateral films, while with a barium swallow the indentation of the esophagus is seen on its anterior wall. Surgical reanastomosis of the aberrant vessel is the treatment for this problem, although there may be persistent cartilaginous deformity of the airway postoperatively, making the course of recovery stormy (Park et al., 1971) (Figs. 66B–5 and 66B–6).

Individual Cartilage Deformity. As has been mentioned, abnormal formation or even absence of tracheal cartilage often occurs in patients with vascular abnormalities with resultant respiratory problems. However, isolated deformities also occur (Holinger et al., 1952) and can result similarly in dyspnea and cyanosis. Absence or deformity of the rings leads to poor support of these segments, a situation that can be seen endoscopically as localized flaccidity of the tracheal wall. With growth of the child and with increase in lumen size, usually the symptoms gradually disappear (Fig. 66B–7). In contrast, patients with complete rings have increasing severity of symptoms, especially with respiratory infections (Greene, 1976). Noisy respirations, retractions, and cyanosis occur; radio-

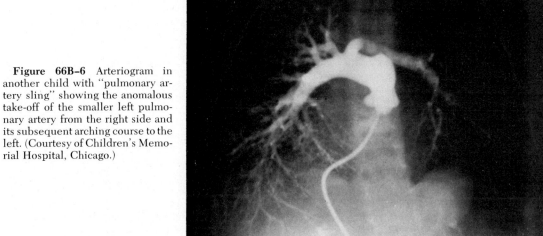

Figure 66B-6 Arteriogram in another child with "pulmonary artery sling" showing the anomalous take-off of the smaller left pulmonary artery from the right side and its subsequent arching course to the left. (Courtesy of Children's Memorial Hospital, Chicago.)

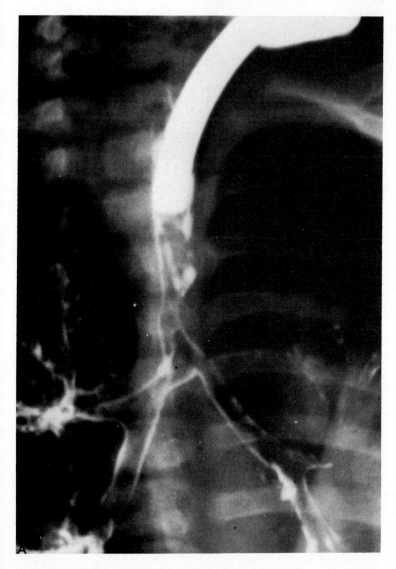

Figure 66B-7 Tracheograms of a three month old child with absence of lower tracheal ring showing the localized lumen change of the trachea from inspiration (A) to expiration (B). Tracheostomy was necessary for aspiration of pent-up secretions. (Courtesy of Children's Memorial Hospital, Chicago.)

Illustration continued on the following page

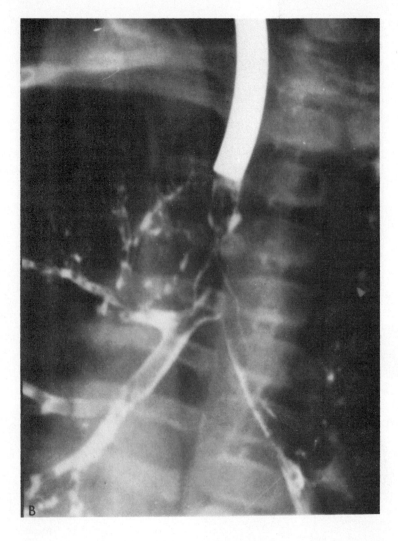

Figure 66B–7 *Continued* See Legend on preceding page.

graphs may show narrowing. With careful airway management, including tracheostomy in proximal involvement, the patient may be relieved of obstruction by further growth. However, the prognosis is frequently grim.

Tracheal Enlargement

Trachiectasis has been described by Soulas and Mounier-Kuhn (1949) as occurring on a congenital basis, usually in association with bronchiectasis or other organomegaly. It is a rarely recognized defect.

Tracheal Evagination

Tracheogenic Cysts. These cysts are similar to bronchogenic cysts and are thought to originate from evaginations of the primitive tracheal bud (McManus et al., 1971). (Because of their embryologic relation to the esophagus, they may contain elements of esophageal structures.) They are lined with columnar or cuboidal epithelium and may contain other elements of the tracheobronchial wall. The contents vary in lucency from clear to opaque and may be infected. The location may be anywhere along the trachea to the carina; direct connection to the trachea is usually absent, in contrast to bronchogenic cysts (Fig. 66B–8). The individual may be asymptomatic through adulthood; however, large cysts or those that are infected will give rise to early symptoms of stridor, wheezing, cyanosis, or coughing. The location of the cyst determines the associated signs; for instance, carinal cysts may cause bilateral

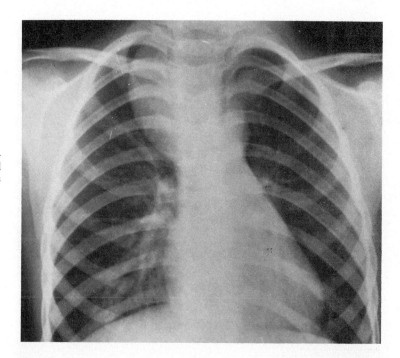

Figure 66B–8   Large cyst adjacent to trachea in a four year old child. (Courtesy of Children's Memorial Hospital, Chicago.)

wheezing, while posteriorly located cysts may result in impingement on the esophagus and deviation of this structure. Lateral ones may deviate the trachea or compress adjacent lung tissue (Miller et al., 1953). The location of some of these cysts is suggestive of pulmonary artery sling because of distortion of both the esophagus and the trachea (Fig. 66B–9). Diagnosis is made from the presence of radiographic evidence of a cystic structure of the mediastinum, but this may require oblique views, tomography, esophagography, or even bronchography to demonstrate, although the last is a risky test in cases of severe airway compression (Grafe et al., 1966). Bronchoscopy may be necessary to define the airway distortion as being extraluminal but must be done very cautiously to avoid any increase in obstruction from traumatic edema. Treatment consists of surgical excision, which defines the lesion and relieves any compression from the cyst.

Fistulas.   Tracheoesophageal fistula is a common congenital malformation of the newborn airway. It occurs as a faulty development and differentiation of the trachea from the esophagus and consequently can be located anywhere along the length of the trachea or even on the main bronchi, but frequently appears at the midtrachea level. The primary symptom is production of a profuse amount

of pharyngeal secretions and is noticeable within minutes of delivery. Those children with a proximal attachment of the esophagus (and distal blind pouch) have severe mucous problems without air in the intestines and may develop fatal airway problems if fed. The least symptomatic of the patients with fistulas are those with intact esophageal lumens but with a connection to the trachea — the "H" type of fistula — where fluid may flow readily into the stomach and only small amounts are diverted into the trachea to cause symptoms. These children may not be diagnosed for a considerable period of time if the connection is very small. However, once suspicion is aroused by presence of the "excess mucus," the diagnosis is made on the basis of inability to advance a catheter beyond the upper esophagus or by the result of esophagography. In the latter test, care must be taken to avoid spillage of contrast material because of its irritating effect. Therefore, only 1 to 5 cc of a thin, radiopaque material is introduced through a small feeding tube positioned in the esophagus distal to the larynx. With this tube in place, the material may be immediately removed by suction following the procedure with little chance of aspiration. In the "H"-type fistula, the examination may need to be repeated to show a small or high tract. Occasionally, bronchoscopy is necessary

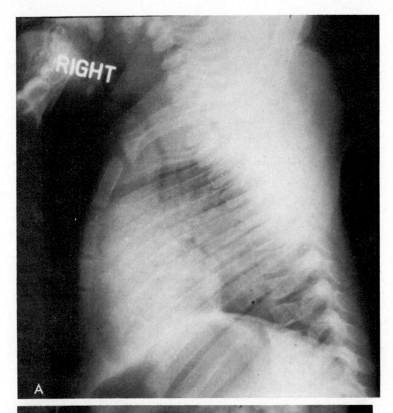

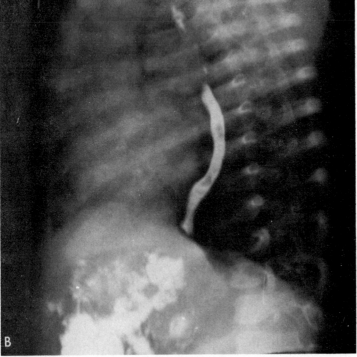

Figure 66B–9 Cyst causing deviation of both the trachea (*A*) and esophagus (*B*) in a young child. (Courtesy of Children's Memorial Hospital, Chicago.)

to identify the tiny opening in the trachea, indicated at the point of V-shaped folds of the membranous wall. Methylene blue placed in the esophagus may also be seen seeping into the trachea at this spot. Correction is by surgery, followed by dilatation of the anastomosis should it stenose. The patient will continue to show a dimple of varying depth

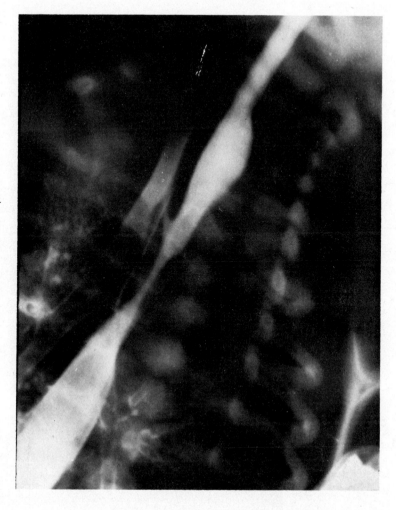

Figure 66B–10 "H" type tracheo-esophageal fistula in a three day old child. Contrast material has passed from the esophagus cephalically through the tiny fistula to enter the trachea and outline the bronchial tree. (Courtesy of Children's Memorial Hospital, Chicago.)

in the trachea, marking the site, and most will have a barking cough for months following the procedure from residual flaccidity of the membranous wall (Fig. 66B–10).

Abnormal Bifurcation

Tracheal Bronchus. This is a rather common occurrence and is identified in approximately 3 per cent of adult bronchograms according to Harris (1958). The location of the bronchus is above the level of the carina on the lateral wall, almost always on the right. The bronchus may be complete, serving the entire upper lobe. Rarely is it associated with tracheal stenosis (Maisel et al., 1974). It may be completely asymptomatic and discovered only incidentally when the tracheobronchial tree is examined for difficulties elsewhere. Problems, if present, are related to obstructions or infections, such as emphysema, atelec-

tasis, and persistent or recurrent pneumonia. The lumen of the anomalous bronchus may be seen endoscopically, appearing at first to be a dimple or small diverticulum on the lateral tracheal wall. However, the orifice can also appear widely patent and be easily visualized distally. Bronchography may be necessary for complete definition of the anomaly. Treatment is not necessary unless there is a disease, at which time excision may become necessary (Fig. 66B–11).

Anomalous Morphology. This may refer to a simple tracheal lobe but may be more significant. Both upper lobes may exit simultaneously from the trachea, which then bifurcates distally to the right and left. The distal bronchi may or may not have anomalous formations. The babies may have multiple anomalies of varying severity (Holinger et al., 1956). Treatment is dependent on the severity of the anomaly and on manifestation of symptoms (Fig. 66B–12).

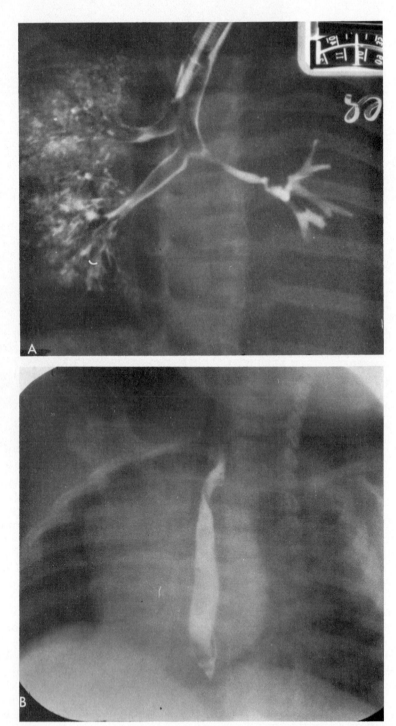

Figure 66B–11   Tracheal bronchus to right upper lobe seen on bronchogram, which also shows stenosis of the left main bronchus (*A*). Patient also has aberrant right subclavian artery seen on esophagogram (*B*). (Courtesy of Children's Memorial Hospital, Chicago.)

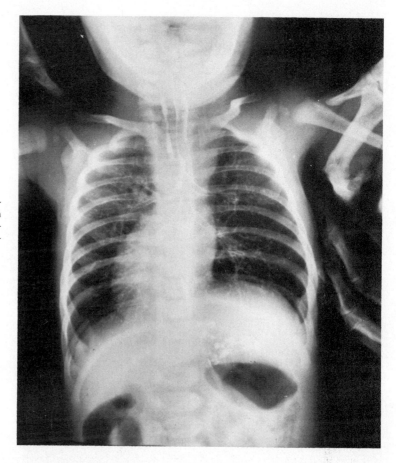

Figure 66B–12 Abnormal tracheal bifurcation in a child with dextrocardia. (Courtesy of Children's Memorial Hospital, Chicago.)

ANOMALIES OF BRONCHI

Agenesis or Atresia

Congenital absence of one bronchus occurs more frequently than tracheal agenesis and is not incompatible with life. The chest may be symmetric, although the trachea is deviated; the left lung is said to be absent more frequently than the right (Evans, 1948). Many patients are noted at birth to have some respiratory difficulty, cyanosis, or both. Chest films show opacity, which may not be complete if there is herniation of the opposite lung via the mediastinum (Holinger, 1961) (Fig. 66B–13). Breath sounds can be heard over the herniated area. Differentiation of this condition must be made from atelectasis secondary to the presence of mucus or a meconium plug; this can be accomplished by bronchoscopy, which must, however, be done with caution because of the patient's poor respiratory reserve. Other congenital anomalies may coexist, giving these babies a tenuous chance for survival. There is no treatment.

Bilateral agenesis is extremely rare; live-born infants with this problem may make gasping efforts to breathe before dying (Kissane, 1975).

Localized atresia of a bronchus is also very rare, although the actual incidence may be greater than is apparent since many patients are totally asymptomatic. The process usually is discovered on routine chest films in older age groups; however, the youngest symptomatic patient had tachypnea at birth. Typically, a small radiodensity is seen near the hilum with distal hyperinflation. The process is most frequently seen in the left upper lobe (Oh et al., 1976). Treatment is by resection of the involved area if the condition is causing severe compression of surrounding lung. At surgery an atretic bronchus is usually found with dilatation and mucus collection just beyond the bronchial closure. Distal to this mucocele is hyperinflation of the area supplied by that bronchus, a condition that is thought to be due to lateral air drift through the alveolar pores.

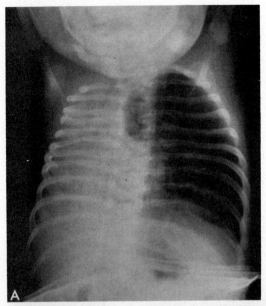

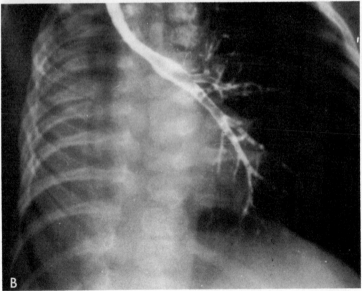

Figure 66B–13 Agenesis of the right lung in a one month old child. The trachea and mediastinal structure deviate to the right; there are also rib and vertebral anomalies (*A* and *B*). (Courtesy of Children's Memorial Hospital, Chicago.)

Constriction

Fibrous Strictures

Webs. Webs can occur in bronchi of any size. They appear as delicate mucous membrane diaphragms partially occluding the lumen. Symptoms will depend on the size of the residual orifice and vary from an occasional wheeze to severe obstruction. Treatment is by simple rupture by an advancing bronchoscope or, in the smaller bronchi, by forceps dilatation (Wallace, 1945).

Fibrous Bronchostenosis. This is a much more severe constriction involving the entire wall of the bronchus along a greater length. It is frequently associated with other anomalies of the area, such as vascular anomalies with deformity of the neighboring bronchus (Chang et al., 1968). While minor variations involving small bronchi may result in only intermittent localized problems such as right middle lobe recurrent pneumonia, major stenosis of a main bronchus may cause enough difficulty to necessitate resection and end-to-end anastomosis of the bronchus (Fig. 66B–14).

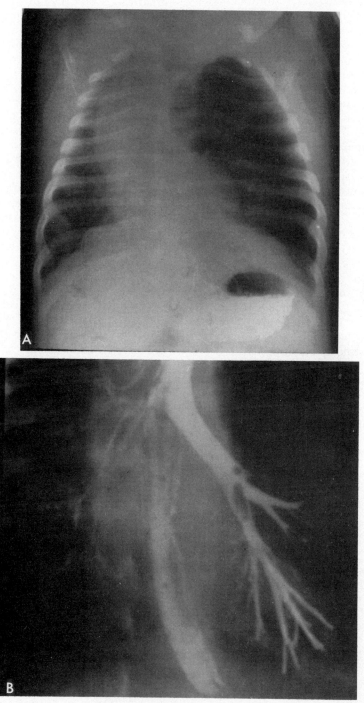

Figure 66B-14 Emphysema of the left upper lobe (A) secondary to stenosis of the bronchus to the upper segment (B). (Courtesy of Children's Memorial Hospital, Chicago.)

Absence or Deformity of Bronchial Cartilages

Bronchomalacia. This condition usually appears, along with tracheomalacia, as a generalized involvement of the tracheobronchial tree. The lumen on inspiration is of normal caliber, but on expiration there is marked diminution of lumen size, which may result in an expiratory wheeze. Symptoms become worse when secretions are increased or thickened as the result of a respiratory infection, since they then are more difficult to expel because of the malacic narrowing. Treatment consists of the administration of mucolytic agents; rarely is aspiration necessary. Growth of the child eventually resolves the problem as size increases and supporting tissues mature.

Hypoplasia. Hypoplasia of bronchial cartilage occurs in segmental bronchi and here results in local collapse with exhalation. The involved area acts as a one-way valve to allow air to enter but not to exit a bronchus. The resultant trapping of air causes hyperaeration of the distal lung with compression of normal adjacent lung and possibly even herniation of the emphysematous tissue across the mediastinum. The process may be minimal in effect but more often occurs so quickly that it causes progressive respiratory embarrassment. Surgery to remove the emphysematous lobe is curative, since the neighboring compressed lung tissue soon expands and resumes its function (Lincoln et al., 1971).

Changes Associated with Vascular Anomalies. Compression, distortion, and defective cartilages have been mentioned already in relation to tracheal problems; they are seen as well in the bronchi (Fig. 66B–15).

Bronchial Enlargement

Congenital Bronchiectasis. The congenital form of this condition can be difficult to distinguish from the acquired variety, but in the congenital type trouble may be present from shortly after birth: cough, respiratory distress, repeated episodes of pneumonia, and persistent atelectasis are some of the presenting signs. The suspected congenital origin is confirmed if an anomalous formation of vasculature or of the bronchial tree is found upon performance of an exploratory operation. On microscopic examination of a specimen of bronchial tissue, abnormalities of development of the bronchial wall, including cartilage deficiency, are found (Poradowska, 1972; Wayne and Taussig, 1976). Treatment is medical control of infection, reduction of viscosity of secretions, improvement of secretion clearance by postural drainage with physiotherapy, and surgical removal of diseased areas unimproved by medical management.

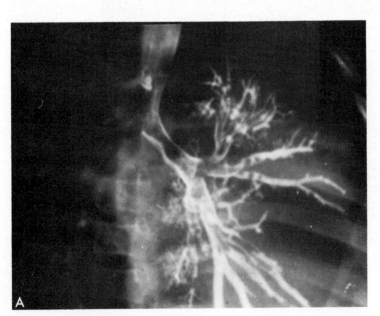

Figure 66B–15 Bronchograms of left side showing, on inspiration (*A*), slight indentation of the main bronchus from an anomalous pulmonary artery. On expiration (*B*) there is marked narrowing of the same area. (Courtesy of Children's Memorial Hospital, Chicago.)
Illustration continued on the opposite page.

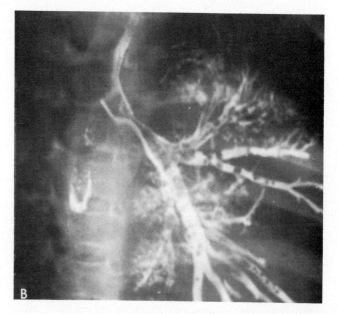

Figure 66B–15 *Continued*   See legend on the opposite page.

Kartagener Syndrome. This syndrome also involves bronchiectasis along with situs inversus, sinusitis, and absent frontal sinuses. Recently found to be part of this syndrome is defective ciliary motility, which compounds the problem (Eliasson et al., 1977) (Fig. 66B–16).

Bronchial Evaginations or Outgrowths

Bronchogenic Cysts.   Bronchogenic cysts arise from the bronchi in the same manner as tracheogenic cysts from the trachea, as previously described. Here also the cysts are lined by respiratory epithelium, and the walls may

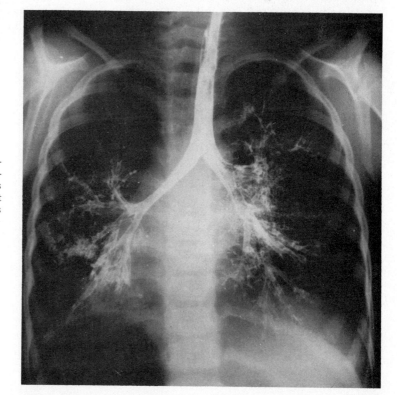

Figure 66B–16 Kartagener syndrome in a four year old child evidenced on bronchogram by situs inversus and bronchiectasis of right lower lobe. (Courtesy of Children's Memorial Hospital, Chicago.)

contain any elements of normal bronchial wall. They are filled with clear to cloudy material and may be multiloculated. The contents may become infected even if not in communication with the air passages, and those with bronchial connections can have an air-fluid level. Cysts in association with distal bronchi may be surrounded by pulmonary parenchyma. Many are asymptomatic until the patient reaches adulthood, but infants with cysts may present with dyspnea, cyanosis, wheezing, coughing, and a fever (McManus et al., 1971). Investigation of these problems, as with tracheogenic cysts, includes obtaining chest radiographs, an esophagogram, and a bronchogram. Angiography may be necessary if the differential diagnosis cannot be made from sequestered lung by the foregoing examinations. When symptomatic, surgical excision of the cyst is recommended, since mortality otherwise is high (Buntain et al., 1974) (Fig. 66B–17). A perhaps related congenital anomaly is that of cystic adenomatoid malformation. In these patients, multiple cysts of varying size occur and involve one or two lobes of one lung. There is a bronchial connection with proliferated terminal bronchioles forming cysts lined with respiratory epithelium (Aslam et al., 1970). In contrast to bronchogenic cysts, there may be little cartilage in the adenomatoid cyst walls. The pathologic changes produce compression of the normal lung with resultant respiratory distress of increasing severity. Surgical removal of the cyst allows for normal expansion of the lung and relief of symptoms (Fig. 66B–18).

Fistulas. Communications between the esophagus and the main bronchi occur as well as do fistulas to the trachea, as described earlier. Additionally, congenital bronchobiliary fistulas may occur (Sane et al., 1971). In one patient it was associated with a tracheoesophageal fistula (Kalayoglu and Olcay, 1976). Symptoms are coughing and respiratory distress, sometimes including coughing up bile-stained material. Diagnosis is made on the basis of both bronchoscopy and bronchography results, since either procedure alone may fail to show the fistula. Bile-stained material is visible coming from a bronchial opening, which is then outlined by contrast materials, delineating the source and direction of the fistula. Treatment is by surgical excision.

Abnormal Bifurcation

As mentioned in the discussion of the tracheal lobe, there are frequent anomalies of lobation that may be completely asymptoma-

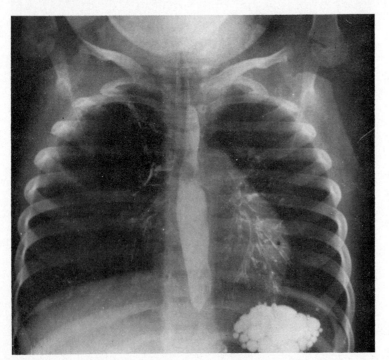

Figure 66B–17 Cyst of the right upper lobe associated with a tracheal bronchus. (Courtesy of Children's Memorial Hospital, Chicago.)

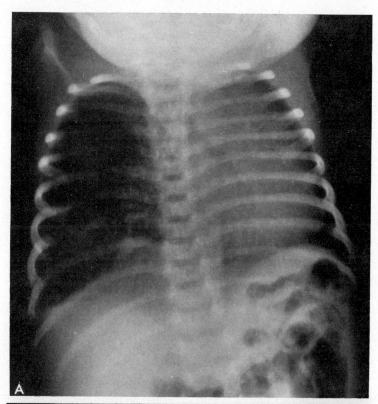

Figure 66B–18 Cystic malformation of right middle and lower lobes in a nine day old infant. (Courtesy of Children's Memorial Hospital, Chicago.)

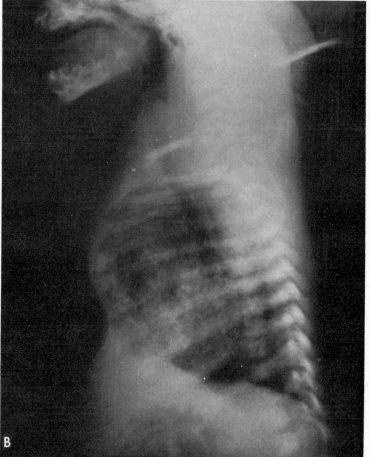

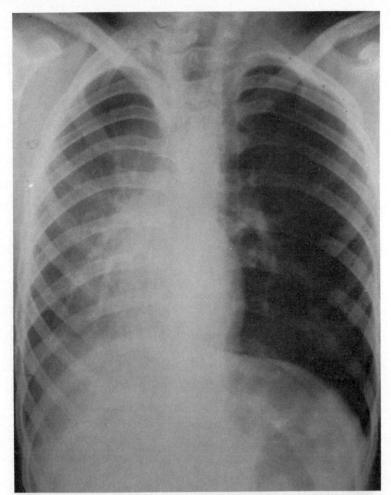

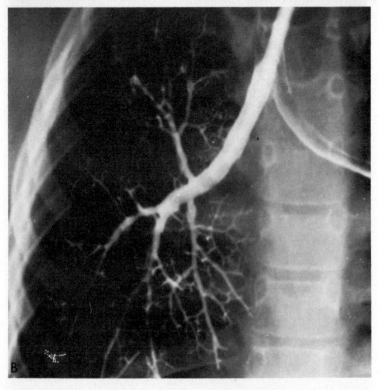

Figure 66B–19 Congenital absence of the right upper and middle lobes seen in bronchography of a nine year old girl; (A) chest film, (B) bronchogram. (Courtesy of Children's Memorial Hospital, Chicago.)

tic or that may cause problems severe enough to warrant resection. Regularly, the differentiation of the living tissue is into three lobes on the right and two on the left. As the bronchi branch further into segments, the distal branching becomes less regular in all areas (Bloomer et al., 1960). To complicate matters further, the arteries and veins are even more irregular. Smaller bronchi may be less numerous than usual, may branch into the usual number but in an unusual location, or may be more numerous than expected (Nagaishi, 1972) (Fig. 66B–19). No difficulty may arise from these altered branchings. However, should disease occur that requires resection of the lung, the surgeon's problems

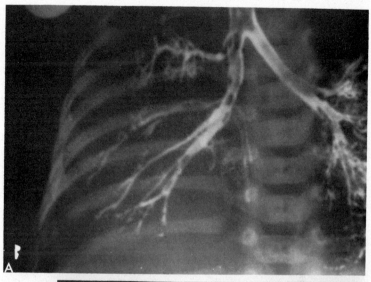
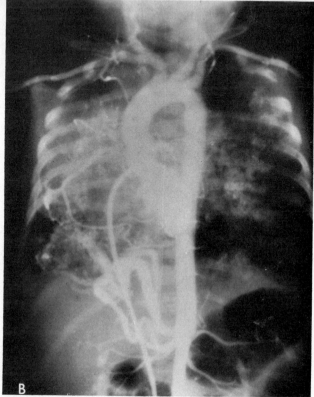

Figure 66B–20 Bronchogram (A) and arteriogram (B) delineating sequestration of the right lower lobe. (Courtesy of Children's Memorial Hospital, Chicago.)

increase in segmental resections. Additionally notable is the association of this anomaly with other anomalies, such as scimitar syndrome and polysplenia or asplenia with cardiac malformations (Dehner, 1975).

Anomalous Attachments

Sequestered Lung. This is a term used to describe lung tissue unattached to the bronchial system that has circulation from major vessels other than the pulmonary artery, usually the aorta. This tissue may be surrounded by normal lung tissue (intralobar sequestration) or may be completely separate from it, including having a separate pleural covering (extralobar sequestration) (DeParedes et al., 1970). In both instances, the

predominant location of this anomaly is on the left side and in the lower lobe area. In the case of extralobar sequestration, there are frequently associated diaphragmatic defects that may be noted first, with the sequestration found only at surgery for repair of the diaphragm. Respiratory distress and recurrent infections are usually found in these children's histories. Diagnosis is based on chest radiograph findings of opacity of the lower lobe, which clears to cystic areas after treatment with antibiotics. Bronchoscopy and bronchograms indicate the lack of bronchial connection and the displacement of adjacent lung tissues. Angiography will confirm the diagnosis by showing the anomalous arterial supply. Surgical resection is necessary with care taken to find and control the vascular supply (Fig. 66B–20).

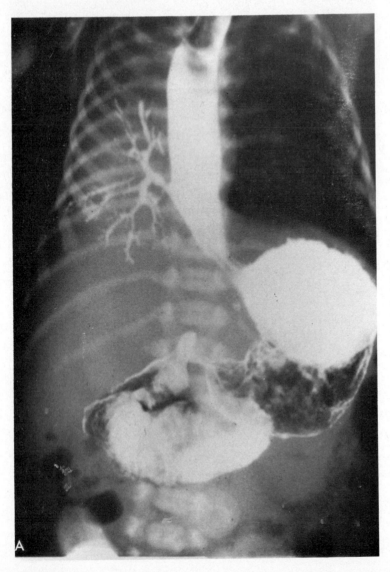

Figure 66B–21 Origin of the right main bronchus from the esophagus. (*A*) anteroposterior view, (*B*) lateral view. (Courtesy of Children's Memorial Hospital, Chicago.)

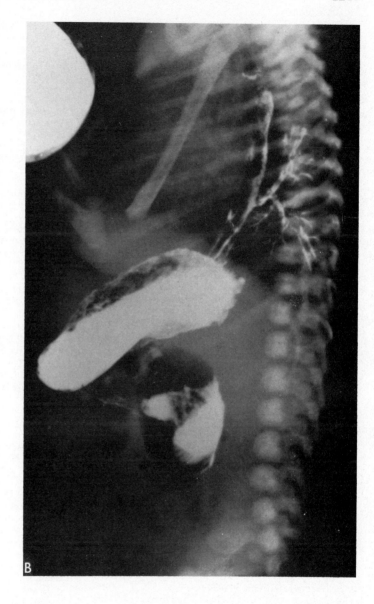

Figure 66B–21 *Continued* See legend on the opposite page.

Gastrointestinal Tract Attachments. Connection of anomalous lung tissue to the gastrointestinal tract has also been found. These are felt by some to be related to sequestered lung, described before, since they have the obvious gut connection that sequestered lobes no longer retain (Gerle et al., 1968). Anatomically, the lobe takes its origin from the lower esophagus or stomach via a bronchus that contains cartilage fragments and is lined by respiratory epithelium; the blood supply is via the aorta. In these children, symptoms may be gastrointestinal as well as respiratory. Treatment is surgical removal (Nikaidoh and Swenson, 1971) (Fig. 66B–21).

SELECTED REFERENCES

Avery, M. E., and Fletcher, B. D. 1974. The Lung and Its Disorders in the Newborn Infant, 3rd ed. Philadelphia, W. B. Saunders Co.
An excellent, comprehensive text dealing with normal physiology as well as pathologic conditions.

Holinger, P. H. 1961. Clinical aspects of congenital anomalies of the larynx, trachea, bronchi and oesophagus. J. Laryngol. Otol., 75:1–44.
Clear illustrations, both endoscopic and radiographic, make this review of the author's clinical experience a valuable source of information.

Kissane, J. 1975. Pathology of Infancy and Childhood, 2nd ed. St. Louis, The C. V. Mosby Co.
This is an overview of pediatric pathology with concise explanations of tracheobronchial conditions.

REFERENCES

Aslam, P. A., Korones, S. B., Richardson, R. L., Jr., et al. 1970. Congenital cystic adenomatoid malformation with anasarca. J.A.M.A., *212*:622–624.

Avery, M. E., and Fletcher, B. D. 1974. The Lung and Its Disorders in the Newborn Infant, 3rd ed. Philadelphia, W. B. Saunders Co.

Baxter, J. D., and Dunbar, J. S. 1963. Tracheomalacia. Ann. Otol. Rhinol. Laryngol., *72*:1013–1023.

Bloomer, W. E. 1960. Surgical Anatomy of the Bronchovascular Segments. Springfield, IL, C C Thomas.

Buntain, W. L., Isaacs, H., Jr., Payne, V. C., Jr., et al. 1974. Lobar emphysema, cystic adenomatoid malformation, pulmonary sequestration, and bronchogenic cyst in infancy and childhood: A clinical group. J. Pediatr. Surg., *9*:85–93.

Cantrell, J. R., and Guild, H. G. 1964. Congenital stenosis of the trachea. Am. J. Surg., *108*:297–305.

Chang, N., Hertzler, J. H., Gregg, R. H., et al. 1968. Congenital stenosis of the right mainstem bronchus: A case report. Pediatrics, *41*:739–742.

Dehner, L. P. 1975. Pediatric Surgical Pathology. St. Louis, The C. V. Mosby Co., p. 196.

DeParedes, C. G., Pierce, W. S., Johnson, D. G., et al. 1970. Pulmonary sequestration in infants and children: A 20-year experience and review of the literature. J. Pediatr. Surg., *5*:136–147.

Eliasson, R., Mossberg, B., Camner, P., et al. 1977. The immotile-cilia syndrome: A congenital ciliary abnormality as an etiologic factor in chronic airway infections and male sterility. N. Engl. J. Med., *297*:1–6.

Evans, W. A. 1948. Congenital obstructions of the respiratory tract. Am. J. Roentgenol. Radium Ther. Nucl. Med., *62*:177–184.

Fearon, B., and Shortreed, R. 1963. Tracheobronchial compression by congenital cardiovascular anomalies in children: Syndrome of apnea. Ann. Otol. Rhinol. Laryngol., *72*:949–969.

Gerle, R. D., Jaretzki, A., III, Ashley, C. A., et al. 1968. Congenital bronchopulmonary-foregut malformation: Pulmonary sequestration communicating with the gastrointestinal tract. N. Engl. J. Med., *278*:1413–1419.

Grafe, W. R., Goldsmith, E. I., and Redo, S. F. 1966. Bronchogenic cysts of the mediastinum in children. J. Pediatr. Surg., *1*:384–393.

Greene, D. A. 1976. Congenital complete tracheal rings. Arch. Otolaryngol., *102*:241–243.

Harris, J. H., Jr. 1958. The clinical significance of the tracheal bronchus. Am. J. Roentgenol. Radium Ther. Nucl. Med., *79*:228–234.

Holinger, P. H. 1961. Clinical aspects of congenital anomalies of the larynx, trachea, bronchi and oesophagus. J. Laryngol. Otol., *75*:1–44.

Holinger, P. H., and Johnston, K. C. 1957. Clinical aspects of congenital anomalies of the trachea and bronchi. Dis. Chest, *31*:613–621.

Holinger, P. H., Johnston, K. C., and Basinger, C. E. 1950. Benign stenosis of the trachea. Ann. Otol. Rhinol. Laryngol., *59*:837–859.

Holinger, P. H., Johnston, K. C., Parchet, V. N., et al. 1952. Congenital malformations of the trachea, bronchi and lung. Ann. Otol. Rhinol. Laryngol., *61*:1159–1180.

Holinger, P. H., Zimmerman, A. A., Parchet, V. N., et al. 1956. A correlation of the embryonic development of the trachea and lungs with congenital malformations. Adv. Otorhinolaryngol., *3*:1–39.

Holinger, P. H., Zimmerman, A. A., and Schild, J. A.

1972. Tracheobronchial tree malformations. *In* Ferguson, C. F., and Kendig, E. L., Jr. (eds.) Pediatric Otolaryngology, Vol. 2, 2nd ed. Philadelphia, W. B. Saunders Co., p. 1286.

Joshi, V. V. 1969. Tracheal agenesis. Am. J. Dis. Child., *117*:341–343.

Kalayoglu, M., and Olcay, I. 1976. Congenital bronchobiliary fistula associated with esophageal atresia and tracheo-esophageal fistula. J. Pediatr. Surg., *11*:463–464.

Kissane, J. 1975. Pathology of Infancy and Childhood, 2nd ed. St. Louis, The C. V. Mosby Co. pp. 471–53.

Leape, L. L. 1973. Silastic tracheal stent as an aid in decannulation. J. Pediatr. Surg., *8*:717–721.

Lincoln, J. C. R., Deverall, P. B., Stark, J., et al. 1969. Vascular anomalies compressing the oesophagus and trachea. Thorax, *24*:295–306.

Lincoln, J. C. R., Stark, J., Subramanian, S., et al. 1971. Congenital lobar emphysema. Ann. Surg., *173*:55–62.

McManus, W. F., Davis, W. C., and Sellers, R. D. 1971. Bronchogenic cyst arising from the trachea in an adult. Am. Surg., *37*:555–557.

Maisel, R. H., Fried, M. P., Swain, R., et al. 1974. Anomalous tracheal bronchus with tracheal hypoplasia. Arch. Otolaryngol., *100*:69–70.

Miller, R. F., Graub, M., and Pashuck, E. T. 1953. Bronchogenic cysts: Anomalies resulting from maldevelopment of the primitive foregut and midgut. Am. J. Roentgenol. Radium Ther. Nucl. Med., *70*:771–785.

Moes, C. A. F., Izukawa, T., and Trusler, G. A. 1975. Innominate artery compression of the trachea. Arch. Otolaryngol., *101*:733–738.

Nagaishi, C. 1972. Functional Anatomy and Histology of the Lung. Baltimore, University Park Press, p. 15.

Nikaidoh, H., and Swenson, O. 1971. The ectopic origin of the right main bronchus from the esophagus. J. Thorac. Cardiovasc. Surg., *62*:151–160.

Oh, K. S., Dorst, J. P., White, J. J., et al. 1976. The syndrome of bronchial atresia or stenosis with mucocele and focal hyperinflation of the lung. Johns Hopkins Med. J., *138*:48–53.

Park, C. D., Waldhausen, J. A., Friedman, S., et al. 1971. Tracheal compression by the great arteries in the mediastinum. Arch. Surg., *103*:626–632.

Peison, B., Levitsky, E., and Sprowls, J. J. 1970. Tracheoesophageal fistula associated with tracheal atresia and malformation of the larynx. J. Pediatr. Surg., *5*:464–467.

Poradowska, W. 1972. Surgical Lung Diseases in Childhood. Warsaw, Polish Medical Publishers.

Potts, W. J., Holinger, P. H., and Rosenblum, A. H. 1954. Anomalous left pulmonary artery causing obstruction to the right main bronchus: Report of a case. J.A.M.A., *155*:1409–1411.

Sane, S. M., Sieber, W. K., and Girdany, B. R. 1971. Congenital bronchobiliary fistula. Surgery, *69*:599–608.

Smith, E. I. 1957. The early development of the trachea and esophagus in relation to atresia of the esophagus and tracheoesophageal fistula. Contrib. Embryol., *245*:43–57.

Soulas, A., and Mounier-Kuhn, P. 1949. Bronchologie: Technique endoscopique et pathologie trachéobronchique. Paris, Masson & Cie, p. 623.

Wallace, J. E. 1945. Two cases of congenital web of a bronchus. Arch. Pathol., *39*:47–48.

Wayne, K. S., and Taussig, L. M. 1976. Probable familial congenital bronchiectasis due to cartilage deficiency (Williams-Campbell syndrome). Am. Rev. Respir. Dis., *114*:15–22.

Chapter 67

INFECTIONS OF THE LOWER RESPIRATORY TRACT

Martha L. Lepow, M.D.

GENERAL FEATURES

Infections of the respiratory tract constitute the most common cause of morbidity and mortality in infants and young children. In this chapter, infections of the larynx, trachea, bronchi, bronchioles, and lungs will be considered.

Etiologic agents of disease, which include anatomic predisposition to infection, are age-related. For example, the upper airway in a young child is quite small, and obstruction may be a great problem. For children, ages one to three years is the period of most frequent acquisition of a number of respiratory viruses (Cherry, 1973) and bacteria such as pneumococci and *Haemophilus influenzae* type B (*H. influenzae* B). Frequently, the first experience with these agents leads to more severe disease than reexposure later in childhood, and upper and lower portions of the respiratory tract are affected. Table 67–1 is a listing of the more common ones and the anatomic sites of predilection. It is apparent that the same infectious agent may infect more than one site. As the various disorders are described according to anatomic site of infection, further reference will be made to Table 67–1.

CROUP

Incidence and Epidemiology

This is a syndrome characterized by inspiratory stridor, cough, and hoarseness with varying degrees of respiratory distress. Anatomic location of the infection is one of the most important factors in predicting the outcome of the illness, and a supraglottic (epiglottic) infectious process is by far the more serious, although subglottic infections are far more common. Etiology differs according to the anatomic site (Table 67–1). Epiglottitis, which is almost always bacterial (*H. influenzae* type B) accounts for 5 to 10 per cent of croup infections, and viral croup constitutes 90 to 95 per cent of all croup cases in reported series (Rabe, 1948; Lockhart and Battaglia, 1977). *H. influenzae* B epiglottitis is sporadic and occurs at any time of the year, although it is seen most commonly in winter and spring. Viral croup, which affects the larynx and subglottic region, is frequently epidemic, and outbreaks occur in spring and autumn. Epiglottitis affects a broader age range of children (from two to eight years), whereas viral croup affects infants from six months to two years of age.

The incidence of *H. influenzae* B epiglottitis is difficult to ascertain since the disease is not reportable. As in determining the incidence of *H. influenzae* B meningitis, data are best collected from large hospitals and based upon positive blood cultures. Since only 50 to 75 per cent of patients with epiglottitis have positive blood cultures, the actual number of cases may be greater than the number reported. It appears to be more common in the northeastern part of the country than in the South, but confirmed data are difficult to find. There are some clues that *H. influenzae* B epiglottitis may have a different pathogenesis

Table 67–1 ASSOCIATION OF ETIOLOGIC AGENT WITH ANATOMIC SITE IN
CHILDHOOD RESPIRATORY INFECTION

Anatomic Site	Bacteria	Virus	Other
Nose (sinuses)	β-hemolytic streptococci *Pneumococcus* *H. influenzae* B *S. aureus*	Rhinoviruses Influenza A and B	
Pharynx and tonsils	β-hemolytic streptococci *Gonococcus*	Adenoviruses Parainfluenza 1, 2 Coxsackie and ECHO viruses	

Larynx
  Epiglottic
 	
  Subglottic
	H. influenzae B
	C. diphtheria
		
		Parainfluenza 1, 2
		Influenza A and B
		Rubella
		Varicella	

Bronchi and bronchioles	*H. influenzae* B *Pneumococcus*	Respiratory syncytial Adenoviruses Parainfluenza 1, 2, 3 Rhinoviruses	

Lung and pleura	*Pneumococcus*
	H. influenzae B
	Beta-hemolytic
	  streptococci
	K. pneumoniae
	Anaerobic bacteria (abscess)
		Respiratory syncytial
		Adenoviruses
		Parainfluenza 3
		Influenza A and B
		Rubella
		Varicella
		Psittacosis
		Cytomegalovirus
			
			M. pneumoniae
			M. tuberculosis
			Q. fever
			Fungi
			Pneumocystis carinii
			Chlamydia
			  trachomatis

from meningitis since the affected children are older and seasonal distribution is different. There may be anatomic factors and socioeconomic factors (Sell and Karzen, 1973) that also contribute to the distribution of this disease.

Acute Epiglottitis

Clinical Features. Acute bacterial epiglottitis usually has a sudden onset and a rapidly progressive course. Typically, the child may develop a high fever with respiratory distress, drooling, and painful swallowing. The illness may quickly progress to respiratory obstruction.

Inspection of the pharynx reveals a cherry-red or edematous epiglottis. Manipulation of the pharynx with a tongue depressor or swabs should be avoided unless the examiner is prepared either to intubate or to perform a tracheostomy because such manipulation may result in complete obstruction of the trachea. A lateral radiograph of the nasopharynx should be obtained for an assessment of the retropharyngeal space and the remainder of the upper airway, as well as for documentation of edema of the epiglottis (Fig. 67–1). A professional person capable of intubating the child should accompany the patient to the radiology department. Any physician seeing a patient with epiglottitis should consider it a medical emergency and as soon as possible should arrange to have an artificial airway created either by a tracheostomy or by nasotracheal intubation (Schuller and Birck, 1975). The method that is selected depends upon the expertise of the staff caring for the patient. Intubation requires the constant availability of personnel capable of reintubating should the patient extubate prematurely. On the other hand, a tracheostomy requires continuous attention to be sure the secretions are cleared. This is especially important in the very small child in whom the tube may easily become occluded, resulting in asphyxia.

Laboratory Features. The most common etiologic agent is *H. influenzae* type B, although pneumococci or beta-hemolytic streptococci have also been implicated. Laryngotracheitis due to *Corynebacterium diphtheriae* may occasionally occur, and a membrane may be visible. Over 50 per cent of cases due to *H. influenzae* type B will have an associated pneumonia or other extralaryngeal site of inflammation (Molteni, 1976). Bacteremia occurs in over 50 per cent of these patients; thus, blood cultures should always be obtained from them. In these patients, the white blood cell count will usually be elevated, and the differential count will show a predominance of polymorphonuclear leukocytes.

Management. Once an artificial airway has been placed, it should remain until spasm and edema have subsided and infection is under control. This usually requires two to three days. The clinical state of the patient should determine when extubation should occur. Antibiotics should always be used. Ampicillin, 150 to 200 mg per kg per day, is the drug of choice. Because some strains of *H. influenzae* B are resistant to ampicillin, treatment should also include chloramphenicol, 100 mg per kg per day for 7 to 10 days, until the antibiotic susceptibility of the offending organisms is known, according to the most recent recommendation of the Committee on Infectious Disease of the American Academy of Pediatrics (1976). Recurrences of this illness are very uncommon. Disease control with a polysaccharide vaccine against *H. influenzae* B is a distinct possibility in the near future.

Acute Subglottic Croup

Acute subglottic croup is also called acute laryngotracheobronchitis and may follow an upper respiratory tract infection or fall into the category of "spasmodic croup," which will be described later.

Etiology and Epidemiology. This type of croup is almost always viral in etiology (Table 67–1). Parainfluenza and influenza viruses

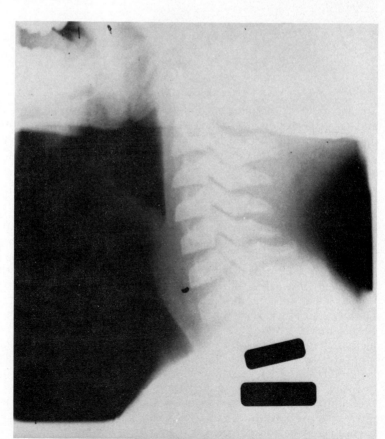

Figure 67–1 Epiglottitis with massive swelling of the epiglottis and a ballooned hypopharynx.

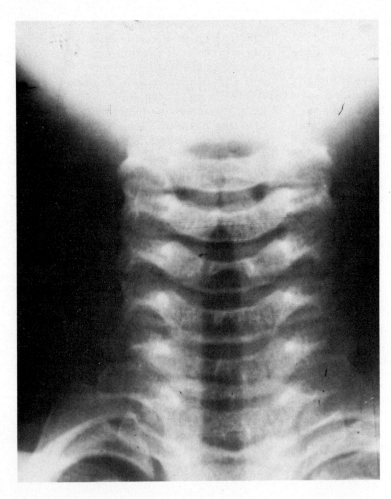

Figure 67–2 Subglottic croup showing ballooned hypopharynx and subglottic narrowing.

are frequent pathogens, although measles and varicella and other viral agents can cause similar symptoms.

Parainfluenza virus-induced croup frequently occurs in clusters of cases in the spring and fall. It occurs primarily in young children one to three years of age, in contrast to acute epiglottitis, which occurs in older children, and is generally benign. There may be involvement of the larynx, trachea, bronchi, and bronchioles (Fig. 67–2). Occasionally, interstitial pneumonia occurs.

Clinical Features. The patient usually has a low-grade or moderate fever, and upper respiratory symptoms are common. Respiratory distress of varying degrees with increased rate and respiratory effort is common. Inspiratory stridor, hoarseness, a barking cough, and expiratory rhonchi occur frequently. The larynx may be involved predominantly, or the lower airway may be involved as well. Although many children can be managed as outpatients, any child with stridor at rest will probably benefit from observation in a hospital setting. If there are retractions and restlessness or a respiratory rate over 30, admission becomes mandatory. Intervention may be required to maintain a patent airway.

Restlessness may be a sign of hypoxia, as is tachycardia. Blood gases should be measured if there is any question of impending respiratory failure, of which cyanosis will be a late sign. Rarely, a child will develop significant upper airway obstruction with evidence of respiratory failure, which necessitates tracheostomy or intubation.

Laboratory Features. White blood cell counts in these cases are usually within the normal range, with differential counts appropriate for the age of the patient. Throat cultures usually do not reveal significant bacterial pathogens. Viral cultures can be done for appropriate respiratory agents. If respiratory failure ensues, the PO_2 will be low, while the PCO_2 would be expected to be normal or high.

Management. Treatment consists of

maintaining adequate hydration and cold humidification. There have been a number of studies of the use of corticosteroids in viral croup. These have included several double-blind studies with varying doses and preparations, ranging from methylprednisolone, 0.1 mg per kg body weight every six hours for four doses (Eden and Larkin, 1964), to dexamethasone, 0.1 to 1.0 mg per kg body weight every six hours for up to eight doses (Skowton et al., 1966; Eden et al., 1967). Since the course of the illness is likely to be short and the need for airway intervention is rare, it is difficult to determine what role, if any, steroids might play. In none of the studies was the effect of steroid administration striking.

There are experimental data from work with monkeys that show a positive effect from administration of a single large dose (5 to 6 mg per kg body weight) of dexamethasone phosphate in treating postintubation laryngeal edema (Biller et al., 1970). This suggests that a larger dose might be important in resolving viral croup. Since prophylactic steroids are most likely to be useful when given before edema ensues, and since, in viral croup, edema has occurred and may be at its maximum when other symptoms commence, it is unlikely that a well-controlled study can be done on the effects of steroids on croup.

The widespread use of racemic epinephrine in viral croup was stimulated by the publication by Adair et al. (1971) of a 10 year favorable experience with intermittent positive pressure breathing (IPPB) with racemic epinephrine. Those authors stated that the routine use of racemic epinephrine diluted 1:8 with water and administered with IPPB for 15 minutes in patients with croup eliminated the need for tracheostomy for these problems during a period of several years.

Since that time, in double-blind studies, positive (Gardner et al., 1973; Singer and Wilson, 1976) and negative (Taussig et al., 1975) effects have been reported. It has still not been determined whether the immediate effectiveness of the treatment might be due to nebulization of moisture. All investigators agree that there is a beneficial effect acutely but that repeat doses are usually needed from 30 minutes to six to eight hours later. A prospective study comparing nebulized water and racemic epinephrine should be done.

Since the apparent beneficial effect of racemic epinephrine may be short-lived and since marked rebound may occur one to two hours later (Taussig et al., 1975), such a

treatment is best done in the hospital. Antibiotics are usually not indicated. The usual course of the disease is three to five days, but this type of croup is frequently recurrent.

Spasmodic Croup

This type of croup may be a variant of viral croup but is characterized by a sudden onset, frequently during sleep, with or without preceding upper respiratory tract infection, with significant inspiratory stridor, and with respiratory distress. It may be recurrent. The major pathophysiologic process is spasm of the larynx. The symptoms are frequently relieved by inducing vomiting with one tablespoon of ipecac. Children with this syndrome are commonly between one and three years old, and the disease is rarely seen in older children. Cold, humid air is helpful, and the symptoms usually subside spontaneously.

Laryngitis

Inflammation and edema of the larynx are manifestations of croup. The younger the infant, the greater the likelihood of the edema's producing obstruction. The term "laryngitis" refers to hoarseness without obstructive symptoms. In older children and adults, laryngitis is more common than croup. Laryngitis is almost always viral. Subacute or chronic laryngitis are more common in older children and adults and may be an extension of an acute laryngitis attack. Physical examination may reveal a hyperemic pharynx, and inflammatory edema of the larynx may be seen by laryngoscopy. Treatment includes resting of the vocal cords if possible. The presence of trauma, tumor, or congenital defects should be ruled out in chronic laryngitis, especially in infants.

Diphtheria

This is an acute infectious disease caused by C. diphtheriae, characterized by local growth of the organism in the respiratory tract and by systemic manifestations, which are due to absorption and spread to exotoxin. Owing to widespread immunization in temperate areas where the disease is most prevalent, clinical diphtheria is relatively uncommon.

The portal of entry is most commonly in

the respiratory tract, and local bacterial growth with toxin production leads to tissue necrosis with bleeding. As epithelium degenerates, a serosanguinous exudate develops, which produces a membrane-like cover over the area. Bloody nasal discharge occurs frequently. A pseudomembrane may be visible in the nose or over the tonsils, soft palate, larynx, or tracheobronchial tree. A membrane over the lower respiratory tract may produce obstruction and respiratory failure. Fever is low-grade and malaise is common. Systemic effects on the heart, liver, kidney, and brain are later sequelae, occurring 10 to 14 days after onset of the symptoms.

The diagnosis should be made clinically and confirmed by specific bacterial smears and cultures from the membrane on Löffler's or tellurite media.

Other processes that may produce a pseudomembrane and thus mimic diphtheria include infectious mononucleosis, in which atypical lymphocytes will appear in the peripheral blood and a heterophil test will have positive results. Streptococcal pharyngitis is usually limited to the tonsils. Blood dyscrasias associated with granulocytopenia may result in membranous tonsillitis as well. Ulcerative pharyngitis due to herpes simplex or herpangina should be considered in the differential diagnosis. Prevention is best accomplished by immunization according to approved schedules. The treatment for respiratory obstruction is provision of an artificial airway; systemic therapy includes antitoxin, 20,000 to 60,000 units IM or IV, and 600,000 units of procaine penicillin per day for 10 days, or erythromycin, 40 mg per kg per day in divided doses for 10 days. Carriers are treated by penicillin therapy.

Angioneurotic Edema

This is usually acute and affects older children, rarely infants. It is the most severe manifestation of systemic allergy due to foreign proteins such as bee stings. Obstruction occurs in the subglottic area, and symptoms will respond to epinephrine and antihistamines.

Retropharyngeal Abscess

Occasionally, this may present as respiratory obstruction. If the posterior pharyngeal wall is palpated, a mass, sometimes fluctuant, may be outlined. A lateral radiograph of the neck will show an increased soft tissue density between the pharynx and the vertebrae.

ACUTE BRONCHITIS

Clinical Features

This syndrome is characterized by a cough, which may be dry or spasmodic, and which later becomes productive of cloudy or yellow-green sputum. The child may have a fever. Coarse rhonchi or inconstant rales may be heard. This illness is frequently an extension of an upper respiratory infection.

Treatment is symptomatic, and antibiotics are usually not indicated. Cold, humid air may relieve distress. Antihistamines and antitussive agents should be used in moderation, since coughing may be an important mechanism in clearing the airway. Chronic bronchitis is an uncommon sequel to an upper respiratory infection in the absence of underlying disease.

Laboratory Features

In the differential diagnosis, pertussis is characterized by paroxysmal cough with vomiting and sometimes cyanosis, usually in the absence of fever or specific physical signs in the lungs. Several adenoviruses, especially types 5 and 12, can cause an illness that mimics pertussis. Nasopharyngeal cultures planted on Bordet-Gengou medium or testing of nasopharyngeal smears with fluorescent antipertussis antibody may be helpful in establishing the diagnosis. Acute and convalescent sera from patients suspected of having pertussis may be tested for an increase in pertussis agglutinins. Erythromycin, 50 mg per kg per day, is the present treatment of choice with ampicillin, 100 mg per kg per day, being an alternative in pertussis.

Adenovirus can be isolated from throat swabs or sputum in appropriate cell cultures. Studies that demonstrate an increase in antibody in response to the presence of adenovirus group antigen between acute and convalescent sera may also be useful. *Mycoplasma pneumoniae*, another potential cause of bronchitis, more commonly extends to the lung and will be covered in the section on pneumonia.

Bronchitis with wheezing that is reversible with bronchodilators by definition indicates asthma, which is appropriate to mention at this point but is beyond the scope of this chapter to discuss.

BRONCHIOLITIS

Clinical Features

Bronchiolitis is an acute illness mainly occurring in young infants in whom the major site of inflammation and obstruction is the small bronchiole (Reynolds, 1972; Holdaway et al., 1967). The major symptom is prolongation of expiration with expiratory wheezing. There may be a low-grade fever. Other clinical features include tachypnea, intercostal retraction, and sometimes cyanosis. Auscultation reveals fine rales, a prolonged expiratory phase, and a wheeze. A chest radiograph may show hyperinflation of the lungs, atelectasis, or both. Frequently differentiation between bronchiolitis and bronchial asthma is difficult, and, indeed, asthma may occur later on in life in patients who have had bronchiolitis during the first two years of life (Zweiman, 1971; Simon and Jordan, 1967). If the patient is atopic, there is a higher incidence of subsequent asthma.

Pathophysiology

Pathologically, bronchiolar obstruction is caused by edema, peribronchiolar cellular infiltrate, and mucous plugs. The process may progress to cause atelectasis with intrapulmonary shunts and poor perfusion. Oxygen should be used liberally. Humidification of air will help relieve dryness of the upper airway. Hypoxia and hypercarbia may occur and may occasionally progress to respiratory failure. Under these circumstances, intubation and mechanical ventilation should be instituted. Cardiac failure is exceedingly uncommon in the absence of underlying heart disease. Dehydration is important and requires fluid replacement.

Etiology

Viruses, especially respiratory syncytial virus (Simon and Jordan, 1967), are major etiologic agents of this syndrome. The mechanism of disease production may be in part hypersensitivity to the virus in the case of respiratory syncytial virus, with the bronchioles representing the target organ of antigen–antibody reactions. *M. pneumoniae* and *H. influenzae* species are less frequent causes.

Laboratory Features

White blood cell counts and differential counts are usually normal in this illness. Results of viral cultures may be positive in up to 50 per cent of bronchiolitis cases, with respiratory syncytial virus being the most common pathogen cultured, especially during epidemic periods in the spring and fall in temperate regions. In the patient who is atopic, a determination of IgE concentration may be helpful in predicting the possibility of asthma occurring subsequent to the infection (Polmar et al., 1972).

Management

In infants less than one year old, the principal pathophysiologic process of asthma, bronchospasm, would be a minor component in bronchiolitis. In the slightly older child, in whom asthma is a possibility, a judicious trial of epinephrine, 0.01 cc per kg of 1:1000 concentration, not to exceed 0.3 cc subcutaneously and repeated once in 20 minutes, would be indicated. If there is a positive response, aminophylline 5 mg per kg IV should be given every six hours. The blood level of aminophylline one hour after a dose should be 10 to 15 mg per 100 cc, and the lowest level (4 to 6 hours after a dose) should not be less than 10 mg per 100 cc. Short-term hydrocortisone administration, 2 to 4 mg per kg, may be helpful if spasm seems to be prominent, but in general corticosteroids have not been shown to be effective in bronchiolitis (Dabbous et al., 1966). Antibiotics are not indicated unless pyogenic complication is present.

PNEUMONIA

Definition

Pneumonia is a clinical syndrome characterized by elevation of temperature, cough, and increased respiratory rate with rales on auscultation. An infiltrate will be found on the radiograph, and its character will vary with age of the patient, anatomic location of the infiltrate, and its etiology (Moffet, 1975).

Anatomic Location, Etiology, and Age

It is important to attempt to define the etiology of pneumonia by several parameters, including the history of progression of the illness and its anatomic location, since there is a large number of possible etiologic agents and management of the resulting illnesses may differ. Beyond the neonatal period, pyogenic bacteria account for only a small percentage of cases of pneumonia, while viruses and *M. pneumoniae* predominate as pathogens (Denny et al., 1971; Lepow et al., 1968).

Lobar or Segmental Consolidation

The etiology of this type of pneumonia is most commonly bacterial, due to *Pneumococcus* or *Klebsiella*, with the former being most common. At times, *H. influenzae* type B, beta-hemolytic *Streptococcus*, *Staphylococcus aureus*, and *M. pneumoniae* may be primary. *Klebsiella* and staphylococci may cause pneumatoceles. Staphylococcal pneumonia will often result in bronchopleural fistulae and pleural effusion or empyema. *Klebsiella pneumoniae* will produce bulging of fissures along with pneumatoceles. It mainly occurs in infants or immunologically compromised children. Children rarely will expectorate sputum so that the diagnosis is presumptive unless the results of deep tracheal or transtracheal aspirates (Kalinske et al., 1967; Klein, 1969), lung puncture, or pleural fluid cultures are positive or the presence of a bacteremia is documented (see the section on laboratory tests).

Pleural Effusion

If pleural effusion is present, usually *Pneumococcus*, group A *Streptococcus*, *Staphylococcus*, or *Mycobacterium tuberculosis* is involved. *M. pneumoniae* can rarely cause pleural effusion. Physical findings when pleural fluid is present include decreased lung excursion, increased dullness, and decreased breath sounds on the involved side. The character of any drainage is very important for diagnosis and therapy.

Bronchopneumonia (Including Interstitial — Diffuse)

The etiology of this disease is mainly viral, due to adenovirus, respiratory syncytial virus, or influenza virus (see Table 67–1) in infants and young children. *M. pneumoniae* becomes a significant pathogen in the school-age child.

In hosts compromised immunologically as a result of primary immunodeficiency or as a result of chemotherapy for malignancy, *Pneumocystis carinii*, or cytomegalovirus, herpes simplex and giant cell pneumonia due to measles virus must be considered in the differential diagnosis. Physical findings are usually minimal, with fever and tachypnea being the most common signs. Radiographs will show diffuse or focal infiltrates that are peribronchiolar in location. Blood gas determinations will reveal evidence of alveolar capillary block.

Although bacteria less commonly cause interstitial pneumonia, bacterial pneumonia will usually be more sudden in onset and more rapidly progressive. Viral pneumonia, except for that caused by influenza and *M. pneumoniae*, will usually be slower in onset and more slowly progressive and with fewer systemic signs than bacterial pneumonia. Recently, *Chlamydia trachomatis* has been implicated in interstitial pneumonia in young infants (Beem and Saxon, 1977).

Diagnostic Studies

White blood cell counts in children may be increased in bacterial disease with increased polymorphonuclear leukocytes. Throat cultures for bacteria are not useful. Blood cultures are of help when positive and should always be obtained if bacterial or fungal pneumonia is considered possible. If pleural fluid is obtained, a cell count, protein and sugar determinations, and smears and cultures for pyrogens, fungi, and *M. tuberculosis* should be done. A tracheal or transtracheal aspirate is useful if a single organism is found and polymorphonuclear leukocytes are present. The most direct information is derived from lung puncture, but this is usually reserved for difficult cases, especially when the child fails to respond to therapy or in an immunologically compromised host in whom *Pneumocystis carinii* or cytomegalovirus infection is suspected.

Viral cultures of tracheal aspirates or throat swabs may be helpful. If cytomegalovirus is suspected, urine as well as sputum should be tested for the presence of the virus by inoculation into an appropriate tissue culture or examination of urine for inclusion-bearing cells. Acute and convalescent serologic studies for viruses, *M. pneumoniae* and cold agglutinins for *M. pneumoniae* may also be helpful, especially when epidemics are occurring.

Treatment of Lobar or Segmental Pneumonia with or without Pleural Effusion

A general principle is to treat as presumptive bacterial pneumonia any infiltrates that are lobar or segmental in distribution. These patients should be given an antibiotic selected on the basis of the most likely etiologic agent (McCracken and Eichenwald, 1974). A specific diagnosis can be made only if the patient has a bacteremia or positive culture from pleural fluid or lung.

If pneumococci or beta-hemolytic streptococci are presumptive etiologic agents, treatment with penicillin, 100,000 units per kg per day, is sufficient (Table 67–2). *Staphylococcus aureus* would require a penicillinase-resistant

Table 67–2 RECOMMENDED ANTIBIOTICS FOR TREATMENT OF PNEUMONIA ACCORDING TO ETIOLOGY

Organism	Antibiotic
S. aureus	Methicillin Oxacillin Cephalosporins
S. pneumoniae Beta-hemolytic streptococci	Penicillin
H. influenzae B	Ampicillin or chloramphenicol
K. pneumoniae	Aminoglycoside
M. pneumoniae	Erythromycin
Lung abscess	Penicillin Clindamycin Chloramphenicol

antibiotic, such as methicillin or oxacillin, and *Klebsiella* would be treated with an aminoglycoside drug.

Aspiration Pneumonia

This type of pneumonia could be bacterial, mechanical, or chemical in etiology. Small objects, i.e., toys or peanuts, that are inadvertently aspirated may result in recurrent pneumonia. Bronchoscopy is indicated if there is any suspicion of mechanical obstruction associated with aspiration, such as a persistent wheeze (Law and Kosloske, 1976). Usually, the patient will not require therapy with ingestion of hydrocarbon or aspiration of gastric secretions.

Uncommon Organisms Resulting in Pneumonia in Normal Persons

Rarely, some persons become exposed to histoplasmosis or coccidioidomycosis, which may result in pulmonary processes that mimic viral infections or malignancies. Appropriate skin and serologic tests should be performed on these patients, and they should have smears and a culture of sputum or a lung biopsy taken as well.

Tuberculosis

The management of *M. tuberculosis* is beyond the scope of this chapter. In high-risk children, such as those who have household exposure and then develop pneumonia, tuberculin testing and gastric aspirate cultures should be done routinely. Routine tuberculin tests should be done one or two times in the first five years of life. An enlarged unilateral hilar node seen on the radiograph, with or without infiltrate, should raise a suspicion of primary pulmonary tuberculosis.

Lung Abscess

This may be primary, as a complication of pneumonia, or secondary to aspiration or other obstruction (foreign body). If the sputum smells foul, anaerobes are probably the cause. Otherwise, aerobic pyogenic organisms are the most likely cause.

Bronchoscopy may be necessary, regardless of etiology, for diagnosis and treatment and possible drainage. Penicillin is the drug of choice, but clindamycin or chloramphenicol could be used in the patient with penicillin allergies.

BRONCHIECTASIS

Definition

Dilation of bronchi may be congenital, owing to a postnatal arrest in development. Acquired bronchiectasis results most frequently from antecedent infection, such as pertussis, rubeola, or recurrent pneumonia. In addition, the presence of a foreign body or enlarged hilar nodes may contribute to the condition. A triad described by Kartagener in 1933 consists of sinusitis, bronchiectasis, and situs inversus. Occasionally, it is familial.

Patients with asthma, cystic fibrosis, hypogammaglobulinemia, sinusitis, tuberculosis, and repeated pulmonary infections may develop bronchiectasis. In patients without underlying disease, bronchiectasis is more likely to be reversible.

Pathogenesis and Pathology

Obstruction of bronchi is most important. In areas that are atelectatic, secondary to obstruction, bronchial secretions favor both aerobic and anaerobic growths. The greatest damage is to the cartilage of the bronchi. Columnar cells are replaced by cuboidal ones, and cilia are scanty. The left lower lobe is most frequently involved, with the right middle lobe being second in this respect.

Clinical Features. The onset may be acute or more insidious. The most frequent symptom is cough, which is variably productive. Hemoptysis comes from erosion of the bronchial wall. The presence of a fever is variable, and dyspnea is a late feature.

Radiographic Findings. Persistence of atelectasis and failure of the chest radiograph to return to normal after appropriate therapy are important signs. Bronchoscopy would be indicated for patients with localized atelectasis. Bronchograms are useful, but not in the presence of an acute exacerbation.

Treatment. Medical management includes postural drainage and other mechanisms of enhancing pulmonary toilet to decrease obstruction and atelectasis. Prompt treatment of exacerbations with antibiotics is recommended, but controversy exists about the continuous administration of antibiotics to children since so many of the illnesses are viral. Bronchoscopy followed by surgical treatment may be indicated with segmental disease if it is not controlled medically after an appropriate period of chemotherapy.

SELECTED REFERENCES

Cherry, J. D. 1973. Newer respiratory viruses: Their role in respiratory illness of children. Adv. Pediatr., 20:225.

This reference offers to the reader a review of the interrelationships among bacteria, viruses, and mycoplasma in the etiology of common respiratory illnesses. Experimental approaches are considered, and therapy can be approached more scientifically.

Moffet, H. L. 1975. "Pneumonia Syndromes" in Pediatric Infectious Diseases. Philadelphia, J. B. Lippincott Co., p. 102.

This is a recent reference and uses the problem-oriented approach to the issue of pneumonia. It has a complete reference list.

Reynolds, E. O. R. 1972. Bronchiolitis. *In* Kendig, E. L., Jr. (Ed.) 1972. Disorders of the Respiratory Tract in Children, Vol. 1, Pulmonary Disorders. Philadelphia, W. B. Saunders Co., p. 223.

This chapter offers a comprehensive view of the clinical laboratory and epidemiologic aspects of this disease of infancy.

Zweiman, N. 1971. Patterns of allergic respiratory disease in children with a past history of bronchiolitis. J. Allergy Clin. Immunol., 48:283.

This paper reviews the past history of bronchiolitis as an adjunct to predicting the possibility of asthma occurring later in life. In contrast to some other investigators, the author's data support the concept that bronchiolitis is a distinct disease without bronchospasm.

REFERENCES

Adair, J. C., Ring, W. H., Jordan, W. S., et al. 1971. Ten-year experience with IPPB in the treatment of acute laryngotracheobronchitis (croup). Anesth. Analg., 50:649.

Beem, M. O., and Saxon, E. M. 1977. Respiratory-tract colonization and a distinctive pneumonia syndrome in infants infected with Chlamydia trachomatis. N. Engl. J. Med., 296:306.

Biller, H. F., Harvey, J. E., Bone, R. C., et al. 1970. Laryngeal edema, an experimental study. Ann. Otol. Rhinol. Laryngol., 79:1084.

Cherry, J. D. 1973. Newer respiratory viruses: Their role in respiratory illness of children. Adv. Pediatr., 20:225.

Committee on Infectious Diseases of the American Academy of Pediatrics. 1976. Current status of ampicillin-resistant *Hemophilus influenzae* type B. Pediatrics, 57:417, p. 4.

Dabbous, I. A., Tkachyk, J. S., and Stamm, S. J. 1966. A double-blind study on the effects of corticosteroids in the treatment of bronchiolitis. Pediatrics, 37:477.

Denny, F. W., Clyde, W. A., Jr., and Glezen, W. P. 1971. *Mycoplasma pneumoniae* disease: Clinical spectrum, pathophysiology, epidemiology, and control. J. Infect. Dis., 123:74.

Eden, A. N., Kaufman, A., and Yu, R. 1967. Corticosteroids and croup: A controlled double-blind study. J.A.M.A., 200:403.

Eden, A. N., and Larkin, V. D. 1964. Corticosteroid treatment of croup. Pediatrics, 33:768.

Gardner, H., Powell, K. R., Roden, V. J., et al. 1973. The evaluation of racemic epinephrine in the treatment of infectious croup. Pediatrics, 52:52.

Holdaway, D., Romer, A. C., and Gardner, P. S. 1967. The diagnosis and management of bronchiolitis. Pediatrics, 39:924.

Kalinske, R. W., Parker, R. H., Brandt, D., et al. 1967. Diagnostic usefulness and safety of transtracheal aspiration. N. Engl. J. Med., 276:604.

Kartagener, M. 1933. Zur Pathogenese der Bronchiektasien; Bronchiektasien bei Situs viscerum inversus. Beitr. z. Klin. d. Tuberk., 83:489.

Klein, J. O. 1969. Diagnostic lung puncture in the pneumonias of infants and children. Pediatrics, 44:486.

Law, D., and Kosloske, A. M. 1976. Management of tracheobronchial foreign bodies in children: A re-evaluation of the postural drainage and bronchoscopy. Pediatrics, 58:262.

Lepow, M. L., Ballassanian, N., Emmerich, J., et al. 1968. Interrelationships of viral, mycoplasmal, and bacterial agents in uncomplicated pneumonia. Am. Rev. Resp. Dis., 97:533.

Lockhart, C. H., and Battaglia, J. D. 1977. Croup (laryngotracheal bronchitis) and epiglottitis. Pediatr. Ann., 6:262.

McCracken, G. H., Jr., and Eichenwald, H. F. 1974. Antimicrobial therapy: Therapeutic recommendations and review of newer drugs: Part 1, Therapy of infectious conditions. J. Pediatr., 85:297.

Moffet, H. L. 1975. "Pneumonia Syndromes" in Pediatric Infectious Disease. Philadelphia, J. B. Lippincott Co.

Molteni, R. A. 1976. Epiglottitis: Incidence of extraepiglottic infection. Report of 72 cases and review of the literature. Pediatrics, 58:526.

Polmar, S. H., Robinson, L. D., Jr., and Minnefor, A. B. 1972. Immunoglobulin E in bronchiolitis. Pediatrics, 50:279.

Rabe, E. F. 1948. Infectious croup. IV. *Hemophilus influenzae* type B croup. Pediatrics, 2:559.

Reynolds, E. O. R. 1972. Bronchiolitis. *In* Kendig, E. L., Jr. (Ed.) Disorders of the Respiratory Tract in Children, Vol. 1, Pulmonary Disorders. Philadelphia, W. B. Saunders Co., p. 223.

Schuller, D. E., and Birck, H. G. 1975. The safety of intubation in croup and epiglottitis: an 8-year follow-up. Laryngoscope, 85:33.

Sell, S. H. W., and Karzen, D. T. (Eds.) 1973. *Hemophilus influenzae*. Nashville, Vanderbilt University Press, pp. 215, 248, 262.

Simon, G., and Jordan, W. S., Jr. 1967. Infectious and allergic aspects of bronchiolitis. J. Pediatr., 70:533.

Singer, O. P., and Wilson, W. J. 1976. Laryngotracheobronchitis: Two years' experience with racemic epinephrine. Can. Med. Assoc. J., 115:132.

Skowton, P. N., Turner, J. A., and McNaughton, G. A. 1966. The use of corticosteroid (Dexamethazone) in the treatment of acute laryngotracheitis. Can. Med. Assoc. J., 94:528.

Taussig, L. M., Castro, O., Beaudry, P. H., et al. 1975. Treatment of laryngotracheobronchitis (croup): Use of intermittent positive-pressure breathing and racemic epinephrine. Am. J. Dis. Child., 129:790.

Zweiman, N. 1971. Patterns of allergic respiratory disease in children with a past history of bronchiolitis. J. Allergy Clin. Immunol., 48:283.

Chapter 68

NONINFECTIOUS DISORDERS OF THE LOWER RESPIRATORY TRACT

Donald B. Hawkins, M.D.

INTRODUCTION

"Noninfectious disorders of the lower respiratory tract" is a very broad subject. To discuss all the conditions that might be included would result in too long a chapter, with duplication of subjects that are covered in other sections. Therefore, this chapter is devoted to a discussion of noninfectious disorders that fall into three categories: alterations of intrathoracic dynamics, responses of the lung to injury or other forms of stress, and complications of mechanical ventilation. Also included is a discussion of several rare idiopathic disorders of the lower respiratory tract.

ALTERATIONS OF INTRATHORACIC DYNAMICS

Several conditions that alter the dynamics of respiration are encountered frequently in pediatric otolaryngology. These are emphysema, atelectasis, pneumomediastinum, and pneumothorax. They are related to a variety of diseases or injuries, and their occurrence and their management affect the patient's prognosis.

Emphysema

Emphysema is defined as a swelling or inflation due to the presence of air. The term, with various clinical or anatomic modifiers, is used to denote several different conditions. In adults, idiopathic pulmonary emphysema is a chronic disease, usually associated with smoking and chronic bronchitis, which may progress to respiratory insufficiency. Chronic emphysema is rare in children; occasionally it develops in patients with asthma or cystic fibrosis of the pancreas. Congenital lobar emphysema refers to distention of one or more lobes secondary to a congenital anomaly of a large airway that prevents adequate egress of air. This may be from extrinsic compression, intrinsic narrowing, or, more commonly, a defect in the cartilage of the involved bronchus. Compensatory emphysema refers to distention of one or more lobes to fill in the space left by collapse, removal, or agenesis of a portion of the lung. Mediastinal emphysema, synonymous with pneumomediastinum, means the accumulation of air within the mediastinum. Subcutaneous emphysema refers to the presence of air beneath the skin. Pulmonary interstitial emphysema refers to air within the interstitial areas of the lung, usually a complication of mechanical respiration. Distention of one or more lobes secondary to obstruction of bronchi on expiration is called obstructive emphysema.

Obstructive emphysema is the most common variety encountered in pediatrics. It may be acute or chronic, localized or generalized. The generalized variety is characterized by the diffuse pulmonary hyperinflation seen with bronchiolitis or asthma. Localized obstructive emphysema can result from obstruction within the bronchial lumen, from extrinsic compression of a bronchus, or from bronchomalacia, as in congenital lobar emphysema. Causes of intraluminal obstruction include foreign body, mucosal edema, mucous plug, granulation tissue and scarring from infection or trauma, and, rarely in children, tumors. Extrinsic compression results from mediastinal or hilar lymph nodes, cysts or tumors, or anomalous blood vessels.

Aspirated foreign bodies are the most common causes of localized obstructive emphysema and should be suspected initially in all cases, except perhaps in very young infants. The ball valve effect of a bronchial foreign body was well described by the Jacksons (1959): Inspiratory dilatation of the obstructed bronchus allows air to pass by the foreign body, whereas expiratory contraction of the bronchus around the object traps the inspired air within the obstructed portion of lung. Among the causes of extrinsic compression, enlarged tuberculous lymph nodes is the most common at our institution. Obstructive emphysema is a not-too-rare part of the initial presenting picture of primary pulmonary tuberculosis in young children.

The symptoms and physical signs vary among patients. Some children are remarkably asymptomatic with large emphysematous lobes. This is especially true in patients with slowly developing extrinsic compression. In general, however, physical signs vary with the extent of emphysema. With mild air trapping the child may be asymptomatic or may only have a cough. With severe hyperinflation, the child may exhibit severe respiratory distress, especially if the emphysematous lung has filled one hemithorax and has her-

niated over to the other side. Breath sounds are diminished or absent over the obstructed lung. Localized wheezing may be heard on inspiration or on expiration, which may be prolonged. The diagnosis is made by chest radiograph, which demonstrates the hyperlucent inflated lung. This is shown more dramatically on expiration. Often it is necessary to obtain radiographs on both inspiration and expiration (Fig. 68–1). On inspiration, both sides inflate, and the difference may not be noticeable. On expiration, the obstructed portion of lung does not empty; it appears hyperlucent in comparison to the deflated normal lung. The heart and mediastinum shift toward the normal side. Fluoroscopy will demonstrate impaired motion of the diaphragm on the involved side and is useful in diagnosing the young child who will not cooperate for inspiratory and expiratory films.

Treatment is directed to the condition causing the emphysema. This is discussed in other chapters dealing with those conditions.

Atelectasis

Atelectasis literally means imperfect expansion. In clinical descriptions, the term is most often synonymous with collapse of one or more segments or lobes of the lung. This can be classified, according to etiology, as obstructive or nonobstructive atelectasis.

Obstructive atelectasis may result from extrinsic compression or intrinsic occlusion of a bronchial lumen. The causes are the same as those listed for localized obstructive emphy-

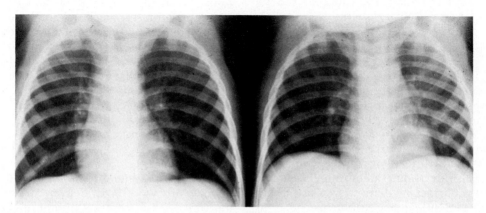

Figure 68–1 Obstructive emphysema of the right lung secondary to foreign body in the right mainstem bronchus. Chest radiograph taken on inspiration (left) shows symmetrical inflation of both lungs; on expiration (right), hyperlucency of the right lung and shift of the mediastinum to the left are demonstrated.

sema; the difference is the degree of obstruction. Emphysema results from partial bronchial obstruction that allows air to enter but which impedes the egress of air on expiration. Atelectasis is the result of total bronchial occlusion that prevents air from entering the obstructed portion of lung. Air that is trapped within that portion of lung is absorbed into the circulation; oxygen is absorbed in a few minutes, while nitrogen takes several hours. As the remaining air is absorbed, the obstructed lobe or segment collapses. For a period of time, the involved lung continues to be perfused with blood, creating a ventilation/perfusion abnormality. This is usually transient in children, especially with bronchopulmonary infections, in which mucosal edema and mucous plugs occlude small bronchi. Atelectasis may result from a long-present foreign body, especially from those, such as nuts, that produce a mucosal reaction. Mucous plugs associated with asthma can produce a picture identical to that of aspirated foreign bodies: partial obstruction creating emphysema, leading to total obstruction and atelectasis. Postoperative atelectasis is usually due to mucous plug obstruction in combination with nonobstructive factors discussed next.

Nonobstructive atelectasis results from insufficient pulmonary surfactant or inadequate expansion of the thorax. Surfactant is the surface tension-lowering substance present in the alveolar lining layer. It is a complex mixture of proteins and phospholipids. The predominant phospholipid is lecithin, the molecules of which are arranged so that they form a highly compressible, tension-lowering film. Without surfactant, alveolar inflation would be determined according to the La Place relationship for a sphere:

$$\text{Pressure} = \frac{(2)\ (\text{Surface tension})}{\text{Radius}}$$

On expiration, when both alveolar radius and pressure are low, surface tension would promote collapse of alveoli. The presence of a substance that lowers alveolar surface tension prevents this occurrence. Surfactant deficiency is the cause of diffuse atelectasis associated with hyaline membrane disease of neonates. Surfactant deficiency also plays a role in the pulmonary problems, such as shock lung or inhalation of noxious gases, in which the alveolar lining film and cells are damaged. Limited expansion of the chest may result from discomfort, as after injuries or after surgery; it may also result from either congenital or acquired neuromuscular dysfunction.

Except in cases of massive atelectasis causing severe dyspnea, the symptoms of atelectasis are the same, with perhaps slight accentuation, as those of the underlying condition. The diagnosis is usually made by chest radiograph, the collapsed portion having increased density and sometimes a contracted appearance with concave lines. The adjacent lung may appear hyperlucent, demonstrating compensatory emphysema. Right upper lobe atelectasis is common in recumbent infants; in older children, the right middle and both lower lobes are more often affected.

Treatment of atelectasis is directed toward the underlying disease. Atelectasis associated with pulmonary infections in childhood usually clears with the infection. Chest physiotherapy and postural drainage aid in clearing mucus from the obstructed bronchus. Bronchoscopy and removal of mucous plugs are indicated if atelectasis is impeding the child's recovery or if it persists after clearing of the infection. If a foreign body is the suspected cause, early bronchoscopy is indicated. Long-standing atelectasis of months or years duration that is unresponsive to medical treatment and bronchoscopy may require surgical resection if it is a site of repeated infections.

Pneumomediastinum and Pneumothorax

Pneumomediastinum (PM) and pneumothorax (PT) may develop from any condition causing a break in the wall of the air or food passages within the neck or thorax. Subcutaneous emphysema is often associated with pneumomediastinum and pneumothorax.

Spontaneous PT is rare in children; it occurs occasionally with acute asthma. The most common causes of PM and PT in children are artificial respiration, surgical procedures in the neck, injuries occurring during endoscopy or endotracheal intubation, perforating foreign bodies, and injuries to the neck or chest.

Although PM and PT may be found in the neonate after a difficult delivery or with pulmonary diseases such as hyaline membrane disease or meconium aspiration, most cases are secondary to artificial respiration. For example, the incidence of PT in hyaline membrane disease without respirator management is less than 5 per cent, whereas it is 20 per cent with mechanical respiration (Ogata et al., 1976). The initial break in the airway with artificial ventilation is rupture of an alveolus producing pulmonary interstitial emphysema. Air dissects along the perivascular and peribronchial spaces to the mediastinum. If enough air leaks from the alveolus, it can dissect through the superior mediastinum into the subcutaneous tissues of the neck. It can also break through into the pleural space and produce PT.

Tracheostomy is the most common surgical procedure causing PM and PT. The mechanism for production of PM and PT during tracheostomy was first demonstrated as early as 1882 (Champneys). If an opening is made in the pretracheal fascia, air may be drawn into the mediastinum with inspiratory expansion of the chest. This is more likely to occur if the patient is struggling for breath and the longer the interval is between opening into the pretracheal area and incision into the trachea. If sufficient air enters the mediastinum, it will break through into the pleural

cavity, resulting in PT. Another potential cause of PT is injury to the pleural apices, which on inspiration often reach into the hyperextended neck of a child undergoing tracheostomy. Insertion of a bronchoscope or endotracheal tube to establish an airway prior to tracheostomy diminishes, but does not eliminate, the possibility of developing PM and PT (Forbes et al., 1947; Rabuzzi and Reed, 1971; Hawkins and Williams, 1976). Since PT usually develops as an extension of PM after tracheostomy, PM alone is a more frequent complication. It is often asymptomatic and is noted only on the postoperative radiograph (Fig. 68–2). Cervical subcutaneous emphysema develops if the skin incision is sutured snugly around the tracheal cannula; air exiting the trachea around the cannula on expiration cannot escape through the skin. If enough air accumulates, it may dissect subcutaneously up into the face or down over the chest; it may also dissect into the mediastinum.

Perforation of the esophagus during esophagoscopy will result in PM. This is more likely to occur while removing a sharp for-

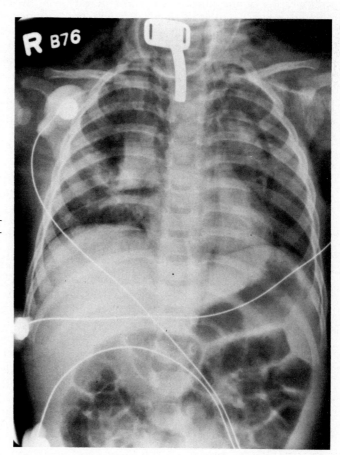

Figure 68–2 Asymptomatic pneumomediastinum and subcutaneous emphysema secondary to tracheostomy.

eign body or while dilating an esophageal stricture. The trachea or a bronchus may rarely be perforated during bronchoscopy for removal of a foreign body or for biopsy. This may lead to rapid development of tension pneumothorax, initially manifested by a drop in blood pressure and difficulty ventilating the patient. The hypopharynx may be perforated during attempted endotracheal intubation, especially when done under emergency conditions (Wolff et al., 1972; Hawkins, 1974). Air leaks into the cervical subcutaneous layer, the mediastinum, and occasionally into the pleural space. The initial symptom may be rapidly developing respiratory distress secondary to tension pneumothorax.

Sharp foreign bodies lodged in the esophagus may perforate its wall, resulting in PM. Penetrating injuries to the neck or chest and some blunt injuries may lacerate or rupture the hypopharynx, esophagus, larynx, or trachea.

Pneumomediastinum alone seldom causes significant symptoms, even though a large amount of mediastinal air can be seen on radiographs of the chest. Symptoms of PT depend on its extent; a small PT will be asymptomatic, whereas a large one results in severe respiratory distress. Limited respiratory excursions may be noted on the side of the chest in which the PT has developed. Breath sounds are diminished over an area of PT. A peculiar sound, referred to as the mediastinal crunch, may be heard by auscultation over the mediastinum in patients with PM. This sound may not be identified, however, and is not necessary for the diagnosis. The symptoms may be predominantly those of the condition causing PM or PT, for instance, substernal and back pain occurring after esophageal dilatation. A chest radiograph revealing PM in this case would confirm the diagnosis of esophageal perforation.

Mild PT that does not compromise the patient's respiration requires no treatment. It is allowed to be resorbed. The patient should be watched closely and should have serial radiographs to detect any increase in pleural air. If the PT is large, it must be drained. In some cases, one needle aspiration is sufficient; in other cases a chest tube must be inserted for continuous closed drainage until the air leak into the pleural cavity seals. In patients with rapidly developing tension PT and increasing respiratory distress, prompt needle aspiration of pleural air may be lifesaving. A chest tube should be inserted in these patients at the time of initial needle aspiration.

Pneumomediastinum without pneumothorax usually requires no specific treatment. Its presence, however, may indicate that there is an underlying condition that needs treatment. For example, a patient with PM secondary to esophageal perforation would need prompt thoracotomy and mediastinal drainage, not for the PM but for suppurative mediastinitis. Very rarely, massive PM may produce respiratory and circulatory distress; needle aspiration of the mediastinum may be helpful in these rare cases.

RESPONSE OF THE LUNG TO INJURY OR OTHER FORMS OF STRESS

Progressive respiratory distress is a frequent complication of severe injury or other forms of stress. A confusing number of terms, including adult respiratory distress syndrome, progressive pulmonary insufficiency, posttraumatic lung, shock lung, and others, have been used to describe this pulmonary reaction to various forms of stress. Conditions known to have resulted in pulmonary insufficiency include severe injuries, hypotensive episodes resulting from hemorrhagic, gram-negative, or endotoxic shock, inhalation of noxious gases, aspiration of gastric acid or irritating fluids, drowning, pulmonary fat emboli, oxygen toxicity, damage to the central nervous system or spinal cord, fluid overload, and congestive heart failure.

The pulmonary changes in association with this variety of initiating factors appear to represent a common response of the lung to injury (Pruitt et al., 1975; Powers et al., 1972). Disruption of alveolar epithelium occurs with loss of surfactant activity, resulting in atelectasis, decreased functional residual capacity, and hypoxemia from intrapulmonary shunting of blood. Damage to pulmonary capillary endothelium results in protein-rich interstitial and alveolar edema formation. The end result in patients who do not survive is the development of heavy, "liver-like," almost airless lungs resembling those of neonates dying of hyaline membrane disease. Microscopic changes vary from an expanded interstitium containing protein-rich fluid to fibrotic thickening of pulmonary septa. Alveoli and distal airways contain fluid and hyaline membranes, and the parenchyma shows varying degrees of vascular engorgement and hemorrhage.

Shock Lung

Shock lung is the term used to define a syndrome of progressive pulmonary insufficiency that develops after severe nonthoracic injury or a profound hypotensive episode. Often developing in patients without known pulmonary disease, the syndrome consists of a triad: intrapulmonary shunting with hypoxemia, diminished pulmonary compliance, and chest radiographic findings consistent with bilateral pulmonary edema (Sladen, 1976). Shock lung is a life-threatening condition that has been responsible for up to 70 per cent of shock-related deaths (Bredenberg et al., 1969). It has also been known by other terms, such as "wet lung" and "posttraumatic lung."

Progression of the disease can be divided into four phases (James, 1975). First is the hypotensive episode and resuscitation. The duration and severity of hypotension often correlate with the frequency of onset of shock lung. During this initial phase, the Po_2 can be maintained by increasing the inspired oxygen concentration. The second phase is that of circulatory stabilization. The patient is often lucid but is tachypneic. Increasing intrapulmonary shunting leads to declining Po_2. This leads to the third phase of progressive pulmonary failure, during which the Po_2 is markedly lowered and the Pco_2 begins to rise. The fourth phase is one of severe hypoxia, hypercarbia, and acidosis leading to ventricular arrhythmia and death.

Chest radiographs taken immediately after the episode of shock may not indicate impending development of shock lung, but those taken several hours later will show changes that have been correlated with pathologic findings (Ostendorf et al., 1975). The earliest radiographic changes consist of widened segmental vessels with fuzzy surface contours, most obvious in the upper midchest. These changes are followed by a diffuse, veil-like cloudiness of varying density, which may progress to complete opacification of the lung fields. The enlarged vascular shadows correlate with early pathologic findings of perivascular edema and dilatation of pulmonary lymphatics. The veil-like cloudiness correlates with histologic findings of interstitial edema. Diffuse alveolar atelectasis also contributes to this radiographic appearance. The dense opacification is associated with formation of intra-alveolar edema, and a final parahilar butterfly shadow on radiographs correlates with the pulmonary edema of cardiac failure.

Pulmonary vasoconstriction secondary to shock results in hypoxic damage to pulmonary vascular endothelium and to alveolar epithelium. Microthrombi form within the smaller pulmonary vessels. Injury to the type II alveolar epithelial cells results in deficient surfactant production, which leads to unstable alveoli, atelectasis, and decreased functional residual capacity. Blood perfusing nonventilated portions of lung creates an intrapulmonary right-to-left shunt with resulting hypoxemia. Increased vascular permeability results in perivascular and interstitial edema, then intra-alveolar edema.

Transfusion of large quantities of blood is a feature many patients with shock lung have in common. For this reason, emboli from microaggregates that form in stored blood have been implicated as causative agents. Studies on canine lungs (Geelhoed and Bennett, 1975) showed that pulmonary injury similar to that seen with shock lung develops in lungs perfused with stored blood but not in those perfused with fresh blood. This affect was not eliminated by depth filtration designed to remove microaggregates, leading the authors to infer that a toxic serum-borne factor may be etiologic in shock lung syndrome.

As mentioned earlier, a chest radiograph taken shortly after the hypotensive episode may not indicate impending shock lung. Expiratory wheezes heard in a tachypneic patient who is recovering from shock are almost pathognomonic of early shock lung. Serial measurements of blood gases, functional residual capacity, and tidal volume can be diagnostic and prognostic; early in the disease, arterial Po_2 ranges from 50 to 60 mm Hg; Pco_2 varies from 20 to 30 mm Hg. The pH may be normal or alkalotic. Later, the Po_2 drops, the Pco_2 rises, and the pH becomes acidotic. The most significant early findings are decrease in Po_2 in spite of increased inspired oxygen and a decrease in functional residual capacity.

For any patient who appears to be developing shock lung, the earlier treatment is begun, the better the results will be.

1. Place the patient in a high semi-Fowler position. He should be repositioned and turned frequently.
2. Vital signs should be monitored. Blood gases, tidal volumes, and functional residual capacity, as well as hemoglobin and hematocrit levels, should be measured serially. The patient should be weighed two to three times daily to assess fluid volume.
3. Regulate intravenous fluid administration so that effective circulation is maintained without increasing the risk of pulmonary extravasation. Serum salt-poor albumin or low molecular weight dextran will enhance the colloidal osmotic pressure of the pulmonary circulation and diminish pulmonary edema formation. Diuretics, such as furosemide or ethacrynic acid, are sometimes used in conjunction with intravenous colloids.
4. Administer oxygen in concentrations necessary to maintain the arterial Po_2 between 60 and 90 mm Hg.
5. Regulate the patient's breathing. Continuous positive airway pressure (CPAP) will prevent alveolar collapse on expiration, increasing the surface area for gas exchange, decreasing intrapulmonary shunting of blood, and diminishing formation of intra-alveolar edema. A positive pressure volume-cycled respirator, using positive end-expiratory pressure (PEEP), will be necessary if alveolar hypoventilation is present. Both require endotracheal intubation or tracheostomy. Because of decreased pulmonary compliance in shock lung, the effects of CPAP and PEEP on venous filling and cardiac output are negligible.
6. Take cultures of sputum and tracheal secretions. Consider administration of broad-spectrum antibiotics.
7. Administer steroids, dexamethasone, or methylprednisolone. The value of steroids has been considered mainly that of reversing the shock state rather than a direct effect upon the lung. James (1975) states that steroids must be given early after the shock-producing event to be effective and uses the following regimen: dexamethasone (4 mg per kg) or methylprednisolone (30 mg per kg) given as a bolus in 100 cc of normal saline over a 10 minute period. The same dose is repeated in 4 hours. If the patient's condition deteriorates, the dose is repeated again in 12 hours, but no further doses are given.

Sladen (1976), on the other hand, reported data indicating that methylprednisolone was effective in reversing the shock lung syndrome when given in a dose of 30 mg per kg every 6 hours for 48 hours.

Respiratory Complications of Burns

Pulmonary complications develop in 20 to 25 per cent of patients with major burns. Up to 85 per cent of those with pulmonary complications die of respiratory failure, the most common cause of death in burn patients.

The incidence of respiratory complications can be correlated with the extent and location of burns and especially with a history of being burned in an enclosed space. Ninety-five per cent of patients with inhalation injuries have associated face and neck burns (Pruitt et al., 1975). Only a small percentage of patients with head and neck burns suffer inhalation injury, however. Except with patients inhaling steam, direct thermal injury to the respiratory tract is rare and is almost unheard of below the larynx in surviving patients. Only one of 697 patients at Brooke Army Hospital demonstrated evidence of heat injury below the glottis, and this was limited to the subglottic area and upper trachea (Pruitt et al., 1970). One reason for this is the efficiency of the upper airway in cooling hot air passing through it. Also, a blast of hot air induces reflex closure of the vocal cords, protecting the lower airway. The supraglottic larynx, however, is still exposed to the thermal insult. Although it is protected from heat injury, the lower airway is affected by inhalation of smoke and noxious chemicals of incomplete combustion. The result is a chemical tracheobronchitis and alveolitis.

Respiratory complications of burns can be divided into three main categories according to the time of onset (Achauer et al., 1973). Although useful for discussion purposes, there is obviously some overlap between categories. The first group is composed of patients with respiratory distress developing within the first 24 hours. This is due to inhalation of heat, carbon monoxide, and noxious chemicals. Heat injury to the larynx will result in edema formation with varying degrees of obstruction and inspiratory stridor. An especially treacherous aspect of this condition is the formation of edematous blebs in the supraglottic larynx. These may prolapse between the vocal cords, producing sudden airway obstruction. Carbon monoxide poisoning is the major immediate cause of death in fires (Parks, 1976). Except in smokers, the normal blood level of carboxyhemoglobin is less than 1 per cent. A level over 20 per cent is considered serious, and levels of 30 per cent or more lead to confusion and coma. Levels over 60 per cent are usually lethal. In most surviving cases of inhalation injury, carboxyhemoglobin levels are between 15 and 25 per cent. Oxygen administered to burn patients lowers the carboxyhemoglobin level rapidly; its half-life is about 4 hours in patients breathing room air but only 30 minutes in those breathing 100 per cent oxygen. Inhalation of noxious chemicals results in mucosal edema of the larynx, trachea, or bronchi, which may manifest itself early or after a "clear period" of up to 24 hours. Obstruction of small airways by peribronchiolar edema and by sloughing of mucosa may result in tachypnea with wheezing. Tracheal and bronchial casts of necrotic mucosa may create significant airway obstruction.

The second category is made up of patients who are relatively asymptomatic for one or two days and then develop respiratory distress with dyspnea, tachypnea, hypoxemia, and cyanosis. Pulmonary infiltrates, diffuse or patchy, appear on radiographs; the radiographic picture usually lags behind the clinical picture, however. Atelectasis, ventilation/perfusion abnormality, pulmonary edema, and pneumonia are common in these patients. The course is usually progressive and may require mechanical ventilation. Myocardial depression and pneumonia contribute to the high mortality rate.

The third group of patients are those who escape serious inhalation injury but who develop late complications, such as pneumonia or pulmonary embolus.

Although the circumstances are different, the result within the alveoli from smoke inhalation is similar to that of shock lung. Injury to the alveolar epithelium results in a deficiency of surfactant with resultant atelectasis, intrapulmonary shunting of blood, and hypoxia. Pulmonary vasoconstriction develops in response to hypoxia. Injury to pulmonary capillary endothelium leads to interstitial and intra-alveolar edema.

Since radiographic changes lag behind the clinical progression of inhalation injury, they may be of little predictive value in the earliest stages. Xenon lung scans are useful for this purpose (Pruitt et al., 1975). Following intravenous injection, 95 per cent of the xenon is cleared in a single passage through normal lungs. Delay of gas clearance has been well correlated with subsequent evidence of inhalation injury.

Patients with suspected inhalation injury must be observed closely for obstruction from edema, sloughed mucosa, or bronchospasm. Examination of the larynx by indirect or direct methods should be done on admission and later as indicated. Moist oxygen is administered. Bronchodilators and mucolytic agents are sometimes used. Steroids are advocated by some (Achauer, 1973; Pruitt et al., 1975), but not by others (Parks, 1976). If bronchial debris and casts cannot be cleared by coughing or suction, bronchoscopy is indicated. For upper airway obstruction from burns, endotracheal intubation is preferred to tracheostomy. Edema of inhalation injury usually peaks at 48 hours, then begins to recede, and the endotracheal tube can usually be removed after 5 days. An exception would be a patient with known severe heat damage to the larynx, in whom an indwelling tube would increase the damage. Other indications for tracheostomy would be difficulty keeping the tracheobronchial tree clear by other means and for long-term respirator management. The chief objection to tracheostomy in burned patients is an increased incidence of pulmonary sepsis (Eckhauser et al., 1974).

For management of the bronchopulmonary component of inhalation injury, in addition to the measures mentioned above, continuous positive airway pressure breathing or positive pressure mechanical ventilation with PEEP may be necessary. Antibiotics, determined to be appropriate by frequent tracheal cultures, are used to combat pulmonary infection. Details of fluid management in burns are beyond the scope of this chapter, but excessive fluid administration may be a contributing factor in development of pulmonary edema.

Some patients who recover from inhalation injury have residual pulmonary function defects, such as decrease in forced vital capacity and maximum breathing capacity. Some also develop bronchiectasis.

Aspiration

Hydrocarbons such as kerosene are notorious for the chemical injury they may produce in the lungs. Although a portion of hydrocarbons absorbed from the gastrointestinal tract is excreted via the lung, experimental and clinical studies have shown this to be an insignificant factor in chemical pneumonitis resulting from their ingestion (Foley et al., 1954; Baldachin and Melmed, 1964). Because of its low surface tension, ingested kerosene is easily aspirated, and pulmonary damage is the result of aspiration.

Instillation of small amounts of kerosene into the tracheas of animals produces a hemorrhagic, necrotizing brochopneumonia with pulmonary edema and hyaline membrane formation. Absorption of large amounts from the alimentary tract may result in cerebral depression. In actual clinical experience, however, kerosene is relatively nontoxic by the oral route, and pulmonary damage does not develop unless it is aspirated. For this reason, gastric lavage is contraindicated, and vomiting should not be induced.

Management of kerosene ingestion should be conservative, consisting of observation and serial radiographs of the chest. Whether or not prophylactic antibiotics are used depends upon the views of the treating physician. In the occasional case with severe aspiration, aggressive treatment of the pulmonary component with oxygen, and even with mechanical ventilation, may be necessary.

Aspiration of gastric contents is a hazard with any patient who is vomiting. It is also likely to occur in patients with swallowing dysfunction, such as cricopharyngeal achalasia (Reichert, 1977), disorders of laryngeal sphincteric function, or congenital anomalies such as H-type tracheoesophageal fistula, laryngotracheal cleft, or hiatal hernia (Lorin, 1975). Aspiration is a particular hazard in patients undergoing anesthesia, as well as in those who are semicomatose or debilitated from various causes, those who are oversedated, and those restrained in a supine position.

Aspiration of vomitus may produce two types of problems (McCormick, 1975; Ruggera and Taylor, 1976). Aspiration of solid material may obstruct the airways. Large particles can obstruct the larynx and trachea, resulting in asphyxia and death, or smaller particles may obstruct lobar or segmental bronchi. The second type of problem is the result of aspiration of gastric acid. The hydrogen ion concentration and the volume of the aspirate determine the extent of pulmonary injury, with hydrogen ion concentration being the major factor. Aspirated gastric con-

tents with pH of less than 2.5 can severely injure pulmonary capillary endothelium and epithelium of the distal airways. Mendelson (1946) emphasized this danger, so a severe reaction with high mortality from aspiration of gastric fluid of pH below 2.5 is known as the Mendelson syndrome. Amounts of acid aspirate of 25 cc or more are sufficient to injure the lungs.

Radiographs of the chest reveal scattered, soft, irregular densities. The lower lobes are most often involved, the right side more so than the left. The left upper lobe is least often involved. The right upper lobe may be involved in any supine patient.

Recurrent aspiration of small amounts may be difficult to diagnose but can be suspected from the radiographic picture in a child with recurrent pulmonary infections. The patient should be evaluated for possible swallowing dysfunction. Cineradiography and endoscopy will often be necessary in this evaluation.

Aspiration may cause immediate circulatory collapse, but the onset of severe illness often follows a latent period of several hours. Symptoms of tachycardia, tachypnea, and wheezing develop and may progress to severe distress with cyanosis. In a patient not known to have aspirated, the cause of these symptoms may not be recognized initially. Aspiration should certainly be suspected when respiratory distress develops in a patient known to have vomited within the previous eight hours. It should also be suspected, even without a known history of vomiting, in patients falling within the categories that are prone to aspiration. Direct laryngoscopy and bronchoscopy may be both diagnostic and therapeutic. Frothy serosanguinous fluid in the tracheobronchial tree would be diagnostic of pulmonary edema. If an endoscopist is not immediately available, endotracheal intubation and suction may obtain the same information. Determination of the pH of tracheal secretions may be diagnostic if done before pulmonary edema develops; pulmonary edema has been shown to neutralize aspirated acid within 10 minutes. Persistent hypoxemia develops in spite of inspired oxygen in high concentrations, indicating the presence of a ventilation/perfusion abnormality secondary to atelectasis and intrapulmonary shunting of blood. The P_aCO_2 may be low, normal, or high, depending on the severity of acid aspiration and the resulting pulmonary insufficiency. Radiographs of the chest show widespread pulmonary infiltration, often more severe in the lower lobes and on the right side. Radiographic findings, however, will lag behind the clinical symptoms.

The current therapy for aspiration of gastric contents, outlined by McCormick (1975) and Ruggera and Taylor (1976), is as follows.

1. Tilt the patient's head down and place the patient on the right side. The right lung is more likely to be affected, so this position may protect the left lung. Suction the upper airway and oxygenate the patient.
2. Perform bronchoscopy to remove solid material and to determine pH of the aspirate. Liquid aspirate spreads to the lung periphery immediately, so bronchoscopy serves little purpose in its removal. Lavage is contraindicated; it may worsen the pulmonary injury by further spreading the acid; it is also relatively ineffectual in neutralizing the acid reaction.
3. Oxygen should be administered, and if spontaneous respiration is inadequate, mechanical ventilation with PEEP will be required. This may be necessary for one to seven days until regeneration of alveolar epithelium permits a resumption of surfactant function and capillary endothelial integrity is restored.
4. Administer sodium bicarbonate to correct acidosis.
5. Hypovolemia results from loss of plasma into the lungs. Plasma or plasma substitutes are administered to correct this while monitoring central venous pressure.
6. Aminophylline is given to combat bronchospasm.
7. Antibiotics are given to combat secondary infection.
8. Corticosteriods are given for 48 to 72 hours.

Controversial subjects in the previous outline are the ineffectiveness of pulmonary lavage and the effectiveness of steroids (Hamilton, 1976).

The seriousness of gastric acid aspiration is emphasized by the data reported by Cameron et al. (1973). Of 47 patients with documented aspiration, the overall mortality was 62 per cent. If only one lobe was involved as shown by radiograph, the mortality was 41 per cent; if two or more lobes were involved on one or both sides, the mortality was 90 per cent.

Antibiotics, steroids, and ventilatory assistance were used in various combinations, but none seemed to change the outcome effectively.

COMPLICATIONS OF MECHANICAL VENTILATION

Trauma From Endotracheal Tubes

Laryngeal and tracheal injury from prolonged intubation is being seen more frequently now that many patients are recovering from illnesses requiring mechanical ventilation. Although airway stenosis develops in only a small percentage of children undergoing mechanical ventilation, when it does develop it is a serious problem.

The factors responsible for airway obstruction from endotracheal tubes are trauma during insertion of the tube, duration of intubation, size of the tube in relation to size of the larynx, composition of the tube, shape of the tube, chemical irritants on the tube, motion of the tube within the larynx or of the larynx against the tube, and characteristics of the cuff. For any one case of stenosis, probably two or more factors are responsible. Duration of intubation is the most important factor. For instance, if any of the other factors is active, the longer the tube remains in place, the greater the trauma will be.

The proper position for the cuff of an endotracheal tube is within the trachea. High-pressure cuffs have been a cause of numerous cases of tracheal stenosis (Grillo, 1969, 1973). Low-pressure cuffs now available should cause fewer problems. If the endotracheal tube is not in far enough, the cuff may be within the subglottic or glottic larynx; in this case, it could cause laryngeal stenosis. In most instances, however, tracheal stenosis is due to trauma from the cuff, whereas laryngeal stenosis is due to trauma from the tube itself. Uncuffed tubes seldom, if ever, result in stenosis below the subglottic area enclosed by the cricoid cartilage. Cuffed endotracheal tubes should not be used until at least late childhood unless absolutely necessary for ventilation. At any age, for that matter, cuffs should not be used unless they are needed.

Endotracheal tubes used in children should be composed of polyvinyl chloride (PVC), the most suitable plastic material currently available (Guess, 1970). Tubes of PVC mold to the contour of the airway at body temperature; they are soft and less irritating to the larynx and trachea than tubes of rubber or other plastics. For protection of the larynx, tubes should not fit snugly in the larynx. A leak should be audible around the tube when positive pressure is applied.

For prolonged intubation, only tubes of uniform diameter should be used. Cole tubes, with the distal 3 cm narrower than the proximal portion, can be tolerated for brief periods, such as during surgical anesthesia. They should not be used for prolonged intubation because the shoulder at the junction of distal and proximal portions can severely damage the larynx (Brandstater, 1969; Hawkins, 1978).

Of course, endotracheal tubes should be inserted with as little trauma as possible. Once inserted, they should not be changed unless they become occluded or are accidentally removed.

Endotracheal tubes that are sterilized with ethylene oxide may contain a residue of this gas that is toxic to human tissues (Stetson and Guess, 1970). Dissipation of ethylene oxide depends on the type of material that was sterilized, the temperature at which it is stored, and the type of wrapping material that is used. Generalizations of time after sterilization before an endotracheal tube is safe to use are difficult to make but should be several days, at least. Another problem with ethylene oxide is that it reacts with free chloride ions in PVC to form another toxic product, 2-chloroethanol (chlorohydrin). This source of laryngeal trauma is eliminated by the use of disposable PVC endotracheal tubes.

Laryngeal stenosis secondary to intubation may develop at the glottic or subglottic levels, or both. Subglottic stenosis begins as granulation tissue forming in ulcerations within the cricoid ring. This granulation tissue matures into fibrous scar tissue, which narrows the subglottic lumen. Glottic stenosis usually results from scarring in the interarytenoid area. This is the area on which the tube exerts maximum pressure (Dwyer et al., 1949; Harrison and Tonkin, 1968; Lindholm, 1969; Hengerer et al., 1975). The stenosis may be in the form of a fibrous band between the arytenoid vocal processes or more extensive scarring (Fig. 68–3), each of which limits abduction of the vocal cords. Scarring in this area may be surprisingly difficult to identify initially; this can lead to a misdiagnosis of

vocal cord paralysis. If the problem is found to be a scar tissue band between the arytenoid vocal processes (Fig. 68–3, bottom illustration), dividing this band may be all that is necessary to restore an adequate airway. If the scarring is more diffuse, as in the middle and top illustrations of Figure 68–3, correction may be more difficult. Division of discrete portions of scar, followed by separation of the vocal cords by passing laryngeal dilators or bronchoscopes, may need to be repeated several times before an adequate airway is established. Many cases of subglottic stenosis can be corrected by frequent dilatations without stenting. There is some doubt as to the value of stents in laryngeal stenosis resulting from intubation. The success of endoscopic management of both glottic and subglottic stenosis in children and adults seems to depend on severity of the scarring, starting dilatations early while the scar tissue is less dense, and how frequently and persistently the dilatations are repeated (Hawkins, 1977). In some cases, it may not be possible to

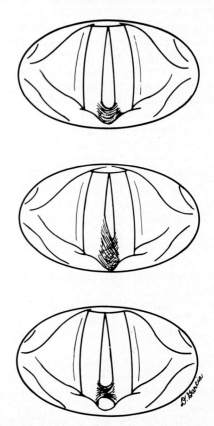

Figure 68–3 Three varieties of interarytenoid scarring causing glottic stenosis. (From Hawkins, D. B. 1977. Glottic and subglottic stenosis from endotracheal intubation. Laryngoscope, 87:339–346.)

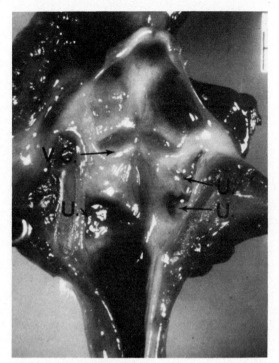

Figure 68–4 The larynx of a neonate intubated 29 days. VC, vocal cord; U, ulceration. Ulcerations are shown bilaterally in the cricoid area beneath the arytenoids and extending up to the right arytenoid cartilage. (From Hawkins, D. B. 1978. Hyaline membrane disease of the neonate. Laryngoscope, 88:201–224.)

establish an adequate airway by endoscopic methods; external laryngeal surgery may be required. The appropriate age for external laryngeal surgery in children is a controversial subject at the present time.

The length of time an endotracheal tube can be left in place without resulting in stenosis of the larynx varies with each situation. So many factors are involved that each patient must be considered individually. General guidelines can be developed, however, based on factors relating to stenosis discussed in earlier paragraphs and on changes in the larynx with growth. Neonates tolerate extended periods of intubation with PVC tubes (Conner and Maisels, 1977), yet autopsy examinations have revealed a high incidence of cricoid ulceration (Fig. 68–4) in larynges of neonates dying after prolonged intubation (Hawkins, 1978). This shows that PVC tubes do injure the larynx; the neonate's tolerance of long periods of intubation must be due to resiliency of their cricoid cartilages.

Laryngeal cartilages of neonates, upon gross examination, seem softer and more pliable than those from older children. Rigidity of cartilage is determined by its matrix, which is made up of proteoglycans and collagen tissue. Proteoglycan content changes from a high concentration at birth of highly soluble chondroitin-4-sulfate to a high concentration of less soluble, more protein-laden keratan sulfate in adulthood. As cricoid cartilage grows, its matrix increases in amount, becoming less hydrated, more fibrous, and more rigid. As shown in Figures 68–5 and 68–6, the cricoid cartilage of the neonate, and especially of the premature neonate, is hypercellular with little intervening matrix. The scant matrix is smooth, stains pale, and looks like a gel. By one year of age (Fig. 68–7) the cricoid cartilage looks more solid than that of a neonate. The cells are more organized, and the matrix stains more deeply, indicating less water content. This appearance of increasing firmness progresses with increasing age. By five years, a developing fibrous stroma can be

Figure 68–5 Cricoid cartilage of an 800 gm neonate with small, randomly distributed cells lying close together. The matrix is scant, pale-staining, and smooth. × 120. (From Hawkins, D. B. 1978. Hyaline membrane disease of the neonate. Laryngoscope, 88:201–224.)

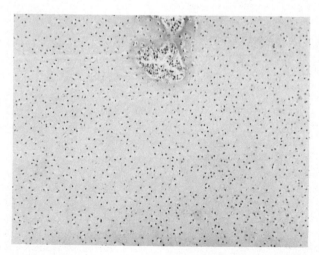

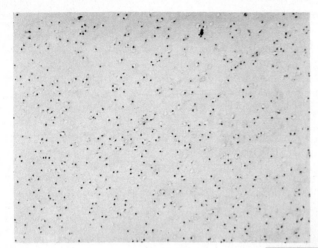

Figure 68–6 Cricoid cartilage of a 3000 gm neonate, still hypercellular but with more matrix than in Figure 68–5. × 120. (From Hawkins, D. B. 1978. Hyaline membrane disease of the neonate. Laryngoscope, 88:201–224.)

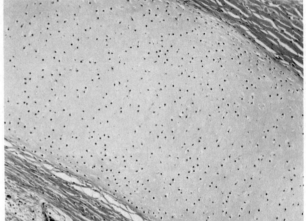

Figure 68–7 Cricoid cartilage from a 1 year old, from a thinner portion of cartilage. Matrix stains more deeply, lacunae are arranged in a more orderly fashion, and the cartilage looks more solid than in Figures 68–5 and 68–6. × 120. (From Hawkins, D. B. 1978. Hyaline membrane disease of the neonate. Laryngoscope, 88:201–224.)

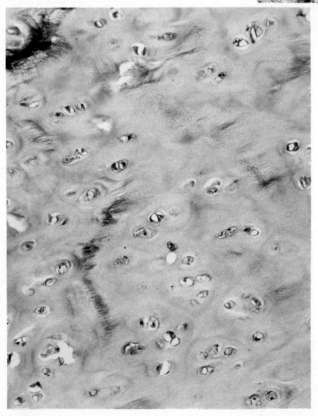

Figure 68–8 Cricoid cartilage from a 14 year old. The cells are widely separated by an abundant matrix that stains deeply basophilic and has a demonstrable fibrous stroma. The lacunae are large and have distinct capsules. × 120. (From Hawkins, D. B. 1978. Hyaline membrane disease of the neonate. Laryngoscope, 88:201–224.)

detected in an abundant matrix. By 10 years the fibrous stroma is obvious, and by the age of 14 years (Fig. 68–8) the predominant feature is an abundant, deeply staining matrix with a definite fibrous stroma. Neonatal cricoid cartilage looks like a different structure from that of a 14 year old.

Clinical experience has shown that normal neonatal larynges can tolerate extended periods of up to several months of intubation. The resiliency of the neonatal larynx, however, cannot be duplicated in older patients. The older the patient, the shorter the duration of intubation probably should be. Prolonged intubation of neonates can be measured in weeks, but intubation of older children should still be measured in days.

Children below five years of age with normal larynges can probably tolerate 14 days of intubation with little risk of laryngeal stenosis. Those under one year can probably tolerate slightly longer periods. In patients over five years of age, shorter periods of intubation are advisable; five to seven days may be an appropriate time. Toward the end of these periods, tracheostomy should be considered seriously if the patient still needs ventilatory support. Intubation of inflamed larynges or those known to be stenotic should be of as brief duration as possible.

As mentioned earlier, many factors are involved, and each patient must be considered individually. For instance, an intubated child who is restless will sustain laryngeal injury more easily than a child who is motionless. Tracheostomy should be done earlier in a restless patient.

Bronchopulmonary Dysplasia

Bronchopulmonary dysplasia (BPD) is the term introduced in 1967 by Northway and colleagues to describe a disease of chronic pulmonary insufficiency developing in neonates with severe hyaline membrane disease who had received positive pressure ventilation with high oxygen concentrations for at least several days. Subsequently, it has also been described following mechanical ventilation for conditions other than hyaline membrane disease. The reported incidence varies widely, from 17 to 36 per cent of low birth weight infants who survive artificial ventilation (Watts et al., 1977). It probably represents the end result of severe pulmonary disease, with superimposed injury from high

concentrations of oxygen administered by positive pressure through an endotracheal tube (Stocks and Godfrey, 1976). Microscopic changes in the lungs of infants dying of BPD resemble those observed in lungs of laboratory animals dying of oxygen toxicity. A high concentration of inspired oxygen is not the only factor, however; BPD has not been reported in lungs of neonates ventilated by negative pressure respirators, even with high oxygen concentrations. The incidence of BPD has been shown to diminish after respirator adjustments lowering peak airway pressures and using slow respiratory rates. The most important factor in pathogenesis of BPD appears to be the use of high peak airway pressures (Reynolds and Taghizadeh, 1976).

The pathologic changes in BPD consist of bronchial and terminal airway damage with repair by hyperplasia, metaplasia, and fibrosis. The principal pathologic changes found in the lungs are obliterative airway disease, interstitial fibrosis, persistent collapse, diminished alveolization, emphysematous coalescence of alveoli, thickening of alveolar basement membranes, and evidence of pulmonary hypertension.

The radiographic changes as the disease progresses are as follows: Stage I (Fig. 68–9) shows moderately severe hyaline membrane disease, i.e., a diffuse, fine, reticulogranular pattern with prominent bronchial air shadows creating an air bronchogram. Stage II radiographs (Fig. 68–10) show nearly complete opacification of all lung fields. Stage III (Fig. 68–11) is characterized by multiple small, round, radiolucent areas distributed throughout both lungs, alternating with areas of irregular density. This gives the appearance of a sponge. These cystic-appearing areas increase in size and number, and the lungs become increasingly hyperexpanded as the process reaches Stage IV (Fig. 68–12). As resolution progresses, the cystic areas are replaced by hyperlucency at the bases and streaky infiltration extending toward the apices (Fig. 68–13).

Infants with BPD may be respirator-dependent for weeks or months and may die of pulmonary insufficiency, with or without cor pulmonale. Even after they are weaned from the respirator, they may require higher than atmospheric oxygen levels for extended periods of time to prevent cyanosis. Those who survive have frequent respiratory infections during their first two years of life.

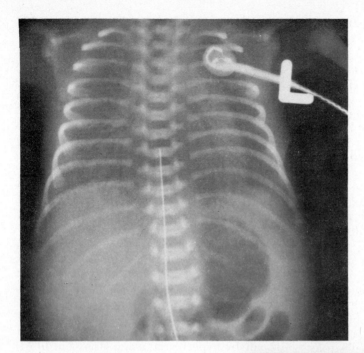

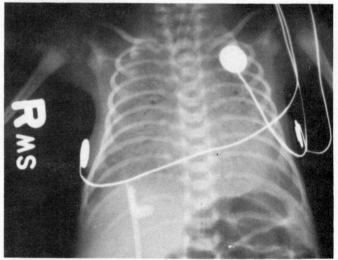

Figure 68–9 Chest radiograph of stage I bronchopulmonary dysplasia, or moderately severe hyaline membrane disease, demonstrating a fine reticulogranular pattern in all lung fields with exaggeration of bronchial air columns creating an air bronchogram. (From Hawkins, D. B. 1978. Hyaline membrane disease of the neonate. Laryngoscope, 88:201–224.)

Figure 68–10 Chest radiograph from stage II bronchopulmonary dysplasia. The diffuse granularity has become more dense, giving a "whiteout" appearance to the lungs. The air bronchogram is prominent on the right side.

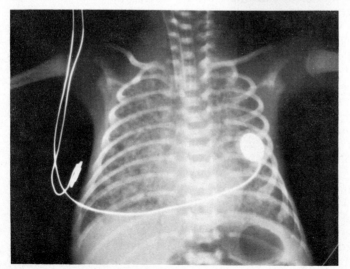

Figure 68–11 Chest radiograph of stage III bronchopulmonary dysplasia with multiple small cystic areas scattered throughout both lungs alternating with areas of increased density.

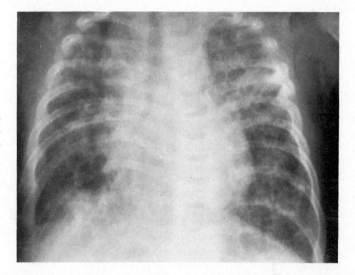

Figure 68–12 Chest radiograph of early stage IV bronchopulmonary dysplasia, demonstrating enlarging cystic spaces and some basilar overexpansion.

MISCELLANEOUS CONDITIONS

The following paragraphs are devoted to brief descriptions of several rare idiopathic disorders of the lower respiratory tract that those interested in pediatric otolaryngology should be aware of. For more detailed descriptions, the reader is referred to Nelson's Textbook of Pediatrics (Vaughan et al., 1979) or Kendig's Disorders of the Respiratory Tract in Children (1977).

Pulmonary Hemosiderosis

This term is used to describe several conditions characterized by abnormal hemosiderin deposits in the lungs resulting from diffuse alveolar hemorrhage. This may be due to primary pulmonary disease or secondary to cardiac disease that produces a chronic increase in pulmonary capillary pressure, such as mitral stenosis. Another form of secondary pulmonary hemosiderosis is that associated with collagen disease or diffuse vascular disorders.

There appear to be three types of primary pulmonary hemosiderosis.
1. Idiopathic pulmonary hemosiderosis begins in late childhood or early adulthood with episodes of cough, hemoptysis, wheezing, and dyspnea. It is associated with iron deficiency anemia that is refractory to treatment. Approximately 50 per cent of these patients die of acute pulmonary hemorrhage or respiratory failure within five years of the onset of symptoms.

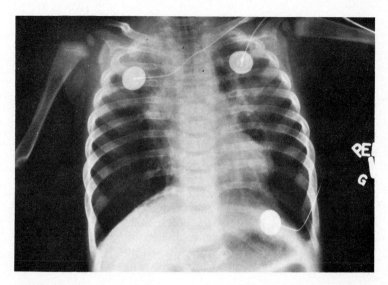

Figure 68–13 Chest radiograph of late stage IV bronchopulmonary dysplasia showing basilar emphysema and fibrotic changes in the upper lobes.

2. Primary pulmonary hemosiderosis with myocarditis: The clinical picture in this type is similar to that of the idiopathic form with the addition of clinical, radiographic, and electrocardiographic signs of myocarditis.
3. Primary pulmonary hemosiderosis with glomerulonephritis (Goodpasture syndrome): more common in young adults than in children, the pulmonary symptoms of this form are identical to those of the idiopathic variety. These patients, however, have progressive renal disease that is usually the cause of death.

Some children with primary pulmonary hemosiderosis were found to be sensitive to cow's milk, and they improved when cow's milk was removed from their diets. However, other patients with pulmonary hemosiderosis have not been sensitive to cow's milk and did not improve with its removal from their diets.

Desquamative Interstitial Pneumonitis

This condition, classified as a collagen disease, usually occurs in adults, but it has been reported in children. Symptoms consist of progressive dyspnea, nonproductive cough, and weight loss without fever. Radiographs of the lungs reveal poorly defined hilar densities and a ground-glass appearance in both bases. The basic pathologic manifestations are massive proliferation and desquamation of the epithelium of distal air passages and thickening of their walls. Treatment with corticosteroids arrests the disease in most patients.

Idiopathic Diffuse Interstitial Fibrosis of the Lung (Hamman-Rich Syndrome)

Also more common in adults, this disorder has been reported in children. It is a progressive disease leading to death from pulmonary insufficiency resulting from interstitial fibrosis and thickening of the alveolar-capillary membrane. Symptoms begin with dyspnea, first only with exercise but later even at rest, cough with hemoptysis, anorexia, and weight loss, progressing to right-sided cardiac failure. Radiographic findings are progressive granular mottling or small nodular densities throughout the lungs. Therapy is symptomatic only. Corticosteroids afford some symptomatic relief but do not alter progression of the disease.

Pulmonary Alveolar Proteinosis

This disorder usually presents before one year of age with cough, dyspnea, and sometimes with gastrointestinal symptoms. Chest radiographs reveal a fine, diffuse infiltrate radiating from the hilus to the periphery. The diagnosis is made by lung biopsy revealing alveoli distended by fine, granular, eosinophilic material that stains positively with periodic acid–Schiff stain. Some patients with this disorder are also immunologically deficient. There is no effective treatment; most children die of respiratory failure within one year of the onset of symptoms.

Pulmonary Alveolar Microlithiasis

This disease is characterized by the formation of tiny calcium carbonate stones within pulmonary alveoli. The mechanism by which the stones are formed is not known; the patients appear to have no identifiable metabolic abnormalities. Radiographic examination shows fine granular densities scattered throughout the lungs. The appearance has been likened to that of an overfilled bronchogram.

The disease begins in childhood, progresses slowly, and the patients usually die of cardiopulmonary failure in mid-adult life.

REFERENCES

Achauer, B. M., Allyn, P. A., Furmas, D. W., et al. 1973. Pulmonary complications of burns. Ann. Surg., 177:311.

Baldachin, B. J., and Melmed, R. N. 1964. Clinical and therapeutic aspects of kerosene poisoning: a series of 200 cases. Brit. Med. J., 2:28.

Brandstater, B. 1969. Dilatation of the larynx with Cole tubes. Anesthesiology, 31:378.

Bredenberg, C. E., et al. 1969. Respiratory failure in shock. Ann. Surg., 169:392.

Cameron, J. L., Mitchell, W. N., and Zuidema, G. D. 1973. Aspiration pneumonia. Clinical outcome following documented aspiration. Arch. Surg., 106:49.

The author wishes to express his appreciation to Emily Kahlstrom, M.D., and Eithne MacLaughlin, M.D., Assistant Professors of Pediatrics, Respiratory Disease Division, University of Southern California School of Medicine, for reviewing portions of this chapter and offering very helpful advice.

Champneys, F. H. 1882. Mediastinal emphysema and pneumothorax in connection with tracheotomy. Med-Chir Trans., 47:75.

Conner, G. H., and Maisels, M. J. 1977. Orotracheal intubation in the newborn. Laryngoscope, 87:87.

Dwyer, C. S., Kronenberg, S., and Saklad, M. 1949. The endotracheal tube: a consideration of its traumatic effects. Anesthesiology, 10:714.

Eckhauser, F. E., Billote, J., Burke, J. F., et al. 1974. Tracheostomy complicating massive burn injury. Am. J. Surg., 127:418.

Foley, J. C., Dreyer, N. B., Soule, A. B., Jr., et al. 1954. Kerosene poisoning in young children. Radiology, 62:817.

Forbes, G. B., Salmon, G., and Herweg, J. C. 1947. Further observations on post-tracheotomy mediastinal emphysema and pneumothorax. J Pediatr., 31:172.

Geelhoed, G. W., and Bennett, S. H. 1975. "Shock lung" resulting from perfusion of canine lungs with stored bank blood. Ann. Surg., 41:661.

Grillo, H. C. 1969. The management of tracheal stenosis following assisted respiration. J. Thorac. Cardiovasc. Surg., 57:52.

Grillo, H. C. 1973. Reconstruction of the trachea: experience in 100 consecutive cases. Thorax, 28:667.

Guess, W. L. 1970. Plastics for tracheal tubes. Int. Anesthesiol. Clin., 8:805.

Hamilton, W. K. 1976. Aspiration pneumonitis — a continuing problem. West. J. Med., 125:384.

Harrison, G. A., and Tonkin, J. P. 1968. Prolonged endotracheal intubation. Br. J. Anaesth., 40:241.

Hawkins, D. B., Seltzer, D. C., Barnett, T. E., et al. 1974. Endotracheal tube perforation of the hypopharynx. West. J. Med., 120:282.

Hawkins, D. B. 1977. Glottic and subglottic stenosis from endotracheal intubation. Laryngoscope, 87:339.

Hawkins, D. B. 1978. Hyaline membrane disease of the neonate — prolonged intubation in management — effects on the larynx. Laryngoscope, 88:201–224.

Hawkins, D. B., and Williams, E. H. 1976. Tracheostomy in infants and young children. Laryngoscope, 86:331.

Hengerer, A. S., Strome, M., and Jaffe, B. F. 1975. Injuries to the neonatal larynx from long-term endotracheal tube intubation and suggested tube modification for prevention. Ann. Otol., Rhinol. Laryngol. 84:764.

Jackson, C. 1959. Foreign bodies in the air and food passages. In Jackson, C., and Jackson, C. L. Diseases of the Nose, Throat, and Ear, 2nd ed. Philadelphia, W. B. Saunders Co., p. 842.

James, P. M. 1975. Treatment of shock lung. Ann. Surg., 41:451.

Kendig, E. L. 1977. Disorders of the Respiratory Tract in Children, 3rd ed. Philadelphia, W.B. Saunders Co., pp. 538–552.

Lindholm, C. E. 1969. Prolonged endotracheal intubation. Acta Anaesth. Suppl., 33:1.

Lorin, M. I. 1975. Mechanical defense mechanisms of the respiratory system. In Scarpelli, E. M. Pulmonary Physiology of the Fetus, Newborn, and Child. Philadelphia, Lea and Febiger, p. 220.

McCormick, P. W. 1975. Immediate care after aspiration of vomit. Anaesthesia, 30:658.

Mendelson, C. L. 1946. Aspiration of stomach contents into lungs during obstetric anesthesia. Am. J. Obstetr. Gynecol., 52:191.

Northway, W. H., Rosan, R. C., and Porter, D. Y. 1967. Pulmonary disease following respiratory therapy of hyaline membrane disease — bronchopulmonary dysplasia. N. Engl. J. Med., 276:357.

Ogata, E. S., Gregory, G. A., Kitterman, J. A., et al. 1976. Pneumothorax in the respiratory distress syndrome. Pediatrics, 58:177.

Ostendorf, P., Birzle, H., Vogel, W., et al. 1975. Pulmonary radiographic abnormalities in shock. Radiology, 115:257.

Parks, S. 1976. Inhalation injury in burn patients. West. J. Med., 124:244.

Powers, S. R., Jr., Burdge, R., Leather, R., et al. 1972. Studies of pulmonary insufficiency in non-thoracic trauma. J. Trauma, 12:1.

Pruitt, B. A., Flemma, R. J., DiVincenti, F. C., et al. 1970. Pulmonary complications in burn patients. A comparative study of 697 patients. J. Thorac. Cardiovasc. Surg., 59:7.

Pruitt, B. A., Erickson, D. R., and Morris, A. 1975. Progressive pulmonary insufficiency and other pulmonary complications of thermal injury. J. Trauma, 15:369.

Rabuzzi, D. D., and Reed, G. F. 1971. Intrathoracic complications following tracheotomy in children. Laryngoscope, 81:939.

Reichert, T. J., Bluestone, C. D., Stool, S. E., et al. 1977. Congenital cricopharyngeal achalasia. Ann. Otol., Rhinol., Laryngol., 86:603–613.

Reynolds, E. O. R., and Taghizadeh, A. 1976. Pathogenesis of bronchopulmonary dysplasia following hyaline membrane disease. Am. J. Pathol., 82:241.

Ruggera, G., and Taylor, G. 1976. Pulmonary aspiration in anesthesia. West. J. Med. 125:411.

Sladen, A., 1976. Methylprednisolone. Pharmacologic doses in shock lung syndrome. J. Thorac. Cardiovasc. Surg., 71:800.

Stetson, J. B., and Guess, W. L. 1970. Causes of damage to tissues by polymers and elastomers used in the fabrication of tracheal devices. Anesthesiology, 33:635.

Stocks, J., and Godfrey, S. 1976. The role of artificial ventilation, oxygen, and CPAP in the pathogenesis of lung damage in neonates. Pediatrics, 57:352.

Vaughan, V. C., McKay, R. J., and Behrman, R. E. 1979. Nelson Textbook of Pediatrics, 11th ed. Philadelphia, W. B. Saunders Co., pp. 1148–1248.

Watts, J. L., Ariangno, R. L., and Brady, J. P. 1977. Chronic pulmonary disease in neonates after artificial ventilation. Pediatrics, 60:273.

Wolff, A. P., Kuhn, F. A., and Ogura, J. H. 1972. Pharyngo-esophageal perforations associated with rapid oral endotracheal intubation. Ann. Otol., Rhinol. Laryngol., 81:258.

Chapter 69

NEUROGENIC DISEASES OF THE LARYNX

Douglas D. Dedo, M.D.
Herbert H. Dedo, M.D.

INTRODUCTION

Isolated neurologic disorders of the upper respiratory and gastrointestinal tracts are unusual in the pediatric population. However, unilateral and occasionally bilateral recurrent nerve paralysis is seen in the newborn or infant. It may be a manifestation of a multiple-system anomaly, or, if there is no apparent cause, it presumably is due to stretching of the recurrent laryngeal nerves at delivery. Early detection of these neurogenic disorders is based upon a high index of suspicion and is important to prevent catastrophes during periods of acute respiratory embarrassment.

CLINICAL SYMPTOMS

Acquired or congenital neurogenic laryngeal disorders affect one or all of the normal functions of the larynx. An abnormal cry or voice, respiratory obstruction, and difficulty swallowing are the symptoms of altered laryngeal function. A neonate with a weak or absent cry may have a laryngeal anomaly whether or not respiration is impaired. Unilateral vocal cord paralysis tends to produce a more breathy and weak cry than bilateral vocal cord paralysis. In the latter, the cry is normal, but significant airway obstruction is ordinarily present; expiratory air passing through the glottis with the cords in a median or paramedian position will produce a normal cry and voice, even though both cords are paralyzed. A muffled cry usually signifies a problem of pharyngeal origin, such as a vallecular cyst, lingual thyroid, or pharyngeal abscess.

Stridor, the harsh respiratory sound produced when air passes a partially vibrating obstruction (the vocal cords), is the most frequent symptom of children with cord paralysis for which parents seek advice (Cavanaugh, 1955). When the stridor is associated with a normal cry, the commonest cause (confirmed by direct laryngoscopy) is congenital laryngomalacia (soft cartilage or floppy epiglottis). Unilateral or bilateral vocal cord paralysis, laryngotracheobronchitis, web, foreign body, cricoarytenoid joint fixation, and tumor must be ruled out in these stridorous patients.

Abnormal deglutition is frequently associated with disorders of the larynx. Drooling, recurrent choking, and aspiration of pharyngeal secretions suggest either a developmental anomaly of the laryngopharynx, such as a posterior cleft larynx or a tracheoesophageal fistula, or a peripheral or central lesion of the ninth or tenth cranial nerves. Pharyngeal and vocal cord paralysis have been reported to occur together (Holinger, 1961).

ETIOLOGY OF LARYNGEAL PARALYSIS

Laryngeal paralysis may be congenital or acquired in the neonate or infant, but in older children, as in adults, trauma is the usual cause. The following outline lists the myriad sources of laryngeal paralysis in children.

A. Neonate and infant
  1. Congenital
    a. Central nervous system
      (1) Cerebral agenesis
      (2) Hydrocephalus
      (3) Encephalocele
      (4) Meningomyelocele
      (5) Meningocele
      (6) Arnold-Chiari malformation
      (7) Nucleus ambiguus dysgenesis
      (8) Associated multiple congenital anomalies
        (a) Mental retardation
        (b) Mongolism
        (c) Other cranial nerve palsies
    b. Peripheral nervous system
      (1) Congenital defect in peripheral nerve fiber at neuromuscular junction, as in myasthenia gravis
      (2) Platybasia
    c. Cardiovascular anomalies
      (1) Cardiomegaly
        (a) Interventricular septal defect
        (b) Tetralogy of Fallot
      (2) Abnormal great vessels
        (a) Vascular ring
        (b) Dilated aorta
        (c) Double aortic arch
        (d) Patent ductus arteriosus
        (e) Transposition of the great vessels
    d. Associated with other congenital anomalies
      (1) Tumors or cysts of mediastinum (bronchogenic cyst)
      (2) Malformation of the tracheobronchial tree
      (3) Esophageal malformation
        (a) Cyst
        (b) Duplication
        (c) Atresia
        (d) Tracheoesophageal fistula
      (4) Diaphragmatic hernia
      (5) Erb palsy
      (6) Cleft palate
      (7) Laryngeal anomalies
        (a) Laryngeal cleft
        (b) Subglottic stenosis
        (c) Laryngomalacia
  2. Acquired
    a. Trauma
      (1) Birth injury
      (2) Postsurgical correction of cardiovascular or esophageal anomalies

    b. Infectious
      (1) Whooping cough encephalitis
      (2) Polyneuritis
      (3) Polio encephalitis
      (4) Diphtheria
      (5) Rabies
      (6) Syphilis
      (7) Tetanus
      (8) Botulism
      (9) Tuberculosis
    c. Supranuclear and nuclear lesions
      (1) Kernicterus
      (2) Multiple sclerosis
B. Older child and adolescent — etiology similar to most adult series — traumatic following:
  1. Thoracic or head and neck surgery
  2. External neck trauma
  3. Intubation for general anesthesia

Congenital

Vocal cord paralysis is the second most common laryngeal anomaly of the neonate. (The commonest is laryngomalacia.) Unilateral or bilateral paralysis together account for approximately 10 per cent of all congenital laryngeal lesions (Holinger et al., 1976). The majority of these infants have multiple congenital defects. Table 69–1 summarizes the various congenital disorders of the nervous system that have been reported with vocal cord paralysis. Since the larynx is not routinely examined in these patients, the vocal cord paralysis may remain undiagnosed for a long period of time.

The Arnold-Chiari malformation is frequently seen with hydrocephalus, meningocele, and myelomeningocele (cervical, lumbar, or sacral) (Graham, 1963). The anatomy of the malformation is illustrated in Figure 69–1. The medulla and cerebellum protrude

Table 69–1 DISORDERS OF THE NERVOUS SYSTEM SEEN WITH VOCAL CORD PARALYSIS

Hydrocephalus
Meningomyelocele
Arnold-Chiari malformation
Meningocele
Encephalocele
Cerebral agenesis
Nucleus ambiguus dysgenesis
Neuromuscular disorders
Myasthenia gravis

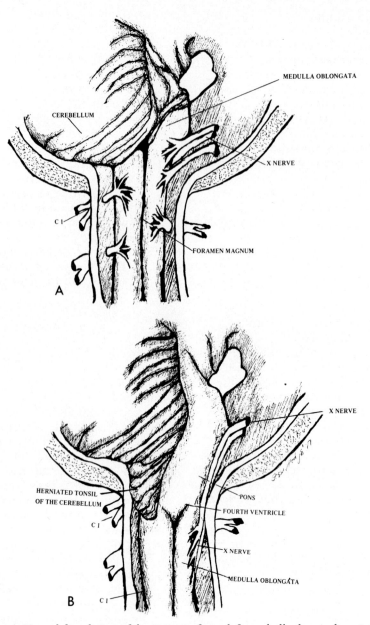

Figure 69–1 *A*, Normal dorsal view of the posterior fossa; left cerebellar hemisphere is in place and right cerebellar hemisphere is removed.
   B, Arnold–Chiari malformation showing herniation and inferior displacement of brain stem with subsequent abnormal course of vagus nerves, superiorly through foramen magnum to exit via jugular foramen.

through the foramen magnum into the spinal canal so that the tenth cranial nerves exit the brain stem in the spinal canal. The abnormal course of the vagal nerves — traveling superiorly through the foramen magnum to exit via the jugular foramen — leaves them vulnerable to injury. The subsequent caudal displacement of the brain stem by increasing intracranial pressure stretches the vagi and causes tenth cranial nerve, and therefore recurrent nerve and vocal cord, paralysis.

Other developmental anomalies of the central nervous system, such as encephalocele, cerebral agenesis, mental retardation, and nucleus ambiguus dysgenesis, have been reported with vocal cord paralysis.

Vocal cord paralysis with or without other bulbar palsies has been described with other progressive congenital and acquired neuro-muscular disorders (Holinger, 1961; Priest et al., 1966; Hart, 1970). Benign congenital hypotonia, Werdnig-Hoffmann disease, leukodystrophy, and Charcot-Marie-Tooth disease have all been complicated by laryngeal paralysis. Unfortunately, the causal relationship between the disease and the paralysis has not been defined.

Myasthenia gravis is a disease affecting all age groups. It is characterized by weakness and abnormal fatigability of skeletal muscles. The return of normal muscle strength after fatigue is prolonged. Neonatal myasthenia gravis may present with bulbar symptoms. These children, whose mothers have myasthenia gravis, are noted to have marked inability to suck or swallow (Stuart, 1963). An absent or weak cry and facial weakness are also common symptoms. Tracheotomy is performed on those infants unable to swallow or to cough effectively.

Congenital or juvenile myasthenia gravis affects those children with normal mothers. While the presenting symptom is usually ptosis of the eyelids, they may also present with dysphagia or dysphonia. These symptoms occur because of weak pharyngeal and tongue muscles (Maxwell and Locke, 1968). The diagnosis is established by the use of anticholinesterase drugs.

Skeletal malformations may damage the peripheral cranial nerves. Platybasia is a flattening of the base of the skull on the cervical spine. Subsequent stretching of the cranial nerves may produce vocal cord paralysis. The diagnosis is readily made with skull radiographs (Merritt, 1963).

A wide variety of congenital cardiovascular anomalies has been associated with vocal cord paralysis. Although the left recurrent nerve is more vulnerable to injury than the right because of its longer course, right vocal cord paralysis has been seen with cardiovascular defects. Cardiomegaly secondary to an interventricular septal defect or tetralogy of Fallot may stretch the left recurrent nerve. Abnormalities of the great vessels, such as a vascular ring, dilated aorta, double aortic arch, transposition, and patent ductus arteriosus, have all been associated with vocal cord paralysis (Holinger, 1961).

The intimate embryologic development of the laryngopharynx, esophagus, and tracheobronchial tree from the third, fourth, fifth, and sixth visceral arches accounts for the associated congenital anomalies in these structures. Esophageal cysts, duplication or atresia of the esophagus, diaphragmatic hernia, and tracheoesophageal fistula have been reported with laryngeal paralysis. Bronchogenic cysts of the mediastinum and tracheobronchial malformations have also been complicated by vocal cord paralysis. Similarly, congenital defects of the larynx, including subglottic stenosis, laryngomalacia, and laryngeal clefts (Cohen, 1975), may have associated unilateral or bilateral vocal cord paralysis. Several other congenital disorders and syndromes, such as mongolism, arthrogryposis multiplex congenita (Cohen and Isaacs, 1976), and cleft palate, have been reported with laryngeal paralysis as one facet of the anomaly.

Acquired

The acquired neurogenic lesions of the larynx in the pediatric patient may be divided into three broad categories: traumatic, infectious, and miscellaneous. Injury to the recurrent laryngeal nerves at birth has been implicated. For a significant number of pediatric patients with vocal cord paralysis, as in any adult series, no apparent cause of the problem can be found. It has been suggested that in these cases the recurrent nerves have been unavoidably stretched during delivery, as with a breech presentation with twisting and stretching of the neck to deliver the head. Hyperextension of the neck to the right or left in the vertex position to rotate and deliver the shoulders may also produce recurrent laryngeal nerve injury. The anatomy of the recurrent laryngeal nerves makes them vulnerable to injury as they course around the subclavian artery on the right and the aorta on the left. During delivery the vessels provide counter traction against the nerves, thus stretching them, with subsequent paralysis, which may be temporary or permanent. Tracheotomy is usually necessary for bilateral but not for unilateral paralysis.

Surgical correction of many of the thoracic and cardiovascular anomalies may be complicated by injury to the recurrent laryngeal nerves. Since vocal cord paralysis has been reported following repair of patent ductus arteriosus, tracheoesophageal fistula, and other similar anomalies, preoperative visualization of the larynx to determine vocal cord mobility is useful.

Antibiotics and immunizations (vaccinations) have greatly reduced the infectious types of vocal cord paralysis. Whooping cough encephalitis, polio, diphtheria, rabies, tetanus, syphilis, and botulism have been sources of laryngeal paralysis that are fortunately rarely seen in present-day pediatric practice (Cavanaugh, 1955). Any bacterial or viral encephalitis may be complicated by bulbar paresis. Similarly, an ascending paralysis, as in the Guillain-Barré syndrome will occasionally involve the bulbar nuclei with subsequent laryngeal or chest paralysis, or both, requiring cuffed tracheotomy and assisted ventilation for several days or weeks. Infectious mononucleosis has a neurologic complication rate of 1 to 2 per cent. Meningoencephalitis and peripheral neuritis with pharyngeal and laryngeal paralysis have been reported with mononucleosis (Montandon et al., 1956).

Idiopathic vocal cord paralysis occasionally follows a viral infection (Graham, 1962) and is usually in the form of a peripheral neuritis similar to Bell palsy. Return of vocal cord mobility in two to six months can occur. In unusual cases tracheotomy is necessary to relieve the airway obstruction.

Tumors of the central nervous system may present with bulbar paralysis. Ross and Chambers (1957) reported a case of an infant with a chondroma at or near the nucleus ambiguus that caused laryngeal nerve paralysis. Similar paresis from a spongioblastoma multiforme of the right cerebellar hemisphere confluent with the pons and medulla has also been reported (Jackson and Jackson, 1937).

A broad category of miscellaneous causes for acquired neurogenic disorders includes those diseases in which the laryngeal nerve may be involved along its anatomic course (Rontal and Rontal, 1977). The supranuclear areas and nuclei may be involved in kernicterus and multiple sclerosis. Holinger (1961) reported a case of mediastinitis secondary to an esophageal foreign body that caused bilateral recurrent nerve paralysis.

In adolescence, the incidence of vocal cord paralysis decreases, and the causes reflect those of most adult series. In this age group, the most frequent cause of vocal cord paralysis is trauma to the recurrent laryngeal nerves. In addition, head and neck or thoracic surgery may be complicated by a postoperative vocal cord paralysis. Blunt neck trauma from motor vehicle accidents may generate forces sufficient to stretch or even to avulse the recurrent laryngeal nerves, with subsequent vocal cord paralysis. Postintubation vocal cord paralysis, the pathogenesis for which numerous hypotheses have been proffered, usually resolves spontaneously over a six month period.

DIAGNOSIS AND MANAGEMENT

In the neonate, the diagnosis of a vocal cord paralysis is frequently overlooked because of a more severe associated central nervous system or cardiovascular anomaly. A newborn or infant with an airway problem, feeding difficulties, weak or absent cry, deglutition abnormalities, or known anomaly of the esophagus, heart, or central nervous system should have a laryngeal examination.

Direct laryngoscopy without anesthesia is the method of choice to evaluate vocal cord mobility. With oxygen and pediatric endotracheal tubes available for immediate assistance, the laryngoscope blade is carefully placed in the vallecula and tilted forward. Laryngeal movement must be evaluated during inspiration and phonation or crying. This is often difficult because of cyanosis, apnea, and the cardiac status of the infant. Administration of oxygen throughout the examination may be necessary. After assessment of laryngeal movement, the blade is placed under the epiglottis to examine the configuration of the vocal cords, anterior commissure, and subglottic surface. In children with severe dyspnea, a tracheotomy tray, in addition to the endotracheal tubes, should be ready for immediate use. If there is no apparent pathologic condition to explain the stridor or partial upper airway obstruction, direct laryngoscopy under general anesthesia should be done. Subglottic lesions not visible with direct laryngoscopy when the child is awake are sometimes visible only through the cords when they are fully relaxed.

Paralysis of the recurrent laryngeal nerve results in the affected cords lying in a paramedian position. When both the recurrent and superior laryngeal nerves are paralyzed, the vocal cord lies in the intermediate position (Dedo, 1970).

When other congenital anomalies of the respiratory or digestive systems are suspected, bronchoscopy and esophagoscopy should be part of the management protocol.

The appropriate radiologic studies are largely determined by the presence or absence of other congenital anomalies. Posterior, anterior, and lateral radiographs of the chest and neck can be helpful. Skull films and dye studies of the larynx, trachea, esophagus, and cardiovascular system may be required to document and evaluate associated defects (Kahn et al., 1977).

TREATMENT

The initial treatment of a child with a neurogenic disorder of the larynx is primarily symptomatic. Maintenance of the airway and adequate nutrition are of prime importance. Cavanaugh (1955) and Holinger (1961) reported a 50 per cent incidence of tracheotomy in children with bilateral vocal cord paralysis; the incidence of tracheotomy for unilateral vocal cord paralysis was 20 per cent. Once the condition of the patient is stabilized, the search for the cause of the paralysis may proceed. A diagnosis is usually obvious in 90 per cent of the cases, while the remaining 10 per cent are classified as idiopathic.

Once the diagnosis of a laryngeal paralysis has been made and the etiology investigated, the patient must be carefully followed over the next several weeks to months. Cavanaugh (1955) and Holinger (1961) both reported spontaneous resolution of the paresis in a few cases. Bluestone et al. (1972) emphasized the importance of close cooperation between the neurosurgeon and the otolaryngologist in treating children with the Arnold-Chiari malformation secondary to myelomeningocele. In these children, when the increased intracranial pressure was corrected by a shunt within 24 hours of onset of the vocal cord paralysis, reversal to normal vocal cord mobility was seen to occur up to two weeks later. A delay in diagnosing the increased intracranial pressure and subsequent laryngeal paralysis could result in irreversible vocal cord paralysis. Because of the possibility of spontaneous recovery for any vocal cord paralysis, six months to a year should elapse before any definitive therapy is planned.

Correction of an incompetent glottis in unilateral recurrent laryngeal paralysis or tracheal decannulation after relieving the airway obstruction in bilateral vocal cord paralysis are the two major treatment problems in these children. The optimal age for .either procedure is unknown. Priest and colleagues (1960) have successfully performed the classic Woodman and Pennington (1976) procedure in children 5, 6, and 14 years of age with bilateral vocal cord paralysis. Similarly, Teflon injection has been used by one of the authors (H. Dedo) in a nine year old female to correct an incompetent glottis due to laryngeal nerve paralysis following open heart surgery.'

Unfortunately, the management of these children is complex and not limited to the realm of the otolaryngologist. For instance, parent instruction in maintaining a "oo" sized tracheotomy in an infant cannot be taken for granted. In this case, we have found the Jackson metal double-cannula tracheotomy tubes to be best tolerated. Because of the associated pharyngeal paralyses, a gastrostomy is often necessary.

The associated central nervous system or cardiovascular anomalies make many of these patients chronic nursing problems, never able to be discharged from the hospital.

PROGNOSIS

The acquired forms of vocal cord paralysis have a more favorable outcome than those of congenital origin. The latter are dependent upon the survival rate of the underlying central nervous system or cardiovascular anomaly. Unilateral vocal cord paralysis involves the left more commonly than the right because of its longer course and associated cardiac anomalies; the prognosis is also poorer for left-sided than for right-sided paralysis. In general, the right paresis is an isolated finding with laryngeal function being found ultimately to be good.

Bilateral vocal cord paralyses have the worse prognosis. The children who require a tracheotomy for obstruction and who do not die of their other anomalies generally cannot be decannulated. The exception is the child with a traumatic delivery in whom the paralysis resolves spontaneously four to six months after birth.

SELECTED REFERENCES

Cavanaugh, F. 1955. Vocal palsies in children. J. Laryngol. Otol., 69:399.

This important work was one of the first to draw attention to vocal cord paralysis in children. The author reviews the case reports in the literature through 1955 and then adds several cases of her own. It is an article referenced by all authors writing on pediatric vocal cord paralysis.

Holinger, P. H. 1961. Clinical aspects of congenital anomalies of the larynx, trachea, bronchi, and esophagus. J. Laryngol. Otol., 75:1–44.

A perspective of the relative incidences of the different anomalies of the upper airway is gained from this excellent paper. A large series of vocal cord paralyses with management and long-term follow-up is presented.

REFERENCES

Bluestone, C. D., Delerme, A. N., and Samuelson, G. H. 1972. Airway obstruction due to vocal cord paralysis in infants with hydrocephalus and meningomyelocele. Ann. Otol., 81:778.

Cavanaugh, F. 1955. Vocal palsies in children. J. Laryngol. Otol., 69:399.

Laryngol., 84:747.

Cohen, S. R., and Isaacs, H., Jr. 1976. Otolaryngological manifestations of arthrogryposis multiplex congenita. Ann. Otol. Rhinol. Laryngol., 85:484.

Dedo, H. H. 1970. Paralyzed larynx: Electromyographic study in dogs and humans. Laryngoscope, 80:1455.

Graham, M. D. 1963. Bilateral recurrent laryngeal nerve paralysis associated with upper respiratory infection. J. Laryngol. Otol., 76:535.

Hart, C. W. 1970. Functional and neurological problems of the larynx. Otolaryngol. Clin. North Am., 3:609.

Holinger, L. D., Holinger, P. C., and Holinger, P. H. 1976. Etiology of bilateral abductor vocal cord paralysis — a review of 389 cases. Ann. Otol. Rhinol. Laryngol., 85:428.

Holinger, P. H. 1961. Clinical aspects of congenital anomalies of the larynx, trachea, bronchi, and esophagus. J. Laryngol. Otol., 75:1.

Jackson, C., and Jackson, C. L. 1937. Larynx and Its Diseases. Philadelphia, W. B. Saunders Co., p. 289.

Kahn, A., Baran, D., Sephl, N., et al. 1977. Congenital stridor in infancy, Clin. Pediatr., 16:19.

Maxwell, S., and Locke, J. L. 1968. Voice and myasthenia gravis. Laryngoscope, 78:1902.

Merritt, H. H., 1963. A Textbook of Neurology. Philadelphia, Lea and Febiger, p. 424.

Montandon, Rauch, S., and Reytan 1956. Mononucleosis, Guillain Barré syndrome and paralysis of the posterior cricoarytenoid muscle. Acta Otolaryngol., 46:35.

Priest, R. E., Ulvestad, H. S., Van de Water, F., et al. 1960. Arytenoidectomy in children. Ann. Otol. Rhinol. Laryngol., 69:869.

Rontal, M., and Rontal, E. 1977. Lesions of the vagus nerve: Diagnosis, treatment and rehabilitation. Laryngoscope, 87:72.

Ross, D. E., and Chambers, D. C. 1957. Recurrent laryngeal nerve paralysis occurring in the infant, Am. J. Surg., 94:513.

Stuart, W. D. 1963. Otolaryngological aspects of myasthenia gravis. Laryngoscope, 1973:112.

Woodman, D., and Pennington, C. L. 1976. Bilateral abductor paralysis. Ann. Otol. Rhinol. Laryngol., 85:437.

Chapter 70

INJURIES OF THE LOWER RESPIRATORY TRACT

William Alonso, M.D.
James Holliday, M.D.

INTRODUCTION

Trauma of the lower respiratory tract is uncommon in children but shows considerable variation in its incidence and etiology when it does occur. A convenient clinical classification of laryngotracheal injuries divides these into the internal type of injury and the external type of injury. Internal trauma includes iatrogenic complications, such as from intubation and the use of catheters and endoscopes. Other examples of internal trauma include inhalation of toxic substances, thermal damage, ingestion of caustics, and aspirated foreign bodies. Most instances of external trauma in children have been related to playground accidents or vehicular injuries. Less frequently, injury to the larynx and trachea may occur after a tracheotomy or from assaults with projectiles and sharp objects (Murphy et al., 1966) (Figs. 70–1 and 70–2).

INCIDENCE

Infants under two years of age almost exclusively develop internal injuries of the laryngotracheal complex (Holinger and Schild, 1972). The majority of these injuries are the sequelae of prolonged endotracheal intubation, and the remainder of the injuries in this age group are associated with the aspiration of foreign bodies and various iatrogenic mishaps (Holinger and Schild, 1972). A discussion of the problem of foreign body aspiration is included in Chapter 71. Between the ages of 2 and 12 years prolonged intubation and foreign body aspira-

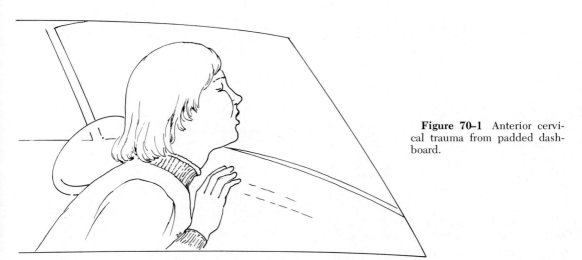

Figure 70–1 Anterior cervical trauma from padded dashboard.

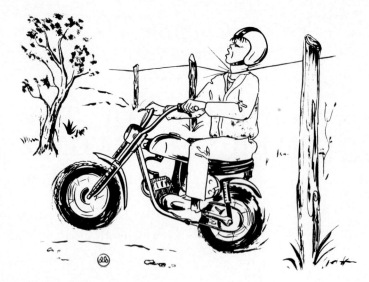

Figure 70–2 Neck trauma in a mini-biker. (From Alonso, W. A., Caruso, V. G., and Roncace, E. A. Minibikes, a new factor in laryngotracheal trauma. Ann. Otol. Rhinol. Laryngol. 82:800–804, 1973.)

tion continue to figure prominently as causes of trauma (Holinger and Schild, 1972). However, as the child approaches puberty, vehicular injuries begin to take their toll (Fitz-Hugh and Powell, 1970; Holinger and Schild, 1972). Among adolescents, the most common type of injury is an external injury usually associated with a vehicular accident (Fitz-Hugh and Powell, 1970). Certain anatomic features are significant underlying factors in the type of laryngotracheal injury to be expected in children of different ages. In the infant and young child, the larynx is positioned relatively high in the neck compared with its placement in the adolescent or young adult, and the head of the younger child is also proportionately more prominent in relation to the neck and trunk than in older children, thus providing more protection for the neck. The mandible is a formidable shield against injury of the anterior neck. The elasticity and flexibility of the younger child's laryngeal cartilages is another protective feature against crushing injuries or fractures; however, since the intercartilaginous connecting membranes are not fully mature until adulthood, they are more prone to rupture in children. Another key variable, especially in the infant and young child, is the relative diameter of the laryngeal and tracheal airway. Although older children and adults can tolerate restrictions of the airway lumen of up to 50 per cent of normal, this would cause serious respiratory embarrassment in the infant or young child. This restricted airway would be especially problematic in the subglottic region encompassed by the ringlike, nonyielding cricoid cartilage (Fig. 70–3). More anatomic information about this region can be obtained from Chapter 59.

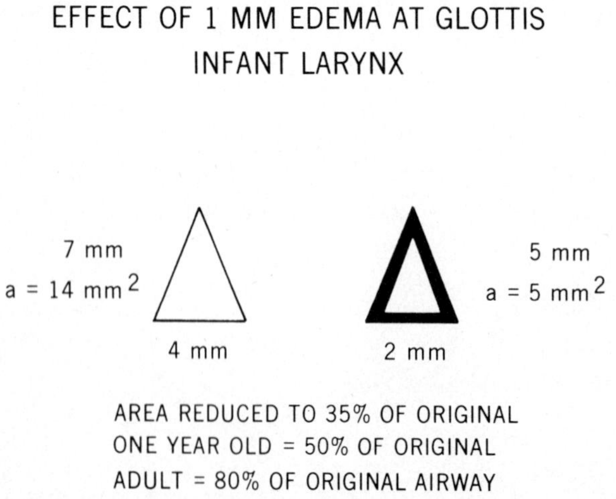

EFFECT OF 1 MM EDEMA AT GLOTTIS
INFANT LARYNX

7 mm

$a = 14$ mm^2

4 mm

5 mm

$a = 5$ mm^2

2 mm

AREA REDUCED TO 35% OF ORIGINAL
ONE YEAR OLD = 50% OF ORIGINAL
ADULT = 80% OF ORIGINAL AIRWAY

Figure 70–3 Effect of 1 mm edema at glottis. (Courtesy of Dr. Marshall Nathan.)

PATHOPHYSIOLOGY OF INJURIES

As a model for internal injuries, the sequelae of endotracheal intubation deserve special attention. Experimentally, even the gentle passage of an endotracheal tube by a skilled operator results in extensive damage to the respiratory epithelium, including loss of cilia (Hilding, 1971). Prolonged friction between an indwelling tube and the surrounding respiratory mucosa will eventually lead to erosion of the mucosa (Grillo, 1970; Hilding, 1971; Lindholm, 1969). Breakdown of the mucosa results in the exposure of underlying cartilage and pathogens (usually *Staphylococcus aureus* and *Pseudomonas aeruginosa*) may invade the debilitated cartilage, which may lead to necrosis and replacement of cartilage by granulation tissue (Glenn et al., 1975). This process eventually leads to fibrous deposition and stenosis. The principal variables of pathogenic significance in this case are duration of intubation, the size of the tube, presence of an inflated cuff, constant motion in the tube, presence of infection subglottically, and the chemical composition of the tube (Glenn et al., 1975; Grillo, 1970). Serious, underlying systemic illness and episodes of hypotension also contribute to the complications of intubation.

Damage due to erosion from an inflated cuff is of a much greater magnitude than the superficial mucosal changes from a tracheotomy alone. Occasionally, tracheoesophageal fistulas and innominate artery rupture develop after cuff erosion (Glenn et al., 1975; Grillo, 1970). Symptoms of airway obstruction may appear within 48 hours but usually are seen within 2 to 6 weeks after extubation. However, airway obstruction may become clinically symptomatic up to 90 days after extubation (Table 70–1) (Glenn et al., 1975; Grillo, 1970).

The widespread use of automobiles and the growing popularity of motor-powered recreational vehicles has given rise to increased numbers of severe head and neck injuries (Alonso et al., 1973; Alonso et al., 1974; Fitz-Hugh and Powell, 1970; Holinger and Schild, 1972). However, severe injuries of the head and neck are less common in children than in adults because children under 16 years of age generally do not operate automobiles or motor-powered recreational vehicles. Furthermore, the reduced speed limit and the availability of passive restraints, such as seat belts, shoulder straps, and air bags, can be expected to reduce the overall incidence of serious injuries due to automobile accidents. Some anatomic features of the head and neck in children, as discussed in a previous paragraph, offer significant protection for the cervical area. Despite the generally lower incidence of vehicular injury in children, some indulgent parents have provided their youngsters with a variety of recreational, motor-powered vehicles with disastrous results for their health (Alonso et al., 1973; Alonso et al., 1974). Included among these vehicles are minibikes, trail bikes, go-carts and snowmobiles. Some of these "toys" can generate velocities of up to 50 miles per hour, and numerous instances have been recorded of children injuring their necks after unexpected contact with non-yielding environmental hazards such as cables, tree branches, and fences (Alonso et al., 1973).

The biodynamics of laryngotracheal injury in children after blunt trauma to the neck are similar to those in adults (Nahum and Seigel, 1967). Briefly, the victim and the vehicle are moving at the same speed prior to impact. After collision and momentary deceleration, inertial forces bring the victim forward and hyperextend the neck. The vulnerable anterior cervical structures, including the larynx and upper trachea, are forced against the unyielding cervical vertebrae. Owing to the resiliency of the pediatric larynx and its protected position higher in the neck, this rarely results in a fractured larynx, as usually occurs in an adult, but laryngotracheal disruption occurs more commonly, a result of the immaturity of the intercartilaginous connecting membranes and ligaments (Alonso et al., 1974). Sometimes shearing forces separate the soft tissue from the cartilage, allowing prehyoid laryngotracheal hemorrhage and intralaryngeal hematoma to occur, particularly at the level of the true vocal cords. After a laryngotracheal disruption, other contiguous structures may be injured. Commonly, there is injury of one or both recurrent

Table 70–1 FACTORS CONTRIBUTING TO INTERNAL LARYNGOTRACHEAL INJURY FOLLOWING INTUBATION

Duration of intubation
Tube size
Inflated cuffs
Presence of infection
Constant motion of the tube
Systemic illness and episodes of hypotension
Chemical composition of the tube

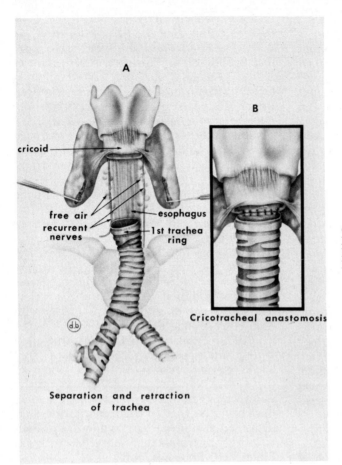

Figure 70–4 Laryngotracheal disruption. (From Alonso, W. A., Caruso, V. G., and Roncace, E. A. Minibikes, a new factor in laryngotracheal trauma. Ann. Otol. Rhinol. Laryngol., 82:800–804, 1973.)

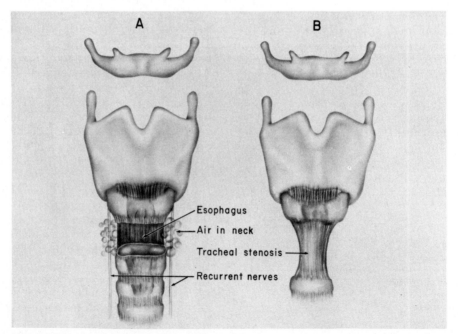

Figure 70–5 Laryngotracheal disruption *(A)*. Note proximity of recurrent nerves with the sequelae of inadequate repair *(B)*.

laryngeal nerves and occasionally tears in the tracheoesophageal wall (Alonso et al., 1974). In addition to vocal cord paralyses and traumatic tracheoesophageal fistulas, arytenoid cartilage dislocations and cricoid cartilage fractures may be observed. Rarely, injuries to the great vessels and cervical spine are seen. As a consequence of a laryngotracheal disruption, air can easily dissect the paratracheal spaces to produce a unilateral or bilateral tension pneumothorax, or aeromediastinum (Figs. 70–4 and 70–5).

DIAGNOSTIC TECHNIQUES

History and Physical Examination

Careful history will usually provide clues about the type and extent of the suspected injury. Exposure to toxic chemicals or smoke inhalation result in diffuse edema of the larynx and tracheobronchial tree, producing stridor, hoarseness, or cough (Fearon, 1972). Similarly, the ingestion of a caustic or an acid

results in severe laryngeal edema with airway obstruction and marked odynophagia. After prolonged intubation some prediction of the extent and location of an injury can be made. After nasotracheal or orotracheal intubation, damage is likely to be found in the posterior commissure of the larynx or in the subglottic area and may be anything from a posterior commissure granuloma to a stricture.

Following decannulation after a tracheotomy, certain types of injuries may be present. If the surgeon removed tracheal cartilage during the pediatric tracheotomy, some degree of anterior wall tracheomalacia may develop. Occasionally, extensive granulations may form at the superior edge of the tracheotomy stoma and may partially obstruct the tracheal airway. If a tracheotomy tube with an inflated cuff was inserted, stenosis may develop 1 or 2 cm distal to the tracheotomy stoma. Symptoms of dyspnea, stridor, or difficulty in clearing secretions may develop immediately after extubation or may be delayed by as much as 90 days (Grillo, 1970) (Fig. 70–6).

Site of Stricture

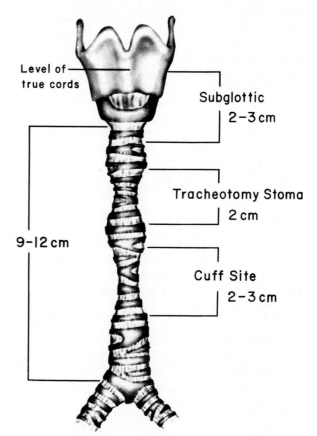

Level of true cords

Subglottic 2–3 cm

Tracheotomy Stoma 2 cm

9–12 cm

Cuff Site 2–3 cm

Figure 70–6 Internal laryngotracheal trauma and stricture formation.

Table 70–2 STRUCTURES AT RISK DURING EXTERNAL LARYNGOTRACHEAL INJURY

Pharynx
Esophagus
Thyroid cartilage
Hyoid bone
Arytenoid cartilage
Vocal cords
Recurrent laryngeal nerves
Cricoid cartilage
Trachea
Thyroid gland
Great vessels in the neck
Cervical vertebrae

As with any serious injury, attention is first directed towards stabilizing the patient by establishing an airway and insuring adequate alimentation. Emergency intubation and nasogastric tube insertion may be mandatory. The initial examination should rule out any neurologic deficits and, specifically, any suggestion of cervical spine injury. The traditional treatment priority with a victim of trauma in multiple areas is followed. It may be difficult and counterproductive to attempt a mirror examination of the pharynx and larynx in a struggling youngster.

Careful information gathering may alert the examining physician to the presence of a blunt, external, laryngotracheal injury (Table 70–2). If the observer is aware that the child struck his or her neck during an automobile collision or after riding a recreational vehicle, the examiner will look carefully for the signs and symptoms of impending airway obstruction. Disturbances of voice, respiration, or deglutition may appear in laryngotracheal injuries. The child's voice may be hoarse, aphonic, or muffled, although it may initially be normal and may deteriorate gradually. Respiration may be labored with a component of inspiratory stridor and retractions, and injuries at the intrathoracic level are usually manifested by expiratory wheezing. The child may cough, with or without expelling blood and may complain of pain while talking or swallowing. Inspection of the injured patient may reveal scars in the neck or lacerations, contusions, and subcutaneous emphysema. It may be difficult to identify and palpate the thyroid eminence and cricoid prominence (Table 70–3).

Diagnostic Tests

In the acute setting, radiographs of the chest and cervical spine should be obtained with the physician present if it is felt to be necessary. If there is a suspicion of a vascular injury, an arteriogram may be necessary. Hypaque or thin barium swallow may be helpful in identifying tears in the pharyngeal and esophageal mucosa although this procedure will not usually identify a tracheoesophageal fistula. If a laryngotracheal disruption is suspected, a tracheotomy is preferred to an endotracheal intubation (loss of palpable continuity of the laryngotrachea is usually a bronchoscopic diagnosis).

Further diagnostic studies are performed on a more elective basis. Lateral soft tissue radiographs or xeroradiographs of the neck may provide valuable information about displaced laryngeal cartilages, soft tissue swelling, and foreign body identification. Xeroradiography, where available, is a tremendous advance in the detailed study of the larynx and trachea. Laryngograms are useful to assess the dynamic functions of the larynx (vocal cord mobility) and to identify false passages. Retrograde tracheograms complement the laryngogram by providing an accurate estimate of tracheal damage. However, definitive study of the larynx and trachea is accomplished with endoscopic techniques and should be done prior to any use of barium (which could confuse any diagnosis). Direct laryngoscopy and bronchoscopy provide an accurate assessment of the type and extent of injury and are mandatory if there is any question about the adequacy of upper airway function. Retrograde tracheoscopy with a direct nasopharyngoscope may be helpful in assessing subglottic and high tra-

Table 70–3 SIGNS AND SYMPTOMS OF LARYNGOTRACHEAL INJURY

Historical background (prolonged intubation, blunt or sharp cervical trauma, time elapsed)

Airway (immediate or progressive respiratory distress, inspiratory stridor, wheezing, suprasternal retractions, cough and hemoptysis, difficulty clearing secretions)

Voice (aphonia, hoarseness, diminished volume, muscles)

Deglutition (dysphagia, odynophagia)

Neck examination (loss of cartilaginous prominences, fullness and crepitus, old tracheotomy scars)

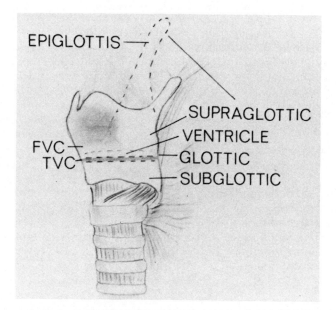

Figure 70–7 Anatomic division of the larynx. FVC = false vocal cords; TVC = true vocal cords.

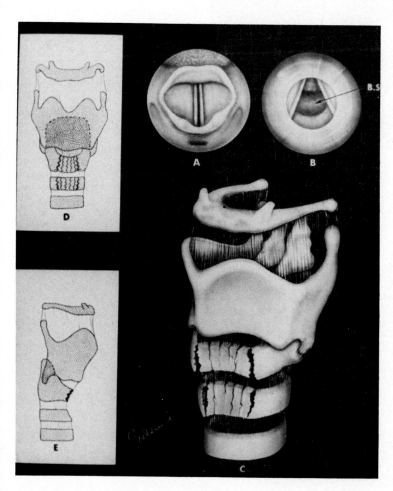

Figure 70–8 Infraglottic laryngeal fracture. (From Ogura, J. and Biller, H. 1971. Reconstruction of the larynx following blunt trauma. Ann. Otol. Rhinol. Laryngol., 80:492–506.)

cheal injuries. Esophagoscopy (rigid or fiberoptic) is performed when indicated on the
basis of a nonbarium esophagogram. Introduction of methylene blue into the trachea at
the completion of tracheobronchoscopic examination followed by esophagoscopy will
identify a suspected T-2 fistula if it is present.

TREATMENT

Emergency treatment of the acute laryngotracheal injury has been discussed under the
diagnostic evaluation section because this intervention takes precedence in a life-threatening situation. Before entering into a detailed discussion of definitive care after a

patient is stabilized, another classification is
useful.

Laryngeal injuries can be separated into
three anatomic divisions (Ogura and Biller,
1971). The first division is the supraglottic,
which includes injuries of the false cords,
arytenoepiglottic folds, preepiglottic space,
epiglottis, and hyoid bone. The second division is the glottic, which includes injuries of
the true cords, arytenoid cartilages, and the
thyroid cartilage. The third division is infraglottic, which includes injuries in the subglottic area involving the cricoid and thyroid
cartilages as well as upper tracheal injuries
(Fig. 70-7). In children, most cases of laryngotracheal trauma involve the infraglottic division (Fig. 70-8), although there are occasional cases of glottic injuries involving

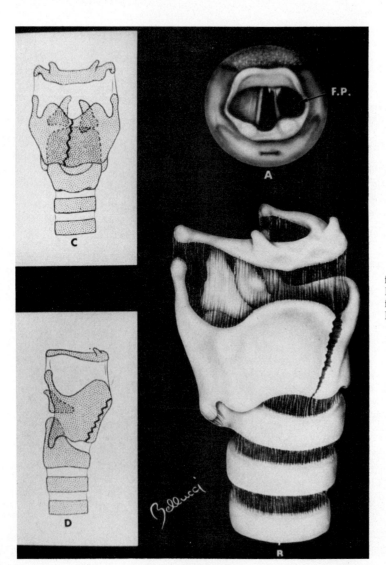

Figure 70-9 Glottic laryngeal
fracture. (From Ogura, J. and Biller,
H. 1971. Reconstruction of the larynx
following blunt trauma. Ann. Otol.
Rhinol. Laryngol., 80:492-506.)

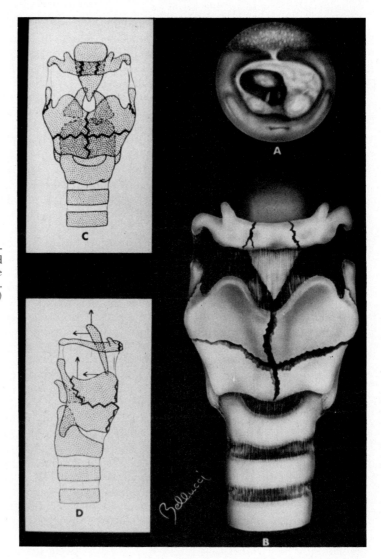

Figure 70–10 Supraglottic laryngeal fracture. (From Ogura, J. and Biller, H. 1971. Reconstruction of the larynx following blunt trauma. Ann. Otol. Rhinol. Laryngol., *80*:492–506.)

fractures of the thyroid cartilage with arytenoid dislocations (Fig. 70–9). Supraglottic injuries are exceedingly rare in the pediatric age group (Fig. 70–10), as most internal injuries following prolonged endotracheal intubation are located at the glottic and infraglottic levels and are more commonly at the latter (Fearon and Ellis, 1971; Grillo, 1970; Holinger et al., 1976; Lindholm, 1969; Striker et al., 1967). Injuries associated with cuffed tracheotomy tubes are usually located at the thoracic inlet of the trachea (Grillo, 1970; Pearson et al., 1968a, b; Yanagisawa and Kirchner, 1964).

After diagnostic study is completed, if the injury appears to be granuloma of the posterior commissure region of the larynx or granulation tissue in the subglottic or high tra-

cheal areas, endoscopic removal is the treatment of choice. Unless otherwise contraindicated, a course of systemic steroids for two or three weeks is helpful in preventing a reappearance of the granuloma or granulation tissue. Generally, these lesions can be handled endoscopically without the necessity of establishing a tracheotomy. Partial or circumferential subglottic and tracheal stenoses are much more difficult to manage. In some cases of partial stenosis, early conservative management with repeated dilatations and simultaneous steroids (long-acting) has been successful (Fearon, 1972; Grillo, 1970). When the degree of stenosis is sufficient to cause airway obstruction, it is mandatory to establish a tracheotomy as distal to the site of stenosis as possible. The fully developed circumferential stenotic lesion is not amenable to conservative management with dilatations (Alonso, 1976; Grillo, 1970). However, in the very young child, it is best to defer open exploration and repair until at least puberty. There is still some uncertainty about the effect of open surgical repair on the developing larynx and trachea, although experimental data suggest that this can be accomplished without sequelae (Calcaterra et al, 1974). By delaying open repair until puberty, the surgeon will have larger structures to work with (Fearon, 1972), and a larger intraluminal diameter will increase the chances of success.

Open exploration of glottic and subglottic stenoses is performed through a horizontal, collar-like incision about the tracheotomy site where possible (Montgomery, 1973). The larynx and trachea are opened through a vertical, midline incision, and scar tissue is excised while every effort is made to preserve mucosa and perichondrium. Bare areas of cartilage are covered with a tissue graft of very thin split skin. An indwelling stent of an inert substance such as Silastic or Teflon is used to hold the graft and maintain a lumen during the healing process (Alonso et al, 1974; Evans, 1975; Grhane, 1971; Montgomery, 1973; Ogura and Biller, 1971; Ward et al., 1977). Indwelling stents are maintained for approximately four weeks where cartilage support and cartilaginous diameter are adequate; otherwise they may need to remain in place for 1 to 12 months. Cases in which little or no mucosa is lost are repaired without stents.

Stenoses involving a subglottic area will benefit from efforts to increase or widen the cricoid space (Alonso et al., 1976; Fearon and Cinnamond, 1976; Ward et al., 1977). Efforts along these lines involve the use of an autograft of cartilage or hyoid bone (Alonso et al., 1976; Fearon and Cinnamond, 1976; Toohill et al., 1976; Ward et al., 1977) (Figs. 70–11 and 70–12). These autografts are especially useful when chondritis has resulted in the resorption of the cricoid cartilage. Partial tracheal stenoses, such as anterolateral defects at a tracheotomy stoma, are correctable by resection and direct end-to-end anastomosis (Alonso, 1976; Grillo, 1970), which requires a wedge resection of the stenotic portion. A complete circumferential tracheal stenosis is handled by sleeve resection of the involved rings and direct end-to-end anastomosis (Alonso, 1976; Grillo, 1970). In the pediatric age group, elasticity of the tracheal rings allows for great mobility, and the essential ingredient in a successful sleeve resection and anastomosis is a tension-free suture line (Dedo and Fishman, 1969; Grillo, 1970; Montgomery, 1973). Laryngeal mobilization by an infrahyoid release of musculature and membranous attachments can result in up to 5 cm (Alonso et al., 1974; Dedo and Fishman, 1969; Montgomery, 1973; Ogura and Biller, 1971) (Fig. 70–13). In the older patient less mobility is possible, so that following laryngeal and tracheal mobilization and sleeve resection, the patient's head is flexed at the time of the anastomosis (Grillo, 1970). Nonabsorbable sutures are first placed in the posterior and posterolateral walls around the

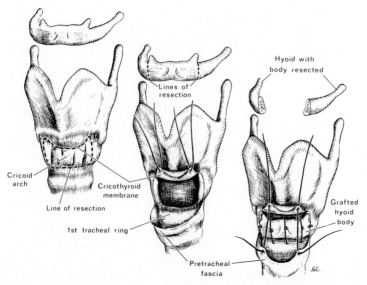

Figure 70–11 Hyoid bone transposition for cricoid arch replacement. (From Alonso, W. A., Pratt, L. L., Zollinger, W. K., et al. Complications of laryngotracheal disruption. Laryngoscope, 84:1276–1290, 1974.)

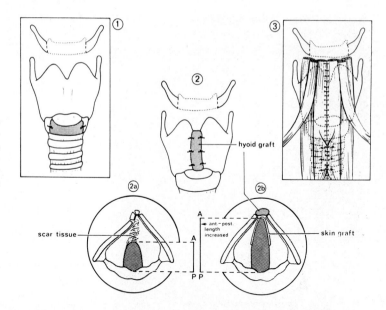

Figure 70–12 Hyoid bone transposition in glottic, subglottic, and tracheal stenoses. (From Alonso, W. A., Pratt, L. L., Zollinger, W. K., et al. Complications of laryngeal disruption. Laryngoscope, *84*:1276–1290, 1974.)

tracheal rings, where possible laterally, with the knots to be tied outside the lumen. It is desirable to tag these sutures and not to tie any until the anterior suture line is completed. While the sutures are being tied, an assistant can further reduce tension at the suture line by crossing the next suture (Grillo, 1970). A tracheotomy is maintained distal to the site of the tracheal anastomosis; within a week after the anastomosis, decannulation is usually possible.

The management of external trauma, whether open or closed, depends on the severity of the injury. After emergency measures have been completed and after adequate diagnostic study, a decision must be made for conservative management or open surgical intervention. Laryngeal injuries consisting primarily of hematomas with minimal mucosal derangement and good preservation of laryngeal architecture can be managed conservatively (Fearon, 1972; Fitz-Hugh and Powell, 1970). This involves maintaining an airway and applying constant humidity, systemic steroids, and antibiotics. After a few days, the edema and hematoma will subside,

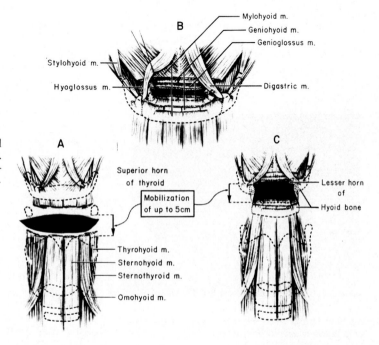

Figure 70–13 Infrahyoid laryngeal release. (From Alonso, W. A., Pratt, L. L., Zollinger, W. K., et al. Complications of laryngotracheal disruption. Laryngoscope, *84*:1276–1290, 1974.)

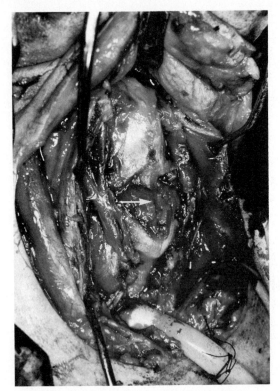

Figure 70–14 Cricothyroid disruption. (Note arrow at site of disruption.)

Table 70–4 COMPLICATIONS ASSOCIATED WITH LARYNGOTRACHEAL DISRUPTION

Tension pneumothorax
Tracheoesophageal fistula
Bilateral vocal cord paralysis
Cervical spine fractures and dislocations
Subglottic stenosis

is employed to repair lacerations of the cords and to reduce arytenoid dislocations. Care is taken to reposition any cartilage fragments and indwelling stents are used to maintain the repositioned tissues. Usually three to four weeks of stenting in acute cases is sufficient. Laryngotracheal disruptions require mobilization and primary anastomosis as described in the discussion of the repair of tracheal stenoses.

It is most important to record the mobility of vocal cords before any cricotracheal dissection is done (Table 70–4). Displaced cartilage fragments impinging on the recurrent laryngeal nerves are elevated to decompress the nerve and encourage a return of function. After nerve interruption, anastomoses may be attempted, but it is generally very difficult if not impossible to identify the nerve endings due to extensive soft-tissue damage and granulation. In fact, harm may follow aggressive exploration.

allowing decannulation. However, extensive injuries involving the laryngotracheal complex require open surgical intervention, preferably within a week after the injury (Alonso et al., 1974; Montgomery, 1973; Ogura and Biller, 1971) (Figs. 70–14 and 70–15). It is desirable to explore immediately and repair the damage in an open wound. The approach through the neck is similar to that described for internal injuries, and a median thyrotomy

RESULTS

Success with the conservative management of less complicated internal injuries has been good (Fitz-Hugh and Powell, 1970; Holinger and Schild, 1972). The endoscopic removal of granulomas and granulation tissue is highly effective. Managing minor stenosis with repeated dilatations and allowing the child to develop avoids unnecessary or intemperate open exploration. However, a complete, circumferential stenosis does not respond to repeated dilatations and may actually be aggravated by this procedure (Grillo, 1970) so that experience with the open repair of glottic and subglottic stenoses in children is limited (Fearon and Cinnamond, 1976; Fitz-Hugh and Powell, 1970; Ward et al., 1977) (Figs. 70–16 and 70–17). Recently, encouraging results have been reported after open explorations and efforts to widen the lumen (Alonso et al., 1976; Fearon and Cinnamond, 1976; Grhane, 1971; Ward et al., 1977). Acute external injuries, open and closed, can be managed successfully if treated within a

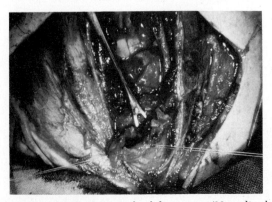

Figure 70–15 Cricotracheal disruption. (Note distal tracheal stump grasped with instrument below and comminuted cricoid fracture above.)

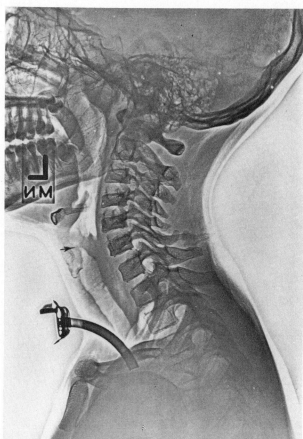

Figure 70–16 Glottic stenosis after external trauma. (Arrow indicates stenosis.)

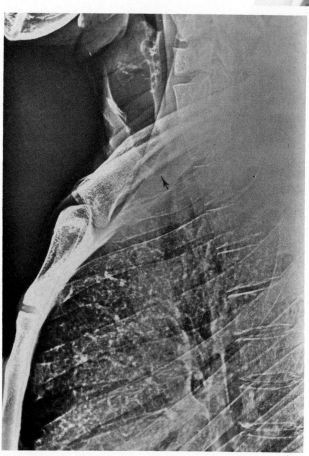

Figure 70–17 Subglottic stenosis after prolonged intubation. (Arrow indicates stenosis.)

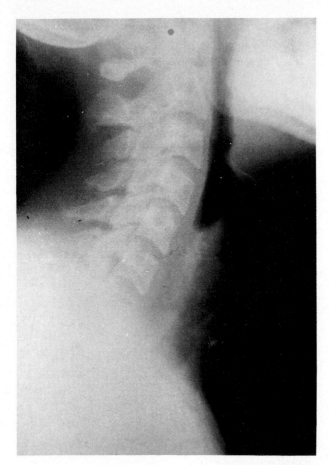

Figure 70–18 Successful bone autograft for subglottic stenosis repair. (Note wire sutures at anastomotic site.)

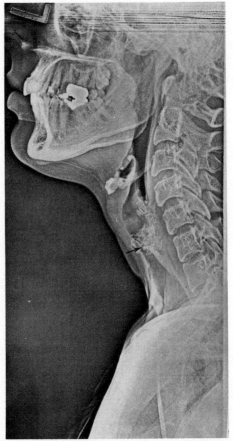

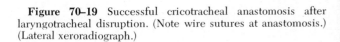

Figure 70–19 Successful cricotracheal anastomosis after laryngotracheal disruption. (Note wire sutures at anastomosis.) (Lateral xeroradiograph.)

few days after the injury. The conservative management of soft tissue injuries and non-displaced cartilaginous fractures yields good results (Fitz-Hugh and Powell, 1970; Ogura and Biller, 1971). Open exploration, resection and anastomosis where indicated are also successful (Figs. 70–18 and 70–19).

COMPLICATIONS

Disorders of voice, airway, and deglutition may develop following cervical trauma. Vocal cord paralysis can be associated with an internal or an external injury, the latter being more common. Following bilateral, recurrent laryngeal nerve palsy, a serious disturbance of voice and airway may occur. However, any attempts at vocal rehabilitation should be postponed for a year, pending the return of vocal cord function. After a year, vocal cord lateralization or laryngeal reinnervation may be considered to improve the airway. Unilateral vocal cord paralysis can be managed with injection of the paralyzed cord with glycerin

one month after trauma, followed by a permanent Teflon-glycerin implant at one year if necessary and speech therapy. The problem of restenosis after open repair is less frequent but very formidable (Fig. 70–20), and usually requires reexploration and prolonged stenting. Unrecognized or improperly treated esophageal laceration or tracheoesophageal injury can result in esophageal stenosis or tracheoesophageal fistula, which requires repeated dilatations, open exploration, or both (Fig. 70–21).

CONCLUSION

Injuries of the laryngotracheal complex are uncommon in the pediatric age group, but, with the growing use of advances in respiratory care (including prolonged intubation and ventilatory assistance), larger numbers of severe internal laryngotracheal complications are developing. Subglottic and tracheal stenoses are more likely to occur following prolonged rather than short-term ventilatory as-

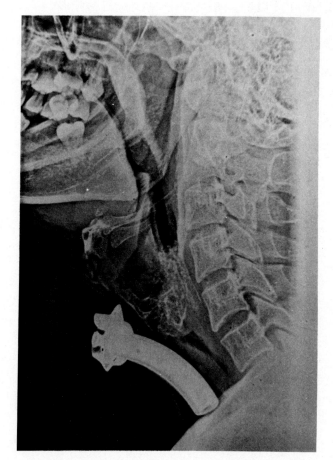

Figure 70–20 Subglottic stenosis after unsuccessful repair of postintubation stricture. (Lateral xeroradiograph.)

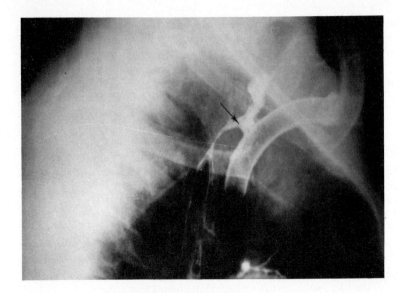

Figure 70–21 Tracheoesophageal fistula after prolonged intubation and mechanical ventilation. (Arrow denotes T-E fistula.) Oblique contrast radiograph.)

sistance, and in the pediatric age group this type of internal laryngotracheal injury is a common cause of lower respiratory tract damage. External, blunt trauma to the neck may cause laryngotracheal disruptions in older children. These mishaps are frequently associated with the use of motor-powered recreational vehicles. However, certain anatomic features peculiar to children render them less susceptible to external, cervical injuries.

Experience in the management of subglottic and tracheal stenosis in children is limited, and a conservative approach is generally advocated to allow the child to grow and therefore improve the success of an open repair. Despite optimal care, some of these children will continue to have serious impairments of voice and airway.

Greater awareness of the hazards of prolonged intubation with assisted respiration in pediatric respiratory units will substantially reduce the number of serious laryngotracheal complications. Stricter control and supervision of children using motor-powered recreational vehicles will reduce the number of serious laryngotracheal injuries.

SELECTED REFERENCES

Grillo, H. C. 1970. Surgery of the Trachea: Current Problems in Surgery. Chicago, Yearbook Medical Publishers Inc., pp. 1–60.
> *This excellent monograph by one of the foremost experts in surgery of the tracheobronchial tree reviews the history, pathogenesis, and repair of acquired lesions of the trachea.*

> *Surgical techniques are especially lucidly described and illustrated.*

Holinger, P. H., and Schild, J. A. 1972. Pharyngeal, laryngeal and tracheal injuries in the pediatric age group. Ann. Otol. Rhinol. Laryngol., *81*:538–545.
> *These authors report one of the most extensive experiences in internal and external pediatric laryngotracheal trauma. The incidence according to age and the etiologic factors are fully described.*

Montgomery, W. W. 1973. Surgery of the Upper Respiratory System, Vol. 2, Chaps. 6 and 8, pp. 373–435, pp. 543–595. Philadelphia, Lea & Febiger.
> *This fine book with many good illustrations provides a comprehensive review of numerous laryngologic techniques as applied to laryngotracheal trauma.*

Ogura, J. H., and Biller, H. F. 1971. Reconstruction of the larynx following blunt trauma. Ann. Otol. Rhinol. Laryngol., *80*:492–506.
> *This outstanding paper, although primarily discussing laryngotracheal injuries in adults, summarizes a very large personal experience. Very useful clinical and anatomic classifications are included, and the work is richly illustrated with examples of cases and drawings of the surgical techniques.*

REFERENCES

Alonso, W. A. 1976. Reconstruction of the cervical trachea. Triological thesis, pp. 1–50. Unpublished data.

Alonso, W. A., Caruso, V. G., and Roncace, E. A. 1973. Minibikes, a new factor in laryngotracheal trauma. Ann. Otol. Rhinol. Laryngol., *82*:800–804.

Alonso, W. A., Pratt, L. L., Zollinger, W. K., et al. 1974. Complications of laryngotracheal disruption. Laryngoscope, *84*:1276–1290.

Alonso, W. A., Druck, N. S., and Ogura, J. H. 1976. Clinical experiences in hyoid arch transposition. Laryngoscope, *86*:617–624.

Calcaterra, T., McClure, R., and Ward, P. H. 1974.

Effect of laryngofissure on the developing canine larynx. Ann. Otol. Rhinol. Laryngol., 83:810–813.

Dedo, H. H., and Fishman, N. H. 1969. Laryngeal release and sleeve resection for tracheal stenosis. Ann. Otol. Rhinol. Laryngol., 78:285–295.

Evans, J. N. G. 1975. Laryngeal disorders in children. In Wilkinson, A. W. (Ed.) Recent Advances in Pediatric Surgery. New York, Churchill-Livingston, Inc., pp. 174–182.

Fearon, B. 1972. Acute airway obstruction. In Ferguson, C. F., and Kendig, E. L. (Eds.) Pediatric Otolaryngology, Vol. 2. Disorders of the Respiratory Tract in Children. Philadelphia, W. B. Saunders Co., Ch. 105, pp. 1183–1213.

Fearon, B., and Ellis, D. 1971. Management of long term airway problems in infants and children. Ann. Otol. Rhinol. Laryngol., 80:669–678.

Fearon, B., and Cinnamond, M. 1976. Surgical correction of subglottic stenosis of the larynx. J. Otolaryngol., 5:475–478.

Fitz-Hugh, G. A. S., and Powell, J. B. 1970. Acute traumatic injuries of the oral pharynx, laryngopharynx and cervical tracheal in children. In Davison, F. W., (Ed.) Otolaryngol. Clin. North Am., Symposium on Pediatric Otolaryngology, 3:375–393.

Glenn, W. W. L., Leibow, A. A., and Lindskog, D. E. 1975. Thoracic and cardiovascular surgery with related pathology. In Trauma to the Chest, 3rd ed. New York, Appleton-Century-Crofts, pp. 104–110.

Grhane, B. 1971. Operative treatment of severe, chronic, traumatic laryngeal stenosis in infants up to three years old. Acta Otolaryngol., 72:134–137.

Grillo, H. C. 1970. Surgery of the Trachea: Current Problems in Surgery. Chicago, Year Book Medical Publishers, Inc., pp. 1–60.

Hilding, A. C. 1971. Laryngotracheal damage during intratracheal anesthesia. Ann. Otol. Rhinol. Laryngol., 80:565–581.

Holinger, P. H., and Schild, J. A. 1972. Pharyngeal, laryngeal and tracheal injuries in the pediatric age group. Ann. Otol. Rhinol. Laryngol., 81:538–545.

Holinger, P. H., Schild, J. A., Kutnick, S. L., et al. 1976. Subglottic stenosis in infants and children. Trans. A.B.E.A., pp. 95–103.

Lindholm, C. E. 1969. Prolonged endotracheal intubation. Acta Anesthesiol. Suppl., 33:

Montgomery, W. W. 1973. Surgery of the Upper Respiratory System. Vol. 2. Philadelphia, Lea & Febiger, pp. 373–435, 543–595, Chaps. 6 and 8.

Murphy, D. A., MacLean, L. D., and Dobell, A. R. C. 1966. Tracheal stenosis as a complication of tracheostomy. Ann. Thorac. Surg., 2:44.

Nahum, A. M., and Seigel, A. W. 1967. Biodynamics of injury to the larynx in automobile collisions. Ann. Otol. Rhinol. Laryngol., 76:781–785.

Ogura, J. H., and Biller, H. F. 1971. Reconstruction of the larynx following blunt trauma. Ann. Otol. Rhinol. Laryngol., 80:492–506.

Pearson, F. G., Goldberg, M., and DeSilva, A. J. 1968a. A prospective study of tracheal injury complicating tracheostomy with a cuffed tube. Ann. Otol. Rhinol. Laryngol., 77:867–882.

Pearson, F. G., Goldberg, M. and DeSilva, A. J. 1968b. Tracheal stenosis complicating tracheostomy with cuffed tubes: Clinical experience and observation from a prospective study. Arch. Surg., 97:380–394.

Striker, T. W., Stool, S., and Downes, J. J. 1967. Prolonged nasotracheal intubation in infants and children. Arch. Otolaryngol., 85:106–109.

Toohill, R. J., Martinelli, D. L., and Janowak, M. C. 1976. Repair of laryngeal stenosis of nasoseptal graft. Trans A.B.E.A., 104–112.

Ward, P. H., Canalis, R., Fee, W., et al. 1977. Composite hyoid sternohyoid muscle grafts in humans. Arch. Otolaryngol., 103:531–534.

Yanagisawa, E., and Kirchner, J. A. 1964. The cuffed tracheotomy tube. Arch. Otolaryngol., 79:80–87.

Chapter 71

FOREIGN BODIES OF THE LARYNX, TRACHEA, AND BRONCHI

Timothy J. Reichert, M.D.

INTRODUCTION

Prior to the 20th century, a foreign body in the lung led to a long and torturous illness frequently ending in death. Motivated by the sight of his patients who suffered from this problem, Chevalier Jackson attempted to devise safe techniques for foreign body removal. In his autobiography, he described his early years as those spent in developing safe bronchoscopy and his later years as those spent in spreading the gospel of safe bronchoscopy. By 1936, Jackson reported that the mortality from foreign bodies had decreased from 24 per cent to 2 per cent and that in 98 per cent of cases bronchoscopic therapy was successful.

The armamentarium and techniques of bronchoscopy have improved much since Chevalier Jackson's time, but improved results of treatment for these patients are also due to better diagnosis of the problem. As Ryland (Clerf, 1936) wrote in 1838, "The diagnosis of the (foreign body) accident claims the most minute attention and we must avail ourselves of every circumstance at all calculated to throw light upon the subject." Familiarity with incidence, pathophysiology, and the signs and symptoms of foreign bodies will facilitate early diagnosis and successful therapy for this problem.

INCIDENCE

Studies of large series of foreign body cases (Jackson, 1951; Holinger, 1962) have re-

vealed that about 70 per cent of all foreign bodies ingested into the food and air passages occur in children; of these, about one third are aspirated and become lodged in the airway.

Age is the most important factor in incidence — children under the age of four years comprise about 55 per cent (Holinger, 1962) of the total number of cases of foreign bodies in the airway. Furthermore, in 1975, children under the age of four also had a higher incidence of accidental deaths from ingestion or inhalation of foreign objects than any other age group. For infants under one year of age, suffocation from ingestion or inhalation of foreign objects was the leading cause of accidental death (National Safety Council, 1976). Thus, for small children, foreign bodies pose a significant health hazard.

The incidence of foreign body ingestion is higher in this age group because children either do not know what belongs in their mouths or cannot adequately manage what goes into their mouths. Infants frequently ingest objects of fascination, such as coins, buttons, and pins. Nuts and other chunky vegetal foreign bodies are frequently aspirated in the two to four year old age group because these children have no molars and cannot chew their food finely. The chunks of food are too large and may cause gagging or cannot readily be moved into the hypopharynx; they are then near the laryngeal inlet when the child inspires. An association has also been noted between the presence of a concomitant upper respiratory infection

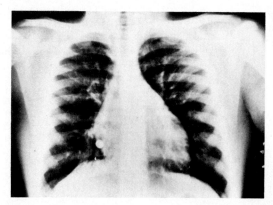
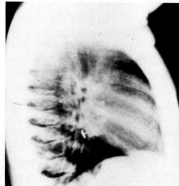

Figure 71–1 A 12 year old boy accidentally aspirated a thumb tack he had carelessly placed in his mouth. The posteroanterior and lateral chest radiographs demonstrate the tack lodged in the right lower lobe orifice.

(URI) and foreign body aspiration. Perhaps the mouth breathing that occurs with the URI interrupts a mouth breathing-swallowing pattern, which makes the child prone to aspiration, or perhaps the normal protective reflexes are interrupted by the URI. Older children are careless and frequently aspirate objects that do not belong in their mouths (Fig. 71–1).

Most foreign bodies pass through the larynx and trachea to become lodged more peripherally in the airway. Foreign bodies are usually caught in the larynx because they

have sharp, irregular edges (Fig. 71–2) or are too large to pass through the larynx. Laryngeal foreign bodies are more common in infants under one year of age. Foreign bodies of the bronchi occur most frequently on the right side because the right mainstem bronchus is larger, has a greater airflow, and diverges from the trachea at a less acute angle than does the left mainstem bronchus.

Aspiration of foreign bodies usually causes significant coughing, choking, gagging, and wheezing in a short time, thus calling attention to the problem. However, about 25 per

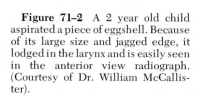

Figure 71–2 A 2 year old child aspirated a piece of eggshell. Because of its large size and jagged edge, it lodged in the larynx and is easily seen in the anterior view radiograph. (Courtesy of Dr. William McCallister).

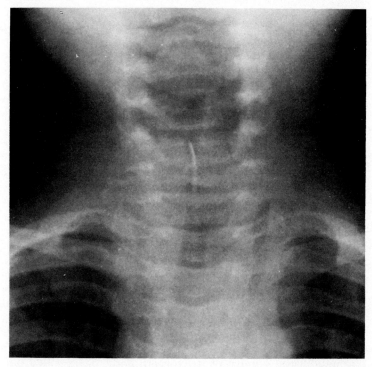

cent of foreign bodies are not detected for more than a week, usually because the ingestion was not witnessed, because there were no symptoms, or because the presence of a foreign body was not suspected when symptoms did appear. Foreign bodies may be the cause of a variety of acute and chronic diseases of the lung and should be considered in differential diagnoses. Also, the physician may be misled into assuming an object has been swallowed and will safely pass through the digestive tract when no signs or symptoms are present. The mucosa of the larynx, trachea, and bronchi rapidly adapts to the presence of foreign objects, and the physician must be aware that symptoms may not appear immediately.

The types of foreign bodies ingested are changing in nature, making diagnosis of the problem more difficult. In Jackson's series of over 4000 cases reported in 1951 (Jackson), there were no plastic foreign bodies, whereas series reported in the 1970s reveal that 6 to 8 per cent of the objects aspirated were plastic (Kim, 1973; Benjamin and Vandalius, 1974; Pyman, 1971). Plastics are inert, and some of the plastics, such as the polyethylenes, have no incorporated radiopaque substances (Pyman, 1972), making them difficult to detect on radiographic examination. Because of their nonirritating and radiolucent qualities, plastics may remain as foreign bodies in the tracheobronchial tree for prolonged periods of time. The history must be carefully obtained or appropriate diagnostic techniques undertaken to determine the cause of the symptoms produced.

PATHOPHYSIOLOGY

The pathophysiology of foreign object aspiration is related to two factors: the type of foreign body and the length of its sojourn in the body. These two factors also dictate the length of the symptomless interval — the time when there are no indications or minimal indications of the presence of a foreign body. Foreign bodies can be classed as (1) nonirritating (plastic, glass, metal), or (2) irritating (bones or vegetal matter, such as peanuts or beans).

When a foreign body is aspirated, initial laryngeal protective reflexes produce coughing, choking, gagging, and wheezing. When those reflexes are quieted, the symptomless interval begins. Frequently, a cough persists throughout the sojourn of the foreign body,

Table 71–1 SYMPTOMS AND SIGNS OF FOREIGN BODIES

Larynx	Trachea	Bronchi
Discomfort, sense of contact	Cough	Cough, at first unproductive
Pain	Asthmatoid wheeze	Expectoration— mucopurulent
Hoarseness	Audible slip	Fever
Croupiness	Tracheal flutter	Hemoptysis
Cough		
Aphonia		
Hemoptysis		
Wheeze		
Dyspnea		
Cyanosis		
Stridor		

although initially it may be very mild. As mucosal reaction to the foreign body increases, more prominent symptoms, signs, and complications begin (these are summarized in Table 71–1).

Foreign bodies of the larynx and trachea usually cause reactions that alter airflow and that are the result of the relatively large size of the foreign body or the edema created by the foreign body. These symptoms are hoarseness, stridor, wheezing, or even dyspnea.

Foreign bodies of the bronchi cause airflow changes first and pulmonic complications later. The early symptoms are from the physical obstruction caused by the foreign body and include distant stridor, wheezing, a cough, and dyspnea. Poor airflow out of an obstructed lung or lobe will result in unequal emptying and will be seen as obstructive emphysema on radiologic examination (Fig. 71–3). Pneumothorax may result either from the obstructive emphysema or from the penetration through a bronchial wall of a sharp foreign body. If incomplete obstruction persists, the impaired outflow of secretions may result in recurrent pneumonia.

If complete obstruction occurs, atelectasis will develop. With prolonged obstruction, the inspissated secretions will dilate the bronchus, resulting in fibrosis and bronchiectasis. Granulation tissue caused by the pressure of the foreign body, eroded bronchiole venules, or erosion of the foreign body into a vessel will produce hemoptysis. Hemoptysis should be a suspicious symptom since it is infrequently caused by bronchitis, asthma, or bronchiectasis (Kurkan et al., 1973). Other childhood causes of hemoptysis — parasitic infections and cystic fibrosis — may readily be ruled out as the source of hemoptysis.

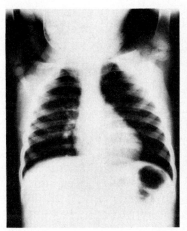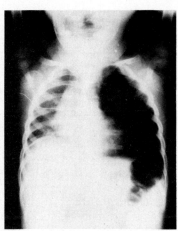

Figure 71–3 A 3 year old aspirated a peanut. The inspiration radiograph is normal, but the expiration radiograph reveals obvious obstructive emphysema on the left side.

Foreign bodies may also cause diffuse bronchospasms that are associated with asthma, or the object may shift from one site in the lung to another to produce confusing changes in symptoms.

Dissolving foreign bodies such as candy may cause a severe, though temporary, chemical tracheobronchitis. Such inflammation may require short-term airway support and intubation (Mearns and England, 1975).

RADIOGRAPHIC ASSESSMENT

Radiographic examination of the extended neck for soft tissue visualization as well as anterior and lateral radiographs of the chest constitute the most efficacious laboratory studies in patients with airway foreign bodies. Also helpful is a lateral chest radiograph with the arms behind the back, the neck flexed, and the head extended to allow for visualization of the entire airway from the mouth to the carina.

Since foreign bodies of the bronchi frequently occlude an orifice of either a mainstem bronchus or a lobar takeoff, a dynamic examination of the lungs is helpful in diagnosis. Videofluoroscopy is best as it has the advantages of fluoroscopy and allows multiple reviews without prolonged radiographic exposure. A dynamic examination such as fluoroscopy allows for evaluation at the time of expiration or inspiration, thus showing a partial obstruction to airflow in a lung that will ventilate completely if given enough time. Inspiratory and expiratory views can be difficult to obtain, and the physician should not hesitate to request repeat films if the first set is not satisfactory. Lateral decubitus films are another means of obtaining a view of the

lung in expiration utilizing body weight to promote expiratory excursion.

The radiographic examination may, however, be misleading if it is normal. The foreign body may not produce sufficient obstruction, or the obstructive phase may not have developed. Kim (1973) noted that obstructive emphysema was evident radiographically in 40 per cent of tracheobronchial foreign bodies, while Baraka (1974) noted normal chest radiographs in 86 per cent of his child patients studied within the first 24 hours but abnormal chest radiographs in 90 per cent of children after 24 hours. Pyman (1971) noted that 88 per cent of patients with a wheeze on physical examination had evidence of air trapping on radiographic examination.

Bronchograms are occasionally helpful in outlining a radiolucent foreign body that is too peripheral for endoscopic visualization. Frequently, only obstruction of a segment of lung is demonstrated because the foreign body has created enough reaction to occlude an orifice. Bronchograms may also be necessary to evaluate and follow bronchiectasis caused by a long-standing foreign body.

HISTORY AND CLINICAL EXAMINATION

If the parent is able to relate a clear description of foreign body aspiration (e.g., he was eating peanuts and he began to choke and cough), the history is simple; however, the history may be very unclear. Initial symptoms may involve changes in voice, such as hoarseness or aphonia, or merely a persistent wheeze or recurrent pneumonia.

The physical examination will be interpret-

Table 71–2 PULMONIC SYMPTOMS DUE
TO A FOREIGN BODY IN THE
ESOPHAGUS

Aspiration leading to pneumonia
Tracheal compression
Laryngeal inflammation leading to stridor
Tracheoesophageal fistula

ed correctly if the physician remembers (1) the symptomless interval and (2) the variety of pathologic changes a foreign body may provoke.

Laryngeal foreign bodies produce changes in vocal quality — hoarseness, aphonia, or stridor — that are sudden and striking. Tracheal foreign bodies usually cause significant airway distress if they are large, and an audible slap and palpable wheeze as the foreign body moves from the glottis to the carina. Sharp tracheal foreign bodies embedded in tracheal mucosa may produce only a mild cough or hemoptysis. Lastly, bronchial foreign bodies produce a cough and a wheeze or decreased air entry in the involved lung or lobe. If pneumonitis or bronchiectasis supervenes, then the results of the physical examination will be dominated by symptoms of those disease processes.

The proximity of the larynx, trachea, and esophagus enables foreign bodies of the food passages to produce three varieties of symptoms referable to the airway, as noted in Table 71–2. Large esophageal foreign bodies may compress the trachea and cause a cough, wheeze, and dyspnea. Obstruction of the esophagus by a foreign body may also lead to aspiration. Lastly, esophageal foreign bodies that are undiagnosed for a long time may erode through the wall of the esophagus and trachea to produce a fistula, airway obstruction, and hemoptysis (Yee, 1975).

MANAGEMENT

Therapy for foreign bodies generally is composed of endoscopic examination and removal. The primary physician may withhold consultation for endoscopy unless there is strong evidence of a foreign body. Endoscopy, however, should be considered a form of physical examination (inspection) and is, therefore, a diagnostic as well as therapeutic technique. If the history or physical findings are suspicious, endoscopic examination may

be indicated to establish the diagnosis and to provide relief of symptoms.

Removal of foreign bodies is best performed in an operating suite where a trained team and complete equipment are available. Treatment on the street or in the emergency room should be attempted only in the most desperate cases of respiratory obstruction. Careful assessment of the emergency situation must be made; frequently, after the initial bout of coughing, choking, and gagging, the child will be able to breathe well enough for transport to a hospital.

If the foreign body is impacted in the hypopharynx or larynx and is causing total respiratory obstruction, the Heimlich maneuver (forceful compression of the epigastrium) should be attempted (Heimlich, 1975). An emergency tracheotomy may be necessary if the Heimlich manuever is not successful. Attempts at digital retrieval of foreign bodies from the pharynx may lead to impaction of the foreign object in the larynx or esophagus and are therefore discouraged. Backslapping at home or in the emergency room to dislodge an endobronchial foreign body should also be discouraged, for it may result in dislodgment of the bronchial foreign body and accidental impaction of the object in the larynx, precipitating respiratory obstruction.

In order to avoid an endoscopic procedure, conservative treatment of endobronchial foreign bodies is tempting. Physical therapy, humidity, and bronchodilators may induce spontaneous expulsion of the foreign body. Such conservative therapy, however, sacrifices control of the airway during the removal of the foreign body from the air passages. When the size, numbers, shape, and composition of the foreign body are unknown, and if an endobronchial foreign body becomes impacted in the larynx or precipitates laryngospasm, the results of such lack of control may be disastrous. Thus, the "conservative" method of treatment, because of the risks it entails, is in reality a radical mode of therapy. With endoscopic control the airway will not be compromised, and the foreign body will be removed completely, surely and safely.

Endoscopy may be performed as an emergency or as an elective procedure. Emergency endoscopy is preferred only in those children with laryngeal foreign bodies or foreign bodies in the tracheobronchial tree that are causing airway obstruction. Potentially hazardous foreign bodies such as beans, which have strong hydroscopic properties and which will swell to a large size, should be removed on an emergency or semiemergency basis. Although the child may have few symptoms (the symptomless interval) when he or she presents, airway obstruction may rapidly ensue when the bean swells.

Elective examination and treatment allow for the necessary forethought and planning that contribute to safe foreign body removal. Duplicate foreign bodies can be obtained and used on a mannequin board to solve the particular problems a foreign body may present. Practice with duplicates also refreshes the physician in the necessary techniques and results in a smoother procedure. Dr. Holinger stated in 1961: "if two hours are spent in such preparation, the safe endoscopic removal may take only two minutes. But if only two minutes are taken for preparation, the endoscopist may find himself attempting makeshift ineffective procedures for the next two hours."

Anesthesia

General anesthesia is used in the removal of almost all foreign bodies of the airway. The relaxation obtained in the anesthetized patient reduces trauma to the subglottic area and allows a longer time for the manipulation of foreign bodies. The monitoring and ventilatory support provided by the anesthetist are also helpful in providing safety for the patient during the procedure. However, with two teams — the endoscopic team and the anesthesia team — sharing the airway, good communication is essential. Both teams should know what the other team is doing and what the plans will be to inspect, manipulate, and remove the foreign body while simultaneously ventilating the patient. If the endoscopic procedure is diagnostic in intent — examination for stridor — the anesthetist should be informed if a foreign body may be present.

In preparation for the endoscopic procedure, the endoscopist and the anesthetist should evaluate the chest radiograph for underlying pulmonary pathologic conditions. If prominent evidence of pathologic processes is present or if a degree of respiratory obstruction exists, measurements of arterial blood gases may be helpful in determining the respiratory status of the patient.

Medication of the patient with atropine 0.02 mg per kg of body weight or a minimum of 0.15 mg is given intramuscularly approximately a half hour prior to the procedure. Anesthesia is induced by mask using halothane and oxygen; nitrous oxide is not used because it may produce apnea. All patients are monitored with an electrocardiogram, a precordial stethoscope, blood pressure cuff, and thermometer. Within 6 to 10 minutes following induction of anesthesia, the endoscopist exposes and sprays the larynx with a 2 per cent solution of lidocaine. The endoscopist should expose the larynx in case the foreign body is present in the larynx or hypopharynx.

The bronchoscope is inserted, and the tracheobronchial tree is then inspected while the patient is ventilated and anesthetized through the bronchoscope side arm. Spontaneous respirations are maintained, and a closed system is created using an eyeglass to occlude the proximal end of the bronchoscope; alternatively, intermittent thumbing of the bronchoscope may be performed to create a closed system. If bradycardia or other evidence of hypoxia appears, priority for management must be given to the anesthetist, and adequate ventilation must be established.

Instruments

Instruments should be selected to accomplish three tasks: (1) ventilation, (2) visualization, and (3) manipulation. The conventional open tube endoscopes allow for the best ventilation, but the new rod lens systems provide superior visualization of the airway. Open tube systems and rod lens systems may be used interchangeably, although the excellent visualization obtained with the rod lens systems is nullified when copious secretions or bleeding cover the distal lens.

A good selection of forceps must be available to allow for manipulation of the object. Figure 71–4 shows several basic types of forceps — grasping, rotating, and globular object. Many types of forceps have been designed to aid in the safe extraction of a wide variety of foreign bodies, and a number of forceps of the types suggested in Table 71–3 should be available and in working order. Since almost all forceps are designed for use through an open tube system, the rod lens

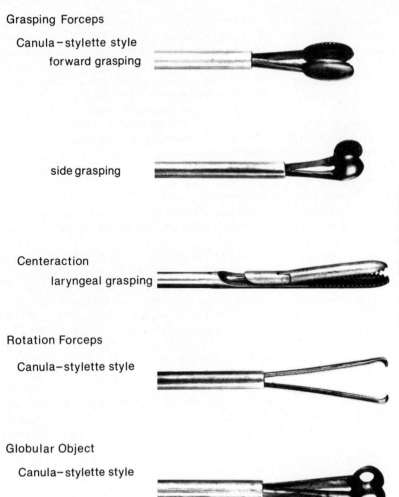

Grasping Forceps

Canula–stylette style
        forward grasping

        side grasping

Centeraction
        laryngeal grasping

Rotation Forceps

Canula–stylette style

Globular Object

Canula–stylette style

Figure 71–4 Three basic types of forceps are shown. Grasping forceps are the first type and are designed to seize and hold an object. Rotation forceps are the second type and permit a jagged (chicken bone) or pointed (safety pin) foreign body to dangle. The third type, a globular object or ball-bearing forceps, is used to grasp smooth, round objects, such as beads or pearls.

systems are limited in the removal of foreign objects. Only one small forceps, an alligator forceps, is available for use in conjunction with the rod lens system.

For a particular foreign body, the forceps are selected and tried with a duplicate foreign body on a mannequin board. The forceps should be smooth in operation, and the jaws should close completely when the forceps handles are closed. The shaft of the forceps must be straight to provide proper visualization and to prevent friction between the forceps and the lumen of the tube. Two varieties of forceps should be available for removal of any foreign body. Although a forceps may be chosen that is apparently best suited for the foreign body extraction, unexpected circumstances may arise after the procedure is underway and may require the use of a second variety of forceps.

Table 71–3 SUGGESTED FORCEPS FOR REMOVAL OF LARYNGEAL AND TRACHEOBRONCHIAL FOREIGN BODIES

Laryngeal Forceps	Bronchoscopic Forceps	
	Cannula-stylette style	Center-action style
Alligator	Side curved	Alligator
Rotation	Forward grasping	Rotation
	Rotation	Peanut
	Ball-bearing	
	Peanut	

Technique

For the removal of a foreign body, a laryngoscope, laryngeal forceps, an appropriate bronchoscope, bronchoscopic forceps, and open-tip suctions should be available. Appro-

Table 71–4 SUGGESTED ENDOSCOPE SIZES FOR INFANTS AND CHILDREN

Age	Laryngoscopes (Jackson Number)	Bronchoscopes
Newborn to 3 months	Newborn	3.5 mm × 25 cm
4 to 6 months	9	3.5 mm × 25 cm
7 to 12 months	9	3.5 mm × 30 cm or 4.0 mm × 30 cm
1 to 2 years	11	3.5 mm × 30 cm or 4.0 mm × 30 cm
3 years	11	4.0 mm × 30 cm
4 years	12	4.0 mm × 35 cm or 5.0 mm × 30 cm
5 to 7 years	12	5.0 mm × 35 cm
8 to 12 years	12	5.0 mm × 35 cm or 6.0 mm × 35 cm or 7.0 mm × 40 cm

Adapted from Holinger, P. H., Schild, J. A., and Weprin, T. C., 1970. Pediatric laryngology. Otolaryngol. Clin. North Am., 3:625.

priate endoscope sizes are suggested in Table 71–4. Foreign bodies of the larynx may be lost in the tracheobronchial tree, or tracheobronchial foreign bodies may be lost in the larynx, and the endoscopist should be prepared to remove the foreign body from either area if necessary. In addition, the endoscopist must be able to secure the airway with a bronchoscope if it becomes occluded with a foreign body.

Laryngeal foreign bodies are best removed with a spatula tip laryngoscope. After the patient is well anesthetized, the laryngoscope is inserted first into the vallecula so as not to dislodge the intralaryngeal foreign body; then, if better visualization is needed, the epiglottis is elevated.

Tracheobronchial foreign bodies also require a methodical, careful approach. The tracheobronchial tree should be completely inspected, as multiple foreign bodies may be present. Inspection should begin with the anticipated normal lung, and all secretions should be removed to insure optimal respiratory function when the pathologic side is inspected. When a foreign body is seen, its shape, position, and space available for forceps should be assessed. The open-tip suction may be used to remove secretions from around the foreign body so that the observer may better identify the shape and position of the object and the forcep spaces available. Suction is inadequate to hold foreign bodies and should not be utilized for removal.

Forcep spaces — the spaces where the blades of the forceps may be safely placed — may be obliterated if granulations are present or if the surrounding mucosa is swollen. If granulations are present proximal to the foreign body, the bronchoscope may be pushed past the granulations, or the granulations may be removed. It is better to push beyond the granulations because their removal may result in bleeding that obscures the foreign body and makes manipulation difficult. If bleeding makes manipulation unsafe, the endoscopist should desist and should remove the foreign body in a second procedure.

Vegetable foreign bodies such as peanuts must be grasped lightly to avoid fragmentation. Use of a "peanut forceps" with light, soft blades facilitates such gentle handling. In grasping round or globular foreign bodies, the blades must pass beyond the axis before they are closed; an improper grasp, shown in Figure 71–5, will result in the loss of the foreign body. Pointed foreign bodies require identification of the point and then protection of the point. If the point is embedded, the shaft should be grasped and pushed distally to disengage the point. Once the point is seen it must be ensheathed by pushing the bronchoscope tip over it to protect it.

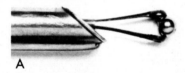
A

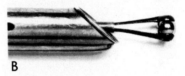
B

Figure 71–5 Improper grasp of a ball bearing is shown in *A*; blades were closed before they had passed far enough around the foreign body. Passing the blades beyond the axis of the foreign body, however, results in a secure grasp, as seen in *B*.

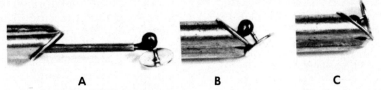

Figure 71–6 Use of the bronchoscope tip to manipulate a tack after the point has been grasped is demonstrated. In *A*, the tack is grasped; in *B*, the tip of the bronchoscope is rotated 180 degrees and used to rotate the tack to a position where it is better sheathed and protected, as seen in *C*.

Use of the bronchoscope tip as shown in Figure 71–6 will facilitate endobronchial manipulation. Once the foreign body is grasped it must be protected with the tip of the bronchoscope. Such protection prevents the foreign body from being stripped from the forceps at the glottis as it is removed. Traction must be along the axis of the forceps shaft with the index finger aiding in identifying closure of the forceps tips, as shown in Figure 71–7. The forceps and bronchoscope are then grasped as one unit with the left hand, and removal is accomplished in one smooth motion.

Loss of the foreign body after it is grasped indicates an improper grasp, improper selection of forceps, or improper sheathing of the object. If the foreign body is lost in the larynx, the laryngoscope and laryngeal forceps should be used for removal. If immediate removal cannot be accomplished, then the foreign body should be carried down to its original position and the airway should be reestablished.

Rod lens bronchoscopes may also be used for foreign body work. The rod lens systems allow excellent visualization of the foreign body to assess its position and shape. If appropriate, the small alligator forceps may be used to grasp the foreign body and bring it up to the mouth of the bronchoscope. If the small alligator forceps is not an appropriate forceps, the rod lens system may be removed and conventional open tube techniques and

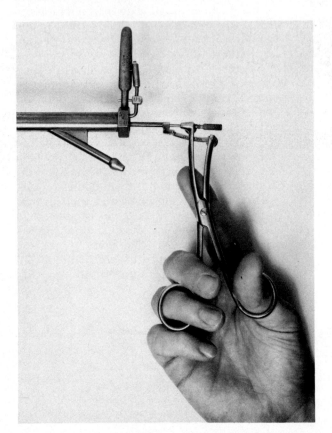

Figure 71–7 Proper handling of the forceps handle is demonstrated in this figure. The index finger is used to aid in assessment of closure of the forceps blade and is also used to direct traction along the axis of the forceps shaft after the foreign body is grasped.

forceps used. Basic principles of inspection, visualization, forceps space, and sheathing are all followed regardless of the type of system used. The rod lens system also allows for accurate placement of a Fogarty catheter beyond an impacted foreign body. The balloon may then be inflated and pulled proximally, thus removing the impacted foreign body by pulling it up ahead of the balloon. Using baskets or other loops to grasp foreign bodies under direct visualization with the rod lens systems is tempting, but such techniques should be discouraged until they are thoroughly tested in laboratory animals.

The flexible fiberoptic endoscopes occupy too much of the airway for use in children, and no instruments are available to use with them for removal of a foreign body.

SUMMARY

Foreign bodies continue to challenge physicians caring for children. New techniques, new instruments, and wider training enable physicians to remove foreign bodies safely. However, the challenge is most significant in the diagnostic stage of the foreign body's sojourn. To remove the foreign body before it may create atelectasis, pneumonia, or bronchiectasis is the goal of the otolaryngologist.

The diagnosis requires a thorough understanding of the pathophysiology and symptoms associated with a foreign body in the airway. In addition, the physician must be aware of the advantages and pitfalls of radiologic diagnosis of this problem.

Parents and other physicians should also be educated to prevent exposure of children to situations and objects that create a risk of foreign body aspiration. Since suffocation from foreign bodies is a major cause of accidental death in children, efforts should be concentrated on that age group.

SELECTED REFERENCES

Heimlich, H. J. 1975. A life saving maneuver to prevent food choking. J.A.M.A., *234*:398–401.
   This article describes a most important life saving maneuver to prevent deaths from foreign bodies obstructing the airway.

Jackson, C., and Jackson, C. L. 1936. Diseases of the Air and Food Passage of Foreign Body Origin. Philadelphia, W. B. Saunders Co.

The author wishes to acknowledge the assistance of Beverly Gestring in the preparation of this manuscript and Dr. Gabriel Tucker for his valuable advice.

This is the classic text on diagnosis and treatment of foreign bodies. Though out of print, many medical libraries have copies. The text contains a superb set of tables describing various foreign bodies with data regarding removal and the complications encountered.

Kim, I. G., Brunsitt, W. M., Humphrey, A., et al. 1973. Foreign bodies in the airway: a review of 202 cases. Laryngoscope, *83*:347–354.
   Dr. Kim provides an excellent analysis of a trial of symptoms and signs produced by airway foreign bodies.

REFERENCES

Baraka, A. 1974. Bronchoscopic removal of inhaled foreign bodies in children. Br. J. Anesth., *46*:124.

Benjamin, B., and Vandalius, T. 1974. Inhaled foreign bodies in children. Med. J. Aust., *1*:355.

Brown, T. C. K. 1973. Bronchoscopy for removal of foreign bodies in childhood. Anesth. Int. Care, *1*:521.

Clerf, L. H. 1936. Historical notes on foreign bodies in the air passages. Am. Med. Hist., *8*:547–552.

Fine, A., and Abram, L. E. 1971. Asthma and foreign bodies. Ann. Allergy, *29*:217.

Gross, S. E. 1854. A Practical Treatise of Foreign Bodies in the Air Passages. Philadelphia, Blarchard and Lea.

Heimlich, H. J. 1975. A life saving maneuver to prevent food choking. J.A.M.A., *234*:398.

Holinger, P. H. 1962. Foreign bodies in the food and air passages. Trans. Am. Acad. Ophthalmol. Otolaryngol., *66*:210.

Holinger, P. H., Schild, J. A., and Weprin, T. C. 1970. Pediatric laryngology. Otolaryngol. Clin. North Am. *3*:625.

Jackson, C., and Jackson, C. L. 1936. Diseases of the Air and Food Passage of Foreign Body Origin. Philadelphia, W. B. Saunders Co.

Jackson, C., and Jackson, C. L. 1951. Bronchoesophagology. Philadelphia, W. B. Saunders Co.

Kim, I. G., Brunsitt, W. M., Humphrey, A., et al. 1973. Foreign bodies in the airway: a review of 202 cases. Laryngoscope, *83*:347–354.

Kurkan, E. U., Williams, M. A., and LeRoux, B. T. 1973. Bronchiectasis consequent upon foreign body retention. Thorax, *28*:601.

Linton, J. S. A. 1957. Long standing intrabronchial foreign bodies. Thorax, *12*:164.

Mark, M. 1971. Significance of recurrent hemoptysis in allergic asthma. Clin. Pediatr., *10*:479.

Mearns, A. J., and England, P. M. 1975. Dissolving foreign bodies in the trachea and bronchi. Thorax, *30*:461.

National Safety Council. 1976. Accident Facts.

Pasquariello, P. S., and Kean, H. 1975. Cyanosis from a foreign body in the esophagus. Clin. Pediatr., *14*:223.

Pyman, C. 1971. Inhaled foreign bodies in childhood. Med. J. Aust., *1*:62.

Pyman, C. 1972. Radiolucent foreign bodies. Aust. Pediatr. J., *8*:166.

Slim, M. S., and Yacoubian, H. D. 1966. Complications of foreign bodies in the tracheobronchial tree. Arch. Surg., *92*:388.

Yee, K. F., Schild, J. A., and Holinger, P. H. 1975. Extraluminal foreign bodies in the food and air passages. Ann. Otol. Rhinol. Laryngol., *84*:619.

Chapter 72

TUMORS OF THE LARYNX, TRACHEA, AND BRONCHI

Allan B. Seid, M.D.
Robin Cotton, M.D.

This chapter deals with tumors of the larynx, trachea, and bronchi. Nonspecific inflammatory tumors or "granulomas" that occur commonly in the airway will not be included in the discussion.

Tumors of the larynx, trachea, and bronchi are relatively rare in children. The presentation of these tumors is usually due to the mechanical obstruction of the airway. Thus, symptoms of cough, hoarseness, and wheezing may occur. With obstruction of the distal airways, collapse or infection of lung parenchymal tissue will occur.

TUMORS OF THE LARYNX
(Table 72–1)

Papilloma

The majority of tumors of the larynx are benign. The commonest of the laryngeal tumors in childhood is the papilloma. In contrast to the usually single adult papilloma, papillomatosis is generally multiple in the child. Papillomas usually originate on the vocal cords; however, they may extend to involve contiguously the walls of the pharynx and also occur apparently isolated from the main laryngeal mass on the palate and uvula. Papillomas may also grow down the tracheobronchial tree, or they may be seeded by implantation at endoscopy.

Holinger commented that papillomas had never been encountered in the esophagus below the cricopharyngeus (Holinger et al., 1970). Nuwayhid and colleagues (1977), however, recently reported a case with endoesophageal papillomas. Miller reported an additional three cases of papillomatosis occurring in the esophagus. These three cases all occurred in adults (Miller et al., 1978).

The specific etiology of papillomas is not known. Papillomas have been transplanted to skin and mucous membrane by a filterable agent, suggesting a viral origin (Ullman, 1923). Electron microscopy has, however, failed to demonstrate conclusive inclusion bodies or other signs of viruses (Svoboda et al., 1963).

Papillomas appear as irregular warty nodular masses that are usually pink or red in color. The size is variable and may appear as a single pedunculated mass or as a blanket covering the endolarynx and occluding the airway. Microscopically, the papilloma is definitely neoplastic and not just a chronic inflammatory condition (Holinger et al., 1970). The tumor consists of vascular connective tissue cores covered by multiple layers of stratified squamous epithelium. There is no invasion of the basement membrane. There is no histologic difference between the adult and childhood tumors.

Spontaneous regression of juvenile papillomatosis may occur at puberty, suggesting an endocrine factor. Manipulations of the hormonal environment by local and systemic hormone therapy have not shown significant benefit.

The tumors have been identified in the newborn. There is no significant difference

Table 72-1 TUMORS OF THE LARYNX

Epithelial
Benign
Squamous cell papilloma
Adenoma
Oncocytic adenoma
Benign mixed tumor

Malignant
Squamous cell carcinoma
Verrucous carcinoma
Spindle cell carcinoma
Adenosquamous carcinoma
Basal cell carcinoma
Malignant melanoma
Adenoid cystic adenocarcinoma
Adenocarcinoma
Malignant mixed tumor

Connective Tissue
Benign
Fibroma
Chondroma
Hemangioma
Leiomyoma
Lipoma
Rhabdomyoma

Malignant
Fibrosarcoma
Chondrosarcoma
Liposarcoma
Angiosarcoma
Rhabdomyosarcoma

Neurogenic
Neurilemoma
Neurofibroma
Chemodectoma
Granular cell myoblastoma

Hematopoietic
Plasmacytoma
Reticulosarcoma
Acute leukemia
Lymphosarcoma

Miscellaneous
Hamartoma
Adenolipoma
Metastatic carcinoma
Lymphangioma

(Modified from Barney, P. L., 1970. Histopathologic problems and frozen section diagnosis in diseases of the larynx. Otolaryngol. Clin. North Am., 3(3):493.)

in incidence by sex or race. However, in a census of 107 cases, Szpurnar (1967) reported that most of the patients were from economically poorer families.

Multiple forms of therapy have been tried. No one form of therapy has been uniformly successful. Topical agents have included caustics, podophyllin (Hollingsworth et al., 1950), and estrogens (Szpurnar, 1967). Systemic medications used have been heavy metals, arsenic, potassium iodide, bismuth compounds, androgens, and tetracyclines (Baker and Hui, 1972).

Autogenous papilloma vaccines, as well as bovine wart vaccines, have been tried without great success (Moffitt, 1959; Gross and Hubbard, 1974; Lyons et al., 1976).

Methotrexate and alkylating agents have been used but with no great success.

Surgical measures are aimed at removing the papillomas while not damaging normal laryngeal structures. Forceps removal using microscopic endolaryngeal technique is still the mainstay of treatment. Cryosurgery and ultrasound have also been used for local control (Birk and Mannhart, 1963).

Thyrotomy with laryngofissure and vein graft to the denuded cords have been advocated with some degree of success in adult patients (Tabb and Kirk, 1962).

Currently, it has been found that the CO_2 laser used in conjunction with the otomicroscope has been extremely useful in controlling papillomas and in avoiding tracheotomy. The use of the laser has minimized bleeding and is associated with very little laryngeal edema. Thus, even in severe cases with significant airway compromise, tracheotomy has been avoided using the CO_2 laser (Strong et al., 1973).

Tracheotomy is to be avoided if at all possible, as it has been found that extension of papillomas into the trachea and bronchi or around the stomal site has occurred.

Irradiation is also not to be used in this condition because of the reported cases of subsequent development of laryngeal cancers (Walsh and Beamer, 1950).

The number of endoscopic removals of tumor may vary from only one to two procedures to one case in which 166 procedures were required over a four year period (Holinger et al., 1970).

With advances in microsurgical technique and the use of the laser, it has been possible to remove papillomas on multiple occasions without causing structural damage to the larynx. This is especially true if the anterior commissure is not violated. If papillomas are encountered crossing the anterior commissure, they should be removed up to but not into or across the commissure. A second delayed attempt is made to remove those papillomas on the adjacent aspect of the commissure after allowing an adequate period for the raw, denuded area to heal. This technique will prevent webbing at the anterior commissure.

In the unusual case in which webbing or structural damage to the larynx occurs, this damage can be repaired by the technique of laryngofissure when the papillomas no longer recur.

Subglottic Hemangioma

Subglottic hemangiomas are true angiomas that cause symptoms of respiratory obstruction by their anatomic situation in the subglottis. These hemangiomas occur in children under the age of one year, and 85 per cent of children present prior to the age of six months. Girls are affected approximately twice as frequently as boys. The presentation is usually that of stridor, and the lesion may mimic the presentation of laryngomalacia, with increased stridor occurring with periods of increased stress (crying) due to vascular engorgement.

The children may also present with hoarseness, dyspnea, failure to thrive, and feeding difficulties. Hemangiomas elsewhere in the skin occur in 40 to 50 per cent of the children. Sweetser (1921) is credited with first noting that subglottic hemangiomas differ from the adult glottic and supraglottic hemangiomas. In adults, the hemangiomas are usually rounded and sometimes pedunculated and may cause hoarseness but relatively little dyspnea. Infantile hemangiomas will cause respiratory obstruction.

Diagnosis of subglottic hemangioma may be made on laryngoscopy and bronchoscopy. The lesion is described as occurring in the immediate subglottic area, and although there is a normal mucosal covering, there may be a bluish discoloration to the mucosa. The endoscopic picture may change frequently. The tumor is asymmetric and usually involves only one side of the subglottis. Endoscopic diagnosis should be performed only with light anesthesia, as straining and coughing may make the tumor more prominent and thus more noticeable.

Histologic diagnosis may be made by biopsy; however, it is felt that this may be unnecessary and even dangerous because of possible hemorrhage.

Radiologic diagnosis, including high kilovolt inspiratory and frontal radiography of the larynx, is a useful technique. Sutton and Nogrady (1973) feel that the radiologic picture is pathognomonic and, thus, that endoscopy is not needed. Leikensohn and colleagues (1976) disagree; they feel that other subglottic conditions, such as papillomas or subglottic stenosis, may have a similar radiographic appearance.

In the evaluation of these children, Feurstein (1973) stresses the need for an electrocardiogram, blood gases, and chest radiograph to detect either the presence of hyperaeration secondary to a chronic respiratory obstructive state or the presence of cardiomegaly associated with high output right heart failure (Feurstein, 1973).

Hemangiomas may spontaneously involute. Lampe and LaTourette (1959) in an article on skin hemangioma state that the majority of hemangiomas are involuting. Involuting hemangiomas are also called strawberry nevus, capillary hemangioma, and vascular nevus. The involuting hemangiomas enlarge rapidly during the first few months of their appearance, but growth rarely continues beyond one year of life and often ceases between six and eight months (Lister, 1938).

Port-wine marks, spider hemangiomas, and true cavernous hemangiomas do not involute spontaneously. It is essential, therefore, to distinguish the involuting from the noninvoluting type of hemangioma. Lesions that enlarge during the first few months of life but cease growing before one year of age will disappear. Hemangiomas that do not grow early in life will usually regress spontaneously. A further group of hemangiomas do present at birth but do not grow for the first or second year of life. These may subsequently enlarge. Thus, it is difficult to differentiate different treatment regimens in children in whom the lesions can spontaneously regress. Leikensohn and colleagues (1976) feel that in a two month old child with a subglottic hemangioma, it is not possible to tell whether the lesion will grow or spontaneously involute without a period of observation.

Hemangiomas have usually been treated with radiation. Ferguson (1970) and Fleck and Tefft (Tefft, 1966) have accumulated long series in which the child with a tracheotomy received three doses of 150 rads to a total of 450 rads. In the child without a tracheotomy, the initial dose is only 25 rads, but the amount is gradually increased until a total of 450 rads has been administered. In the latter group, the dosage is slowly increased so that further subglottic swelling and respiratory obstruction are avoided. Tefft (1966) felt that the average regression time and consequent relief of inspiratory symptoms was nine months. Lampe and LaTourette felt that hemangioma may not be a radiosensitive lesion. In their experience, a single dose of 400 rads almost never produced immediate regression of the hemangioma (Lampe and LaTourette, 1959). Walters (1953) has shown that a dose of 400 rads gives an average reduction of surface area of skin hemangioma that is not statistically significant. An important disadvantage to the use of radiation therapy for subglottic hemangioma is the definite association between thyroid malignancy and anterior neck radiation (Saenger and Silverman, 1960; Refetoff and Harrison, 1975; Braverman, 1975).

A new technique involving intralaryngeal application of beta radiation has been described by Bourne and Taylor (1972).

Katz and Askin (1968) used steroids in the treatment of thrombocytopenia associated with visceral and skin hemangioma and noticed a marked regression in the hemangioma during treatment. Cohen and Wang (1972) reported favorable results in eight of 10 patients with either head and neck or subglottic hemangiomas in whom they had administered prednisone. The two failures occurred in children two and four years of age. Best results were obtained in those treated early.

Steroid therapy may cause growth retardation, spontaneous fractures, glycosuria, and Cushing syndrome. Leikensohn and colleagues (1976) feel that steroid therapy will not replace the need for tracheotomy if there is significant airway intrusion but feel that a trial of steroid therapy for a three week period is appropriate.

Surgical therapy should be attempted, if at all, only after failure of steroid therapy. Calcaterra (1968) feels that surgical removal via thyrotomy is indicated only in those patients with a symptomatic lesion that remains unchanged or has enlarged during a one-year period of observation. Leikensohn and colleagues (1976) feel that observation only must be considered when one is formulating the definitive treatment plan of the young child with subglottic hemangioma.

Malignant Tumors of the Larynx

Malignant tumors of the larynx are infrequent in patients less than 30 years of age. The majority of these lesions are of epithelial origin, such as squamous cell carcinoma.

In a review of malignant disease in the first three decades of life, New and Hertz (1940) reported on one patient with squamous cell carcinoma of the larynx aged two years old. This patient was treated with roentgen x-rays, radium, and diathermy for recurrences but died of her disease. They point out that the prognosis for carcinoma of the larynx in young persons is poor.

Neurofibromatosis

Neurogenic tumors of the larynx are rare. Approximately 19 cases have been reported in the literature. The youngest case reported had its onset at three months of age (Van-Loon and Diamond, 1942). Females have been noted to have a slightly greater incidence than males. Crowe and colleagues (1956) established the incidence of multiple neurofibromatosis to be approximately 1 in 3000 births. Classically, the disease consists of multiple cutaneous visceral nodules, café au lait spots, radiologically demonstrable bone change, and occasionally mental deficiency. There is an increased incidence of pheochromocytoma, visceral and cutaneous neurogenic sarcomas, and acoustic and optic neurinomas. The disease is thought to be familial with variable expressivity. Laryngeal neurofibroma associated with multiple neurofibromatosis (von Recklinghausen's disease) is exceedingly rare. The tumor causes symptoms of dyspnea, dysphonia, and dysphagia. Cummings and colleagues (1969) stress that although neurogenic tumors of the larynx represent a small segment of benign laryngoneoplasms, they should not be discounted. Any submucosal mass in the typical anatomic location of the aryepiglottic fold and false cord should be suspected of being a neurofibroma. They feel that biopsy should be attempted via the endolaryngeal route; however, if any difficulty is encountered during the procedure, then the lesion should be approached externally.

The combination of lateral thyrotomy and complete removal of the lesion appears to be the most direct route and the one least attended by complications. Cummings and colleagues (1969) feel that once the histologic diagnosis of neurofibroma is made, the lesion should be completely removed rather than waiting until the patient develops further symptoms.

TUMORS OF THE TRACHEA

Primary tumors of the trachea are rare. Gilbert and Mazzarella (1953) reported a series of 546 cases of primary tracheal tumors in which 509 (92.1 per cent) occurred in adults and only 37 (7.9 per cent) occurred in infants. They noted a striking difference between tumors that appear in children and in adults. In adults, 49.1 per cent were malignant and only 50.9 per cent were nonmalignant. In children, 93.1 per cent were nonmalignant and only 6.9 per cent were malignant. Of these malignant tumors in the infant, all were sarcomatous and all occurred in girls.

In children, the predominant benign tumors were papilloma in 57.5 per cent, fibroma in 22.5 per cent, and angioma in 15 per cent (Gilbert et al., 1953) (Tables 72–2 to 72–5).

Site of Origin and Symptomatology

Contrasted with the adult, in whom the most frequent site of tumor has been in the lower third of the trachea, in children the commonest site of tumor is usually the upper third of the trachea. Tumors arising in the lower third of the trachea, which may occlude either bronchus, will cause partial or complete atelectasis, as well as wheezing. Tumors in the upper third of the trachea may interfere with vocal cord action, causing hoarseness and stridor. Tumors in the mid third of the trachea may be silent and asymptomatic for prolonged periods.

Papilloma

Papilloma of the trachea or bronchus is most often seen in children or infants as an

Table 72–2   PRIMARY TRACHEAL TUMORS IN CHILDREN AND ADULTS

	Von Bruns, 1898	Krieg, 1908	Lombard and Baldenweck, 1914	D'Aunoy and Zoeller, 1931	Culp, 1938	Gilbert et al., 1952
Carcinoma	31	40	54	91	147	194
Chondroma, osteoma, tracheopathia osteoplastica	29	42	47	65	71	77
Papilloma	33	41	51	59	63	65
Fibroma	23	25	29	33	36	39
Sarcoma	14	21	23	26	31	39
Intratracheal goiter	7	14	19	25	28	32
Adenoma	5	6	6	8	9	14
Angioma	–	–	1	2	2	8
Mixed salivary tumor	–	–	–	2	3	7
Basal-cell carcinoma	–	–	–	–	–	6
Cylindroma	–	–	–	1	1	6
Fibroepithelioma	–	–	–	–	–	5
Lipoma	3	4	5	5	5	5
Amyloid tumor	–	–	1	2	2	4
Lymphoma	2	2	2	3	4	4
Osteogenic sarcoma	–	–	–	–	–	3
Leiomyoma	–	–	–	–	–	2
Endothelioma	–	–	–	1	1	2
Adenosarcoma	–	–	–	–	–	2
Carcinosarcoma	–	–	–	1	1	1
Rhabdomyoma	–	–	–	–	–	1
Oncocytoma	–	–	–	–	–	1
Type histologically undetermined	–	6	14	27	29	29

(Modified from Gilbert, J. G., Mazzarella, L. A., and Feit, L. J. 1953. Primary tracheal tumors in the infant and adult. Arch. Otolaryngol., 58:1–9.)

Table 72–3 INCIDENCE OF PRIMARY TRACHEAL TUMORS IN CHILDREN AND ADULTS

	Children	Adults
Nonmalignant	40 (93.1%)	256 (50.9%)
Malignant	3 (6.9%)	247 (49.1%)
Total	43	503

(Modified from Gilbert, J. G., Mazzarella, L. A., and Feit, L. J. 1953. Primary tracheal tumors in the infant and adult. Arch. Otolaryngol., 58:1–9.)

Table 72–5 PREDOMINANT BENIGN PRIMARY TRACHEAL TUMORS IN CHILDREN AND ADULTS

	Children	Adults
Osteochondroma	1 (2.5%)	76 (29.4%)
Papilloma	23 (57.5%)	42 (16.4%)
Fibroma	9 (22.5%)	30 (11.7%)
Angioma	6 (15.0%)	2 (0.78%)

(Modified from Gilbert, J. G., Mazzarella, L. A., and Feit, L. J. 1953. Primary tracheal tumors in the infant and adult. Arch. Otolaryngol., 58:1–9.)

extension of the tumor from the larynx either by direct growth or by implantation. The papillomas may be severe around the carina and may involve the bronchi and bronchioles and extend into the lung parenchyma.

The pathologic course and treatment of tracheobronchial papillomas is the same as that described for laryngeal papillomas. With extensive parenchymal lung destruction, lobectomy or pneumonectomy may be required (Holinger, 1968).

Chondroma, Osteochondroma, and Osteoma

These are cartilaginous and bony tumors that may occur in the trachea and mainstem bronchi. They appear as enlargements of existing tracheal or bronchial cartilages but may be completely separated from normal cartilage rings and are surrounded by their own capsule. The tumors are firm and may be hard as glass when ossified, making bronchoscopic diagnosis by biopsy impossible. The tumors grow very slowly and may cause extensive bronchopulmonary destruction. Potential sarcomatous degeneration may occur. Sessile or pedunculated tumors may be removed by bronchoscopic snare or bronchotomy.

Table 72–4 PREDOMINANT MALIGNANT PRIMARY TRACHEAL TUMORS IN CHILDREN AND ADULTS

	Children	Adults
Sarcoma	3 (100%)	36 (14.5%)
Carcinoma	0	194 (78.5%)

(Modified from Gilbert, J. G., Mazzarella, L. A., and Feit, L. J. 1953. Primary tracheal tumors in the infant and adult. Arch. Otolaryngol., 58:1–9.)

Tracheopathia Osteoplastica

This is a rare condition of the tracheal and bronchial cartilages consisting of multiple small, bony, hard masses projecting into the tracheal lumen. The masses are covered with mucosa and involve only the lateral and anterior walls since they originate from the cartilaginous rings. It has been suggested that they are the result of deposition of multiple anomalous anlagen of cartilaginous tissue endotracheal mucosa.

Clinically, the lesion may be an incidental finding detected on a radiograph or a post-mortem study.

Holinger (1968) reported occasional wheezing, cough, and hemoptysis with gradually increasing dyspnea that may lead to bronchoscopic studies and that demonstrate the characteristic bony spicules. At bronchoscopy, the tracheal surfaces, except for the posterior wall, consist of a massive, irregular, hard, mucosa-covered projection that cannot be removed. The walls are thick and hard, and encroachment on the lumen may be severe enough to embarrass respiration. Serum calcium studies are within normal limits, and radiographs of other bony structures are within normal limits. There is no known therapy. When dyspnea is severe, a bronchoscope forced through the obstructed tracheal lumen may be the only form of assistance. This will mechanically fracture the masses causing the greatest obstruction (Caldarola et al., 1964).

Other Rare Tumors of the Trachea

Cohen and colleagues (1978) have reported a series of rare diseases of the larynx and trachea in the pediatric age group. Included in this report is one case of fibrous histiocytoma of the trachea occurring in a two year old female child. In the same report, a case of solitary plasmacytoma of the larynx and upper trachea was reported in a child with systemic lupus erythematosus of nine years' duration. Nonspecific inflammatory tumors of the bronchi are relatively common. Granulomas and polyps may occur. In addition, although specific inflammatory tumors such as tuberculomas or sarcoid may occur, true primary tumors of the bronchi are rare.

Liebow (1952) classifies primary tumors of the bronchi as epithelial, mesodermal, or of developmental origin. Papillomas and adenomas of the bronchial tree are the only benign epithelial tumors considered. Benign mesodermal tumors consist of vascular tumors, such as hemangiomas, fibromas, lipomas, fibrolipomas, chondromas, osteochondromas, and granular cell myoblastomas. Liebow listed hamartomas as separate tumors of developmental origin and described fibromas, fibrolipomas, and lipomas to be the most common benign tumors of the trachea and bronchi, with papillomas being next in order of frequency. Papillomas of the bronchi may occur as an extension of the tracheobronchial distribution or may occur independently, possibly by implantation. The pathologic process and behavior are the same as those of the papillomas in the larynx and trachea described earlier.

BRONCHIAL ADENOMA

Bronchial adenoma in childhood is a rare condition. A recent review of the literature reveals only 56 cases under the age of 16 years (Wellons et al., 1976). The subject of bronchial adenoma remains a controversial topic with different opinions as to the origin, nomenclature, pathology, and degree of malignancy, as well as forms of treatment. Most of these tumors are found in the major bronchi; however, microscopic lesions strongly suggestive of adenoma have been reported in small branch bronchi and as incidental findings in surgical specimens removed for other causes.

The origin of these tumors has been described as that of embryonic lung buds, oncocytes, or serous or mucinous glands of the main bronchi. Although most frequently seen in women usually in the 30 to 40 year age group, cases have been reported in a child of four years old and with a spectrum between five and 16 years of age.

The tumor causes symptoms by its obstruction of the bronchial airway or by hemoptysis, which occurs in 80 per cent of patients.

The tumor appears as a small, rounded, red lesion seen on bronchoscopy that has broad points of attachment with occasional extension of the tumor through the wall in a dumbbell-shaped fashion. It appears that the histologic pattern may vary in the same slide. Generally, the lumina of the acinus spaces are filled with cells, while in other areas solid sheets of cells are present with little or no dividing stroma. The proximity of cartilage in or near the tumor and its necrosis and subsequent calcification probably account for this observation. Despite the variation in the arrangement of the adenomas, the individual cells are very similar. They have a cuboidal to columnar shape and have a faint eosinophilic granulocytoplasm and round to oval nuclei. The chromatin network is usually fine and scattered. Mitoses are extremely rare. This picture must be differentiated from that of the cylindroma.

Although rare regional lymph node metastases have been reported, these tumors are usually locally invasive. The therapy of adenomas is usually conservative. Endoscopic resection may have to be done if the tumor is entirely intrabronchial. However, in some cases because the tumor is slow-growing and diagnosis is delayed, the long-standing bronchial obstruction may result in irreversible bronchiectasis distal to this tumor. For this reason, segmental resection or lobectomy may be necessary. In some instances, bronchotomy or sleeve resection may be possible.

FIBROMA OF THE BRONCHUS

Fibroma of the bronchus is a slow-growing tumor that usually becomes apparent through symptoms of bronchial obstruction. This is a rare tumor, and the incidence in children is not documented. Holinger (1968) reports that on bronchoscopy, the tumor is seen as a smooth, firm, round, pink to purple mass, sometimes nodular and usually pedunculated. Purulent material from beyond the tumor prevents an accurate bronchoscopic evaluation on the first examination, and, thus, he suggests that repeated bronchoscopic aspirations may be required. Histologically, the tumor consists of closely packed, spindle-shaped cells, some containing considerable fatty tissue. Pedunculated fibromas may be removed by bronchoscopic forceps or snare, and Holinger describes the use of a bronchoscopic resectoscope and the combined cutting and coagulating current to remove the tumor. External surgery may be indicated if the lesion has a long, sessile base, and in cases of long duration with persistent atelectasis and extensive bronchiectasis, surgical excision of the entire diseased area by lobectomy or pneumonectomy may be indicated (Holinger, 1968).

INTRABRONCHIAL LIPOMA

Intrabronchial lipoma occurs usually in adult patients between the fifth and eighth decade and more commonly in men than in women. The incidence, again, is not known in children. The tumor produces respiratory obstruction and pulmonary changes secondary to bronchial obstruction. The ·tumor is described by Holinger as smooth, soft, pale in color, and pedunculated and does not extend beyond the cartilaginous bronchial walls. He reports that the tumor does not bleed as actively as an adenoma on removal, and on histology, the lipoma consists of lobules of fat cells, between which is an interlaced and delicate fibrous stroma. The tissue arises from adipose tissue normally present in the submucosa. Treatment is generally by endoscopic removal.

REFERENCES

Baker, D. C., Jr., and Hui, R. M. 1972. Tumors and cysts of the larynx. *In* Ferguson, C. F., and Kendig, E. L. (Eds.) Pediatric Otolaryngology, Vol. 2. Philadelphia, W. B. Saunders Co.

Birk, J., and Mannhart, H. 1963. Ultrasound for juvenile laryngeal papillomatosis. Arch. Otolaryngol., *77*:603.

Bourne, R. G., and Taylor, R. G. 1972. Treatment of juvenile laryngeal angioma with beta-ray applicator. Radiology, *103*:423–426.

Braverman, L. 1975. Consequences of thyroid radiation in children. N. Engl. J. Med., *202*:204–206.

Calcaterra, T. V. 1968. An evaluation of the treatment of subglottic hemangioma. Laryngoscope, *78*:1956–1964.

Caldarola, V. T., Harrison, E. G., Jr., Clagett, O. T., et al. 1964. Benign tumors and tumor-like conditions of the trachea and bronchi. Transactions of the 44th Annual Meeting of the American Broncho-Esophageal Association. pp. 46–49.

Chang-ho, M. 1977. Laryngeal involvement in von Recklinghausen's disease — a case report and review of the literature. Laryngoscope, *87*(3):35–42.

Cohen, S. R., and Wang, C. 1972. Steroid treatment of hemangiomas of the head and neck in children. Ann. Otol. Rhinol. Laryngol., *81*:584–590.

Cohen, S. R., Landing, B. H., and Isaacs, H. 1978. Fibrous histiocytoma of the trachea. Ann. Otol. Rhinol. Laryngol., Suppl. 52, 87.

Crowe, F., Schull, W., and Neel, J. 1956. Multiple Neurofibromatosis. Springfield, IL., Charles C Thomas.

Cummings, C. W., Montgomery, W. W., and Balogh, K. 1969. Neurogenic tumors of the larynx. Ann. Otol. Rhinol. Laryngol., *78*:76–95.

Ferguson, C. F. 1970. Congenital abnormalities of the infant larynx. Otolaryngol. Clin. North Am., *3*:185.

Feurstein, S. S. 1973. Subglottic hemangioma in infants. Laryngoscope, *83*:466–475.

Gilbert, J. G., Mazzarella, L. S., and Feit, L. J. 1953. Primary tracheal tumors in the infant and adult. Arch. Otolaryngol., *58*:1–9.

Gross, C. W., and Hubbard, R. 1974. Management of juvenile laryngeal papilloma with further observations. Laryngoscope, *84*:1090–1097.

Holinger, P. H. 1968. Benign tumors of the trachea and bronchi. Otolaryngol. Clin. North Am., p. 219, June 1968.

Holinger, P. H., Schild, J. A., and Weprin, L. 1970. Pediatric laryngology. Otolaryngol. Clin. North Am., *3*:625.

Hollingsworth, J. B., Kohlmoos, M. W., and McNaught, R. C. 1950. Treatment of juvenile papilloma of the larynx with resin of podophyllin. Arch. Otolaryngol., *52*:82.

Katz, H. P., and Askin, J. 1968. Multiple hemangiomata with thrombopenia — an unusual case with comments on steroid therapy. Am. J. Dis. Child., *115*:351–357.

Lampe, I., and LaTourette, H. B. 1959. Management of hemangiomas in infants. Pediatr. Clin. North Am., *6*:511–528.

Leikensohn, J. R., Benton, C., and Cotton, R. 1976. Subglottic hemangioma. J. Otolaryngol., *5*:487–491.

Liebow, A. A. 1952. Tumors of the lower respiratory tract. Armed Forces Institute of Pathology, Sec. V, Fascicle 17.

Lister, W. A. 1938. Natural history of strawberry nevi. Lancet, *1*:1429–1434.

Lyons, G. D., Schlosser, J. V., Loustean, R., et al. 1976. Laser surgery and immunotherapy in the management of laryngeal papilloma. Laryngoscope, *88*:1586–1588.

Miller, B. J., Murphy, F., and Lukie, B. E. 1978. Squamous cell papilloma of esophagus. Can. J. Surg., *21*:538–539.

Moffitt, D. P., Jr. 1959. Treatment of laryngeal papillomatosis with bovine wart vaccine. Laryngoscope, *69*:1421.

New, G. B., and Hertz, C. S. 1940. Malignant disease of the face, mouth, pharynx and larynx in the first three decades of life. Surg. Gynecol. Obstet., *70*:163–169.

Nuwayhid, N. S., Ballard, E. T., and Cotton, R. 1977. Esophageal papillomatosis — case report. Ann. Otol. Rhinol. Laryngol., *86*(5):623.

Oparah, S., and Subramanian, V. A. 1976. Granular cell myoblastoma of the bronchus. Report of two cases and review of the literature. Ann. Thorac. Surg., *22*(2):199.

Refetoff, S., and Harrison, T. 1975. Continuing occurrence of thyroid carcinoma after irradiation to the neck in infancy and childhood. N. Engl. J. Med., *242*:171–175.

Saenger, G. L., and Silverman, F. M. 1960. Neoplasia following therapeutic irradiation for benign conditions in childhood. Radiology, *74*:889–904.

Strong, M. S., Jako, G. J., Polyani, T., et al. 1973. Laser surgery in the aerodigestive tract. Am. J. Surg., *126*:529.

Sutton, T. J., and Nogrady, M. B. 1973. Radiologic diagnosis of subglottic hemangioma in infants. Pediatr. Radiol., *1*:211–216.

Svoboda, D. J., Kirshner, F. R., and Proud, G. D. 1963. Electron microscopic study of human laryngeal papillomatosis. Cancer Res., *23*:1084.

Sweetser, T. H. 1921. Hemangioma of the larynx. Laryngoscope, *31*:797–806.

Szpurnar, J. 1967. Laryngeal papillomatosis. Acta Otolaryngol., *63*:74.

Tabb, H. G., and Kirk, R. L. 1962. Vein grafts in management of laryngeal papillomas. Laryngoscope, *72*:1228.

Tefft, M. 1966. Radiotherapeutic management of subglottic hemangioma in children. Radiology, *86*:207–214.

Ullman, E. V. 1923. On the etiology of the laryngeal papilloma. Acta. Otolaryngol., *5*:317.

VanLoon, E. L., and Diamond, S. 1942. Neurofibroma of the larynx. Ann. Otol. Rhinol. Laryngol., *60*:122–126.

Walsh, T. E., and Beamer, P. R. 1950. Epidermoid carcinoma of the larynx occurring in two children with papilloma of the larynx. Laryngoscope, *60*:1110–1124.

Walters, J. 1953. The treatment of cavernous hemangioma. J. Fac. Radiol., *5*:134–140.

Wellons, H. A., Jr., Eggleston, P., Golden, G. T., and Allen, M. S. Bronchial adenoma in childhood — two case reports and review of literature. Am. J. Dis. Child, *130*(3):301–304.

Chapter 73

TRACHEOTOMY

Sylvan E. Stool, M.D.
Ronald Eavey, M.D.

INTRODUCTION

Tracheotomy has enjoyed a long and colorful history. The procedure initially was discussed almost simultaneously by both Galen and Aretaeus in the second century A.D., but neither admitted to performing the operation. The first procedure was attributed to Asclepiades, who practiced in Rome in the second century B.C. The only known indication for such surgery at that time was for "synanche" or "cynanche," which referred to nonspecific inflammatory conditions about the larynx, floor of the mouth, and head. Tracheotomy technique was further defined by Antyllus in the second century A.D., who advised that the *arteria aspera* (trachea) should be divided at the third or fourth ring. In the seventh century, Paul of Aegina recorded that the physician could be aware that the airway had been entered because he would hear a rush of air and loss of the patient's voice. Not until the sixteenth century, however, was the performance of a successful tracheotomy recorded — the Italian physician Antonio Musa Brasovala operated on a near-terminal patient suffering from an abscess of the windpipe.

Nicholas Habicot in 1620 described four successful tracheotomies; one of these, performed on a 14 year old boy, was possibly the first successful pediatric tracheotomy. The youth had attempted to swallow a bag of gold coins to prevent their possible theft, but the bag had become lodged in the esophagus and obstructed the trachea. After performing the tracheotomy, Habicot manipulated the bolus so that the bag passed along the esophagus and eventually was recovered per rectum. In 1766, Caron successfully performed the procedure on a 7 year old boy to remove a bean.

Andree, in 1782, and Chevalier, in 1814, also recorded having performed tracheotomies on pediatric patients.

According to Goodall (1934), only 28 tracheotomies had been reported as being performed prior to 1825. That year Bretonneau published a significant report of a successful tracheotomy in a 5 year old girl with diphtheria, a disease that he defined as a distinct clinical entity. This single pediatric tracheotomy influenced the historical course of the operation: In 1833 Trousseau reported having salvaged 50 of 200 children with diphtheria by performing tracheotomies on them. Trousseau also stressed techniques for postoperative care for the first time. As a result of this successful use of tracheotomy in treating cases of diphtheria, surgical management of airway problems increased in popularity, even though the mortality of the procedure continued to be high and many parents refused to allow surgery to be performed on their children. However, Jackson (1921) demonstrated that the mortality from the procedure itself was actually low when it was properly performed and when postoperative care was adequate; his contributions to tracheotomy history were to diminish complications through good technique and management, thus increasing the desirability of performing the operation. The next impetus to enlarge the scope of the procedure was provided by Galloway (1943) when he reported the usefulness of the procedure for respiratory care of patients with poliomyelitis.

The name given to the procedure of cutting a hole in the trachea is still evolving and is a matter of controversy. Currently, "tracheotomy" and "tracheostomy" are used almost interchangeably, although "tracheotomy" is derived from the Greek word *tome*

Table 73-1 CONDITIONS FOR WHICH TRACHEOTOMY HAS BEEN ADVOCATED

	Allergy	Metabolic	Prophylactic	Degenerative; Idiopathic	Sleep Disorders
Upper Airway Obstruction	Angioneurotic edema Anaphylaxis		Head and neck surgery Neurosurgery Cardiac surgery, etc. Prolonged endotracheal tube placement	Vocal cord paralysis	Pharyngeal musculature collapse Tonsilloadenoidal hypertrophy
Pulmonary Toilet Assisted Ventilation	Asthma	Cystic fibrosis Coma secondary to diabetes, Reye syndrome, uremia, etc. Respiratory distress syndrome		CNS or neuromuscular failure as in Guillain-Barré syndrome, polymyositis, myasthenia gravis, botulism, cardiac arrest, respiratory arrest	

	Congenital	Trauma	Toxic	Infection	Neoplastic
Upper Airway Obstruction	Choanal atresia Macroglossia Cleft palate Pierre-Robin anomaly Laryngomalacia Laryngeal stenosis Vocal cord paralysis Laryngeal webs, cysts Subglottic stenosis Vascular ring Tracheal hypoplasia	Facial injury Oral injury Foreign body Burns (steam, smoke, thermal) Laryngeal edema Recurrent laryngeal nerve injury Laryngeal fracture	Corrosives	Epiglottitis Laryngotracheitis (croup) Gingivostomatitis Diphtheria Retropharyngeal abscess Ludwig's angina Neck cellulitis Tetanus Rabies Plague	Laryngeal tumors Tracheal tumors Tumors of pharynx and tongue: papilloma, hemangioma, lymphangioma, sarcoma
Pulmonary Toilet Assisted Ventilation	Congenital heart disease Congenital heart failure Esophageal atresia secondary to tracheoesophageal fistula Hypoplastic lung secondary to diaphragmatic hernia	Head trauma Crushed chest Shock lung Intrapulmonary hemorrhage Pneumothorax Post-bypass lung	Coma secondary to toxins such as phenobarbital Hydrocarbon lung Aspiration syndromes such as from meconium	Meningitis Encephalitis Brain abscess Pneumonia Bronchiolitis Poliomyelitis	Brain tumors Spinal cord tumors

(to cut), whereas "tracheostomy" is derived from the word *stomoun* (to furnish with an opening or mouth) (Dorland, 1974). Thus, "tracheotomy" implies the performance of a nonpermanent type of surgery in contrast to "tracheostomy," which indicates that the tracheal mucosa is brought into continuity with the skin, probably with the intention of creating a permanent tracheal stoma. However, when the tracheotomy tube is in place for a prolonged time the tract usually becomes epithelialized; thus, a tracheotomy may become a tracheostomy.

INDICATIONS

For 2000 years a tracheotomy was performed only to relieve upper airway obstruction and only when the patient was at the brink of asphyxic death. For the past two generations, however, the procedure has been advocated in a multitude of situations, and indications for its performance may occur even before respiratory distress develops. The indications for creation of an artificial airway (Aberdeen and Downes, 1974) may be divided into three broad categories: (1) airway obstruction, (2) assisted ventilation, and (3) pulmonary toilet. Specific conditions for which the procedure has been advocated are found in Table 73–1. A review of the indications for tracheotomy at Children's Hospital of Pittsburgh for the period 1965 to 1977 reveals that 605 procedures were performed. Airway obstruction was the indication listed for 195 of the procedures, and in 410 cases assisted ventilation and pulmonary toilet were the indications for tracheotomy.

Decision-Making

The decision to perform a tracheotomy is frequently a very complex process in which a number of factors must be considered. An orderly, well-timed procedure utilizing the best assistants and equipment available is always preferred; thus, the surgeon who is confronted with this decision must be aware of the numerous facets involved and must anticipate the course of the patient's illness. This is frequently complicated by the fact that the child who requires an artificial airway may be surrounded by concerned and frightened adults.

It is not possible to provide guidelines that are applicable for each case. The general factors involved in decision-making may be considered as a matrix involving tissue, time, and the team. The *tissue* factors relate primarily to the age of the patient and the origin of the disease. The younger child has a smaller airway; therefore, a minimal amount of swelling of the airway will result in increased obstruction. The younger child may also not have sufficient strength to overcome obstruction and may tire more easily. A disease process that is characterized by acute inflammation may result in rapid obstruction. For example, the child with acute epiglottitis may not appear to have marked airway obstruction, but this is a rapidly progressive disease that frequently requires operative intervention. Thus, it is necessary to consider the *time*. Is the disease process one that is slowly or rapidly progressive, and what has been the sequence of events? In the child who is cyanotic, gasping for air, and in shock, the decision to operate is relatively easy, but the procedure may be different because there might not be time to secure adequate equipment or help. The preferred approach is to anticipate that such events might occur and intervene early, when it is possible to provide an adequate *team* of physicians and nurses. In order to determine the degree of emergency that exists, Douglas and colleagues (1978) proposed using the mnemonic TRACHS shown in Table 73–2. This provides some guidelines

Table 73–2   DEGREE OF EMERGENCY (TRACHS)

	Mild (days)	Moderate (hours)	Severe (minutes)	Extreme (immediate)
Tussive (cough)	occasional	hoarse	bark	bark or depressed
Retractions	absent	suprasternal	supra- and infrasternal	all accessory muscles
Anxiety	calm	anxiety when disturbed	restless	agitated or stuporous
Cyanosis	0	0	in room air	in 40% O_2
Heart rate	less than 120	less than 140	over 140	over 140
Stridor	occasional	inspiratory	inspiratory and expiratory	marked or diminished

for determining whether intervention is indicated immediately or in minutes, hours, or days. Most patients do not fall into such neat classifications, but this is a convenient and orderly method of evaluating the patient.

TRACHEOTOMY TUBES

Not until the time of Fabricius in the sixteenth century was there discussion about use of a cannula in tracheotomy management. The initial tube design was short and straight (Goodall, 1934), while Habicot and others utilized curved metal tubes (some of which were a quarter-circle design not appropriate for tracheal anatomy). The idea of using an inner cannula was conceived by Martine in 1730. It was not until the 1960s that plastic tubes became popular, although some rubber tubes had been used earlier (Stool et al., 1968).

The ideal tracheotomy tube should have several characteristics. It should be soft, pliable, nonreactive, easy to clean and maintain, and available in a number of sizes and lengths. Figure 73–1 shows several of the popular models of tracheotomy tubes that the authors have used and that are available for children in the United States. Other types of tubes are available throughout the world, and many physicians (Gray, 1960) have fabricated their own special designs. Each of the types of tube has distinctive features, and the size and design of the tube used will depend largely upon the indications for tracheotomy (Hatcher et al., 1967; Hawkins and Williams, 1976; Holinger et al., 1965). For instance, when the procedure is performed solely to provide an airway, the tube usually does not have to, and indeed should not, fill the tracheal lumen. However, if it is necessary to use artificial ventilation, then the tube should be of sufficient size to prevent excessive leakage of air. In general, it has usually not been necessary to use cuffed tubes in small children, thus avoiding the hazards of the cuff. In older children who require a cuff, it is advisable to use tracheotomy tubes that require only low pressure.

A critical measurement of the tracheotomy tube is the diameter. The external diameter will determine the size of the tube that may be inserted, but the more critical diameter is the inner or actual airway diameter. According to Gray (1960), the maximum external diameter of a tube for an infant up to six months of age should be 5.0 to 5.5 mm, and from six months to two years of age, 6 to 7 mm. The airway diameter for a child up to six months of age should be 4.0 to 4.5 mm, and from six months to two years, 5.0 to 5.5 mm. The size of the tube to be used when the tracheotomy is performed is usually determined by visualizing the tracheal lumen and ascertaining its size, thus individualizing the size of the tube to be inserted. Usually, this can be gauged by examining the relationship of the previously placed endotracheal tube or bronchoscope to the tracheal wall (Fearon and Whalen, 1967; Friedberg and Morrison, 1974). The manufacturers of plastic tubes usually provide information regarding the inner diameters of

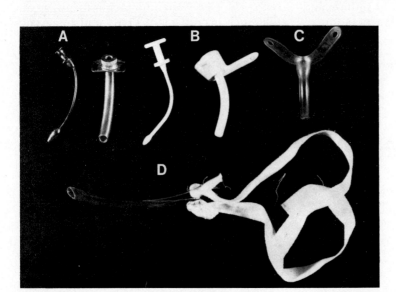

Figure 73–1 Tracheotomy tubes currently used by the authors. *A*, Holinger. *B*, Shiley. *C*, Great Ormand Street, Aberdeen design. *D*, Tube fabricated from an endotracheal tube.

Table 73–3 APPROXIMATE SIZE OF ENDOTRACHEAL AND TRACHEOTOMY TUBES
FOR INFANTS AND CHILDREN
(Based on outer diameter or circumference [French No.])

	Endotracheal*	Shiley	Aberdeen	Holinger
Premature	11–13	00		00
Newborn	14	0	3.5	0
Newborn–3 mos.	15–16	0	3.5	1
3–10 mos.	17	1	4.0	2
10–12 mos.	18	2	4.5	3
13–24 mos.	20	3	5.0	3
2–3 yrs.	22	4	5.0	4
4–5 yrs.	24	4	5.0	4
6–7 yrs.	26	4	5.0	4
8–9 yrs.	28	4	6.0	5
10–11 yrs.	30	6	6.0	6
12 and over	32	6	7.0	6

Usually a larger size tracheotomy than an endotracheal tube may be used because the trachea is larger than the subglottic region. The outer diameter or circumference will determine the size tube that may be used.
*French Number.

the tubes, but as the manufacturers of most metal tubes do not provide this information it may be necessary to use a gauge to determine it. Table 73–3 indicates the approximate sizes of the tubes shown in Figure 73–1, which are suitable for infants and children. Table 73–4 shows the approximate dimensions or gauge equivalents of endotracheal and tracheotomy tubes.

ANESTHESIA

In most pediatric institutions the anesthesiologist is an integral part of a team concerned with the performance of tracheotomies and with the subsequent care of these patients. Although there may have been some controversy in the past regarding the safety of general anesthesia for the child with acute

Table 73–4 APPROXIMATE GAUGE EQUIVALENTS FREQUENTLY USED IN
ENDOTRACHEAL AND TRACHEOTOMY TUBES
(Based on nearest inner diameter measurement)

Endotracheal[1]			Shiley[2]				Aberdeen[3]			Holinger[4]			
ID	OD	FR*	ID	OD	FR	Size	ID	OD	FR	ID	OD	FR	Size
2.0	2.9	8											
2.5	3.5	10								2.5	4.0	13	00
3.0	4.2	12	3.1	4.5	14	00				3.5	5.0	15	0
3.5	4.9	15	3.4	5.0	15	0	3.5	5.0	15	3.5	5.5	17	1
4.0	5.5	16	3.7	5.5	17	1	4.0	6.7	20	4.0	6.0	18	2
4.5	6.1	18	4.1	6.0	18	2	4.5	6.7	20	4.5	7.0	21	3
5.0	6.8	20	4.8	7.0	21	3	5.0	7.3	22	5.0	8.0	25	4
5.5	7.4	22	5.0	8.5	26	4				5.5	9.0	27	5
6.0	8.0	24					6.0	8.7	26	6.0	10.0	30	6
6.5	8.7	26											
7.0	9.5	29	7.0	10.0	30	6	7.0	10.7	32				
7.5	10.0	30											
8.0	10.7	32											

*The French number is arrived at by multiplying the outside diameter in millimeters by 3.
[1]The endotracheal tubes are marked with the internal diameter, usually with the outer diameter, and the length.
[2]The Shiley tube is manufactured by Shiley Laboratories, Irvine, CA. The tube is stamped with the size and inner and outer diameters. The larger sizes are supplied with a low-pressure cuff.
[3]This tube is the Aberdeen design, known also as the Great Ormand Street Tube. It is manufactured by J. G. Franklin & Sons, Ltd., High Wycombe, England. The tube is stamped with the inner diameter.
[4]The Holinger design is manufactured by several companies; therefore, the sizes may vary, and the internal diameter may show considerable variation. These measurements were made on tubes produced by Pilling Company, Fort Washington, PA.

airway obstruction, it is best to use when skilled personnel are available.

There are several decisions that must be made in consultation with the anesthesiologist. Should the child be anesthetized prior to intubation, or is an awake intubation necessary? Should the intubation be performed with a bronchoscope or an endotracheal tube in the airway? In general, it is favorable to employ general anesthesia prior to intubation and after adequate oxygenation. Even with a struggling child the anesthesiologist, using positive pressure, can accomplish some gas exchange. When the child has relaxed, the airway is much easier to manage and intubation is greatly facilitated. Under any circumstance, the surgeon should have a bronchoscope available in the event that direct visualization of the larynx and insertion of a rigid tube are necessary. The usual technique is to oxygenate the child in the position in which he or she is most comfortable. Most often, this is with the patient sitting up or leaning forward. After oxygenation it is usually desirable to provide a route for intravenous medication and then to begin the anesthesia using an anesthetic agent that allows for a high oxygen concentration. In some instances, the anesthesiologist may wish to use muscle relaxants to effect intubation. These should be used with great caution and only after it is certain that the child has an airway that can be ventilated adequately with bag and mask. The management of acute airway problems requires team work between the surgeon and anesthesiologist.

TECHNIQUE

Variations have always existed in the actual surgical technique of tracheotomy (Goodall, 1934; Tucker and Silberman, 1972; Smythe, 1966; Bigler et al., 1954; Pickard and Oropeza, 1971; Lawrence and Bailey, 1971; Gibson and Byrne, 1972; Jaffee, 1963). Prior to the time of Fabricius (sixteenth century) the procedure was often performed with the patient in a sitting position, and skin incisions were transverse. Fabricius, who never performed a tracheotomy, advocated the use of a vertical skin incision, and Heister, in 1718, also recommended a vertical tracheal incision; incisions had been made transversely based on the hippocratic teaching that cartilage would not heal. Trousseau emphasized that the procedure should be done slowly, but Jackson

(1921) published the following description of his technique.

. . . it rests fundamentally on making two incisions, the first of which splits open the entire front of the neck from 'Adam's apple' to the suprasternal notch; the second incision opening the trachea, which has been found by palpation with the left index finger in the pool of blood that fills the wound . . . the trachea being incised by sense of touch instead of sight. . . . The two step, finger-guided operation does not require more than one minute. . . .

While this technique may be appropriate for an adult in severe distress, it hardly seems appropriate to use in children.

The procedure requires prior intubation with a bronchoscope or an endotracheal tube (Marcy and Cook, 1975). Monitoring of the patient is very important. The minimum of equipment should include a precordial stethoscope, blood pressure cuff in place, and, if available, electrocardiographic and temperature monitors. The patient is positioned in the middle of the table (it is important for the surgeon to position the patient), and the shoulders are elevated on a roll so that the neck can be hyperextended. If possible, the anesthesiologist holds the chin with the neck somewhat stretched in order to keep the tissues stable (Fig. 73–2A). The operator palpates the neck to identify the thyroid and cricoid cartilages, which may be very difficult to do in the young child because the structures are soft and the larynx is very high. The trachea is palpated down to the suprasternal notch; the presence of an endotracheal tube or bronchoscope in the trachea greatly facilitates accurate palpation of the airway. Usually, about one finger breadth above the suprasternal notch the trachea turns posteriorly; it is at this point that we advocate placing the opening into the trachea. Thus, a skin incision about 2 cm long is made approximately one finger breadth above the sternal notch. There is still much difference of opinion as to whether a vertical or a horizontal skin incision is preferable; although the horizontal is preferred, the choice probably is not critical. In young infants there is usually a large fat pad present over the trachea, and a portion of this is occasionally removed. Hemostasis of the skin and the fat may be obtained with hemostats or electrocautery; usually, if dissection is careful it is not necessary to tie the superficial vessels, as they will clot spontaneously. The fascial layer beneath the subcutaneous fat is grasped with hemo-

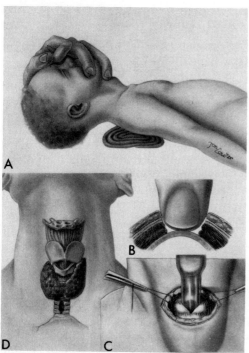

Figure 73–2 Important considerations for tracheotomy technique. *A,* The shoulders are elevated and the neck is hyperextended; the anesthetist holds the chin up and the head is held in the midline. *B,* The trachea is palpated after each layer is incised; palpation is as important as visualization. *C,* Stay sutures are placed in the trachea — usually only two are used; these are placed 1 to 2 mm from the midline and tied 2 to 3 cm from the trachea, and the ends are identified. If additional control of the trachea is indicated, then additional sutures may be placed over the cut edge. *D,* The site of the tracheal incision is below the thyroid isthmus. A vertical incision is used and no cartilage is excised.

monofilament sutures through the tracheal wall, 1 to 2 mm from the midline. By applying traction to the sutures, the trachea may be elevated into the wound; a vertical incision is then made through three or four tracheal rings (Fig. 73–2*D*). Some operators prefer to make the tracheal incision with electrocautery in order to decrease the tendency for the vessels and the mucosa to bleed. Frequently a small incision is made and spread, the previously placed endotracheal tube or bronchoscope is identified, and then the remainder of the trachea is opened with a blunt scissors. To enhance control of the trachea or in case it should be desirable to insert a very large tracheotomy tube, additional sutures can be applied over the edge of the tracheal wall so that the trachea may be pulled into the wound and the edges everted. The tracheotomy tube is inserted by opening the new tracheal stoma with anterolateral traction on the sutures. The tube is then held in place, and the roll is removed from beneath the shoulders. The chest is auscultated to ascertain that the tube has been placed properly. The neck is flexed, and the tracheotomy tube is held in place with tapes tied around the neck to ensure the tube's stability. The chest is again auscultated to ascertain that the mainstem bronchi have not been cannulated. Radiographic examination is then performed to ascertain the exact relationship of the tracheotomy tube to the carina and to assure complete intratracheal passage of the tube.

EMERGENCY TRACHEOTOMY

It is always desirable that a surgical procedure such as a tracheotomy be performed in an orderly and controlled manner. However, in some situations this is not possible, and an emergency tracheotomy may be necessary. A number of special instruments and techniques have been advocated for this procedure, but they have not gained wide acceptance, especially for use in children, because of the potential hazards of perforation and uncontrolled bleeding (Utley et al., 1972; Vilinskas, 1968). The procedure that is advocated for children is a cricothyrotomy. This is accomplished by elevating the shoulders, hyperextending the neck, and palpating the larynx and trachea. The larynx is relatively high in the neck of the young infant and child and may be very difficult to palpate. However, when the larynx is palpated it should be

stats, delivered into the wound, and then opened with scissors in the midline. The fascia is spread and slightly undermined with a hemostat or blunt scissors. A finger can be inserted through the wound and the trachea palpated — tracheotomy is a procedure that is done as much by *palpation* as by direct visualization (Fig. 73–2*B*). It is important that all the layers be incised flush with the wound edge so that there is not a funneling effect as the procedure is performed. The successive layers of fascia and strap muscles are incised in the midline. After each layer is incised, the trachea is *again palpated* to insure its location. With the trachea identified, retractors may be placed in the edge of the wound in order to aid visualization of the trachea. It is preferable to use a stay suture through the trachea wall instead of a hook to deliver the trachea into the wound (Fig. 73–2*C*). This is usually accomplished by applying 000 or 0000 silk or held in the midline with the thumb and index finger; a small incision then may be made in the cricothyroid membrane. A hemostat is inserted to enlarge the incision, and the tube is placed through the incision. If a tracheotomy tube is not available, an endotracheal tube or large catheter may be inserted.

There has been discussion in the literature about the feasibility of using a large-bore needle transtracheally for resuscitation. Hughes et al. (1967) performed an experiment using small dogs in which they were able to ventilate them successfully for an hour with a 13 gauge needle, but they commented that this may be harder to do in a child because definition of the child's trachea is difficult owing to its relatively small size and flexibility. Davies and Belam (1967) advocated performing a minitracheotomy with an intravenous cannula, but only for resuscitation; even as a life-saving method they did not feel that it was the method of choice. Attia et at. (1975) advocated the use of a Teflon cannula, such as is used for administering intravenous medication, and felt that this would be effective for resuscitation when used with high-pressure flows. Oppenheimer (1977) stated that the performance of a needle tracheotomy in children was almost impossible because of the softness of the cartilage and extreme mobility of the trachea of a child. It is obvious that there is a great deal of controversy regarding this mode of resuscitation; however, virtually all the authors state that after attempts at resuscitation with positive pressure or oral intubation have not been successful, it is only logical to try whatever other methods the physician is familiar with to prolong or restore life. In essence, needle tracheotomy seems to be a fairly straightforward, although difficult, procedure. The largest bore needle should be attached to a syringe, inserted through the cricothyroid membrane, and aspirated to insure its placement in the airway. More than one needle can be used if necessary. If positive-pressure oxygen is available it can be used to improve oxygenation, or the syringe itself can provide positive pressure (Jacobs, 1972; Jacoby et al., 1956). Another way to improve the airway under such circumstances is to give the child partial relief from hypoxia to decrease the strong respiratory effort necessary; with such relaxation of effort, soft tissue that has been pulled into the airway may not cause as much obstruction, and the supraglottic airway may improve.

POSTOPERATIVE CARE

A tracheotomy tube bypasses some normal physiologic processes that must then be replicated artificially. In addition, the tracheotomy patient is exposed to unusual hazards, the effects of which must be minimized.

Inspired air that bypasses the nose will not be warmed, filtered, or humidified, so air supplied to the patient by tracheotomy should first be warmed to body temperature and humidified beyond the dew point (when condensation occurs) to prevent tracheal drying, discomfort, and possible infection and obstruction. Tussive action is lost, so tracheal secretions must be artificially suctioned in a fashion that is aseptic and minimally traumatic. Voice communication is forfeited, and the patient must be provided with alternative means of gaining attention and discussing ideas. A bell, buzzer, pencil, and writing pad or other devices should be explained and practiced with the patient to prevent feelings of frustration, isolation, and fear of an emergency.

Micro-organisms and foreign bodies have easier access to a tracheotomized patient's respiratory system than they do to a normal system. Frequent changes of equipment and the use of aseptic technique can minimize the risk of infection. Tracheal trauma can be minimized by gentle suctioning with soft tubing only when necessary. The threat of accidental decannulation should be minimized by appropriate education and practice of all personnel involved in the child's care.

A coordinated approach by the physician, nurses, parents, and patient and constant surveillance and care are required for the child whose new airway is secured only by a tape around the neck. For additional information regarding tracheotomy care, several excellent articles are available (Stool and Tucker, 1972; Schild, 1970; Kaler and Kaler, 1974; Cohen et al., 1977; Stool and Beebe, 1972).

DECANNULATION

Most patients tolerate decannulation uneventfully, but on occasion a tube must be replaced to maintain comfortable ventilation.

Adherence to a few basic guidelines can facilitate a successful routine decannulation. First, the appropriate time for removal of the tube will be determined largely by the underlying pathologic condition. For example, epiglottitis usually resolves quickly, and decannulation can be attempted in a few days, but a tracheotomy performed for a neurologic condition or congenital anomaly might require prolonged cannulation. Second, before the tube is removed, the physician, nurses, and patient should have established a working rapport so that the child feels a minimum of anxiety during the manipulation. Third, when the tube is removed, an increase of 300 per cent in airway resistance will be added to the work of breathing and dead space will double (Baker and Savetsky, 1972). This may frighten the child, especially one who has been cannulated for a prolonged period. To avoid this unpleasant surprise, the patient should have experienced periods of laryngeal breathing prior to final decannulation by maneuvers such as periodic occluding of the tube with the finger, corking the tube, or using progressively smaller-caliber tubes. Fourth, an evaluation of the airway by endoscopy or radiographs is mandatory just before decannulation, both to evaluate the original pathologic condition and also to ascertain whether or not complications have arisen secondary to the presence of the tracheotomy *per se*. Sasaki et al. (1978), in a retrospective review of 123 pediatric tracheotomies, found that decannulation was delayed in 44, usually as a result of mechanical problems such as the occurrence of tracheal granulomas (Fig. 73–3). They emphasized that in 25 per cent of the 44 cases temporary abductor failure, which could be treated by using progressively smaller tubes, was the cause of delayed decannulation. The last consideration is that the actual decannulation should be done in appropriate surroundings. Usually it should take place early in the day in a place that is not frightening to the patient and with resuscitation equipment nearby. A final point to remember is that the longer the cannula is in place, the more likely it is that complications may occur.

Occasionally, a patient will not tolerate decannulation. Infants seem particularly vulnerable; this may be because there is less subglottic area available and, therefore, any reaction to the tube will decrease the lumen size. For instance, a 1 mm circumferential decrease in the tracheal lumen may compromise 50 per cent of the airway in an infant but only 10 to 20 per cent of the airway in an adult. The child's cartilaginous support is not

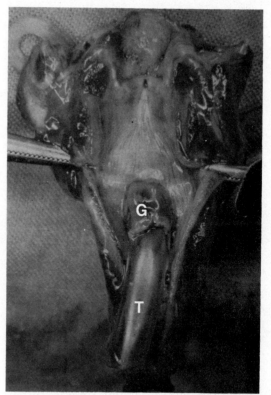

Figure 73–3 A tracheal granuloma found in a patient who expired 10 days postoperatively from central nervous system disease. Any patient who has a tracheotomy tube in place for longer than five to seven days should be investigated for this condition. *G*, granuloma; *T*, tracheotomy tube.

as rigid as an adult's, and increased force of respiration may cause tracheal collapse (Diamant et al., 1961; Wind, 1971). In such instances when a patient cannot be decannulated, alternate approaches are necessary. Techniques such as substituting nasotracheal intubation for tracheotomy for a short period of time have been advocated (MacLachlan, 1969); removing the tube while the patient is sedated is sometimes effective. If there is mechanical obstruction to the trachea, such as from granulation tissue at the tracheotomy site, it obviously should be removed.

Although much has been written about the psychologic factors involved in decannulation, it is the authors' opinion that the majority of the difficulties with decannulation are mechanical. In the past, these may have been difficult to recognize, but with newer radiographic and endoscopic techniques, a more precise diagnosis may be made and, when possible, appropriate therapy instituted.

Table 73–5 OPERATIVE COMPLICATIONS

Hemorrhage — Coagulation defect, vascular anomalies

Air entry — Subcutaneous emphysema, mediastinal emphysema, pneumothorax, air embolus

Anatomic damage — Cricoid cartilage and laryngeal injury, esophageal puncture, recurrent laryngeal nerve injury

Tracheotomy tube problems — Incorrect choice of tube size, faulty placement (false passage into a bronchus)

Respiratory drive cessation — Cardiac and ventilatory arrest secondary to a rapid change in CO_2 tension

COMPLICATIONS

Operative Complications

A number of problems can arise during the operative procedure (Table 73–5). Many times they can be avoided, at least in part, by thoughtful anticipation.

Hemorrhage. The possibility of a coagulation abnormality must be considered in any child who is having a surgical procedure. Besides the obvious clotting defects, such as hemophilia, other clinical examples might be deficient clotting factors in the neonate or in a child with liver disease, or thrombocytopenia in a septic patient or in a child receiving chemotherapy. Accidental hemorrhage might be encountered as a result of vascular anomalies: The aortic arch occasionally can reach the manubrium, and the innominate artery has been reported to overlap the trachea in the neck (Fig. 73–4). The left common carotid may originate from the innominate artery, or an arteria thyroidea may ascend anterior to the trachea. Also, the common carotid artery in a neonate can appear deceptively like the trachea. In addition, the inferior thyroid vein lies anterior to the trachea and may be encountered during tracheotomy (Greenway, 1972). Fortunately, most surgical bleeding is mere capillary oozing, which occasionally will persist but which most often stops spontaneously. Cautious observation is required, however, as an unligated vessel in a hypotensive patient might not bleed until restoration of a normal blood pressure.

Air Entry. Children are especially likely to develop complications during or after tracheotomy. The most common problem is air dissection between the deep and superficial cervical fascia and then into the mediastinum. Goldberg and colleagues demonstrated this mechanism in 1942; Forbes and others (1947) concurred with their theory of the process and demonstrated an appreciable decrease in the incidence of the problem when preoperative intubation and anesthesia were used. Minimal pretracheal fascia dissection should be performed in order to prevent air entry into the thorax. This is especially important when the procedure is done in the absence of an endotracheal tube or bronchoscope in the trachea, as the struggling child may develop high negative intrathoracic pressure and may draw air into the mediastinum through the tracheotomy wound. Pneumothorax may be produced by laceration of the pleural dome. This can usually be avoided if there is careful dissection in the midline with identification of the involved structures. Despite all precautions, however, these complications may still

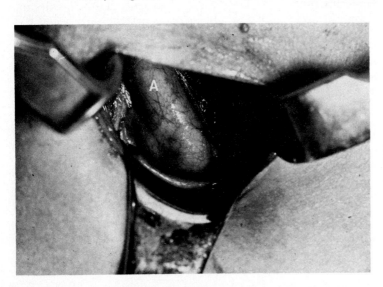

Figure 73–4 An innominate artery (A) overlying the trachea, found during tracheotomy on a newborn. The incision was closed and another one was made above it.

occur, and a postoperative radiograph should be obtained routinely to assess the postoperative status of the chest (Rabuzzi and Reed, 1971).

Anatomic Damage. As emphasized by Jackson (1921), the cricoid cartilage should not be incised because tracheal stenosis commonly occurs after injury to this structure. Laceration of the membranous trachea or esophagus is averted by placement of an endotracheal tube or bronchoscope preoperatively and the use of stay suture tracheal traction during the incision. Injury to the recurrent laryngeal nerve may occur and may not be apparent in the aphonic, tracheotomized patient.

Tracheotomy Tube Problems. As indicated in the description of the surgical technique to be used in tracheotomy, proper choice of the tube size and tube material is extremely important in order to avoid complications. Too small a tube is easily dislodged and produces high airway resistance; too large a tube may cause pressure against the tracheal wall. Care must be taken not to create a false passage or to cannulate a mainstem bronchus.

Respiratory Arrest. Greene (1959) discussed this phenomenon in patients who deteriorated soon after tracheotomy. The problem was attributed to the rapid washout effect of retained CO_2, which resulted in cardiac arrhythmias, hypotension, and loss of ventilatory drive.

Pulmonary Edema. The authors have seen several cases in which pulmonary edema developed following tracheotomy. It is felt that the mechanism for this was the extravasation of fluid through the alveolar wall because of the rapid changes in pressure within the trachea in a child who was hypoxic and hypercarbic and who may have retained secretions. This may be avoided by utilizing continuous positive airway pressure (Galvis et al., 1980).

Postoperative Complications (see Table 73–6)

Hemorrhage. Massive postoperative hemorrhage may be fatal and may occur from days to months following surgery. The most common mechanism is arterial erosion, usually of the innominate artery, either by the tip or the side of the tracheotomy tube (Potondi, 1969). The use of the correct size

Table 73–6 POSTOPERATIVE COMPLICATIONS

Hemorrhage — Wound ooze, tracheal erosion, paratracheal hematoma, tracheoarterial fistula

Air entry — Subcutaneous emphysema, mediastinal emphysema, pneumothorax, pneumopericardium

Anatomic (trachea) damage — Mucosal ulceration, stenosis, dilatation (caused by cuff), malacia, granuloma, crusting, fistulae (tracheocutaneous, tracheoesophageal, tracheopleural), skin-lined tube

Tracheotomy tube problems — Obstruction by crusts or mucous plug, displacement, cuff complications, malposition (false passage into a bronchus, excess tracheal wall pressure), difficult decannulation

Infection — Wound infection, neck cellulitis, perichondritis, tracheobronchitis, pneumonia, mediastinitis, lung abscess

Deglutition difficulty — Dysphagia, odynophagia, aspiration

Cosmesis — Tracheotomy scar, keloid

Laryngeal disuse

Delayed decannulation

tube will help to avoid this catastrophe. This complication may be heralded by pulsation of the tube, by prior, less significant episodes of bleeding, or both. If bleeding persists or is very marked, it is mandatory that the tube be changed and endoscopy utilized for evaluation of the bleeding site. Treatment consists of tamponade produced either by the inflated cuff of an endotracheal tube or by digital compression of the artery between the posterior sternum and a finger driven into the pretracheal area, followed by median sternotomy (Mathog et al., 1971).

Air Entry. In addition to the problems previously mentioned, air can enter the pleural space from high inflation pressures if the patient is on a respirator or is overzealously bagged by hand. This is a common finding even in neonates who have never been tracheotomized but are on a ventilator via an endotracheal tube. Inflation pressures cause alveolar rupture. The leaking alveolar air dissects along perivascular and perilymphatic channels back to the hilum from where it can spread. Such complications have also been reported to occur spontaneously even after decannulation (Lehmann, 1974).

Tracheal Lesions. The literature is generously supplied with reports of tracheal lesions that occur after tracheotomy (Harley, 1971; Samaan, 1970; Davidson et al., 1971;

Johnson and Stewart, 1975; Louhimo et al., 1971; Schloss, 1972; Harley, 1972; Bain, 1972; Westgate and Roux, 1970). Many factors can contribute to such lesions: decreased vascular perfusion at the time of operation, cartilage excision, use of an inordinately large tube or a cuffed tube, mucosal edema, infection, systemic debility, tube motion, tube material, the original indication for tracheotomy, and length of intubation. These lesions result in fibrosis with subsequent stenosis of the trachea and other problems. The exact incidence of stenosis after decannulation is unknown because investigations are not routinely carried out in asymptomatic patients, and a severe degree of narrowing is required to elicit symptoms (to a 3 to 4 mm lumen in adults). A follow-up study by Friman (1976) revealed that 69 of 70 patients had evidence of stenosis on lateral radiographic views of the trachea, and 25 of the 70 had narrowing as seen in the anteroposterior view. Dane and King (1975) report in a prospective study that 16 per cent of their patients developed asymptomatic stomal site stenosis and 16 per cent developed asymptomatic cuff site

stenosis. Freeland et al. (1974) showed that marked tracheal and cricoid dimension abnormalities occur in children tracheotomized for longer than seven days but that the dimension remained normal in those cannulated for less than one week. There are several methods to evaluate the size of the trachea; it should be done routinely prior to decannulation by endoscopy or radiographic methods and sometimes by the use of pulmonary function tests. Any child who develops evidence of stenosis should be evaluated by endoscopic examination of the larynx, trachea, and bronchi. Another interesting complication in children still cannulated is tracheal collapse at the tip of the tracheotomy tube, which on a chronic basis produces bronchitis and emphysema (Murphy and Popkin, 1971).

The most common tracheal lesion is granulation at the superior aspect of the tracheotomy site, as shown in Figure 73–3. This may be considered as a consequence of the procedure rather than a complication. The radiographic appearance of this lesion before and after removal is shown in Figure 73–5. A number of techniques are available to ac-

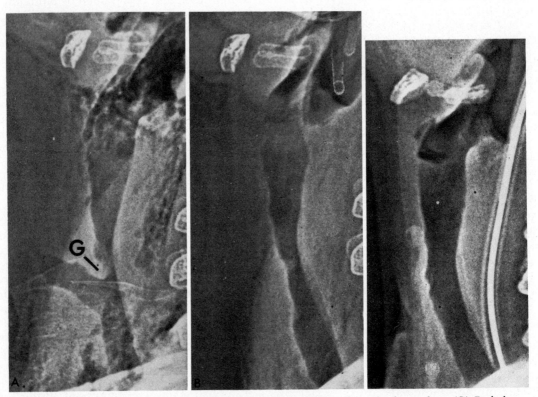

Figure 73–5 *A,* A xerogram of the trachea showing the usual site of a tracheal granuloma (G). Both the immediate postexcision appearance *(B)* and the appearance after seven weeks *(C)* are demonstrated. (Photograph courtesy of Lyon Greenberg, M.D., and John Scott, M.D.)

complish removal of this tissue. Small soft masses may be removed endoscopically with forceps or suction. Larger masses are removed by visualizing the tumor endoscopically and inserting a small skin hook through the tracheotomy stoma so the mass may be pulled into the tract and amputated with a scissors. Electrocautery can also be employed to remove or amputate the mass. When the granuloma has epithelialized or is very fibrous, it may be necessary to excise the entire epithelialized tract along with the mass.

Tracheotomy Tube Problems. Obstruction of the artificial airway by crusts and plugs can be avoided by proper humidification of inspired air and by dedicated nursing care. If an obstruction occurs because the tube becomes displaced in the immediate postoperative period, it can be replaced by applying traction on the stay sutures to identify the trachea.

Infection. Whenever an incision is made into the trachea that communicates with the external environment, local inflammation and infection will ensue. This may be considered as much a consequence of the procedure as a complication. However, there are some instances in which this poses a special problem: Burn patients may be especially prone to bacteremia and infection (Eckhauser et al., 1974). Rogers and Osterhout reported a pneumonia rate of 15 per cent in patients with tracheotomy (1970), and prophylactic antibiotics did not seem to suppress the infection rate in that series. In many instances organisms such as pseudomonas and staphylococcus are recovered from the tracheotomy wound. It is often difficult to determine whether these organisms are colonizers or whether they may be responsible for infection.

Deglutition Difficulties. Although it is not often appreciated, a tracheotomy tube can interfere with swallowing and can result in dysphagia and aspiration. Bonanno (1971) postulates that the tube serves to anchor the trachea to the strap muscles of the neck. The suprahyoid musculature is tethered, and normal laryngeal excursion is hindered. Also, aerophagia (Rosnagle and Yanagisawa, 1969) may develop, which may result in gastric dilatation with subsequent respiratory problems. It is felt that the pressure sensations in the throat may encourage the swallowing, which results in gastric dilatation. Insertion of a nasogastric tube and changing of the tracheotomy tube may alleviate this condition. Lastly, aspiration was detected in 69 per cent

of 61 patients by means of blue dye placed on the tongue that was later noted to be aspirated through the tracheotomy tube (Cameron et al., 1973).

Cosmesis. Scars may develop after tracheotomy whether a transverse or horizontal incision is utilized. The degree of scarring depends greatly on the length of time the tube has been in place and the type of tube that has been utilized. With any patient in whom the cannula has been in place for several weeks, the tract may become epithelialized with subsequent development of a tracheocutaneous fistula. In the young child this does not pose a physiologic hazard; it may have some psychologic import, and it is usually desirable after the child reaches school age to revise the wound if the tracheocutaneous fistula persists or if there is an unsightly scar.

Aphonia. A serious problem for the child in the immediate postoperative period is the inability to communicate and to express distress. There has been some concern as to whether tracheotomized children would develop adequate verbal communication skills; however, in the authors' experience if there are no other neurologic defects the children who have had tracheotomies do not seem to encounter undue difficulty with speech development.

HOME CARE

It is not possible to decannulate all patients on whom a tracheotomy has been performed. Therefore, it is necessary to make suitable provisions for prolonged tracheotomy care. Properly trained, skillfully counseled parents can provide excellent nursing care. Their personal attention and diligent nursing care can more than compensate for the sophistication of the hospital setting, and the advantages of continuity of care and decreased risk of cross-infection are obvious. In addition, the financial burden of prolonged hospitalization and its accompanying emotional strain are considerably lessened. There is also a tremendous advantage gained in not separating the child from his or her family. Home care may not be feasible for every patient who must endure a prolonged period of tracheotomy breathing; however, it should be considered, and an ultimate decision should be made at the discretion of the physician in concert with the parents, nursing staff, social workers, and family physician.

Prior to discharge of the patient, the parents must be trained in the use of equipment, tracheotomy care, early detection of complications, and emergency techniques. The facilities of the home must be arranged and necessary equipment obtained. Family responsibilities should be assigned and the instruction of the parents should be organized. The physician or his or her designate must become both a teacher and a counselor, promoting total patient management, instilling the parents with knowledge and confidence, and providing support for a difficult adjustment. A nurse specialist who may be available in many institutions is the ideal person to accomplish this transition, provide patient counseling, and maintain the necessary contacts with the hospital and physician.

Training for home care usually begins with explaining to the parents the anatomic structures involved in the tracheotomy and breathing through it. The parents need to visualize the esophagus and trachea as two separate tubes that involve eating and breathing. The reasons for accumulation of secretions in the trachea should be explained. The parents should be made aware of the importance of moisture and warmth in the inspired air and should have some basic understanding of the function of ciliary activity in removing secretions from the trachea. Their natural fears of having to irrigate the trachea, provide suction, and perform percussion may be overcome with experience and the realization that these are not necessarily painful experiences for the child.

Ideally, this instruction should last for several days within the hospital, where the parents can practice under the supervision of nurses and the physician. It is important that both parents participate in the hospital training rather than one parent receiving training from the other after the child returns home. If possible, it is helpful for the parents to spend a 24 hour period in complete charge of their child in the hospital before the child's discharge. In addition, it is advantageous to have the parents speak to the parents of other tracheotomized children who have been on a home care program. The importance of this opportunity cannot be overemphasized, as the parents can obtain much information and confidence from such an experience.

Equipment

All necessary equipment purchased should be on hand and should be tested prior to the child's discharge from the hospital. An area that is well-lighted should be available. It is desirable to have all the equipment on one table near the child's bed, and a dust-free environment is preferred, with animals and other furry or fuzzy objects removed.

Suction Machine. A variety of suction machines is available. They usually cost from $150 to $400 to purchase or about $35 per month to rent. In general, it is desirable for the suction machine to require little maintenance, weigh 16 to 20 pounds, be small enough to occupy less than one square foot of space, and be portable. There should be a pressure gauge and a regulator valve to maintain optimal suction, and an overflow trap or valve should be attached to prevent moisture from entering the pump. Necessary accessories for the suction machine that should be available are an ample length of tubing (preferably translucent or rubber) with appropriate connectors — preferably of transparent plastic so that there is a means of observing the quantity and quality of the mucus aspirated. The suction machine should have an adapter so that it can be easily connected to household current. A spare connector and adapter should be available at all times.

Emergency Suction. It is important to have portable emergency suction available. A number of these machines are marketed that provide a trap. Usually a mouthpiece is available so that suction can be provided by the parent.

Catheters. It is necessary to use a size that fits the tracheotomy tube. Whistle tip catheters are preferred. The catheters may be plastic or rubber, disposable or reusable. Rubber catheters are softer; therefore, they cause less tissue damage. The plastic catheters frequently are disposable; however, since the catheters will be used on only one patient, it is usually possible to clean them adequately with soap and water and store them in a clean jar or tray for reuse.

Tracheotomy Tubes. The tracheotomy tubes that the child will use at home should be inserted several days prior to discharge. The family should have at least two tracheotomy tubes of the same style available. In addition, it is wise to have one tracheotomy tube of the same style but of smaller size available. The tubes are usually washed with soap and water and, depending upon the type of tube that is being used, sterilized by soaking or boiling in water after each use.

Tracheotomy Tape. Cotton twill tape can usually be purchased at the notions counter of variety or department stores. It is important that a good quality tape be used.

Bandage Scissors. It is important to have a bandage scissors, preferably with a blunt end, to cut the tape.

Humidifier. A number of fairly inexpensive mist humidifiers are available. One of these should be kept in the child's room and adequate humidity should be maintained at all times. It is important to clean these periodically. In addition to the room humidifier, it is desirable that humidification for the entire house be provided if this is at all feasible. Although this is occasionally fairly expensive, proper humidification will decrease the tendency for other members of the family to have upper respiratory tract infections and will provide a more healthful atmosphere for the child.

Syringes. Syringes or droppers are necessary to drop saline into the tracheotomy tubes in order to liquefy the secretions. The size of syringe used will depend upon the age of the child.

Normal Salt Solution. A normal saline solution may be made by mixing two teaspoons of noniodized salt in one quart of boiled water.

Intercom. A good portable intercom system is available for as little as $60 from any electronics or radio store. The microphone may be placed in the child's room while the auxiliary end may be placed anywhere in the house or even outdoors. This is an item that may be of immense value, as it permits the attendant to detect if the child is in distress without constantly being present in the patient's room. Since the child is unable to cry with a tracheotomy, it is frequently desirable to attach small bells to the bed or to the infant's shoes, as these will make noise if the infant is in distress and moves about in the bed.

Nursing Technique

Irrigation. The intervals for irrigation depend upon the individual child's needs. These are often related to the age of the child and the duration of the tracheotomy. The intervals usually lengthen as the child grows older and as he or she develops a more efficient cough reflex. Usually when the child first goes home, the hospital routine of irrigation every three or four hours is followed, but the child may rapidly adapt to the family routine and sleep through the night.

Suction Technique. Whenever possible, the child should be encouraged to cough and clear accumulated mucus. However, when suctioning is necessary, the catheter should be inserted past the end of the tracheotomy tube. The catheter is usually occluded so suction is not applied as it is inserted; it is then withdrawn slowly with a rotating motion, using suction to clear the airway. The catheter should be rinsed in saline solution after each aspiration. The duration of suctioning should be not more than 30 seconds as the child may become hypoxic if it is prolonged.

Percussion. Usually when the child first goes home, chest physiotherapy is continued on the same routine as it was in the hospital. However, after a child develops a strong cough reflex, percussion usually becomes necessary less frequently if at all.

Changing The Tube. This is probably the most traumatic problem of the home program. It is mandatory that at least two adults be present when the tube is changed. It is especially important when the child first goes home and as the child becomes older and stronger and may resist the tube change. Parents can expect the child to become tense and cough or cry as a normal protest. The frequency of changing the tube will depend upon the child's age, the amount of secretions, and the type of tube used. With most of the newer silicone rubber tubes, weekly changes are sufficient. It behooves the parent to discover the best time to change the tube. Generally, it is advisable to avoid meal times. Occasionally, it is desirable to arouse the child from a deep sleep and change the tube before he or she fully awakens. The tube change is accomplished by having one of the parents position the child so that the neck can be seen clearly. Good lighting is essential. The child can be wrapped in a towel or sheet to restrain the arms and legs, and the shoulders should be elevated to hyperextend the neck. All the necessary equipment for the tube change should be available as well as emergency equipment. The tube is removed by cutting the tape holding the tube and allowing the child to cough it out, or it may be removed by the attendant. The new tube is quickly inserted. It is important that a smaller tube be readily available in case the tube of the same size as that which was removed cannot be reinserted. It is also desirable to have an emergency, small and longer tube, such as an endotracheal tube, available to establish an airway if the tracheotomy tube cannot be inserted. In children who resist the tube change by tightening their neck muscles, it may be necessary to use a length of catheter as a guide for insertion of the tube; about a six inch length of catheter is inserted into the stoma, which will usually cause the child to cough, thus relaxing the neck muscles. The tracheotomy tube to be inserted can then be threaded over this catheter and the catheter guide removed.

Skin Care. Usually after a tracheotomy has been established the area will epithelialize, and minimal skin care is necessary. However, areas of irritation may develop beneath the tube. These can usually be cleaned with cotton balls and a preparation containing hexachlorophene (pHisoHex). Occasionally antibiotic ointment is desirable, and, in some cases, if granulation tissue develops around the tube, antibiotic ointments with steroids are of value. The care of the tube will depend upon the material from which it is constructed; however, as soon as the tube is removed, it is usually wise to clean it with pipe cleaners and to soak it in germicide solution, or if the tube is made of metal to boil it for five minutes.

Adjustment to Tracheotomy

The physicians must help the parents accept the tracheotomy and its aftercare responsibilities. Despite adequate explanations prior to surgery and obvious airway improvement postoperatively, the initial appearance of the newly tracheotomized child is a shock to the parents. Their fear is eased through adequate explanations, which many times must be repeated and reinforced. The child's loss of voice can cause extreme emotional distress, and the parents must be reassured that it is not permanent. When the child goes home, it is important to emphasize that care of the child should be shared by all members of the family and that a certain amount of emotional stress is inevitable for a task that requires 24 hours a day, 7 days a week.

It is important to emphasize to the family that relatives and friends may not understand the operation and that they may ask questions that seem indiscreet. Usually, the adjustment occurs rapidly and satisfactorily. It is important that the child should attempt to live as normal a life as possible. There should be little restriction on active play, although obviously the child should be watched around sandboxes and swimming pools.

Helpful Hints

During bathing it is important that the child not be permitted to submerge himself or herself, and during hair washing water must be kept from the tracheotomy. Spray attachments for the faucet are valuable for rinsing the hair.

Clothing. Turtleneck sweaters and blouses may not be advisable, but thin scarves or loosely knit bibs may be of value, especially on windy days, to prevent particles from entering the trachea.

Feeding. Feeding by breast, bottle, or spoon is usually a problem. However, when the child begins to feed himself or herself, a small bib over the neck may keep food from falling into the tracheotomy tube.

Sleeping. If possible, the parents should maintain their normal sleeping arrangements and should install a portable intercom between the child's room and their own. Bells attached to the child's bed or to the child's limbs will usually warn of distress. The reason for this is that the child in respiratory distress will not lie quietly but will thrash around and create noise from the attached bells.

Traveling. It is possible to carry an aspirator or a hand suction unit when traveling. Usually the aspirator can be connected to the current of service stations, toll booths on expressways, or other business establishments. For traveling on airplanes, permission forms from physicians may be required, and permission from the airline may be necessary.

Schooling. Children with tracheotomies may attend public schools, but each child should be considered as an individual problem. Parents may need a letter from the physician stating that the child may attend school. In most instances, this is sufficient, although a call to the school nurse by the physician may be necessary.

Entertainment. It is important that a third person be trained to take care of the child. One of the major difficulties that parents have is the inability to leave home for entertainment purposes. The physician should encourage the family to entertain and seek entertainment as they normally would. As the child adapts to the tracheotomy, the care of the tracheotomy becomes more routine, and it is usually possible for parents to assume a more normal lifestyle.

Detection of Complications. Complications of tracheotomy may be evidenced by changes in the color and consistency of the mucus. Unusual sounds may herald difficulty because of airway obstruction, with coughing or wheezing if there is a foreign body in the tracheobronchial tree. Unusual odors may arise from the wound site if the tube needs to be changed, and irritation around the skin with development of granuloma or bleeding may be due to irritation from the tracheotomy tube or superficial skin infections.

Emergency Procedures

It is important that adequate preparation for emergencies be made prior to the child's discharge from the hospital. The community police department, fire department, or ambulance or rescue squad should be contacted to ascertain the best source of equipment and personnel in case there is a respiratory emergency. Telephone numbers for the best sources of this equipment should be posted in plain view near the home telephone. The names of the emergency physician and the residents in otolaryngology or pediatrics services in the hospital should be available to the parents, and the child's doctor's telephone numbers should be posted in several places throughout the house. If the child lives a fair distance from the hospital, it is wise to have several local physicians know about the child so that they might respond in case of emergency. Spare keys to the family's car should be located near the door to save time in the event that the keys are misplaced. The parents should be taught mouth-to-mouth resuscitation as well as provided with a large catheter or endotracheal tube that may be inserted into the stoma for resuscitation.

Electric failure may present some problems. It is necessary, therefore, to have emergency suction equipment available, and, in some instances, it is advisable to notify the local electric company that the residents should be on a priority panel in case of power failure. Parents should know where emergency power is available; in many communities the fire department has a mobile generator that is adaptable to house current.

Checklist for Home Care

The steps to arranging for home care are: (1) instruct parents in tracheotomy techniques, (2) notify referring physicians and other agencies that the patient is to be discharged, (3) arrange home care service contacts such as a visiting nurse and have agencies evaluate the home for its ability to care for the child, (4) assemble appropriate equipment, (5) have parents provide tracheotomy care within the hospital setting, (6) evaluate and arrange for emergency care, and (7) arrange for appropriate follow-up care after discharge.

REFERENCES

Aberdeen, E., and Downes, J. J. 1974. Artificial airways in children. Surg. Clin. North Am., 54:1155–1170.

Attia, R. R., Battit, G. E., and Murphy, J. D. 1975. Transtracheal ventilation. J.A.M.A., 234:1152–1153.

Bain, J. A. 1972. Late complications of tracheostomy and prolonged endotracheal intubation. Int. Anesthesiol. Clin., Fall, 225–244.

Baker, D. C., and Savetsky, L. 1972. Decannulation problems in infants. Ann. Otol. Rhinol. Laryngol., 81:555–557.

Bigler, J. A., Holinger, P. H., Johnston, K. C., et al. 1954. Tracheotomy in infancy. Pediatr., 13:476–485.

Bonanno, P. C. 1971. Swallowing dysfunction after tracheostomy. Ann. Surg., 174:29–33.

Cameron, J. L., Reynolds, J., and Zuidema, G. D. 1973. Aspiration in patients with tracheostomies. Surg. Gynecol. Obstet., 136:68–70.

Cohen, S. R., Eavey, R. D., Desmond, M. S., et al. 1977. Endoscopy and tracheotomy in the neonatal period. Ann. Otol. Rhinol. Laryngol., 86:577–583.

Dane, T. E. B., and King, E. G. 1975. A prospective study of complications after tracheostomy for assisted ventilation. Chest, 67:398–404.

Davidson, I. A., Cruickshank, A. N., Duthie, W. H., et al. 1971. Lesions of the trachea following tracheostomy and endotracheal intubation. Proc. Roy. Soc. Med., 64:26–30.

Davies, I. J., and Belam, O. H. 1967. Mini-tracheostomy. Practitioner, 199:76–77.

Diamant, H., Kinnman, J., and Okmian, L. 1961. Decannulation in children. Laryngoscope, 71:404–414.

Dorland's Illustrated Medical Dictionary, 25th ed. 1974. Philadelphia, W.B. Saunders Co., p. 1626.

Douglas, G. S., Hoskins, D., and Stool, S. E. 1978. Tracheotomy in pediatric airway management. ENT J., 57:55–70.

Eckhauser, F. E., Billtoe, J., Burke, J. F., et al. 1974. Tracheostomy complicating massive burn injury: A plea for conservatism. Am. J. Surg., 127:418–423.

Fearon, B., and Whalen, J. S. 1967. Tracheal dimensions in the living infant. Ann. Otol. Rhinol. Laryngol., 76:965–974.

Forbes, G. B., Salmon, G., and Herweg, J. C. 1947. Further observations on post-tracheotomy, mediastinal emphysema and pneumothorax. Pediatr., 31:172–194.

Freeland, A. P., Wright, J. L. W., and Ardran, G. M. 1974. Developmental influences of infant tracheostomy. J. Laryngol. Otol., 88:927–936.

Friedberg, J., and Morrison, M. D. 1974. Pediatric tracheotomy. Can. J. Otolaryngol., 3:147–155.

Friman, L., Hedenstierna, G., and Schildt, B. 1976. Stenosis following tracheostomy. Anesthesia, 31:479–493.

Galloway, T. C. 1943. Tracheotomy in bulbar poliomyelitis. J.A.M.A., *123*:1096–1097.

Galvis, A. G., Stool, S. E., and Bluestone, C. D. 1980. Pulmonary edema following relief of acute upper airway obstruction. Ann. Otol. Rhinol. Laryngol., *89*:124–128.

Gibson, R., and Byrne, J. E. T. 1972. Tracheotomy in neonates. Laryngoscope, *82*:643–650.

Goldberg, J. D., Mitchell, N., and Angrist, A. 1942. Mediastinal emphysema and pneumothorax following tracheotomy for croup. Am. J. Surg., *56*:448–454.

Goodall, E. W. 1934. The story of tracheotomy. Br. J. Child. Dis., *31*:167–273.

Gray, L. P. 1960. Infant tracheostomy. J. Laryngol. Otol., *74*:145–154.

Greene, N. M. 1959. Fatal cardiovascular and respiratory failure associated with tracheotomy. N. Engl. J. Med., *261*:846–848.

Greenway R. E. 1972. Tracheostomy: Surgical problems and complications. Int. Anesthesiol. Clin., *10*:151–172.

Harley, H. R. S. 1971. Laryngotracheal obstruction complicating tracheostomy or endotracheal intubation with assisted respiration. Thorax, *26*:493–533.

Harley, H. R. S. 1972. Ulcerative tracheo-oesophageal fistula during treatment by tracheostomy and intermittent positive pressure ventilation. Thorax, *27*:338–352.

Hatcher, C. R. Abbott, O. A., Logan, W. D., Jr., et al. 1967. Tracheostomy in infancy and childhood. South Med. J., *60*:411–415.

Hawkins, D. B., and Williams, E. H. 1976. Tracheostomy in infants and young children. Laryngoscope, *86*:331–340.

Holinger, P. H., Brown, W. T., and Maurizi, D. G. 1965. Tracheostomy in the newborn. Am. J. Surg., *109*:771–779.

Hughes, R. K., Davenport, C., and Williamson, H. 1967. Needle tracheostomy — further evaluation. Arch. Surg., *95*:295–296.

Jackson, C. 1921. High tracheotomy and other errors — the chief causes of chronic laryngeal stenosis. Surg. Gynecol. Obstet., *32*:392–398.

Jacobs, H. B. 1972. Emergency percutaneous transtracheal catheter and ventilator. J. Trauma, *12*:50–55.

Jacoby, J. J., Hamelberg, W., Ziegler, C. H., et al. 1956. Transtracheal resuscitation. J.A.M.A., *162*:625–628.

Jaffee, I. S. 1963. Tracheostomy in infancy. Laryngoscope, *73*:1336–1343.

Johnson, D. G., and Stewart, D. R. 1975. Management of acquired tracheal obstructions in infancy. J. Pediatr. Surg., *10*:709–717.

Kaler, J., and Kaler, H. 1974. Michael had a tracheostomy. Am. J. Nurs., *74*:852–855.

Lawrence, R. A., and Bailey, B. J. 1971. A review of experience in pediatric tracheotomy. South. Med. J. *64*:1049–1055.

Lehmann, W. B. 1974. Bilateral pneumothorax five days after tracheotomy decannulation. Ann. Otol. Rhinol. Laryngol., *83*:128.

Louhimo, I., Grahne, B., Pasila, M., and Suutarinen, T. 1971. Acquired laryngotracheal stenosis in children. J. Pediatr. Surg., *6*:730–737.

MacLachlan, R. F. 1969. Decannulation in infancy. J. Laryngol. Otol., *83*:991–1003.

Marcy, J. H., and Cook, D. R. 1975. Pediatric anesthesiology. *In* Practice of Surgery, Chap. 22. Hagerstown, MD, Harper and Row.

Mathog, R. H., Kenan, P. D., and Hudson, W. R. 1971. Delayed massive hemorrhage following tracheostomy. Laryngoscope, *81*:107–119.

Murphy, D. A., and Popkin, J. 1971. Tracheal collapse in tracheostomized infants: Resistance in reference to flow rates in a variety of tracheostomy tubes. J. Pediatr. Surg., *6*:314–323.

Oppenheimer, P. 1977. Needle tracheotomy. ORL Digest, *39*:9–10.

Pickard, R. E., and Oropeza, G. 1971. Tracheotomy in premature infants. Laryngoscope, *81*:418–422.

Potondi, A. 1969. Pathomechanism of hemorrhages following tracheotomy. J. Laryngol. Otol., *83*:475–484.

Rabuzzi, D., and Reed, G. F. 1971. Intrathoracic complications following tracheotomy in children. Laryngoscope, *81*:939–946.

Rogers, L. A., and Osterhout, S. 1970. Pneumonia following tracheostomy. Am. Surg., *36*:39–46.

Rosnagle, R. S., and Yanagisawa, E. 1969. Aerophagia: An unrecognized complication of tracheotomy. Arch. Otolaryngol., *89*:537–539.

Samaan, H. A. 1970. Benign tracheal stenosis. Br. J. Surg., *57*:909–913.

Sasaki, C. T., Gaudet, P. T., and Peerless, A. 1978. Tracheostomy decannulation. Am. J. Dis. Child., *132*:266–269.

Schild, J. A. 1970. Tracheostomy care. Int. Anesthesiol. Clin., *8*:649–654.

Schloss, M. D. 1972. Laryngeal and tracheal complications following prolonged intubation and tracheostomy. Can. J. Otolaryngol., *1*:135–140.

Smythe, P. M. 1966. Tracheotomy for the neonate. Int. Anesthesiol. Clin., *44*:427–434.

Stool, S. E., and Tucker, J. 1972. Larynx, trachea and endoscopy. *In* Brennemann's Practice of Pediatrics. Chap 48. Hagerstown, MD, Harper and Row.

Stool, S. E., Campbell, J. R., and Johnson, D. G. 1968. Tracheostomy in children: The use of plastic tubes. J. Pediatr. Surg., *3*:402–407.

Stool, S. E., and Beebe, J. K. 1973. Tracheotomy in infants and children. Current Problems in Pediatrics, Vol. III, No. 5. Chicago, Year Book Medical Pub.

Tucker, J. A., and Silberman, H. D. 1972. Tracheotomy in pediatrics. Ann. Otol. Rhinol. Laryngol., *81*:818–824.

Utley, J. R., Singer, M. M., Roe, B. B., et al. 1972. Definitive management of innominate artery hemorrhage complicating tracheostomy. J.A.M.A., *220*:577–579.

Vilinskas, J., and Schweizer, R. T. 1968. The needle tracheostomy: Re-evaluation. Med. Times, *96*:1218–1222.

Westgate, H. D., and Roux, K. L. 1970. Tracheal stenosis following tracheostomy: Incidence and predisposing factors. Anesth. Analg., *49*:393–401.

Wind, J. 1971. Reflections on difficult decannulation. Arch. Otolaryngol., *94*:426–431.

Chapter 74

INTENSIVE CARE OF RESPIRATORY DISORDERS

Antonio G. Galvis, M.D.
Jessica K. Lewis, M.D.

This chapter presents practical information for the physician managing the intensive care of respiratory illness; techniques for diagnosis and evaluation of specific disease entities are presented elsewhere. It is hoped that the following information may serve as a useful guideline in caring for a child with a severe respiratory disorder.

ASSESSMENT OF RESPIRATORY DISTRESS

In order to manage adequately those respiratory disorders that require intensive care, the physician must be able to evaluate accurately the severity of the respiratory distress. The accurate assessment and appropriate prompt treatment of respiratory distress will decrease the morbidity and mortality rates of the condition and prevent a child from slipping subtly into a catastrophic state.

Clinical Evaluation

Respiratory failure is a common clinical end-state of a variety of illnesses. Children with respiratory distress resulting from neuromuscular, cardiac, airway, or pulmonary parenchymal pathology will have many common clinical manifestations.

The observer's initial overall impression of a child with respiratory distress can yield valuable information. A child with decreased *activity*, who does not relate to the environment, who does not respond to pain, and who shows decreased muscle tone, is in immediate need of respiratory assistance. As hypercarbia and hypoxia affect brain function, the patient passes from the stage of restlessness to lethargy and finally to coma.

Observation of the *facies* of a child with severe respiratory embarrassment also can be helpful. Quite often small infants express anxiety in their wide-eyed, frightened facies. Central cyanosis that does not clear with 40 per cent oxygen by inhalation is either cardiac in origin or represents a severe pulmonary pathologic condition. If respiratory causes for cyanosis exist, such cyanosis is an ominous sign, and the child should be monitored carefully. Other clinical signs of respiratory embarrassment that may be noted in the face are flaring of the nasal alae, head bobbing, diaphoresis, use of accessory neck muscles of respiration, and "fish-mouth" breathing.

Chest expansion is an important index in gauging the severity of respiratory distress. With obstruction of the airways, the expiratory phase of respiration becomes prolonged, and the respiratory cycle is no longer regular. Retractions of the intercostal and subcostal muscles can be seen clearly in infants and small children, since their chest walls are elastic and readily reflect changes in intrathoracic pressures. The resting respiratory rate is a sensitive index of pulmonary function and should be measured with the child asleep and undisturbed. Newborns have a rate of about 40 to 50 breaths per minute; this decreases with age, so that a two year old has a rate of about 20 breaths per minute. With respiratory distress, tachypnea, which increases minute ventilation to improve gas exchange, is a major compensatory mechanism.

Observation of the *abdomen* and chest movements together during the respiratory cycle can be used as a clinical index of diaphragmatic function and of the severity of respiratory distress. In a patient with a history of birth trauma, a thoracic operation, or neurologic disorders, the possibility of phrenic nerve palsy with diaphragmatic paralysis should be considered as a cause of respiratory distress. If the paralysis is unilateral, a rocking type of movement of the chest and abdomen will be visible with inspiration. As the chest expands, the abdomen will paradoxically be sucked inward and upward, and on the side of the paralysis the lower anterolateral costal margin will expand outward. This inward movement is most evident in the supine position, where the action of gravity assists displacement of the abdominal contents and the flaccid diaphragm into the thorax, resulting in more marked paradoxic movement of the abdominal wall and further ventilatory embarrassment.

Noises generated by severe respiratory disorders are well-known to the clinician. Stridor will be discussed elsewhere in this text. (Chap. 64). No discussion of respiratory failure would be complete without a mention of grunting respirations. The grunt signifies closure of the glottis, with the patient creating a positive expiratory pressure in order to stabilize his or her alveoli and small airways

(Harrison, 1968). The importance of the grunt cannot be overlooked. If an artificial airway is inserted into a patient without also providing some positive airway pressure during expiration, the patient's degree of oxygenation may deteriorate rapidly. Bradycardia, hypotension, or both are late signs presaging respiratory arrest.

Laboratory Evaluation

Many complex and detailed methods of assessing pulmonary function are available, but these tests are often dependent on the patient's putting forth effort and are too cumbersome to be carried out on the small, critically ill child. Assessment of these patients should be limited mainly to the evaluation of basic laboratory data (Table 74–1).

The single most important test of respiratory efficiency remains the measurement of *arterial blood gas* levels. The sample may be obtained by arterial puncture, digital artery stick, or arterialized capillary stick. A capillary sample should be drawn from a free-flowing stab wound of the toe, heel, or finger warmed to 37° C and free of air bubbles. It must be cautioned, however, that measurements of these parameters in patients with hypoperfusion generally will be inaccurate because of peripheral vascular stasis. Values for Pco_2 and pH in capillary samples will closely approximate those in arterial samples, but the Po_2 values will be unreliable above 60 mm Hg. A direct arterial sample will be necessary

Table 74–1 APPROXIMATE NORMAL LABORATORY VALUES FOR RESPIRATORY ASSESSMENT

Parameter	Newborn Infant	Older Infant and Child
Respiratory frequency (breaths/minute)	40–60	20–30 (to 6 years) 15–20 (over 6 years)
Tidal volume (ml/kg)	5–6	7–8
Arterial blood pH	7.30–7.40	7.30–7.40 (to 2 years) 7.35–7.45 (over 2 years)
Pco_2 (mm Hg)	30–35	30–35 (to 2 years) 35–45 (over 2 years)
HCO_3 (mEq/l liter)	20–22	20–22 (to 2 years) 22–24 (over 2 years)
Po_2 (mm Hg)	60–90	80–100
Heart rate (beats/minute)		100–180 (to 3 years) 70–150 (over 3 years)
Blood pressure (mm Hg) Systolic	60–90	75–130 (to 3 years) 90–140 (over 3 years)
Diastolic	30–60	45–90 (to 3 years) 50–80 (over 3 years)

if the Pa_{O_2} value must be determined. When serial measurements are necessary, an indwelling arterial line should be placed in a radial, temporal, or dorsalis pedis artery (Galvis et al., 1972). Even in small infants, arterial lines can be placed percutaneously with a No. 22 gauge Teflon catheter; however, when this is not technically feasible, the catheter may be inserted via an arterial cutdown.

Transcutaneous oxygen monitoring, a technique developed within the past seven years, is reliable, safe, and extremely useful during initiation of respiratory assistance and during the adjustments necessary when prolonged respiratory assistance is mandatory. Monitoring is accomplished by means of transcutaneous sensor, a polarographic cell modeled after the Clark cell, which is used in blood gas analyzers. The time needed to stabilize a child and the number of blood samples that are taken are greatly reduced. The information obtained with this system has had a profound effect on patterns of care, especially in those patients who are very unstable and in whom it is difficult and risky to maintain an indwelling catheter (Huch, 1976).

Even more important than obtaining a satisfactory sample is the interpretation of the arterial blood gas results. By strictest definition, hypoxia is a Pa_{O_2} of less than 90 mm Hg, but for practical purposes no serious tissue hypoxia exists when the Pa_{O_2} is maintained at a level above 50 mm Hg. The level of Pa_{O_2} varies normally with age and follows a bell-shaped curve, with the highest values in the teenage years and the lowest values at the extremes of life. Thus, a newborn normally has a Pa_{O_2} of about 70 mm Hg, as does a 60 year old adult; a 7 year old child and a 45 year old man would both be expected to have a Pa_{O_2} of about 90 mm Hg (Mansell, 1972). The real significance of the Pa_{O_2} is in its relation to the fractional concentration of inspired oxygen ($F_I O_2$), which is an indicator of the efficiency of oxygenation.

The *alveolar–arterial gradient for oxygen* (A–aD_{O_2}) is a reflection of ventilation–perfusion inequality, venous admixture, diffusion barriers, or a combination of these (Bates et al., 1971). Complex formulas are used to determine the A–a gradient, but a simplified approximation of the A–aD_{O_2} can be used at any $F_I O_2$ and rapidly determined at the patient's bedside. The "rule of seven" can be used to calculate the inspired oxygen tension ($P_I O_2$) so

that the $P_I O_2$ in millimeters of mercury is equal to the per cent of O_2 multiplied by seven. Thus, for 40 per cent O_2, the $P_I O_2$ is 40×7 or 280 mm Hg. The A–aD_{O_2} is the alveolar tension of O_2 minus the arterial tension of O_2. Thus, A–aD_{O_2} (per cent $O_2 \times 7$ – Pa_{CO_2}) – Pa_{O_2}. Stated another way, the A–$aD_O \approx F_I O_2 \times 7 - (Pa_{O_2} + Pa_{CO_2})$ when the alveolar tension of O_2 (PA_{O_2}) is derived from the alveolar–air equation, $PA_{O_2} = PI_{O_2} - (PA_{CO_2} \times 1/R)$ when R (which is the respiratory quotient) is one (Graef and Cone, 1974).

As an example, if a patient has a Pa_{O_2} of 65 mm Hg and a Pa_{CO_2} of 40 mm Hg while ventilating with an $F_I O_2$ of 0.4 or 40 per cent O_2, then the A–$aD_{O_2} = 40 \times 7 - (65 + 40) = 175$ mm Hg. Thus, although the value of 65 mm Hg for the Pa_{O_2} is adequate, the patient's Pa_{O_2} should have been close to 200 to 215 mm Hg when he was breathing 40 per cent O_2.

When interpreting the A–a gradient, normal right-to-left shunts of 5 to 10 per cent secondary to the thebesian veins and bronchial circulation must be subtracted. Of course, other factors, such as intracardiac right-to-left shunts, can also affect the A–a gradient. When hemodynamic states are normal, however, the A–a gradient can be used as a reflection of pulmonary efficiency.

The degree of *hemoglobin oxygen saturation* is an important index to follow in respiratory distress and becomes especially significant when dealing with high concentrations of oxygen. In general, a saturation of about 85 per cent will be sufficient to maintain normal cellular metabolism. However, many factors can alter the oxyhemoglobin dissociation curve. For instance, acidosis shifts the curve to the right and alkalosis to the left. Thus, alkalosis will have a detrimental effect on the ability of hemoglobin to give up oxygen to the tissues. Although acidosis is beneficial for oxygen unloading, greater degrees of acidosis (pH less than 7.25) can have a deleterious effect on pulmonary vasculature and systemic vascular resistance.

In carbon monoxide poisoning, hemoglobin saturation cannot accurately be judged from the Pa_{O_2} value because of the strong affinity of carbon monoxide for hemoglobin. Thus, in cases of carbon monoxide poisoning, the exact blood level of carbon monoxide must be determined since the concentration of carbon monoxide will describe the degree to which the oxyhemoglobin dissociation curve is shifted to the left of normal. To improve the oxygen-carrying capacity of blood in cases of severe respiratory insufficiency, the hemoglobin level should be maintained at a minimum of 13 grams per cent by means of transfusions of fresh, packed red cells. In addition, an increase in the concentration of 2,3-diphosphoglycerate (2,3-DPG) will maximize oxygen release at the tissue level by decreasing the affinity of hemoglobin for oxygen. These factors are particularly important to remember when dealing with premature and small infants of less than 6 months of age, since fetal hemoglobin has lower concentrations of 2,3-DPG than does adult hemoglobin (Delivoria-Papadopoulous et al., 1971).

The $Paco_2$ remains the best indicator of alveolar ventilation but must be evaluated in relation to the minute ventilation. Assuming a constant rate of CO_2 production, there is an inverse relationship between the volume of alveolar ventilation and the $Paco_2$; thus, if the minute ventilation doubles, the $Paco_2$ is decreased by 50 per cent. In cases of hypercarbia, the physician must determine whether the elevated Pco_2 is acute or chronic. If the Pco_2 is elevated in the presence of a normal plasma bicarbonate level and acidosis, the respiratory problem is acute and demands immediate care. However, if the Pco_2 is elevated, but the pH is normal and the bicarbonate level is elevated, the patient probably has pulmonary disease of longer standing, which requires less critical evaluation and treatment.

The *pH* of arterial blood is significant as a measurement of respiratory acidosis or alkalosis. With respiratory acidosis resulting from hypoventilation, hypertension develops secondary to the release of catecholamines. If this condition is not relieved promptly, hypotension ensues; because of the continous release of catecholamines, marked peripheral vasoconstriction and lactic acidosis can develop. Hypercarbia will cause an increase in cerebral blood flow with the potential complication of increased intracranial pressure. However, the most life-threatening pH alteration occurs with profound circulatory collapse and respiratory failure. In this condition, severe respiratory and metabolic acidosis develop rapidly. As tissue perfusion fails, the pH falls below 7.0, and epinephrine and norepinephrine are released at increased rates; however, they are unable to act upon the heart, the peripheral blood vessels dilate, and cardiac rhythmicity is also impaired (Fenn and Bahn, 1965).

Another laboratory value useful to measure in the acutely ill patient with respiratory insufficiency is the *mixed venous* Pao_2. If a patient has a pulmonary artery catheter in place, then comparison of the mixed venous partial O_2 tension (P_{VO_2}) and Pao_2 is helpful in estimating the adequacy of tissue oxygen tension. Normally P_{VO_2} should be about 30 to 40 mm Hg. If the value is much lower, either the oxygen supply to the tissues has been reduced or there has been an increase in the demand of tissues for oxygen (Finch and Lenfant, 1972).

Other simple pulmonary function tests can be used to assess the patient when more than arterial blood gases are needed. The *inspiratory effort* is a good gauge of ventilatory reserve and is especially useful in pediatrics since no cooperation is needed from the patient. The inspiratory effort is a measure of the maximal subatmospheric pressure that the patient is able to generate against an occluded airway during a 10 to 20 second test. Generally speaking, if the inspiratory effort is greater than −20 cm H_2O, a patient has the neuromuscular capability to breathe spontaneously.

Measurements of *tidal volume* and *vital capacity* also can serve as guides for intervention in respiratory distress or for weaning from ventilatory support. Normally a patient's vital capacity is about five times the tidal volume. When the vital capacity approaches three times the tidal volume, a patient's reserve of ventilatory effort and ability to cough deeply are seriously impaired. For example, as the vital capacity of a patient with neuromuscular disease falls below three times the tidal volume, the patient must be watched carefully; as the vital capacity approaches tidal volume, the patient will require ventilatory support (Bendixen et al., 1965).

Roentgenographic examination of the chest is invaluable in assessing respiratory distress. A number of life-threatening conditions are readily diagnosed by this means. The presence of extrapulmonary air, massive effusions, lung collapse, and pulmonary edema can all be diagnosed by chest radiographs. In addition, the tip of the endotracheal or tracheostomy tube can be visualized to determine its optimal placement about the midtrachea. Radiographs are also helpful in severe respiratory disorders: Dynamic inspiratory and expiratory films may assess normal diaphragmatic position and may demonstrate evidence of pulmonary air trapping from an airway obstruction.

RESPIRATORY CARE

A few basic principles of respiratory care apply to all patients with pulmonary disease. For instance, if a child with upper airway obstruction with an endotracheal tube in place is left unattended and no basics of respiratory care are provided, pulmonary secretions soon will accumulate, atelectasis will result, ventilation–perfusion inequalities will follow, and finally there will be life-threatening hypoxia. Although management of the intensely ill child will vary somewhat depending on whether the respiratory distress is secondary to congestive heart failure or follows a thoracic operation or distal airway obstruction, certain unalterable principles of sound respiratory care will be common to all patients.

Patients in respiratory failure require frequent turning and *repositioning* to prevent compression atelectasis, vascular congestion, and unilateral pulmonary edema of the dependent lung. Patients with respiratory distress should be nursed in a semi-sitting position as much as possible in order to maximize the functional residual capacity and to allow the diaphragm to perform at optimal efficiency. In the supine position the hydrostatic forces of the abdomen are transmitted to the chest by pushing the diaphragm higher into the chest and decreasing the functional residual capacity. Furthermore, in the supine position the hydrostatic pressure of the abdominal contents is greatest posteriorly near the spine, so that pulmonary ventilation is directed first to the upper lung, where hydrostatic forces are less, and the dependent lung perfusion increases markedly owing to the forces of gravity. The result is ventilation-perfusion mismatching and consequent hypoxia. Although it is often technically difficult to assume, the prone position can improve ventilation of dependent areas of the lung by minimizing the encroachment of intra-abdominal contents on the thoracic space (Froese and Bryan, 1974).

The rationale for the use of *physical therapy* is the loosening of pulmonary secretions that would otherwise increase airway resistance and promote atelectasis (Mellins, 1974). Even a small mucous plug can decrease the radius of a child's distal airway by one half and increase the resistance 16 times, resulting in a marked increase in the work involved in breathing and oxygen consumption. Therefore, physical therapy is essential at least twice every eight hours for patients who have abundant secretions or who are unable to remove secretions from their airways spontaneously. An essential element of pulmonary physical therapy is vigorous chest cupping with the patient placed appropriately to drain each major lobe bronchus. Also useful in loosening secretions is vibration of the chest, either with a mechanical vibrator or by a manual "vibratory squeeze." These maneuvers are carried out by placing one hand over each side of the chest; with mechanical vibrator or opposing hand the chest is simultaneously vibrated and squeezed after a deep inspiration. If the patient has an artificial airway, this deep inspiration can be accomplished manually by using an Ambu bag. With repetitive vibratory squeezes, air in the lung forces secretions up and out of the small airways into the major bronchi where they can be reached by suction catheters.

If the patient can cough up the secretions loosened by physical therapy, then *suctioning* of the oral pharynx is sufficient. However, when the patient cannot force the secretions to the pharynx, direct tracheal suctioning is necessary. If a patient is intubated, hyperoxygenation with a bag and 100 per cent O_2 for three to five minutes should be carried out through the endotracheal tube. Gentle bagging is required to promote adequate ventilation past the mucous plugs without driving the plugs deeper into the distal airways. Using the single-glove sterile technique, 1 to 5 cc of sterile saline (depending on the age of the child), with no preservative added, is instilled through a catheter into the trachea and aimed at either mainstem bronchus by turning the head to the contralateral side (Williams and Galvis, 1974). The catheter used to instill the saline should be disposable and small in diameter so that it will reach as distally into the airways as possible. Now the patient is again bagged with oxygen, and the vibratory squeeze is employed every other breath for a total of 10 ventilatory cycles in an attempt to liquefy the mucus with saline. The suction catheter is then inserted past the tip of the endotracheal tube, and suction of about 15 mm Hg is applied to the catheter. If possible, the suction catheter should have a diameter less than 50 per cent of the diameter of the airway, with side and end holes. As the catheter is withdrawn rapidly, a twisting motion should be applied to enhance removal of secretions that may be clinging to the bronchial mucosa. The entire procedure is repeated with the head turned to the opposite side in an attempt to enter the other mainstem bronchus. Care should be taken to hyperoxygenate the patient prior to each instillation of saline and suctioning. If at any time the patient becomes dusky or bradycardiac, the procedure must immediately be stopped and the patient must be manually ventilated with 100 per cent O_2 until his or her clinical condition is stable. However, in the great majority of instances, any clinical deterioration usually is related to technical difficulties and not to the suctioning procedure itself.

If an artificial airway is not in place, safe, direct suctioning of the trachea can be carried out as well. The basic difference is that a catheter less than 30 per cent of the diameter of the airway is introduced into the trachea under direct laryngoscopy and left in place. The patients, usually infants, are given 100 per cent O_2 by mask and bag for at least three to five minutes before and after introduction of the catheter and saline instillation. The catheter usually induces coughing, which facilitates removal of secretions. The vibratory squeeze is performed with the catheter in place. Intermittent suction is then carried out through the catheter. This procedure should be repeated until secretions are markedly diminished as determined by auscultation. This method of suctioning is helpful, particularly in avoiding prolonged or repeated intubation in patients who might require an airway only for management of their secretions or during the critical first 24 to 48 hours after extubation. When a patient's trachea has been extubated, mobilization of secretions is often hampered by an ineffective cough, inability to approximate the vocal cords, subglottic edema, and tracheitis secondary to repeated suctioning and possible bacterial colonization of the tracheobronchial tree. If suctioning is needed more than twice in an eight hour period or for more than several days to maintain clear airways, reinsertion of the endotracheal tube may be necessary (Galvis et al., 1974).

Whenever oxygen or a mixture of gases is administered or when the natural humidifiers (the nose and nasopharynx) are bypassed by an artificial airway, these gases must be at least 70 per cent saturated with water vapor for adequate *humidification*. If the mucociliary blanket is exposed to gases that are less than 70 per cent saturated with water vapor, ciliary activity becomes impaired (Toremalm, 1961). It is important to realize that 70 per cent saturation refers to the relative humidity

at body temperature. This amounts to a total water content of approximately 30 mg per liter of air. At room temperature, 70 per cent relative humidity would describe an atmosphere with only 15 mg per liter, which at body temperature would give only 30 per cent relative humidity. What is important to proper functioning of the mucociliary escalator is the absolute water content, not the relative humidity, which refers to different water contents at different temperatures. Thus, a bubble humidifier provides 90 per cent relative humidity to the atmosphere within the chamber, but the temperature within the chamber is only 12° C. This produces a water content of only 10 mg water per liter of air and would offer no more than 20 per cent relative humidity when the air is heated to body temperature (Cushing et al., 1965).

Scientific data fail to support the widespread use of mist in respiratory therapy. Theory supports the use of a highly humid or mist atmosphere in the therapy of upper airway disease, but little benefit would appear to be derived from such therapy in diseases of the smaller airways and the lung parenchyma, since the amount of water that can be presented to these areas of the lung is negligible, and the problem of increased airway resistance is great.

Too often the importance of *systemic hydration* is either overlooked or overstressed. For instance, current recommendations for the treatment of asthma in children universally include administration of fluids as well in excess of those necessary for homeostasis. Although it is widely assumed that this step will help loosen secretions and make them less viscid, there are no studies to support this assumption. Vigorous fluid therapy may have two deleterious effects: an increase in the microvascular hydrostatic pressure and a decrease in the plasma colloid osmotic pressure. Both of these effects favor pulmonary edema formation, which is further enhanced when very high negative pleural pressures are transmitted to the interstitial space. Certainly, many patients in respiratory failure may be dehydrated when first seen, and their fluid deficits must be replaced. Thereafter, it would seem prudent to maintain the patient in as near normal water balance as possible (Stalcup and Mellins, 1977).

Many of the physiologic alterations present in acute respiratory failure occur as a result of hypoxia. *Oxygen* is therefore the most important therapeutic agent in managing this condition. Like any other drug, oxygen must be ordered and administered with care, and its effects must be observed carefully. By monitoring arterial blood gases, the Pao_2 should be maintained in the range of 60 to 90 mm Hg consistent with the lowest F_1O_2 possible. In newborns, slightly lower values of Pao_2, between 50 and 80 mm Hg, should be accepted in order to limit the risks of retrolental fibroplasia. In certain cases of carbon monoxide poisoning or severe metabolic alkalosis, the oxyhemoglobin dissociation curve is shifted to the left; simply measuring the Pao_2 in these cases is not sufficient to determine the degree of hypoxia. A more exact measurement of hemoglobin saturation is needed. In the majority of patients it is sufficient to monitor the Pao_2 every 30 to 60 minutes while significant physiologic and therapeutic changes are occurring. The F_1O_2 ideally should be maintained at 0.4 to 0.5, since there has been no evidence provided to indicate that oxygen toxicity occurs as a result of inspired oxygen concentrations in these ranges. However, if sufficient respiratory embarrassment is present to require an F_1O_2 of 0.6 or greater to maintain an acceptable Pao_2 and there is not a right-to-left intracardiac shunt, hypoxia often can be ameliorated by the judicious use of continuous distending airway pressure (CDAP) breathing.

The delivery of oxygen should be carried out with a blender system so that oxygen concentrations from 21 to 100 per cent can be selected. Frequent measurement of the oxygen concentration delivered to the patient should be carried out with an analyzer. The delivered oxygen should be warmed to at least 30° C and fully humidified so that it will provide approximately 70 per cent humidity at body temperature (Graff, 1975).

After the concentration, humidity, and temperature of the oxygen have been adjusted, many methods of delivery to the patient are available. In the small infant, the oxygen hood is a useful method of oxygen delivery that maintains a relatively constant environmental oxygen concentration. Indications for a mist tent are limited, and its use should be relegated to the delivery of moderate levels of inspired oxygen to an occasional restless child who will not permit any apparatus near his or her face. Face masks are commonly used in pediatric patients over the age of one year for delivery of oxygen. Nasal prongs have not been widely used in children, although occa-

sionally combative patients find the prongs much less threatening than a face mask. The disadvantages of this system are that the oxygen cannot be analyzed accurately or fully humidified.

Other means of oxygen therapy might be considered only when standard methods have failed to correct the hypoxia. Real indications for hyperbaric oxygenation rarely are seen in children; moreover, only a few major centers have the hyperbaric chambers to provide this mode of therapy. Another method of dealing with intractable hypoxemia is the use of an extracorporeal bypass with a membrane lung. At the moment, the complications of bleeding and the problems of selecting cases that might respond make this treatment modality more of research than of clinical interest.

Oxygen toxicity is a complex problem and is considered a genuine iatrogenic disease. Few well-documented cases of pure oxygen toxicity can be found in the literature; too often the evidence for oxygen toxicity is clouded by the underlying pulmonary process that necessitated the use of oxygen therapy, the numerous metabolic derangements of the critically ill patients, and the inaccuracy of the pathologic sample. However, oxygen toxicity does exist at high oxygen tensions and can be demonstrated in the lung, eye, brain, and kidney (Balentine, 1966). Pulmonary oxygen toxicity warrants attention because it is the symptom most commonly encountered in clinical practice, but the dangers of oxygen toxicity must be evaluated *vis-a-vis* the knowledge that sometimes oxygen therapy in high concentrations must be used clinically, since the effects of hypoxia are well established and drastic while the effects of oxygen toxicity still need to be fully elucidated.

The following statements can be made from currently available data: (1) there is no evidence that pulmonary oxygen toxicity develops with an F_1O_2 of 0.4 to 0.5, regardless of the duration of exposure; (2) no significant pulmonary toxicity occurs in patients breathing 100 per cent O_2 for less than 24 hours; (3) no evidence exists to imply that patients with underlying pulmonary disease develop oxygen toxicity faster than patients with normal lungs (Winter and Smith, 1972). In order to minimize the degree of any oxygen toxicity that may occur, the F_1O_2 should be kept as low as possible. No evidence exists to suggest that supranormal arterial oxygen tensions are beneficial, except in those instances where the pulmonary vasculature may be hyper-reactive to rapid decreases in F_1O_2. Every mode of therapy possible should be used to decrease the concentration and duration of oxygen administration, including optimal treatment of the underlying disease process, decreasing the shunt fraction and A–a gradient, maximizing effective ventilatory support, and appropriate treatment of abnormal metabolic states.

ASSISTED VENTILATION

Assisted ventilation can be considered a method of tiding a patient over a period of respiratory failure until the acute process has resolved. Since serious pulmonary disorders are associated with the majority of critically ill patients regardless of the underlying pathologic condition involved, the use of ventilators has become common in the intensive care unit. Little physiologic information is available on respiratory failure in children, but much information can be extrapolated from work done in newborns and adults. The management of assisted ventilation is based on physiologic knowledge; modifications in management can be made depending on the equipment and other resources available.

The first method of assisted ventilation to be discussed is spontaneous *continuous distending airway pressure* (CDAP) *breathing*. With this system, no ventilator is necessary. Often, this mode of therapy can be carried out without intubation of the trachea. Many variations of CDAP are available, but two methods mainly are applicable for children.

The first is nasopharyngeal CDAP. This is a modification of the nasal prongs, which were first widely used in newborns (Kattwinkel et al., 1973). An endotracheal tube is placed through the nostril to the level of the uvula in the posterior pharynx, and a constant flow of humidified oxygen and air is provided through the inhalation arm of the T-piece with the CDAP apparatus at the exhalation arm. CDAP may be delivered via commercially available values or by underwater immersion of the exhalation arm of a T-piece apparatus. The only major accessories necessary when setting up spontaneous CDAP are a constant source of a humidified mixture of gases, a method of providing resistance to exhalation, a reservoir, and a nonrebreathing circuit (Galvis and Benson, 1973). Care must be taken to secure the

nasopharyngeal tube in place just like an endotracheal tube and to insert a nasogastric tube to relieve gas that might accumulate in the stomach. If high levels of CDAP are required, or if CDAP cannot be maintained because the patient is crying excessively, then CDAP must be carried out through an artificial airway, either an endotracheal or a tracheostomy tube.

CDAP improves oxygenation by increasing the functional residual capacity and, possibly, by stabilizing the small airways and decreasing airway resistance (Gregory et al., 1975). With CDAP, the alveoli and small airways remain open during exhalation; perfusion of nonventilated areas of the lung is minimized, and less right-to-left shunting occurs. The other major benefit of CDAP results from the fact that the patient must be able to maintain his or her own respirations in order to use this method. Thus, the patient uses his or her own peripheral and central chemoreceptors, sets his or her own respiratory pattern, and uses the intercostal muscles and particularly the diaphragm; this helps to maintain adequate ventilation of basilar areas and avoids extremes of lung inflation and deflation, which may deplete the surfactant system.

The second method of ventilatory assistance is with *mechanical ventilators*. Ventilators can be classified according to how they end the inspiratory cycle. Thus, there are three basic types of ventilators: volume-limited, pressure-cycled, or time-cycled.

A volume-limited ventilator, e.g., Emerson, MAI, or Bournes, delivers a preset tidal volume. The resultant airway pressure depends on the mechanical properties of the ventilator and tubing and lung compliance. One advantage of a fixed volume ventilator is that despite changes in pulmonary compliance or resistance, the preset tidal volume will be delivered.

A pressure-cycled ventilator, e.g., Bird Mark VII or Bennett PR-2, ends the inspiratory phase when a predetermined pressure in the circuit of the ventilator is reached. However, the pressure in the alveoli that determines tidal volume is different from the cycling or airway pressure and even in normal lungs can vary by as much as 30 per cent. Thus, the tidal volume will decrease if the airway resistance increases or if the lung compliance decreases.

A time-cycled, flow-generated ventilator, e.g., Baby Bird or Bournes BP200, effectively is volume-cycled, since it supplies a fixed pattern of flow for a fixed time. Both the inspiratory (I) and expiratory (E) duration are independently adjustable, so that the I:E ratio can be preset. Because of the constant flow, the time-cycled ventilator is useful in weaning the patient to spontaneous breathing. In addition, the peak proximal airway pressure can be limited; thus, this type of ventilator can be used either as a pressure-limited or volume ventilator (Muskin et al., 1969).

The gap between controlled and spontaneous ventilation can be filled by intermittent mandatory ventilation (IMV) and by synchronized intermittent mandatory ventilation (SIMV). IMV permits the patient to breathe spontaneously with positive pressure breaths intermittently delivered by the ventilator. With this method, the patient benefits from the use of the respiratory muscles. The ventilator is used almost as a sigh mechanism, to help to inflate the lung fully intermittently, and to prevent atelectasis. The process of weaning is simplified, since the rate of the ventilator is gradually lowered while the patient takes over more and more of his or her own work of breathing (Kirby, 1975). With SIMV, positive pressure breaths are delivered *in phase* with the patient's own spontaneous ventilation. Thus, theoretically, SIMV has all the advantages of IMV plus the benefit of minimal elevation of intrathoracic pressure, which could compromise venous return and promote extrapleural air leaks (Shapiro et al., 1976). The "assist" mode of mechanical ventilator is rarely needed in children, but it may be indicated when inspiratory effort is insufficient during the transition from controlled to spontaneous ventilation.

Management of a Patient Requiring Mechanical Ventilation

Table 74–2 gives a glossary of terms used in this section.

Patient Selection. The first and most important step in mechanical ventilation is to decide which patient is an appropriate candidate. Criteria for the selection of patients have been outlined by Downes as respiratory failure in pulmonary, cardiac, or neurologic disease. Exceptions to these guidelines exist in patients with terminal chronic pulmonary disease, such as cystic fibrosis, in whom mechanical ventilation is of questionable value (Downes et al., 1972).

Table 74–2 GLOSSARY OF TERMS

MV	=	Mechanical Ventilation
CV	=	Controlled Ventilation
AV	=	Assisted Ventilation
SB	=	Spontaneous Breathing
IPPV	=	Intermittent Positive Pressure Ventilation
IPPB	=	Intermittent Positive Pressure Breathing
CPPV	=	Continuous Positive Pressure Ventilation
CPPB	=	Continuous Positive Pressure Breathing
PEEP	=	Positive End Expiratory Pressure
EPAP	=	Expiratory Positive Airway Pressure
IPAP	=	Inspiratory Positive Airway Pressure
CDAP	=	Continuous Distending Airway Pressure
IMV	=	Intermittent Mandatory Ventilation
IAV	=	Intermittent Assisted Ventilation
SIMV	=	Synchronized Intermittent Mandatory Ventilation

Airway. Table 74–3 shows specifications for pediatric orotracheal tube selections. The precise procedure to follow in orotracheal intubation has been covered in great detail in the section discussing nasotracheal intubation. Oral intubation is the procedure of choice in an emergency situation. Care must be taken to prevent hypoxia or aspiration while intubation is carried out, and the patient should be immobilized sufficiently to prevent damage to airway structures. If an artificial airway is anticipated to be in place for more than 24 hours, then a nasotracheal tube can be substituted for an orotracheal tube under controlled conditions. Nasotracheal intubation offers the advantages of better fixation of the tube and better access to oral and pharyngeal secretions. In general, the same-sized tube can be used since the diameters of the glottis and of the external nares are about the same. In the intensive care unit most intubations can be carried out with the patient awake or mildly sedated. However, if this cannot be done with ease, then succinylcholine (1 mg per kg) or pancuronium (0.1 mg per kg) can be used as a muscle relaxant, after adequate ventilation has been accomplished with bag and mask.

A tracheostomy should be performed when a patient requires mechanical ventilation for more than a week to minimize the complications of subglottic stenosis; in situations where airways may be compromised by secretions or blood, which impair gas exchange; or where upper airway obstruction or other conditions exist that make intubation from above infeasible.

Cuffed endotracheal or tracheostomy tubes are rarely needed in children. However, a cuffed tube may be necessary to protect

Table 74–3 OROTRACHEAL TUBE SPECIFICATIONS FOR THE
PEDIATRIC AGE GROUP*

Age Group	French Size	Internal Diameter (mm)	15-mm** Connector Size (mm I.D.)	Length (Oral) (cm)†
Newborn (1.0 kg)	11–12	2.5	3.0	10–11
Newborn (1.0 kg)	13–14	3.0	3.0–4.0	11–12
1–6 months	15–16	3.5	4.0	12–13
6–12 months	17–18	4.0	5.0	13
12–18 months	19–20	4.5	5.0	14
18–36 months	21–22	5.0	6.0	15
3–4 years	23–24	5.5	6.0	16
5–6 years	25	6.0	7.0	18
6–7 years	26	6.5	7.0	18
8–9 years	27–28	7.0	8.0	20
10–11 years	29–30	7.5	8.0	22
12–14 years	32–34	8.0	9.0	24

*Average size for age
**15 mm tapered connectors are recommended
†For nasotracheal intubation add 2 to 3 cm in length
Thin-walled, uncuffed, disposable polyvinyl chloride tubes that conform to A.N.S.I. Standard Z-79.1 and the
U.S.P. Animal Implantation Test is recommended.

the airway from aspiration or to provide adequate ventilation when significant air leaks occur around the tube with poor lung compliance, an excessively large trachea, or both. Cuffed tubes are now available for infants,* but care should be taken to use low inflation pressures so that as much tracheal damage as possible is avoided. Also important is the prevention of unnecessary tracheal pressure by the tip of the artificial airway. This may lead to complications, such as mucosal erosion, granuloma formation, or tracheomalacia. Anteroposterior and lateral chest radiographs are invaluable in helping to assess proper position of the artificial airway in the trachea.

Respiratory Therapy. Basic respiratory care is especially important for a patient on mechanical ventilation, since the patient's degree of illness negates many of the normal physiologic, protective, and clearing mechanisms.

Regardless of the etiology of respiratory insufficiency, certain priorities exist in ventilating children: (1) strive for optimal Pao_2 without circulatory impairment; (2) maintain the P_{aCO_2} within 5 mm Hg of what is normal for the patient without using dangerously high airway pressures; and (3) provide optimal patient comfort and safety.

In the patient with normal lungs, almost any ventilator can be used successfully. Heavy or stiff lungs, which usually are found in patients with postoperative atelectasis, with pneumonia, or with congestive heart failure, are characterized by a low functional residual capacity (FRC), decreased compliance, venous admixture, and a large physiologic dead space-to-tidal volume ratio (V_D/V_T). In these cases, treatment should be directed to correction of the low FRC and its underlying cause. Positive end expiratory pressure (PEEP) may be life-saving. In the presence of obstructive lung disease special consideration should be given to the high FRC, abundant secretions, and increased airway resistance. Although the proper use of mechanical ventilation is of utmost importance in the management of respiratory failure, there is no magic in the ventilator. It is one of the most important tools available when respiratory failure occurs or is imminent, but it is only a tool. Success depends on its proper use and in treating the underlying condition.

Choice and Use of Ventilators. The most commonly used mechanical ventilators are volume-limited and time-cycled ventilators, since they provide reliable ventilation in the presence of both increased airway resistance (airway disease) and decreased compliance (stiff lungs). These two types of ventilators are available in pediatric models; an adult ventilator can be used, however, when a pediatric one is not available by decreasing the size of the tubing and connectors (mechanical

*American Hospital Supply, McGaw Park, IL 60085

dead space), increasing the rate, and adjusting the tidal volume to account for compression volume losses.

When using a volume ventilator, the *initial* tidal volume should be set at about 10 to 15 cc per kg (normal tidal volume for a child is about 5 to 8 cc per kg) to use up the mechanical dead space of the ventilator, the increased (V_D/V_T) of the patient, and the compression volume of the ventilator. Although respiratory rates vary with age, a rate between 15 and 20 breaths per minute should be selected by adjusting the inspiratory and expiratory times or on the rate dial, depending on the type of ventilator. The F_IO_2 should be selected with prior knowledge of the patient's oxygenation needs. Initially the F_IO_2 is set at 1.0 to determine the A–a gradient and then rapidly lowered to a level determined by physiologic criteria. Usually, 2 cm H_2O PEEP should be added to simulate the normal resistance of the glottis during exhalation; higher levels should be selected if the patient has a low FRC or if the oxygen requirements are excessive.

When using a time-cycled ventilator (e.g., Baby Bird), the flow should be set initially at 1 liter per kg, which will approximate three times a normal minute ventilation. The rate should be set again at between 15 and 20 breaths per minute, as determined solely by the inspiratory and expiratory times. An inspiratory-to-expiratory ratio (I:E) of 1:2 or 1:3 is usually chosen, but this can be varied depending upon the pulmonary pathologic condition that is present. Some authors advocate the use of an I:E ratio of 2:1 or 4:1, which may improve oxygenation by forcing open collapsed alveoli (Herman and Reynolds, 1973). The resulting airway pressure, generated by the volume delivered and the patient's lung compliance, can be limited, if desired, to prevent increases in intrathoracic pressure. The F_IO_2 and PEEP settings should be adjusted as discussed under volume ventilators.

The true test of the effectiveness of mechanical ventilation is its clinical and physiologic effects on the patient. The patient must be examined immediately after placement on the ventilator for adequate and bilateral chest expansion. Lateral inspection of the child's thorax gives the best information about chest excursion. After allowing 10 to 15 minutes for stabilization, arterial blood gases must be drawn to determine the effectiveness of ventilation. The Pco_2 is a direct result of minute ventilation, which is determined by rate and tidal volume. If the PEEP setting is too high, hypercarbia may result owing to ventilation of dead space as the ideal FRC is surpassed, and it may decrease cardiac output by decreasing venous return. Depression of renal plasma flow and urine flow have been observed as well. (The latter may be partly mediated by the release of antidiuretic hormone.) The desired P_aO_2 is determined by the F_IO_2, PEEP, and tidal volume. Frequent evaluation of the patient must be coordinated with necessary adjustments of the ventilator (Galvis et al., 1976).

Sedation. If a patient is "fighting" the ventilator so that coordination does not exist between the ventilator and the patient, problems may arise from inadequate ventilation and acute elevations in airway pressure. First, it should be determined that no mechanical difficulties exist in the ventilator or artificial airway and that the patient's clinical status has not altered significantly. Only then may the patient be sedated in order to allow assisted ventilation to be effective. Morphine (0.1 mg per kg) or diazepam (0.1 mg per kg) can be used for this purpose. In some instances, morphine has the added benefit of vasodilation of the pulmonary vasculature, which may improve pulmonary vascular resistance and decrease oxygen consumption; however, it should be used with caution if hypovolemia is suspected.

Neuromuscular Blockade. If sedation and appropriate settings on the ventilator have failed to provide coordinated, controlled ventilation, then a neuromuscular blockade may be employed to assure adequate ventilation. The use of pancuronium (0.1 mg per kg) or d-tubocurarine (0.3 mg per kg) as an initial dose is recommended. The frequency of the doses should be titrated to the patient's response. With repeated doses, the interval between doses is prolonged, and the patient should be examined prior to each injection. Pancuronium is preferred when extreme tachycardia is not a problem. d-Tubocurarine has the side effect of producing hypotension secondary to peripheral vasodilation from histamine release and sympathetic ganglionic blockade (Goodman and Gilman, 1975). Occasionally, the vasodilation of d-tubocurarine can be beneficial, especially when it affects the pulmonary vasculature or when profound increases in peripheral systemic resistance exist. The use of muscle relaxants in young infants is rarely indicated and should be reserved for extreme cases of respiratory failure. Neuromuscular blockades should be used only with close observation and meticulous monitoring, since accidental disconnection of the patient from the ventilator or extubation could be catastrophic in these circumstances.

Weaning. Techniques for discontinuation of mechanical ventilation vary with institutions and patient populations. However, criteria for weaning patients should be based on clinical, physiologic, and ventilator factors.

Clinically the patient should have demonstrated improvement in the basic disease process that caused respiratory failure and should be stable with a minimal amount of support. For example, inotropic drugs should no longer be necessary for cardiovascular regulation. The patient should be alert, with good gag and cough reflexes to insure protection of the airway. Muscle tone must be adequate to support spontaneous respiration. Pulmonary secretions should be minimal so that the endotracheal tube will not be needed for pulmonary toilet. Finally, the chest radiograph should demonstrate no significant pathology such as pneumonia, atelectasis, pulmonary edema, or the presence of extrapleural air.

Certain physiologic measurements are helpful in determining when to wean a patient. The arterial blood gases should be as normal as possible, consistent with reversibility of the patient's underlying pathologic state. The inspiratory effort should be at least -20 cm H_2O to provide adequate ventilatory mechanics; and the V_D/V_T should be 0.6 to assure adequate ventilation. The A–a gradient, assuming there is no significant right-to-left shunting, should be less than 300 mm Hg with the F_IO_2 under toxic levels (F_IO_2 less than 0.5).

When these criteria for the patient and the ventilator have been met, a trial of IMV or SIMV is indicated in order that the patient may assume more and more of the work of breathing. As the mechanical ventilator input on the work of breathing is decreased, the patient must be evaluated clinically and by arterial blood gas determinations. Clinically, there should be no signs of respiratory failure, and the patient should be breathing comfortably. The arterial blood gases should remain at about the same levels as previously. If the trend is for the P_aO_2 to fall and the P_aCO_2 to rise, the patient still requires assisted

ventilation. The process of weaning a patient from the ventilator is basically one of trial and error. The physician must be in attendance at each step in the withdrawal of ventilation support!

When the IMV or SIMV rate is at a minimum and the patient is continuing to do well, a trial of spontaneous ventilation with the artificial airway in place can be attempted. The F_IO_2 should now be increased approximately 0.1 in anticipation of the ventilation-perfusion inequality that usually results as the ventilator is discontinued. This trial of spontaneous ventilation should be evaluated in a manner similar to evaluation of the SIMV or SIMV trial. Usually a period of 1 to 12 hours of spontaneous ventilation is sufficient to determine the feasibility of extubation. When a patient no longer requires mechanical ventilation but still needs PEEP for oxygenation, he or she can be weaned from the ventilator to spontaneous CDAP breathing, and then the level of CDAP reduced gradually as the patient improves.

Complications of Mechanical Ventilation. Complications of mechanical ventilation have been discussed by various authors (Downes et al., 1972; Bendixen, 1965). An awareness of potential complications allows prevention and prompt treatment should they arise.

Airway obstruction can occur secondary to edema, stenosis, or granuloma and can be lessened by the use of appropriately sized, tissue-compatible endotracheal tubes that are left in place no longer than one week before a tracheostomy is performed. Infection of the tracheobronchial tree and pulmonary parenchyma can be minimized by meticulous respiratory care and by strict adherence to aseptic techniques when handling the airway and the respiratory equipment. The pulmonary complications of inspissated secretions, atelectasis, oxygen toxicity, and extrapleural air can be lessened by adequate humidification, delivery of nontoxic levels of inspired oxygen, and avoidance insofar as possible of excessive airway pressures. If the ventilator is checked frequently and methodically, mechanical problems such as air leak, valve malfunctions, kinked tubing, and delivery of dry gases can be avoided.

Appropriate fluid therapy for the patient on mechanical ventilation is often overlooked. Frequently, the assessment of the fluid status of a patient in respiratory failure poses a real problem since hypotension, cardiac failure, sepsis, malnutrition, renal disease, or excessive fluid losses often are also present. While the patient is on assisted ventilation, retention of pulmonary water is a common complication and is usually secondary to a relative fluid overload because of decreased insensible loss through the lung and a rise in the production of antidiuretic hormone (Sladen et al., 1968). With positive pressure ventilation, left arterial volume may fall when airway pressures transmitted to the alveoli are greater than left atrial filling pressures. The vagus senses this fall in vascular volume and signals the pituitary to increase its output of antidiuretic hormone. In addition, there is a fall in cardiac output and the glomerular filtration rate, a shift in renal cortical perfusion to the juxtamedullary glomeruli, and an increase in aldosterone secretion. These renal and left atrial volume changes account for a positive water and sodium balance. Thus, diuresis and fluid restriction to reverse pulmonary edema must be titrated against hypovolemia and borderline low cardiac output (Moylan et al., 1975).

The addition of PEEP can complicate fluid management even further. PEEP causes a reduction in ventricular filling pressure with a subsequent fall in cardiac index and stroke volume. These hemodynamic changes will persist without apparent compensation while the patient is on PEEP and can be reversed by blood volume replacement. However, with discontinuation of PEEP, hypervolemia may become evident and may precipitate cardiac failure in the face of marginal right ventricular function (Qvist et al., 1975). Little evidence exists to show that venous return is with levels of PEEP less than 5 cm H_2O. Thus, while a child receives mechanical ventilation, frequent assessments of electrolyte levels, in addition to vascular pressures, are mandatory to maintain optimal oxygen carrying capacity and cardiovascular hemodynamics in the presence of changing airway pressures and PEEP. In addition, adequate nutrition, maintained orally or parenterally, is important in order to maintain normal total protein levels, which minimize pulmonary capillary and alveolar transudation of fluid into the pulmonary interstitium.

Inability to Wean. Every physician who has managed a patient on mechanical ventilation for respiratory failure has been faced with the problem of inability to wean the patient from the ventilator. The incidence of failure to wean has been lessened with the advent of IMV and SIMV, but it still exists; the most common cause is the failure to resolve the underlying problem that precipitated the respiratory failure. Other mechanisms include decreased muscle strength from diaphragmatic paralysis, chest wall pathology, or poor nutrition. Such patients may not be able to sustain adequate respirations. The use of PEEP or CDAP may mask diaphragmatic paralysis, and the chest radiograph may show the diaphragm in a functional position for inspiration (Oh et al., 1974). Increased work of breathing secondary to lowered pulmonary compliance or increased airway resistance can also be a cause of failure to wean. Low pulmonary compliance can be a result of acute pulmonary disease or more chronic problems, such as bronchopulmonary dysplasia and pulmonary fibrosis. Increases in airway resistance can be secondary to bronchospasm or airway obstruction, such as are seen in tracheal stenosis or tracheomalacia. Obstruction can also result from retained secretions, as occurs in tracheitis, bronchitis, or pneumonitis, and may make discontinuation of mechanical ventilation very difficult. The final causes of inability to wean are increased ventilatory requirements as a result of pulmonary diseases with increased V_D/V_T, inadequate cardiac output, or an increased metabolic rate, as in the febrile patient (Feeley and Hedley-Whyte, 1975).

The intensive care of respiratory disorders is founded on a logical, analytical evaluation of clinical and physiologic factors. A reasoned approach for the management of critically ill patients in respiratory failure can be based on sound diagnostic and therapeutic criteria.

NASOTRACHEAL INTUBATION

The oral route in the newborn is generally recommended for assisted ventilation, but after this period the nasal route offers the following advantages: (1) it is more stable and easier to tape in place; (2) its particular position in the trachea is more physiologic by descending directly into the trachea with less curvature; (3) there is less to-and-fro motion; (4) attachment to the ventilator is easily accomplished; (5) it allows better suctioning of the mouth and oropharynx; and (6) since less gagging occurs the tube is more easily tolerated. The disadvantages of nasal intubation are that (1) it is slightly more difficult to perform and often causes epistaxis; (2) occasionally, adenoid tissue may be traumatized and portions may be carried into the trachea; (3) sometimes it is necessary to use a smaller tube; (4) it may cause pressure necrosis of the turbinates and alae nasi, particularly in patients in prolonged hypoperfusion states; and (5) it has been implicated in cases of otitis media.

Equipment for Nasotracheal Intubation

All the necessary equipment should be available so that the procedure can be performed expeditiously. This is especially important if the procedure is to be performed with the aid of muscle relaxants. The items prepared should include the following: (1) a working laryngoscope; (2) three sizes of endotracheal tubes; (3) tape for fixation of the tube; (4) tincture of benzion, USP; (5) suction catheters that will pass easily through the tubes; (6) at least one relatively large catheter to aspirate nasal and oral secretions readily; (7) a small basin with sterile saline to moisten the catheter tip; and (8) a pair of Magill's forceps.

Technique of Intubation

Although the procedure has not been standardized, the following description appears to conform to the usual practice. The child is placed in a supine position and the head is elevated on a folded towel. The operator stands at the head and suctions the nasal airway, posterior pharynx, and the gastric contents. The child is then oxygenated by bag and mask with 100 per cent oxygen. The operator must be certain that adequate ventilation can be maintained by observing the chest expansion under positive pressure. If an orotracheal tube has previously been inserted it should not be removed. Instead the tape is loosened and the tube is moved to the left side of the mouth and held firmly by an assistant while ventilation is maintained with 100 per cent oxygen. At this time a dose of atropine 0.01 mg per kg is administered intravenously and followed two to four minutes later by the standard dose of 1 mg per kg of succinylcholine to provide muscle relaxation. If the trachea is not intubated an "awake" intubation should be attempted; however, in some instances children have sufficient strength to resist the introduction of the laryngoscope, and intubation with a

muscle relaxant is indicated. In any case the physician must be certain of his or her ability to maintain ventilation with positive pressure by bag and mask before a muscle relaxant is administered. A sterile, polyvinyl chloride nasotracheal tube should be selected for size and length according to Table 74–3 (see p. 1348). The larger of the two nares is intubated, and the tube is advanced until it reaches the posterior nasopharynx. At this point the child's head is held in extension by the assistant placing his or her hands firmly on the lateral aspects of the face and temples and simultaneously holding the shoulders down by pressing on the midclavicular area with the heel of the hands or the wrists to prevent arching of the back. Then, the appropriate laryngoscope blade is inserted to the right of the midline of the mouth in order to avoid the upper incisor teeth (if present) and to displace the tongue toward the left. As the blade is advanced carefully, the oropharynx, the hypopharynx, and the upper end of the esophagus are exposed in succession. The glottis lies anterior to the esophagus, or above it as the patient is lying supine. To bring the glottis into view, the left hand, which is holding the laryngoscope, steadies the head, and the whole floor of the mouth is raised by lifting the laryngoscope in the direction of the handle. The epiglottis will then be seen, and by elevating the tip of the epiglottis, the vocal cords are exposed and the tube is then advanced under direct vision. With smaller children it may be helpful to depress the larynx in order to visualize the glottis. This can be done simply by compressing the hyoid bone with the little finger of the hand that is holding the laryngoscope or by an assistant. Most often the end of the tube can be seen advancing toward the esophagus; the Magill's forceps may be used to grasp the end of the tube, thereby aligning the tube. It is helpful to have an assistant advance the tube at the nose; the operator watches the tube descend through the glottis. If the child has an orotracheal tube in place, once the nasal tube has been grasped at the end the former is removed, and the nasal tube is held with the Magill's forceps and threaded into the larynx. The child is then ventilated and oxygenated (bag-to-tube). The chest is auscultated to ensure that both lungs have been ventilated. (Distinct, loud breath sounds over the stomach indicate that the tube is probably in the esophagus, in which instance the tube is then withdrawn, the patient is ventilated with mask and bag, and the tube is reinserted into the trachea.)

Fixation of the Nasotracheal Tube

Once the tube has been inserted the correct distance into the trachea, it is marked at the level to the nostril. This procedure avoids inadvertent withdrawal or advancement of the endotracheal tube. A chest roentgenogram is obtained to confirm the position of the tube. The tip of the tube should always be about midtrachea. To tape the tube in place, tincture of benzoin is applied liberally from ear to ear, over the upper lip, and also over the endotracheal tube segment near the nostril. After the benzoin tincture has fully dried, a one half inch strip of adhesive tape is applied over the benzoin and wrapped tightly around the tube. To fix the tube more securely, a second piece of "Micropore" surgical tape 1 inch wide could be used to reinforce the first tape. Occasionally it is necessary to retape the tubes but not to change them.

SUGGESTED RESPIRATORY CARE PROGRAM

A significant source of postoperative morbidity in infants and children is the atelectasis, infection, or both that result from the inadequate removal of secretions. In any child who has had surgery and particularly in those who are receiving artificial ventilation, a regular program of meticulous pulmonary care is essential. The following guidelines are suggested.

1. Change the infant's position from side to side every two hours. If possible, change from supine to prone every two hours.
2. With the patient in slight Trendelenburg position, carry out forceful percussion of all sides of the chest with a "cupped" hand or, even better, with a specially adapted infant anesthesia mask, size 0. This should be adapted with inflated borders without head strap hooks and fitted with a rubber stopper to seal off the adapter opening. This maneuver helps to dislodge the secretions and promotes bronchial drainage and should be done every four hours.
3. Use a mechanical vibrator on all sides of the chest after cupping. The Panabra-

tor has proved useful because of its long handle and electrical safety features (Matushita Electronic Works, Ltd.)

4. Then if the child is not breathing deeply, attempt to ventilate him with a bag and mask for one minute.
5. Suction the oropharynx and nasopharynx briefly (less than 15 seconds) every four hours after the preceding chest physiotherapy. This procedure can be rather difficult to perform in an infant who requires an ambient O_2 of more than 40 per cent; in this case it is advisable to increase the child's oxygen environment for 5 minutes prior to chest physiotherapy.

If a child has an endotracheal tube or a tracheostomy tube in place, the preceding routine is modified as follows.

1. Percuss;
2. Vibrate;
3. Hyperventilate with 100 per cent O_2 (or the prescribed F_IO_2 for ventilation);
4. Using sterile gloves, introduce a sterile catheter through the endotracheal tube or tracheostomy and suction any secretions present in the major airway — limit suction to 10 to 20 seconds;
5. Hyperventilate with 100 per cent O_2 again (or the prescribed F_IO_2 for hyperventilation) for a few breaths to a volume close to the child's vital capacity;
6. Using sterile gloves, reintroduce a sterile catheter gently into the airway. Place the catheter deeply into the tracheobronchial tree, and while removing it upwards instill 1 to 3 ml of saline through the catheter until the full amount is finished. Normal saline without preservative must be used;
7. Again hyperventilate with 100 per cent O_2 (or the prescribed F_IO_2 for hyperinflation) to a large volume for a few breaths, and maintain peak pressures momentarily; follow this with the forceful application of pressure (squeezing) with one hand or a vibrator to the anterior and lateral aspects of the chest on exhalation only. The sudden release of pressure in the airway helps to express secretions into the larger airways, from which they can be suctioned;
8. Suction again for 10 to 20 seconds, rotating the catheter as it is removed upwards;
9. Send the tracheal aspirate for smear, culture, and sensitivity tests daily or at least twice a week;

10. Check breath sounds before and after tracheal toilet.

Repeat the above procedure if necessary.

If a cuffed endotracheal tube or tracheostomy tube is used (high-volume, low-pressure cuff), the following steps are necessary.

1. Deflate the cuff for five minutes every one to two hours;
2. Inflate the cuff until the pilot balloon is fully expanded;
3. Allow the cuff pressure to equilibrate to the ambient pressure and reseal the cuff vent. Cuff pressures above the ambient pressure should be specifically ordered.

REFERENCES

Balentine, J. D. 1966. Pathologic effects of exposure to high oxygen tensions. N. Engl. J. Med., 275:1038.

Bates D. V., Macklem, P. T., and Christie R. V. 1971. Respiratory Function in Disease, Philadelphia, W. B. Saunders Co., pp. 61–67.

Bendixen, H. H., Egbert, L. D., Hedley-Whyte, J., et al. 1965. Respiratory Care, 5th ed. Saint Louis, C. V. Mosby Co., pp. 51–52.

Bryan, C. 1974. Comments of a devil's advocate. Am. Rev. Respir. Dis., Suppl., 110:143.

Cushing, I. E., Miller, W. F., and Safar, P. 1965. Nebulization Therapy in Respiratory Therapy. Philadelphia, F. A. Davis Co., p. 188.

Delivoria-Papadopoulous, M., Ronevic, N. P., and Oski, F. A. 1971. Postnatal changes in oxygen transport of term, premature and sick infants: The role of adult hemoglobin and red cell, 2,3-dephosphoglycerate. Pediatr. Res., 5:235.

Downes, J. J., Fugencio, T., and Raphaelly, R. 1972. Acute respiratory failure in infants and children. Pediatr. Clin. North. Am., 19:423.

Feeley, T. W., and Hedley-Whyte, J. 1975. Weaning from controlled ventilation and supplemental oxygen. N. Engl. J. Med., 292:903.

Fenn, W. O., and Rahn, H. 1965. Handbook of Physiology, Sec. 3: Respiration. Baltimore, The Williams and Wilkins Co., p. 1297.

Finch, C. A., and Lenfant, C. 1972. Oxygen transport in man. N. Engl. J. Med., 286:407.

Froese, A. B., and Bryan, A. C. 1974. Effects of anesthesia and paralysis on diaphragmatic mechanics in man. Anesthesiology, 41:242.

Galvis, A. G., and Benson, D. W. 1973. Spontaneous continuous positive airway pressure (CPAP). Breathing in the management of acute pulmonary edema in infants. Clin. Pediatr., 12:265.

Galvis, A. G., Donahoo, J. S., and White. J. J. 1976. An improved technique for prolonged arterial catheterization in infants and children. Crit. Care Med., 4:166.

Galvis, A. G., White, J. J., and Oh, K. S. 1974. A bedside washout technique for atelectasis in infants. Am. J. Dis. Child., 127:824.

Galvis, A. G., White, J. J., and Gordon, D. H. 1976. Continuous dynamic monitoring of pressure and flow patterns during assisted ventilation. J. Pediatr. Surg., 11:307.

Goodman, L. S., and Gilman, A. 1975. The Pharmacological Basis of Therapeutics, 5th ed. New York, Macmillan, pp. 601–615.

Graef, J. W., and Cone, T. E. L. 1974. Manual of Pediatric Therapeutics, Boston, Little, Brown & Co., p. 413.

Graff, T. D. 1975. Humidification: Indications and hazards in respiratory therapy. Anesth. Analg., 54:444.

Gregory, G. A., Edmunds, L. H., Kitterman, J. A., et al. 1975. Continuous positive airway pressure and pulmonary and circulatory function after cardiac surgery in infants less than three months of age. Anesthesiology, 43:426.

Harrison, V. C., Heese, H. deV., and Klein, M. 1968. The significance of grunting in hyaline membrane disease. Pediatrics, 41:549.

Herman, S., and Reynolds, E. O. R. 1973. Methods of improving oxygenation in infants mechanically ventilated for severe hyaline membrane disease. Arch. Dis. Child., 48:612.

Huch, R., Huch, A., Albani, M., et al. 1976. Transcutaneous PO_2 monitoring in routine management of infants and children with cardiorespiratory problems. Pediatrics, 57:681.

Kattwinkel, J., Fleming, A. A., and Keaus, M. H. 1973. A device for administration of continuous positive airway pressure by the nasal route. Pediatrics, 52:130.

Kirby, R. R. 1975. Is intermittent mandatory ventilation a satisfactory alternative to assisted and controlled ventilation? American Society of Anesthesiologists Annual Meeting, Chicago, IL, Oct. 11–15, 1975.

Mansell, A., Bryan, C., and Levison, H. 1972. Airway closure in children. J. Appl. Physiol., 33:711.

Mellins, R. B. 1974. Pulmonary physiotherapy in the pediatric age group. Am. Rev. Respir. Dis., Suppl., 110:137.

Moylan, F. M., O'Connell, K. C., Todres, I. D., et al. 1975. Edema of the pulmonary interstitium in infants and children. Pediatrics, 55:783.

Muskin, W. W., Rendell-Baker, L., Thompson, P. W., et al. 1969. Automatic Ventilation of the Lungs, 2nd ed. Philadelphia, F. A. Davis Co., pp. 102–155.

Oh, K. S., Stitik, F. P., Galvis, A. G., et al. 1974. Radiological manifestations in patients on continuous positive-pressure breathing. Radiology, 110:627.

Qvist, J., Pontoppidan, H., Wilson, R. S., et al. 1975. Hemodynamic responses to mechanical ventilation with PEEP. Anesthesiology, 42:45.

Shapiro, B. A., Harrison, R. A., Walton, J. R., et al. 1976. Intermittent demand ventilation (IDV): A new technique for supporting ventilation in critically ill patients. Respir. Care, 21:521.

Sladen, A., Laver, M. B., and Pontoppidan, H. 1968. Pulmonary complications and water retention in prolonged mechanical ventilation. N. Engl. J. Med., 279:448.

Stalcup, S. A., and Mellins, R. B. 1977. Mechanical forces producing pulmonary edema in acute asthma. N. Engl. J. Med., 297:592.

Toremalm, N. G. 1961. Air flow patterns and ciliary activity in the trachea after tracheostomy. Acta Otolaryngol., 53:442.

Williams, M. L., and Galvis, A. G. 1974. Pulmonary complications in infants. Surg. Clin. North Am., 54:1137.

Winter, P. M., and Smith, G. 1972. The toxicity of oxygen. Anesthesiology, 37:210.

Section VI

THE NECK

Chapter 75

EMBRYOLOGY AND ANATOMY

Joseph P. Atkins, Jr., M.D.

William M. Keane, M.D.

INTRODUCTION

The neck is a complex region that is the passageway for communication between the head and the trunk. The tremendous variety of pathologic conditions that may present in this region make an understanding of the embryology and anatomy of the neck a vital part of the otorhinolaryngologist's armamentarium. In this chapter, special emphasis will be given to the embryology of the major vessels, nerves, muscles, and the thyroid and parathyroid glands. The surface anatomy of the neck with reference to the triangles of the neck and lymphatic drainage will be discussed. The fascial planes and related spaces will receive special attention.

THE EMBRYOLOGIC DEVELOPMENT OF THE ARTERIES OF THE NECK

Bilateral symmetry is a fundamental principle in the embryologic development of the body. In accordance with this principle, the arteries constitute initially a paired symmetrical system that is altered during subsequent development by the fusion or atrophy of their various parts.

As the heart is displaced caudally and the pharyngeal arches are formed, six pairs of pharyngeal arteries develop in successive fashion. Not all six pairs of pharyngeal vessels are present at the same time. The mandibular and hyoid arch vessels disappear before the fifth and sixth pharyngeal arch vessels have differentiated.

As can be seen in Figure 75–1, the pharyngeal arch arteries arise ventrally from the aortic sac and terminate laterally in the dorsal aorta of the corresponding side. At a more caudal level, the two dorsal aortae fuse to form a single midline dorsal aorta. The initial arrangement of the arch vessels is subsequently transformed during development. The first and second pharyngeal arch vessels disappear at about the time the third and fourth arch vessels mature and increase in size. The remnant of the first arch artery is the maxillary artery, and the stapedial artery (when present) represents a remnant of the second arch. The ventral portions of the first and second arch vessels may also contribute to the development of the external carotid artery (Fig. 75–1) (Arey, 1974; Crelin, 1976).

The third pharyngeal arch vessels differentiate into the internal carotid arteries. The fourth arch vessels form the arch of the aorta on the left side and contribute to the proximal aspect of the subclavian artery on the right. The left subclavian artery arises by hypertrophy of a branch of the left dorsal aorta (Fig. 75–1) (Langman, 1969).

Abnormalities of the great vessels are among the commonest developmental anomalies. With the growth of the body and changes in the vascular patterns, certain channels may persist that normally undergo regression, or vessels that normally persist may disappear. In most cases, these variations have little effect on function, and circulation is not impaired. In some cases, however, variations in the aortic arch development may be of greater clinical significance. For instance, the persistence of the right and left fourth arches and dorsal aortic root results in

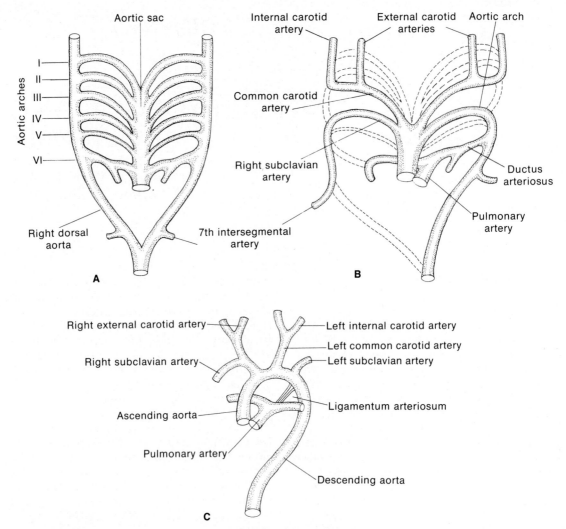

Aortic sac

I
II
Aortic arches
III
IV
V
VI

Right dorsal
aorta

7th intersegmental
artery

A

Internal carotid
artery

External carotid
arteries

Aortic arch

Common carotid
artery

Right subclavian
artery

Ductus
arteriosus

Pulmonary
artery

B

Right external carotid artery

Left internal carotid artery

Left common carotid artery

Right subclavian artery

Left subclavian artery

Ascending aorta

Ligamentum arteriosum

Pulmonary artery

Descending aorta

C

Figure 75–1 *A,* Aortic arches before transformation into definitive vascular pattern. *B,* Aortic arches after transformation. *C,* The great arteries in the adult. (After Langman, J. 1969. Medical Embryology: Human Development — Normal and Abnormal. Baltimore, Williams & Wilkins.)

a structure called an "aortic ring," which may compress the trachea and esophagus. The resulting interference with swallowing may require ligation of one of the two arches.

Another arch abnormality that produces clinical symptoms is the development of the right subclavian artery from the arch of the aorta. In this case, the vessel passes from the dorsal aortic root across the midline behind the esophagus. It may then exert pressure sufficient to interfere with swallowing, although usually not as great as is seen in cases of aortic ring malformation. A variety of other abnormalities in the development of the branchial arch vessels may be encountered and are discussed further in major embryologic texts (Patten, 1968; Jaffe, 1972).

EMBRYOLOGIC DEVELOPMENT OF THE MUSCLES OF THE NECK

The muscles of the body are developed from mesoderm. Segmentation of the para-axial mesoderm into somites is followed by their subsequent differentiation into the myotome, which gives rise to the muscle mass; the dermatome, which gives rise to integumentary tissues; and the sclerotome, which gives rise to the axial skeleton. Unlike the voluntary musculature of other parts of the body, most of the segmental musculature of the neck is formed by the differentiation of branchial arch mesenchyme, with some contributions from the cervical somites. The extensor musculature of the back of the neck is formed from the epiaxial divisions of the cervical myotomes. The hypoaxial portions of these myotomes form the scalene, the prevertebral, geniohyoid, and the infrahyoid muscles (Patten, 1968).

In general, the muscles of branchiomeric origin retain the innervation characteristic of the arch. Therefore, the muscles that are derived from the mesenchyme of the mandibular arch are supplied by fibers of the trigeminal nerve. This group would include the muscles of mastication and the mylohyoid, anterior belly of the digastric, tensor veli palatini, and tensor tympani muscles. The third arch gives rise to the stylopharyngeus muscle and part of the constrictor group of the pharynx. Their innervation is by the glossopharyngeal nerve. The primordial muscle masses of the fourth and fifth arches give rise to the muscles of the larynx and part of the pharyngeal constrictors. These muscles are, therefore, innervated largely by the vagus nerve. The precise development of the sternocleidomastoid and trapezius muscles is difficult to prove. Most feel that this muscle group is formed primarily from branchiomeric tissue but that the migration of muscle cells from the occipital somites contributes to part of this development. The innervation of these muscles is from the spinal accessory nerve. The infrahyoid muscles of the anterior aspect of the neck are of somitic origin. These muscles are innervated by a branch of the hypoglossal nerve with fibers from the first and second cervical nerves. Early in embryologic development, the infrahyoid muscle mass was closely associated with the mass that gives rise to the diaphragmatic musculature. This helps to explain the origin of their innervations from the cervical nerves (Langman, 1969).

THE EMBRYOLOGY OF THE THYROID AND PARATHYROID GLANDS

The thyroid gland presents early in embryologic development as a thickening of the endoderm of the floor of the pharynx in the midline between the first and second pouches, near the portion that becomes the tuberculum impar. This tissue mass forms a diverticulum with a bilobed, flask-like appearance. This thyroid primordium soon begins to descend, but a thin connection, the stalk-like thyroglossal duct, remains attached to the buccal cavity. This point of attachment marks the origin of the thyroid gland and may be seen in the adult as the foramen caecum. When the thyroid primordium de-

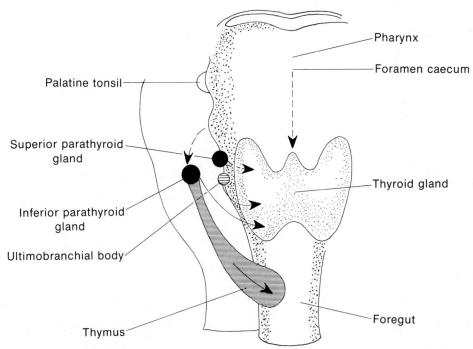

Figure 75–2 The migration of the thymus, parathyroid glands, and ultimobranchial body. The thyroid gland descends from the level of the foramen caecum to the level of the first tracheal ring. (After Langman, J. 1969. Medical Embryology: Human Development — Normal and Abnormal. Baltimore, Williams & Wilkins.)

scends, it consists of two lobes extending to either side of the midline with only a narrow isthmus of tissue joining them medially. This tissue mass reaches the level of the laryngeal primordium at about the seventh week of gestation. The thyroglossal tract is normally obliterated, but when it persists may predispose to the formation of thyroglossal duct cysts. Accessory thyroid tissue may be found along the path of migration of the thyroid gland. When the primordial thyroid fails to descend, it may persist in the tongue musculature as a lingual thyroid (Fig. 75–2) (Patten, 1968; Langman, 1969).

Two pairs of parathyroid glands develop from separate pouches. One pair is derived from the third and the other from the fourth pharyngeal pouch. They are frequently designated as parathyroids 3 and parathyroids 4. At the seventh week of development, the parathyroid primordia free themselves from the parent pouches and move caudally. Although they initially move in close association with each other, parathyroids 3 remain attached to the thymus and migrate further caudally than do parathyroids 4. Occasionally during their migration, fragmentation of the parathyroid tissue may take place, resulting in the formation of accessory parathyroid glands. Parathyroids 4 usually become adherent to the thyroid capsule and may become embedded in the substance of the thyroid gland (Fig. 75–2). Further details of the embryology and developmental abnormalities of the thyroid and parathyroid are discussed in Chapter 78.

SURFACE ANATOMY OF THE NECK

The neck may be divided into an anterior region, the cervix, and a posterior region, the nucha. The nuchal division is more properly related to the back and is represented by the vertebral column with its paravertebral musculature. The cervical division is of greater interest to the otolaryngologist. When viewed from the lateral aspect, it has a quadrilateral outline. It is bounded superiorly by the mandible and mastoid process, inferiorly by the clavicle, anteriorly by the median line of the neck, and posteriorly by the anterior border of the trapezius muscle.

Triangles of the Neck

The sternocleidomastoid muscle is a prominent landmark in the neck and divides it into

anterior and posterior parts or triangles as it courses from the mastoid tip to the medial aspect of the clavicle (Fig. 75–3).

The *posterior triangle* is bounded posteriorly by the trapezius muscle, anteriorly by the sternocleidomastoid muscle, and inferiorly by the middle third of the clavicle. Its floor is formed by the deep layer of the deep cervical fascia, which covers the scalene, levator scapulae, and splenius capitus muscles. Its roof is the superficial layer of the deep cervical fascia (Fig. 75–3).

The most important contents of the posterior triangle are the subclavian artery, brachial plexus, spinal accessory nerve, and posterior cervical lymph nodes. The omohyoid muscle crosses the posterior triangle and divides it into a superior occipital triangle and an inferior subclavian triangle (Gray, 1959; Pernkopf, 1963).

The *anterior triangle* is bounded posteriorly by the sternocleidomastoid muscle, anteriorly by the midline of the neck, and superiorly by the lower border of the mandible. Its floor (deep border) is formed by the mylohyoid, hyoglossus, and parts of the thyrohyoid and pharyngeal constrictor muscles. Its roof (superficial border) is formed by the superficial layer of the deep cervical fascia and the platysma muscle. The anterior triangle is crossed by the digastric, stylohyoid, and omohyoid muscles, which subdivide this area into smaller triangles: the submandibular, carotid, submental, and inferior carotid triangles. The common, external, and internal carotid arteries; the internal jugular vein; the laryngeal, pharyngeal, vagal, and recurrent laryngeal nerves; the submandibular gland; and lymphatic tissue are the chief contents of this triangle (Fig. 75–3).

LYMPH NODES OF THE NECK

The lymph nodes of the neck include five main groups: submandibular, submental, superficial cervical, anterior cervical, and deep cervical nodes (Fig. 75–4) (Gray, 1959; Hollingshead, 1974).

The submandibular nodes are found beneath the body of the mandible in the submandibular triangle and are chiefly superficial to the submandibular gland. Small lymph nodes are sometimes found on the undersurface of the submandibular gland. These nodes drain the cheek, the medial canthal region, the lateral aspect of the nose, the upper lip, the gingiva, and the anterolateral

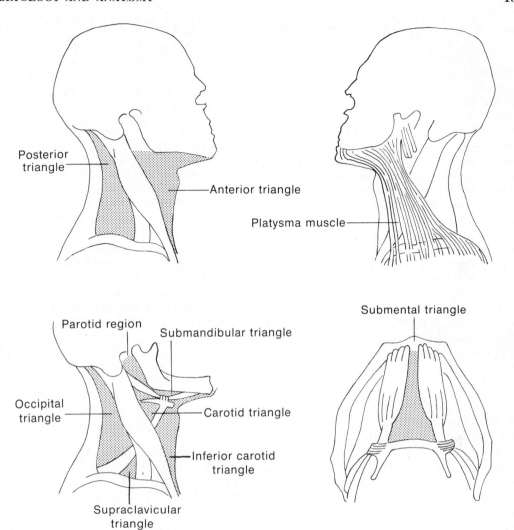

Figure 75–3 Triangles of the neck.

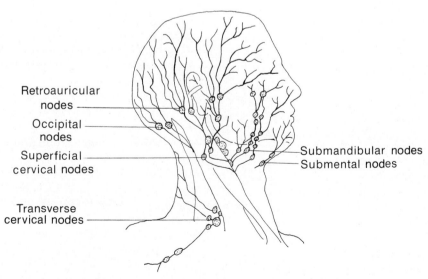

Figure 75–4 Superficial lymph nodes of the head and neck.

aspect of the tongue. The submandibular nodes drain subsequently into the superior deep cervical nodes.

The submental nodes may be found between the anterior bellies of the digastric muscles. These nodes drain the central aspect of the lower lip and floor of the mouth and the mobile tongue. The submental nodes drain subsequently into the submandibular nodes and into the deep cervical node group at the level of the cricoid cartilage.

The superficial cervical nodes lie adjacent to the external jugular vein and superficial to the sternocleidomastoid muscle. These nodes drain the inferior aspects of the auricular and parotid regions and drain subsequently into the superior deep cervical nodes (Fig. 75–4).

The anterior cervical nodes lie ventral to the larynx and trachea and serve to drain the lower part of the larynx, the thyroid gland, and the cervical aspect of the trachea. Efferents from this node group pass deeper into the deep cervical nodes, which are large and numerous and lie along the carotid sheath from the base of the skull to the root of the neck. The deep cervical nodes are frequently divided into two groups: the superior deep cervical nodes and the inferior deep cervical nodes (Fig. 75–5).

The superior deep cervical nodes lie deep to the sternocleidomastoid muscle and in close association with the internal jugular vein and spinal accessory nerve. These nodes drain the occipital region, the back of the neck, the auricle, most of the tongue, the larynx, thyroid gland, trachea, nasopharynx, nasal cavities, palate, and esophagus. They also receive efferent vessels from a major portion of the other nodes of the head and neck (Figs. 75–5 and 75–6).

The inferior deep cervical nodes lie deep to the sternocleidomastoid muscle in the supraclavicular area and are in close proximity to the brachial plexus and subclavian vein. This inferior node group drains the back of the scalp and neck as well as part of the pectoral region. The inferior deep cervical nodes receive lymphatic drainage from the superior deep cervical nodes. The deep cervical node groups on the right side form a large lymphatic vessel, the jugular trunk, which joins the venous system at the junction of the internal jugular and subclavian veins. On the left side, the jugular trunk joins the thoracic duct (Fig. 75–5).

The retropharyngeal nodes represent an important nodal chain in the pediatric patient. Infection and subsequent suppuration in these nodes causes retropharyngeal abscess formation. These nodes lie in the buccopharyngeal fascia, behind the upper part of the pharynx and anterior to the cervical vertebrae; they drain the nasal cavities and the nasopharynx. Efferents from this group pass to the superior deep cervical nodes (Fig. 75–6).

It is important to understand the position of the lymph nodes relative to the fascial layers and compartments of the head and neck. The lymphatic system drains three areas of infection in the head and neck. Subsequent suppuration and necrosis in the involved node may lead to the accumulation of purulent material, which may spread

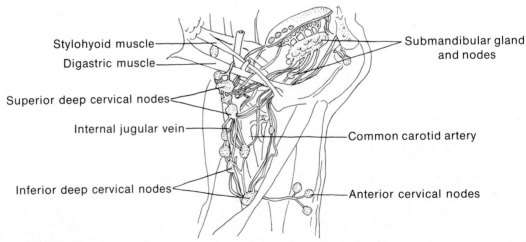

Figure 75–5 Deep cervical lymph nodes of the neck. (After Gray, H. 1959. Anatomy of the Human Body, 27th ed. Philadelphia, Lea & Febiger.)

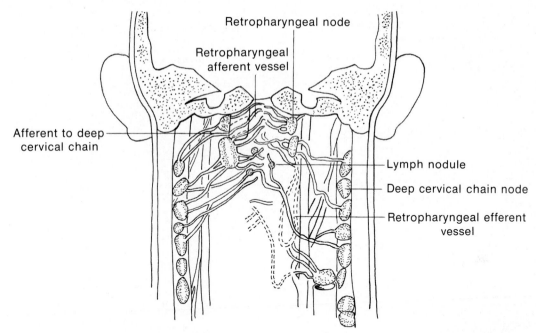

Figure 75–6 Retropharyngeal nodes. (After Gray, H. 1959. Anatomy of the Human Body, 27th ed. Philadelphia, Lea & Febiger.)

through one or more continuous fascial compartments. Thus, infections that originate from one site in the skin or in the pharynx may subsequently spread to involve specific lymphatics of the neck with subsequent deep neck infection.

A knowledge of the anatomy of the cervical fascia is essential to the understanding of the pathophysiology and treatment of infectious and noninfectious diseases of the head and neck.

FASCIAL LAYERS OF THE NECK

Cervical Fascia

The neck is enveloped by two basic fascial layers, the superficial and deep cervical fasciae. These fascial layers both unite and separate various important structures. In so doing, certain fascial planes and compartments are formed.

By understanding the contents of these spaces together with their position in the neck and their relationships to other structures, the differential diagnosis of a neck mass may be made more easily, and potential complications from deep neck infections may be anticipated. The surgeon must be fully familiar with these structures and their relationships

if the surgical approach to and drainage of deep neck infections is to be effective (Hollingshead, 1974).

The superficial cervical fascia surrounds the neck and is continuous with the superficial fascia of the pectoral, deltoid, and back regions inferiorly and the fascia of the muscles of facial expression superiorly. Within this layer are the thin sheets of platysma muscle as well as the external jugular vein and superficial lymph nodes. The more important deep cervical fascia is in three layers: a superficial investing layer, a middle pretracheal layer, and a deep prevertebral layer (Fig. 75–7).

The superficial layer of the deep cervical fascia completely surrounds the neck like a stocking. Posteriorly it is attached to the spinal processes of the cervical vertebra and ligamentum nucha. It passes forward and divides to ensheath the trapezius muscle and then forms a single layer as it passes over the posterior triangle of the neck. After dividing again to ensheath the sternocleidomastoid muscle, the fascia continues across the neck as a single layer to join the corresponding layer of the opposite side in the anterior midline. The superficial layer is attached to the hyoid bone in the anterior triangle and is divided into suprahyoid and infrahyoid portions. The suprahyoid portion splits to envelop the

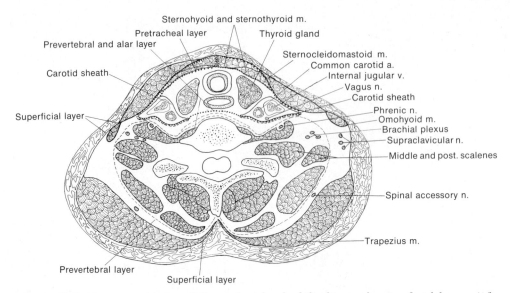

Figure 75–7 Transverse section of the neck at level of the larynx showing facial layers. (After Hollingshead, W. H. 1974. Textbook of Anatomy, 3rd ed. Hagerstown, Harper & Row.)

submandibular and parotid glands. Between these two glands, the fascia unites to form a strong membranous process, the stylomandibular ligament, which attaches to the hyoid bone at the angle of the mandible and the styloid process. Thus, the superficial layer of the deep cervical fascia separates the submandibular and parotid glands from each other and from the rest of the neck. The superficial layer continues superiorly to ensheath the posterior body of the mandible. Its medial extension ensheaths the internal and external pterygoid muscles.

The infrahyoid portion of the superficial layer of the deep cervical fascia splits inferiorly to attach to the anterior and posterior aspects of the manubrium, where it forms the suprasternal space of Burns. This space contains the anterior jugular veins with their communicating veins and a few lymph nodes (Fig. 75–7).

The middle or pretracheal layer of the deep cervical fascia is composed of two layers, a superficial muscular layer and a deep visceral layer. The more superficial muscular layer ensheathes the strap muscles — the sternohyoid, sternothyroid, thyrohyoid, and omohyoid muscles. The deeper visceral layer surrounds the trachea, thyroid gland, and esophagus. Both layers are attached to the thyroid cartilage superiorly and extend downward to the posterior aspect of the sternum, where they blend with the tissue between the pericardial sac and great vessels and with that of the sternum. The lateral

aspect of this layer contributes to the formation of the carotid sheath before fusing with the outer superficial fascial layer. The posterosuperior portion of this visceral fascial layer envelops the constrictor muscles of the pharynx and the buccinator muscles and attaches to the base of the skull, forming the anterior aspect of the retropharyngeal space. This portion of the visceral layer is also referred to as the buccopharyngeal fascia (Fig. 75–7) (Anson and McVay, 1971).

The deep or prevertebral layer of the deep cervical fascia, like the superficial layer, begins in the posterior midline and completely surrounds the neck. As the fascial layer proceeds forward from the ligamentum nuchae and the cervical spine, it covers the prevertebral musculature, forming the floor of the posterior cervical triangle, and covers the brachial plexus and subclavian artery. After attaching to the transverse process of the cervical vertebra, this fascial layer splits into two layers in front of the vertebral column, forming the danger space. Both layers of this prevertebral fascia originate at the base of the skull, but the anterior layer fuses with the fascia of the esophagus in the superior mediastinum, forming the posterior wall of the retropharyngeal space. The posterior lamina continues further down through the mediastinum to the coccyx. An anterior extension of this layer to the carotid sheath, called the alar fascia, separates the retropharyngeal space from the pharyngomaxillary space (Fig. 75–7).

The Carotid Sheath. The carotid sheath is the condensation of fascia that invests the carotid artery, internal jugular vein, and vagus nerve. It has contributions from all three layers of the deep cervical fascia. The cervical sympathetic trunk lies behind the sheath superficial to the prevertebral fascia. The carotid sheath extends from the base of the skull through the pharyngomaxillary space, superficial to the deep layer of the deep cervical fascia, into the superior mediastinum (Fig. 75–7).

POTENTIAL NECK SPACES

It is important to remember that although the interfascial spaces of the neck are shown as being anatomically absolute and distinct, almost all these spaces may communicate with each other by way of defects in fascial integrity produced by perforating vessels and nerves, developmental aberrations, or by destruction secondary to a disease process. For this reason, variations in the clinical behavior of certain diseases of the head and neck may take place (Levitt, 1970; Hollingshead, 1974).

The hyoid bone serves as a point of attachment for the fascial layers and as such divides the fascial spaces into a suprahyoid and infrahyoid group. Those spaces whose ensheathing fascia are not bound to the hyoid run through the entire length of the neck. Insofar as these fascial layers limit the spread of infection, the hyoid bone represents an important structure in the control of certain diseases.

Spaces Extending Through the Entire Length of the Neck

Retropharyngeal Spaces

The retropharyngeal space may be divided anatomically into three separate spaces: the retroesophageal, prevertebral, and danger spaces (Figs. 75–7 and 75–8).

The retroesophageal space lies between the middle layer of the deep cervical fascia anteriorly and the prevertebral layer of the deep cervical fascia posteriorly. It extends from the base of the skull superiorly into the superior mediastinum at the level of T_1, where the middle and deep layers fuse. This space contains the retropharyngeal lymph nodes, which are typically present in children under the age of 4 years. Infection in the adenoids, nasal cavities, nasopharynx, and posterior ethmoid sinuses may spread via lymphatics to involve these nodes. Nodal necrosis may result in abscess formation within this retroesophageal space.

The prevertebral space is located between the prevertebral layer of the deep cervical fascia and the bodies of the cervical vertebrae. Extending from the base of the skull along the spinal column to the coccyx, this potential space allows for the spread of infection from the neck to the psoas muscle. Tuberculosis involving the cervical vertebrae with extension into this space was seen prior to the development of effective tuberculosis therapy (Figs. 75–7 and 75–8).

The danger space lies within the two layers of the prevertebral fascia and extends from the base of the skull downward through the

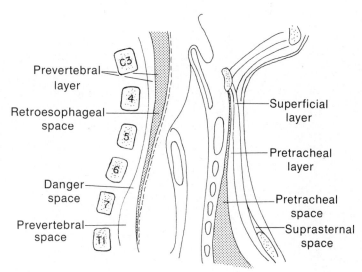

Figure 75–8 Longitudinal section through the neck showing spaces and fascial layers. (After Hollingshead, W. H. 1974. Textbook of Anatomy, 3rd ed. Hagerstown, Harper & Row.)

mediastinum. Infection within this space may spread as far inferiorly as the diaphragm. The close relationship of this potential space to the prevertebral, retroesophageal, and lateral pharyngeal spaces may allow for infection in the pharynx to spread into the mediastinum or beyond. The potential danger of infection in this area is great.

The Vascular Space. The visceral vascular space is the potential space within the carotid sheath and extends from the base of the skull into the superior mediastinum. Because all three layers of the deep cervical fascia contribute to the formation of this space, infection in any other fascial space may ultimately involve this space. Thrombosis of the internal jugular vein and erosion of the carotid artery represent serious complications of infection within the carotid sheath; it is thus most important that the clinician recognize and treat carotid space infections (Figs. 75–7 and 75–8).

Suprahyoid Spaces

The Submandibular Space. The submandibular space is divided by the mylohyoid muscle into the sublingual space superiorly and the submaxillary space inferiorly. The submandibular gland extends into and communicates with both of these spaces. The central compartment of the submaxillary space, which is medial to the anterior belly of the digastric muscle, is termed the submental space (Fig. 75–9).

The entire submandibular space is bound above by the mucosa of the floor of the mouth, laterally and anteriorly by the mandible, posteriorly and inferiorly by the intrinsic muscles of the base of the tongue and hyoid bone, and inferiorly by the superficial layer of the deep cervical fascia.

The submandibular gland protrudes around the posterior border of the mylohyoid muscle to enter and become a passageway between the superior sublingual compartment and the inferior submaxillary compartment. Infection in the submental space may spread freely beneath the anterior belly of the digastric muscle and into the submaxillary space and then via the submandibular gland into the sublingual space. Because of this free intercommunication, these spaces should be considered as a single unit.

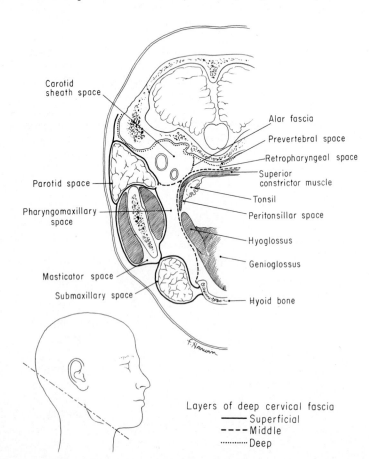

Carotid sheath space
Alar fascia
Prevertebral space
Retropharyngeal space
Superior constrictor muscle
Parotid space
Tonsil
Peritonsillar space
Pharyngomaxillary space
Hyoglossus
Genioglossus
Masticator space
Submaxillary space
Hyoid bone

Layers of deep cervical fascia
——— Superficial
- - - - Middle
·········· Deep

Figure 75–9 Oblique section through the neck. (From Everts, E. C., and Echevaria, J. *In* Paparella, M. M., and Shumrick, D. A. 1973. Otolaryngology. Philadelphia, W. B. Saunders Co.)

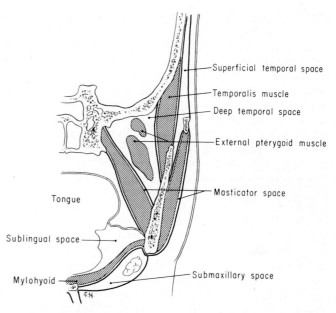

Superficial layers of deep cervical fascia
—— Superficial

Figure 75–10 Coronal section through head. (From Everts, E. C., and Echevaria, J. *In* Paparella, M. M., and Shumrick, D. A. 1973. Otolaryngology. Philadelphia, W. B. Saunders Co.)

This concept was discussed by Ludwig, and multispace infection is the hallmark of Ludwig angina (Fig. 75–9).

The Pharyngomaxillary Space. The pharyngomaxillary space is a clinically important space and has also been called the parapharyngeal or lateral pharyngeal space. This lateral, cone-shaped potential space has its base along the sphenoid bone at the base of the skull and its apex at the hyoid bone. It is bounded medially by the buccopharyngeal fascia, which covers the superior constrictor muscle. Its lateral limit is formed by the superficial layer of the deep cervical fascia covering the mandible, by the internal pterygoid muscle, and by the deep lobe of the parotid. The pterygomandibular raphe limits it anteriorly, and the prevertebral fascia limits it posteriorly. The styloid process and its attachments divide this space into two compartments, an anterior muscular compartment and a posterior neurovascular compartment. The posterior compartment contains the carotid sheath and cranial nerves nine through twelve. The anterior compartment contains no vital structures and extends upward between the lateral wall of the pharynx and the medial surface of the internal pterygoid muscle (Fig. 75–10).

The pharyngomaxillary space communicates with several other spaces in the neck. The inferomedial submandibular space, the posteromedial retropharyngeal space, the lateral parotid and masticator spaces, and the posterior carotid sheath all communicate with the parapharyngeal space and as such may influence the spread of infection in the head and neck. The adenoids, tonsils, nasal cavities, and paranasal sinuses represent sources of infection in this space. Mastoid infection may progress to a coalescent mastoiditis and may erode through the mastoid tip at the digastric ridge and spread into this space, producing a Bezold abscess (Fig. 75–10).

The Masticator Space. The masticator space is anterior and lateral to the pharyngomaxillary space. It contains the masseter muscle, the internal and external pterygoid muscles, the ramus of the mandible, the tendon of the temporalis muscle, and the inferior alveolar neurovascular bundle. The space is bounded by the superficial layer of the deep fascia, which divides around the mandible. The outer layer surrounds the masseter muscle and attaches to the zygoma. The inner layer ensheathes the internal and external pterygoid muscles. These two layers then reunite around the posterior and anterior bodies of the mandibular ramus. Infections in this space most commonly arise from molar teeth, but infection in the region of the zygoma, temporal bone, or mandible may also spread to this space (Fig. 75–9).

The Parotid Space. The parotid space is formed by the superficial layer of the deep cervical fascia as it splits to enclose the parotid gland. The space is separated from the submandibular space inferiorly by the stylomandibular ligament. Connective tissue septa radiate from the surface of the capsular sheath into the surrounding connective tissue. Similar septa perforate the gland itself and internally bind the gland to its capsule. The medial aspect of this parotid capsule is incomplete and allows direct communication of the parotid space with the pharyngomaxillary space. Infections in the parotid space, therefore, pose a significant threat, as they may spread readily into the pharyngomaxillary space and then to the prevertebral space (Fig. 75–10) (Levitt, 1970; Beck, 1955).

The Peritonsillar Space. The peritonsillar space lies between the capsule of the faucial tonsil medially, the superior constrictor muscle laterally, and the tonsillar pillars anteriorly and posteriorly. Infection in this space may spread into the pharyngomaxillary space, and involvement of the carotid sheath with subsequent thrombosis of the internal jugular vein may occur (Fig. 75–10).

The Anterior Visceral Space. This pretracheal portion of the visceral compartment is bounded by the visceral fascia, which surrounds the trachea from the thyroid gland superiorly to the anterior portion of the mediastinum at the level of the arch of the aorta inferiorly. This space communicates freely with the posterior visceral space. Penetration of the cervical esophagus by instruments or a foreign body may cause infection in this space with subsequent extension into the mediastinum (Figs. 75–7 and 75–8).

The fascial layers and compartments in the infant do not differ significantly in anatomy from those of the adult. The fascia of the infant may be somewhat thinner and less well-developed than that of the adult, but the fascial layers and compartments contain the same structures and have the same anatomic relationships as do those of the adult. The less well-developed neck musculature of the infant and child may not supply the same degree of support as is found in the adult and so may be more prone to displacement and distortion from disease processes that expand in volume with time. Infection in the deep neck spaces may therefore interfere with breathing and swallowing to a greater degree in the child than in the adult. It should also be remembered that the fascial layers may become quite thickened and well-defined in response to chronic infection so that what

may represent a flimsy layer of fascia in the uninfected neck may become a thickened fascial layer that serves as an effective barrier to the spread of infection in response to chronic infection in this area.

SELECTED REFERENCES

Anson, B. J., and McVay, C. B. 1971. Surgical Anatomy, 5th ed. Philadelphia, W. B. Saunders Co.
  A surgical anatomy text with fine illustrations and a discussion of the anatomy of the neck that relates well to the surgical approach to pathologic processes in this region.

Crelin, E. S. 1976. Development of the upper respiratory system. Clin. Symp., *28*:4.
  Clear and concise review that covers comparative anatomy as well as embryology of the head and neck. Also instructive drawings by Dr. Frank Netter.

Levitt, G. W. 1970. Cervical fascia and deep neck infections. Laryngoscope, *80*:409.
  A frequently cited paper that discusses well the fascial spaces with reference to deep neck infections.

Patten, B. M. 1968. Human Embryology, 3rd ed. New York, McGraw-Hill.
  A clear presentation of human embryology with fine illustrations.

REFERENCES

Anson, B. J., and McVay, C. B. 1971. Surgical Anatomy, 5th ed. Philadelphia, W. B. Saunders Co.

Arey, L. B. 1974. Developmental Anatomy; A Textbook and Laboratory Manual of Embryology, 7th ed. Philadelphia, W. B. Saunders Co.

Beck, A. L. 1955. Surgical approaches to deep neck infection. Ann. Otol. Rhinol. Laryngol., *64*:91,

Crelin, E. S. 1976. Development of the upper respiratory system. Clin. Symp., *28*:4.

Everts, E. C., and Echevaria, J. 1973. The Pharynx and Deep Neck Infections. *In* Paparella, M. M., and Shumrick, D. A. (Eds.) Otolaryngology, Vol. 3, Philadelphia, W. B. Saunders Co.

Gray, H. 1959. Anatomy of the Human Body, 27th ed. Philadelphia, Lea and Febiger Co.

Hollingshead, W. H. 1974. Textbook of Anatomy, 3rd ed. Hagerstown, Harper and Row.

Jaffe, B. F. 1972. The branchial arches — normal development and abnormalities. *In* Ferguson, C. F. and Kendig, E. L. (Eds.) Pediatric Otolaryngology, Vol. 2, Chap. 99, Philadelphia, W. B. Saunders Co.

Langman, J. 1969. Medical Embryology: Human Development — Normal and Abnormal, 2nd ed. Baltimore, Williams and Wilkins.

Levitt, G. W. 1970. Cervical fascia and deep neck infections. Laryngoscope, *80*:409.

Patten, B. M. 1968. Human Embryology, 3rd ed. New York, McGraw-Hill.

Pernkopf, E. 1963. Atlas of Topographical and Applied Human Anatomy, Vol. 1. Philadelphia, W. B. Saunders Co.

Chapter 76

METHODS OF EXAMINATION

Jose A. Lima, M.D.
Edward R. Graviss, M.D.

The cervical region consists of a complex of muscles, blood vessels, nerves, glands, lymph nodes, and lymphatic channels, in addition to the vital midline structures, such as the spinal column, the pharynx, the larynx, and the esophagus. In a relatively small cross-sectional area, these important organs are located within a short distance of each other. This compact arrangement of structures permits early diagnosis of disturbances since minimal changes in shape or volume in the affected cervical area become evident and lead the individual to seek treatment soon after the changes become noticeable. It is of fundamental importance for the physician to be familiar with the anatomy of the cervical facial planes, compartments, and organs prior to the diagnosing of disease in this area. Chapter 75 covers this subject in detail.

The child's neck is not a miniature adult neck, and the difference between the two must be recognized by the examiner. Accumulations of fat in the superficial cervical fascial compartment are prominent until the age of nine months, when the neck begins to slenderize. Fat resorption is maximal during the second year of life. Small changes in the necks of newborn infants, as opposed to those seen in the necks of older children, are, therefore, poorly perceived by inspection and can only be diagnosed adequately by careful palpation.

The cartilaginous framework of the infantile larynx is less prominent and located higher in the neck than is the adolescent larynx.

The diagnosis of problems in the neck should begin with the taking of a history and should be followed by a physical examination and performance of diagnostic procedures when indicated by the history and physical.

HISTORY

The organized collection of data is of crucial importance for arriving at a diagnosis. This information may be obtained directly from an older child or from the parent of a younger child. The diagnosis can be strongly suspected on historical information alone in 50 per cent of cases. The questioning should be conducted to determine the chief complaint, the time and mode of onset of the problem, the duration of the symptoms, their severity and exact location, and progression of symptoms. The character of pain, when present, and the response of pain to medication are also useful items of information. A family history and a discussion of the case with the referring physician can also provide the diagnostician with valuable information.

The several basic types of pathologic conditions found in the cervical area present different characteristics that can be used as clues to their diagnosis. Congenital lesions are frequently obvious at birth. However, some may only become noticeable later in life; for instance, branchial cleft cysts may go unnoticed until the cyst becomes secondarily infected. Inflammatory processes may be chronic or acute. Granulomatous diseases of the neck are usually characterized by a chronic course often accompanied by an intermittent, low-grade fever. Acute bacterial infections are generally of sudden onset and are accompanied by pain or discomfort, inflammatory signs, and high fever. Asymptomatic neck masses of neoplastic origin can frequently become very large without having significant symptoms. Pain that may be associated with such neoplasms in the late stages may be the result of invasion of neural tissue or sudden hemorrhage into the center of the neoplasm. Neck tumors may grow considerably before interfering with air or food passage. Occasionally a cervical neoplasm can lead to airway obstruction by extrinsic compression of the trachea or by directly interfering with the nerve supply to the larynx.

Environmental factors contributing to diseases in children should be sought. Radiation therapy to the neck is associated with an increased risk of thyroid carcinoma in later years. Diphenylhydantoin (Dilantin), a widely used anticonvulsive medication, can promote cervical lymphadenopathy that resembles neoplastic disorders of the lymphatic system. In areas of the United States where large numbers of recent immigrants may settle, the examiner should be suspicious of the presence of tropical diseases, which may manifest themselves by causing cervical lymphadenopathy.

Periodic tender swelling in the neck during meals may indicate obstruction of the ducts of the salivary glands by stricture or stones. The enlargement of a neck mass during exertion or crying may represent the filling of vascular channels secondary to diminished venous return, indicating the presence of a hemangioma. Laryngoceles, although uncommon in children, may also distend during crying or straining (Chap. 78).

EXAMINATION

Perhaps the most important factor in a successful examination is the establishment of good rapport between physician and child. It is surprising how much cooperation one can obtain from a young child once a good relationship is initiated and the child learns to trust the examiner. Every procedure should be explained carefully to the child, who will then become less anxious as he or she knows what to expect.

Inspection

Good light is an important prerequisite to performing the physical examination and can be obtained with the head mirror or the headlight. The inspection should start by the systematic identification of normal landmarks: the jaw, the sternocleidomastoid muscles, the clavicles, and the cartilaginous framework of the larynx and trachea. Asymmetry and deformities, the presence of neck masses, vascular marks, abnormal pulsations, or discolorations of the skin should be recorded. Scars, fistulas, abnormalities of neck motion, and changes in neck masses caused by swallowing, tongue protrusion, and lowering of the head are important. For instance, masses attached to the thyroid gland tend to move with deglutition or tongue protrusion. Thyroglossal duct cysts are also mobile with tongue protrusion since they are connected to the hyoid bone. Cavernous hemangiomas tend to increase in size when the head is lowered as a result of increased venous congestion in their vascular spaces (Chisholm et al., 1959).

Palpation

The examiner's hands should be clean, dry, and moderately warm. Palpation is better performed with the palmar surface of the finger tips, while the opposite hand exerts gentle control of the head motion. The location of a neck mass can have diagnostic and prognostic importance and should always be recorded. Thyroglossal duct cysts almost invariably occur in the midline, whereas branchial cleft cysts occur in the lateral neck.

The mobility of a cervical mass may also be important in establishing a diagnosis. Sebaceous cysts are firmly attached to the epidermis, and one is unable to roll the skin over their surfaces. In contrast, benign soft tissue masses are almost never attached to the skin or deeper structures and are usually mobile. Primary cancers or metastatic lesions can be fixed by invasion of skin and adjacent organs. Shape and regularity of masses are also important characteristics. Lesions can be diffuse or localized, regular or irregular. Degenerative lesions of the salivary glands, such as those seen in Sjögren syndrome, tend to be diffuse, whereas neoplasms are more localized. Irregularity is suggestive of malignancy.

The consistency of a mass (soft, rubbery, woody, cystic, bag of worms, fluctuating, or pulsatile) can also provide the diagnostician with valuable information. Lipomas are usually soft and localized, generally independent of the remaining adipose tissue. Benign lymph nodes are rubbery, well defined, and mobile. Advanced malignancies can be woody and hard because of rapid growth. Cysts have a typical "cystic" consistency, denoting the interface between solid and liquid. Cavernous hemangiomas may be felt as a "bag of worms" owing to the presence of calcified particles (phleboliths) in the mass. Abscesses are tender, fluctuating swellings. Air in the neck secondary to trauma to the airway or lung is characterized by a crepitant sensation on palpation (Chap. 80).

Tenderness is an important characteristic, often but not always associated with an inflammatory process. Pulsation in a neck mass can indicate the presence of an aneurysm or a carotid body tumor. However, masses adjacent to the carotid artery may transmit the anteroposterior pulsation of the vessel without being vascular themselves. Palpating the mass sidewise and gently pulling it away from the artery may disclose the nonpulsatile nature of the lesion (Chap. 81).

The different cervical organs should be palpated in a sequential order (Chap. 77).

Salivary Glands

The parotids are not usually palpable in normal children, but the Stensen duct can occasionally be palpated against the masseter muscle in a slender child. Unilateral enlargement of the gland by tumor or inflammatory, metabolic, or degenerative disease will cause facial asymmetry. When the tail of the parotid gland is enlarged, there may be lateral displacement of the earlobe on the side of the lesion. Parotid neoplasms in children are usually benign lymphangiomas or hemangiomas. These are usually soft and diffuse. The presence of a solid mass in the parotid area is somewhat alarming, since most of the solid tumors of this area in children are malignancies. The examination of the parotid gland should be completed by the internal examination of the parotid duct. In acute parotitis, pus can be expressed from the parotid duct orifice near the second molar by external massage of the gland.

The submandibular gland as well as the submental triangle should be examined by bimanual techniques. One gloved index finger is inserted intraorally over the sublingual space while the opposite finger exerts gentle rotary pressure upon the gland externally (Fig. 76–1). This maneuver allows a three-dimensional evaluation of the gland. Likewise, the presence of stones in the sub-

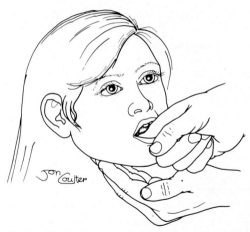

Figure 76–1 Bimanual palpation of the submandibular gland. The right index finger palpates the contents of the submandibular triangle intraorally while gentle external pressure is exerted by the left hand. Stones in the parenchyma of the gland or in the ductal system are easily felt by the examining finger in this manner.

mandibular duct can easily be ascertained by this technique (Chap. 51).

Lymph Nodes

Lymphadenopathy in childhood is common and usually indicates benign hyperplastic processes. Large nodes in the posterior triangle should, however, be regarded suspiciously since such nodes have been demonstrated to have a higher incidence of malignancy than nodes in other locations. The enlargement of a single node to greater than 3 cm or the presence of a hard, nontender node much larger than any other should also be regarded suspiciously, particularly if such a node fails to diminish in size after a trial with antibiotic therapy.

A thorough examination of the upper respiratory and digestive tract may reveal the primary source of a neoplasm. Multiple nodal enlargement associated with inflammatory changes that cause them to be matted together or the presence of a draining sinus associated with chronic lymphadenopathy is suggestive of a granulomatous, fungal, or tuberculous process (Pollock et al., 1978). Delphian nodes, midline lymph nodes located in front of the trachea, are in children commonly associated with thyroiditis and less commonly with thyroid carcinoma (Chap. 79).

Sternocleidomastoid Muscle

The sternocleidomastoid muscles are the most prominent muscles in the neck. The carotid sheath, containing the carotid artery, internal jugular vein, and vagus nerve, is located behind this muscle. In the newborn, an asymmetry of the sternocleidomastoid muscles characterized by a unilateral mass usually reflects the presence of congenital torticollis, a disorder the etiology of which is still much debated.

Thyroid Gland

The thyroid gland consists of two lobes connected by the isthmus, which lies in front of the second or third tracheal ring. In about one third of children there is a pyramidal lobe extending upward from the isthmus. This lobe represents the remnant of the thyroglossal duct. The normal thyroid is not easily palpable, but a small goiter or thyroid nodule can frequently be felt readily by the examiner. The thyroid gland is best palpated with the patient sitting and the examiner standing behind him or her (Fig. 76–2). The isthmus is normally palpable 1 cm below the cricoid cartilage, and the lobes are located lateral to the trachea underneath the sternocleidomastoid muscle. A slight retraction of this muscle with one hand will permit the fingertips of the other hand to outline the surface of the lobe as it is demonstrated in Figure 76–2. If the patient is asked to swallow, the gland will be felt to move upward. Nodules situated inside the gland will likewise move upward with the swallowing motion. In general, diffuse enlargement of the thyroid gland in children represents thyroiditis, par-

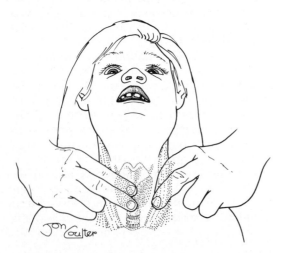

Figure 76–2 Palpation of the thyroid gland. The examiner stands behind the patient. A slight retraction of the sternocleidomastoid muscle away from the midline with one hand permits the other hand to outline the surface of the lobe.

ticularly Hashimoto thyroiditis (Gould et al., 1977). Thyroid cancer in children is uncommon, except when the neck has been irradiated. Increased incidences of papillary and other histologic types of carcinoma of the thyroid gland have been observed in children who underwent irradiation of the neck (Altman and Schwartz, 1978; Prior and Silberstein, 1977) (Chap. 79).

Auscultation

Since obstruction of the carotid arteries in children and adolescents is uncommon, most of the vascular sounds heard in the neck are heart murmurs transmitted upwards. Occasionally, however, children with diffuse toxic goiters will present a systolic bruit over the thyroid area.

Auscultation of the neck is a very important part of the evaluation of children with upper airway obstruction. The characteristics of the stridor combined with the quality of the cry or voice can lead to the determination of the nature of the disease causing the obstruction.

ANCILLARY METHODS OF EXAMINATION

Radiography

Radiographic evaluation of the neck cannot be separated from the evaluation of the airway or of the cervical spine and face. The lateral projection of the neck should be done in a neutral or extended position, and the frontal projection should be performed so that the chin appears superimposed over the occiput. The radiographs must be made during inspiration in order to reproduce normal anatomic patterns accurately (Brodeur et al., 1980).

Air in the hypopharynx and trachea is a natural contrast agent. The vocal cords are at the level of the inferior portion of the pyriform sinuses, between the lower border of the second cervical vertebra (C2) and the lower border of C3 in the infant. The larynx in a 16 year old will have migrated inferiorly and is usually located between C4 and C5. The cricopharyngeal muscle delineates the upper extent of the esophagus. On an esophagogram the cricopharyngeal muscle can be seen anterior to C3 in the infant. With growth, the cricopharyngeus migrates until it reaches the adult level at C5. Air in the hypopharynx outlines the anterior portion of the retropharyngeal space, which is bordered posteriorly by the vertebral bodies. Fatty densities on the radiograph represent the subcutaneous fat found in the neck. It is not possible to identify muscle, blood vessels, nerves, or glands using standard radiographic techniques.

The retropharyngeal space in the infant and young child has caused many diagnostic problems (Chisholm et al., 1959; Pinto and Becker, 1977). The space is thicker in the child than in the adult, partially owing to the fact that the cartilage of the vertebral bodies anterior to their ossified centers is of the same radiographic density as the soft tissues. The soft tissues themselves are very expandable. The normal extent of the prevertebral soft tissue in an infant is less than the size of one vertebral body; however, these soft tissues can expand to the size of three vertebral bodies during forceful expiration such as occurs with crying. By adolescence, the upper limit of normal has decreased to one third the size of the vertebral body.

In children over six months of age, normal adenoids should create a minimum of 5 mm of soft tissue density. Enlarged adenoids can impinge upon the superior aspect of the retropharyngeal space, and enlarged palatine tonsils will create rounded densities that protrude into the center of the oropharyngeal air column. It is important to evaluate these normal structures during inspiration, as it is difficult on an expiration film to differentiate a normal retropharyngeal space from one containing an abscess or one with diffuse cellulitis, myxedema, or neoplastic involvement (Maguire et al., 1965). When there is any doubt concerning the retropharyngeal space, fluoroscopic evaluation during a single inspiratory effort should resolve the problem.

Most retropharyngeal abscesses do not initially contain the "pathognomonic bubble of air." Infrequently, gas can be identified within the esophagus during a lateral neck examination, but this normal variant should not be confused with air in a retropharyngeal abscess. A repeat examination should demonstrate air having cleared the esophagus because of normal esophageal peristalsis. Persistent retention of gas within the cervical esophagus should alert the examiner to a possible esophageal foreign body. A contrast esophagogram will demonstrate such a foreign body. Air in the external ear or in the apex of the lung can also simulate the presence of air in the prevertebral space.

Radiographic studies are helpful when calcifications are present in the neck. Calcifications anterior to the trachea may be suggestive of papillary carcinoma of the thyroid. Calcifications of the lymph nodes in the lateral neck are sometimes observed in tuberculous lymphadenitis.

The cartilaginous structures of the larynx are seldom calcified at birth. However, the body of the hyoid bone is ossified at birth. The greater horn of the hyoid bone ossifies at a very early age, but the lesser horn has a variable ossification pattern. Both the greater and the lesser horns can project over the airway, and the separate ossification center of the lesser horn can be mistaken for an opaque foreign body, such as a chicken bone or fish bone. In addition, the stylohyoid ligament can ossify to such an extent as to project over the pharynx or cervical soft tissues to create the appearance of a foreign body.

The spinal column can also be evaluated in neck radiography. Abnormal curvatures, slippage of vertebrae, and degenerative or traumatic changes can be easily identified on lateral and posteroanterior films of the neck.

A special roentgenographic technique, magnification, allows for the more accurate visualization of small or closely approximated structures in the neck. With this technique, small or faintly opaque foreign bodies are more easily identified than by standard radiographic techniques (Brodeur et al., 1980).

In the frontal projection, high kilovoltage filtered radiography can decrease the radiation absorption of the ossified cervical spine while enhancing delineation of the airway. This technique increases the likelihood of recognition of foreign bodies in the airway but decreases the examiner's ability to detect opaque objects within the soft tissues (Maguire et al., 1965; Shovis, 1977).

Xeroradiography is a photoelectric method of presenting a roentgenographic image. The usefulness of the method lies in its ability to enhance the outlines of soft tissues, thus aiding in the evaluation of these structures for the presence of abnormalities. Xeroradiography is superior to conventional plain lateral roentgenograms for demonstration of airway abnormalities, soft tissue tumors, and calcified structures. The degree of radiation to which xeroradiography exposes the subject varies depending on the technique employed but is usually 6 to 100 times that of conventional neck radiography. For this reason, this technique should not be used in children.

Esophagogram

The barium swallow is a time-honored diagnostic test for evaluating a patient for the presence of extraluminal pathologic conditions of the upper digestive tract. Since the study of swallowing disturbances and esophageal lesions is covered in Chapters 42 and 53 of this book, it will not be discussed here. However, esophagograms have proved useful in assessing patients for the presence of other disorders of the neck.

An esophagogram may demonstrate displacement of the retropharyngeal, hypopharyngeal, or cervical esophageal areas caused by tumor masses or inflammatory lesions and abscesses. Large thyroid goiters are also known to cause deviation of the cervical esophagus laterally. Accumulation of contrast medium in the soft tissue of the prevertebral space may be an indication that a post-traumatic fistula secondary to a penetrating foreign body is present. In the young child, both fluoroscopy and a barium swallow may be necessary to complete the examination of the neck.

Sialography

Sialography involves the injection of an oil-based contrast medium into the parotid or submandibular ducts so that the ductal systems will appear opaque on radiographic examination. It is diagnostic for stones, strictures, salivary fistulas, and recurrent parotitis. Sialography may also be helpful in determining whether a mass is intraglandular or extraglandular. Intraglandular masses will produce parenchymal opacification and will deform and displace components of the canalicular system. Puddling of contrast medium within the gland and disruption of the ducts are suggestive of malignant invasion of the ducts. In cases of salivary gland diseases of degenerative nature, such as Sjögren syndrome, it is common to find sialectasis, which is characterized by localized saccular dilatation in the gland ductal system.

Arteriography

Standard angiography is receiving special attention in the diagnosis of masses in the neck occurring in children. Arteriography can be performed by percutaneous carotid puncture or the retrograde femoral approach. The latter is much more commonly used today. Lesions such as hemangiomas, chemodectomas, nasopharyngeal angiofibromas, and arteriovenous malformations may readily be diagnosed by this method (Overhold et al., 1978). The procedure is an alternative to obtaining a biopsy specimen of these highly vascular tumors.

On arteriography, cavernous hemangiomas display large venous lakes containing phleboliths. Chemodectomas, nasopharyngeal angiofibromas, and capillary hemangiomas display staining in the capillary phase of the study. Arteriovenous malformations may often clinically and radiologically simulate hemangiomas; such malformations are characterized by large feeding vessels and show prompt filling of large draining veins during the arterial phase. They occur more commonly in the brain but can also occur extracranially.

Arteriography can aid in the preoperative evaluation of vascular tumors, as this technique can determine the extent, location, and degree of intracranial invasion of these tumors. In the last decade, techniques have been developed by which tumors can be embolized angiographically. A large variety of materials, including plastic, gelatin sponges (Gelfoam), metal, china, and muscle have been employed for occlusion of feeding vessels. Vascular thrombosis distal to the embolic material results in diminution of tumor vascularity. Lesions such as neurilemomas can be differentiated from chemodectomas by the lack of capillary vascular stain blush during arteriography of the former. Carotid body tumors present in the capillary stage of the study as densely stained masses separating the external carotid from the internal carotid artery. These tumors also tend to be multicentric, and angiography is helpful in detecting the hidden foci. Arteriography is also of assistance in the evaluation of patients who sustained neck trauma and are suspected of having suffered vascular injury.

Computerized Tomography

It has become common to evaluate a child with neurologic symptoms by computerized tomography (CT) because this noninvasive technique can demonstrate differences in the densities of different intracranial structures, consequently allowing the diagnosis of intracranial diseases (Pinto and Becker, 1977). Although computerized body scanning equipment is useful in visualizing the cervical area, it is even more helpful in evaluating the brain, orbit, and sinuses. Transverse sectional images of cervical structures can be obtained by this method, and the relationship of these structures can be studied in a way not previously possible (Gould et al., 1977). A large hemangioma in the neck of a newborn can be seen in the CT scan shown in Figure 76–3.

Vascular tumors, such as chemodectomas and angiomas, become more visible when the patient has been given an intravenous injection of iodinated contrast material to enhance the observability before the scan is performed. Contrast scanning can also be used to determine the extent of these lesions prior to their surgical excision.

Computerized tomography requires the child to be motionless for successive periods of five seconds until the required number of images has been obtained. It is therefore desirable to sedate young children for this procedure. CT scanning will probably prove to be more useful in the assessment of neck masses as faster scanners with improved spatial resolution are developed. Figure 76–3 illustrates a cervical hemangioma displacing the trachea and esophagus in a newborn child.

Ultrasonography

Ultrasonography, like CT scanning, is a relatively new method of visualizing structures within the body. When ultrasonography of the neck is performed, high-frequency sound waves are passed through the neck, and their reflective and refractive patterns are evaluated. Since the sound waves do not create ionizing radiation, ultrasonography is considered to be the safest and least invasive method of evaluating the neck. In addition, sedation is rarely required for this test. B-mode, gray-scale scanning and real-time imaging allow the examiner to make anatomic projections of the neck in a transverse or longitudinal plane. The initial images are viewed on a television monitor, with hard copies being made on Polaroid or radiographic films.

Ultrasonic examination of a normal neck demonstrates vascular structures as linear, echo-free areas. With real-time imaging, arteries will pulsate and veins will change size with respiration. Real-time, high-resolution imaging has been used in the evaluation of arterial diseases in adults. This type of imaging is excellent for evaluating small lesions in a child's neck.

Ultrasonography is used to evaluate mass lesions or nodules in the neck (Goldberg et al., 1975), such as that in the thyroid gland shown in Figure 76–4. Purely cystic lesions can be differentiated from solid masses by this method. Some lesions are complex (both cystic and solid). Since ultrasonic examination basically makes abnormal structures visible rather than delineating normal structures, it is appropriate to talk about the ultrasonic patterns of pathologic lesions.

Hematomas can initially be very sonolucent but may then give the appearance of complex

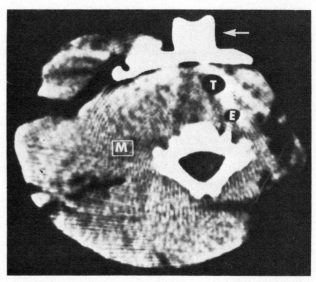

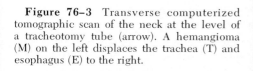

Figure 76–3 Transverse computerized tomographic scan of the neck at the level of a tracheotomy tube (arrow). A hemangioma (M) on the left displaces the trachea (T) and esophagus (E) to the right.

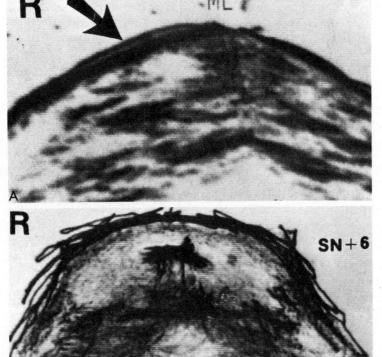

Figure 76–4 *A,* Ultrasonogram showing echo-free nodule in the right lobe of the thyroid gland (white area below the skin) of a 13 year old girl from whom a colloid nodule was subsequently removed. ML, midline; R, right. *B,* Ultrasonogram showing diffuse goiter in a seven year old girl. R, right; SN+6, section 6 cm above the level of the sternal notch. (Courtesy of Dr. Arnold Shkolnik.)

lesions as the clot liquefies during clot resolution. Adenopathy, when inflammatory, presents as a solid lesion, but should an abscess form, the lesion becomes complex with cystic components. Lymphomas may appear as relatively echo-free masses that simulate cystic structures because of their homogenous cellular nature. Differentiation may be made by the lack of posterior wall enhancement and increased transmissibility that are seen in true cystic structures (Yeh and Wolf, 1977). Hemangiomas and lymphangiomas may evidence complex patterns with multiple small cysts in an echogenic area.

Ultrasonic scanning of the thyroid gland has become a valuable tool in the evaluation of the cold nodule. If a cold thyroid nodule appears to be cystic on ultrasound examination, a cyst puncture and needle aspiration can be performed, sparing the patient surgical procedures. Solid nodules must, however, be removed surgically.

The vascular structures in the neck can be well visualized with high-resolution, real-time scanning. The neck vessels can be evaluated for patency, thrombus formation, atheromatous plaques, and arteriovenous malforma-

tions. The ultrasonic examination of the neck must be evaluated in light of several factors. Most important is the type of equipment and its ability to provide adequate spatial resolution. Lesions smaller than the spatial resolution of the ultrasound unit, obviously, cannot be evaluated. This must be coupled with the skill of the ultrasonographer, who must literally "paint a picture" with the ultrasound transducer. Many artifacts can be introduced into the images if the unit is not accurately tuned and adjusted.

Nuclear Medicine

The thyroid gland is easily evaluated by isotope examinations. Radioactive iodine as a tracer agent is handled by the gland as normal iodine and is incorporated into the thyroxin molecule. The evaluation of thyroid function by radioactive iodine uptake has been supplanted by the evaluation of T_3 and T_4 levels in the serum. If radioactive iodine is used in children, a short half-life isotope such as ^{125}I or ^{123}I should be used. Although ^{131}I is readily available in most nuclear medicine departments, it should not be used in children because of the high radiation dose to the thyroid gland (1.5 rads per μCi ^{131}I) caused by its β-particle emission.

In the last decade, [99m] technetium has totally replaced radioactive iodine for scanning of the thyroid gland. Technetium administered in the form of sodium pertechnetate is concentrated within the thyroid gland by the same trapping mechanism that stores iodine, but the isotope is not incorporated into the precursors of thyroxin. Thyroid scanning is useful in evaluation of thyroid nodules. Nonfunctioning "cold" nodules are demonstrated as filling defects within the image of the gland. Functioning nodules are demonstrated as a very hot area of activity, which may be the only area of activity visualized within the neck. If only the nodules concentrate the radioactive isotope, stimulation of the thyroid gland by thyroid stimulating hormone (TSH) must be performed and the patient rescanned. Following TSH stimulation, a normal thyroid gland will appear as such with the autonomous thyroid nodule evident in the normal tissue.

The salivary glands also concentrate iodine and sodium pertechnetate and can be viewed scintigraphically. However, such scintigraphic studies of salivary glands are of limited usefulness since the results are nonspecific (Fiori-Ratti et al., 1977). Degenerative diseases such as Sjögren disease are characterized by decreased uptake of radioisotope by the salivary glands. Any neoplastic or inflammatory mass that destroys or displaces the gland will show decreased uptake in that area. The exception to this rule is a Warthin tumor which (rare in children), can concentrate the isotope.

Technetium diphosphonate is a bone scanning agent that makes evident structures in the cervical spine. This agent will be taken up in any area of necrosis or calcification within the soft tissues of the neck. Neuroblastomas are known to take up bone scanning agents even when calcification of these entities cannot be demonstrated radiographically.

[67]Gallium has been used in the evaluation of inflammatory processes and of lymphomas (Teates and Hunter, 1975). Because it is more useful in demonstrating abnormalities of this sort in the chest and the abdomen than in the neck and requires a relatively high radiation dose, its use is discouraged in children.

Needle Aspiration

Obtaining a biopsy specimen by needle aspiration is a valid alternative to performing surgery to obtain such a specimen in order to diagnose a neck mass. Needle aspiration can be efficiently performed under local anesthesia in the outpatient unit, and the procedure takes only a few minutes. Any mass of unclear nature, particularly if it is bigger than 3 cm in diameter, is the only mass, and is nontender, should be regarded with suspicion and investigated. If thorough endoscopy of the upper airway and food passages fails to demonstrate a primary source of the mass enlargement, it is in order to proceed with the aspiration biopsy under local or general anesthesia.

Some 40 years ago, Martin and Ellis (1930) popularized a technique in which a minute incision was made in the skin adjacent to the neck mass and a 16 or 18 gauge needle attached to a syringe was utilized under vacuum aspiration to obtain a plug of tissue from the depth of the lesion. The resulting specimen is histologically processed like any other surgical specimen. This method identifies metastatic lesions very accurately, but it is criticized by many in that it may allow the seeding of tumor cells in the needle track.

More recently, a method for obtaining biopsy specimens by aspirating with a fine needle was developed and widely used in Scandinavian countries. This technique is, in general, the same as that of Martin and Ellis (1930) except that a fine (18 to 22 gauge) needle attached to a 20 cc disposable syringe in a syringe holder is used to obtain the specimen (Fig. 76–5). As the mass is punctured by the needle, the syringe piston is withdrawn slightly in order to create a vacuum inside the syringe. The needle is then moved back and forth within the mass without completely withdrawing it. The vacuum in the syringe is then released before the needle is withdrawn from the lesion. The specimen retrieved inside the needle may be divided into several samples for bacteriologic studies and cytologic smears. The cytologic smears are prepared and stained by the Papanicolaou method. Expertise in analyzing the cytologic specimen is required, but in experienced hands, a fairly high degree of accuracy of diagnosis may be expected. No convincing evidence has been presented that shows that this fine needle biopsy method leads to tumor seeding.

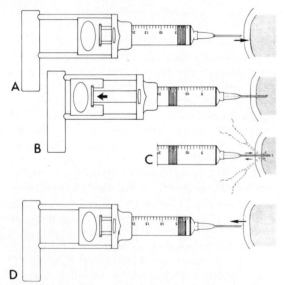

Figure 76–5 Technical aspects of the aspiration biopsy technique. *A*, The needle is introduced into the mass, which is firmly grasped by the fingers. *B*, Vacuum pressure is applied to the syringe. *C*, The needle is moved back and forth within the mass and in different directions without completely withdrawing it. *D*, With the needle still in the mass, the vacuum in the syringe is released, and the needle containing the specimen is then withdrawn. (Modified from Frable, W. J. 1976. Thin needle aspiration biopsy. Am. J. Clin. Pathol., 65:168.)

SUMMARY

The successful diagnosis of diseases of the neck in children depends on a sound knowledge of the anatomy of this region and upon the realization that the child's neck is different from the adult neck both structurally and in the spectrum of pathologic conditions that may present in this area.

History and physical examination alone will lead to a correct diagnosis in the majority of cases. Ancillary methods of diagnosis that are available to confirm or establish the diagnosis in more complex cases may be used. Among the advances in the diagnosis of cervical pathologic conditions, two new tools present an excellent potential and deserve special mention: computerized tomography and diagnostic ultrasound.

REFERENCES

Altman, A. J., and Schwartz, A. D. 1978. Diagnosis of Cancer in Childhood in Malignant Diseases of Infancy, Childhood and Adolescence. Philadelphia, W. B. Saunders Co., p. 18.

Brodeur, A. E., Silberstein, M. D., and Graviss, E. R. 1980. Direct microfocus magnification: Its many advantages in pediatrics. Am. J. Dis. Child., 134:245–249.

Caffey, J. P., and Baker, D. A. 1978. Pediatric X-ray Diagnosis. Chicago, Year Book Medical Pub.

Chisholm, T., Spencer, B. J., and McFarland, F. A. 1959. Visible lesions of the neck in children. Pediatr. Clin. North Am., 6(4):1011–1022.

Cole, T. B., and Baylin, G. 1973. Radiographic evaluation of prevertebral space. Laryngoscope, 83:721–732.

Fiori-Ratti, L., DeCampora, E., and Senin, U. 1977. Sequence scintigraphy: A morphological and functional study of the salivary glands. Laryngoscope, 87(7):1086–1094.

Frable, W. J. 1976. Thin needle aspiration biopsy. Am. J. Clin. Pathol., 65:168–182.

Goldberg, B. B., Pollock, H. M., Capitanio, M. A., and Kirkpatrick, J. A. 1975. Ultrasonography: An aid in the diagnosis of masses in pediatric patients. Pediatrics, 56(3):421–428.

Gould, L. V., Cummings, C. W., Rabuzzi, D. D., et al. 1977. Use of computerized axial tomography of the head and neck region. Laryngoscope, 87(8):1270–1276.

LeBoeuf, G., and Ducharme, J. R. 1966. Thyroiditis in children. Diagnosis and management. Pediatr. Clin. North Am., 13:19–42.

Maguire, G. H., Beique, R. A., and Rotenburg, A. D. 1965. Selective filtration: The practical approach to high-kilovoltage radiography. Radiology, 85:343–351.

Martin, H. E., and Ellis, E. F. 1930. Biopsy by needle puncture and aspiration. Ann. Surg., 92:169–181.

McCook, T. A., and Felman, A. H. 1979. Retropharyngeal masses in infants and young children. Am. J. Dis. Child., 133:41–43.

Overhold, S. L., Gado, M., Sessions, D. G., and Ogura, J. H. 1978. Angiography in the diagnosis and management of extracranial vascular lesions of the head and neck. Laryngoscope, 88:1769–1783.

Pinto, R. S., and Becker, M. H. 1977. Computed tomography in pediatric diagnosis. Am. J. Dis. Child., 131:583–592.

Pollock, P. J., Koontz, F. P., Viner, T. F., et al. 1978. Cervicofacial actinomycosis. Arch. Otolaryngol., 104:491.

Principato, J. J., and Liebowitz, M. 1971. Lateral x-ray film of neck in otorhinolaryngology. Arch. Otolaryngol., 93:505–510.

Prior, J. A., and Silberstein, J. S. 1977. Head, face and neck. *In* Prior, J. A., and Silberstein, J. S. (Eds.) Physical Diagnosis, 4th ed. St. Louis, The C. V. Mosby Co., p. 83.

Shovis, T. L. 1977. Noninvasive evaluation of the pediatric airway: A recent advance. Pediatrics, 59:872–880.

Teates, C. D., and Hunter, J. G., Jr. 1975. Gallium scanning as a screening test for inflammatory lesions. Radiology, 116(2):383–387.

Winship, T., and Rosvoli, R. V. 1961. Childhood thyroid carcinoma. Cancer, 14:734–743.

Wolf, B. S., Nakagawa, H., and Yeh, H. C. 1977. Visualization of the thyroid gland with computed tomography. Radiology, 123:368.

Yeh, H. C., and Wolf, B. S. 1977. Ultrasonography and computed tomography in the diagnosis of homogeneous masses. Radiology, 123:425–428.

Chapter 77

NECK MASSES

Mark May, M.D.

Victor L. Schramm, Jr., M.D.

Neck masses in children are common but result from a variety of causes; because the etiology of a neck mass encompasses such a wide range of possibilities, a systematic approach to the differential diagnosis of neck masses is essential. The physician must be familiar with a wide variety of causes of neck masses and must reach a final diagnosis of the cause of a particular mass by assessing the patient's history, physical condition, the results of laboratory tests, and other pertinent data. This chapter attempts to provide some guidelines for the physician faced with assessing the origin and determining a diagnosis for neck masses.

Each clinician must begin the investigation of a neck mass by examining the patient's history for occurrences of local or systemic diseases and the taking of significant medications; further information is derived from the physical examination of the appearance, location, and characteristics of the neck mass.

The diagnosis is frequently established based on findings from the history and physical examination. Confirmation of the diagnosis may require hematologic tests, urinary analysis, serologic skin tests, or radiographic evaluation, or needle aspiration biopsy or culture of the mass may be necessary. Biopsy specimens for frozen section evaluation should be obtained in such a way that simultaneous definitive surgical extirpation is possible, if indicated. Above all, if the diagnosis is not certain, multiple therapeutic trials or prolonged periods of observation are not indicated. A search for a more definitive diagnosis should be instituted as soon as there is reasonable doubt.

The chronology of the patient's symptoms and information obtained from the patient's history may suggest a diagnosis to the physician. Some normal neck structures may appear to be abnormal, and occasionally a mesenchymal malignancy may be noted at or soon after birth and may be confused with a congenital anomaly. Masses associated with local or regional infection may be either inflammatory or congenital neck masses. A history of trauma suggests that a neck mass could be a hematoma, although the clinician should be aware that incidental trauma is a particular hazard in childhood (Krugman, 1976). Masses of recent onset that are enlarging and painful suggest an inflammatory process, although hemorrhage into a neoplastic mass may mimic benign disease. A mass enlarging rapidly (over a period of one to two months) is frequently malignant, whereas a slowly enlarging mass is usually a benign neoplasm or congenital anomaly. Masses that fluctuate in size suggest benign inflammatory adenopathy or low-grade inflammation of a congenital cyst. A mass that fluctuates with eating is likely to be related to a salivary gland infection or a sialocele (Table 77–1).

Congenital neck lesions frequently may be diagnosed by physical examination. Although congenital masses are present from birth, they may not be recognized as masses until later childhood or even until adulthood.

Table 77–1 DIAGNOSIS BY HISTORY

History	Type of Mass
Present from birth	Congenital
Associated with infection	Congenital, inflammatory
Associated with trauma	Hematoma
Enlarging in size	
slowly, over 6 months or more	Congenital or benign
rapidly over 2 months	Malignant
recent onset and painful	Inflammatory
Enlarging and becoming tender with eating	Salivary gland infection

(From May, M. 1976. Neck masses in children: Diagnosis and treatment. Pediatr. Ann., 5:8.)

They may enlarge slowly or become infected and present as acute inflammatory masses. A branchial cleft cyst, when it is not infected, will present as a soft mass anterior to the sternocleidomastoid muscle. First branchial cleft derivatives may present below the earlobe or as cord-like masses along the anterior sternocleidomastoid muscle, ending in a subcutaneous nodule of cartilage. If the branchial cleft cyst becomes infected, the patient will usually present with a red, tender diffuse or fluctuant mass anterior to or beneath the sternocleidomastoid muscle. The pathognomonic sign of a branchial cleft anomaly is the presence of a fistula located along the anterior border of the sternocleidomastoid muscle. The cutaneous orifice of a second or a third branchial cleft fistula will often retract with swallowing since the cleft communicates with the pharynx directly or by fibrous attachment.

Thyroglossal duct cysts arise from the thyroid anlage that descends during fetal life from the foramen cecum at the base of the tongue. For this reason, thyroglossal duct cysts are most frequently found midline at or below the level of the hyoid arch. Like branchial cleft cysts, they may not be noticed until secondary infection causes their enlargement. Dermoid cysts or lymph nodes located near the midline may be differentiated from thyroglossal duct cysts with swallowing or tongue protrusion. Rarely, an adenocarcinoma may originate in the thyroglossal duct (Widstrom, 1976).

Cystic hygroma is usually a multilocular, fluid-filled swelling located in the lateral neck. These lesions are usually present at birth or are noted by the end of the first or

Table 77–2 PHYSICAL CHARACTERISTICS OF CONGENITAL LESIONS

Cystic hygroma — Diffuse, compressible, enlarges with straining, transilluminates

Hemangioma — Similar to cystic hygroma, lesions are more limited in size, bluish hue, may decrease in size with time

Branchial cleft cyst — May retract with swallowing, cystic, located along anterior border of sternocleidomastoid muscle, may have a mucus-producing fistula

Thyroglossal duct cyst — Retracts with protruding tongue, cystic or solid, usually located at level of hyoid in midline, may have a fistula

Esophageal diverticulum — Findings similar to those for laryngocele except that it is found in paratracheal area, usually on left side; may be associated with dysphagia and aspiration; diagnosis confirmed by esophagogram

Dermoid cyst — Midline, doughy, cystic, nontender, does not transilluminate

Teratoma — Same as dermoid cyst; calcifications or tooth remnants may be noted on radiograph; should be suspected in a rapidly enlarging solitary cervical mass in infancy

Venous malformation — Diffuse, compressible, may be multiple, enlarges with straining, palpable phleboliths, may increase in size with time

Laryngocele — May be associated with muffled voice, air–fluid level noted on radiograph, compressible, transilluminates, gurgles on compression, increases in size with straining, located in region of thyrohyoid membrane just lateral to midline

(From May, M. 1976. Neck masses in children: Diagnosis and treatment. Pediatr. Ann., 5:8.)

Table 77–3 DIAGNOSTIC CHARACTERISTICS

Consistency	Number
Soft	Solitary
Firm/hard	Multiple
Indurated	Generalized
Cystic	Diffuse
Compressible	

Color	Dynamic
Red	Heat
Bluish	Tender
Transilluminates	Pulsatile
	Bruit
Mobility	Fluctuation
Mobile	Strain
Fixed	Cough
Skin or deep	Eating
Superior or inferior	Position change
	Swallow
	Tongue protrusion

(From May, M. 1976. Neck masses in children: Diagnosis and treatment. Pediatr. Ann., 5:8.)

second year of life. A diagnosis may be established by physical examination since these masses are diffuse, soft, compressible, painless, and usually can be transilluminated (Saijo, 1975).

Hemangiomas are congenital, vascular anomalies that are noticed at birth or during the first year of life. The diagnosis is usually established by the appearance of a bluish mass that increases in size with straining or crying. The hemangioma will usually regress spontaneously but may occasionally enlarge and compromise the airway.

A variant of the hemangioma, one that does not regress, is the congenital venous anomaly. These present most commonly in the area of the parotid gland or midline of the neck. The venous malformation may intermittently become painful and tender when thrombosis in the thin-walled venous channels occurs. Venous malformations may be diagnosed subsequent to thrombosis by the calcification of the thrombus, which may then be palpated or demonstrated radiographically as a phlebolith.

Dermoid cysts and teratomas may be noted at any age. The dermoid cyst is more common than the teratoma and presents as a smooth, doughy, midline-cervical mass (McAvoy, 1976). The teratoma is frequently more irregular, firm, and laterally placed (Rundle, 1976). A teratoma may contain calcifications that can be detected radiographically.

A laryngocele is an air-containing cyst that arises from the laryngeal ventricle as a mucosal pocket between the anterior aspects of the true and false vocal cords. When infected or when the neck of the laryngocele is obstructed, the cyst becomes fluid-filled and is known

Table 77–4 DIAGNOSIS OF NECK MASSES BY PHYSICAL CHARACTERISTICS

Characteristic	Possible Diagnosis
Bluish hue, enlarges with straining, compressible	Hemangioma, venous malformation
Pulsatile, bruit, compressible	Vascular: arteriovenous malformations, glomus tumors
Enlarges upon straining	Cystic hygroma, hemangioma, laryngocele, venous malformation
Painful and swells with eating	Salivary gland, esophageal diverticulum
Generalized adenopathy	Infectious mononucleosis, lymphoma, cat-scratch fever, mucocutaneous lymph node syndrome, sinus histiocytosis
Red, tender, warm	Inflammatory
Toxic	Suppurative adenitis, deep neck-space abscess
Nontender, soft, discrete, attached to skin	Epidermoid inclusion cyst, keloid
Nontender, soft, discrete, deep to skin	Lipoma, fibroma, neurofibroma
Nontender, cystic	Congenital lesions
Transilluminates	Cystic hygroma
Mass along anterior border of sternocleidomastoid fistula, retracts with swallowing	Branchial cleft cyst
Midline mass that retracts with protruding tongue	Thyroglossal duct cyst
Multiple	Infection (adenitis), lymphoma
Solitary firm mass	Congenital lesions, thyroid, parathyroid, salivary gland tumors, carotid body tumor, neurofibroma, chondroma, dermoid cyst, lymphoma
Nontender, fixed, hard, matted, rubbery, rapidly enlarging, more than 4 cm, deep to sternocleidomastoid muscle	Malignancy — mesenchymal in origin
Mobility limited, superior-inferior	Congenital cyst, malignancy attached to carotid sheath

(From May, M. 1976. Neck masses in children: Diagnosis and treatment. Pediatr. Ann., 5:8.)

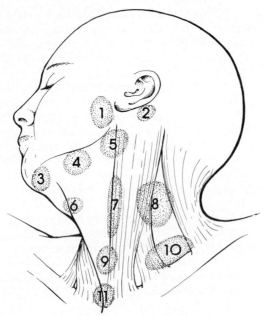

Figure 77–1 Diagnosis of neck masses by location (see Table 77–5). (From May, M. 1976. Neck masses in children: Diagnosis and treatment. Pediatr. Ann., 5:8.)

as a laryngopyocele. These masses present in the neck only after they have dissected out of the larynx along the superior laryngeal nerves and vessels. They then present as masses at the lateral aspect of the thyrohyoid membrane. A laryngocele will frequently in-

crease in size with straining or crying. A laryngopyocele is a doughy, tender, fluctuant mass located in the same area.

Esophageal diverticula very rarely occur in children, but when they do they exhibit findings similar to those for a laryngocele except that the mass is located in the paratracheal area (usually on the left). The characteristics of congenital lesions are summarized in Table 77–2, and their specific management is detailed in the following chapter.

The physical characteristics of a neck mass as assessed by inspection, palpation, and auscultation aid greatly in narrowing the diagnostic possibilities. The methods of examination are presented in Chapter 76. The color, consistency, mobility, and number of neck masses, among other criteria, are useful in establishing some diagnostic probabilities. The characteristics of neck masses that may be helpful in establishing their pathogenesis are listed in Table 77–3. Once the various characteristics are noted, they may be combined to suggest a diagnosis, such as those given in Table 77–4. For example, a compressible, lateral neck mass that enlarges with straining and has a bluish hue is likely to be a hemangioma, whereas a mass that is compressible but is pulsatile and is associated with a bruit is more likely an arteriovenous malformation or glomus tumor.

Certain neck masses have a predilection for

Table 77–5 DIAGNOSIS OF NECK MASSES BY LOCATION (see Fig. 77–1)

Area 1: Parotid (Preauricular)

Congenital
  Cystic hygroma, hemangioma, venous malformation

Inflammatory
  Lymphadenitis — secondary to upper face and anterior scalp infections (discrete, mobile, warm, tender)
  Parotitis (diffuse, indurated, tender parotid gland)
    Viral — puncta red, secretions clear
    Bacterial — puncta normal, secretions purulent
  Granuloma
    Tuberculosis and sarcoidosis

Traumatic — sialocele

Neoplastic
  Benign – pleomorphic adenoma
  Malignant – mucoepidermoid carcinoma
    Lymphoma (Hodgkin disease simulates parotid tumor in 6% of parotid masses)

Idiopathic
  Sjögren syndrome—puncta normal, sialogram shows "bunch of grapes" pattern
  Caffey-Silverman syndrome — puncta normal, secretions normal, sialogram normal, radiographs of

mandible show thickening and separation of periosteum

Area 2: Postauricular

Congenital
  First branchial cleft — cystic, inflamed, or both

Inflammatory
  Lymphadenitis — discrete, tender — secondary to posterior scalp inflammation

Area 3: Submental

Congenital
  Thyroglossal duct cyst
  Cystic hygroma
  Dermoid cyst
  Venous malformation

Inflammatory
  Lymphadenitis — secondary to perioral, anterior oral, or nasal cavity inflammation

Neoplastic
  Thyroglossal duct adenocarcinoma

Table continued on opposite page

Table 77–5 DIAGNOSIS OF NECK MASSES BY LOCATION (see Fig. 77–1) (Continued)

Area 4: Submandibular

Congenital
  Cystic hygroma, hemangioma

Inflammatory
  Lymphadenitis — secondary to cheek and/or midoral cavity inflammation
  Submandibular gland
    Sialadenitis — tender, indurated submandibular gland, purulent secretions from puncta, stone may or may not be palpable
    Cystic fibrosis — gland enlarged

Neoplastic tumor
  Pleomorphic adenoma, mucoepidermoid carcinoma, adenoid cystic carcinoma

Area 5: Jugulodigastric (Tonsil node)

Normal structures
  Transverse process of C2
  Styloid process

Congenital
  First or second branchial cleft, hemangioma, cystic hygroma

Inflammatory
  Lymphadenitis — secondary to oropharyngeal inflammation

Neoplastic
  Parotid tumor
  Mesodermal neoplasm

Area 6: Midline Neck

Normal structures
  Hyoid, thyroid isthmus, thyroid cartilage

Congenital
  Thyroglossal duct cyst, dermoid cyst

Inflammatory
  Lymphadenitis

Area 7: Anterior Border Sternocleidomastoid Muscle

Normal structures
  Hyoid, thyroid cartilage, carotid bulb

Congenital
  Branchial cleft, I, II, III, (IV rare), laryngocele hemangioma, lymphangioma

Metabolic
  Dilantin-induced adenopathy (Green, 1975)

Neoplastic
  Neurilemmoma — can be moved from side to side but not up and down
  Carotid body tumor — same as neurilemmoma but with palpable or audible bruit and angiographic blush
  Lymphoma
  Sarcoma

Area 8: Spinal Accessory

Neoplastic
  Lymphoma
  Metastatic (from nasopharynx)

Inflammatory
  Lymphadenitis (secondary to nasopharyngeal inflammation)

Area 9: Paratracheal

Thyroid, parathyroid, esophageal diverticulum, metastatic (e.g., renal to thyroid)

Area 10: Supraclavicular

Normal structure
  Fat pad, pneumatocele from apical lobe — defect in Gibson fascia, prominent mass with Valsalva maneuver (Devgan, 1976)

Congenital
  Cystic hygroma

Neoplastic
  Lipoma
  Lymphoma
  Metastasis
    Left side
    Lung (all but right upper lobe), esophagus from structures below diaphragm — renal, testicular
    Right side
    Esophagus, right upper lobe

Area 11: Suprasternal

Thyroid, lipoma, dermoid, thymus, mediastinal mass

(From May, M. 1976. Neck masses in children: Diagnosis and treatment. Pediatr. Ann., 5:8.)

a particular neck location. For purposes of this discussion, we divide the neck into eleven areas, as shown in Figure 77–1. Within each area, congenital or acquired masses may be found. Diagnostic possibilities suggested by the location of the mass are outlined in Table 77–5.

The relative frequency of neck masses in children can now be put into perspective: up to 90 per cent of such neck masses are be-

nign. Although the major portion of benign neck masses are inflammatory, they do not all have common bacterial and viral etiologies, and care must be taken to differentiate the less common inflammatory causes (Olley, 1977; Mair, 1977). The diagnosis and management of inflammatory neck masses are discussed in Chapter 76. Mesenchymal derivatives account for 90 per cent of benign and malignant neck neoplasms. The type of pri-

Table 77–6 MALIGNANT NECK MASSES IN CHILDREN ACCORDING TO AGE

Newborn	Privileged Immunity	Neuroblastoma, Rhabdomyosarcoma
1–6	Neuroblastoma, leukemia	Lymphosarcoma*, rhabdomyosarcoma
7–13	Hodgkin disease*	Lymphosarcoma*, thyroid cancer
14–21	Hodgkin disease*	Lymphosarcoma*, epidermoid cancer

*Hodgkin disease and lymphosarcoma account for 55 per cent of all pediatric head and neck malignancies.
(From May, M. 1976. Neck masses in children: Diagnosis and treatment. Pediatr. Ann., 5:8.)

mary neck malignancy varies with age (Table 77–6). The newborn is considered to be immune to this type of neck mass, although neuroblastomas and rhabdomyosarcomas are occasionally seen at a very early age. Children through age six most commonly develop neck masses secondary to neuroblastomas or leukemia; lymphosarcomas and rhabdomyosarcomas may also result in the development of neck masses in these children, although not as frequently. For children between 7 and 13 years of age, Hodgkin disease is the most common malignant neck neoplasm followed in frequency by lymphosarcomas (Traggis,

1975) and thyroid cancer. After 14 years of age children most frequently develop neck masses associated with Hodgkin disease and lymphosarcomas (Goepfert et. al., 1977), although the first significant incidence of epidermoid carcinoma metastasizing to the cervical lymph nodes is also noted at this age. Malignancies develop more frequently in salivary glands or thyroid masses in children than they do in adults: 50 per cent of parotid tumors and submandibular gland tumors are malignant in children, and thyroid nodules in children under 10 years of age have up to an 80 per cent incidence of malignancy. Metasta-

Table 77–7 DIFFERENTIAL DIAGNOSIS OF NECK MASSES IN CHILDREN IN APPROXIMATE ORDER OF FREQUENCY

Normal Cervical Masses

Mandible	Lateral process of C2
Mastoid tip	Lateral process of C6
Greater cornu of hyoid and thyroid	Styloid process, carotid bulb

Congenital Masses

Common	*Uncommon*	*Rare*
Cystic hygroma	Dermoid cyst	Laryngocele
Hemangioma		Esophageal diverticulum
Branchial cleft cyst		Teratoma
Thyroglossal duct cyst		

Inflammatory Masses

Very Common	*Very Rare*
Cervical adenitis (viral or bacterial)	Actinomycosis
	Cytomegalovirus infection
Common	Leptospirosis
Suppurative adenitis	Brucellosis
Toxoplasmosis	Tularemia
Mononucleosis	Leprosy
Uncommon	*Extremely Rare*
Submandibular or parotid sialadenitis	Sinus histiocytosis
Lateral pharyngeal abscess	Mucocutaneous lymph node syndrome
Cervical tuberculosis	Caffey-Silverman syndrome
Sarcoidosis	
Rare	
Syphilis	
Cat-scratch fever	

Table continued on opposite page

Table 77–7 DIFFERENTIAL DIAGNOSIS OF NECK MASSES IN CHILDREN IN APPROXIMATE ORDER OF FREQUENCY (Continued)

Noninflammatory, Benign Superficial Masses

Uncommon

Epidermoid inclusion cyst	Neurofibroma
Lipoma	Keloid
Fibroma	Ranula (intraoral mucocyst)

Noninflammatory, Benign Deep Masses

Uncommon

Salivary glands (Mair, 1977)	Hematoma

Extremely Rare

Sternocleidomastoid muscle (spasm, fibroma, hematoma, torticollis)
Neurilemmoma
Paraganglioma
  Carotid bifurcation
  Jugular
  Vagal
Chondroma
Diphenylhydantoin-induced lymphoid hyperplasia
Thyroid
Parathyroid

Malignant Masses

Most Common Cause

Lymphosarcoma	Hodgkin disease

Less Common and Varying with Age (see Table 77–6)

Neuroblastoma	Epidermoid carcinoma
Leukemia	Salivary gland malignancies
Rhabdomyosarcoma	Melanoma
Fibrosarcoma	Metastatic
Thyroid malignancies	Thyroglossal duct adenocarcinoma

(From May, M. 1976. Neck masses in children: Diagnosis and treatment. Pediatr. Ann., 5:8.)

tic malignant melanoma is frequently misdiagnosed when the disease occurs in children (Shanon, 1976). A listing of the differential diagnosis of pediatric neck masses in their approximate order of frequency is given in Table 77–7.

Therapy for these diseases, particularly in the malignant neoplasms, is constantly being modified and improved (Chap. 77). However, therapeutic success can be expected only when the treatment is appropriate for the disease state. The clinical evaluation must involve systematic categorization of symptoms and signs in order to arrive at an accurate diagnosis.

REFERENCES

Devgan, D. K. 1976. Apical pneumatocele. Arch. Otolaryngol., 102(2):121–123.

Goepfert, H., et al. 1977. Soft-tissue sarcoma of the head and neck after puberty. Arch. Otolaryngol., 103(6):365–368.

Green, D. A. 1975. Localized cervical lymphadenopathy induced by diphenylhydantoin sodium (Dilantin). Arch. Otolaryngol., 101:446–448.

Krugman, M. E. 1976. The sternomastoid "tumor" of infancy. J. Otolaryngol., 5(6):523–529.

Mair, I. W. 1975. Cervical mycobacterial infection. J. Laryngol. Otol., 89(9):933–939.

Mair, I. W. 1977. Heterotopic cervical salivary glands. J. Laryngol. Otol., 91(1):35–40.

McAvoy, J. M. 1976. Dermoid cysts of the head and neck in children. Arch. Otolaryngol., 102:529–531.

Olley, S. F. 1977. Suppurative cervical adenitis caused by opportunist mycobacterium. Br. J. Oral Surg., 14(3):257–263.

Rundle, F. W. 1976. Cervical teratoma. J. Otolaryngol., 5(6):513–518.

Saijo, M. 1975. Lymphangioma — a long-term follow-up study. Plast. Reconstr. Surg., 56(6):642–651.

Shanon, E. 1976. Malignant melanoma of the head and neck in children. Arch. Otolaryngol., 102:244–247.

Traggis, D. 1975. Non-Hodgkin's lymphoma of the head and neck in childhood. J. Pediatr., 87:933–936.

Widstrom, A. 1976. Adenocarcinoma originating in the thyroglossal duct. Ann. Otol. Rhinol. Laryngol., 85:286–290.

Chapter 78

DEVELOPMENTAL ANOMALIES OF THE NECK

Collin S. Karmody, M.D.

The neck represents an area where complex embryonic events occur. It is, therefore, not surprising that anomalies of development of the neck structures are common. They are usually obvious but are sometimes difficult to diagnose and at times even more difficult or dangerous to treat. As anomalies might primarily affect any embryonic tissue layer of the neck, they will be described according to tissue systems. We will discuss, in order, anomalies of the skeletal system, muscles, and skin; blood vessels and lymphatics; and the branchial apparatus.

SKELETAL ANOMALIES

Skeletal anomalies are due to one or a number of the following mechanisms: (1) failure of differentiation, (2) defective segmentation, (3) failure of fusion of ossification centers, (4) failure of migration, (5) supernumerary parts, or (6) structural defects or deformities.

Anomalies of the Cervical Vertebrae

Only selected pertinent anomalies will be discussed.

Congenital Synostosis of the Cervicothoracic Vertebrae (Klippel-Feil Syndrome). This is a rare malformation in which there is congenital fusion of two or more cervical vertebrae (Shoul and Ritvo, 1952) (Fig. 78–1). The vertebral bodies are often widened and flattened, and cervical spina bifida is common. The disorder results

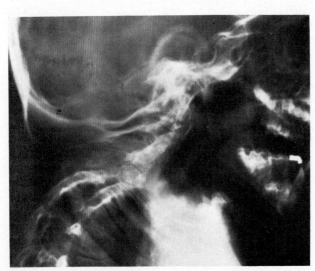

Figure 78–1 A roentgenogram of a three year old child with Klippel-Feil syndrome. The bodies of the cervical vertebrae are fused, and the neck is shortened. There was gross limitation of lateral motion of the neck.

1386

from failure of segmentation of the mesodermal somites during the third to eighth week of fetal life. Females are more often affected, but there is no definite pattern of inheritance. Clinical manifestations vary according to the severity of the deformity, and milder deformities might be diagnosed incidentally. More severe deformities, however, give the impression of a very short neck with a head sitting directly on the thorax (Klippel and Feil, 1912). There is usually marked limitation of motion of the cervical spine, but flexion and extension, which take place at the atlanto-occipital joints, are unrestricted. Webbing of the lateral soft tissues of the neck is not uncommon, and there is frequently a torticollis. Other congenital anomalies of the skeleton might be associated, such as the Sprengel deformity, cervical ribs, scoliosis, and kyphosis. Anomalies of soft tissues in other parts of the body have been reported, for instance, cleft palates or intraventricular septal defects. A sensorineural hearing loss occurs in 30 per cent of patients with the Klippel-Feil syndrome.

The treatment for this syndrome is passive stretching exercises to maintain maximum mobility. Surgical efforts are directed towards improvement of appearance and function. Pterygium colli can be alleviated by a Z-plasty.

Congenital Fusion of the First Cervical Vertebrae and Occiput (Occipitalization of the First Cervical Vertebrae). Weakness and ataxia of the lower extremities and occasionally of the upper extremities are the usual primary complaints in this syndrome. Headache, neck pains, and numbness might also occur. In addition, there is frequent blurring of vision, diplopia, dizziness, dysphagia, and hoarseness.

The diagnosis of this disorder is established by features of the roentgenograms, although tomography might also be necessary to define the problem. Intracranial anomalies, such as the Arnold-Chiari malformation and posterior dural bands, might be associated with fusion of the first cervical vertebra and occiput. The treatment of this problem is posterior laminectomy and spinal fusion. Occipitalization of the first cervical vertebra is a common finding in achondroplasia.

Separate or Absent Odontoid Process. A separate odontoid process might be congenital or traumatic. In both cases the disorder might be associated with severe neurologic disturbances, and at least half of those suffer-

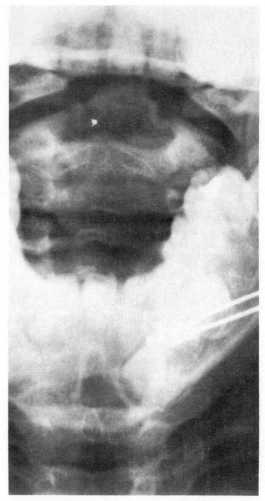

Figure 78–2 A transoral view of the upper cervical vertebrae of a five year old child shows absence of the odontoid process.

ing from this problem have neurologic deficits. Clinically, however, there might be a wide range of symptoms. When the problem is congenital there is usually a history of mild trauma with symptoms and signs out of proportion to the degree of trauma. There might be pain and stiffness of the neck, transient signs of spinal cord compression, or even quadriplegia. Congenital lack of development of the odontoid process sometimes also occurs (Fig. 78–2).

Congenital Absence of the Pedicles and Articular Facets of the Cervical Spine. These disorders usually occur together and are compatible with normal life. Most patients are asymptomatic. The significance of this anomaly lies in the fact that it must be differentiated in diagnosis from erosive lesions.

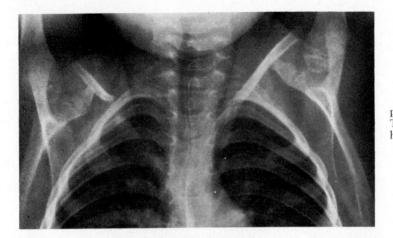

Figure 78-3 A roentgenogram of a patient with cleidocranial dysostosis. The medial half of the right clavicle has failed to develop.

Acro-osteolysis. Individuals with acro-osteolysis show straightening of the cervical spine with dense intervertebral discs.

Anomalies of the Clavicle

Mutational Dysostosis (Cleidocranial Dysostosis). Cleidocranial dysostosis is a congenital disorder of the skeleton characterized by imperfect ossification of bones formed in membranes. Bones preformed in cartilage, however, are also affected (Fitchet, 1929). The disease usually becomes evident in the first two years of life, when the child typically presents with a large head and a small face. The clavicle might be totally or partially missing (Fig. 78-3), and as a result the shoulders are narrow and can be adducted so that they almost meet in the midline (Fig. 78-4). The condition causes little functional disability. Cleidocranial dysostosis is sometimes associated with bilateral mixed hearing losses (Jafee, 1968).

Congenital Pseudarthrosis of the Clavicle. This is a rare, nonfamilial anomaly that results from failure of normal ossification of the clavicle (Aldred, 1963). Clinically there is a mass just lateral to the middle of the clavicle, usually discovered soon after birth. The deformity increases with growth and might become unsightly, in which case a bone grafting procedure is performed. The clinical significance of this problem is primarily cosmetic, and the differential diagnosis from other disorders, notably neoplasms, must be made.

Anomalies of the Scapula — Scapula Elevata (Sprengel Deformity)

The scapula begins as a cervical appendage, then descends to the upper posterior thorax towards the end of the third fetal month. If, however, it fails to descend from the neck, the result is an abnormally high scapula known as the Sprengel deformity (Engel, 1943).

In the Sprengel deformity the scapula is small, distorted, and might be attached to the cervical vertebrae by fibrous tissue, cartilage, or even bone (omovertebral bone). The musculature of the shoulder girdle is usually defective, and the trapezius muscle is sometimes weak or absent. There might be other associated anomalies, for instance absence or fusion of ribs, the presence of cervical ribs, spina bifida, or a hypoplastic clavicle.

There is no propensity as to sex, and the condition is usually unilateral. The Sprengel deformity is diagnosed at birth because the scapula is high, sometimes as high as the fourth cervical vertebra, and is tilted forward.

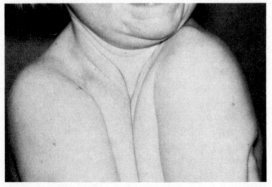

Figure 78-4 This is the patient shown in Figure 78-3 with cleidocranial dysostosis. There is excessive adduction of the shoulders.

Early passive and active stretching of the musculature is useful in increasing function and mobility of the abnormal scapula. Various surgical maneuvers have also been described for repositioning the scapula inferiorly.

ANOMALIES OF THE CERVICAL MUSCLES

Congenital Muscular Torticollis. Congenital muscular torticollis involves unilateral contracture of the sternocleidomastoid muscle, thus tilting the head toward the side of the shortened muscle and rotating the chin towards the opposite side. The immediate cause is fibrosis within the sternocleidomastoid muscle with subsequent contracture and shortening of the muscle fibers. Experimental evidence suggests venous occlusion as the cause of the fibrosis (Lidge et al., 1957).

The deformity may be noted at birth or may become evident thereafter. Within the first 10 days of life a nontender, fibrous "tumor" becomes palpable in the substance of the muscle (Fig. 78–5). This mass progresses to maximum size in a month and then regresses, leaving a contracted muscle. The head then becomes tilted to the ipsilateral side, and the chin becomes tilted upwards to the contralateral side. Untreated, the condition causes developmental asymmetry of the face and ocular imbalance. Soon after diagnosis is made, the muscle must be passively stretched by exercises four to six times daily. If conservative management fails, surgery is indicated. Surgery consists of division or par-

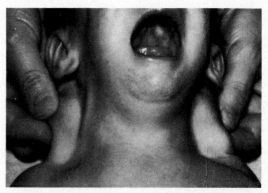

Figure 78–6 A 10 month old child with Turner syndrome: the pterygium colli are being stretched by the examiner's fingers.

tial excision of the sternal and clavicular heads of the sternocleidomastoid muscle and postoperative splinting of the neck.

Other Developmental Anomalies of the Cervical Muscles. The sternocleidomastoid and trapezius muscles are developmentally related and might be simultaneously deficient. Occasionally the trapezius muscle is absent as an isolated defect.

ANOMALIES OF THE SKIN

Developmental abnormalities of the skin of the neck might be localized or might be part of a generalized ectodermal defect.

Pterygium Colli (Wing Neck). A pterygium is a flat fold of skin and connective tissue that extends from the region of the mastoid process to the point of the shoulder. Pterygia are found in the following conditions: Turner syndrome, Leopard syndrome, Noonan syndrome, and multiple pterygium syndrome.

XO Syndrome (Turner Syndrome). Turner syndrome involves monosomy of the sex chromosomes. The classical features of Turner syndrome are short stature, pterygium colli, absence of sexual maturation, and a broad, shield-like chest with widely spaced nipples (Turner, 1938) (Fig. 78–6). Aortic stenosis is a frequently associated anomaly.

Multiple Lentigines (Leopard) Syndrome. Leopard syndrome is inherited as an autosomal dominant and is characterized by the presence of numerous lentigines on the neck and trunk, electrocardiographic defects, hypertelorism, pulmonary stenosis, abnormalities of the genitalia, retardation of

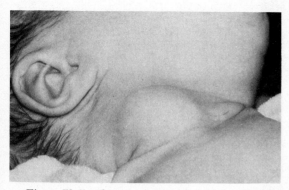

Figure 78–5 This two week old child developed a firm mass in the right sternocleidomastoid muscle five days after birth. The mass was very firm, nontender, and was not enlarging. It represented a "fibrous tumor," which is the first stage in the development of congenital muscular torticollis.

growth, and sensorineural deafness. Individuals with this syndrome commonly have pterygium colli as well.

Turner Phenotype with Normal Karyotype (Noonan Syndrome). The Noonan and Leopard syndromes have many features in common, such as hypertelorism, small stature, pulmonary stenosis, and abnormal electrocardiograms. In addition, individuals with both syndromes may have pterygium colli. Noonan and Turner syndromes are phenotypically similar (Noonan, 1968).

Multiple Pterygium Syndrome. In this syndrome, folds of skin occur across the angles of most of the joints, such as the posterior aspect of the knee joints, the elbows, and the metacarpophalangeal joints. In addition, prominent pterygium colli usually occur (Aarskog, 1971).

Anomalous cervical skin is found with the following generalized abnormalities.

Cutis Laxa (Generalized Elastolysis). This condition is characterized by hanging skin, hernias, and various diverticula. His-

tologically there is absence or marked diminution of elastic fibers (Robinson and Ellis, 1958).

Dyskeratosis Congenita (Zinsser-Engman-Cole Syndrome). In this syndrome, reticular atrophy of the skin occurs along with pigmentation about the time of puberty. In addition, dystrophy of the nails and oral leukoplakia are seen. The skin changes are prominent on the face, neck, and chest.

Cutis Hyperelastica (Ehlers-Danlos Syndrome). This syndrome involves hyperelasticity of the skin, skin hemorrhages, loose jointedness, and the occurrence of cutaneous pseudotumors and subcutaneous spherules (Beighton, 1972). There are many variations of this syndrome. In 15 to 20 per cent of patients hernias are noted, and 25 per cent of patients with this syndrome have epicanthal folds.

Pseudoxanthoma Elasticum (Grönblad-Strandberg Syndrome). This syndrome is inherited as an autosomal recessive disease and involves alterations of the skin, gastroin-

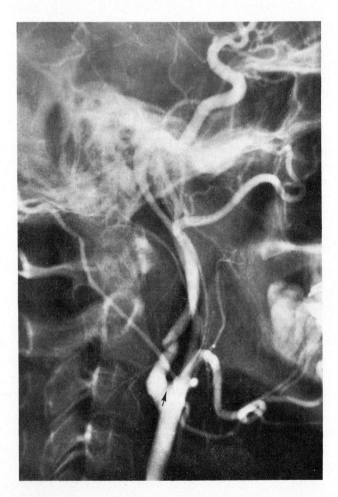

Figure 78–7 This is the carotid angiogram of a 23 year old woman with a parapharyngeal tumor. The carotid bifurcation is unusually high, at the level of the angle of the mandible.

testinal hemorrhages, weak peripheral pulses, and failing vision. The skin is thickened, and raised, flat, yellow papules appear around the mouth, neck, axilla, and groin. Changes may appear in the third or fourth year of life but usually present in the second decade.

ANOMALIES OF THE BLOOD VESSELS AND LYMPHATICS

Arterial Anomalies. The development of the arterial system of the neck has been adequately described in Chapter 75 and will not be repeated here. Arterial anomalies in the neck consist mainly of abnormalities of the carotid and subclavian systems. The vertebral system is rarely involved. There are only three anomalies that occur in the neck that are of importance in clinical practice: high bifurcation of the common carotid artery, left-sided origin of the right subclavian artery, and left-sided origin of the innominate artery.

High bifurcation of the common carotid artery (Fig. 78–7) is not rare and is usually not of significance except when a chemodectoma

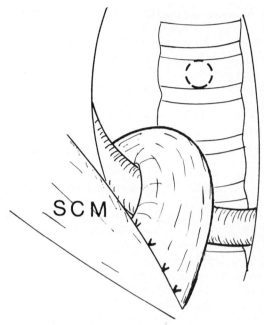

Figure 78–9 Explanatory diagram of the surgical maneuver performed on the patient described in Figure 78–8. The sternohyoid muscle was detached from the hyoid. The muscle was then looped around the innominate artery, and its free end was firmly sutured to the lower sternocleidomastoid muscle (SCM). A tracheostomy was placed at the second tracheal ring.

develops or when there are penetrating wounds of the neck.

When the right subclavian artery arises from the left side of the aortic arch it usually runs posterior to the esophagus or between the esophagus and trachea, in which position it might compress the trachea, resulting in respiratory difficulty. The treatment is to ligate and section the vessel.

The innominate artery sometimes arises from the left side of the aortic arch and then runs upwards and to the right into the neck before bifurcating. In this position the vessel is unusually high and might be directly in the path of a tracheostomy (Fig. 78–8), or it might be liable to erosion by placement of a tracheostomy tube. If this situation is encountered during tracheostomy, the vessel can be ligated and sectioned, a maneuver that might cause hemiplegia. Alternatively, the sternohyoid muscle can be detached from the hyoid bone and the free end passed between the vessel and the trachea, then sutured to the lowest point of the sternal head of the sternocleidomastoid muscle so as to form a tissue barrier and downward sling for the innominate artery (Fig. 78–9).

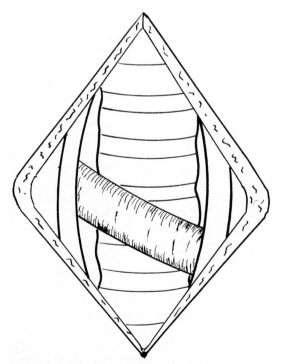

Figure 78–8 Diagram of findings at tracheostomy in a three year old girl with multiple congenital anomalies. The innominate artery is at the level of the third and fourth tracheal rings.

Venous Anomalies. Significant anomalies of the venous system are uncommon. Alonso and Chambers (1970) described a patient with an anomaly of the external jugular vein that presented as a cystic mass at the anterior border of the sternocleidomastoid muscle. The external jugular vein joined the internal jugular vein lateral to the carotid artery in a siphon-like confluence. The mass disappeared on ligation of the external vein.

Anomalies of the Lymphatic System

Cystic Hygroma (Lymphangioma). Although there is a question as to whether or not lymphangiomas are developmental, neoplastic, or hamartomatous, we shall discuss them as though they were developmental anomalies. Lymphangiomas and cystic hygromas have been classified into three groups, of which cystic hygromas are but one type. Histologically, however, it is difficult to differentiate between a lymphangioma and a cystic hygroma. It would, therefore, seem rational to reconsider them as variations of a single entity (Bill and Summer, 1965).

The lymphatic vessels develop as spaces in embryonic tissue. These coalesce to form definitive channels that drain into the venous system. If there is regional failure of connection to the rest of the lymphatic system, the spaces continue to expand to form a soft, progressively enlarging mass. This is a lymphangioma or cystic hygroma. Hygromas are most common in the head and neck and might be present at birth or might present in

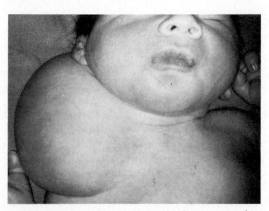

Figure 78–10 This photograph shows a newborn child with a large cystic hygroma that involves the entire length of the right neck and the right upper chest. Fortunately, this mass did not extend to the trachea or pharynx and was successfully excised. (Courtesy of Paul Mellish, M.D.)

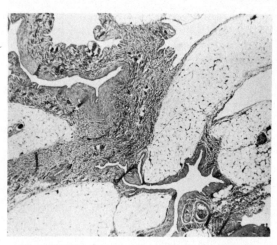

Figure 78–11 Photomicrograph of a lymphangioma removed from the shoulder of a three year old child. There are large spaces lined by delicate strands of endothelium. In addition, there are thin-walled vessels without muscular layers that are lined by a single layer of flat endothelium.

young adulthood. Congenital cystic hygromas can be of substantial size (Fig. 78–10), involving the full thickness of the neck from the skin to the mucosal surfaces of the mouth, base of the tongue, larynx, and pharynx. They might cause respiratory obstruction.

When there are anomalous developments of the vascular spaces, all three elements — arteries, veins, and lymphatics — are frequently simultaneously involved. Therefore, lymphangiomas are not uncommonly associated with angiomatous malformations. A single mass might contain abnormal lymphatics and blood vessels — a lymphangiohemangioma.

A lymphangioma is a soft, smooth, nontender mass of almost fat-like consistency, grey and edematous-looking where it involves a mucosal surface. Lymphangiomas and cystic hygromas are asymptomatic except for cosmesis or where there is infection or spontaneous hemorrhage. Where there are angiomatous elements, the dilated vessels are usually easily visible on the skin and surface of the lesion, and, where there is involvement of the oral mucosa, bleeding frequently occurs. Pure cystic hygromas are the only cervical masses that transilluminate. Histologically hygromas and lymphangiomas consist of widely dilated lymphatic spaces whose walls vary in thickness from very thin to very thick (Fig. 78–11). Dilated, thin-walled blood vessels compose a variable part of the mass.

The treatment of lymphangiomas is surgical excision. This is not always easy because of lack of definition between the hygromatous mass and normal tissue. A number of other approaches to therapy have been tried — these have usually taken the form of trying to create fibrosis in the lesion and have varied from the passage of suture material through the lesion, to the injection of sclerosing agents, to radiation therapy.

ANOMALIES OF THE BRANCHIAL APPARATUS

The embryology of the neck is discussed in detail in Chapter 75.

By the end of the fourth week of embryonic life, four branchial arches are visible externally. The fifth and sixth arches are rudimentary. The branchial apparatus consists of grooves, arches, and pouches and is the anlage of many structures in the head and neck (Albers, 1963). Anomalies of each component may occur together with, or independent of, anomalies of the other components, and they may be inherited (Karmody and Feingold, 1974).

Anomalies of the First Branchial Groove

Anomalies of the first branchial groove (cleft) are uncommon and result from either nondevelopment, maldevelopment, or duplication of the groove. These anomalies can be divided into four broad categories — aplasia, atresia, stenosis, and duplication anomalies (Fig. 78–12).

Aplasia Anomalies. Aplasia of the external auditory canal occurs with nondevelopment of the first branchial groove. There may be associated varying degrees of deformity of the pinna. Clinically the condyle of the mandible is immediately anterior to the mastoid process, a condition that is easily defined by palpation.

Aplasia anomalies of the first groove are frequently associated with anomalies of the first branchial arch, such as in mandibulofacial dysostosis (Treacher-Collins syndrome).

Alternatively, the derivative (external auditory canal) does not develop, but the groove persists as a tract. The external point of the persistent groove presents either as a birthmark-like lesion, a cyst, or as an external sinus, which may be inferior to the pinna (Fig. 78–13), near the angle of the mandible, along the mandible, or occasionally in the submandibular triangle. The tract runs from

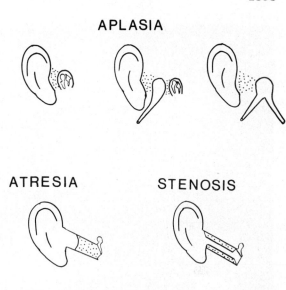

APLASIA

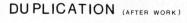

ATRESIA   **STENOSIS**

DUPLICATION (AFTER WORK)

TYPE 1   TYPE 2

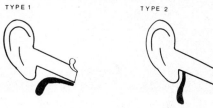

Figure 78–12 Diagrammatic representations of the anomalies of the first branchial groove. All these anomalies might be associated with either a fully formed or a deformed pinna.

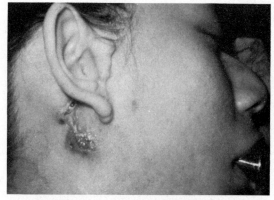

Figure 78–13 This 23 year old woman had been deaf in the right ear since birth. The right pinna had always been small and cup-shaped, and there was no external auditory canal. Also since birth she had had a small opening on the skin inferior to the lobule that frequently drained clear to yellow material. Two weeks prior to presentation she had developed an acute infection in this area. The line of the tract can be clearly seen extending superiorly from the angle of the mandible to the expected position of the external auditory canal.

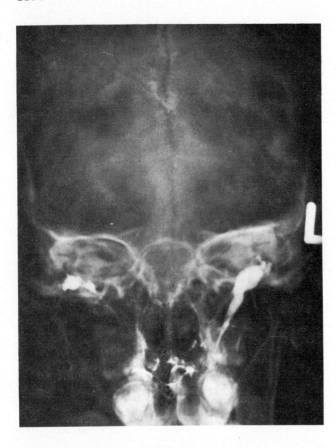

Figure 78–14 A contrast roentgenogram of a four year old boy demonstrates a fistulous communication between an external opening, the cavity of the middle ear, and the eustachian tube. This is a rare case of true fistulization of the first branchial groove.

the skin to the expected position of the external auditory canal, where it ends as a blind pouch (Fig. 78–12). Rarely, the tract communicates with the middle ear cleft to form a fistula (Fig. 78–14). The pinna might be fully formed but is usually small and cup-shaped or might even be absent (Fig. 78–15).

Atresia Anomalies. In atresia anomalies, the external ear canal is present, but the lumen has failed to develop. The canal is closed by either a mass of bone, fibrous tissue, or a mixture of both. The degree of atresia varies considerably.

Stenosis Anomalies. In stenosis anoma-

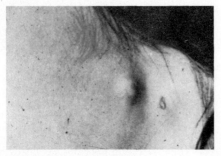

Figure 78–15 The pinna of this three year old girl is represented by a small mass of tissue. Posterior to this is a sinus with a mucoid discharge.

lies, the external auditory canal is present, and its lumen has developed but is narrow. The size of the lumen varies from almost normal to the width of a thread. Stenosis occurs in the cartilaginous or bony canal and sometimes simultaneously in both.

Duplication Anomalies. When there is duplication of the first branchial groove, the external auditory canal usually develops completely, but in addition, there is persistence of a tract that extends from the skin of the upper neck to the external auditory canal. Again this may present externally as a birthmark-like lesion, a cystic mass, or as an external sinus. Work (1972) and Work and Proctor (1963) classify duplication anomalies into two types. Type I (Fig. 78–12) they consider to be of ectodermal origin and to be a duplication of the membranous external auditory canal. Characteristically these lesions are medial to the concha and extend to the postauricular crease. They pass superior to the facial nerve, parallel to the normal external auditory canal, and finally end in a blind sac at the level of the mesotympanum. Microscopically, the tract is lined by keratinizing squamous epithelium. Type II (Fig. 78–12) anomalies are considered to be duplications of the membranous external auditory canal and pinna and are of ectodermal and mesodermal (cartilaginous) origin. The tract presents at the level of the angle of the mandible, runs upwards, either lateral or medial to the facial nerve, and may end inferior to the membranous external auditory canal or may open into the canal. The middle ear is normal.

All the anomalies that result from persistence of the first branchial groove usually present after infection, when an inflamed cystic mass develops on the upper neck. Incision or spontaneous rupture of this mass results in an external sinus, which might be the site of recurrent infection (Fig. 78–13). Treatment will depend upon the degree of problem this anomaly presents to the patient. Surgical excision is the method of choice. In all cases, the facial nerve must be identified first and the tract then followed carefully from its external opening to prevent damage to the nerve. The standard incision for a parotidectomy should be used, and the tract can sometimes be delineated by injecting methylene blue into the external opening.

Where there is a duplication anomaly and if the tract opens into the external auditory canal, after excision of the tract, the canal should be split inferiorly and packed open to heal by second intention.

Anomalies of the Second Branchial Groove

Persistence of the second branchial groove might present in one of three ways: as a cyst, as a sinus, or as a fistula. Because second groove anomalies are by far the commonest, these are the lesions that are colloquially known as branchial cysts, sinuses, or fistulae.

Branchial Cleft Cysts. Failure of obliteration of the cervical sinus results in the persistence of an epithelium-lined space. If the cervical sinus is completely trapped without an external or internal opening, the closed space forms a cystic mass. These cysts are commonest in children from birth to age 10. They are lined by squamous-type epithelium with lymphoid tissue in the wall of the cyst (Fig. 78–16). Occasionally the cysts become evident in middle adult life. This late onset

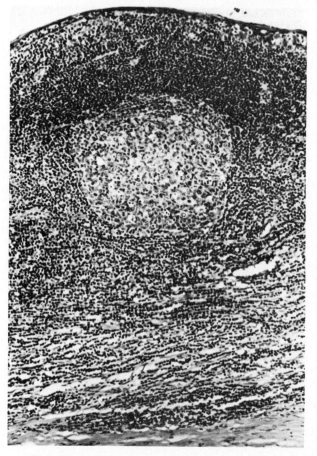

Figure 78–16 Photomicrograph of the wall of a branchial cleft cyst. At the top of the picture there is a thin layer of flat squamoid epithelium. There are numerous lymphocytes and a well-defined germinal center. At the bottom is a thin outer layer of fibrous tissue.

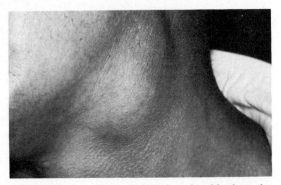

Figure 78–17 This mass developed suddenly in the left upper neck of this 43 year old man. The mass was nontender, cystic, and mobile. Its posterior third was deep to the upper sternocleidomastoid muscle

suggests an alternative theory of derivation, that is, persistence of epithelial rests in lymphoid tissue in the neck.

The usual position of a second groove cyst is high in the lateral neck with the posterior segment of the cyst deep to the anterior border of the sternocleidomastoid muscle (Fig. 78–17). This is a very characteristic presentation and facilitates easy diagnosis. These cysts usually present spontaneously, probably as a result of acute or subacute infection. Differential diagnosis seldom presents problems. A few other cystic masses may present in this area: aneurysms of the carotid artery, which are pulsatile, or Warthin tumors (cystadenoma lymphomatosum) of the parotid or submandibular salivary glands.

Branchial cleft cysts are usually treated by surgical excision, preferably at a time when they are not infected. If the infection is severe, then treatment with antibiotics is necessary. Vigorous therapy is indicated to prevent the necessity for surgical drainage before excision.

For excision, an incision is made in the skin crease overlying the cystic mass and extending to at least midway across the width of the sternocleidomastoid muscle. Care is taken to avoid damage to the greater auricular nerve. With soft tissue dissection the cyst is easily identified. If there has not been recent infection, the cyst is easily dissected from the surrounding tissues. Dissection is facilitated by careful hemostasis and by gentle maneuvering to keep the cyst intact. These cysts lie on the lateral aspect of the carotid bifurcation, and occasionally there is a tract that extends from the posterior aspect of the cyst upward to between the external and internal carotid arteries (Fig. 78–18). This tract

should be followed and might even extend through the constrictor muscles into the tonsillar fossa, where it should be divided and ligated.

Second Branchial Groove Sinus. A sinus from the second branchial groove usually presents as a small stoma along the line of the anterior border of the sternocleidomastoid muscle that frequently discharges a mucoid secretion (Fig. 78–19). Sometimes the external opening is represented by a dimple or by a pigmented spot, and the stoma might be at the level of the hyoid bone or lower. If the persistent space is a derivative of only the branchial groove, then there is usually a comparatively short tract.

Second groove sinuses are easily treated by excision. The sinus should first be investigated for position and depth by contrast radiog-

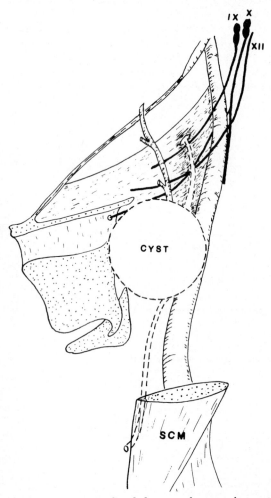

Figure 78–18 Stylized diagram showing the position of a cyst of the second branchial cleft. Outlined by broken lines are the tracts that are sometimes associated with anomalies of the second branchial cleft. SCM = sternocleidomastoid muscle.

Figure 78–19 This is the anterior neck of a four year old girl who was born with bilateral draining pits along the outer edge of the middle section. There was mucoid discharge from both pits. These represented second branchial groove sinuses that did not communicate with the pharynx. The sinuses were 4 cm in length and were excised.

raphy. At the time of surgery, dissection is facilitated by filling the tract with a color contrast material such as methylene blue. An incision is made around the external opening, and the tract is removed by sharp and blunt dissection. The tract tends to run upwards and medially towards the bifurcation of the common carotid artery.

Second Branchial Groove Fistula. The anatomic relationships of congenital branchial fistulae are constant because of their derivation during embryologic development (Frazer, 1923). For instance, all congenital fistulae with internal openings in the oropharynx and hypopharynx run lateral to the hypoglossal nerve (Simpson, 1969).

Second branchial groove fistulae develop if the second branchial groove and the second branchial pouch communicate. The external opening is usually along the anterior border of the sternocleidomastoid muscle in the lower third of the neck, and the internal upper opening is in the tonsillar fossa and is frequently related to the posterior tonsillar pillar (Rudberg, 1954). The fistulous tract ascends from the lower neck upwards and medially, penetrates the platysma, then runs between the external and internal carotid arteries lateral to the hypoglossal and glossopharyngeal nerves to enter the pharynx in the area of the tonsillar fossa (Fig. 78–20). These openings are sometimes visible on oral

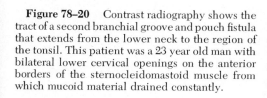

Figure 78–20 Contrast radiography shows the tract of a second branchial groove and pouch fistula that extends from the lower neck to the region of the tonsil. This patient was a 23 year old man with bilateral lower cervical openings on the anterior borders of the sternocleidomastoid muscle from which mucoid material drained constantly.

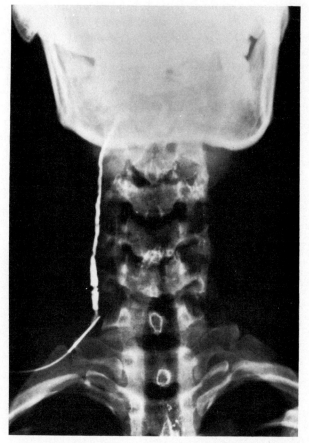

examination. The fistulae discharge a clear to yellow mucoid secretion, and the tract might tend toward recurrent infection. Treatment is dictated by cosmesis and by the severity of any infection, but these fistulae sometimes are present for a lifetime without causing significant problems.

Second groove and pouch fistulae are easily demonstrated radiologically after filling with radiopaque material via the lower end of the tract. Surgical excision is the only method of treatment that has been consistently successful, although other methods, such as the injection of sclerosing solutions, have been tried. Surgery is accomplished after defining the tract with the injection of a color contrast material such as methylene blue. An incision is made around the external opening, and by sharp and blunt dissection the tract is carefully dissected upwards and medially. A second incision higher in the neck is necessary. The tract is delivered through this, and the superior part of the dissection is completed. As the fistulous tract runs between the carotid arteries, care must be taken not to damage either of these vessels or the hypoglossal or glossopharyngeal nerves. An alternative method of removing the fistula by stripping has been described recently (Taylor and Bicknell, 1977). The method is similar to the technique used for stripping varicose veins from the legs.

Anomalies of the third branchial groove are rare. A fistula of the third branchial apparatus has its external opening low on the anterior border of the sternocleidomastoid muscle. The tract courses superiorly and medially, superficial to the vagus nerve and the common carotid artery. It then loops over the hypoglossal nerve, inferior to the glossopharyngeal nerve, runs downwards and medial to the carotid arteries, and pierces the thyrohyoid membrane to open in the pyriform sinus.

The treatment of a third branchial fistula is by surgical excision as described for fistulae of the second groove and pouch.

Anomalies of the Branchial Pouches

First Branchial Pouch. The first branchial pouch contributes to the developing eustachian tube and middle ear cleft. Significant anomalies of the first pouch are rare, but minor anomalies are common in association with first branchial arch aberrations. Agenesis of the eustachian tube and middle ear cleft has not been described in humans. Rarely, there is anomalous communication between the first branchial groove and the first pouch derivatives where an external sinus is in continuity with the middle ear cleft and eustachian tube (Fig. 78–14).

Second Branchial Pouch. The second branchial pouch is involved in the development of the palatine tonsils. The pouch, however, sometimes persists as an internal sinus. This is a blind tract of varying depths within or close to the palatine tonsil and might be a factor in recurrent tonsillitis (Fig. 78–21).

Third and Fourth Branchial Pouches. The third branchial pouch contributes to the thymus gland and to the inferior parathyroid, and the fourth pouch to the superior parathyroid glands. Failure of development of the pouches results in the absence of these structures (DiGeorge syndrome). The syndrome, characterized by absence of the thymus and parathyroid glands, involves neonatal tetany and impaired cellular immunity but with an intact humoral immunologic system. Rarely, the third pouch

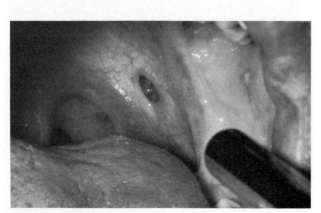

Figure 78–21 A 28 year old man complained of recurrent sore throat. On examination there was a clean opening in the left anterior tonsillar pillar that communicated with the blind tract that ran through the tonsil and ended at the level of the base of the tongue. This probably represents a second branchial pouch sinus.

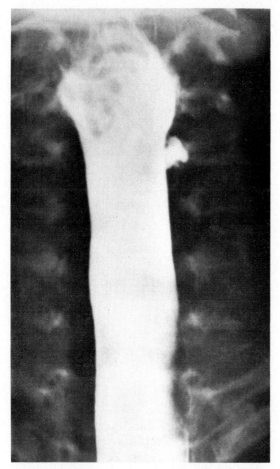

Figure 78–22 A seven year old girl presented with a recurrent abscess in the anterior neck for which numerous surgical maneuvers had been performed. A barium swallow demonstrated a fistulous tract from the left pyriform sinus. This was a congenital anomaly and represented an internal sinus from the third branchial pouch that had caused local infection.

persists as a cul-de-sac from the pyriform sinus (Fig. 78–22). If this sac becomes infected, it might fistulize with a straight course to the skin of the anterior neck. A tract then develops that runs directly from the skin to the pyriform sinus.

Anomalies of the Branchial Arches

The embryology and the facial anomalies of the branchial arches have been discussed elsewhere in this book and, therefore, will not be repeated here. The only such anomalies that will be discussed are thyroglossal duct cysts and anomalies of the lower branchial arch cartilages.

Thyroglossal Duct Cysts. The thyroid gland is not strictly a derivative of the branchial arches. It begins from a median thickening in the floor of the embryonic pharynx just caudal to the tuberculum impar. The thickening forms the thyroid diverticulum, which descends to the front of the neck, but a connection to the foramen cecum of the tongue persists as the thyroglossal duct. By the eighth week of embryonic life the bilobed thyroid gland has attained its final position in front of the trachea. The upper end of the thyroglossal duct usually disappears, but the tissue around the lower end sometimes persists as the pyramidal lobe of the thyroid gland. The duct, however, might persist as thyroglossal duct cysts anywhere from the foramen cecum to the thyroid gland. If a cyst becomes infected and ruptures on the skin, a thyroglossal duct sinus results. During the descent of the thyroid gland and the thyroglossal duct, the second branchial arch grows forward, and its cartilage (Reichert), which eventually becomes the hyoid bone, comes into close relationship with the thyroglossal duct. The hyoid bone might completely surround the duct or might displace the duct forward so that the duct lies anterior to the hyoid bone, or the duct might end at the hyoid bone. Therefore, if excision of the thyroglossal duct becomes necessary, the tract of the duct must be dissected free of the hyoid bone, or a block of the central bone must be taken to ensure that the duct is completely removed.

Thyroglossal duct cysts are more common in children but can present in adult life. They are usually in the midline of the neck inferior to the hyoid bone. Frequently, however, they are lateral and superior or much inferior to the hyoid bone. The possible locations of thyroglossal duct cysts are shown in Figure 78–23, and their actual locations in 72 patients are listed in Table 78–1 (Ward et al., 1970).

The treatment of thyroglossal duct cysts is excision. A horizontal incision is made over the mass. The soft tissues of the neck are divided, and the cystic mass is identified and carefully dissected from the surrounding tissue, taking great care to prevent its rupture. There is usually a tract that runs to the central body of the hyoid bone. This is dissected free but left attached to the hyoid bone. The upper ends of the sternohyoid and the thyrohyoid muscles are released from the central 2 cm of the body of the hyoid bone,

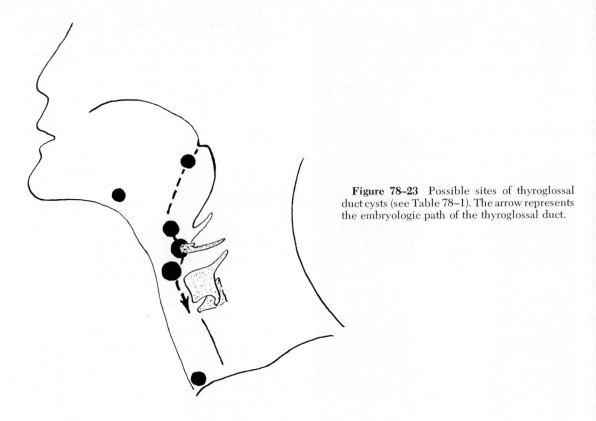

Figure 78–23 Possible sites of thyroglossal duct cysts (see Table 78–1). The arrow represents the embryologic path of the thyroglossal duct.

and the hyoid bone is divided 1 cm from the midline on both sides. A block of tissue from the central hyoid to the foramen cecum of the tongue is then cored from the substance of the tongue. The upper end of this core is clamped and ligated superiorly at the level of the foramen cecum, thus insuring complete removal of the thyroglossal duct. This method was first described by Sistrunk (1928) and is the method of choice for total excision of a thyroglossal duct cyst. Any lesser technique might result in the development of a draining sinus postoperatively.

Table 78–1 LOCATION OF THYROGLOSSAL DUCT CYSTS IN 72 PATIENTS

Location	Number
Lingular	0
Submental	2
Suprahyoid	18
Transhyoid	2
Infrahyoid	45
Suprasternal	5

(From Ward, P. H., Strahan, R. W., Acquarilli, M., et al. 1970. The many faces of cysts of the thyroglossal duct. Trans. Am. Acad. Ophthalmol. Otolaryngol., 74:310.)

Anomalies of the Branchial Arch Cartilages

Most of the branchial arch cartilages disappear except for those parts that contribute to bony structures or ligaments. Occasionally, however, remnants of arch cartilages persist as small, triangular masses deep to the skin along the anterior border of the sternocleido-

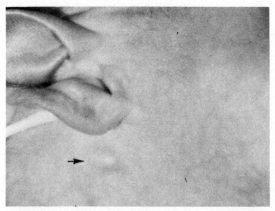

Figure 78–24 The small mass (arrow) inferior to the lobule of the ear was firm and contained a triangular mass of cartilage — the remnant of a branchial arch cartilage.

mastoid muscle (Fig. 78–24). These present only cosmetic problems and are easily removed.

SELECTED REFERENCES

Aarskog, D. 1971. Pterygium syndrome. Birth Defects, 7(6):232–234.
> This paper provides an excellent review of pterygia and of the syndromes in which they occur.

Jafee, I. S. 1968. Congenital shoulder–neck–auditory anomalies. Laryngoscope, 78:2119–2139.
> This article presents a useful, clear review of shoulder–neck anomalies.

Simpson, R. A. 1969. Lateral cervical cysts and fistulas. Laryngoscope, 79:30–58.
> This good review of branchial cysts and fistulae contains superb illustrations.

Ward, P. H., Strahan, R. W., Acquarelli, M., et al. 1970. The many faces of cysts of the thyroglossal duct. Trans. Am. Acad. Ophthalmol. Otolaryngol., 74: 310.
> This paper presents in a concise and orderly manner the embryology, clinical manifestations, and anatomic distributions of thyroglossal duct cysts.

Work, W. D. 1972. Newer concepts of first branchial cleft defects. Laryngoscope, 82:1581–1593.
> A classic paper on duplication anomalies of the first branchial cleft. Excellent anatomic descriptions are included.

REFERENCES

Aarskog, D. 1971. Pterygium syndrome. Birth Defects, 7(6):232–234.

Alberts, G. D. 1963. Branchial anomalies. J.A.M.A., 183:399–409.

Aldred, A. J. 1963. Congenital pseudarthrosis of the clavicle. J. Bone Joint Surg., 45B:312–319.

Alonso, W. A., and Chambers, R. G. 1970. Aberrant jugular vein simulating a cervical cyst. Laryngoscope, 80:244–248.

Beighton, P. E. 1972. The Ehlers-Danlos Syndrome. London, Heinemann Medical Books, Ltd.

Bill, A. H., and Summer, D. S. 1965. A unified concept of lymphangioma and cystic hygroma. Surg. Gynecol. Obstet., 120:79.

DiGeorge, A. M. 1968. Congenital absence of the thymus and its immunologic consequences: concurrence with congenital hypoparathyroidism. In Bergsma, D., and Good, R. A. (Eds.), Birth Defects: Original Article Series. Immunologic deficiency diseases in man, 4(1):116. The National Foundation – March of Dimes, New York.

Engel, D. 1943. The etiology of the undescended scapula and related syndromes. J. Bone Joint Surg., 45:613–625.

Fitchet, S. M. 1929. Cleidocranial dysostosis: hereditary and familial. J. Bone Joint Surg., 11:838–866.

Frazer, J. E. 1923. Nomenclature of disease states caused by certain vestigial structures of the neck. Br. J. Surg., 11:131–136.

Jafee, I. S. 1968. Congenital shoulder–neck–auditory anomalies. Laryngoscope, 78:2119–2139.

Karmody, C. S., and Feingold, M. 1974. Autosomal dominant first and second branchial arch syndrome — ? A new inherited syndrome. Malformation Syndromes. Birth Defects: Original Article Series. The National Foundation, March of Dimes, New York, 10(7):31–40.

Klippel, M., and Feil, A. 1912. Anomalie de la colonne vertebrale par absence des vertebres cervicales: cage thoracique remontant jusqua la base du crane. Bull. Soc. Anat. Paris, 87:185–188.

Lidge, R. T., Bechol, R. C., and Lambert, C. N. 1957. Congenital muscular torticollis. Etiology and pathology. J. Bone Joint Surg., 39A:1165–1182.

Noonan, J. A. 1968. Hypertelorism with Turner phenotype: a new syndrome with associated congenital heart disease. Am. J. Dis. Child., 116:373.

Robinson, H. M., and Ellis, F. A. 1958. Cutis laxa. Arch. Dermatol., 77:656–665.

Rudberg, R. D. 1954. Congenital fistulae of the neck. Acta Otolaryngol. Suppl., 116:271–283.

Shoul, M. L., and Ritvo, M. 1952. Clinical and roentgenological manifestations of the Klippel-Feil syndrome (congenital fusion of the cervical vertebrae brevicollis). Am. J. Roentgenol., 68:369.

Simpson, R. A. 1969. Lateral cervical cysts and fistulas. Laryngoscope, 79:30–58.

Sistrunk, W. E. 1928. Technique of removal of cysts and sinuses of the thyroglossal duct. Surg. Gynecol. Obstet., 46:109.

Taylor, P. H., and Bicknell, P. G. 1977. Stripping of branchial fistulae, a new technique. J. Laryngol. Otol., 91(2):141–149.

Turner, H. H. 1938. A syndrome of infantilism, congenital webbed neck, and cubitus valgus. Endocrinology, 23:566–574.

Ward, P. H., Strahan, R. W., Acquarelli, M., et al. 1970. The many faces of cysts of the thyroglossal duct. Trans. Am. Acad. Ophthalmol. Otolaryngol., 74:310.

Work, W. P., and Proctor, C. A. 1963. The otologist and first branchial cleft anomalies. Ann. Otol. Rhinol. Laryngol., 72:548–562.

Work, W. D. 1972. Newer concepts of first branchial cleft defects. Laryngoscope, 82:1581–1593.

Chapter 79

CERVICAL ADENOPATHY

Stephen I. Pelton, M.D.

INTRODUCTION

Cervical adenopathy occurs frequently in childhood. Often it is associated with upper respiratory tract symptoms, pharyngitis, or one of the many exanthems of childhood. In order to develop a diagnostic approach to pediatric patients with cervical adenopathy, it is necessary to categorize the disease into three major presentations: the child with acute adenitis accompanied by fever and toxicity, the child with cervical adenopathy without systemic signs, and the child with cervical adenopathy as a manifestation of an illness presenting with generalized lymph node enlargement. Each of these presentations suggests a different etiology of the adenopathy that must be approached differently by the physician.

In the child with acute illness, that is, one presenting with swelling, erythema, tenderness of the cervical lymph nodes, and fever, the adenopathy often is due to an infectious agent. The differential diagnosis of such lesions includes bacterial adenitis (staphylococcus, streptococcus, *Yersinia pestis* (formerly *Pasteurella pestis*), *Francisella tularensis* (formerly *Pasteurella tularensis*), viral adenitis (Epstein-Barr virus, cat-scratch disease), adenitis due to protozoa (*Toxoplasma gondii*), and fungal adenitis (candida). Children in a second group may present with a cervical mass and minimal or absent systemic signs and symptoms. The diagnoses considered for these children must include tuberculosis, atypical tuberculosis, toxoplasmosis, hypersensitivity reactions, tumors, and cysts.

In the third group of children are those who have cervical adenitis as part of a well-described systemic illness, such as measles, rubella, mucocutaneous lymph node syndrome, or malignancy.

This chapter concentrates on the etiology of cervical adenopathy when it is one of the significant manifestations of a disease such as scrofula, suppurative adenitis, or a particularly prominent part of a clinical syndrome (such as mucocutaneous lymph node syndrome). The history, the associated signs, and the confirmatory laboratory tests that are associated with specific pathogens or clinical syndromes will be emphasized.

SUPPURATIVE ADENITIS

Staphylococcal and Streptococcal Disease

The infant or toddler presenting with fever, symptoms of upper respiratory tract disease, and an enlarging neck mass is encountered frequently in practice. The history may reveal that an upper respiratory tract infection with coryza, sore throat, or an earache has preceded the onset of a swelling in the neck by days or as long as several weeks; usually the interval is less than seven days. Otitis media and pharyngitis are the most common associated findings, although impetigo, carious teeth, or scalp abrasions are not uncommon.

The sites most often involved are the submandibular and anterior cervical nodes (Scobie, 1969); however, the submental, posterior cervical, and preauricular and postauricular nodes are sometimes affected. The bacterial etiology has changed dramatically since the earliest large series reported by Powers and

Table 79–1 ETIOLOGY OF CERVICAL ADENOPATHY (1944–1974)

	Powers and Boisvert, 1944	Dajani et al., 1963	Wright, 1967	Scobie, 1969	Barton and Feigin, 1974
			(per cent of cases)		
Staphylococcus aureus	17	12	50	67	36
Hemolytic streptococci	79	44	10	7	26
Staphylococcus aureus and hemolytic streptococci		3			3
Anaerobic peptostreptococci					5
Fungi			3		
Enteric bacteria			7		3
Mycobacterium		6		0.5	1.5
Francisella tularensis					1.5
Sterile		35	21		24

Boisvert (1944). Initially, more than 75 per cent of the cases were attributed to group A streptococci. Later studies (Barton and Feigin, 1974; Wright, 1967) have established that an increasing percentage of cases are due to *Staphylococcus aureus* (Table 79–1). No clinical distinctions have been found that would guide the physician in distinguishing between these two pathogens. Cultures from the upper respiratory tract often grow one or the other pathogen but are not completely reliable in indicating the causative bacterial organism. Aspirates of cervical nodes have recovered *S. aureus* from patients whose throat cultures yielded group A betahemolytic streptococcus, and group A streptococcus has been isolated from patients who did not have this pathogen in cultures of the nasopharynx or throat (Danjani et al., 1963).

Needle aspiration of the largest or most fluctuant node is the only reliable method of establishing a specific bacterial diagnosis. The indications the author uses for this procedure are fever and toxicity requiring hospitalization; an infant less than six weeks of age in whom the bacteriology may include enteric bacilli; the child who fails to improve (who has persistent fever, toxicity, pain, or tenderness); the child with an underlying altered immune status (due to malignancy or chemotherapy with immunosuppressive agents); and finally, the child whose history suggests that an unusual pathogen may be the cause of the illness. To perform needle aspiration of a node, the overlying skin is cleaned with povidine-iodine, and then a local anesthetic is injected. A sterile needle is inserted into the most fluctuant or largest node, and the syringe is aspirated. If no purulent material is obtained, 1 to 2 ml of sterile 0.85 per cent

NaCl is injected, and the aspiration is repeated. In about two thirds of cases, positive cultures are obtained from both fluctuant and nonfluctuant cervical nodes. Most investigators have reported no complications from this procedure. No laboratory tests (such as complete blood cell count, hematocrit, or erythrocyte sedimentation rate) other than needle aspiration have been helpful in distinguishing between disease of staphylococcal and that of streptococcal origin.

Based on our present level of knowledge regarding the bacteriology of cervical adenitis and the fact that staphylococci are frequently resistant to penicillin, a penicillinase-resistant penicillin should be the initial antibiotic used in the management of children with acute cervical adenitis. If a needle aspiration has been performed, any change in therapy should be determined by the results of cultures and sensitivity tests. A 7 to 10 day course of therapy will be adequate for resolution of fever and local signs of inflammation in most patients. Although enlarged nodes may still be present at the end of therapy, they can be expected to regress over a period of weeks. When fluctuance is present, incision and drainage will result in a more rapid resolution of symptoms and signs of inflammation.

Unusual Pathogens

Three bacterial species that may produce acute cervical adenopathy should be considered as etiologic agents when the history and physical findings are appropriate. *Plague,* an acute bacterial infection caused by *Y. pestis,* is characterized by fever and acute regional lymphadenitis. The sylvatic rodent is the reservoir of plague in this country, and the disease is usually spread by infected fleas or by handling of infected animal tissues. The common form, bubonic plague, is not spread from person to person, although the pneumonic form may be spread among humans by infected droplets. The disease begins with inoculation of the infecting organism at the site of the flea bite and spreads to regional lymph nodes. An inflammatory response follows, and enlarged lymph nodes, lymphedema, and hemorrhagic necrosis ensue. Septicemia often is present during this stage of the illness. The onset is usually acute, with fever, headache, prostration, and the simultaneous development of the bubo. Although the most common sites are the inguinal and femoral lymph nodes, cervical disease has been reported. The bubo varies in size from 1 to 10 cm in diameter and is characterized by excruciating pain with erythema of the overlying skin.

An increasing number of cases of plague have been reported in the United States during the last 10 years (Palmer et al., 1971); this is probably related to increased travel in the Southwest, communal living, and immigration from Vietnam. The diagnosis of plague can be suspected when travel to the Southwest or contact with rodents, prairie dogs, squirrels, or chipmunks is reported. The diagnosis can be confirmed by smear and culture of the bubo. The gram stain usually reveals polymorphonuclear leukocytes and gram-negative coccobacillary forms. Cultures of the aspirate and blood are usually positive for *Y. pestis*. In the absence of positive cultures, a serologic diagnosis can be made by the hemagglutination technique. A fourfold or greater rise in titer of antibody to *Y. pestis* or a single specimen with a titer of 1:16 or greater is diagnostic.

Therapy with streptomycin (15 mg per kg IM every 12 hours for 10 days) or chloramphenicol (25 mg per kg IV as a single dose followed by 15 mg per kg IV every 6 hours for 10 days) results in defervescence within 72 hours. The bubo usually recedes, although incision and drainage may be indicated if enlargement or fluctuance occurs (Butler et al., 1977).

Infection with *F. tularensis* results in a clinical syndrome characterized by enlargement of lymph nodes, malaise, weakness, and fever. In 50 per cent of patients the axillary nodes are enlarged, whereas the cervical and inguinal nodes are affected in 30 per cent and 10 per cent of cases, respectively (Klock et al., 1973). Cutaneous ulcers are the hallmark clinical findings. Most lesions are found on the hands and fingers and are painful (Young et al., 1969). Children often present with oropharyngeal disease (Levy et al., 1950). Exudative tonsillitis accompanied by cervical adenopathy that is unresponsive to penicillin is the most common presentation. This disease is clinically indistinguishable from exudative pharyngitis due to other causes (Tyson, 1976).

Tularemia is contracted by contact with an infected rabbit or arthropod. During the past ten years, large outbreaks have been reported in Vermont and Utah, although the rural South remains the major endemic area in the United States. *F. tularensis* often can be recovered from the ulcer or from the regional lymph node. Serologic (agglutination) tests are usually positive during the second or third week of illness. A fourfold or greater rise in the antibody or a titer of more than 1:160 is presumptive evidence of disease.

Streptomycin is the antibiotic of choice for therapy of infections due to *F. tularensis*; 0.5 to 1.0 gm IM every 12 hours for 10 days is the dose most frequently employed. The patient's temperature usually returns to normal within a few days; however, the lymph nodes may continue to enlarge, and surgery may be necessary for drainage. Alternative antibiotics are tetracycline and chloramphenicol. Recurrence of symptoms is not uncommon, and a second course of therapy with streptomycin, tetracycline, or chloramphenicol may be necessary.

Brucellosis is usually a disease of domestic animals — cattle, swine, goats, and sheep. In the United States the disease in humans generally is acquired by dermal contact with infected animals, although epidemics due to the ingestion of unpasteurized milk still occur. At present the disease remains an occupational hazard of veterinarians, meatpacking plant employees, and livestock producers (Busch and Parker, 1972).

The initial manifestations of brucellosis are usually insidious in nature: Fever, headache, weakness, myalgia, and other nonspecific symptoms are present. On occasion the illness is more acute, with high fever, lethargy, and hepatosplenomegaly. In children the disease is seldom of the severe toxic type but rather of the mild, possibly self-limited, form (Street et al., 1975). Controversy continues as to whether this presentation is characteristic of the age group or of the causative agents, *Brucella abortus* or *Brucella suis*, which are more common in this country than *Brucella melitensis*.

Cervical adenopathy is present in about half of the patients. Other manifestations of brucellosis include splenomegaly, orchitis, and arthralgia. Often the diagnosis is suspected only after a complete evaluation for fever of unknown origin has been fruitless. The pathology of the nodes is nonspecific, showing epitheloid cells, giant cells of the foreign body and Langerhans types, and granuloma. The most practical method of confirming a suspected diagnosis is the agglutination reaction. A titer of 1:320 or greater suggests active disease and usually is found by the second or third week of illness (Street et al., 1975).

The organism itself can be cultured from the blood or bone marrow. In a study of a large series of patients, Spink (1952) found that 50 per cent of the patients had blood cultures positive for *Brucella*. Other laboratory tests are nonspecific. Leukopenia and leukocytosis both have been reported. Hepatocellular enzymes often are elevated, especially with the toxic form of illness due to *B. melitensis*. The acute form of brucellosis must be distinguished from typhoid fever, infectious mononucleosis, and malaria.

Most patients recover spontaneously with bed rest. The course of the illness can be shortened and the complications reduced by administration of tetracycline (500 mg orally every six hours for 21 days). In addition, streptomycin (1 to 2 gm daily IM for two weeks) is recommended for more serious cases. Relapse is not uncommon and may respond to a second course of therapy. The use of steroids remains controversial and, at least in children, does not seem to be indicated.

Actinomyces produce two types of clinical syndromes that are manifested by cervical swelling. The first is a chronic, progressive illness characterized by induration and trismus and resulting finally in draining sinus tracts. The second type is an acute process characterized by suppuration and abscess; trismus may also be present.

Actinomyces are usually saprophytic organisms that may be part of the normal flora of the mouth or may be found in soil or grasses.

Trauma or the eruption of a tooth, especially a molar, may create the conditions conducive to tissue damage, invasion, and suppuration. A peculiar characteristic of this infection is the presence of an abscess between tissue planes and beneath the skin as a primary manifestation; involvement of the lymph nodes is only secondary. The agent most often responsible for human infection is *Actinomyces israelii*. The diagnosis can be suspected when the gram stain reveals either the filamentous or the gram-positive diphtheroid form. The diagnosis can be confirmed by use of fluorescent antibody techniques (Hartley and Schatten, 1973).

Therapy usually requires incision and drainage. Penicillin (10 to 20 million units IM or IV daily for two to three weeks followed by oral penicillin for up to three months) is usually successful. Alternative antibiotic regimens of ampicillin, lincomycin, or cephalothin in comparable doses also have given satisfactory results.

TUBERCULOUS ADENITIS

The pathogenesis, diagnosis, and treatment of cervical lymph node infection due to *Mycobacterium tuberculosis* or atypical mycobacteria remains controversial. Each study of a large series of cervical inflammatory masses still reports that 1 to 10 per cent of cases are tuberculous, with an increasing number of cases due to atypical mycobacteria (Dajani et al., 1963; Wright, 1967).

Cervical adenopathy due to *M. tuberculosis* usually presents with minimal, if any, systemic signs or symptoms. About 10 per cent of cases may present as one of the variants, so-called "Asian tuberculosis," manifested by high fever and disseminated lymph node enlargement. Kent (1967) reported a painless node or group of nodes to be the most common presentation. Only 10 per cent in his series had fever, and about an equal number had swollen and tender nodes. Involvement of one group of nodes was found in more than 80 per cent of patients (Kent, 1967); anterior cervical, posterior cervical, superclavicular, and submandibular nodes were the most common sites of infection.

The relative importance of spread from local oropharyngeal and pulmonary sources has never been completely determined. Nevertheless, for therapeutic purposes, this ques-

Table 79–2 DISTINGUISHING CHARACTERISTICS OF CERVICAL INFECTION DUE
TO *MYCOBACTERIUM TUBERCULOSIS* AND ATYPICAL MYCOBACTERIA

	M. tuberculosis	Atypical mycobacteria
Location	usually bilateral with multiple groups	usually unilateral; submandibular
Family contact with TB	positive	negative
Chest radiograph	parenchymal disease	normal
PPD-S	≥ 10 mm	< 5 mm
PPD-G	< 5 mm	≥ 10 mm
Symptoms	variable	absent

tion remains an important one. All investigators have reported a high incidence of abnormal chest radiographs with evidence of hilar adenopathy, parenchymal lesions, or blunting of the costophrenic angle in patients with proven disease; these observations suggest that hematogenous spread at the time of pulmonary infection is the most common pathogenesis (Kent, 1967). Other investigators have regarded the tonsils, the gingiva, or both as the likely source of infection, with direct spread through the lymphatics. When tonsillar tissue has been studied histologically, lesions compatible with tuberculosis were found in 9 per cent (Kendig and Wiley, 1955) to 47 per cent of cases (Wilmot et al., 1957). Although this controversy has not been completely resolved and both routes of infection probably play a part, most patients have evidence of active or inactive disease at another site (usually pulmonary).

Studies conducted during the past 10 years have shown that an increasing percentage of tuberculous nodes are caused by atypical mycobacteria. The majority of patients present with a single affected node, usually posterior and inferior to the angle of the mandible, and without systemic signs or symptoms (Chapman and Guy, 1959). The node may be freely movable or attached to the skin. The overlying skin is often erythematous but without increased heat; occasionally drainage from a sinus tract is present. When the causative agent is an atypical strain of mycobacteria, fewer than 5 per cent of patients have bilateral involvement. Chest radiographs are normal in 90 per cent of cases proved by culture to be due to atypical mycobacteria (Salyer et al., 1968).

Although the distinction between disease due to atypical mycobacteria and that due to *M. tuberculosis* ultimately rests on the results of the culture, several epidemiologic, clinical, and laboratory clues are available for differentiation (Table 79–2). A history of contact with a known case of tuberculosis is critical in making the distinction. Although the absence of such a contact does not confirm the diagnosis of disease due to atypical mycobacteria, about 50 per cent of children with cervical disease secondary to infection with *M. tuberculosis* have an identifiable contact. The routine laboratory tests (complete and differential blood cell counts and erythrocyte sedimentation rate) are not helpful. A chest radiograph that shows hilar, pleural, or parenchymal disease strongly supports the diagnosis of infection with *M. tuberculosis* (Black and Chapman, 1964). In all the series of patients with cervical disease due to atypical strains of mycobacteria, the paucity of instances of pulmonary disease was notable.

The skin tests of *M. tuberculosis* (purified protein derivative [PPD]-S) and for atypical mycobacterial (PPD-B, PPD-G) are probably the most reliable tests for distinguishing disease due to atypical mycobacteria from that due to *M. tuberculosis*. Tuberculin skin testing with 0.0001 mg of PPD-S almost always will be positive for patients with cervical disease due to *M. tuberculosis* and often will be negative for patients with disease due to atypical strains of mycobacteria. The reagins PPD-B (prepared from the Battey strain of atypical mycobacteria) and PPD-G (prepared from a scotochromogenic strain) usually give a larger reaction than does PPD-S in patients with cervical disease due to atypical strains. In most reported series, the correlation between reactivity to PPD-S or PPD-B and the results of cultures has been extremely good (Smith et al., 1965).

The distinction between cervical infection due to *M. tuberculosis* and that due to atypical mycobacteria is important because of the relative resistance of atypical strains to most antituberculosis drugs.

Antituberculosis therapy has been found to be successful in treating disease due to *M.*

tuberculosis. Before the introduction of isoniazid (INH) and streptomycin, recurrence rates of 1 to 43 per cent were reported with surgical therapy alone (Dowd, 1916); the chance of recurrence depended on the extent of the disease at the time of diagnosis. Among patients with oropharyngeal lesions and isolated ipsilateral cervical enlargement, only 1 per cent had recurrences, but among patients with massive node involvement in the neck, 43 per cent had recurrences.

Since the advent of effective chemotherapy, medical therapy alone has been advocated (Hooper, 1972) for treatment of patients with infection due to *M. tuberculosis*. Kent (1967) reported successful treatment with isoniazid and para-aminosalicylic acid of 35 to 36 patients who completed at least an 18 month course of antituberculosis therapy with at least these two drugs. At present, surgery limited to the obtaining of a diagnostic biopsy specimen is appropriate when infection due to *M. tuberculosis* is suspected (Ord and Matz, 1974). Excisional surgery should be reserved for patients with cold abscesses or impending breakdown of skin and for patients who have pathologic or bacteriologic support for the diagnosis of *M. tuberculosis* and have failed to respond adequately to medical management. Once antituberculosis therapy is begun, the usual course of illness is regression over a three month period with virtually complete reduction in size of the lymph nodes within six months. Therapy should consist of isoniazid plus para-aminosalicylic acid, streptomycin, or ethambutol. The duration of therapy has not been evaluated adequately in controlled trials, but since at least 50 per cent of patients will have pulmonary or other organ system involvement, a minimum of 18 months appears to be appropriate.

The role of tonsillectomy for treatment of disease due to *M. tuberculosis* remains controversial. No studies have proved that tonsillectomy alters the course of the illness (Hooper, 1972).

The results of chemotherapy alone for therapy of disease due to atypical mycobacteria have been unsatisfactory. Surgical excision of the affected node and overlying skin is the procedure of choice. Less extensive procedures, such as incision and drainage or curettage, have resulted in persistent draining sinuses in more than 50 per cent of cases (Davis and Comstock, 1961).

Most patients infected with atypical mycobacteria have received a combination of surgical and medical therapy. Salyer and colleagues (1971) reported successful treatment of 47 patients by surgical excision and a two-drug chemotherapeutic regimen (isoniazid and para-aminosalicylic acid, ethambutol, or streptomycin). Although results of surgery have been successful, excision is not always possible or cannot always be done without complications and should not be attempted when other structures, especially the facial nerve, cannot be isolated from the infected nodes. Salyer and others (1971) reported an 8 per cent incidence of paralysis of the mandibular branch of the facial nerve. Since isoniazid, para-aminosalicylic acid, and streptomycin generally are inactive against atypical mycobacteria *in vitro* (even though they have been used widely), other agents should be tried. Mandell and Wright (1975) described four patients who were treated successfully with rifampin alone. The therapy was well-tolerated, and complete resolution occurred within 11 months.

Excision of the affected node remains the treatment of choice when disease due to atypical mycobacteria has been diagnosed and complete removal is possible. Limited experience with rifampin suggests that it may be an effective adjunct to therapy when excision is not possible for a period of four to six months after surgery.

NONBACTERIAL ADENITIS

Toxoplasmosis

The diagnosis of toxoplasmosis should be considered in children with cervical adenopathy. In some series, 5 to 8 per cent of patients with cervical adenopathy were found to have toxoplasmosis (Siim, 1960).

Cervical adenopathy is the most commonly acquired form of this disease. The adenopathy may be part of the total clinical presentation of fatigue, myalgia, weakness, and fever, or may be an isolated presentation. Physical examination usually reveals slightly tender, firm nodes without inflammation of the surrounding tissue. The form of toxoplasmosis that is limited to lymphadenopathy classically has a benign course and is believed not to progress to the more severe form of the disease, which is characterized by cardiac involvement, infection of the central nervous system, pneumonia, or chorioretinitis (Karlan and Baker, 1972).

The diagnosis of toxoplasmosis should be suspected in patients with nonspecific symptoms, adenopathy with lymphocytosis, atypical lymphocytes, and a negative heterophile reaction. The disease is acquired by inoculation of the encysted form of *Toxoplasma gondii*. These oocysts are excreted in the feces of domestic cats. The diagnosis is confirmed by serologic testing (either the Sabin-Feldman dye test or an indirect fluorescent antibody test). An antibody titer of 1:1024 is diagnostic of active infection, while a titer of 1:256 or 1:512 is equivocal (Karlan and Baker, 1972). The titer usually begins to rise two weeks after exposure and reaches a maximum level four to six weeks later. It falls slowly over a period of months. The histopathology is suggestive of toxoplasmosis when eosinophilic histiocytes are found; however, this finding in itself is not diagnostic (Smith et al., 1970; Butler, 1969).

Treatment for the disease usually is not indicated when it is limited to lymphadenopathy. If the more serious manifestations are present (i.e., central nervous system involvement or myocardial disease), a sulfonamide plus pyrimethamine is the most effective therapy.

Cat-Scratch Disease

Adenopathy limited to a single node or a chain of nodes at a single site is the hallmark of cat-scratch disease. Such nodes are usually tender and are found most often in the extremities. Cervical adenopathy has been reported in 20 per cent of the cases studied (Margileth, 1968). The onset has been described as being variably acute or slowly progressive; adenopathy develops 5 to 50 days after the patient experienced the initial cat scratch. The acute onset is characterized by fever (101 to 106°F), malaise, and headaches. The slowly progressive form often presents without systemic signs or symptoms and with only a progressively enlarging node. In either form of the disease, multiple sites of adenopathy are distinctly uncommon (Margileth, 1968).

In about 95 per cent of cases, the history of a cat scratch (92 per cent) or other animal scratch (3 per cent) can be obtained. The primary lesion (papule, pustule, or conjunc-

tivitis) will be found distal to the regional bubo but is frequently in a healing state at the time of presentation. Supportive evidence for the diagnosis is obtained from the cat-scratch skin test. Although the procedure is not standardized, a safe preparation can be made from aspirated pus by use of the process described by McGovern and colleagues (1955). Although these preparations vary in activity and a positive test in itself indicates only sensitization in the recent or distant past, most authors agree that cat-scratch disease can be excluded if a skin test with two different antigens of proven potency are negative both initially and after four weeks. The skin test involves intracutaneous injection of 0.1 ml of antigen. An area of more than 5 mm of induration is considered positive, an area of less than 4 mm is negative, and those between 4 and 5 mm are equivocal. Since the etiologic agent of this disease remains unknown, specific therapy is unavailable. Antibiotics have proved ineffective. Needle aspiration can be valuable to relieve pain if suppuration has occurred, and repeated aspirations have been employed for symptomatic relief in some cases. Obtaining a biopsy specimen is indicated only when there is substantial doubt about the diagnosis. Spontaneous recovery within two months is the rule in the majority of cases.

Infectious Mononucleosis

Infectious mononucleosis is an acute, self-limited, usually benign illness caused by infection with the Epstein-Barr virus. Commonly, infectious mononucleosis is manifested by involvement of the cervical nodes in conjunction with generalized adenopathy or pharyngitis or, less often, as an isolated finding. Review of the records of 203 patients with infectious mononucleosis showed that 23 (11 per cent) had either anterior or posterior cervical adenopathy without generalized adenopathy (Baehner and Shuler, 1967).

The nodes generally are not tender or suppurative and rarely exceed 3 cm in size. Other manifestations of infectious mononucleosis include exudative tonsillitis, splenomegaly and/or hepatomegaly, and rash. These physical findings may occur in any combination. The diagnosis of infectious mononucleosis should be suspected in any child with the symptoms or signs just described. The white blood cell count is often diagnostic: 90 per cent of patients have a white blood cell count of 5000 to 20,000 with more than 25 per cent atypical lymphocytes. Specific tests confirm the diagnosis. A heterophile antibody titer of 1:128 or more that does not change more than one tube after absorption with guinea pig erythrocytes is specific. The mononucleosis slide test provides a rapid slide agglutination technique for diagnosis. For this test, serum is absorbed with either guinea pig kidney or beef erythrocytes, to which Morse erythrocytes are then added. If agglutination appears only in the serum absorbed with guinea pig kidney or is greater in the serum absorbed with guinea pig kidney, the test is positive and the diagnosis is confirmed.

Although infectious mononucleosis has been reported to occur infrequently in children younger than three years, use of a recently developed immunofluorescent test for antibody to Epstein-Barr virus has demonstrated that the illness is more common in this age group than was previously suspected. The clinical manifestations are usually less specific: Diarrhea, vomiting, otitis media, and fever are the most prominent symptoms. Lymphadenopathy was distinctly uncommon in children younger than one year of age who had an antibody response to Epstein-Barr virus (Tamir et al., 1974). In infants, isolated cervical adenopathy is not likely to be due to Epstein-Barr virus, but with older children this infection must be included in the physician's consideration.

The sore throat associated with infectious mononucleosis usually lasts five to ten days, and the fever subsides after one to four weeks. Full recovery, including resolution of the adenopathy, usually occurs within six weeks, but a few patients may have prolonged lethargy. The most serious complications are splenic rupture or subcapsular hemorrhage, respiratory insufficiency secondary to tonsillar edema, and central nervous system infection producing aseptic meningitis, encephalitis, monoplegia, or Guillain-Barré syndrome.

Symptomatic treatment with limited activity and maintenance of hydration is usually all that is required. Steroids have been used with success in patients with impending respiratory insufficiency or prolonged fever, but use of these drugs should be limited to severe cases because they have not been shown to alter the course of hepatic or central nervous system complications. Hospitalization should be reserved for patients with jaundice, anemia, thrombocytopenia, central nervous system manifestations, or laryngeal edema.

In patients in whom the heterophil reaction is negative, investigation for the presence of cytomegalovirus infection is warranted. Cervical adenopathy, fever, tonsillitis, and atypical lymphocytosis have been reported in association with cytomegalovirus infection in one patient (Stern, 1968).

Mucocutaneous Lymph Node Syndrome

Mucocutaneous lymph node syndrome (MLNS) has recently been recognized with increasing frequency in the continental United States. The Center for Disease Control (CDC) has established diagnostic criteria for identifying cases based on the presence of typical signs and symptoms and the exclusion of other syndromes. Five of the following are required for the diagnosis (CDC, 1976): (1) fever lasting at least five days that is unresponsive to antibiotics, (2) bilateral conjunctivitis, (3) dryness, redness, and fissuring of the lips or erythema of the oropharyngeal mucosa, (4) erythema or induration of the hands and feet with desquamation beginning at the fingertips, (5) a polymorphous exanthem of the body without vesicles, and (6) acute, nonpurulent enlargement of the cervical lymph nodes.

The etiology of this disease as yet remains unknown. Seven thousand cases have been reported from Japan, and clusters of cases in Hawaii and New York as well as isolated cases throughout the continental United States have been reported since 1967 (CDC, 1976). The pathology resembles infantile periarteritis nodosa with swelling of the endothelial cells of the postcapillary vesicles and hyperplasia of the reticuloendothelial cells within lymph nodes (Fujiwara and Hamashima, 1978; Riley, 1976).

Laboratory findings in MLNS are nonspecific. The white blood cell count is often elevated, as is the erythrocyte sedimentation rate. The alpha two globulin level and the platelet count usually increase in the second week of illness. No diagnostic test is available, however, and scarlet fever, leptospirosis, and Stevens-Johnson syndrome must be considered in patients presenting with a clinical picture of MLNS.

There is no specific therapy for MLNS. The mortality in the larger series has been reported to be 1 to 2 per cent with coronary thrombosis as the cause of death. Investigators have employed salicylates or prednisone, but there have been no controlled studies, and the efficacy of these agents in preventing morbidity and mortality is unknown.

WHEN TO OBTAIN A BIOPSY SPECIMEN

The patient with fever, toxicity, and an enlarged cervical mass requires immediate evaluation. A careful history and thorough examination will often reveal likely diagnostic considerations and will suggest the laboratory tests most likely to be fruitful. Needle aspiration and collaboration with the microbiology laboratory will often identify a specific pathogen in these cases.

A child with asymptomatic cervical swelling represents a different problem. Since many respiratory illnesses are associated with cervical lymphadenopathy that may persist for periods of time after the symptoms have resolved, the clinician must decide when to initiate a rigorous evaluation of a cervical mass. In reviewing a large series of cervical masses, Moussatos and Baffes (1963) found some predictors of "serious" disease. Age, sex, and duration of symptoms were not reliable indications for excluding malignant tumors, but they found that most benign cervical masses were located anterior to the sternocleidomastoid muscle, while malignant tumors were either found in the posterior cervical triangle or both anterior and posterior to the sternocleidomastoid muscle.

Branchial cleft and thyroglossal duct cysts are almost exclusively located anterior to the sternocleidomastoid muscle. Both of these may intermittently become infected and drain purulent material. On occasion they have been misdiagnosed as tuberculous nodes. The presence of movement when the tongue is protruded characterizes a thyroglossal duct cyst. A third diagnostic consideration is cystic hygromas, which are classically located in the lower portion of the neck, anterior to the sternocleiodomastoid muscle. These three diagnostic possibilities are rarely associated with systemic signs or symptoms, such as weight loss, anemia, or pallor.

Neoplasms in the neck usually are located in the posterior cervical triangle and enlarge during a period of observation. In those that represent metastasis (lymphoma, lymphosarcoma, or Hodgkin disease), a primary lesion is usually evident.

When the clinician is confronted with the presence of systemic illness and an asymptomatic cervical mass located posterior to the sternocleidomastoid muscle, malignancy must be considered, and a biopsy specimen should be obtained early. The findings of Lake and Oski (1978) support the association of weight loss, hepatosplenomegaly, and arthralgia or anemia (hemoglobin less than 10) with malignancy. When the patient is well and the mass is stable in size and is located in the anterior triangle, a course of observation and diagnostic evaluation can precede surgical exploration of the mass.

The value of close follow-up of patients whose biopsy specimens are nondiagnostic is confirmed by Lake and Oski (1978): 18 per cent of patients whose biopsy specimens were nondiagnostic later proved to have a definable disease. A second biopsy specimen, often from additional nodes, from patients with persistent or recurrent symptoms led to the appropriate diagnosis. Although nondiagnostic reactive hyperplasia usually suggests benign antigenic stimulation, in a small number of patients lymphoreticular disease will declare itself.

SELECTED REFERENCES

Barton, L. L., and Feigin, R. D. 1974. Childhood cervical lymphadenitis: A reappraisal. J. Pediatr., 84:846–852.

Lake, H. M., and Oski, F. A. 1978. Peripheral lymphadenopathy in childhood. Am. J. Dis. Child., 132:357–359.

Margileth, F. M. 1968. Cat scratch disease: Nonbacterial regional lymphadenitis. Pediatrics, 42:803–818.

Moussatos, G. H., and Baffes, T. G. 1963. Cervical masses in infants and children. Pediatrics, 32:251–256.

Salyer, K. E., Votteler, T. P., and Forman, W. G. 1971. Cervical adenitis in children due to atypical mycobacteria. Plast. Reconstr. Surg., 47:47–53.

REFERENCES

Baehner, R. L., and Shuler, S. E. 1967. Infectious mononucleosis in childhood. Clinical expressions, serologic findings, complications, prognosis. Clin. Pediatr., 6:393–399.

Barton, L. L., and Feigin, R. D. 1974. Childhood cervical

lymphadenitis: A reappraisal. J. Pediatr., *84*:846–852.

Black, B. G., and Chapman, J. S. 1964. Cervical adenitis in children due to human and unclassified mycobacteria. Pediatr., *33*:887–893.

Busch, L. A., and Parker, R. L. 1972. Brucellosis in the United States. J. Infect. Dis., *125*:289–294.

Butler, J. J. 1969. Non-neoplastic lesions of lymph nodes of man to be differentiated from lymphomas. Natl. Cancer Inst. Monogr., *32*:233–255.

Butler, T., Mahmound, A. A. F., and Warren, K. S. 1977. Algorithms in the diagnosis and management of exotic diseases. XXV. Plague. J. Infect. Dis., *136*:317–320.

Center for Disease Control 1976. Mucocutaneous lymph node syndrome — United States. Morbidity & Mortality Weekly Report, *25*:157–158.

Center for Disease Control 1978. Kawasaki Disease — United States. Morbidity & Mortality Weekly Report, *27*:9.

Chapman, J. S., and Guy, L. R. 1959. Scrofula caused by atypical mycobacteria. Pediatrics, *23*:323–331.

Dajani, A. S., Garcia, R. E., and Wolinsky, E. 1963. Etiology of cervical lymphadenitis in children. N. Engl. J. Med., *268*:1329–1333.

Davis, S. D., and Comstock, G. W. 1961. Mycobacterial cervical adenitis in children. J. Pediatr., *58*:771–778.

Dowd, C. N. 1916. Tuberculosis of the cervical lymphatics. A study of six hundred and eighty-seven cases. J.A.M.A., *67*:499–502.

Fujiwara, H., and Hamashima, Y. 1978. Pathology of the heart in Kawasaki disease. Pediatrics, *61*:100–107.

Hartley, J. H., Jr., and Schatten, W. E. 1973. Cervicofacial actinomycosis. Plast. Reconstr. Surg., *51*:44–47.

Hooper, A. A. 1972. Tuberculous peripheral lymphadenitis. Br. J. Surg., *59*:353–359.

Karlan, M. S., and Baker, D. C. 1972. Cervical lymphadenopathy secondary to toxoplasmosis. Laryngoscope, *82*:956–964.

Kendig, E. L., and Wiley, W. M., Jr. 1955. The treatment of tuberculosis of the superficial cervical lymph nodes in children. J. Pediatr., *47*:607–613.

Kent, D. C. 1967. Tuberculous lymphadenitis: Not a localized disease process. Am. J. Med. Sci., *254*:866–874.

Klock, L. E., Olsen, P. F., and Fukushima, T. 1973. Tularemia epidemic associated with the deerfly. J.A.M.A., *226*:149–152.

Lake, A. M., and Oski, F. A. 1978. Peripheral lymphadenopathy in childhood. Am. J. Dis. Child., *132*:357–359.

Levy, H. B., Webb, C. H., and Wilkinson, J. D. 1950. Tularemia as a pediatric problem. Pediatrics, *6*:113–121.

Mandell, F., and Wright, P. F. 1975. Treatment of atypical mycobacterial cervical adenitis with rifampin. Pediatrics *55*:39–43.

Margileth, A. M. 1968. Cat scratch disease: Nonbacterial regional lymphadenitis. The study of 145 patients and a review of the literature. Pediatrics, *42*:803–818.

McGovern, J. J., Kunz, L. J., and Blodgett, F. M. 1955. Nonbacterial regional lymphadenitis ("cat-scratch fever"). An evaluation of the diagnostic intradermal test. N. Engl. J. Med., *252*:166–172.

Moussatos, G. H., and Baffes, T. G. 1963. Cervical masses in infants and children. Pediatrics, *32*:251–256.

Ord, R. J., and Matz, G. J. 1974. Tuberculous cervical lymphadenitis. Arch. Otolaryngol., *99*:327–329.

Palmer, D. L., Kisch, A. L., Williams, R. C., Jr., et al. 1971. Clinical features of plague in the United States: The 1969–1970 epidemic. J. Infect. Dis., *124*:367–371.

Powers, G. F., and Boisvert, P. L. 1944. Age as a factor in streptococcosis. J. Pediatr., *25*:481–503.

Riley, H. D., Jr. 1976. Mucocutaneous lymph node syndrome (Kawasaki disease). J. Infect. Dis., *134*:302–305.

Salyer, K. E., Votteler, T. P., and Dorman, G. W. 1968. Surgical management of cervical adenitis due to atypical mycobacteria in children. J.A.M.A., *204*:1037–1040.

Salyer, K. E., Votteler, T. P., and Dorman, G. W. 1971. Cervical adenitis in children due to atypical mycobacteria. Plast. Reconstr. Surg., *47*:47–53.

Scobie, W. G. 1969. Acute suppurative adenitis in children: A review of 1964 cases. South. Med. J., *14*:352–354.

Siim, J. C. 1960. Clinical and diagnostic aspects of human acquired toxoplasmosis. *In* Human Toxoplasmosis, E J N A Munksgaard Forlag, Copenhagen, Denmark, pp. 53–79.

Smith, D. H., Doherty, R. A., and deLemos, R. A. 1965. Unclassified mycobacterial infection and disease in children residing in Massachusetts. J. Pediatr., *67*:759–767.

Smith, J. M., McCulloch, W. F., and Davis, J. R. 1970. A case of toxoplasmic lymphadenitis in an adult with a description of the biopsied lymph nodes. Am. J. Med. Sci., *260*:184–191.

Spink, W. W. 1952. Some biological and clinical problems related to intracellular parasitism in brucellosis. N. Engl. J. Med., *24*:603–610.

Stern, H. 1968. Isolation of cytomegalovirus and clinical manifestation of infection at different ages. Br. Med. J., *1*:665–669.

Street, L., Jr., Grant, W. W., and Alva, J. D. 1975. Brucellosis in childhood. Pediatrics, *55*:416–420.

Tamir, D., Benderly, A., Levy J., et al. 1974. Infectious mononucleosis and Epstein-Barr virus in childhood. Pediatrics, *53*:330–335.

Tyson, H. K. 1976. Tularemia: An unappreciated cause of exudative pharyngitis. Pediatrics, *58*:864–866.

Wilmot, T. J., James, E. F., and Reilly, L. V. 1957. Tuberculous cervical adenitis. Lancet, *2*:1184–1187.

Wright, N. L. 1967. Cervical infections. Am. J. Surg., *113*:379–386.

Young, L. S., Bicknell, D. S., Archer, B. G., et al. 1969. Tularemia epidemic: Vermont, 1968. Forty-seven cases linked to contact with muskrats. N. Engl. J. Med., *280*:1253–1260.

Chapter 80

INJURIES OF THE NECK

Bruce W. Jafek, M.D.
Thomas J. Balkany, M.D.

INTRODUCTION

It has been conservatively estimated that 50,000 children per year are permanently disabled by injuries and that an additional 2 million are temporarily incapacitated. The number of severe injuries in children grows yearly owing to the increase in size of this segment of the population, the increase in nonfatal vehicular trauma, and the advances in lifesaving and rehabilitation techniques (Dietrich, 1954).

The majority of injuries occur to children between the ages of two and seven, the time of transition between total parental protection and adequate education for self-preservation. Approximately 10 to 15 per cent of serious injuries in children are neck injuries, resulting most frequently from automobile accidents (Haller and Talbert, 1973).

GENERAL PRINCIPLES

Pediatric injuries differ generally from those in the adult, not only in the nature of the injuries sustained but also in the emotional reaction of the patient to trauma and often in the management and response to therapy. For example, apparently minor blood loss assumes major importance owing to the child's relatively small total blood volume; fluid replacement with large volumes of cold blood or other fluids may lead to proportionately greater loss of body heat, as may prolonged exposure during emergency management; the problems are legion.

Minor Neck Injuries

The most common neck injuries seen in children are minor soft tissue injuries resulting from a force of relatively large mass and low velocity (Gregory, 1966). As the velocity of the applied force increases, the severity of resultant injury increases as a function of its square, as does the possibility of occult injury to underlying structures. Secondary missiles may be produced by disrupted soft tissue and bone, and the resultant "cone of injury" is increased.

Gunshot wounds at close range may produce their effects by blast injury as well as by missile injury.

Major Neck Injuries

Major neck injuries in the pediatric age range are most common in the aerodigestive system (pharynx, esophagus, larynx, and trachea) and are discussed elsewhere (Chaps. 52 to 54 and 67). Other serious injuries are less common and include those of the major blood vessels, spine, spinal cord, and peripheral nerves that pass through the neck. Significant injuries of the endocrine glands of the neck or thoracic duct are extremely rare.

In addition to their anatomic and etiologic classification, injuries of the neck may be categorized clinically into one of four types according to the immediacy of the treatment requirements (Jones, 1966):

1. Those injuries that interfere with vital physiologic function: airway injuries, hemorrhage, and shock;
2. Those injuries that are severe but not immediately life-threatening;
3. Those injuries whose severity is occult, requiring additional evaluation or observation to determine the correct therapy; and
4. Those injuries that are minor and superficial in character.

Early diagnostic and treatment efforts must avoid converting a lesser injury to one of greater severity.

Anatomic Differences Between Children and Adults

In addition to the general factors mentioned previously, several anatomic differences between pediatric and adult head and neck structures should be kept in mind, as they contribute to a different spectrum of injuries in children.

1. The child's larynx is located much higher in the neck, largely beneath the protection of the mandible, and is less frequently injured. Descent of this structure occurs gradually and is complete by early adulthood.
2. The child's head is proportionately larger, relative to the rest of the body, than the adult's. The supporting neck structures are therefore more susceptible to sudden acceleration or deceleration injuries due to "whipping" of the unrestrained head. These structures, however, have more elasticity, allowing greater compensation without serious injury.
3. The child's total weight is less, meaning that a lesser force will be applied to the neck, or body, in deceleration or acceleration injuries (as in automobile accidents) with more rapid dissipation of the force.
4. The younger child's bones contain a greater percentage of cartilage, allowing proportionately more give, resulting in less breaking of the bones. Fractures are therefore less frequent than in the adult.
5. The types of risks to which the child is exposed are different. For example,

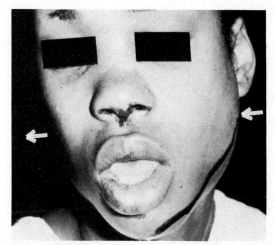

Figure 80–1 16 year old girl shot with .22 caliber bullet. Arrows show entrance (left neck) and exit (right neck) wounds. Complications, including hematomas of the neck and oropharynx, odontoid fracture, left internal carotid artery occlusion with cerebral infarct, and epistaxis, demonstrate multisystem involvement of serious neck injuries.

blunt trauma is responsible for 80 to 90 per cent of serious external cervical injuries in children as compared to the adult in whom penetrating injuries are more common (Haller and Talbert, 1973)

Multisystem Involvement

Figures 80–1 and 80–2 illustrate the multiplicity of systems that may be involved in severe neck trauma and the necessity of being aware of other possible injuries.

INITIAL DIAGNOSTIC APPROACH

The general approach to a child with major trauma and neck injury should include rapidly obtaining a history sufficient to determine

Figure 80–2 "Open-mouth" radiograph shows nondisplaced odontoid fracture (double arrows) and retained bullet fragment (single arrow on left).

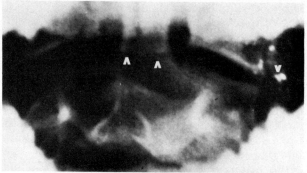

(as certainly as possible) the degree and type of injury and any serious coexistent medical problems, followed by sequential emergency management, including the following measures:

1. Rapid, thorough evaluation of the extent of injury;
2. Immediate treatment of life-threatening conditions (resuscitation);
   a. Airway control with intubation or tracheotomy and ventilation
   b. Control of hemorrhage
   c. Cardiac resuscitation
   d. Treatment of shock
3. Measurement of vital signs;
4. Immobilization of the head and neck for evident or suspected cervical injuries;
5. Indwelling urethral catheter.

In completing a thorough preliminary physical examination, specific evaluation relative to injuries of the neck should include the following.

Soft Tissue Injuries. The nature of the injury (laceration of skin, depth of penetration, velocity of injuring force, contamination, subcutaneous emphysema, hematoma formation or swelling, or devitalized or missing tissue) should be documented. High-velocity missile injuries are often accompanied by a surrounding "cone" of tissue injury that may not be immediately apparent.

Upper Aerodigestive Injuries. These are usually accompanied by cervical subcutaneous emphysema, hemoptysis, and dysphagia or hoarseness but may remain undiagnosed in the presence of other serious injuries. They are covered in detail in Chapters 52–54 and 67.

Neurologic Injuries. Flaccidity or rigidity of all extremities, deep and superficial reflexes, and response to pinprick or noxious stimuli should be checked. The injury may produce a paresis (partial loss of function) or paralysis (complete loss of sensorimotor function) of the involved part. The initial neurologic deficit should be documented carefully in order to monitor progression.

Vascular Injuries. In addition to inspection and palpation of the major vessels of the neck (arterial as well as venous), pulsation in the peripheral branches (superficial temporal, facial and ophthalmic by ophthalmoscopy) should be checked. Peripheral pulses should be followed closely, when occult injury to the major arteries is suspected, if neck

exploration is not elected immediately. Doppler monitoring may be helpful in these cases.

Osseous Injuries. The initial examination should be kept to a minimum, attempting only to elicit point tenderness with the child's neck stabilized, until a complete neurologic examination and radiologic evaluation of the cervical vertebrae can be performed. The child's neck should not be manipulated unless absolutely necessary until the evaluation is complete in order to avoid iatrogenic injury to the spinal cord. These precautions are especially important (and occasionally overlooked) when the neck injury is complicated by an acute airway problem.

Glandular Injuries. Endocrine abnormalities as the result of tissues loss or shock may become apparent as a late manifestation of the acute cervical injury but are quite uncommon.

Adjacent Areas. Low-velocity missiles (such as pistol bullets and flying glass) may be deflected by deep neck structures and may end up in the head or chest. Injury to these adjacent areas must be considered in all penetrating wounds of the neck.

Notification and a progress report to the child's parents or other next of kin should be done as soon as possible following the injury and at appropriate intervals during its acute management.

SPECIFIC CERVICAL INJURIES

Upper Aerodigestive Injuries

Injuries of the upper aerodigestive tract (larynx, trachea, pharynx, and esophagus) are discussed in Chapters 52–54 and 67.

Soft Tissue Injuries

The terminology regarding soft tissue injuries is not always clear, so a brief review is appropriate.

An *abrasion* is a superficial wound produced by friction (large mass, low-velocity injury dissipating energy tangentially). A *contusion* is a deeper injury with tissue damage (primarily vascular) without surface disruption. A *laceration* is a tissue disruption. Consideration should be given to penetration of underlying structures in evaluating the consequences of a laceration. A *puncture wound* may extend to some depth with minimal surrounding tissue damage, whereas *gunshot wounds* with a similar entrance laceration may produce their effects at some distance owing to the surrounding cone of injury, the production of secondary missiles of bone or missile fragments, or by ricochet.

In the management of lacerations or abrasions of the neck, the child's current tetanus immunization status should be obtained. Depending on previous immunization status, age, and type and extent of injury, tetanus prophylaxis can then be undertaken (Fulginiti, 1976).

1. Tetanus immunization should be recommended in the unimmunized individual (three doses of 0.5 ml adjuvent tetanus toxoid each).
2. Tetanus prophylaxis is unnecessary in the immunized child with a clean laceration.
3. Tetanus toxoid (0.5 ml intramuscularly) is recommended for the immunized child with a lesser injury to the aerodigestive system if a booster has not been given in five years. Immunoglobulin is not necessary except in the unimmunized individual, who should be fully immunized as soon as possible.
4. In severe injuries involving gross extensive contamination or massive devitalization of tissue, a booster should be given along with 250 to 500 units of human tetanus immunoglobulin (Hyper-tet). .

Deeper *abrasions* should be scrubbed under local or general anesthesia to remove all foreign material. Foreign bodies such as wood should be meticulously searched for and removed. Greases can be removed more easily if a mild detergent is added. Organic iodine solutions such as povidone-iodine will not cause additional tissue injury and are excellent cleaning solutions. The aqueous solutions of 0.5 to 1.0 per cent are suitable and less irritating than the tincture (Harvey, 1975). Hydrogen peroxide is irritating and is not recommended.

Lacerations should be cleaned of clots and foreign materials, scrubbed with aqueous iodine-iodide solution, and irrigated carefully. Local anesthesia (1 per cent xylocaine with 1:100,000 epinephrine) is recommended, but general anesthesia may be required for more extensive lacerations.

Once the laceration has been cleansed, devitalized tissue should be conservatively debrided with a scissors or sharp scalpel back to clean, bleeding tissue. The wound edges should be at right angles, and the closure should be planned to lie in natural skin lines wherever possible.

The depths of the laceration should be reevaluated prior to closure for injury to the underlying major structures. Once this has been accomplished, the deeper tissues should be approximated with absorbable sutures in layers. The skin is next closed with evenly placed, nonabsorbable, monofilament sutures. Smaller lacerations can often be closed with a running subcuticular suture, which can be removed more easily in the small child. In either case, the skin edges should be reapproximated accurately with slight eversion. Interrupted sutures can be removed from the neck after 4 to 5 days with tape reinforcement for another 3 to 4 days.

Primary closure of cervical lacerations can be accomplished as long as 12 to 18 hours following injury because of the excellent blood supply of the neck. Beyond that time, or in grossly contaminated wounds, closure should be delayed for 72 hours. The laceration can then be sutured loosely or closed with adhesive strips if clean. Subsequent scar revision will probably be required.

Neck scars, in general, may widen slightly in children owing to their increased tissue elasticity, and the parents should be forewarned of this.

Animal bites and human bites may be closed following copious irrigation and cleansing. Tetanus prophylaxis is usually indicated. Animal bites should be reported, and the animal should be observed for rabies. Antirabies serum should be given immediately when there is any suspicion of the disease in the animal, and vaccine should be started at the first sign of rabies in the biting animal (Jones, 1966).

Neurologic Injuries

Pediatric cervical neurologic injuries can be divided into those of the peripheral nerves and those of the central nervous system (cervical spinal cord).

Peripheral nerve injuries are usually caused by penetrating or lacerating trauma. Injuries to the cervical vertebrae or the skull may result in paresis or paralysis, which may be permanent (as in those due to crushing or laceration) or temporary (concussive).

A useful description of the types of peripheral nerve injuries was given by Seddon: *neurapraxia* describes an intact nerve with physiologic block (complete recovery expected); *axonotmesis* implies division of an axon only with intact supporting structures (partial spontaneous recovery); *neurotmesis* characterizes division of both neural and supporting elements (division of the entire nerve) (Seddon, 1954).

Peripheral nerve function, including the brachial and cervical plexuses, phrenic nerve (proximal branch of the cervical plexus), and regional cranial nerves (nine, ten, eleven, and twelve), is first checked systematically.

Cranial nerve injuries are often overlooked and may offer important information as to the nature and location of deeper injuries. They may be checked quickly as follows: glossopharyngeal (nine), soft palate rises in the midline with an intact gag reflex; vagus (ten), intact vocal cord function without hoarseness; spinal accessory (eleven), intact trapezius, sternocleidomastoid muscle function; and hypoglossal (twelve), intact tongue motion without fasciculation.

Injuries to the cervical plexus, formed by the ventral primary divisions of the upper four cervical nerves, may produce sensory or motor deficits. The sensory deficits may occur over the posterior scalp (lesser occipital branch), auricle (greater auricular branch), or anterior neck and chest (cervical cutaneous and supraclavicular branches). Deep muscular branch deficits may be more obvious (phrenic branches) or less obvious depending upon the extent of total involvement.

In clean, open injuries, severed or lacerated nerves should be debrided and repaired primarily (neurorrhaphy) using interrupted, fine, unreactive sutures to reapproximate the perineurium meticulously (Onné, 1962). Microsurgical techniques have provided a useful adjunct to this type of repair and are advocated (Smith, 1964).

Secondary repair may be necessary when the injury is extensively contaminated or seen after a delay. In this case, the nerve end should be tagged at the time of initial exploration, and the repair should be accomplished with meticulous reapproximation of the perineurium or by graft 21 days later (Clark and Grossman, 1966).

"Banding" the anastomotic site with nonabsorbable materials (for instance, polyethylene tubing) to prevent fibrous ingrowth and disruption and to decrease the inflammatory reaction is advocated by some, but further experimental evaluation is necessary before the technique can be accepted as routine (Kline, 1964).

Where there is an extensive area of dehiscence, especially in a motor nerve, an expendable regional sensory nerve, such as the greater auricular nerve, may be interposed as an autograft to facilitate the anastomosis without tension.

The differential diagnosis between division of the peripheral nerve and "concussion" (physiologic block or neurapraxia) is usually made at the time of exploration when there is a coexisting laceration. In blunt injuries electromyographic testing is helpful, but the results are positive only after a delay of two weeks or more when denervation potentials are seen. Changes of denervation can be seen within 48 hours with galvanic nerve excitability testing.

Expectant observation of a peripheral nerve injury is indicated if the skin is intact unless there is progression of the injury or delayed recovery (Clark and Grossman, 1966).

The treatment of brachial plexus injuries is also expectant except when there is progression of the injury or if the insulting injury was to the middle third of the clavicle where direct bony impingement on the nerve may be expected and should be relieved. Otherwise, little benefit can be expected from neurolysis or exploration (Clark and Grossman, 1966).

Partial division of a nerve should be repaired *without* interrupting the intact segment by freshening the divided bundle ends and carefully reapproximating the perineurium with fine, interrupted sutures (Clark and Grossman, 1966). The incidence of neuroma and causalgia is increased relative to repair of a completely divided nerve, but the functional result is improved by not interrupting intact nerve fibers (Hoopes and Jabaley, 1973).

Cervical spinal cord injuries in children are fortunately uncommon. They may occur as the result of direct penetration (less common) or by indirect violent displacement. Displacement injuries may cause injury either through dislocation or by transient cord compression.

Direct injury of the spinal cord may result in partial or complete transection. Complete transection of the cord is more likely by this mechanism than by closed injury (Black, 1973). The extent of the injury is proportional to the velocity of the missile producing the injury and the angle at which the force is delivered to the cord.

Bullets or other high-velocity missiles may cause injury to the spinal cord by striking it directly, with resultant concussion or laceration of the cord; secondarily, by producing missiles composed of splintered fragments of vertebra or other bone; or indirectly through the concussive effects of the cylinder of transmitted energy.

Stab wounds, being of lower velocity, tend to injure only the directly penetrated cord substance, although there may be adjacent areas of contusion, edema, or hematoma formation with resultant deficits. The most common injury is a hemisection of the cord with a resultant Brown-Séquard syndrome (distal ipsilateral hemiplegia and hyperesthesia with contralateral hemianesthesia), but complete transection of the cord may occur. Secondary injury to the cord due to compression by fragments of dislodged lamina or vertebral body is less common.

Closed injuries to the spinal cord are of two types; those accompanied by bony injury or dislocation and those resulting from violent vertebral column displacements without obvious fracture or displacement.

Injuries accompanied by bony fractures are the most common (Clark and Grossman, 1966). Injury may occur to the vertebral body, lamina, or pedicle, resulting in bony fragments being driven into or across the cord. Soft tissue injuries to the intervertebral disc or connecting ligaments, sometimes accompanied by avulsion injuries of the vertebrae, are less common.

In either case, plain radiologic studies may be unrevealing, as fracture fragments may be too small to be seen, or compression of the cord may be by the nonradiopaque parts of the vertebral column (Clark and Grossman, 1966).

Violent, sudden, extreme extension of the cervical spine does not usually result in dislocation owing to the strength of the ligamentous attachments. The dorsal cord and its dorsal cervical division, however, may be injured owing to compression by the ligamentum flavum and the edges of the laminae and pedicles. The characteristic neurologic picture of this problem includes a motor loss that is more severe in the upper than in the lower extremities (acute central cervical cord injury) (Schneider, 1962).

Severe flexion of the cervical spine, on the other hand, tends to produce more severe injury of the ventral columns. Dislocation with anterior displacement of the superior vertebral body on the inferior is more common than the reverse. Injury to the cord, then, occurs by compression of the cord between the posterior (superior) lamina and anterior (inferior) intervertebral body. Posterior herniation of the intervertebral disc may also occur (Clark and Grossman, 1966).

Rotatory injuries are uncommon. They result from marked lateral displacement of the cervical spinal columns or rotatory acceleration of the head or body relative to the other. Injury of the cord usually results from direct shearing or tearing. Herniation of the disc into the vertebral foramina or externally to compress nerve roots or allow compression of the entire cord is uncommon.

Combined craniospinal injuries occasionally occur, with the cervical spine serving as a fulcrum for the relatively heavy head. When due to direct impact on the vertex of the head, as in falls or football injuries, these are usually fatal (Davis et al., 1971).

Regardless of the mechanism of injury, the cervical spinal cord undergoes the same general types of pathologic change as does the brain in response to direct or indirect trauma (Clark and Grossman, 1966). Laceration, contusion, hematomas, edema, or concussion may result.

The *signs and symptoms of cervical spinal cord injuries* may be complex in the case of partial cord involvement or may result in profound physiologic change if transection occurs.

The cord serves as the main neural connection between the brain and body, so complete interruption results in complete distal sensory and motor loss. Autonomic dysfunction also occurs with loss of bowel and bladder control, sweating, and vasomotor tone. Males may also exhibit priapism.

The motor loss is usually obvious, with paralysis of all muscles below the level of injury. In high cervical injuries, paralysis of the intercostal muscles results in poor respiratory and cough reflex. The fourth cervical vertebra is of major importance here, with a 50 per cent mortality rate in the first 30 days with injuries at or above this level, as compared to 19 per cent for injuries below this level (Clark and Grossman, 1966).

The autonomic loss may be more subtle. Urinary retention with bladder distension occurs. More serious is the loss of vasomotor tone with resultant vasodilatation and blood pressure reduction, termed *neurogenic shock.* Orthostatic hypotension may compound the problem and hyperpyrexia may also result, owing to the loss of sweating, if the patient remains exposed to an unusually warm environment; similarly, hypopyrexia may result if cold exposure continues, owing to the heat loss from peripheral vasodilatation. Peripheral to the injury, the patient is warm and dry to the touch, with vasodilatation.

Sensory loss can be verified by testing the response to light touch, temperature sensation, and pain. Deep tendon reflexes are initially absent ipsilaterally (flaccid paralysis, or *spinal shock*) but later are hyperactive (spastic paralysis) owing to loss of modulating inhibitions from higher centers.

The emergency treatment of a child with a *suspected* cervical spinal injury should include immobilization on a flat, firm stretcher without moving the spine. Sedation may be necessary to get the child to cooperate but should be delayed as long as possible in order not to mask coexistent injuries.

Movement prior to definitive evaluation should be done only while stabilizing the neck, preferably with traction along the spinal axis.

Physical examination should include evaluation of the strength and motion of all four extremities. Cervical injury levels can be evaluated by asking the child to flex the elbows (biceps, fifth cervical), extend the elbows (triceps, seventh cervical), and squeeze the examiner's fingers (finger flexors, eighth cervical). Injuries above the fifth cervical vertebra produce major intercostal denervation with paradoxic movement of the chest and abdomen.

The biceps, triceps, and radial reflexes are tested to evaluate motor loss further. Distal reflexes may also be recorded to further document the extent of cord injury, including the plantar reflex (Babinski), which is usually flexor in the acute phase.

Sensory integrity can be evaluated rapidly using cotton and a safety pin. By comparing "sharp" and "dull" using the pin and light touch using the cotton, levels of sensory loss can be determined. These should be sketched on the patient with a pen or other marker, as well as recorded in the chart with the time of examination.

Catheterization and nasogastric drainage may be required but are usually deferred until the definitive evaluation, including radiographs, has been completed.

Evaluation for other injuries is completed prior to radiographic evaluation in order to get complete radiographic information at the time of initial study, as well as to determine the need for treatment of more acute injuries (as in airway obstruction which requires tracheotomy).

Once the initial physical evaluation has been completed, radiographs of the appropriate spinal segments should be obtained. Two points are important: (1) the spinal cord level does *not* correspond to the vertebral body level, and (2) radiographs even tomograms, may *not* show certain linear vertebral fractures with underlying injury. Lateral films are obtained prior to the cervical spine series in order to check for imminent cord transection.

Movement of the child onto and on the radiograph table should be done with care in order to avoid iatrogenic extension of the cord injury.

Anteroposterior and lateral views are ordinarily required to evaluate the cervical spine, with tomography or contrast studies to visualize more subtle or spinal canal injuries.

Neurologic or neurosurgical consultation is indicated early in the case of cord or major neurologic (brachial plexus) injury. Evaluation and treatment can then be coordinated, with the service responsible for treating the major injury assuming primary care.

Spinal cord injury, like any severe stress, may trigger a poorly understood neurohumoral mechanism that results in gastric ulceration, followed by hemorrhage or perforation. Prevention of stress ulceration includes the use of antacids during the initial phase with careful monitoring of vital signs and stool guaiacs (Clark, 1971).

Animal investigations suggest that there is some slight benefit to be gained from the intramuscular administration of corticosteroids for one to two weeks following spinal cord injury. Additional research in this area is indicated (Black and Markowitz, 1971).

When a child presents in the emergency room with major trauma and a suspected cervical spinal cord injury, the following sequence of attention to the injuries is suggested:

1. Vital signs, resuscitation, sandbags to stabilize neck;
2. Rapid evaluation of the problem, including search for associated injuries;
3. Head-halter traction for evident or suspected cervical injuries;
4. Consideration for intravenous cortico-

steroids with subsequent maintenance by an intramuscular route for one to two weeks; antacids and possibly an anticholinergic agent to protect the gastric mucosa against stress ulceration;

5. Request for specialty consultations as indicated;
6. Indwelling urethral catheter;
7. Detailed clinical evaluation;
8. Radiographic evaluation;
9. Skeletal traction for cervical injuries;
10. Lumbar puncture to test for spinal block (Queckenstedt test);
11. Decision as to further management (decompressive laminectomy, for example);
12. Supportive care in respiratory function, nutrition, skin, bladder function, gastrointestinal function, and rehabilitation (Black, 1973).

Definitive operative treatment of cord injuries is not ordinarily delegated to the otolaryngologist or pediatrician and is hence beyond the scope of this chapter. Reduction of cervical dislocation, laminectomy, and cord decompression, or extensive rehabilitative measures may be required. Decompression is warranted when there is (1) progression of the neurologic deficit, (2) manometric (Queckenstedt) or myelographic block, or (3) radiographic evidence of bone fragments (or disc, with contrast studies) projecting into the spinal canal (Black, 1973). For additional discussion of these modalities, the reader is referred to standard orthopedic, neurosurgical, or physical medicine texts.

Osseous (Cervical Vertebral) Injuries

Fractures or dislocations of the cervical spine are rare in children except in cases of extreme violence (Blount, 1955). In fact, Tachdjian (1972) states that "small children (less than eight years old) may be tied in knots without fracturing the cervical spine." Compared to similar injuries in adults, cervical spine injuries in children are less likely to cause cord transection and are less likely to result from whiplash injury. They occur more frequently as the result of diving accidents or football injuries. Radiographic evaluation is somewhat more difficult because of the presence of apophyses, asymmetrical growth centers, or points of fusion and congenital anomalies. Comparison of the radiographs to age-related standards is recommended (Rogers, 1942). The treatment is generally the same as in the adult except for somewhat accelerated healing.

The neurologic evaluation (see previous section) and examination for point tenderness often provide an indication of the site of injury, if other signs of external trauma are absent.

Prevention of extension of neurologic (spinal cord or peripheral nerve) injury and repair of the existing injury, if possible, are the goals of management of the vertebral injury. *Spinal cord injury must be assumed until there is definite proof that none has occurred.* Concomitant injury to the cord may be expected in 25 per cent of cases of severe injury to the cervical spine. Irrevocable cord damage and death may occur by careless handling of the child with cervical vertebral injury and resultant instability. The greatest permanent injury caused by injury to the cervical spine is due to the associated injury to the spinal cord.

The main objectives of the physical examination of the cervical vertebrae are observation for evidence of external trauma (points of missile penetration, for instance), neurologic evaluation (see previous section), and careful palpation of the spine for areas of point tenderness.

If a cord injury or vertebral injury is suspected, the child should be immobilized in the supine (horizontal) position and the head stabilized with sandbags.

Anteroposterior and lateral radiographic views of the entire cervical spine with special attention to areas of suspected injury are indicated. Oblique views requiring rotation of the neck are contraindicated until anteroposterior and lateral films have ruled out gross fracture or dislocation. Certain areas are notoriously difficult to visualize, such as the first and seventh cervical vertebrae. Tomography may be required as well as contrast studies (myelography) where internal compromise of the cord by soft tissue (intervertebral disc) is suspected.

Cervical sprains, dislocations, or fracture–dislocation combinations may be identified and require early orthopedic or neurosurgical consultation. Temporary skin traction is indicated until proper positioning can be secured with skeletal traction, bracing, or both. Open reduction and arthrodesis may be required if closed reduction and stabilization are unsuccessful.

A brief discussion of specific types of injuries follows.

Peripheral nerve root injuries may be expected in 25 per cent of severe injuries to the cervical spine, and are usually due to fracture or dislocation of the vertebral body or posterior displacement of the intervertebral disc. Initially, traction is indicated with possible subsequent exploration.

Compression fracture of the cervical vertebral body without dislocation is apparent as a wedge-shaped deformity of the vertebral body. The injury usually occurs with a direct blow on the head and is rarely unstable. Stabilization with a cervical collar is indicated to decrease pain. The same fracture *with dislocation* requires skeletal traction until the dislocation has been reduced and stability has been achieved.

Anterior dislocation of the cervical spine is likely to be associated with cord injury, if complete. *Subluxation* (incomplete dislocation with articular facets in partial contact) may remain following spontaneous reduction of a complete dislocation, or it may be present as the only injury. Both usually require skeletal traction, with open reduction reserved for those cases that will not reduce or stabilize.

Complete unilateral dislocation of the cervical spine may occur with severe torsional forces and may require open reduction if traction is unsuccessful (Fig. 80–3). Unilateral subluxation is more common in children and may occur spontaneously during sleep. It usually responds to traction followed by neck collar stabilization. Subluxation may be extremely difficult to see on radiographs, but persistent pain and spasm relieved by traction is highly suggestive of the diagnosis.

Posterior dislocation of the cervical spine is fortunately rare and is usually accompanied by major spinal cord damage.

Comminuted fractures usually occur as the result of a heavy blow to the top of the head, which delivers disc pressure from above and below to the vertebral body, causing comminution. Severe injury to the cord often results from posteriorly displaced body fragments. Traction followed by immobilization is usually indicated with open exploration in cases of concomitant neurologic injury. Involvement of the atlas (first cervical vertebra) and axis (second cervical vertebra) includes the unusual *spontaneous atlantoaxial dislocation* secondary to an upper respiratory tract infection in children and *fracture dislocations* (Berkheiser and Seidler, 1931). The former usually requires traction followed by brace immobilization. In the latter, the most common type of fracture is of the odontoid process of the axis

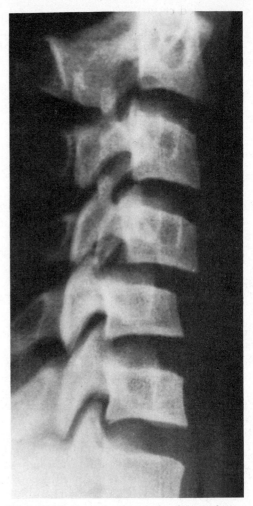

Figure 80–3 Lateral radiographs of cervical spine of 14 year old injured in trampoline accident. Unilateral fracture and dislocation of cervical fourth and fifth vertebrae are seen. Quadriplegia developed with greater involvement of lower extremities (acute central cervical cord injury).

with anterior dislocation of the atlas on the axis, as might occur when the child dives into shallow water or is thrown out of an automobile and lands on his or her head (Figs. 80–4 and 80–5) (Tachdjian, 1972). Traction followed by immobilization is usually sufficient, but open fixation may be necessary, especially if the nerve supply is compromised.

Cervical sprain is usually accompanied by a dull aching pain in the back of the neck, which may be diffuse or discrete. Radiographic findings are, of course, negative, and the treatment is limited to cervical collar immobilization, heat, and analgesics.

It is fortunate that the upper cervical spinal canal has considerable space in excess of that

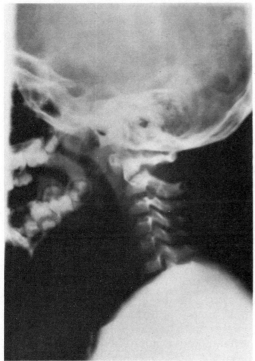

Figure 80–4 Lateral cervical spine radiographs of 5 year old boy injured in diving accident show fracture of odontoid process with slight displacement. Neurologic findings were absent.

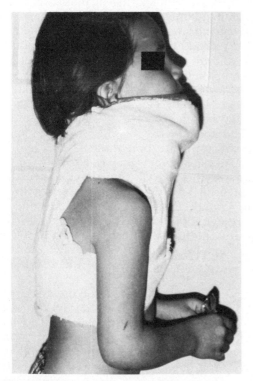

Figure 80–5 Minerva cast applied to patient provides excellent cervical stabilization.

needed by the cord so that a fracture or a dislocation may have fairly marked displacement without more serious neurologic sequelae. Less fortunate, however, is the fact that this may obscure the diagnosis of severe vertebral instability, especially in the comatose patient, and thus lead to a delayed cord injury.

The preceding statements refer to the more common closed vertebral injuries. Open injuries usually require open debridement and exploration. For additional detailed management, the reader is referred to the references listed at the end of the chapter or to other standard neurosurgical or orthopedic texts.

Vascular Injuries

Obvious injuries to major cervical vessels dictate open exploration as soon as possible. When the injury is suspected but not immediately confirmed, or when the site of injury remains obscure, arteriography is indicated (May et al., 1975).

Acute management includes direct pressure to control bleeding, establishment of a large-bore intravenous line, and replacement of lost blood. Vital signs should be monitored closely and blood must be drawn for type and cross-match, initial hematocrit, and appropriate chemistries. The wound should *not* be probed in the emergency room.

Once the child has been stabilized and evaluated, open exploration with control of the bleeding is indicated. The tract of injury is followed to its depth with a systematic examination of each structure in or adjacent to the tract. The bleeding site is identified, and vascular control is secured proximally and distally by passing umbilical tapes around the vessel. Clots are evacuated next, and the wound is thoroughly cleansed and evaluated. The cut vessel edges are freshened, and vascular repair or ligation is accomplished.

Injuries to the internal and common carotid, subclavian, and innominate arteries should be repaired if at all possible. Although it has been stated that the mortality and morbidity rates due to carotid (common or internal) ligation are low in younger patients, the opposite has also been said to be true. In addition, of course, statistics apply only to large groups of patients and cannot be used in an individual case.

Arteriorrhaphy of the common or internal

carotid artery may be accomplished relatively easily using interrupted 4-0 Tevdec sutures in the cleanly penetrating, sharp-missile wound of the neck (for instance that made by a knife) but gets progressively more difficult with more contamination or tissue loss.

Where compromise of the vessel lumen is a potential problem with simple closure, a patch graft of autogenous vessel or synthetic material may be required. More extensive injuries may require a graft, again of autogenous vessel or synthetic material. Autograft vein interposition (using the internal jugular, for instance) is superior to synthetic grafting in contaminated wounds (Rutherford, 1973).

Specific problems include the following. (1) An internal or external shunt (Javid) may be required during carotid arteriorrhaphy, although partial occlusion with a curved vascular (Satinsky) clamp may be possible. (2) Operative manipulation in the region of the bifurcation should be preceded by infiltration of the bulb with 1 per cent lidocaine to avoid reflex hypotension due to stimulation of the carotid pressor receptors. If this occurs inadvertently, atropine can reverse the effects of such stimuli. (3) Injury to the vertebral artery can be controlled only with great difficulty. Arteriorrhaphy is usually impossible (and unnecessary owing to extensive collateral flow), and control can be established only by pressure, bone wax, and suture ligation. (4) Control of subclavian or innominate hemorrhage may be established with difficulty and may require resection of the medial third or entire clavicle, head of the sternocleidomastoid muscle, or splitting the superior sternum (manubrium). The sternal incision may be carried laterally into the third intercostal space to avoid opening the full mediastinum unnecessarily and may be closed with stainless steel wire. (5) Lacerated major veins of the neck, aside from the effects of hemorrhage, introduce the risk of air embolism. Prompt pressure (either in the emergency room or subsequently in the operating room) and putting the patient in a slight reverse Trendelenburg position should prevent the occurrence of air embolism. (6) The internal jugular vein may be repaired if it has been ligated unilaterally without sequelae. Other venous bleeders are ligated with silk.

Glandular Injuries

The *thyroid gland* is a richly vascular structure, and compromise of its endocrine status due to trauma is extremely uncommon. When there has been major tissue loss in this region, however, signs of hypothyroidism should be sought by history (symptoms such as tiredness, constipation, or dull hair), as well as through appropriate blood studies.

When injury of the gland is seen at the time of neck exploration, devitalized tissue should be debrided and hemostasis secured. The recurrent nerves should be evaluated as carefully as possible, as should the parathyroid glands. Traumatic loss of the entire thyroid would undoubtedly result in major vascular (carotid) and airway (trachea) injury, and survival in the acute stage would be unlikely.

Simultaneous injury to all *parathyroid glands* would be most uncommon owing to their separate distribution in the neck. A substernal position of these glands is not uncommon, and total loss would undoubtedly lead to major vascular and airway injury with probable immediate death of the child. If a parathyroid gland is identified in a devitalized area of the neck, it should be reimplanted in an adjacent muscle.

Salivary gland injuries should be handled by debridement, control of bleeding, and drainage of the wound. The *submandibular gland* can be removed, sparing, if intact, the marginal mandibular branch of the facial and the lingual and hypoglossal nerves. Treatment of *parotid gland* injuries is not a consideration of cervical injuries except where the tail of the parotid extends into the neck. Here the preceding principles of debridement of devitalized tissue, hemostasis, and drainage should be followed.

Thoracic Duct. Wounds in the left lower neck near the junction of the internal jugular and subclavian veins may cause injury to the thoracic duct as well. Injury to this structure is identified by pooling of lymph (chyle) in the wound. Simple ligation of the duct is sufficient, but this may be difficult as the identification of the duct may be a problem. Additionally, it may enter the vein as several tributaries, each of which must be identified, if injured, and ligated.

Injury on the right side of the neck may also injure a thoracic duct that uncommonly occurs on that side. Identification and ligation of the duct are again the treatments of choice.

Closure. All neck wounds should be drained if the pharynx, esophagus, or trachea was injured or if there was significant devitalization of tissue. The laceration should be closed in layers, reapproximating divided muscles. Where there is extensive surface tissue loss, appropriate flaps can be rotated in for closure. A sliding local flap (cervical or chest) is usually sufficient with split thickness (0.015 inch) skin closure of the donor site if necessary (this is uncommon).

Antibiotics are given when there has been extensive devitalization, contamination, or entry into the aerodigestive system. Tetanus immunization is carried out according to the previous indications and schedule.

Complications. Late complications include infection, fistula (salivary or digestive), vascular occlusion, or bleeding, as well as other specific problems related to the structure indicated. These are uncommon if emergency treatment and diagnostic evaluation have been meticulous and if care is given according to the preceding principles.

PENETRATING WOUNDS OF THE NECK

Penetrating wounds of the neck may be caused by gunshot, knife, or impalement with a variety of objects during play or vehicular trauma. Penetrating wounds frequently cause injuries to vascular, nervous, visceral, and bony structures of the neck, as described in the preceding section on specific cervical injuries. Vascular injuries are the most common cause of death following penetrating wounds of the neck. Reported mortality rates vary from 3 per cent (May et al., 1975) to 40 per cent (Shirkey, 1963).

Although traditionally all penetrating neck wounds were explored surgically (Fogelman and Stewart, 1956; Patman et al., 1964), recent experience has shown that selective surgical exploration is equally effective in dealing with major complications while eliminating unnecessary surgery. Indications for immediate exploration include evidence of active bleeding (epistaxis, hemoptysis, expanding hematoma) and vascular occlusion (loss of pulse, progressive central nervous system deficit).

Other patients may undergo further diagnostic evaluation to determine the need for exploration when stable. Injury of certain neurologic structures is often associated with occult but significant injury of juxtaposed vascular structures: the hypoglossal nerve affects the facial artery and vein; the Horner syndrome affects the carotid artery; and the glossopharyngeal, vagus, and accessory nerves affect the jugular vein and the internal carotid artery. Arteriography is indicated with such neurologic deficits. Arteriography is also undertaken if vascular injury is strongly suspected but not apparent on examination (as with bruit, aneurysm, or location of the wound near a major vessel).

A dye-contrast pharyngoesophagogram and endoscopy are performed if aerodigestive tract involvement is suspected (as with accompanying crepitus, dyspnea, stridor, or dysodynophagia). The decision to explore or not to explore is then made on the basis of the diagnostic studies and the condition of the patient.

Practically speaking, penetrating wounds of the upper and lower thirds of the neck are more difficult to explore and statistically less dangerous than those of the middle third. Most deaths from penetrating wounds are in the middle third of the neck.

Vascular injuries are ideally treated by primary repair. Experience has shown, however, that the external carotid artery and internal jugular veins may be ligated and divided without significant morbidity. The patency of the internal and common carotid arteries, however, must be preserved. Up to 1.5 cm of damaged carotid artery may be resected with subsequent primary anastomosis. For larger defects, vein interpositions are superior to Dacron or other allografts.

Lacerations of the hypopharynx or esophagus should be closed and drained externally. When they are eight hours old, drainage alone must suffice owing to necrosis of tissue.

SELECTED REFERENCES

Matson, D. D. 1969. Neurosurgery of Infancy and Childhood. 2nd ed. Springfield, IL, Charles C Thomas Pub.

An older text that was completely revised from the original monograph. It considers in greater detail management peculiar to infancy and childhood. Succinctly written, it is a good reference for common problems.

May, M., Chadaratana, P., West, J. W., et al. 1975. Penetrating neck wounds: selective exploration. Laryngoscope, 85:57.

This article reviews 223 penetrating neck wounds to justify selective exploration. It contains an excellent discussion of indications for exploration with a 3 per cent mortality rate, as well as a thorough review of the literature.

Rang, M. 1974. Children's Fractures. Philadelphia, J. B. Lippincott Co.

An excellent review of pediatric fractures with a recent listing of pertinent references.

Zuidema, G. D., Rutherford, R. B., and Ballinger, W. F. 1979. The Management of Trauma, 3rd ed. Philadelphia, W. B. Saunders Co.

This recent review of entire spectrum of trauma contains specific review of pediatric trauma (see Haller and Talbert, 1973). Good review of general management with consideration of potential associated injuries.

REFERENCES

Ballinger, W. F., Rutherford, R. B., and Zuidema, G. D. 1973. *The Management of Trauma*, 2nd ed. Philadelphia, W. B. Saunders Co.

Berkheiser E. J., and Seidler, F. 1931. Nontraumatic dislocations of the atlantoaxial joint. J.A.M.A., *96*:517.

Black P., and Markowitz, R. S. 1971. Experimental spinal cord injury in monkeys: Comparison of steroids and local hypothermia. Surg. Forum, *22*:409.

Black, P. 1973. Injuries of the vertebral column and spinal cord: Mechanisms and management in the acute phase. *In* Zuidema, G. D., Rutherford, R. B., and Ballinger, W. F. (Eds.). The Management of Trauma. 2nd ed. Philadelphia, W. B. Saunders Co.

Blount, W. P. 1955. Fractures in Children. Baltimore, Williams & Wilkins Co., p. 207.

Clark, K., and Grossman, R. G. 1966. Trauma to the nervous system. *In* Shires, G. T. (Ed.) 1966. Care of the Trauma Patient. New York, McGraw-Hill.

Clark, W. K. 1971. Stress ulceration. Clin. Neurosurg., *18*:426.

Davis, D., Bohlman, H., Walker, A. E., et al. 1971. The pathological findings in fetal craniospinal injuries. J. Neurosurg., *34*:603.

Dietrich, H. F. 1954. Prevention of childhood accidents. J.A.M.A., *156*:929.

Fogelman, M. J., and Stewart, R. D. 1956. Penetrating wounds of the neck. Am. J. Surg., *91*:581.

Fulginiti, V. A. 1976. Immunizations. *In* Kempe, C. H., Silver, H. K., and O'Brien, D. (Eds.) Current Pediatric Diagnosis and Treatment, 4th ed. Los Altos, CA, Lange Medical Pub.

Gregory, C. F. 1966. General considerations peculiar to the type of injury sustained. *In* Shires, G. T. (Ed.). Care of the Trauma Patient. New York, McGraw-Hill.

Haller, J. A., and Talbert, J. L. 1973. Trauma and the child. *In* Ballinger, W. F., Rutherford, R. B., and Zuidema, G. D. (Eds.). The Management of Trauma. 2nd ed. Philadelphia, W. B. Saunders Co., p. 719.

Harvey, S. C. 1975. Antiseptics and disinfections. *In* Goodman, L. S., and Gilman, A. (Eds.). The Pharmacological Basis of Therapeutics, 5th ed. New York, Macmillan.

Hoopes, J. E., and Jabaley, M. E. 1973. Soft tissue injuries of the extremities. *In* Ballinger, W. F., Rutherford, R. B., and Zuidema, G. D. (eds.). The Management of Trauma, 2nd ed. Philadelphia, W. B. Saunders Co., p. 510.

Jones, R. C. 1966. Initial Care of the Trauma Patient. *In* Shires, G. T. (Ed.) Care of the Trauma Patient. New York, McGraw-Hill, p. 187.

Kline D. G. 1964. The use of a resorbable wrapper for peripheral nerve repair, experimental studies in chimpanzees. J. Neurosurg., *21*:737.

Matson, D. D. 1969. Neurosurgery of Infancy and Childhood. 2nd ed. Springfield, IL, Charles C Thomas Pub.

May, M., Chadaratana, P., West, J. W., and Ogura, J. H. 1975 Penetrating neck wounds: selective exploration Laryngoscope, *85*:57

Onné, L. 1962. Recovery of sensibility and sudomotor activity in the hand after nerve suture. Acta Chir. Scand., Suppl. 300.

Patman, D. R., Poulos, E., and Shires, G. T. 1964. The management of civilian arterial injuries. SGO *118*:725.

Rang, M. 1974. Children's Fractures. Philadelphia, J. B. Lippincott Co.

Rogers, W. A. 1942. Treatment of fracture-dislocation of the cervical spine. J. Bone Joint Surg., *24*:245.

Rutherford, R. B. 1973. Peripheral vascular injuries. *In* Ballinger, W. F., Rutherford, R. B., and Zuidema, G. D. (Eds.). The Management of Trauma. 2nd ed. Philadelphia, W. B. Saunders Co., p. 528.

Schneider, R. C. 1962. Surgical indications and contraindications in spine and spinal cord trauma. Clin. Neurosurg., *8*:157.

Seddon, H. J. (Ed.) 1954. Peripheral Nerve Injuries. Medical Research Council, Her Majesty's Stationery Office, London.

Shirkey, A. L., Beall, A. C., Jr., and DeBakey, M. E. 1963. Surgical management of penetrating wounds of the neck. Arch. Surg., *86*:955.

Smith, J. W. 1964. Microsurgery of peripheral nerves. Plast. Reconstr. Surg., *33*:317.

Tachdjian, M. O. 1972. Pediatric Orthopedics, Philadelphia, W. B. Saunders Co., 1972.

Zuidema, G. D., Rutherford, R. B., and Ballinger, W. F. 1979. The Management of Trauma, 3rd ed. Philadelphia, W. B. Saunders Co.

Chapter 81

TUMORS OF THE NECK

Eugene N. Myers, M.D.

Kenneth B. Skolnick, M.D.

An appreciation of the importance of malignancy in the pediatric population is obtained by reviewing the leading cause of death among children aged 1 to 14 years in the United States in 1974, as compiled by the Department of Vital Statistics. In this survey, cancer is second to accidents as a leading cause of death and constitutes 11.3 per cent of all deaths of children in their age group. To the otolaryngologist, the significance of these figures lies in the fact that greater than one of every four pediatric malignancies involves the head and neck region (Sutow, 1964).

Malignancies in the head and neck region in the pediatric population differ significantly from malignancies in this region in adults.

In adults, epidermoid carcinoma constitutes the great majority of these cancers. In childhood, lymphoma and sarcoma are more common, and epidermoid carcinomas are a rarity. Consequently, the clinical presentation, pathologic signs, evaluation, and therapy of neck tumors in the pediatric population are considerably different than the way adult tumors of this region are treated. Two large surveys of head and neck cancer in children discuss the major tumors that present in this region (Sutow, 1964; Jaffe and Jaffe, 1973) (Table 81–1). Lymphomas of the Hodgkin and non-Hodgkin variety and rhabdomyosarcomas are by far the most common, and the remaining large variety of uncommon tumors that may present in this region make

Table 81–1 INCIDENCE OF MALIGNANCIES OF THE HEAD AND NECK IN CHILDREN: SUMMARY OF TWO REPORTS

	Sutow, 1964	Jaffe and Jaffe, 1973	Total
Malignant lymphomas	53	97	150
Rhabdomyosarcoma	30	20	50
Thyroid carcinoma	15	9	24
Fibrosarcoma	4	11	15
Neuroblastoma	3	9	12
Squamous cell carcinoma	4	7	11
Malignant melanoma	3	4	7
Ewing sarcoma	4	3	7
Parotid malignancies	3	2	5
Hemangiopericytoma	1	2	3
Hemangioendothelioma	1	2	3
Osteogenic sarcoma	1	2	3
Malignant teratoma	2	1	3
Malignant Schwann cell tumor	–	2	2
Miscellaneous	8	5	13
TOTAL	132	176	308

(Adapted from Sutow, W. W. 1964. Cancer of the head and neck in children. J.A.M.A., *190*(5):414–416, and Jaffe, B. F., and Jaffe, N. 1973. Head and neck tumors in children. Pediatrics, *51*(4):731–740.)

pediatric head and neck tumors a diagnostic and therapeutic challenge.

This chapter will consider the primary and metastatic malignant tumors that present as neck masses and that are not dealt with elsewhere in this text. The clinical presentation will be discussed first, followed by the pathogenesis of the tumors. Specific diagnostic studies will be recommended, and the modes of therapy will be reviewed.

A malignant tumor of the neck generally presents as a painless, enlarging neck mass. The only complaint may be the presence of a mass or "lump" in the neck. Symptoms, if present, are usually secondary to the impingement on local anatomy of a mass lesion in the neck and are referable to the larynx, the airway, or the upper digestive tract. If the larynx or hypopharynx is disturbed by a mass lesion, hoarseness or a change in quality of the voice might occur. When the hypopharynx is involved, the patient may complain of difficult or painful swallowing. If the mass is large enough or invasive, the airway may become compromised, causing stridor or airway obstruction. If the tumor is invasive, bleeding may occur, and the patient may present with hemoptysis. Systemic symptoms are also common with lymphomas (the most common neck malignancies in children) and include weight loss, fever, anorexia, lethargy, and weakness.

The evaluation of suspected neck tumors begins with a thorough physical examination with special emphasis on the head and neck region. Otoscopy that reveals a unilateral middle ear effusion and an examination of the nasopharynx for masses may uncover an unsuspected primary tumor. Examination of the nasal cavity may also help to locate a lesion originating in the nose or paranasal sinuses. A thorough examination of the oral cavity must be performed, and indirect laryngoscopy should be attempted in the cooperative young child. A complete examination of the neck with emphasis on all lymph node chains in the anterior and posterior triangles must be performed. A thorough palpation of the thyroid gland should be done to evaluate this area.

Radiologic investigation may be indicated, depending on the lesion and the symptomatology. Routine sinus and lateral neck radiographs are useful in locating and characterizing a primary lesion in these regions. Tomography of the head and neck region aids in defining the extent of bony involvement of many head and neck tumors. If the

neck tumor is thought to be associated with systemic involvement, a chest radiograph, intravenous pyelogram, lymphangiogram, and skeletal surveys may be advisable. Thyroid scan and uptake are indicated when a mass is palpated in this gland.

Other laboratory investigations, such as a complete blood count with differential, urinalysis, liver and kidney function tests, thyroid studies, and cerebrospinal fluid evaluation, should be done. Bone marrow biopsies are generally recommended when one suspects lymphoreticular malignancy.

Excisional or incisional biopsy of the neck lesion may ultimately be necessary to diagnose the lesion and differentiate it from the much more frequent benign disorders that affect the head and neck region. These benign disorders and a differential diagnosis of neck tumors were presented in an earlier chapter.

LYMPHORETICULAR TUMORS OF THE NECK

Lymphomas are the third most common cancer in children under 15 years of age, following only leukemia and central nervous system cancer. They are the most common group of head and neck solid tumors, constituting about 50 per cent of head and neck malignancies in the pediatric age group. Lymphomas present to the head and neck surgeon as extranodal disease involving the tonsils, nasopharynx, salivary glands, maxilla, maxillary sinus, or tongue, or they present as nodal disease affecting the cervical lymph nodes.

Lymphoreticular malignancies comprise both Hodgkin and non-Hodgkin lymphomas. The latter is a diverse group of reticuloendothelial tumors, which includes lymphosarcoma, reticulum cell sarcoma, and Burkitt lymphoma. Solid lymphoreticular malignancies are uncommon in childhood, with only 700 new cases occurring annually; 300 of these are Hodgkin lymphomas, and 400 are non-Hodgkin lymphomas (Wollner, 1976).

Hodgkin Lymphoma

Clinical Presentation

Hodgkin disease usually presents to the otolaryngologist as a cervical nodal mass. In more than 80 per cent of children with Hodgkin disease, cervical or supraclavicular adenopathy is present, and upper cervical node presentation is three to four times more likely than supraclavicular node presentation (Tan et al., 1975; Schnitzer et al., 1973). When nodal presentation occurs, unilateral presentation is seen 85 per cent of the time (Tan et al., 1975). Extranodal presentation in the head and neck region is unusual for childhood Hodgkin lymphoma. Outside the head and neck region, other areas of adenopathy are axillary, inguinal, femoral, and epitrochlear (Hays, 1975).

About one third of the patients with Hodgkin lymphoma have systemic symptoms, which include weight loss, night sweats, and inexplicable fever. In childhood, Hodgkin disease, pruritus, nocturnal perspiration, or Pel-Ebstein fevers are rare.

Nine per cent of all Hodgkin lymphomas occur in children under 15 years of age (Donaldson et al., 1976), and the average age of pediatric presentation is 10 years old. Presentation prior to age five years is reported as rare, with the frequency of Hodgkin lymphoma increasing with increasing age in childhood. A male-to-female preponderance of about two to one is reported (Tan et al., 1975; Schnitzer et al., 1973; Donaldson et al., 1976; Parker et al., 1976; Norris et al., 1975; Jenkin et al., 1975; Garwicz et al., 1974; Blinova and Kolygin, 1973; Young et al., 1973; Pitcock et al., 1959).

Pathology

The histopathologic classification of Hodgkin disease that is currently utilized is the Rye Modification of the Lukes and Butler Histological Classification (Lukes et al., 1966) (Table 81–2). Reed-Sternberg cells must be present to make a diagnosis of Hodgkin disease, but they are not pathognomonic since they may be seen in other disorders. In North America, the most frequent histology seen is nodular sclerosis followed by mixed cellularity and lymphocytic predominance. Lymphocytic depletion in childhood Hodgkin lymphoma is rare (Tan et al., 1975; Norris et al., 1975; Jenkin et al., 1975; Garwicz et al., 1974;

Table 81–2 HISTOLOGIC CLASSIFICATION OF HODGKIN DISEASE

Lymphocytic predominance
Nodular sclerosis
Mixed cellularity
Lymphocytic depletion

Table 81–3 CLINICAL STAGING CLASSIFICATION OF HODGKIN DISEASE

Stage I: Involvement of a single lymph node region (I) or of a single extralymphatic organ or site (I_E).

Stage II: Involvement of two or more lymph node regions on the same side of the diaphragm (II) or localized involvement of extralymphatic organ or site and of one or more lymph node regions on the same side of the diaphragm (II_E). An optional recommendation is that the numbers of node regions involved be indicated by a subscript (e.g., II_3).

Stage III: Involvement of lymph node regions on both sides of the diaphragm (III), which may also be accompanied by localized involvement of an extralymphatic organ or site (III_E) or by involvement of the spleen (III_S), or both (III_{SE}).

Stage IV: Diffuse or disseminated involvement of one or more extralymphatic organs or tissues with or without associated lymph node enlargement. The reason for classifying the patient as Stage IV should be identified further by defining the site by symbols.

(Data from Carbone, P. P., Kaplan, H. S., Musshoff, K., et al. 1971. Report of the committee on Hodgkin's disease staging classification. Cancer Res., 1860–1861.)

Kolygin and Fedoreeu, 1976). The usefulness of this classification as a prognostic indicator has been shown. Lymphocytic predominance has the best prognosis, followed by nodular sclerosis, which has a favorable prognosis, and mixed cellularity, which shows a less favorable prognosis. Lymphocytic depletion has a poor prognosis, but, fortunately, this pathologic condition is rare in childhood.

In 1971, the Ann Arbor Clinical Staging Classification was adopted and has proved to be a useful classification. In this scheme, there are four steps of progressive severity and worsening prognosis. Constitutional symptoms of fever, night sweats, inexplicable loss of 10 per cent of the body weight, or a combination of these symptoms worsen the prognosis. Such constitutional symptoms are denoted in the classification by affixing the suffix "B" after the Roman numeral for the stage. Under this scheme, pathologic staging is also done and is denoted separately from the clinical staging (Carbone et al., 1971) (Table 81–3).

Evaluation

In evaluating the child with Hodgkin disease, routine laboratory tests, such as a complete blood count and differential, urinalysis, liver function tests, measurement of serum copper, chest radiographs, and bone marrow tests, should be performed. Studies that have not been shown to be rewarding are routine skeletal surveys, intravenous pyelograms, and gastrointestinal series. Surgical staging by exploratory laparotomy with splenectomy, liver biopsy, and node biopsies is generally advocated (Hays, 1975; Donaldson et al., 1976; Norris et al., 1975; Jenkin et al., 1975; Kolygin and Fedoreeu, 1976; Filler et al., 1975). This results in more accurate staging. Studies have shown that surgical staging changed the clinical stage in 31 to 48 per cent of the children studied (Tan et al., 1975; Kolygin and Fedoreeu, 1976; Filler et al., 1975). Although splenectomy may increase the risk of fatal infectious diseases, it has the advantage of improving the patient's tolerance to subsequent therapy as well as improving the accuracy of staging. Involvement of the spleen or splenic hilar lymph nodes was proved in 39 per cent of children who underwent exploratory laparotomy (Kolygin and Fedoreeu, 1976).

Therapy

The mainstays of therapy for Hodgkin lymphoma are well accepted today to be subtotal radiation therapy for early stages and chemotherapy for later stages. This is performed after accurate histologic classification, clinical staging, and pathologic staging. Radiation therapy is commonly utilized for stages I, II, and IIIA, whereas for stages IIIB and IV a combination chemotherapeutic regimen is utilized, with or without radiation therapy. This regimen most commonly consists of cycles of a nitrogen mustard (mechlorethamine hydrochloride), oncovine, procarbazine, and prednisone. This is the well-known MOPP therapy. Therapeutic toxicity includes nausea, vomiting, anorexia, alopecia, and decreased hematopoietic function. In addition to the possibility of increased potential for the occurrence of future malignant solid tumors, altered bone growth may be seen with high-dose radiation therapy in children. Neuropathy is a well-known complication of oncovine therapy and is closely monitored during the treatment regimen.

Non-Hodgkin Lymphoma

Clinical Presentation

Non-Hodgkin lymphoma of childhood differs significantly from its adult counterpart. In childhood, it is generally a rapidly progressive disease with a poor prognosis that differs from the adult form by its rapid and progressive onset, diffuse histology, and poor response to therapy. Non-Hodgkin lymphoma clinically presents with peripheral nodal involvement, particularly of the cervical lymph nodes. In 80 per cent of children with this tumor, symptoms are present for less than one month. Cervical adenopathy occurs as the primary presenting symptom in 11 to 35 per cent of these patients (Bailey et al., 1961; Dargeon, 1961; Sullivan, 1962). A persistent, painless, enlarging mass in the neck is the usual complaint. Constitutional complaints, including fever, malaise, anorexia, weight loss, night sweats, and bone and joint pain, are common. A male-to-female preponderance for this malignancy is well-documented: the ratio is approximately three to one (Bailey et al., 1961; Dargeon, 1961; Wollner et al., 1976, Murphy et al., 1975; Glatstein et al., 1974; Jones and Klingberg, 1963; Rosenberg et al., 1958). Childhood non-Hodgkin lymphoma occurs one third of the time in the 7 to 10 year old age group and rarely presents prior to age 2 years (Murphy et al., 1975). An increased incidence is reported to occur in the 3 to 5 year old age group and also in the 9 to 11 year old age group (Jones and Klingberg, 1963).

Pathology

A variety of classifications and nomenclature have been suggested for the non-Hodgkin lymphoma. Presently, Rappaport's classification is commonly used and is well-accepted (Wollner, 1976). It divides the non-Hodgkin lymphoma into diffuse and nodular patterns and then further subdivides them by the predominant cell type as lymphocytic, histocytic, mixed, or undifferentiated. The degree of differentiation is further described as poorly differentiated or well-differentiated. In childhood non-Hodgkin lymphoma, diffuse pathology predominates, while the nodular variety is uncommon. Diffuse histiocytic, diffuse lymphocytic poorly differentiated, and diffuse undifferentiated are the most common histologic classifications described (Wollner, 1976; Murphy et al., 1975; Glatstein et al., 1974).

Clinical staging for the non-Hodgkin lymphoma has been disappointing. Although the staging adopted at the Rye, New York, Symposium in 1965 has been well-accepted for the Hodgkin lymphomas, a satisfactory clinical staging protocol of proven merit has not been universally accepted for non-Hodgkin lymphomas. Presently, variations of the Rye classification are being utilized.

Evaluation

The diagnosis of non-Hodgkin lymphoma in the child who presents with cervical adenopathy is usually made by lymph node biopsy but is often suspected prior to biopsy by the persistence of the adenopathy and the commonly present constitutional symptoms. Unfortunately, widespread disease and associated symptoms are often present on initial examination. Complete evaluation of the child to determine the extent of the disease begins with a hematologic evaluation. A complete blood count and differential is done to check for a leukemic pattern of disease and also to establish a baseline in case of future leukemic transformation, an occurrence that has been reported in 14.6 to 52.2 per cent of childhood non-Hodgkin lymphomas (Bailey et al., 1961; Sullivan, 1962; Jones and Klingberg, 1963). Bone marrow biopsy and aspira-tion of multiple sites have also been recommended for routine evaluation. Liver and kidney function tests should be performed, as should lumbar puncture and cerebrospinal fluid evaluation for protein, sugar, cytology, and cell count to diagnose early central nervous system involvement. Such an involvement could be generalized in the meninges, a focal central nervous system lesion, or a combination of the two. Chest radiographs and a skeletal survey are routinely ordered to determine the possibility of metastases. Additional studies are indicated depending upon the child's symptomatology and other organ systems involved. Exploratory laparotomy is not advocated presently since this may delay early aggressive therapy.

Therapy

Non-Hodgkin lymphoma is a rapidly progressive disease usually associated with a high mortality. A variety of treatment regimens and radiation therapies have been attempted in the past with discouraging results, a situation the reverse of that encountered in the

Table 81–4 TREATMENT PROTOCOL FOR NON-HODGKIN LYMPHOMA

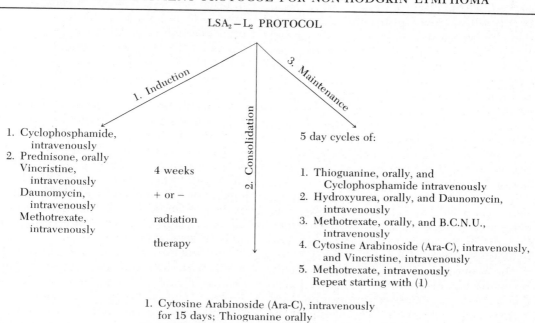

LSA_2–L_2 PROTOCOL

1. Induction

3. Maintenance

2. Consolidation

1. Cyclophosphamide, intravenously
2. Prednisone, orally
   Vincristine, intravenously
   Daunomycin, intravenously
   Methotrexate, intravenously

4 weeks

+ or −

radiation

therapy

5 day cycles of:

1. Thioguanine, orally, and Cyclophosphamide intravenously
2. Hydroxyurea, orally, and Daunomycin, intravenously
3. Methotrexate, orally, and B.C.N.U., intravenously
4. Cytosine Arabinoside (Ara-C), intravenously, and Vincristine, intravenously
5. Methotrexate, intravenously
   Repeat starting with (1)

1. Cytosine Arabinoside (Ara-C), intravenously for 15 days; Thioguanine orally
2. L-Asparaginase, intravenously
   Methotrexate, intravenously
   B.C.N.U., intravenously

(From Wollner, N., Burchenal, J. H., Lieberman, P. H., et al. 1976. Non-Hodgkin's lymphoma in children. Cancer, 37:126.)

treatment of Hodgkin disease. Recently, however, an early, aggressive, and intensive multiple-drug protocol has had excellent results, with 76 per cent of the patients surviving free of disease for over 25 months median observation time (Wollner, 1976; Wollner et al., 1975). There are three phases of treatment with this regimen, beginning with an induction phase. This is followed by a consolidation phase, and finally a maintenance phase is instituted that is continued for two to three years depending on the initial staging (Wollner, 1976) (Table 81–4). It is hoped that the initial promising results of this protocol will be further substantiated.

THYROID CARCINOMA

Clinical Presentation

Pediatric thyroid carcinoma, once quite rare, has taken on a greater importance since its association with radiation to the head and neck in infancy and childhood has been recognized (Duffy and Fitzgerald, 1950). When specifically investigated, 46 to 80 per cent of children with thyroid carcinoma had previous head and neck irradiation (Winship and Rosvoll, 1970; Harness et al., 1971). Such irradiation was used primarily in the treatment of benign disorders, such as enlarged thymus and hypertrophied tonsils and adenoids, before its association with thyroid carcinoma was recognized. Other disorders for which irradiation was given, with subsequent development of thyroid carcinoma, include hemangioma, acne, eczema, other benign skin lesions, and tumors of the central nervous system. Following such standards of treatment for benign disorders, an increase in cases of pediatric thyroid carcinoma began to appear in the middle 1940s with a peak incidence in the late 1950s. A subsequent decline followed the cessation of radiation therapy for the aforementioned benign conditions (Winship and Rosvoll, 1970).

The most common presentation for pediatric thyroid carcinoma is a cervical nodal mass that persists or enlarges despite antibiotic therapy. This occurred in 63 per cent of the cases seen (Harness et al., 1971), the nodal mass having been present for an average of more than two years. The second most common presentation is a palpable mass within the thyroid gland itself, with or without nodal disease. Hoarseness secondary to recurrent laryngeal nerve involvement or airway obstruction due to a mass lesion or invasive carcinoma may be present with extensive disease.

The average age of presentation is about 9.4 years, with a female preponderance not nearly as great as is seen in adult thyroid carcinoma (Winship and Rosvoll, 1970). Approximately 80 per cent of the children have been found to have unilateral or bilateral cervical metastases, and up to 20 per cent develop pulmonary metastases (Harness et al., 1971). Bony metastases are initially present in less than 2 per cent of children with this type of tumor and ultimately develop in an additional 2 per cent (Winship and Rosvoll, 1970). It is important in all these cases to investigate the possibility of history of head and neck irradiation.

Pathology

The four principal types of thyroid carcinoma are papillary, follicular, medullary, and anaplastic. The great majority of pediatric thyroid carcinomas are of the mixed papillary, follicular type; about 72 per cent of pediatric thyroid carcinomas will have papillary elements (Winship and Rosvoll, 1970). The tumors are cystic or solid, and it is not unusual for cystic nodal metastases to be mistaken on initial gross examination for branchial cleft cysts. Microscopically, one sees a papillary axial stroma covered with epithelium. Follicles may or may not be present, and a varying degree of anaplasia of cells may be present.

Follicular carcinoma is the second most common pediatric thyroid malignancy and may be characterized by follicles ranging from those bizarre in shape and form to those with normal-appearing acini. The diagnosis is more easily made when there is marked anaplasia or invasiveness or when the follicular pattern is found in a lymph node. Occasionally, the diagnosis is difficult to make with a well-differentiated tumor.

The final two carcinomas of the thyroid are rare. Medullary carcinoma arises from the parafollicular cells and may secrete calcitonin. Chemical assays for this product are useful diagnostically and for following the patient postoperatively for recurrence. Occasionally, this tumor is associated with a multiple endocrine adenomatosis. In such a case, one would see a pheochromocytoma and occasionally submucosal neuromas associated with a medullary carcinoma. Histologically, round to spindle-shaped cells are seen, characteristically separated by an amyloid stroma. The finding of a pheochromocytoma or family history of similar disease completes the syndrome.

Anaplastic carcinoma is quite rare and is universally considered fatal. Histologically, the cells are undifferentiated and are small or large in size. Invasion outside the capsule of the thyroid gland is common.

Evaluation

A palpable, nonfunctioning nodule of the thyroid in children should be considered malignant unless proved otherwise. Masses of the thyroid gland should be evaluated by thyroid function tests. If a family history of pheochromocytoma or medullary carcinoma is obtained, calcitonin blood levels should be drawn. Arteriograms and intravenous pyelograms may be indicated to evaluate the possibility of a pheochromocytoma. A thyroid scan and update are always indicated for palpable disease within the thyroid. Although iodine 131 is readily available and of low cost, it delivers a significant radiation dose to the thyroid. Consequently, technetium 99M as the pertechnetate ion is recommended for such tests today because of its low beta emission (Hayek and Stanbury, 1971).

A so-called "cold" nodule arouses suspicion of malignancy. Lymph node metastases, if not readily palpable, may be seen on scanning. Chest radiographs are indicated to identify pulmonary metastases, and bone scans or skeletal surveys might be indicated, depending upon symptomatology and pathology. The definitive diagnosis of thyroid carcinoma or nodal metastases is made by biopsy. If the disease is in one lobe of the thyroid gland, an adequate biopsy would be a thyroid lobectomy.

Therapy

Once a diagnosis of thyroid malignancy has been made, a subtotal or total thyroidectomy should be performed because of the potential for multifocal disease and also for the possibility of subsequent therapy with radioactive iodine 131. The major potential complications of a total or near-total thyroidectomy include recurrent laryngeal nerve injury and permanent hypoparathyroidism. These complications should be minimized by careful and meticulous surgery. A modified neck dissection with preservation of the sternocleidomastoid muscle, spinal accessory nerve, and internal jugular vein should be performed for cervical node involvement. The classic radical neck dissection should usually be avoided because of the general lack of involvement of the sternocleidomastoid muscle, spinal accessory nerve, and internal jugular vein. A prophylactic or elective neck dissection is not indicated in the cases without palpable nodes. Thyroid replacement and suppression therapy should be instituted after surgery, and postoperative scanning is mandatory. Iodine 131 therapy for persistent disease should be instituted as necessary.

RHABDOMYOSARCOMA

Clinical Presentation

Rhabdomyosarcoma is the most frequently seen soft tissue sarcoma in children: it constitutes 5 to 18 per cent of solid carcinomas in children (Exelby, 1974; Hornback and Shidnia, 1976; Jaffe et al., 1973).

The median age of presentation for all locations varies from 5 to 7 years of age (Exelby, 1974; Hornback and Shidnia, 1976; Donaldson et al., 1973; Mahour et al., 1967). Head and neck presentation is seen throughout the entire pediatric age group but is more common in the younger ages (Exelby, 1974; Miller and Dalager, 1974). The sex ratio for head and neck presentation is 1.2 males to females, which is in contrast to the more marked male predominance of rhabdomyosarcoma of other locations (Miller and Dalager, 1974). In the pediatric age group, the two most common regions of presentation are the genitourinary tract and the head and neck regions (Hornback and Shidnia, 1976; Miller and Dalager, 1974). The order of frequency of presentation within the head and neck is orbit, nasopharynx, parotid gland, and the neck (Exelby, 1974). The initial complaint with neck presentation is an enlarging, painless mass with other symptoms proportionate to the impingement of the mass on local anatomic structures. Metastases to nodes in the neck also occur, with the initial complaint dependent upon the location of the primary head and neck tumor.

Pathology

Rhabdomyosarcoma is a malignant tumor of the rhabdomyoblast that may present as either a grape-like mass or a solid mass. The latter is most common in the head and neck region. Rhabdomyosarcomas have been classified by Horn and Enterline (1958) into four subgroups: pleomorphic, embryonic, alveolar, and botryoid, a morphologic variant of embryonic. Whereas pleomorphic is the most common rhabdomyosarcoma in adulthood, the embryonic variant is most often seen in pediatric head and neck rhabdomyosarcomas.

Grossly, these tumors have been described as pink, purple, or gray, and soft in consistency. Histologically, they have been noted to resemble muscles of the 7 to 10 week old embryo in that they consist of spindle cells that have eosinophilic cytoplasm. These cells are small and can be rounded. Cross or longitudinal striations are often seen, and they are carefully inspected, although the absence of these does not preclude the diagnosis. Occasionally, the cells contain peripherally arranged vacuoles. The nuclei are ovoid and most often centrally placed. The histologic diagnosis is not readily made and can be confused easily with osteosarcoma, myxoma, and neuroblastoma.

Rhabdomyosarcoma behaves as an aggressive, infiltrating malignancy and metastasizes early. The initial spread is often lymphatic to

Table 81–5 RHABDOMYOSARCOMA – INTERGROUP PROTOCOL GROUPING

(In this system, the grouping is decided upon by the surgeon in the operating room and later confirmed by the pathologist and pediatrician.)

Group   I   A. Localized disease completely resected, confined to muscle or organ of origin

B. Localized disease completely resected, contiguous involvement, infiltration outside the muscle or organ of origin

Group II   A. Grossly resected tumor with microscopic residual disease but no evidence of regional lymph node involvement

B. Regional lymph nodes involved but all disease completely removed

C. Regional lymph nodes involved, grossly resected, but evidence of microscopic residual

Group III   A. Incomplete resection or biopsy with gross residual disease

Group IV   A. Distant metastatic disease present at onset

(From Hornback, N. B., and Shidnia, H. 1976. Rhabdomyosarcoma in the pediatric age group. Am. J. Roentgenol., *126*(3):543.)

the lung, liver, bone, or brain. A clinical staging for rhabdomyosarcoma has been advocated by the Intergroup Rhabdomyosarcoma Protocol Committee (Hornback and Shidnia, 1976) (Table 81–5).

Evaluation

Rhabdomyosarcoma involving the neck may be a primary lesion or metastatic from elsewhere in the head and neck. A meticulous head and neck evaluation is necessary in the routine history and physical examination. Following a satisfactory histologic diagnosis, evaluation for metastases and tests for staging are performed. Routine laboratory tests include complete blood count, platelets, liver function tests, chest radiographs, bone marrow biopsy skeletal survey, and skull and sinus radiographs. Polytomography may be necessary to evaluate the extent of any head and neck primary tumor. Arteriograms, a brain scan, bone scan, and lumbar puncture may also be performed, depending on the individual's symptomatology.

Therapy

The treatment of rhabdomyosarcoma has changed significantly in the past decade. Poor therapeutic results with high mortality early in the course of therapy demonstrated that major ablative surgery by itself was not successful in treating this malignancy. A two year survival rate one decade ago of 10 to 30 per cent was not unusual (Exelby, 1974; Donaldson et al; 1973; Masson and Soule, 1965). In the search for improved, successful therapeutic regimens, radiation therapy was introduced. The positive results were found to be augmented by actinomycin D, and vincristine and cyclophosphamide were found to decrease the occurrence of metastases. Consequently, a combined, aggressive therapeutic regimen is currently advocated: Wide local excision, except in cases in which cosmetic deformity, mutilation, or loss of function will occur, is followed by postoperative radiation therapy of 5000 to 6000 rads by a supervoltage machine. Concurrently, chemotherapy with cycles of vincristine, actinomycin D, and cyclophosphamide is instituted. Although significant side effects may develop, a two year survival rate of greater than 70 per cent has been reported with less extensive surgical procedures (Exelby, 1974; Jaffe et al., 1973; Donaldson et al., 1973; Sessions et al., 1973; Malpas et al., 1976; Heyn et al., 1974; Kilman et al., 1973; Holton et al., 1973; Ehrlich et al., 1971; Grosfeld et al., 1969; Pratt, 1969).

FIBROSARCOMA

Clinical Presentation

Fibrosarcoma is a mesenchymal malignancy that is uncommon as a neck tumor in the pediatric population. In two studies of fibrosarcoma in infants and children, 10 cases out of a total of 33 cases had head and neck involvement. In only two of these was cervical node involvement present (Bizer, 1971; Conley et al., 1967; Stout, 1962). In a recent study of pediatric fibrosarcoma of the head and neck region, 6 of 11 cases did not involve the neck. The remaining five cases were specified as involving the soft tissues of the head and neck region. The clinical presentation of this malignancy generally is that of a slowly enlarging, painless mass in the neck. This may be present at birth or may develop at any time during childhood. There is no specific sex predilection or symptomatology that would suggest this particular malignancy.

Pathology

The histopathologic diagnosis of the mesenchymal tumors has been and continues to be a challenge to the pathologist. Significant difficulty can be encountered in differentiating a variety of lesions from fibrosarcoma. Lesions such as fibroma, fibromatosis, pseudosarcomatis fascitis, and desmoids have occasionally confused the diagnosis. The rarity of this particular neoplasm further compounds the problem for the pathologist.

Prognostically, fibrosarcomas are presently classified as well-differentiated or poorly differentiated. This is determined by the number of mitotic figures, the cellular uniformity and atypia, and the characteristics of the stroma. Special strains can be utilized to facilitate the classification (Stout, 1962; Swain et al., 1974; Hays et al., 1970). These tumors are invasive, and localizing encapsulation does not occur. The poorly differentiated varieties are prone to metastasize. As expected, the well-differentiated fibrosarcomas that are superficially located have a better prognosis. Metastatic disease is usually by hematogenous spread with metastases occurring in the lung, abdomen, or bone; an 18 per cent incidence of such spread has been reported (Conley et al., 1967). Regional lymph node metastases of fibrosarcomas from all locations

have been reported to occur in from 4 to 11 per cent of cases (Bizer, 1971; Stout, 1962), but in one series reporting on head and neck fibrosarcomas, no cervical lymph node metastases were noted (Conley et al., 1967). Trauma has been speculated to be one etiologic factor, and although in occasional cases an antecedent history of physical trauma is present, this has never been proved. Radiation therapy, clinically and experimentally, has been shown to be an etiologic factor.

Evaluation

There are no specific laboratory tests one can utilize in making a preoperative, suggestive diagnosis of fibrosarcoma. An examination to rule out metastases should include chest radiographs and a skeletal survey. An intravenous pyelogram may be helpful, depending on the specific symptomatology, and a complete blood count and urinalysis are routinely done preoperatively. The diagnosis is ultimately made on the basis of an examination of permanent histopathologic sections.

Therapy

With the knowledge that these tumors are locally invasive, do not possess a limiting capsule, and rarely involve cervical nodes, a wide-field local resection is advocated (Swain et al., 1974; Hays et al., 1970; Swain et al., 1976). Radical neck dissection for prophylactic reasons is not indicated but may be necessary to obtain an adequate margin of resection (Swain et al., 1974). Although radiation therapy generally has not had satisfactory results for complete irradication of lesions (Bizer, 1971; Conley et al., 1967; Goldman and Hardcastle, 1969), there is some evidence that it may be useful for palliation of symptoms (Bizer, 1971; Swain et al., 1974; Swain et al., 1976). Chemotherapy has not, as of yet, been proved to be successful for the treatment of fibrosarcomas. The prognosis is poor for the poorly differentiated, deeply invasive fibrosarcoma.

NEUROBLASTOMA

Clinical Presentation

Neuroblastoma is a malignant, solid tumor arising from the sympathetic nervous system or its anlage. It is a rare malignancy but is seen relatively commonly as an infant and childhood tumor. Neuroblastoma constitutes

approximately 10 per cent of malignant neoplasms in childhood and is probably the most
frequent malignant solid tumor in the
younger pediatric population (deLorimier et
al., 1969; Evans, 1972; Harrison et al., 1974;
Evans et al., 1976).

Retroperitoneal presentation occurs involving the adrenal gland or abdominal sympathetics in 63 per cent of cases. Presentation
to the head and neck surgeon may occur as a
cervical mass in 2 to 8 per cent of cases
(deLorimier et al., 1969; Horn et al., 1956;
Bodian, 1959; Gross et al., 1959; Young et al.,
1970). This may represent a primary tumor
arising from the cervical sympathetics, a metastatic deposit from the usual abdominal origin, or a direct extension from the thorax. In
the neck, neuroblastoma presents as a painless, solid mass that may arise high or low in
the neck along the sympathetics. It may present as a metastatic deposit in the Virchow
node, suggesting an abdominal primary
tumor. As with other mass lesions of the neck,
symptoms are referable to the larynx, pharynx, and esophagus with possible symptoms
of dysphagia, odynophagia, hoarseness, or
airway obstruction. Involvement of the cranial nerves may result in neurologic deficits.
Peculiar to the involvement of the sympathetics in the neck, a Horner syndrome with
ptosis, myosis, and anhidrosis would be suggestive of the diagnosis of neuroblastoma.

The majority of cases present in infancy or
early childhood, with 46 per cent occurring
prior to the age of 2 years and 83 per cent
prior to the age of 7 (deLorimier et al., 1969).
Unfortunately, dissemination occurs early,
with approximately 70 per cent of the cases
presenting with metastatic disease (Evans et
al., 1976; Bodian, 1959; Gross et al., 1959;
Sutow, 1958). Skeletal metastases have a uniformly fatal prognosis.

Pathology

Neuroblastomas are solid, fleshy, gray or
pink tumors, often with areas of necrosis,
hemorrhage, or calcification. These tumors
are infiltrative, with blood vessel invasion
occurring commonly. The individual cells are
small, round, or elongated with hyperchro-
mic nuclei. The malignant cells can grow in
an irregular cluster or in an organized fashion. Characteristic rosettes and clusters
around the neurofibril help in establishing
the diagnosis (Horn et al., 1956; Gross et al.,
1959).

Clinical staging, although not widely utilized, has been proposed. Tumors confined
to the site of origin would be Stage I. Stage II
lesions would not cross the midline but might
involve regional lymph nodes. Stage III disease extends across the midline, while Stage
IV involves remote disease.

Evaluation

Neuroblastomas in the neck must be differentiated from other malignancies and
from benign conditions, such as cysts, lymphomas, hematomas, benign lymphadenopathy, cystic hygromas, and thyroid abnormalities. Routine laboratory investigations should
include complete blood count and differential, chest radiographs, a skeletal survey, and
an intravenous pyelogram. A measurement
of urinary catecholamines, vanillylmandelic
acid, and cystathionine would be helpful in
the diagnosis of neuroblastoma, for they are
elevated in up to 75 per cent of the cases seen
(Evans et al., 1976; Young et al., 1970; Evans
et al., 1971; Helson et al., 1972). Neck radiographs may show stippled calcification
(Young et al., 1970), and enlargement or
destruction of intervertebral foramina may
be seen on oblique spine films when the
primary tumor is in the paravertebral area.
An intravenous pyelogram may show involvement of the adrenal glands or the retroperi-
toneum. When these studies are negative,
one can conclude that the neck lesion is the
primary one. The ultimate diagnosis, of
course, is the histologic diagnosis made at the
time the biopsy specimen is obtained.

Therapy

The natural history of neuroblastoma is
variable from patient to patient. In general,
neuroblastoma is a highly invasive malignancy that spreads by both lymphatic and hematologic pathways. Multicentricity has been
speculated to occur in certain cases (Dargeon,
1962; Voorhess and Gardner, 1962), while
benign transformation and spontaneous regression and cure are well-documented in
sporadic cases (deLorimier et al., 1969; Evans
et al., 1976; Gross et al., 1959). The accepted
treatment of choice is surgical extirpation if
possible. The tumor is quite radiosensitive,
and radiation therapy is generally used postoperatively. High-dose vitamin B therapy has
been reported to be successful (Sutow, 1958),
but more recent studies with this therapy

have not been encouraging (Evans, 1971). Chemotherapy is an accepted treatment for widespread disease (Evans, 1972), but evidence for increased survival rates after such therapy has not been proved to be significant (Evans et al., 1976); cyclophosphamide with vincristine is the most commonly used chemotherapeutic regimen (Evans, 1972; Evans et al., 1976; Thurman et al., 1964; Pinkel et al., 1968). Factors related to increased survival and curability of this type of tumor are presentation prior to the age of 2 years, increased differentiation of the tumor, surgical extirpation of the entire tumor, and the absence of skeletal metastases. A better prognosis is usually seen when the tumor arises from extranodal sites such as in the neck.

SQUAMOUS CELL CARCINOMA

Squamous cell carcinoma of the neck in childhood is a rarity and is uncommon as a head and neck malignancy, occurring in only 7 of 178 pediatric head and neck malignant tumor cases reported in one series (Jaffe and Jaffe, 1973). This is in contrast to squamous cell carcinoma in the adult population, where it is the most common head and neck malignancy.

The clinical presentation of this tumor is similar to that of other neck malignancies: a painless, enlarging mass. This may be the only presenting complaint, or symptoms may be related to a primary lesion. Eighty per cent of the visceral squamous cell carcinomas in childhood are located in the pharynx or oral cavity, with about half of these occurring in the nasopharynx or pharynx (Moore, 1958). A careful investigation for the primary tumor site is in order in these cases. A unilateral middle ear effusion or cranial nerve involvement would suggest a nasopharyngeal primary lesion. Other appropriate signs or symptoms would suggest an oral cavity lesion, maxillary sinus lesion, or involvement of the larynx. After exhaustive investigations have failed to discover a primary lesion, one should cautiously suspect that the neck node is the primary lesion, realizing that an occult primary lesion may still be present.

Management of squamous cell carcinoma of the neck in childhood does not differ greatly from that of the adult. Therapy is directed towards the primary lesion and will generally involve surgical en bloc resection, radiation therapy, or both. Chemotherapy may play a role for palliation in advanced cases.

MALIGNANT MELANOMA

Malignant melanoma of the neck is extremely rare in childhood (Shanon et al., 1976; Conley and Pack, 1963; Olbourne and Harrison, 1974) and can present as a primary skin lesion or a metastatic nodal deposit. Its behavior and management do not differ from those of its adult counterpart. Clinical signs suggesting a primary malignant melanoma are rapid growth, satellitosis, ulceration, crusting, and the presence of or change in pigmentation of a skin lesion. This must be differentiated from the more common spindle or epithelial cell nevus, commonly known as the benign juvenile melanoma, which may present in a similar fashion (Trozak et al., 1975).

The histopathologic diagnosis of a malignant melanoma as differentiated from juvenile melanoma was elucidated by Spitz (1948) and Allen and Spitz (1963). Malignancy is suggested by anaplasia and increased cellular pleomorphism. Tissue invasion and mytosis further substantiate the diagnosis. The degree of invasion as described by Clark (1969), is helpful prognostically and therapeutically (Donnellan et al., 1972). Five levels of invasion are described, ranging from superficially located tumors not penetrating the basement membrane to tumors that spread into the subcutaneous tissues.

The principles of management of childhood melanoma are similar to these of the adult form. When possible, a total excisional biopsy should be performed to allow for a definite histopathologic diagnosis. When the diagnosis is confirmed, a wider and deeper reexcision is indicated; reconstruction with either a skin graft or a local flap may be necessary. When clinical signs of nodal involvement are present, an en bloc resection with radical lymph node dissection is necessary. The efficacy of an elective lymph node dissection is controversial today (Trozak et al., 1975; Southwick, 1976; Knutson et al., 1972; Simons, 1972; Lerman et al., 1970; Harris et al., 1925). Chemotherapy and immunotherapy are useful adjuncts when the disease has spread, whereas radiation therapy is generally considered to have a limited role in treatment of malignant melanoma (Conley and Pack, 1963), although reports of the radiosensitivity of this tumor have been described (Hellriegel, 1963).

HEMANGIOPERICYTOMA

The hemangiopericytoma is an extremely rare pediatric neck tumor that was first described in 1942 by Stout and Murry as originating from the capillary pericytes of Zimmermann. The tumor is reported to occur in the head and neck region in 16 to 33 per cent of cases (Enzinger and Smith, 1976; Walike and Bailey, 1971) and to be present in the pediatric population in 10 per cent of all cases of its occurrence (Kauffman and Stout, 1960). Neck presentation, although unusual, occurred in 5 of 88 children with hemangiopericytoma documented by the Armed Forces Institute of Pathology (Hyams, 1977).

This type of tumor generally presents as a painless, enlarging mass that is soft in consistency. There is no age specificity in the pediatric population, and it may present as a congenital tumor. Radiologic evaluation is not specific except on angiographic studies in which a vascular tumor is seen. The diagnosis is made following surgical biopsy.

The hemangiopericytoma has been confused with a variety of other tumors, including hemangioendothelioma, glomus tumor, fibrous histiocytoma, vascular leiomyoma, neurilomyoma, and Kaposi sarcoma (Enzinger and Smith, 1976; Kauffman and Stout, 1960). Histologically, spindle-shaped cells with enlarged nuclei that are tightly condensed around prominent vascular spaces are seen. Mytotic figures are rare. It is essential to the diagnosis that a reticulum stain be done to demonstrate normal-appearing vascular endothelial cells with the tumor cells present in an extravascular position. Malignancy is difficult to determine but is suspected with increased mytotic activity or necrosis. The potential for malignancy is higher in the older age groups of the pediatric population; congenital lesions are commonly benign irrespective of a malignant-appearing histology (Enzinger and Smith, 1976; Kauffman and Stout, 1960).

The recommended treatment of this tumor is wide local excision (Enzinger and Smith, 1976; Walike and Bailey, 1971; McMaster et al., 1975) and life-long observation. Radiotherapy and chemotherapy are generally unrewarding (Enzinger and Smith, 1976), although occasionally successful treatment with each modality has been reported (Cohen et al., 1972). Metastases can occur locally or by hematologic spread with an overall metastatic rate of 50 per cent being reported (Walike and Bailey, 1971; Backwinkel and Diddams, 1970; Cook et al., 1974).

HEMANGIOENDOTHELIOMA

Malignant hemangioendothelioma is another rare vascular tumor that may present in the neck in the pediatric population. Three of 18 pediatric cases reported in the literature prior to 1960 occurred as a head and neck primary lesion (Kauffman and Stout, 1958). Like the hemangiopericytomas, hemangioendotheliomas present as painless, enlarging neck masses without other specific symptomatology.

Histopathologically, the cell of origin is the vascular endothelial cell. The major criteria for diagnosis are the occurrences of prolific, atypical endothelial cells more in number than are necessary to line the vessel, and the propensity of these cells to form anastomosing networks of vascular tubes with a reticulum fiber framework (Stout, 1943). The tumor may be single or multicentric (Sull and Brown, 1972) and must be differentiated from its benign counterpart. Silver reticulum stain easily differentiates the hemangioendothelioma from the hemangiopericytoma, as in the former the cell of origin is within the reticulum sheath of the vessel, and individual cells are not surrounded by reticulum fibers.

Wide local excision is presently recommended for treatment of this tumor. Metastases can occur, and spread is usually by hematogenous routes, although lymphatic spread is known to occur (Kauffman and Stout, 1960; Sull and Brown, 1972). When excision is incomplete or when palliation is desired, radiation therapy is recommended, although these tumors are relatively radioresistant.

SELECTED REFERENCE

Jaffe, B. F., and Jaffe, N. 1973. Head and neck tumors in children. Pediatrics, 51(4):731–740.
The authors have compiled a series of 178 pediatric head and neck malignant tumors. They have discussed the presentation, evaluation, and therapy of these malignancies. This article is an excellent overview of this topic.

REFERENCES

Allen, A. C., and Spitz, S. 1963. Malignant melanoma: A clinicopathological analysis of the criteria for diagnosis and prognosis. Cancer, *6*:1–45.

Backwinkel, K. D., and Diddams, J. A. 1970. Hemangiopericytoma: A report of a case and comprehensive review of the literature. Cancer, *25*:896–901.

Bailey, R. J., Burgert, E. O., and Dahlin, D. C. 1961. Malignant lymphoma in children. Pediatrics, *28*:985–992.

Bizer, L. A. 1971. Fibrosarcoma: Report of 64 cases. Am. J. Surg., *121*:586–587.

Blinova, G. A., and Kolygin, B. A. 1973. Clinical and morphological correlation of Hodgkin's disease in children. Tumori, *59*:409–418.

Bodian, M. 1959. Neuroblastoma. Pediatr. Clin. North Am., *6*(2):449–472.

Carbone, P. P., Kaplan, H. S., Musshoff, K., et al. 1971. Report of the committee on Hodgkin's disease staging classification. Cancer Res., 1860–1861.

Clark, W. H. 1969. Histogenesis and biologic behavior of primary human malignant melanoma of the skin. Cancer Res., *29*:705.

Cohen, Y., Lichtig, C., and Robinson, E. 1972. Combination chemotherapy in the treatment of metastatic hemangiopericytoma. Oncology, *26*:180–187.

Conley, J., and Pack, G. T. 1963. Melanoma of the head and neck. Surg. Gynecol. Obstet., *116*:15–28.

Conley, J., Stout, A. P., and Healey, W. V. 1967. Clinicopathologic analysis of 84 patients with an original diagnosis of fibrosarcoma of the head and neck. Am. J. Surg., *114*:564–569.

Cook, C., Kakos, G. S., and Roberts, S. 1974. Hemangiopericytoma: A case report and rationale for aggressive therapy. Cancer, *34*:1830–1833.

Dargeon, H. W. 1961. Lymphosarcoma in children. Am. J. Roentgenol., *85*(4):729–732.

Dargeon, H. W. 1962. Neuroblastoma. J. Pediatr., *61*(3):456–471.

deLorimier, A. A., Bragg, K. U., and Linden, G. 1969. Neuroblastoma in childhood. Am. J. Dis. Child., *118*:441–450.

Donaldson, S. S., Castro, J. R., Wilbur, J. J., et al. 1973. Rhabdomyosarcoma of head and neck in children: Combination treatment by surgery, irradiation, and chemotherapy. Cancer, *31*:26–35.

Donaldson, S. S., Glatstein, E., Rosenberg, S. A., et al. 1976. Pediatric Hodgkin's disease (II). Cancer, *37*:2436–2447.

Donnellan, M. J., Seemayer, T., Huvos, A. G., et al. 1972. Clinicopathologic study of cutaneous melanoma of the head and neck. Am. J. Surg., *124*:450–455.

Duffy, B. J., and Fitzgerald, P. J. 1950. Cancer of the thyroid in children: A report of 28 cases. J. Clin. Endocrinol., *10*:1296–1308.

Ehrlich, F. E., Haas, J. E., and Kiesewetter, W. B. 1971. Rhabdomyosarcoma in infants and children: Factors affecting long-term survival. J. Pediatr. Surg., *6*(5):571–577.

Enzinger, F. M., and Smith, B. H. 1976. Hemangiopericytoma: An analysis of 196 cases. Hum. Pathol., *7*(1):61–82.

Evans, A. E., D'Angio, G. J., and Koop, C. E. 1976. Diagnosis and treatment of neuroblastoma. Pediatr. Clin. North Am., *23*(1): 161–170.

Evans, A. E., D'Angio, J. D., and Randolph, J. 1971. A proposed staging for children with neuroblastoma. Cancer, *27*(2):374–378.

Evans, A. E. 1972. Treatment of neuroblastoma. Cancer, *30*:1595–1599.

Exelby, P. R. 1974. Management of embryonal rhabdomyosarcoma in children. Surg. Clin. North Am., *54*(4):849–857.

Filler, R. M., Jaffe, N., Cassady, J. R., et al. 1975. Experience with clinical and operative staging of Hodgkin's disease in children. J. Pediatr. Surg., *10*(3):321–328.

Garwicz, S., Landberg, T., and Akerman, M. 1974. Malignant lymphomas in children. Acta Paediatr. Scand., *63*:673–678.

Glatstein, E., Kim, H., Donaldson, S. S., et al. 1974. Non-Hodgkin's lymphoma (IV). Cancer, *34*:204–211.

Goldman, N. C., and Hardcastle, B. 1969. Fibroma of the parapharyngeal space. Laryngoscope, *80*:1809–1815.

Grosfeld, J. L., Clatworthy, H. W., and Newton, W. A. 1969. Combined therapy in childhood rhabdomyosarcoma: An analysis of 42 cases. J. Pediatr. Surg., *4*(6): 637–645.

Gross, R. E., Farber, S., and Martin, L. W. 1959. Neuroblastoma sympatheticum: A study and report of 217 cases. Pediatrics, *23*(6):1179–1191.

Harness, J. K., Thompson, N. W., and Nishiyama, R. H. 1971. Childhood thyroid carcinoma. Arch. Surg., *102*:278–284.

Harris, M. N., Roses, D. F., Culliford, D. A., et al. 1925. Melanoma of the head and neck. Ann. Surg., *82*(1):86–91.

Harrison, J., Myers, J., Rowen, M., et al. 1974. Results of combination chemotherapy surgery and radiotherapy in children with neuroblastoma. Cancer, *34*(3):485–490.

Hayek, A., and Stanbury, J. B. 1971. The diagnostic use of radionuclides in the thyroid disorders of childhood. Semin. Nucl. Med., *1*(3):334–344.

Hays, D. M., Mirabal, V. Q., Karlan, M. S., et al. 1970. Fibrosarcoma in infants and children. J. Pediatr. Surg., *5*(2):176–183.

Hays, D. M. 1975. The staging of Hodgkin's disease in children reviewed. Cancer, *35*(Suppl.):973–978.

Helson, L., Fleisher, M., Bethune, V., et al. 1972. Urinary cystathionine, catecholamine, and metabolites in patients with neuroblastoma. Clin. Chem., *18*(7):613–615.

Hellriegel, W. 1963. Radiation therapy of primary and metastatic melanoma. Ann. NY Acad. Sci., *100*:131–141.

Heyn, R. M., Holland,, R., Newton, W. A., et al. 1974. The role of combined chemotherapy in the treatment of rhabdomyosarcoma in children. Cancer, *34*:2128–2142.

Holton, C. P., Chapman, K. E., Lackey, R. W., et al. 1973. Extended combination therapy of childhood rhabdomyosarcoma. Cancer, *32*:1310–1316.

Horn, R. C., and Enterline, H. T. 1958. Rhabdomyosarcoma: A clinicopathological study and classification of 39 cases. Cancer, *11*:181–199.

Horn, R. C., Koop, C. E., and Kiesewetter, W. B. 1956. Neuroblastoma in childhood. Lab. Invest., *5*:106–119.

Hornback, N. B., and Shidnia, H. 1976. Rhadomyosarcoma in the pediatric age group. Am. J. Roentgenol., *126*(3):542–549.

Hyams, V. 1977. Personal communication.

Jaffe, N., Filler, R. M., Farber, S., et al. 1973. Rhabdomyosarcoma in children: Improved outlook with a multidisciplinary approach. Am. J. Surg., 125:482–487.

Jaffe, B. F., and Jaffe, N. 1973. Head and neck cancer in children. Pediatrics, 51(4):731–740.

Jenkin, R. D. T., Brown, T. C., Peters, M. V., et al. 1975. Hodgkin's disease in children. Cancer, 35(Suppl.): 979–990.

Jones, B., and Klingberg, W. G. 1963. Lymphosarcoma in children. J. Pediatr., 63:11–20.

Kauffman, S. L., and Stout, A. P. 1960. Hemangiopericytoma in children. Cancer, 13(4):695–710.

Kauffman, S. L., and Stout, A. P. 1958. Malignant hemangioendothelioma in infants and children. Cancer, 11(6):1186–1196.

Kilman, J. W., Clatworthy, H. W., Newton, W. A., et al. 1973. Reasonable surgery for rhabdomyosarcoma: A study of 67 cases. Ann. Surg., 178(3):346–351.

Knutson, C. O., Hori, J. M., and Watson, F. R. 1972. Melanoma of the head and neck: A review of 87 cases. Am. J. Surg., 124:543–550.

Kolygin, B. A., and Fedoreeu, G. A. 1976. Exploratory laparotomy and splenectomy in the diagnosis of Hodgkin's disease. J. Surg. Oncol., 8:345–349.

Lerman, R. I., Murray, D., O'Hara, J. M., et al. 1970. Malignant melanoma of childhood: A clinicopathologic study and a report of 12 cases. Cancer, 2436–449.

Lukes, R. J., Craver, L. F., Hall, T. C., et al. 1966. Report of the nomenclature committee. Cancer Res., 26(1):1311.

Mahour, G. H., Soule, E. H., Mills, S. D., et al. 1967. Rhabdomyosarcoma in infants and children: A clinicopathologic study of 75 cases. J. Pediatr. Surg., 2(5):402–409.

Malpas, J. S., Freeman, J. E., Paxton, A., et al. 1976. Radiotherapy and adjuvant combination chemotherapy for childhood rhabdomyosarcoma. Br. Med. J., 1:247–249.

Masson, J. K., and Soule, E. H. 1965. Embryonal rhabdomyosarcoma of the head and neck: Report on 88 cases. Am. J. Surg., 110:585–591.

McMaster, M. J., Soule, E. H., and Ivins, J. C. 1975. Hemangiopericytoma: A clinicopathologic study and long-term followup of 60 patients. Cancer, 36:2232–2244.

Miller, R. W., and Dalager, N. A. 1974. Fatal rhabdomyosarcoma among children in the United States. Cancer, 34:1897–1900.

Moore, C. 1958. Visceral squamous cancer in children. Pediatrics, 21:573–581.

Murphy, S. B., Frizzera, G., and Evans, A. E. 1975. A study of childhood non-Hodgkin's lymphoma. Cancer, 36:2121–2131.

Norris, D. G., Burgert, E. O., Cooper, H. A., et al. 1975. Hodgkin's disease in children. Cancer, 36:2109–2120.

Olbourne, N. A., and Harrison, S. H. 1974. Malignant melanoma of childhood. Br. J. Plast. Surg., 27:305–317.

Parker, B. R., Castellino, R. A., and Kaplan, H. S. 1976. Pediatric Hodgkin's disease (I). Cancer, 37:2430–2435.

Pinkel, D., Pratt, C., Holton, C., et al. 1968. Survival of children with neuroblastoma treated with combination chemotherapy. J. Pediatr., 73(6):928–931.

Pitcock, J. A., Bauer, W. C., and McGavran, M. H. 1959. Hodgkin's disease in children. Cancer, 12:1043–1051.

Pratt, C. B. 1969. Response of childhood rhabdomyosarcoma to combination chemotherapy. J. Pediatr., 74(5):791–794.

Rosenberg, S. A., Diamond, H. D., Dargeon, H. W., et al.

1958. Lymphosarcoma in childhood. N. Engl. J. Med., 259:505–512.

Schnitzer, B., Nishiyama, R. H., Heidelberger, K. P., et al. 1973. Hodgkin's disease in children. Cancer, 31:560–567.

Sessions, D. G.., Ragab, A., Vietti, T. J., et al. 1973. Embryonal rhabdomyosarcoma of the head and neck in children. Laryngoscope, 83:890–897.

Shanon, E., Samuel, Y., Adler, A., et al. 1976. Malignant melanoma of the head and neck in children. Arch. Otolaryngol., 102:244–247.

Simons, J. N. 1972. Malignant melanoma of the head and neck. Am. J. Surg., 124:485–488.

Southwick, H. W. 1976. Malignant melanoma: Role of node dissection reappraised. Cancer, 37:202–205.

Spitz, S. 1948. Melanomas of childhood. Am. J. Pathol., 24:591–609.

Stout, A. P. 1943. Hemangioendothelioma: Tumor of blood vessels featuring endothelial cells. Ann. Surg., 118:445–464.

Stout, A. P. 1962. Fibrosarcoma in infants and children. Cancer, 15:1028–1040.

Sull, W. J., and Brown, H. W. 1972. Malignant hemangioendothelioma. Int. Surg., 57(5):417–421.

Sullivan, M. P. 1962. Leukemic transformation in lymphosarcoma in children. Pediatrics, 29:589–599.

Sutow, W. W. 1958. Prognosis in neurobastoma of childhood. Am. J. Dis. Child., 96:299–305.

Sutow, W. W. 1964. Cancer of the head and neck in children. J.A.M.A., 190(5):414–416.

Swain, R. E., Sessions, D. G., and Ogura, J. H. 1974. Fibrosarcoma of the head and neck: A clinical analysis of 40 cases. Ann. Otol. Rhinol. Laryngol., 83:439–443.

Swain, R. E., Sessions, D. G., and Ogura, J. H. 1976. Fibrosarcoma of the head and neck in children. Laryngoscope, 86(1):113–116.

Tan, C., D'Angio, G. J., Exelby, P. R., et al. 1975. The changing management of childhood Hodgkin's disease. Cancer, 35:808–816.

Thurman, W. G., Fernbach, D. J., and Sullivan, M. P. 1964. Cyclophosphamide therapy in childhood neuroblastoma. N. Engl. J. Med., 270(25):1336–1340.

Trozak, D. J., Rowland, W. D., and Hu, F. 1975. Metastatic malignant melanoma in prepubertal children. Pediatrics, 55:191–204.

Voorhess, M. L., and Gardner, L. I. 1962. Studies of catecholamine excretion by children with neural tumors. J. Clin. Endocrinol. Metab., 22:126–133.

Walike, J. W., and Bailey, B. J. 1971. Head and neck hemangiopericytoma. Arch. Otolaryngol., 93:345–353.

Winship, T., and Rosvoll, R. V. 1970. Thyroid carcinoma in childhood: Final report on a 20 year study. Clin. Proc. Children's Hosp. (Washington, D.C.), 26(11):327–348.

Wollner, N. 1976. Non-Hodgkin's lymphoma in children. Pediatr. Clin. North Am., 23(2):371–378.

Wollner, N., Burchenal, J. H., Lieberman, P. H., et al. 1975. Non-Hodgkin's lymphoma in children. Med. Pediatr. Oncol., 1:235–263.

Wollner, N., Burchenal, J. H., Lieberman, P. H., et al. 1976. Non-Hodgkin's lymphoma in children. Cancer, 37:123–134.

Young, R. C., DeVita, Y. T., and Johnson, R. E. 1973. Hodgkin's disease in children. Blood, 42:163–174.

Young, L. W., Rubin, P., and Hanson, R. E. 1970. The extra-adrenal neuroblastoma: High radiocurability and diagnostic accuracy. Am. J. Roentgenol., 108(1):75–91.

Section VII

COMMUNICATION DISORDERS

Chapter 82

ANATOMY AND PHYSIOLOGY OF SPEECH

Stewart R. Rood, Ph.D.

INTRODUCTION

Speech is the most complex behavior of humans; it distinguishes them from other primates. The acoustic properties of human speech, or vocal communication, are directly related to various structural parameters of the vocal tract. The development in humans of a diversity of speech sounds is the result of maturation of the speech mechanism from birth to puberty. This chapter seeks to provide knowledge that will give the reader an understanding of the structures that underlie mature verbal communication by examining three components of the vocal tract: (1) the subglottic component (the tracheobronchial tree and pulmonary system); (2) the glottic component (activity at the level of the vocal cords); and (3) the supraglottic component (the hypopharynx, oropharynx, nasopharynx, and oral and nasal cavities).

An overview of the relationship between speech and the vocal tract is presented. Lastly, some comments and thoughts on the physiologic basis of language are discussed.

THE SUBGLOTTIC COMPONENT OF THE VOCAL TRACT

Phonation and respiration are performed by the same subglottic structures. Historically, respiration has been deemed the primary function, whereas phonation has been termed the "overlaid function," but this is, at the least, a gross oversimplification. Respiration and phonation, although subserved by the same structures, make use of these struc-

tures in different ways. The goal of this section is to describe alterations in respiration that occur during phonation and to identify the relationship between language and changes in the breathing pattern.

Respiration is a complex function that is performed and controlled by several mechanisms — nervous, chemical, muscular, and air pressure. Although the primary stimulus in the regulation of the respiratory cycle is chemical (blood levels of CO_2), this is certainly not the only factor (Lenneberg, 1967). As CO_2 concentration in the blood increases, activation of the inhalation center results in stimulation of the muscles of inhalation, which leads to expansion of the thoracic cavity. Associated with this expansion is a decrease in intrathoracic air pressure. When the air pressure within the thorax falls below that of the atmosphere, air flows into the lungs (Boone, 1971). Airflow ceases as intrapulmonary and extrapulmonary pressures are equalized. As CO_2 blood levels continue to rise, it is felt that an exhalation center is activated, which inhibits the actions of the inhalation center. The muscles of inhalation are relaxed, and air (along with CO_2) is expelled from the lungs by simple elastic recoil of the thoracic cage (Lenneberg, 1967; Lieberman, 1977). The muscles of exhalation are not activated during quiet breathing but are stimulated under specific conditions, such as speech, exercise, and singing. The average adult completes between 13 and 18 respiratory cycles per minute, depending upon physiologic requirements, but the respiration rate also varies with age. It is 40 to 70 cycles per minute at birth, at 5 years of age it is 25

1441

cycles per minute, at 15 years of age it is 20 cycles per minute, and at 30 years of age it is 13 to 18 cycles per minute (Boone, 1971). During quiet breathing, the inhalation phase is more shallow and slightly shorter in duration than the exhalation phase.

The pattern of breathing during quiet (i.e., nonspeech) respiration is altered significantly during speech. In general, the inhalation-exhalation time relationship is changed so that the inhalation is fast and deep and the exhalation is prolonged, with the ratio of inhalation to exhalation changing from 1:2 to 1:20. Thus, respiration is subject not only to reflexive, brain stem control during quiet breathing but also to cortical control during purposeful breathing as in speech, singing, or exercise. Vocal behavior and breathing coexist in a complex, integrative pattern in which the lower respiratory centers and various cortical centers simultaneously influence (regulate) the respiratory cycle (Lenneberg, 1967; DeuPree, 1971).

In considering the chemical stimulus of respiration (Pco_2) according to Lenneberg (1967), "... it is likely that at the beginning of an utterance, CO_2 is retained somewhat longer than during quiet breathing, or as toward the end, when active exhalation takes place, CO_2 is expelled faster than ordinarily." It is obvious, however, that in speaking, humans can tolerate levels of CO_2 that are above the limit of the "normal" range for short periods of time. Since respiration is important to satisfy metabolic requirements, there must be a "controller mechanism" to regulate air exchange during speech (Lenneberg, 1967).

During quiet breathing, the air pressure applied to the vocal folds (subglottal pressure) changes with the changing volume of air in the lungs. During speech, however, subglottal air pressure must remain relatively stable throughout the linguistic unit, whether that be a prolonged phoneme, syllable, or word, until the end when it falls abruptly (Fig. 82–1). To accomplish this, precise coordination between muscles of inhalation and exhalation is prerequisite. During quiet breathing, at the end of the inspiratory phase, the muscles of inhalation suddenly relax, and the elastic recoil inherent within the now-expanded thoracic cage initiates and maintains an uneven, outward flow of air. According to Boone (1971), "It may well be at the peak of inhalation that the normal elastic-

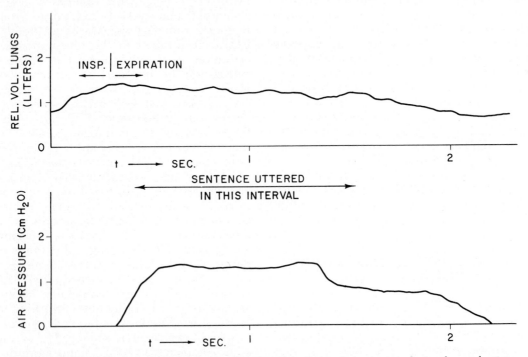

Figure 82–1 The relative volume of air in the lungs and subglottal air pressure during the production of a short sentence. Note the shortened inhalatory phase versus the prolonged exhalatory phase. Also note the maintenance of a relatively stable subglottal pressure throughout the production of the sentence, except at the end of the sentence where the pressure begins to fall. (After Lieberman, P. 1967. Intonation, Perception, and Language. Cambridge, Mass., MIT Press.)

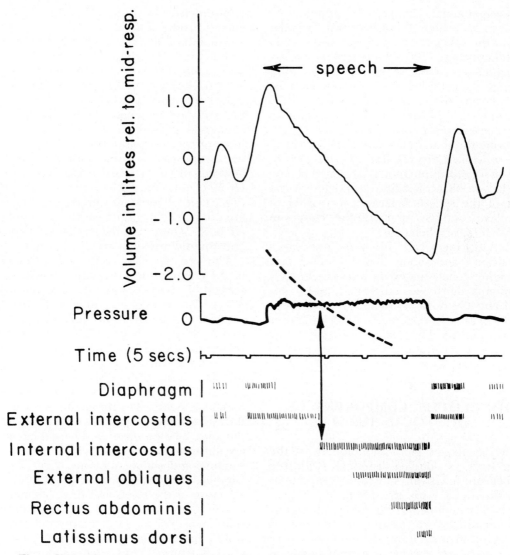

Figure 82–2 The upper two graphs illustrate the relationship between the volume of air in the lungs and subglottal pressure during speech production. Again, note the stable subglottal air pressure maintained throughout the speech act. The dashed line superimposed upon the pressure record represents the effects of simple elastic recoil in exhalation. When the dashed line crosses the subglottal pressure graph, elastic recoil is no longer sufficient to maintain an adequate subglottal pressure for speech. Note that the muscles of exhalation are activated at this point to reestablish the requisite subglottal pressure. (After Ladefoged, P. 1967. Three Areas of Experimental Phonetics. London, Oxford University Press.)

ity of the lungs is sufficient to produce enough subglottal pressure to set the cords to vibrate." However, two conditions must be satisfied during speech: A stable subglottal pressure must be maintained, and the duration of the exhalatory phase must be prolonged at a steady rate of airflow. The elastic recoil mechanism is counteracted by the continued activity of the muscles of inhalation, which at some point in phonation must relax. This point may be when the force of elastic recoil alone is insufficient to maintain a threshold subglottal pressure. Various muscles of exhalation are progressively brought into activity in order to maintain adequate subglottal pressure and to extend exhalation beyond the normal tidal capacity (Boone, 1971). Figure 82–2 illustrates the timing pattern of the various muscles active during speech. They function through an intricate network of intrathoracic pressure receptors and an extensive distribution of muscle spindles throughout the intercostal muscles (Lieberman, 1977).

Developmental changes, in addition to those of growth, are observed in the regulation of the subglottal component of the vocal tract. Lenneberg (1967) wrote that the facility to maintain a stable subglottal air pressure through the complex patterning of the muscles of inhalation and exhalation is "fully developed by the time an infant begins to babble in utterances of multisyllables, roughly during the sixth or seventh month of life." The control of the respiratory cycle to provide energy for phonation is a learned behavior that, in all probability, is initiated at the start of the speech behavior, increasing in complexity and precision with the changes in overall linguistic behavior.

Thus, during speech, breathing undergoes significant alteration. The number of inhalation-exhalation cycles will decrease; inhalation is shortened, quickened, and deepened and the duration of exhalation is prolonged with the respiratory muscles under precise control. The changes observed during speech respiration are independent of any given language.

THE GLOTTIC COMPONENT OF THE VOCAL TRACT

The larynx, or glottic component of the vocal tract, is coupled inferiorly with the trachea and lungs (the subglottic component) and superiorly with the pharynx (the supraglottic component). Physiologically significant anatomic features and the function of the larynx in phonation will be discussed in this section, and various aspects of postnatal laryngeal development will be presented that relate specifically to the role of the larynx in speech production.

The infant, like the adult, must adduct his or her vocal cords in order to initiate phonation. Thus, the larynx is the source of the acoustic energy that is characteristic of all classes of phonatory behavior, from the infant's cry to the singer's aria. The larynx is composed of several cartilages (Fig. 82–3) interconnected by an intricate system of ligaments, muscles, and membranes. The basic anatomy of the larynx is presented in Chapter 59 of this text, but two features that have important physiologic significance and that are often described incorrectly are highlighted here. These are the cricoarytenoid and cricothyroid articulations.

The articular facet of the cricoid member of the cricothyroid articulation has been described as round, oval, or irregular (Fig. 82–4). The facets on the inferior cornu of the thyroid member of the articulation are usually flat, although they have been reported to be concave or convex. Corresponding sets of facets lie in the same plane, and they are directed posterolaterally and inclined inferiorly. The motion of the cricothyroid articulation is dependent upon the geometry of the facets and the ligaments distributed about the joint. The posterior and lateral ligaments are illustrated in Figure 82–5. Although both rotatory and sliding motions have been attributed to the cricothyroid articulation, the structure of the facets and their ligamentous distribution would negate any sliding motion, since, in order to "slide," the thyroid cartilage would have to be disarticulated from the cricoid cartilage. Thus, rotatory motion about an axis placed horizontally through the cri-

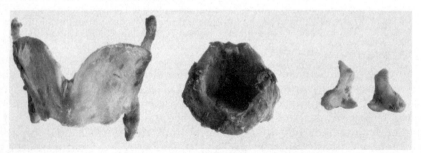

Figure 82–3   The cartilages of an adult larynx. From left to right, the thyroid, cricoid, and paired arytenoid cartilages.

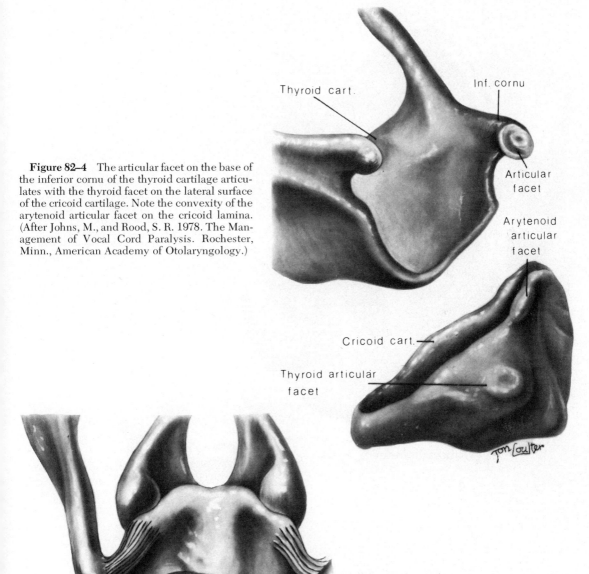

Figure 82–4 The articular facet on the base of the inferior cornu of the thyroid cartilage articulates with the thyroid facet on the lateral surface of the cricoid cartilage. Note the convexity of the arytenoid articular facet on the cricoid lamina. (After Johns, M., and Rood, S. R. 1978. The Management of Vocal Cord Paralysis. Rochester, Minn., American Academy of Otolaryngology.)

Figure 82–5 The distribution of the posterior, anterior, and lateral cricothyroid ligaments. These ligaments limit motion at the cricothyroid joints to a rotatory one. (After Johns, M., and Rood, S. R. 1978. The Management of Vocal Cord Paralysis. Rochester, Minn. American Academy of Otolaryngology.)

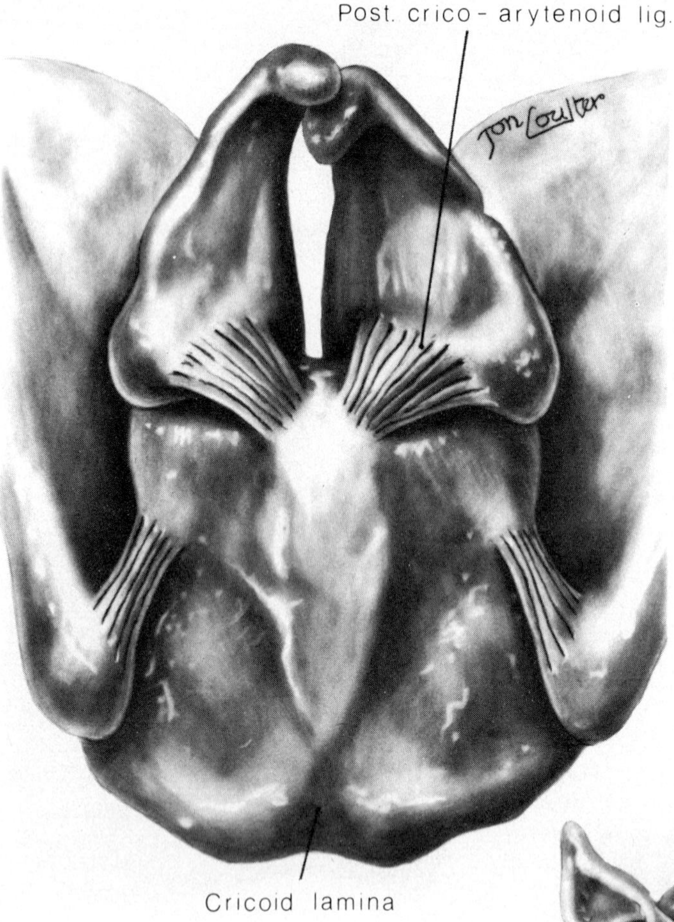

Post. crico - arytenoid lig.

Figure 82–6 The placement of the posterior cricoarytenoid ligament. The motion at the cricoarytenoid articulation is limited by the ligament. (After Johns M., and Rood, S. R. 1978. The Management of Vocal Cord Paralysis. Rochester, Minn. American Academy of Otolaryngology.)

Cricoid lamina

Arytenoid cartilages in abduction

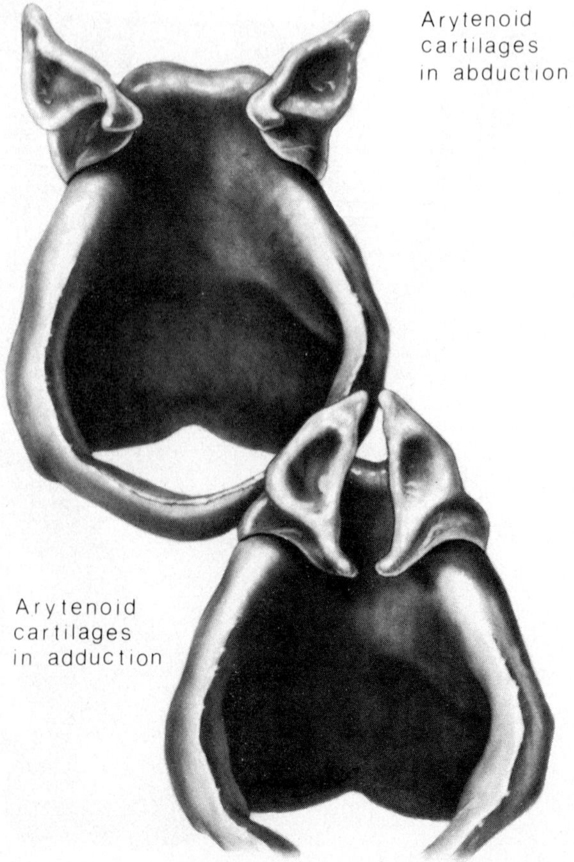

Figure 82–7 The relative positions of the arytenoid cartilages on the cricoid lamina in abduction (top) and adduction (bottom). The arytenoids rock anteriorly to posteriorly on the cricoid lamina to alter vocal cord position. (After Johns, M, and Rood, S. R. 1978. The Management of Vocal Cord Paralysis. Rochester, Minn., American Academy of Otolaryngology.)

Arytenoid cartilages in adduction

cothyroid joint has been described as the only likely motion of this articulation (Maue-Dickson, 1970).

With reference to the cricoarytenoid articulation, the facet on the base of the muscular process of the arytenoid cartilage is described as concave, whereas its fellow on the posterolateral aspect of the cricoid lamina is relatively convex. Maue-Dickson (1970) reported that the cricoid facet is relatively flat along its major axis and convex around it. The arytenoid facet is flat along the corresponding axis and concave around it. Von Leden and Moore (1961) described the distribution of the posterior cricoarytenoid ligaments as illustrated in Figure 82–6. Two axes of motion at the cricoarytenoid joint have been described: The traditional motion shown in many standard anatomy, physiology, and otolaryngology texts is a rotatory motion about the vertical axis through the arytenoid cartilage from apex to base. The second is a rocking motion about the long axis of the articular facet on the cricoid lamina. Maue-Dickson (1970) wrote:

Because of the inclination and angulation of the cricoid facet, rocking motion alone is sufficient to account for approximation of the vocal processes of the arytenoid ... The distance of the vocal processes from their axis of rotation provides the leverage necessary for adduction of the vocal folds.

The gliding motion that has been attributed to the cricoarytenoid joint is minimized by modern investigators. Thus, the inferior and medial rocking motion of the arytenoid, as shown in Figure 82–7, is considered to account for the adduction-abduction movements of the vocal folds (Ardran and Kemp, 1967).

Although the vocal folds are abducted in quiet inhalation, during the inhalatory phase of "speech" breathing the folds are moved more laterally so as to enable a greater volume of air to pass through the glottis. The vocal folds are adducted, and exhalation begins.

Sound production by the vocal folds is a complex function. Much of the pertinent physiologic data available today were published by Müller in the mid-19th century. Müller simulated normal laryngeal physiologic movement in excised human larynges by attaching strings to the cartilages and then manipulating the strings to mimic the forces acting on the cartilages by various muscles of the larynx. He supplied energy to the system by blowing air through the larynges. Van den Berg (1958) replicated Müller's initial work and, based on these experiments, proposed his myoelastic–aerodynamic theory in an attempt to explain the generation of an acoustic signal by the vocal cords. A schematic, coronal view of the larynx is illustrated in Figure 82–8. The force that is applied to the inferior surface of the fold (subglottal pressure) by air forcibly exhaled from the lungs is labeled A. This force would tend to move the previously adducted vocal folds apart but is counteracted by a force produced by muscle contraction (M) acting to stabilize the vocal folds in a horizontal, apposed position (Fig. 82–8).

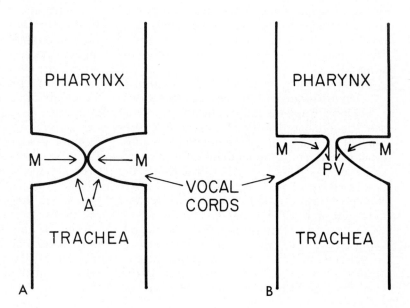

Figure 82–8 *A*, A schematic, coronal section of larynx illustrating the forces active in maintaining cord adduction (M) during the buildup of subglottal pressure (A). *B*, Once the medial edges of the cords are "blown apart," the forces acting on them to resume their opposed position are a pressure effect (PV) and the elastic properties inherent in contracted muscles (M).

When the subglottal pressure (A) becomes greater than M, the folds are blown apart momentarily. The velocity of air flowing through the narrowed glottis (as compared to the velocity of air passing through the wide glottis during nonspeech respiration) is accelerated, producing a partial vacuum (PV) between the medial edges of the vocal folds, which is known as the Bernoulli effect. The edges of the separated cords are "sucked" down and together as a result of this activity. When the cords are blown apart, the medial aspects are spring-loaded (much like a stretched rubber band), and when the increased subglottal pressure (A) is released, the cords tend to resume their previous horizontal position. Thus, once blown apart, the vocal folds will return to their horizontal-apposed position owing to the interaction between PV and M (Kirchner, 1970; Lieberman, 1977). The process repeats itself when the subglottal pressure (A) again becomes greater than M. The cyclical up and down motion of the edge of the vocal cords produces an acoustic signal. It may be seen from this description of phonation that it is dependent upon the interaction of aerodynamic, aerostatic, and muscular forces.

Of prime importance to the efficiency of a vibrating vocal fold system is its ability to sustain undamped movement. If the folds come into contact with any tissue, the limitations imposed upon voice production are significant. According to Ardran and Kemp (1967), " . . . in our view, the laryngeal ventricles are essential to allow the vocal cords to vibrate freely during phonation, undamped by the vestibular false vocal folds." Any tissue that adds mass to the vocal folds (such as a lesion or nodule) or that interferes with their free vibration will produce alterations in voice.

The frequency at which the undamped vocal folds vibrate under "normal" conditions is labeled a fundamental frequency (f_0). This acoustic signal is identified by a listener as the pitch of the voice. The fundamental frequency, hence pitch, is dependent upon several variables: vocal fold length, vocal fold tension, airflow, and subglottal pressure changes. However, the reader must realize that, although these variables are discussed separately, their actual operation within the living larynx involves a complex interaction. In general, most investigators (Hollien and Moore, 1960; Negus, 1962; Kirschner, 1970) have described the relationship between in-creasing anterior–posterior length of the folds and increasing f_0. Grossly, increased vocal fold length is the result of thyroid cartilage rotation about the cricothyroid articulation, accomplished by the action of the cricothyroid muscle. Simultaneously with cricothyroid activity, the lateral cricoarytenoid muscles act to maintain the vocal folds' adducted position (Hardcastle, 1976). Thus, as the folds are elongated, the mass of the vibrating cords is reduced and, therefore, the rapidity with which they can vibrate increases. The second variable operating in fundamental frequency shifts is change in the tension of the thyroarytenoid and vocalis muscles. These muscles are capable of both isotonic and isometric contraction. During the development of isotonic tension, the vocal folds will shorten and thicken, resulting in a slower vibratory pattern and thus a lower f_0. However, if the tension developed in the muscular areas of the vocal folds is isometric, the folds become more taut and rigid, raising the f_0. The rapidity of airflow through the glottis is dependent upon subglottal pressure, and an interaction between subglottal pressure and vocal fold tension appears to exist. Hardcastle (1976) writes:

> When the cords are under isometric tension, a greater subglottal pressure is required to force them apart than when they are relaxed and loose. The greater subglottal pressure will cause an increased rate of airflow through the glottis, thus tending to raise the f_0 and also the intensity of the resulting phonation.

The relative contributions of airflow (subglottal pressure) and vocal fold tension to pitch change vary somewhat with pitch range. In the normal pitch range, both airflow and vocal fold tension control changes in f_0, but at higher pitches the primary mechanism is glottal airflow change, since the vocal folds are already under near-maximum tension. Two additional mechanisms may be functional in pitch change. First, as the pitch continues to rise to approach, but not quite to reach, falsetto, the posterior portion of the vocal folds becomes compressed by the apposed processes of the arytenoid cartilages, and the vibratory area of the folds is shifted anteriorly. Second, there is some evidence to support the thesis that laryngeal tension may also be altered by the contraction of the extrinsic musculature of the larynx. In elevating the thyroid cartilage, vocal fold tension is increased; in depressing the thyroid cartilage toward the cricoid, muscle tension is decreased. Both mechanisms may aid in the production of pitch variations.

In addition to pitch alterations, intensity variations are also an important feature of vocal behavior. Vocal intensities are controlled by changes in laryngeal adductor muscle contractions, which produce changes in glottal resistance and exhalatory force. Increased glottal resistance tends to reduce airflow rates, leading to a reduction in intensity; but given a constant glottal resistance, increased exhalatory force increases the subglottal pressure and airflow rate, thereby raising the intensity of the voice.

Descriptions of the anatomy and physiology of the larynx usually pertain to its adult form, but most functional mechanisms discussed also apply to the immature larynx. Since a neonate is incapable of exercising as precise a control over the larynx as is the adult, the range of his or her vocal output is less, and the changes made are grosser, but the mechanisms of phonation, pitch, and intensity are the same as in the adult.

The structure of the immature larynx is significantly different from that of the mature organ, however; it is not merely a "small adult larynx" but differs from the developed larynx in its shape, relative size, and position in the neck.

The neonatal larynx is approximately 2.0 cm in length (Crelin, 1973) and about the same at its maximum width (the superior aspect of the thyroid cartilage). According to Negus (1962), the larynx is only slightly wider than the lumen of the trachea. The larynx at birth is funnel-shaped (Gedgowd, 1900; Eckenhoff, 1951; Kirschner, 1970), as a result of the posterior tilt of the superior aspect of the lamina of the cricoid cartilage. Eckenhoff (1951) refers to the work of Bayeux, who in the late 19th century reported that "the circumference of the cricoid ring was narrower than that of the trachea or the glottis." The inferiorly directed, funnel-shaped appearance of the lumen gradually diminishes with growth owing to the widening of the cricoid ring and the assumption of a more vertical position of the cricoid lamina. However, Klock (1968) stated that a lateral funnel shape is maintained through puberty.

At birth, the larynx's posterior tilt is such that the subglottic tube extends inferiorly and posteriorly. This angle between the larynx and the trachea is important to keep in mind when intubating an infant for anesthesia. During development, the larynx assumes a straighter, more vertical position, in direct line with the trachea, becoming more angled in relation to the oral and nasal cavities (Negus, 1962; Kirchner, 1970; Crelin, 1973).

The growth of the larynx can be divided into three periods: (1) birth to 3 years of age, (2) 3 years of age to puberty, and (3) puberty. During the first and third periods, the organ undergoes rapid and significant growth, whereas during the second period growth is slow. One of the major changes to occur during development is the expansion of the chamber or internal volume of the larynx. This is attained primarily by the growth and alteration in shape of the major laryngeal cartilages (Figs. 82–9A and 82–9B). As illustrated in Figure 82–10A, the thyroid cartilage in the infant (male and female) is best described as a gradually curving semicircle. The thyroid laminae meet anteriorly at an angle of about 130 degrees (Gedgowd, 1900). With increasing age, the junction angle becomes more acute. By puberty (Fig. 82–10B) the angle has decreased in males (Negus, 1962; Kahane, 1978) and females. The superior and inferior cornua of the cartilage elongate, resulting in a drop of the thyroid laminae from the hyoid bone. The cricoid cartilage at birth is generally the same semioval shape as it is in the adult. The major change that occurs, in addition to overall enlargement, is the movement of the cricoid lamina to a more vertical position, as discussed previously. Generally, the thyroid cartilage enlarges to a greater degree than the cricoid. The arytenoid cartilages undergo little enlargement but change in shape, becoming more mobile coincident with the alteration in their form (Bosma, 1975). Another change is the reduction in the thickness of the submucosa that overlies the minor cartilages, which results in a further increase in the internal volume of the larynx.

The vocal cords are about 3 mm in length at birth, and approximately half of the cord is cartilaginous (vocal process of the arytenoid). Because of the position of the arytenoid cartilage, the neonatal cords are somewhat concave in appearance from above. The cords elongate rapidly during infancy, almost doubling in length by the end of the first year (Kirchner, 1970). No sex differences are noted in the growth rate or absolute length of the cords through the prepubertal period (Klock, 1968; Kahane, 1978), but there is a sudden acceleration in vocal cord length in the pubescent male that is responsible for the

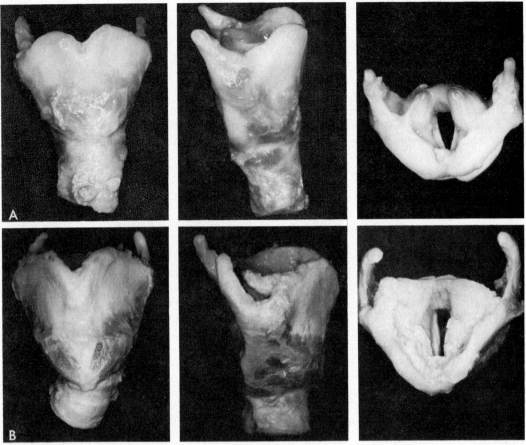

Figure 82–9 Several views of a newborn human larynx (A) and an adult human larynx (B). Note particularly the difference in shape of the thyroid cartilage.

breaks in pitch in adolescent male voices. Adult male vocal cords are 17 to 23 mm in length, and those of the adult female are 12.5 to 17 mm in length. The infantile concavity of the cords lessens with age, owing in part to the stretching of the cords by the anterior inclination of the thyroid cartilage and the somewhat reduced extension of the vocal processes into the cords.

Of the major developmental changes that affect the larynx and are significant for speech (increased mobility of the arytenoids, increased length of the cords, and pitch changes), the most important is the descent of the larynx in the neck. This is a distinctly human event that may be related to the phonation and articulation requirements imposed upon the supraglottic component of the vocal tract by speech (Bosma, 1975). At birth, the inferior margin of the cricoid cartilage lies opposite the third cervical vertebra, while by maturity the lower border of the larynx has descended to lie opposite the seventh cervical vertebra (Noback, 1923).

Negus (1962) wrote that the descent of the larynx is a result of "the alternation of the vertebro-occipital and pituitary angles, together with a downward movement of the tongue into the pharynx."

The descent of the larynx from the nasopharynx and the movement of the larynx to a position that forms an acute angle with the oral cavity makes the adult larynx a less efficient respiratory organ than that of the infant. This adult positioning lessens the volume of air that can traverse a more vertical tube of similar diameter. The position of the larynx in other mammals and in human infants allows for respiration during prolonged feeding. This ability is lost in adults, but elongation of the supraglottic pharynx allows for the development of a large tongue, necessary for humans' articulatory behavior, and an extended resonating cavity, essential for phonation. Thus, some advantages are lost while others are gained during development of the larynx and related areas of the neck from birth to puberty.

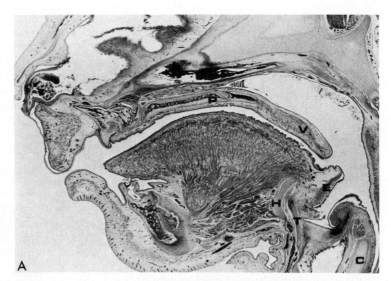

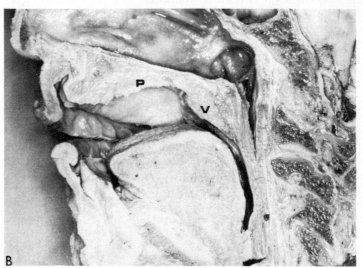

Figure 82–10 A photomicrograph of a sagittal section through the oral cavity of a 20 week old human fetus is shown in A. The tongue at this stage, as in the newborn, rests entirely within the oral cavity; the larynx is high in the neck, so that the epiglottis and velum are capable of apposition. A photograph of a sagittally sectioned human adult cadaver head is shown in B. The tongue has altered its position at this stage. Its anterior two thirds lies within the oral cavity, while its posterior third has descended within the neck to form the anterior wall of the pharynx just below the oral cavity. The larynx has also descended within the neck. P, osseous palate; V, velum; H, hyoid bone; T, thyroid cartilage; E, epiglottis; C, cricoid cartilage.

THE SUPRAGLOTTIC COMPONENT OF THE VOCAL TRACT

The supralaryngeal or supraglottic vocal tract is composed of the pharynx, the oral cavity with its mobile inclusions, and the nasal cavity. These components are illustrated in Figure 82–10.

This part of the vocal tract plays an important role in the production of human speech. According to Lieberman et al. (1972):

Human speech essentially involves the generation of sound by the mechanisms of vocal cord vibration and/or air turbulence, and the acoustic shaping of these sounds by the resonances of the supralaryngeal vocal tract. The shape of the human supralaryngeal vocal tract continually changes during the production of speech.

The newborn upper pharynx is incapable of accomplishing the myriad intricate changes in form that are requisite to the production of speech. Thus, Crelin (1973) wrote that ". . . the development of the pharynx after birth . . . is necessary for the production of the articulate speech of language." This section will discuss the speech-related function of this portion of the vocal tract and the developmental changes specific to the supraglottic area that are fundamental to the maturation of speech behavior.

The importance of the supraglottic vocal tract for the production of speech rests in its being a hollow cylinder capable of continuous alteration in its shape. The primary speech function attributed to this area is that of resonance. Resonance is a phenomenon in which a system oscillates with greatest amplitude for applied frequencies at or near its own natural frequency. The resonant frequency of a system is the frequency at which the maximum response occurs. A column of air, much like the vocal tract, has several or many different resonant frequencies. The vocal tract, or any tube closed at one end and open at the other and consisting of a constant cross-sectional area along its length, has regularly spaced resonant frequencies. When the cross-sectional area varies, however, the resonant frequencies are no longer exact multiples of the first resonant frequency but are irregularly spaced. This latter model represents the pharynx, (including the endolarynx), the cross-sectional area of which differs as a function of the activity of the pharyngeal constrictor muscles. The resonant frequencies produced by the walls of the supraglottic pharynx, having been set into vibration by the acoustic energy emitted at the glottis, are dependent upon the shape and length of the tube. Thus, a graphic illustration of the glottically initiated sound just prior to entry into the oral cavity is a complex wave form, the sum of a number of sinusoidal waves of different frequencies, amplitudes, and phases.

A second function of the supraglottic vocal tract is that of articulation, a subset of resonance. The processes by which the cross-sectional dimensions of the vocal tract and the coupling of various portions of the tract are altered to produce various speech sounds are together termed articulation. The mobile structures that affect the vocal tract are the velum, tongue, mandible, and lips. Three mechanisms are involved in the production of speech sounds. First, the acoustic energy generated at the larynx is altered by the changing shape of the vocal tract, which is the result of the alteration in the resonant characteristics of the tract due to movement of the lips, tongue, and velum. Second, the vocal tract is constricted at some point along its length so that the previously uninterrupted airstream emitted from the lungs during exhalation becomes turbulent as it passes through the constricted area (to produce, for instance, the sounds "sh" or "s"). Third, the airstream may be stopped momentarily and then released as in production of "p" or "b" sounds. The latter two mechanisms of sound production may be employed by the speaker with or without simultaneous glottic activity. A fourth method, the velopharyngeal function, may be invoked to alter the resonance characteristics of the vocal tract. The depression of the velum couples the nasopharynx to the more inferior portion of the pharynx, producing a tube of longer length and differing acoustic characteristics than the tube with the velum elevated.

Resonant frequencies of the vocal tract are called formant frequencies. For each configuration of the tract, i.e., for each speech sound, there is a different pattern of formant frequencies. Again, formant frequencies vary as a function of the geometric characteristics of the entire vocal tract. For example, when the velum is elevated, the primary resonances will be approximately at 500 Hz, 1500 Hz, 3500 Hz, and 4500 Hz (Denes and Pinson, 1973). When the velum is depressed, however, a more complicated tube results, one that is of greater length and greater geometric complexity. Different resonant characteristics, hence different formants, hence different speech sounds, result from the nasal cavity having been added to the system. Thus, the relationship between formant frequency–speech sound production and vocal tract configuration is direct.

In the newborn, the cylindrical pharynx, approximately 4 cm in length, extends from the cranial base to the esophagus. The superior aspect of the nasopharynx rests against the sphenoid and occipital bones and the spheno-occipital synchondrosis. Posteriorly, the pharynx lies against the cervical vertebrae. Anteriorly, the pharynx is incomplete. The nasopharynx is continuous with the choanae of the nasal cavity; the oral pharynx is open to the oral cavity. The laryngopharynx as such is absent in the newborn, as the larynx is located so high in the neck. The lack of a supralaryngeal pharynx severely limits the sound production capabilities of the newborn. The growth of the pharynx reflects alterations in the cranial base and in the vertebral and facial skeleton (Bosma and Fletcher, 1961). Throughout the first year, an increase in the anteroposterior dimension of the pharynx is observed to occur as a result of dorsal displacement due to growth at the spheno-occipital synchondrosis; ventral displacement, with reference to the vertebral column, results from growth at the facial sutures. The ventral growth of the pharynx is a function of differential growth in the craniofacial region and the superior-inferior elongation of the face. The most significant maturational change in the structure of the pharynx is the descent of the larynx in the neck (discussed previously). This gradual movement enlarges the supraglottic pharynx. In addition, the caudal movement of the larynx produces a separation between the epiglottis and the uvula so that a vocal tract with two tubes results, making an adult no longer capable of simultaneous feeding and breathing (Crelin and Netter, 1976). The elongated pharynx is also capable of greater flexibility in the alteration of its size and shape (Negus, 1962). The elongation of the pharynx and a longer supraglottic pharynx alter the acoustic signals emitted from the larynx (resonation).

The greatest changes in structures, their relationships, and their mobility occur in the oral area (Bosma, 1975). In the human newborn, the oral cavity, when the mouth is sealed, is only a potential space; the volume of the cavity is filled by the tongue and palate (Bosma and Fletcher, 1962; Crelin, 1973). As illustrated in Figure 82–10, the tongue is situated entirely within the oral cavity. The organ at this early stage is broad and short, about 4.0 cm in length and 2.5 cm wide (Crelin, 1973). Between the ages of 2 and 4 years, the tongue, owing to elongation of the face and changes in cranial base angle and dimensions, descends into the pharynx. At about 4 years of age, the posterior third of the tongue forms the anterior wall of the supralaryngeal pharyngeal cavity (Fig. 82–10). Bosma (1975) reported that "the tongue elongates apically and it becomes man's most discriminate manipulator."

A second anatomic prerequisite to the maturation of speech behavior is the descent of the hard palate from the cranial base and the subsequent increased mobility of the velum. One of the mechanisms operative in the gradual descent of the hard palate is the remodeling of the cranial base. The basicranium is flat in the newborn human, with no observable marked angulation of the basilar portion of the occipital bone anteriorly to the spheno-occipital synchrondrosis. With maturation, the angulation of the basilar portion of the occipital bone from the base anteriorly to the spheno-occipital synchrondrosis posteriorly increases, resulting in the drop of the hard palate from the cranial base (Laitman and Crelin, 1976). Another mechanism responsible for the descent of the hard palate is growth of the midface and the relative resorptive capabilities of the surfaces of the palate. Enlow (1976) states that "what used to be bony maxillary arch in the child is remodeled to become the expanded nasal region in the adult." The nasal surface of the palate is resorptive (endosteal bone), whereas the oral surface is despository (periosteal)

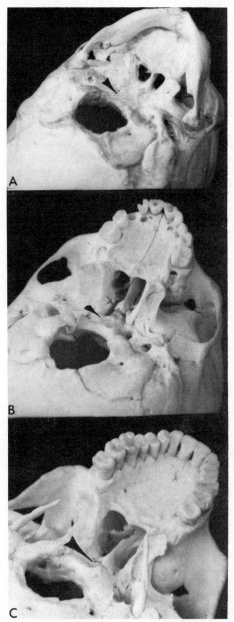

Figure 82–11   An oblique basal view of three human skulls: A, Neonate. B, 5 year old. C, Adult. The basicranium changes from relatively flat at birth to an acute angle in the adult. Also note the descent of the osseous palate from the cranial base.

bone (Enlow, 1976). The relative placement of the velum within the pharynx is controlled by the descent of the osseous palate, and, with the descent of the velum from the cranial base, changes in velar mobility are observed. The levator veli palatini muscle is merely a "tensor" of the palate in infancy, whereas in the adult the muscle becomes a true elevator. Figure 82–11 illustrates the changes in the flexion of the cranial base and the resulting descent of the palatal complex from the cranial base. With the enlargement of the oral cavity and the assumption of a more vertical orientation of the extrinsic muscles of the palate, the velum becomes capable of greater mobility cephalocaudally.

The changes just described occur independently within the same time frame. Apparently, the growth of the spaces of the pharynx, larynx, and oral cavity are not accounted for by skeletal changes. According to Bosma (1975), "these changes in the skeleton are, in turn, unexplained by the familiar mechanisms of skeletal growth and adaptation to imposed mechanical stress." These changes are necessary for the maturation of speech but are not the result of the imposed mechanical stress of speech motor activity, if one considers how delicate these motions are, even compared to the movements associated with feeding.

THE VOCAL TRACT AND SPEECH — AN OVERVIEW

Two periods are identified in the development of speech behavior: First, the appearance of primitive sound production, associated with an anatomically immature vocal tract, and second, the maturation of speech, occurring simultaneously with specific anatomic changes to the vocal tract. Speech may be viewed as an adaptation in respiratory behavior, not the simple imposition of larynx and upper pharynx activities on vegetative respiration. The same motor mechanisms that underlie elementary activities, such as swallowing, are involved in speech, although the changes imposed upon the pharynx are more discriminate in the latter function.

Human speech sounds are the result of the activities of the larynx, which serves as a source of the acoustic signal, and the supraglottic vocal tract, which serves as an acoustic filter. The descent of the larynx in the neck, resulting in an elongated supraglottic pharynx, the descent of the posterior third of the tongue to form a highly mobile anterior pharyngeal wall, and increased mobility of the palate and tongue enable a considerable range of alteration in pharyngeal and oral cavity shape. Speech sounds are the results of changes in the shape and length of the supralaryngeal vocal tract. The human infant is capable of a restricted range of sound production, whereas the adult, in the presence of the anatomic changes that have taken place, is capable of a wide range of sound production. Thus, the development of human speech as the primary vehicle for the unique capacity of humans for verbal communication is directly dependent upon changes in the subglottic, glottic, and supraglottic components of the vocal tract, which are, in themselves, peculiar to humans.

PHYSIOLOGIC BASES OF LANGUAGE

All of what is known about the organization of language within the normal human brain is based upon the study of language performance under conditions of abnormal central nervous system function: brain damage, brain surgery, drug effects on the brain, and electrical stimulation of the exposed brain. Postmortem histologic examination of brains has provided data on the exact locations of lesions. The objective of these studies is to develop a model of how the areas of the brain associated with language communicate and the contribution of each area to language behavior.

In general, according to Penfield and Roberts (1959), " . . . man has devised various means of communication, conveying ideas by means of symbols . . . Associated with the use of words or symbols, a remarkable lateralization and localization of function has appeared in the human brain." The brain at birth, although not a "tabula rasa" with the potential of attaining any arbitrary pattern of organization, may be influenced to alter its normal organization plan leading to area specialization. This is illustrated by studying those children whose central speech and language areas have been damaged early in life but go on to develop normal language function. The plasticity of the human brain decreases with age to a point at which, if a similar lesion pattern were to be created in a mature adult, he or she would evidence severe and probably irreversible speech and language dysfunction (Lenneberg, 1967). Thus, the pattern of lateralization and localization to be presented here will be that hypothesized to exist in the "normal" adult human brain.

The literature on the lateralization of language behavior offers the investigator a consistent, noncontradictory opinion (Penfield and Roberts, 1967; Geschwind, 1972). The areas of the brain concerned with both the interpretation and formulation of language, as differentiated from the motor act of speech or performance, are found within the left cerebral hemisphere regardless of handedness. Again be reminded that the mature adult is being considered here. The motor mechanisms for speech, the actual sound chain, is controlled and directed bilaterally via the pyramidal system with stimuli arising from the anterior margin of the Rolandic fissue, the motor strip.

Cortical and subcortical regions of the left cerebral hemisphere have been identified as language areas. The data here have been obtained from the postmortem study of brains of patients who had suffered from a well-defined language disorder acquired sometime after the normal development of language and speech behavior, i.e., aphasias of varying sorts. According to Penfield and Roberts (1959), these areas of the cortex identified as having language function are:

1. Posterior — a large area in the posterior temporal and posterior-inferior region labeled Wernicke's area;
2. Anterior — an area in the posterior portion of the third frontal convolution, labeled Broca's area; this region is just an-

terior to the caudal end of the motor strip;
3. Superior — a part of the supplementary motor area within the sagittal sulcus, just ventral to the foot portion of the motor strip.

These are illustrated in Figure 82–12. To repeat, the motor mechanism necessary for speech depends upon the mechanism for voice and articulator control found in the prerolandic motor strip of each hemisphere. The ideational mechanism of language is functional in only one hemisphere. The three areas just identified participate in language behavior. These regions are coordinated in some way, probably dependent upon subcortical (thalamic) connections and transcortical channels (arcuate fasciculus).

Geschwind's (1972) model of vocal-verbal language behavior proposes that when a verbal message is received through an auditory channel, the output of the primary auditory cortical area is received by Wernicke's area, where decoding, (comprehension) occurs. If the word is now to be produced, the "pattern is sent on to Broca'a area, where the articulatory form is aroused and passed on to the motor area (prerolandic region) that controls the movement of the muscles of speech,"

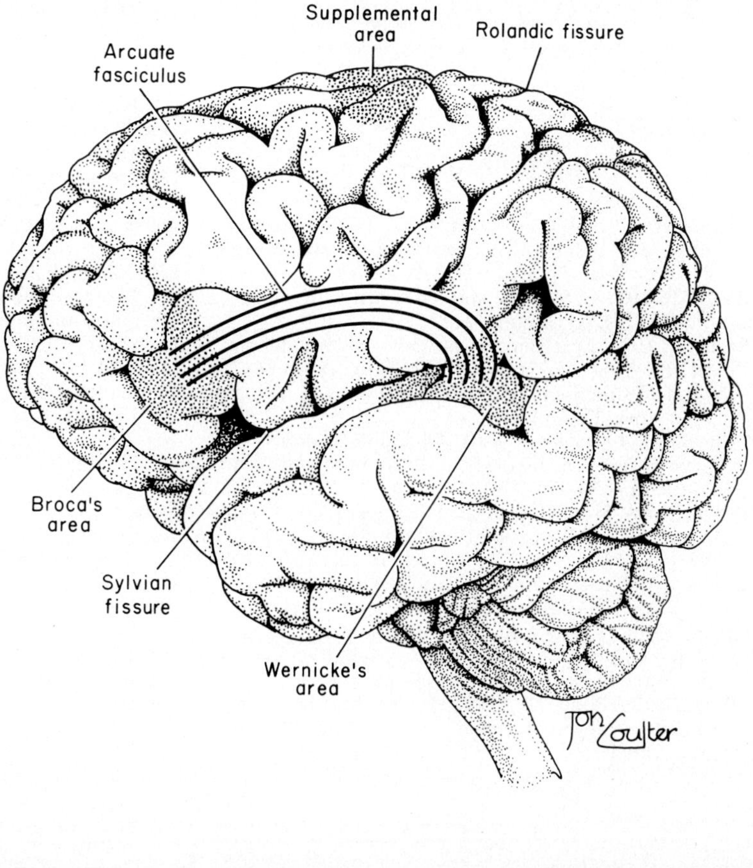

Figure 82–12 A lateral view of the human brain. The relationship between the two primary areas of language control, Broca and Wernicke, is illustrated. Also, note the placement of the supplemental motor area within the sagittal sulcus.

i.e., expression. Damage to any part of the system will produce a characteristic language dysfunction. However, any presentation of the biologic bases of language behavior is hypothetical in that prospective experimentation and animal model work is not possible in dealing with this complex, human function.

SELECTED REFERENCES

Bosma, J. 1975. Anatomic and physiologic development of the speech apparatus. *In* Towers, D. B. (Ed.) Human Communication and Its Disorders. Vol. 3. New York, Raven Press.

An excellent review of the maturational changes in the vocal tract from the neonate period through puberty, coincident with changes in performance capabilities. The chapter succeeds in relating anatomic change to increasing speech sound production competency.

Laitman, J., and Crelin, E. 1976. Postnatal development of the basicranium and vocal tract region in man. *In* Bosma, J. Symposium on the Development of the Basicranium. Bethesda, MD, U.S. Dept. of HEW., PHS, NIH.

The authors trace the development of the pharynx in humans and identify the relationship between changing anatomy and speech behavior. The change in the angulation of the basicranium is highlighted here as specifically related to changes in the volume and mobility of the upper pharynx.

Lieberman, P. 1977. Speech Physiology: Acoustic Phonetics, An Introduction. New York, Macmillan Co., Inc.

An introduction to the anatomic and physiologic parameters underlying speech behavior from respiration through articulation.

REFERENCES

Ardran, G. M., and Kemp, F. H. 1967. The mechanism of changes in form of the cervical airway in infancy. Med. Radiogr. Photogr., *44*:8–9, 26–38.

Boone, D. 1971. The Voice and Voice Therapy. Englewood Cliffs, NJ, Prentice-Hall.

Bosma, J. 1975. Anatomic and physiologic development of the speech apparatus. *In* Towers, D. B. (Ed.) Human Communication and Its Disorders, Vol. 3. New York, Raven Press.

Bosma, J., and Fletcher, S. 1961. The upper pharynx —a review. Part I, embryology and anatomy. J. Speech. Hear. Res., *70*:952–973.

Bosma, J., and Fletcher, S. 1962. The upper pharynx —a review. Part II, physiology. J. Speech Hear. Res., *71*:134–157.

Crelin, E. 1973. Functional Anatomy of the Newborn. New Haven, Yale University Press.

Crelin, E. and Netter, F. 1976. Development of the upper respiratory system. CIBA Clinical Symposia. *28*, Summit, NJ, CIBA Pharmaceutical Co.

Denes, P., and Pinson, E. 1973. The Speech Chain. Bell Telephone Laboratories, Baltimore, MD, Waverly Press, Inc.

Deu Pree, R. 1971. The muscles of voice and speech. *In* Travis, L. E., (Ed.) Handbook of Speech Pathology and Audiology, New York, Appleton-Century-Crofts.

Eckenhoff, J. E. 1951. Some anatomic considerations of the infant larynx influencing endotracheal anesthesia. J. Am. Soc. Anesth., *12*:401–410.

Enlow, D. H. 1976. The prenatal and postnatal growth of the basicranium. *In* Bosma, J. (Ed.) Symposium on the Development of the Basicranium. Bethesda, MD, U.S. Dept. HEW, PHS, NIH.

Gegdowd, V. A. 1900. Anatomical peculiarities of the respiratory organs in children. Unpublished Doctoral Dissertation (translated by S. Polevny). St. Petersburg, Russia.

Geschwind, N. 1972. Language and the brain. Sci. Am., *226*:76–83.

Hardcastle, W. J. 1976. Physiology of Speech Production. New York, Academic Press.

Hollien, H., and Moore, G. P. 1960. Measurement of the vocal folds during changes in pitch. J. Speech Hear. Res., *3*:157–165.

Johns, M., and Rood, S. R. 1978. The Management of Vocal Cord Paralysis. Rochester, MN, American Academy of Ophthalmology and Otolaryngology.

Kahane, J. 1978. A morphological study of the human prepubertal and pubertal larynx. Am. J. Anat., *151*: 11–19.

Kirchner, J. 1970. Pressman and Keleman's Physiology of the Larynx. Rochester, MN. American Academy of Ophthalmology and Otolaryngology.

Klock, L. E. 1968. The growth and development of the human larynx from birth to adolescence. Unpublished Medical Thesis, University of Washington School of Medicine.

Ladefoged, P. 1967. Three Areas of Experimental Phonetics. London, Oxford University Press.

Laitman, J., and Crelin, E. 1976. Postnatal development of the basicranium and vocal tract region in man. *In* Bosma, J. (Ed.) Symposium on the Development of the Basicranium. Bethesda, MD, U.S. Dept. HEW, PHS, NIH.

Lenneberg, E. H. 1967. Biological Foundations of Language. New York, John Wiley and Sons, Inc.

Lieberman, P. 1967. Intonation, Perception, And Language. Cambridge, MA, MIT Press.

Lieberman, P. 1977. Speech Physiology: Acoustic Phonetics. An Introduction. New York, Macmillan Co.

Lieberman, P., Crelin, E. S., and Klatt, D. H. 1972. Phonetic ability and related anatomy of the newborn and adult human, Neanderthal man, and the chimpanzee. Am. Anthropol., *74*:287–307.

Maue-Dickson, W. 1970. Cartilages, ligaments and articulation of the adult human larynx. Unpublished Doctoral Dissertation, University of Pittsburgh.

Negus, V. E. 1962. The Comparative Anatomy and Physiology of the Larynx. New York, Hafner Publ. Co.

Noback, G. J. 1923. The developmental topography of the larynx, trachea and lungs in the fetus, newborn, infant and child. Am. J. Dis. Child., *26*:515–533.

Penfield, W., and Roberts, L. 1959. Speech and Brain-Mechanisms. Princeton, N.J., Princeton University Press.

van den Berg, J. 1958. Myoelastic-aerodynamic theory of voice production. J. Speech Hear. Res., *1*:227–244.

von Leden, H., and Moore, P. 1961. The mechanics of the cricoarytenoid joint. Arch. Otolaryngol., *73*:63–72.

Chapter 83

SCREENING FOR SPEECH AND LANGUAGE DISORDERS

Sharon G. Kulig, Ph.D.

INTRODUCTION

Appreciable understanding of the development of communicative disorders has evolved among those assessing and caring for children, and early symptomatic stages of deviation grow increasingly identifiable. The need for early detection and treatment of communicative disorders is well-recognized, and the practice of screening children for these problems is becoming commonplace in this country.

Physicians in general are among the first professionals to encounter children with communicative disorders (Richardson, 1964; Mullendore, 1965; Light and Walski, 1969; Schave and Ruben, 1971; Kulig and Baker, 1976). Health care providers in particular are in pivotal positions to identify and refer such children to communicative disorders specialists for in-depth evaluation and treatment. It is highly desirable, then, to equip physicians and allied health professionals with the ability to screen children for speech disorders.

The overall goal of this chapter is to teach the reader to identify children six months to six years of age who should be referred to speech pathologists for additional evaluation. Specific instructional objectives of the chapter are to enable the physician to perform the following screening functions:

1. Determine if a child's language is significantly disordered or delayed;
2. Counsel parents of children under four years of age who volunteer concern that their child may be "stuttering,"

3. Determine if a child's articulation is significantly disordered or delayed;
4. Determine if a child exhibits a significant voice deviation; and
5. Determine if a child's speaking ability is compromised by the structure or function of the peripheral speaking mechanism.

AREAS TO BE SCREENED: OPERATIONAL DEFINITIONS

Speech pathology can be considered in terms of five major areas of potential deviation. Disorders of language, articulation, voice, rhythm of speech, and the speaking mechanism are of concern.

Language. For the purposes of this chapter, language disorders will be viewed as involving difficulties with the reception or expression of verbal messages. A child's language status may be viewed in contrast to normative expectancies for his or her chronologic age. One would be concerned, for example, about the four year old youngster who typically converses in two word phrases. Through screening, the physician can determine if a youngster's language is significantly disordered or delayed.

Rhythm of Speech. Stuttering is the most familiar example of a disorder affecting the rhythm of speech. Many nonstuttering preschoolers, however, exhibit repetitions and hesitations in their speech that greatly concern their parents.

Through anticipatory guidance and appropriately counseling parents about the progress of normal speech development, the physician can make this phase of growth less anxiety-arousing for children and their families. In this way, the likelihood that true stuttering will develop may be reduced.

Articulation. Deviant articulation may be viewed as involving unintelligibility in conversational speech and misproductions of the various consonant and vowel sounds of the language. There is a developmental hierarchy for the acquisition of various sounds of the language. A child's articulatory skills must, therefore, be considered in light of normative expectancies for his or her chronologic age.

For example, three year old speakers of English are typically producing correctly such sounds as /m/ (as in *my*), /n/ (as in *no*), /p/ (as in *pie*), /h/ (as in *he*), and /w/ (as in *water*). Three year old children regarded as exhibiting normal articulation may *not* yet have acquired accurate productions of the /s/ (as in *sun*) or the /r/ (as in *red*) sounds, however.

Again, physicians can be of great assistance by (1) making parents aware of age-appropriate behaviors and (2) seeking speech pathology consultation when a need for this is indicated. (Far too often in the past, parents have been encouraged to postpone seeking speech pathology evaluation until their child is six or seven years of age.)

Voice. Examples of voice abnormalities include quality deviations, such as hypernasality (sounds as though the child is speaking "through the nose"), hyponasality ("cold in the nose" quality), breathiness, or hoarseness. Intensity deviations (habitual use of a voice that is excessively "loud" or "soft") and pitch deviations (monopitch or inappropriately high or low pitch) are also of concern.

The physician should be sensitive to vocal deviations in children and should establish a pattern of consultation and referral with a speech pathologist skilled in the identification and treatment of voice disorders.

Speaking Mechanism. Screening for speech disorders also involves examination of the oral peripheral speaking mechanism. The physician must consider the potential influence on speech production exerted, for example, by palatal, tongue, and dental anomalies. Since parents often express concern about the possible restrictiveness of the child's lingual frenulum, the examiner should be able to screen for this problem in particular, as well.

PARENTAL CONCERN AND SCREENING FOR SPEECH AND LANGUAGE DISORDERS

Parental concern, in this writer's opinion, should always be heeded. Many authorities believe that stuttering, for example, may be an extension of normal behavior that was unwittingly reinforced by anxious parents. And as alluded to earlier, too frequently many appropriately concerned parents have been encouraged to postpone seeking needed consultation about their child's speaking or listening skills until the youngster is of school age.

Also of special importance is parental concern regarding a youngster's hearing acuity, for the relationship between hearing and speech is very fundamental. Arrangements for audiologic evaluation should always be undertaken on behalf of any patient suspected of exhibiting a significant speech or language disorder. Health care providers should understand that no child is too young, too uncooperative, or "too retarded" to be referred for evaluation by a certified audiologist specialized in the assessment of children.

OFFICE SCREENING FOR SPEECH DISORDERS

It is probable that screening tests that attempt to consider the several major categories of speech and language disorders will come nearest to meeting the screening needs of health care providers at this time. The notion of screening children for such problems, however, remains relatively new, and only a few appropriate tests to achieve this purpose are available.

It is quite clear that unless a speech screening procedure can be administered readily and efficiently it is unlikely to be used in office practice. The need for the development of practical, comprehensive screening tools that would enable physicians to perform the speech screening functions described previously is great.

It is noted, for example, in Table 83–1, that the *Denver Developmental Screening Test (DDST)* (Frankenburg and Dodds, 1969), insofar as it is concerned with the growth of communicative skills, is primarily focused upon language acquisition. And as its name implies, the concern of the *Denver Articulation*

Table 83–1 SAMPLING OF SPEECH AND LANGUAGE RELATED SCREENING TESTS APPROPRIATE FOR USE BY SPEECH PATHOLOGISTS AND NON-SPEECH PATHOLOGISTS

Title of Screening Test	Age Range	Description of Skills Considered By the Test	Average Administration Time	Author and Distributor
1. *Denver Developmental Screening Test*	Birth to 6 years	Gross motor, Language, Fine motor–Adaptive, Personal–Social	10–25 minutes	Authors: W. R. Frankenburg, J. B. Dodds. Distributor: LADOCA Foundation, East 51st Ave. and Lincoln St., Denver, Colorado 80216
2. *Denver Articulation Screening Exam*	2.5 to 6 years	Articulation	3 minutes	Author: Amelia F. Drumwright, M.A. Distributor: LADOCA Project and Publishing Co., East 51st Ave. and Lincoln Street, Denver, Colorado 80216
3. *Verbal Language Development Scale*	0 to 15 years	Communicative Language Usage	5–10 minutes	Author: Merlin J. Mecham, Ph.D. Distributor: American Guidance Service Inc., 720 Washington Ave. SE, Circle Pines, Minnesota 55414
4. *The Physician's Developmental Quick Screen for Speech Disorders*	6 months to 6 years	Language, Rhythm of Speech, Articulation, Speaking Mechanism, Voice	5 minutes	Author: Sharon G. Kulig, Ph.D., CCC-Sp. Kathryn Ann Baker, M.A., CCC-Sp. Distributor: PDQ Speech Screening Instruments, P.O. Box 2352, Garland, TX 75040
5. *The Classroom Teacher's Quick Screen for Speech Disorders*	6 years to 18 years	Language, Rhythm of Speech, Articulation, Speaking Mechanism, Voice	7 minutes	Authors: Sharon G. Kulig, Ph.D., CCC-Sp. Kathryn Ann Baker, M.A., CCC-Sp. Distributor: Department of Surgery, School of Medicine, The University of North Carolina, Chapel Hill, N.C. 27514
6. *The V-P Competency for Speech Screening Test (Experimental Edition)*	3 years to adulthood	Sign Posts of Velopharyngeal Incompetency for Speech	7 minutes	Authors: Sharon G. Kulig, Ph.D., CCC-Sp. Kathryn Ann Baker, M.A., CCC-Sp. Distributor: Department of Surgery, School of Medicine, The University of North Carolina, Chapel Hill, N.C. 27514

PHYSICIAN'S DEVELOPMENTAL QUICK SCREEN FOR SPEECH DISORDERS (PDQ)
Experimental Edition

FORM 9: To be used with patients from **55 to 60 months of age.** Copyright © 1973 by Sharon G. Kulig, Ph.D. and Kathryn A. Baker, M.A., Child Development Division, Department of Pediatrics, University of Texas Medical Branch, Galveston. The reproduction of any part of this form by mimeograph, hectograph, xerox or in any other way, whether the reproductions are sold or are furnished free for use, is a violation of the copyright law. All rights reserved.

PATIENT'S NAME: _____ RACE: _____ SEX: _____ DATE: _____

IDENTIFICATION NO.: _____ EXAMINER: _____

DATE OF BIRTH: _____ CURRENT AGE: _____ (mos.)

I. LANGUAGE

Directions: Indicate with a checkmark if the patient performs or does not perform the behavior indicated. **Parental report** may be used in lieu of direct observation but should be noted.

Yes   No
( )   ( )   Understands such concepts as longer and larger (see supplemental sheet for stimulus.)
( )   ( )   Can repeat four digits (1/sec.)
( )   ( )   Adjectives usually appear in his speech.
( )   ( )   Four and five word sentences are typical.
( )   ( )   Asks many questions.

(If patient failed ANY of the above, he fails this section of the screening test.)

SCORE: Pass   Fail   (circle one)

II. RHYTHM OF SPEECH
(If the parent or child **"volunteers"** that the child may be "stuttering", the child automatically fails this section of the screening test.)

SCORE: Pass   Fail   (circle one)

III. ARTICULATION

Directions: Have the child imitate your production of each of the following words, **watching** as well as **listening** to his productions. Circle any word in which the underlined sound is misprounced or absent. Record the number of circled words from each word group in the indicated space. Important: Remember to watch the child as he imitates your models.

No. of words
circled   Word Group
_____   1. no   money   pin
_____   2. bed   baby   tub
_____   3. coat   cookie   walk
_____   4. happy   beehive
_____   5. foot   coffee   off
_____   6. pie   puppy   nap
_____   7. go   doggie   egg
_____   8. walk   away
_____   9. man   mommy   game

Yes   No
( )   ( )   The patient's parent asserts that the child's speech is intelligible to listeners unfamiliar with the child's speech patterns. (The patient fails this section of the test if two or more words of ANY word group are circled; or, if his parent answers that the child's speech is not intelligible to listeners who are unfamiliar with the child's speech patterns.)

SCORE: Pass   Fail   (circle one)

IV. SPEAKING MECHANISM

Yes   No
( )   ( )   I believe that the patient's speaking ability is compromised by the structure or function of his speaking mechanism (palatal, breathing, tongue problems, etc. suspected.)

(If the answer to the above question is yes, the patient fails this section of the screening test.)

SCORE: Pass   Fail   (circle one)

V. VOICE

Directions: Based on parental history or your observations of the patient's voice as he verbalized during your administration of the Language and Articulation sections of the screening test, indicate by a checkmark your description of the patient's voice. If more speech sampling is desired, engage the patient in conversation, e.g., What did you have for lunch today? Where's daddy? Did you watch T.V. last night?...What did you see?

1. Typical Quality   normal _____ hoarse _____ (in absence of "a cold")*
                        history of chronic hoarseness _____
                        hypernasal (sounds as though he's "talking through his nose") _____
                        hyponasal (sounds as though he "has a cold" in absence of such findings) _____

2. Typical Pitch   normal _____ significantly low _____ significantly high _____
3. Typical Loudness   normal _____ significantly weak _____ significantly loud _____

(If the patient exhibits a significant voice deviation, he fails this section of the screening test.)

SCORE: Pass   Fail   (circle one)

*If the patient presently exhibits "a cold", a statement regarding typical voice quality must be deferred until resolution of symptoms occurs.

SUMMARY OF RESULTS

If patient has failed ANY of the above sections, he should be referred to a speech pathologist for further evaluation.

                                                                    Date: _____
Referred to: _____

Referred for further evaluation of: Language _____   Rhythm of Speech _____
                                       Articulation N/A   Speaking Mechanism _____
                                       Voice _____

Figure 83–1   Sample PDQ form appropriate for use with children 55 to 60 months of age.

FORM 9 (55 - 60 months)

Screening Exam (DASE) (Drumwright, 1971) is the child's acquisition of the consonant and vowel sounds of the language.

One standardized approach to screening patients for disorders of language, articulation, voice, rhythm of speech, and the speaking mechanism is *The Physician's Developmental Quick Screen for Speech Disorders,* the so-called *PDQ* (Kulig and Baker, 1973a). This test instrument is intended to provide a standardized approach to recognizing and guiding children at risk for speech disorders toward more detailed evaluation. Originally designed for the training of medical students (Kulig et al., 1975), the *PDQ* systematically considers the five possible areas for deviation discussed earlier (Fig. 83–1). For this reason, the *PDQ* will provide the structure for the discussion of screening for speech disorders that follows.

Screening children ranging in age from six months to six years will now be considered in some detail.

SCREENING CHILDREN UNDER SIX YEARS FOR LANGUAGE DISORDERS

Language can be thought of as a symbol system that involves four major components: (1) sounds or phonemes, (2) words or morphemes, (3) syntax or grammar, i.e., those rules that govern the stringing of elements into phrases and sentences and that express relationships within and among phrases and sentences (ASHA, 1978b) and (4) semantics or meaning. For screening test purposes, language skills can be thought of as involving a youngster's ability to make use of what is said to him or her as well as the ability to encode messages into words and sentences so that these might be understood by others. Both receptive (decoding) and expressive (encoding) skills must be considered in language screening. Delayed or disordered language, then, may be reflected by verbalizations, vocabulary, sentence structure, grammar, or sentence lengths that are beneath normative expectancies for a child's age. Table 83–2 presents a sample listing of some of the language skills normally acquired during the first six years of life.

Both receptive (e.g., "is successful when asked to follow directions involving some prepositions") and expressive (e.g., "four and five word sentences are typical") language behaviors are presented in the listing of language skills appearing in Table 83–2. The four major components of language are represented as well: sounds or phonemes (e.g., "uses combinations of sound"), words or morphemes (e.g., "plurals usually appear in his speech"), grammar or syntax (e.g., "converses frequently throughout the day in strings of long, grammatically correct sentences"), and meaning or semantics (e.g., "is successful when asked to point out at least two of the following: shoe, hair, nose, eyes, hand, foot, mouth, pants, diaper, dress").

The language abilities enumerated in Table 83–2 were selected from 174 language behaviors on the basis of their appropriateness as discussed in the developmental literature and confirmed in clinical experience. The rationale for ordering these language items in accord with the various chronologic ages specified in the table is to allow for emergent behaviors and thus reduce false-positive referrals to speech pathologists. For example, the skills ascribed to the 12 month old level, such as "uses combination of sounds," represent minimal expectations, as these behaviors are typically exhibited by infants 6 months of age. Similarly, items appearing in the "13 to 18 months" section, such as "first meaningful word has appeared," are usually performed by the average 12 month old child.

Table 83–3 is intended to serve as a guide for screening children for the acquisition of the language skills enumerated in Table 83–2. A child who cannot perform *all* the language behaviors listed as appropriate to his or her chronologic age as listed in Tables 83–2 and 83–3 is likely to be in need of additional evaluation by a speech pathologist. (A parental report may be used in lieu of direct examiner observation of a behavior, but this should be noted.)

It is well known that documenting a patient's progress with regard to meeting language milestones is a cardinal point when monitoring child development in general. Early referral to a speech pathologist of the patient whose language ability appears to be disordered or delayed is of critical importance, as this relates to the need for in-depth evaluation, family counseling, and early intervention or treatment when a need for these is indicated.

Text continued on page 1469

Table 83–2 SAMPLING OF LANGUAGE SKILLS ACQUIRED DURING THE FIRST
SIX YEARS OF LIFE*

(6 to 12 Months)
   Usually makes some response to voice (smiles or becomes quiet)
   Frequently seeks out speaker
   Has discernible cries to signal hunger, discomfort, or fatigue
   Enjoys making sounds
   Uses combinations of sounds (e.g., "ka-ga," "ng-guh," "puh-puh-puh")

(13 to 18 Months)
   Often understands spoken (not gestured) words, e.g., "bye-bye," "up?", "stop that," "no-no"
   Recognizes own name
   Often appears to be making "statements," using no "real" words
   Often copies sounds produced by caretakers
   First meaningful word has appeared

(19 to 24 Months)
   Is successful when asked to point out at least two of the following: shoe, hair, nose, eyes, hand, food, mouth,
      pants, diaper, dress
   Usually uses voice (with or without gesture) to make wants known
   Is speaking daily two or more true words

(25 to 30 Months)
   Is usually successful when asked to point out two pictured body parts or pictured pieces of clothing: e.g., "point
      to your mouth, foot, shoes, pants"
   Is usually successful when asked to point to pictures of familiar objects; e.g., "point to man"
      (Note: two correct responses or parental reports that such behavior is typical are necessary for passage of
      this item)
   Usually uses phrases and short sentences of at least two words
   Relies more on words to express wants

(31 to 36 Months)
   Is successful when asked to "point to the one who is eating" (drinking, sleeping, running, driving); three correct
      responses or parental reports that such behavior is typical are necessary for passage of this item
   Often uses "you," "me," etc. correctly
   Is successful when asked to name familiar pictures, e.g., dog, tree, ball, airplane, tree, cup, car, man; four correct
      responses or parental reports that such behavior is typical are necessary for passage of this item
   Much of the child's speech is understandable to strangers

   *As considered by the PDQ instrument, in which the rationale is to allow for developing skills as much as possible.

Table 83–2 SAMPLING OF LANGUAGE SKILLS ACQUIRED DURING THE FIRST SIX YEARS OF LIFE (*Continued*)

(37 to 42 Months)

Is usually successful at completing two-part instructions given without intervening pause (e.g., "pick up the penny and give it to mommy.")

Responds successfully when asked his or her name (first and last names), e.g., "What is your name?" "Johnny what?"

Frequently asks simple questions on own initiative

Counts by rote at least to three

(43 to 48 Months)

Is successful when asked to follow directions involving some prepositions (e.g., "put the penny in the cup," "put the penny under the chair," "put the penny on the desk")

Responds successfully when asked his or her name (first and last), e.g., "What is your name?" "Johnny what?"

Plurals usually appear in speech

Past tenses usually appear in speech

Tells of daily activities and experiences

(49 to 54 Months)

Can point correctly to three colors on verbal request, e.g., "show me the red one . . . the blue one . . . the green one" (Ask the child to point to a color on his clothing or a color visible in the room.)

Can imitate production of sentence of eight or nine syllables in length (e.g., "Say this after me, 'I would like to have a little dog.'"

Can count to at least eight

Produces a great deal of conversational speech on a far-ranging variety of topics employing such major parts of speech as nouns, verbs, adjectives, prepositions (e.g., "I went to the circus . . . Grandma took me . . . I saw a lion . . . I ate a hamburger . . . I'm hungry, Daddy . . . Give me my doll . . . Where is Mommy?)

(55 to 60 Months)

Understands such concepts as longer and larger; e.g., sketch a large and a small box and a long and short line for the child to point out to you

Can repeat four digits (one per second)

Adjectives usually appear in speech

Four- and five-word sentences are typical

Asks many questions

(61 to 72 Months)

Has an understanding of numbers — of up to five objects (e.g., after spreading out several pennies, the examiner asks the child to "give me five pennies")

Can correctly identify by name three out of five color samples, e.g., "What color is your shirt?", "What color is your dress?"

Converses frequently throughout the day in strings of long, grammatically correct sentences

Table 83–3 CLINICAL GUIDE TO SCREENING LANGUAGE BEHAVIORS*

6 to 12 Months

Materials Needed:	None
Test Procedure:	Speak to the child in normal conversational voice.
Child should ...	make some response, such as smiling, ceasing to vocalize, altering his breathing or sucking pattern, etc.
Materials Needed:	None
Test Procedure:	Stand outside of the child's visual field and speak to him in normal conversational voice.
Child should ...	turn his head or eyes in the direction from which the voice is coming.
Materials Needed:	None
Test Procedure:	Ask the parent if one can determine from the child's cries whether the child is hungry, tired, in pain, etc.
Child should ...	according to parental report, daily produce distinguishable cries signaling hunger, pain, etc.
Materials Needed:	None
Test Procedure:	Observe the child as he engages in vocalizing.
Child should ...	vocalize extensively. Parental report that such behavior is typical* of the child would also satisfy requirements for passing this item.
Materials Needed:	None
Test Procedure:	Observe the child as he engages in vocalizing.
Child should ...	combine at least two or more different sounds as he vocalizes. Parental report that such behavior is typical of the child would also satisfy requirements for passing this item.

13 to 18 Months

Materials Needed:	None
Test Procedure:	Say to the child "Bye-bye!", "Up?" or "No-no!" (Avoid any accompanying gestures.)
Child should ...	indicate that he understands the spoken words by making an appropriate response such as waving, raising his arms to be picked up, or ceasing an activity. Parental report that such behavior is typical of the child would also satisfy requirements for passing this item.
Materials Needed:	Toy, book, or other interesting object
Test Procedure:	While the child's attention is directed toward a toy, book, or another interesting object, speak a name other than the child's, pause a moment, and then speak the child's own name in a conversational voice.
Child should ...	look toward the speaker or otherwise give evidence that he has recognized his name. Parental report that such behavior is typical of the child would also satisfy requirements for passing this item.
Materials Needed:	None
Test Procedure:	Listen as the child engages in vocalizing.
Child should ...	produce some sentence-like utterances with inflection (although not necessarily using any true words). Parental report that such behavior is typical of the child would also satisfy requirements for passing this item.
Materials Needed:	None
Test Procedure:	Secure the child's attention and repeat a sound or syllable several times, e.g., "ba-ba-ba; puh-puh-puh."

*"Typical" as employed in this table connotes daily observation of the behavior cited.

Table 83–3 CLINICAL GUIDE TO SCREENING LANGUAGE BEHAVIORS (*Continued*)

13 to 18 months (*continued*)

Child should...	respond by imitating or attempting to imitate the examiner's sound-making. Parental report that such behavior is typical of the child would also satisfy requirements for passing this item.
Materials Needed:	None
Test Procedure:	Listen as the child engages in vocalizing.
Child should...	use at least one word appropriately and consistently, e.g., "mama," "dada," "baba" (for bottle), etc. Parental report that such behavior is typical of the child would also satisfy requirements for passing this item.

19 to 24 Months

Materials Needed:	None
Test Procedure:	Instruct the child to "Show me your eyes (nose, mouth, shoe, dress, etc.)"
Child should...	indicate that he understands the spoken instructions by pointing out at least two body parts or pieces of clothing. Parental report that such behavior is typical of the child would also satisfy requirements for passing this item.

25 to 30 Months

Materials Needed:	Toy, book, or other interesting object
Test Procedure:	The child's attention should be directed toward a toy, book, or another interesting object that is held out to him just beyond his reach.
Child should...	vocalize (true words are not necessary) his desire to obtain the item; e.g., while the child is reaching toward the object, he might emit sounds such as "unh unh unh" and thereby employ his voice to signal his desire to obtain the item. Parental report that such behavior is typical of the child would also satisfy requirements for passing this item.
Materials Needed:	None
Test Procedure:	Observe the child as he vocalizes.
Child should...	use at least two words (or word approximations, e.g., tat for cat) appropriately. Parental report that such behavior is typical of the child—consistent daily use of these words in a meaningful way—would also satisfy requirements for passing this item.
Materials Needed:	Supplemental Stimulus Sheet—picture of little boy
Test Procedure:	Present the stimulus sheet to the child and ask him to "Show me his shoes (pants, shirt, etc.)" or "Point to his eyes (mouth, hair, etc.)"
Child should...	indicate that he understands the spoken instructions by pointing out on the sheet at least two named pieces of clothing or body parts. Parental report that such behavior is typical of the child (as they look at books together, for example) would also satisfy requirements for passing this item.
Materials Needed:	Supplemental Stimulus Sheet—pictures of objects
Test Procedure:	Present the stimulus sheet to the child and ask him to "Show me man, show me ball, etc." or "Point to tree, point to dog, etc."
Child should...	indicate that he understands the spoken instructions by pointing out on the stimulus sheet at least two of the objects named. Parental report that such behavior is typical of the child (as they look at books and magazines together, for example) would also satisfy requirements for passing this item.
Materials Needed:	None
Test Procedure:	Observe the child as he talks with his parent.

Table continued on the following page

Table 83–3   CLINICAL GUIDE TO SCREENING LANGUAGE BEHAVIORS (*Continued*)

25 to 30 Months (*continued*)

Child should . . .	demonstrate consistent use of short (at least two word) phrases or sentences, e.g., "mommy up," "go bye-bye," "mommy candy" etc. (The sentences need not be complete or grammatically correct.) Parental report that such behavior is typical of the child—consistent daily use of such phrases or sentences in a meaningful way—would also satisfy requirements for passing this item.
Materials Needed:	None
Test Procedure:	Observe the child as he vocalizes.
Child should . . .	rely primarily on vocalizing, rather than pointing and gesturing, to obtain his needs. Parental report that such behavior is typical of the child would also satisfy requirements for passing this item.

31 to 36 Months

Materials Needed:	Supplemental Stimulus Sheet—pictures of people engaged in activities of daily living
Test Procedure:	Present the stimulus sheet to the child and ask him to "Point to the one who is eating (the one who is driving, etc.)" or "Show me sleeping (running, etc.)"
Child should . . .	indicate that he understands the spoken instructions by pointing out on the stimulus sheet at least three of the activities named. Parental report that such behavior is typical of the child (as they look together at books and magazines, for example) would also satisfy requirements for passing this item.
Materials Needed:	None
Test Procedure:	Engage the child in conversation or observe the child as he talks with his parent.
Child should . . .	evidence meaningful usage of "you" and "me." Parental report that such behavior is typical of the child would also satisfy requirements for passing this item.
Materials Needed:	Supplemental Stimulus Sheet—pictures of objects
Test Procedure:	Present the stimulus sheet to the child, and, pointing to one picture at a time, ask him "What is this?"
Child should . . .	name correctly at least four pictured objects. Parental report that such behavior is typical of the child (as they look at books and magazines together, for example) would also satisfy requirements for passing this item.
Materials Needed:	None
Test Procedure:	Engage the child in conversation or observe him as he talks with his parent.
Child should . . .	speak in such a manner that much of what he says is understandable even by persons unfamiliar with his speech patterns. Parental report that such behavior is typical of the child would also satisfy requirements for passing this item.

37 to 42 Months

Materials Needed:	Small toy or other manipulable small object familiar to the child (e.g., pencil or cup)
Test Procedure:	Instruct the child to "Put the pencil (cup, etc.) on the chair, then give it to mommy." The examiner should *not* accompany the instructions with gestures. He should *not* pause between the instruction "Put the pencil on the chair . . ." and the instruction ". . . then give it to mommy." (The examiner is delivering a two-part instruction; it would be an error to pause and consequently deliver two separate, single instructions to the child.)
Child should . . .	follow your instruction in the order given.
Materials Needed:	None
Test Procedure:	Ask the child "What is your name?" If the child responds by speaking his first name only, e.g., "Johnny," ask "Johnny what?" or "What is your whole name?," etc.

Table 83–3 CLINICAL GUIDE TO SCREENING LANGUAGE BEHAVIORS (*Continued*)

37 to 42 Months (*continued*)

Child should...	respond by giving his first *and* last name. Parental report that such behavior is typical of the child would also satisfy requirements for passing this item.
Materials Needed:	None
Test Procedure:	Engage the child in conversation or observe the child as he talks with his parent.
Child should...	occasionally ask questions on his own initiative; e.g., "What's that?" Parental report that such behavior is typical of the child would also satisfy requirements for passing this item.
Materials Needed:	None
Test Procedure:	Instruct the child to "Count as far as you can!"
Child should...	count on his own "at least to three." The examiner is not asking the child to demonstrate his number concepts in the sense that the child must be able to count actual objects. Rather, the examiner is testing the child's ability to count "by memory" (by rote) only. Parental report that such behavior is typical of the child would also satisfy requirements for passing this item.

43 to 48 Months

Materials Needed:	One small toy or other manipulable small object familiar to the child (e.g., a pencil and a cup)
Test Procedure:	Hand the pencil to the child and instruct him to "Put the pencil on the chair." After the child succeeds (or fails) at completing this task instruct him to "Now put the pencil in the cup." The child may also be instructed to "Put the pencil under the chair." Do not accompany your instructions with gestures.
Child should...	demonstrate his understanding of at least *two* prepositions (on, in, under, in front of, behind or beside, for example) by correctly completing instructions such as the above. Parental report that such behavior is typical of the child would also satisfy requirements for passing this item.
Materials Needed:	None
Test Procedure:	Ask the child "What is your name?" If the child responds by speaking his first name only, e.g., "Johnny," ask "Johnny what?" or "What is your whole name?," etc.
Child should...	respond by giving his first *and* last name. Parental report that such behavior is typical of the child would also satisfy requirements for passing this item.
Materials Needed:	Several identical small objects familiar to the child (e.g., five pencils or five pennies)
Test Procedure:	Holding the objects in your hand, ask the child "What do I have?"
Child should...	display evidence of some usage of plurals; e.g., "You have pencil*s*" or "I want the pencil*s*." Completely correct pronunciation of the "s" sound is not essential for passing this item; a lisped "s" sound, for example, is creditable since this item is concerned with the acquisition of a grammatical concept rather than an articulatory skill. Parental report that the child typically employs plurals in conversational speech even though not always correctly would also satisfy requirements for passing this item.
Materials Needed:	None
Test Procedure:	Engage the child in conversation or observe the child as he talks with his parent.
Child should...	display evidence of some usage of the past tense of verbs. Parental report that the child typically employs the past tense of verbs in conversational speech even though not always correctly would also satisfy requirements for passing this item. ("He felled" or "He hitted me" would be creditable, for example.)
Materials Needed:	None
Test Procedure:	Engage the child in conversation or observe the child as he talks with his parent.
Child should...	converse about his daily activities or experiences. Parental report that such behavior is typical of the child would also satisfy requirements for passing this item.

Table continued on the following page

Table 83–3 CLINICAL GUIDE TO SCREENING LANGUAGE BEHAVIORS (*Continued*)

49 to 54 Months

Materials Needed:	Four objects identical except in color (e.g., pencils or crayons)
Test Procedure:	Instruct the child to "Show me the red (blue, green, yellow, etc.) one."
Child should...	point correctly to at least three of the colored objects.
Materials Needed:	None
Test Procedure:	Instruct the child to "Say this after me: 'I would like to have a little dog.'"
Child should...	be able to imitate production of sentences eight or nine syllables in length such as the above.
Materials Needed:	None
Test Procedure:	Tell the child to "Count as far as you can!"
Child should...	count on his own at least to eight. The examiner is not asking the child to demonstrate his number concepts in the sense that the child must be able to count actual objects. The examiner is testing the child's ability to count by rote only. Parental report that such behavior is typical of the child would also satisfy requirements for passing this item.
Materials Needed:	None
Test Procedure:	Engage the child in conversation or observe the child as he talks with his parent.
Child should...	display evidence of ability to engage in conversational speech concerning a variety of topics (e.g., activities, favorite television programs and stories, pets, etc.). His speech should be characterized by usage of adjectives and prepositions as well as verbs and nouns. Parental report that such behavior is typical of the child would also satisfy requirements for passing this item.

55 to 60 Months

Materials Needed:	Supplemental Stimulus Sheet—pictures of arrows and squares
Test Procedure:	Pointing to the pair of arrows on the stimulus sheet, instruct the child to "Point to the one that is longer." Pointing to the pair of squares on the stimulus sheet, instruct the child to "Point to the one that is larger."
Child should...	correctly identify the arrow that is "longer" and the square that is "larger."
Materials Needed:	None
Test Procedure:	Instruct the child to "Say these numbers after me. Remember—wait until I'm through and then say the numbers exactly the way that I did." The examiner may employ any four numbers he chooses, e.g., 7-3-8-6. It is essential that the numbers be presented at the rate of one number per second.
Child should...	be able to correctly repeat four digits in order as these were presented by the examiner at a rate of one number per second.
Materials Needed:	None
Test Procedure:	Engage the child in conversation or observe the child as he talks with his parents.
Child should...	evidence daily use of adjectives in conversational speech. Parental report that such behavior is typical of the child would also satisfy the requirements for passing this item.
Materials Needed:	None
Test Procedure:	Engage the child in conversation or observe the child as he verbalizes with his parent.
Child should...	produce sentences that are typically four and five words in length. Parental report that such behavior is typical of the child would also satisfy requirements for passing this item.
Materials Needed:	None
Test Procedure:	Engage the child in conversation or observe the child as he talks with his parent.
Child should...	pose questions daily. Parental report that such behavior is typical of the child would also satisfy requirements for passing this item.

Table 83-3 CLINICAL GUIDE TO SCREENING LANGUAGE BEHAVIORS (*Continued*)

61 to 72 Months

Materials Needed:	Eight identical objects (pencils or pennies, etc.) and one sheet of paper
Test Procedure:	Spread out the identical objects beside the paper and instruct the child to "Put five of the pencils (pennies, etc.) on the paper."
Child should ...	evidence a number concept of five by correctly counting out and placing five of the objects on the piece of paper.
Materials Needed:	Four objects identical except in color (e.g., pencils, crayons, buttons, etc.)
Test Procedure:	Pointing to each differently colored object in turn, instruct the child to "Tell me what color this one is."
Child should ...	correctly name at least three of the four color samples provided. Parental report that such behavior is typical of the child would also satisfy requirements for passing this item.
Materials Needed:	None
Test Procedure:	Engage the child in conversation or observe the child as he converses with his parent.
Child should ...	converse daily in strings of grammatically correct, long (at least six words) sentences. Parental report that such behavior is typical of the child would also satisfy requirements for passing this item.

SCREENING FOR DEVIATIONS IN THE RHYTHM OF SPEECH

It is conceivable that an iatrogenic reaction could set in if the attention of previously unconcerned parents becomes focused upon such a feared handicap as stuttering. For this reason, the topic of stuttering is usually best avoided unless a parent spontaneously expresses concern in this regard. The physician is in an excellent position, however, to assist parents who volunteer concern that a young child might be stuttering.

Normal Nonfluency. Between 18 months and 4½ years of age, children may exhibit disruptions in the fluency of their speech. It has been suggested that as many as 90 percent of normal children may exhibit this behavior (Froeschels, 1948). Understandably, repetitions and hesitations in a youngster's speech can frighten parents considerably if they do not understand that this is not unusual among children under four years of age. The physician can provide this usable and reassuring information.

Once parents are informed of and accept the fact the youngsters can be normally nonfluent, referral of children under four years of age for further evaluation of the rhythm of speech does not usually become necessary.

Counseling Parents of Children Younger Than Four Years. Parents verbalizing fears about dysfluency should be told that a child at that age who repeats, prolongs, or hesitates on sounds and words is "not necessarily stuttering." Such interruptions in the speech of very young children might be termed *normal* nonfluencies since they are usually not indications of true stuttering. Parents should be told that some authorities believe that the majority of children exhibit this behavior to some degree.

Parents should be cautioned against applying the label "stutterer" to any child. They should know that interrupting and encouraging their son or daughter to "slow down" or "stop and start over" will not be helpful and could make the child extremely uncomfortable in or even fearful of speaking situations. Similarly, parents should be informed that guessing at or supplying words on which the child is nonfluent will likely be counterproductive. They need to understand that pressuring the child to speak should also be avoided, particularly at this time.

Should parental concern *persist beyond six weeks* despite such counseling, the physician should *immediately* make arrangements for the case to be referred to a speech pathologist for in-depth evaluation.

Referral of Children Above Four Years of Age. The speech clinician should be consulted *without delay* when parents of children older than 4½ years volunteer concern that their child is "stuttering." This recommendation is made because children can become true stutterers in every sense of the word, and the likelihood of true stuttering occurring

Table 83-4 COMPOSITE TABLE SHOWING APPROXIMATE CHRONOLOGICAL AGES* AT WHICH CONSONANT SOUNDS ARE CONSIDERED IN VARIOUS STUDIES, TESTS, OR TEXTS

Sounds	PDQ (Kulig et al., 1973)	Developmental Articulation Test (Hejna, 1955)	Poole, 1934	Johnson, 1950	Language Development Chart**	Communicative Evaluation Chart From Infancy to 5 Years (Anderson, 1963)	Speech & Hearing Check List (Asbed, 1970)	Preschool Language Scale (Zimmerman et al., 1969)	Eisenson, 1972
/n/	43	36	54	48				30	
/h/	43	36	42						
/w/	43	36	42					30	
/p/	43	36	42	36				30	
/m/	43	36	42	36				30	
/b/	55	48	42	36				30	
/k/	55	48	54	48				42	
/f/	55	48	66	60				42	
/g/	55	48	54	48				42	
/y/	67	60	54						
/d/	67	60	54	48				42	
/ng/	67	60	54	48					
much of child's speech intelligible to strangers	31				24	48			24
parent asserts child's speech is intelligible to strangers	37				60	60	60		36–48

*Chronological ages in months.
**Davis, 1938; Irwin, 1947; McCarthy, 1954; Myklebust, 1954; Poole, 1934; Templin, 1957.

increases with advancing chronologic age. (The reader is referred to chapter 85, in which fluency disorders are considered in greater detail.)

SCREENING FOR ARTICULATION SKILLS

For screening test purposes, deviant articulation might be considered to involve misproductions or omissions of consonant or vowel sounds *and* unintelligibility of conversational speech. Although approximately 90 per cent of the speech of a three year old child should be intelligible, there is a developmental hierarchy for the acquisition of consonant and vowel sounds of the language that spans the first seven to eight years of life (Templin, 1952, 1957).

An appreciation of the normal developmental sequence for acquiring the various sounds of the language is basic, then, to screening patients for articulation disorders. The rationale for selection of screening test items is to allow for developing articulation skills as much as possible. Table 83–4 illustrates approximate chronologic ages at which various consonant sounds are uttered as determined by a sampling of studies, tests, or texts. Children who are not producing sounds listed as appropriate to their age according to normative expectations should immediately be referred to a speech and language pathologist for in-depth evaluation.

Figure 83–2 illustrates a sample format for screening articulation in children 61 to 72 months of age. Each consonant sound to be tested at that age level is underlined and tested in the beginning, middle, and final positions of key words. The examiner asks the child to repeat his or her production of each test word and is careful to *watch* as well as to *listen* to the patient's imitation of the test words. The examiner circles any word in which the test sound is mispronounced or absent. When any consonant sound being tested is deviant in two or more word positions, the patient fails the articulation section of the screening test and should be referred to a speech pathologist for further evaluation.

Intelligibility of conversational speech is the "acid test" of articulatory skill. For this reason, any child three years of age and above whose parent asserts that the youngster's conversational speech is *unintelligible* to strangers should also be referred to a speech pathologist for further evaluation.

A Word about Differences vs. Disorders. The physician engaged in screening children for speech disorders will become aware of particular characteristics that may be associated with the speech of some black children. For example, /r/ and /l/ sounds occurring after vowel sounds may not be produced ("soul" may be pronounced "sow"), and the sound /th/ may be produced as a /d/ ("this" may be pronounced "dis"). Similarly, vowels may be produced differently; for example, "floor" may be pronounced "flow;" "hers" may be pronounced "huz" (Houston, 1976).

Black children may similarly utilize rules

III. ARTICULATION

Directions: Have the child imitate your production of each of the following words, **watching** and well as **listening** to his production. Circle any word in which the underlined sound is mispronounced or absent. Record the number of circled words from each word group in the indicated space. Important: Remember to watch the child as he imitates your models.

No. of words circled		Word Group (61 - 66 months)		No. of words circled		Word Group (67 - 72 months)	
_____	1. no	money	pin	_____	1. no	money	pin
_____	2. bed	baby	tub	_____	2. bed	baby	tub
_____	3. coat	cookie	walk	_____	3. coat	cookie	walk
_____	4. happy	beehive		_____	4. happy	beehive	
_____	5. foot	coffee	off	_____	5. foot	coffee	off
_____	6. pie	puppy	nap	_____	6. pie	puppy	nap
_____	7. go	doggie	egg	_____	7. go	doggie	egg
_____	8. walk	away		_____	8. walk	away	
_____	9. man	mommy	game	_____	9. man	mommy	game
				_____	10. yes	yo yo	
				_____	11.	singing	song
				_____	12. day	daddy	bad

Yes   No
( )   ( )   The patient's parent asserts that the child's speech is intelligible to listeners unfamiliar with the child's speech patterns. (The patient fails this section of the screening test if two or more words of ANY word group are circled; or, if his parent answers that the child's speech is not intelligible to listeners who are unfamiliar with the child's speech patterns.)

SCORE: Pass   Fail   (circle one)

FORM 10 (61 - 72 months)

Figure 83–2 Sample format whereby the articulation skills of a child 61 to 72 months of age may be screened.

of a differing grammatical system. Double negatives and the word "ain't" may be used. Habitual action may be expressed with the element "be" as in "he be working." Linking words may be omitted as in "He a bad boy," or the first syllable of certain words may be stressed, for example, *police* (Houston, 1976).

Black children articulating and expressing themselves in this manner are said to be exhibiting pronunciation features of Black English. These children are *not* making errors; rather, they are following regular rules of a consistent sound and grammatical system. A critical part of the examining speech pathologist's role is assuming responsibility for distinguishing between true disorders and differences, as the latter are characteristic of the speaker's linguistic community.

Any child referred to a speech and language pathologist for further evaluation of articulation and language skills will be evaluated by the skilled clinician in terms of what constitutes standard sound and grammatical usage in that particular child's environment. The physician can rely upon the competent speech and language pathologist to assume responsibility for distinguishing "differences" from "disorders."

SCREENING FOR VOICE DISORDERS

Voice disorders can be classified according to problems of quality, pitch, and intensity. Because upper respiratory infections can significantly distort a child's voice, examiners should defer screening patients exhibiting "colds" for voice disorders until resolution of symptoms occurs. Figure 83–3 illustrates a format for screening children for voice disorders.

Hoarseness is a commonly observed deviation of voice quality. In children hoarseness is frequently associated with injurious vocal habits, such as shouting, screaming, and cheering. One investigator, for example, found vocal nodules to be present in 57 per cent of school-aged children referred to otolaryngologists for further evaluation of hoarseness (Shearer, 1972). Hoarseness may also be symptomatic of laryngeal paralysis, congenital laryngeal web, and neurogenic or systemic disease.

Deviations of vocal quality may also result from structural and functional abnormalities in the nasal, oral, and velopharyngeal areas. As suggested earlier, excessive nasal resonance or hypernasality is often a signpost of palatal deviation and velopharyngeal incompetency for speech. Audible nasal escape of air during speech is frequently observed in these cases. Hoarseness, breathiness, and inappropriate pitch level are sometimes found to coexist in the presence of velopharyngeal incompetency for speech as well.

Hyponasality or insufficient nasal resonance is usually due to some obstruction of the nasal or nasopharyngeal passages. Postsurgical and allergic edema, a deviated nasal septum, turbinate hypertrophy, nasal growths such as polyps, enlarged adenoids, and trauma are other possible causal factors of hyponasality. Hyponasality can be observed on the basis of habit pattern as well.

Disorders of vocal pitch may be precipitated by endocrine disorders, the presence of a laryngeal web, or a hearing loss, as the latter is often manifested by monopitch or inappropriate pitch. Habitual functional use of an inappropriate pitch level can constitute vocal misuse and in time can result in structural change as well.

Voices that are inappropriately loud or soft are also suggestive of a possible hearing loss.

V. VOICE

Directions: Based on parental report or your observations of the patient's voice as he verbalized during your administration of the Language and Articulation sections of the screening test, indicate by a checkmark your description of the patient's voice. If more speech sampling is desired, engage the patient in conversation, e.g., What did you have for lunch today? Where's daddy? Did you watch T.V. last night?... What did you see?

1. Typical Quality   normal_____ hoarse_____ (in absence of "a cold")*
                                   history of chronic hoarseness_____
                                   hypernasal (sounds as though he's "talking through his nose") _____
                                   hyponasal (sounds as though he "has a cold" in absence of such findings) _____
2. Typical Pitch   normal_____ significantly low_____ significantly high _____
3. Typical Loudness   normal _____ significantly weak _____ significantly loud _____

(If the patient exhibits a significant voice deviation, he fails this section of the screening test.)

SCORE: Pass   Fail   (circle one)
*If the patient presently exhibits "a cold", a statement regarding typical voice quality must be deferred until resolution of symptoms occurs.

Figure 83–3   Sample format for screening voice disorders.

Similarly, disorders of vocal intensity could be a function of systemic disease, structural deviations, personality characteristics, or noise-polluted environments. (It should be noted that continuous exposure to high noise levels, or "noise pollution," is hazardous to phonation as well as to hearing.)

A detailed discussion of the differential diagnosis of voice dysfunction is not possible within the scope of this chapter. Rather, the purpose here is to heighten the reader's awareness of the importance of screening for likely causal factors of voice disorders.

Those who are not speech pathologists do not typically have appreciable experience with screening children for voice disorders. However, research (Kulig et al., 1975) suggests that encouraging and guiding allied health professionals in screening the vocal quality, pitch, and intensity of patients seen clinically results in the recognition and follow-up of significant voice problems that might not otherwise have been identified.

Interdisciplinary evaluation of vocal deviation by the physician and speech pathologist is in the best interests of their mutual patient. This allows for comprehensive description of the misuse of voice and permits formulation of a plan of management whereby voice therapy might be effectively employed. Patients whose voices appear deviant in pitch, quality, or intensity then should be referred immediately for additional evaluation by a speech pathologist.

SCREENING THE SPEAKING MECHANISM

Speech pathologists tend to be extremely cautious in attributing speech disorders to the structural status of the oral peripheral speaking mechanism: ". . . speaking generally, one is more apt to err in blaming a defect upon oral structure than in referring it to some other cause. The diagnosis of structural causation should therefore be arrived at with great caution" (West et al., 1947).

Nevertheless, the adverse effects potentially imposed upon speech production by factors such as aberrant dental structure; tongue size, shape, and mobility; and the discoordination of breathing for speech must be appreciated. For example, palates may be cleft, restricted in mobility, or insufficient in functional length. Fairly infrequently, lingual frenula are truly restrictive for communicative purposes.

Clinical experience suggests that examination of the lingual frenulum for possible restrictiveness and peroral inspection of the palate and oropharynx are the two areas that should be considered routinely in the screening of speech by non–speech pathologists.

Examining the Lingual Frenulum for "Tongue Tie." Parents frequently ask physicians if a child might be "tongue-tied." The child who is capable of extending the tongue past the central incisors and lips or who accurately says the words "two" and "no" is usually *not* an appropriate candidate for a frenulum release procedure. Most certainly, patients who cannot perform these actions should be referred for additional evaluation by a speech pathologist.

Examining the Palate and Oropharynx. The physician must also be careful to examine the structural and functional adequacy of the patient's palate and oropharynx insofar as these can be examined by peroral inspection. The patient is held to be at risk in the presence of hypernasal voice quality or audible escape of air from the nose during speech which may be the case (1) if the palate does not move symmetrically when the child is instructed to say "ah" vigorously, (2) if the effective length of the palate appears to be unusually short or the oropharynx appears to be atypically deep when the patient is asked to phonate as above, (3) if the uvula is cleft (short or absent), (4) if there is a notch at the juncture of the hard and soft palates, or (5) if there is a change in the coloring of the mucous membrane outlining a submucous cleft. (The reader is referred to the subsequent section of this chapter, which discusses screening for velopharyngeal incompetency for speech in some detail.)

VELOPHARYNGEAL COMPETENCY FOR SPEECH: SOME CONSIDERATIONS

Normal speech production requires a potential for velopharyngeal closure or the ability to separate the oral from the nasal cavity and to impound intraoral breath pressure. Often a lack of velopharyngeal competency for speech is observed in patients exhibiting orofacial disorders—classically, cleft palate. It may also be observed in conditions such as palatal paresis, submucous cleft palate, short effective palatal length, and neuromuscular involvements (cerebral palsy or myasthenia gravis, for example).

THE V-P COMPETENCY FOR SPEECH SCREENING TEST
(THE VPC)
Experimental Edition

PATIENT'S NAME:_____ I.D.#:_____ DATE OF BIRTH:_____

SEX:_____ RACE:_____ CURRENT AGE:_____ DATE OF TESTING:_____

PARENT'S NAME:_____ PATIENT'S CURRENT TELEPHONE NUMBER:_____

PATIENT'S CURRENT ADDRESS:_____ EXAMINER:_____

I.   SPEECH SAMPLE
     Directions: Indicate by checkmark your general impressions of the patient's speech. (Engage the patient in conversation, e.g., "What did you have for lunch today?" "Where's daddy?" "Did you watch TV last night?" "What did you see?" "Do you have a dog or a cat at home?")

YES NO
( )( )   1. The patient's speech is unintelligible.*
( )( )   2. The patient or his parent asserts that his speech cannot be easily understood by strangers.
( )( )   3. The patient's voice is hypernasal (sounds like he's "talking through his nose.")*
( )( )   4. Air can be heard escaping from the patient's nostrils as he speaks.
The patient fails this section of the screening test if any of the above questions are answered "yes".

SCORE: Pass_____ Fail_____ No Response_____

*Parental report may be accepted in lieu of direct observation but should be noted.

Interpretation: A failure on this section may suggest the possibility of velopharyngeal incompetency for speech. The following sections are designed to further delineate areas in which velopharyngeal incompetency for speech may be manifested.

II. ARTICULATION
     Directions: Have the patient imitate your production of each of the following words. Circle any word in which the underlined sound is mispronounced, weakly produced or absent. Be sure to watch as well as listen to the child as he repeats your example.

3 Year Olds		4 & 5 Year Olds		6 Year Olds & Up		
puppy	pepper	puppy	cookie	puppy	button	sister
apple	people	apple	doggie	baby	hot dog	Easter
happy	baby	baby	wagon	chicken	cookie	misty
puppet	bubble	cowboy	coffee	doggie	daddy	wagon
		chicken	muffin	coffee	ice cream	muffin

After the patient has imitated the words on the list appropriate to his age level, make up some sentences for him to repeat containing some of the words that he has just produced in isolation, e.g.,
     3 Year Olds: "Give me apple." (or other 3 word phrases)
     4 Year Olds: "A cowboy eats chicken." (or other 4 word phrases)
     6 Year Olds & Up: "Sister Suzy ate ice cream at Easter."
The patient fails this section if two or more words are circled or if the quality of his articulation deteriorates in connected speech.

SCORE: Pass_____ Fail_____ No Response_____

Interpretation: A failure on this section suggests the possibility of velopharyngeal incompetency for speech. Possible problems include weak production of selected consonant sounds, the substitution of non-speech sounds for consonants (e.g., uh-ee for puppy), or palatal fatigue (as when evidenced by a deterioration of intelligibility when the patient engages over time in conversational speech).

III. VOICE SAMPLING
     Directions: Based on parental report or your observations of the patient's voice as he verbalized during your administration of the Language and Articulation sections of the screening test, indicate by checkmark your description of the patient's voice. If more speech sampling is desired, engage the patient in conversation, e.g., "What did you get for your birthday?" "Where's your car?" "Would you like a cat or a dog?" "What do you like to eat?"

1. Typical Quality   normal_____ hoarse_____ (in absence of a "cold")*
                      history of chronic hoarseness_____
                      breathy_____
                      hypernasal_____ (sounds as though he's "talking through his nose")
                      hyponasal_____ (sounds as though he "has a cold" in absence of such findings)

Figure 83–4   The V-P Competency For Speech Screening Test.

Illustration continued on the opposite page

2. Typical Pitch*   normal_____   significantly low_____   significantly high_____
3. Typical Loudness* normal_____   significantly weak_____   significantly loud_____
The patient fails this section of the screeening test if he exhibits a significant voice deviation.

SCORE: Pass_____ Fail_____ No Response_____

*Note: If the patient presently exhibits a "cold," a condition likely to distort typical voice quality, a statement regarding usual voice quality must be deferred until resolution of symptoms occurs.

Interpretation: Hypernasality or a combination of hypernasality and hyponasality, breathiness, hoarseness, or soft intensity may be signposts of possible velopharyngeal incompetency for speech. These symptoms may occur simultaneously or in isolation.

IIIA. ADDITIONAL TESTING FOR HYPERNASALITY
    Directions: Ask the patient to repeat the words "beat" and "boot." Check below if an appreciable change is observed in the quality of the patient's voice when the examiner gently covers the openings of the patient's nostrils anteriorly with his finger tips.

YES NO		YES NO		YES NO		YES NO	
( )( )	beat	( )( )	boot	( )( )	beat	( )( )	boot

The patient fails this section of the screening test if the quality of his voice changes when the examiner gently covers the openings of the patient's nostrils.

SCORE: Pass_____ Fail_____ No Response_____

Interpretation: A failure of this section suggests the presence of hypernasality, a signpost of possible velopharyngeal incompetency for speech.

IV. NASAL EMISSION
    Directions: Place a cardboard "air paddle" (enclosed in the test kit) beneath the patient's nostrils and ask him to repeat the following words. Indicate with the initial R (right nostril), L (left nostril), or B (both nostrils) is the air paddle moves as the patient produces the test words.

YES NO		YES NO		YES NO	
( )( )	puppy	( )( )	people	( )( )	Easter*
( )( )	apple	( )( )	sister*	( )( )	eggshells*
( )( )	paper	( )( )	lesson*	( )( )	ashtray*
( )( )	pepper	( )( )	ice cream*	( )( )	mushrooms*

The patient fails this section if nasal emission is noted.

SCORE: Pass_____ Fail_____ No Response_____

*Note: Appropriate stimuli only for patients 6 years of age and above.

Interpretation: Nasal escape of air during speech production suggests possible velopharyngeal incompetency for speech.

V. PERORAL INSPECTION OF THE PERIPHERAL SPEAKING MECHANISM
    Velar Structure and Function
    Indicate by checkmark the presence of any of the following conditions:

YES NO QUESTIONABLE		
( )( ) ( )	1.	Velar length inadequate for speech
( )( ) ( )	2.	Velar mobility inadequate for speech
( )( ) ( )	3.	Submucous cleft

The patient fails this section of the screening test if there is a possibility that he may exhibit any of the above.

SCORE: Pass_____ Fail_____ Unobservable due to lack of cooperation_____

Interpretation: Inadequate mobility, insufficient palatal length or submucous cleft are possible etiologies of velopharyngeal incompetency for speech.

    Accompanying Conditions A
    Indicate by checkmark the presence of any of the following conditions:

YES NO QUESTIONABLE			YES NO QUESTIONABLE		
( )( ) ( )	1.	"Cold"	( )( ) ( )	4.	Chronic mouth breathing
( )( ) ( )	2.	Chronic sinus infection	( )( ) ( )	5.	Structural obstruction of
( )( ) ( )	3.	Chronic allergy			nasal passage(s)

The patient fails this section of the screening test if there is a possibility that he may exhibit any of the above. Parental report may be extremely helpful in this regard.

SCORE: Pass_____ Fail_____ Unknown_____
Interpretation: A failure of this section suggests the presence of a condition which may reduce or camouflage symptoms of possible velopharyngeal incompetency for speech.

Figure 83–4 *Continued*

Illustration continued on the following page

Accompanying Conditions B
Indicate by checkmark the presence of any of the following:

YES NO
( )( )   1. Oral nasal fistula(s) (Estimated Size: _____)
( )( )   2. Missing teeth
The patient fails this section of the screening test if he exhibits any of the above.

SCORE: Pass_____ Fail_____ Unobservable due to lack of cooperation_____

Interpretation: A failure of this section suggests the presence of a condition which may contribute to an
exaggerated impression of possible velopharyngeal incompetency for speech.

SUMMARY OF RESULTS

Velopharyngeal competency for speech: Possible velopharyngeal incompetency for speech mani-
                                                 fested by the following:

                     INSUFFICIENT
YES NO QUESTIONABLE   RESPONSE   YES NO   YES NO
( ) ( )   ( )   ( )   ( )( )   articulation   ( )( )   nasal emission
                                                 ( )( )   voice quality   ( )( )   other_____

Description of findings of otoscopic examination:_____

_____

Results of audiometric evaluation:_____

_____

FOLLOW-UP

REFERRED TO:_____   ON:_____
                              speech pathologist   date

Currently in speech therapy?   NAME & ADDRESS OF SPEECH CLINICIAN   ADDITIONAL COMMENTS

        YES NO   _____   _____
        ( )( )
                                _____   _____

COMMENTS:_____

_____

_____

_____

_____

Figure 83–4 *Continued*

Signposts of velopharyngeal incompetency for speech might include hypernasality or excessive nasal resonance, audible escape of air from the nose during speech, articulation errors involving gross sound substitutions for speech sounds, hoarseness, breathiness, and weakened vocal intensity. Standarized speech screening tests can prove useful in training non-speech pathologists to be alert to and to recognize signs of velopharyngeal incompetency for speech.

The V-P Competency for Speech Screening Test. (Kulig and Baker, 1973c). Figure 83–4 is intended to guide those who are not speech pathologists in formulating preliminary impressions of a patient's communicative abilities as these relate to velopharyngeal competency for speech. This teaching guide

was developed shortly after a survey reported (1) that 81 per cent of medical students had never had any clinical experience with cleft palate patients, (2) that some 47 per cent of medical students did not know that a major objective of cleft palate habilitation involved optimizing or improving the patient's capabilities for adequate speech production, and (3) that 21 per cent of students responding omitted the speech pathologist when asked to list professionals who should be involved as members of the cleft palate evaluation and habilitation team (Lass et al., 1973).

The VPC, then, is a study guide; this screening approach is not intended to supplant the in-depth speech evaluation to which every patient suspected of velopharyngeal incompetency is entitled. The VPC format will provide the structure for the discussion that follows concerning signposts of velar inadequacy.

Sampling of Conversational Speech. Engaging the patient in conversational speech (Fig. 83–4, section 1) allows the examiner to screen (1) for general intelligibility, (2) for disorders of vocal quality as this might involve hypernasality or excessive nasal resonance, and (3) for sound distortions occasioned by air escaping from the patient's nostrils during speech. The presence of hypernasality or nasal emission in particular suggests the possibility of velopharyngeal incompetency for speech. The following paragraphs will further examine areas in which inadequate velopharyngeal closure may be manifested.

Articulation Screening. Sometimes, only a few of the sounds in "standard American English" can be produced with little or no difficulty by patients with velopharyngeal incompetency. Such sounds are /m/, /n/, /ng/, and /h/. Conversely, sounds such as those underscored in Figure 83–4 (section 2) may be particularly difficult for patients with velopharyngeal incompetency to produce adequately.

Figure 83–4 (section 2) illustrates a format for screening the articulation of patients suspected of exhibiting velopharyngeal incompetency for speech. The patient is asked to imitate the examiner's productions of chronologically appropriate test words and sentences. (Again, it is stressed that whenever articulatory skills are considered, they must be viewed in light of the patient's developmental age.) The aforementioned sampling of conversational speech and the repetition of test sentences provide helpful examples of the patient's ability to *maintain* adequate velopharyngeal closure as well.

The substitution of nonspeech sounds for consonants (the substitution of "uh-ee" for "*puppy*," for example), an increase in perceived hypernasality, or a deterioration of intelligibility when the patient engages in connected speech over time are symptoms associated with velopharyngeal incompetency for speech.

Voice Screening. The examiner should also record impressions of the patient's vocal quality, pitch, and intensity.

Figure 83–4 (section 3) illustrates a format that encourages the examiner to indicate by a checkmark the presence of normal, hypernasal, hyponasal, hoarse, or breathy voice qualities. The presence of unusually high or unu-

sually low vocal pitch and utilization of inappropriate intensity can similarly be noted in this manner.

Additional Testing for the Detection of Hypernasality. It is known that the action of alternately closing and opening the nostrils of a hypernasal individual during speech production (Fig. 83–5) may exaggerate the perception of distorted resonance. Requiring a patient to repeat test words under nostrils open and nostrils closed conditions helps the examiner to make a judgment as to whether or not hypernasality may be present. Perception of a difference in voice quality when a test word is produced with the nostrils open versus production of the same word when the nostrils are closed is suggestive of hypernasality. This is true because occluding the nostrils of the patient who lacks adequate velopharyngeal closure alters the resonating chamber by creating a cul-de-sac. The resonating chamber becomes an open resonator again once the occlusion is removed; hence a difference in voice quality is perceived.

Figure 83–4 (section 3-A) illustrates the section of the velopharyngeal competency test that requires the examiner to listen for appreciable change in the patient's voice quality during the production of test words under the nostrils closed and nostrils open conditions.

Testing for Nasal Emission of Air During Speech. We are next concerned with the detection of nasal escape of air during speech, another signpost of velopharyngeal incompetency. The patient is again asked to imitate words that should be particularly difficult for patients with inadequate velar function to produce correctly (Fig. 83–4, section 4). The examiner employs a cardboard air paddle (Fig. 83–6) in order to better detect the presence of nasal emission during speech.

Peroral Inspection of the Peripheral Speaking Mechanism. The screener should examine the patient for the presence of submucous clefting, insufficient velar length or marked oropharynx depth, and inadequate mobility of the muscles of the soft palate and pharynx, as these may be associated with velopharyngeal incompetency for speech.

The examiner is also encouraged to indicate by a checkmark the presence of conditions that might reduce or camouflage symptoms of velopharyngeal incompetency. For example, the resonating chamber will be affected by the presence of upper respiratory infection secondary to colds, allergy, or chronic sinus infection, as these can precipi-

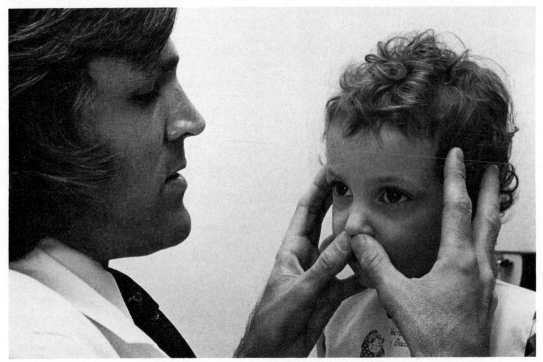

Figure 83–5 The examiner listens for appreciable change in the patient's voice quality during production of test words under the nostrils-closed condition.

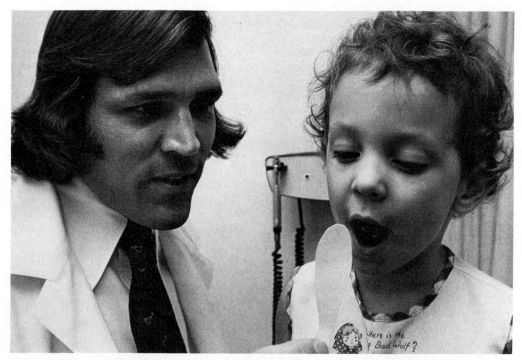

Figure 83–6 The examiner employs a cardboard air paddle in order to confirm the presence of nasal emission during speech.

tate inflammatory swelling of the mucosa and adenoid hypertrophy. Septal deviations and turbinate hypertrophy will also be of concern as these conditions may similarly distort the examiner's impression of abnormal airflow and hypernasal voice resonance.

The examiner must also be alert to conditions that may contribute to an exaggerated impression of nasal emission. This may be created by the patient's inability to direct the airstream effectively due to dental hazards, such as missing teeth or malocclusion. Small oronasal fistulae do not usually affect resonance appreciably nor do they usually precipitate nasal emission of air during speech. Certain types of articulation errors, however (pharyngeal fricatives, for example), may also be misinterpreted as nasal escape.

Hearing Loss with Cleft Palate. The incidence of chronic, fluctuating, bilateral conductive hearing loss is of course extremely high among children with cleft palate. For this reason, the examiner is asked to routinely arrange for otologic and audiologic studies. The reader is referred to Chapter 87, which treats the subject of velopharyngeal incompetency in detail.

CONSULTATION AND REFERRAL

There is little need to screen for speech disorders unless follow-up is possible for additional evaluation and therapy by a speech pathologist when a need for these is indicated. Information regarding the geographic locations, educational backgrounds, and employment affiliations of speech pathologists certified by the American Speech and Hearing Association is available in that organization's annually published directory (ASHA, 1978a). State speech, language, and hearing associations and state speech pathology and audiology licensure boards can also assist health care providers to identify qualified professionals working in their vicinities. University speech and hearing clinics, rehabilitation centers, and public school districts might also provide assistance in this regard.

Finally, it should be remembered that screening is never diagnostic. In the speech screening process, patients are evaluated in terms of whether or not they are *likely* to have speech within normal limits. It is also true that there are few tests of any kind that would not benefit from some sort of modification. The interpretation, then, of screening test results should always be undertaken with caution.

We would much prefer to err in the direction of unnecessarily referring a patient to a speech pathologist than to overlook a child at possible risk for a communicative disorder. Also, the over-referral and under-referral rates of any screening test must always be considered in practical terms. Both rates should be small and in the hoped-for direction — i.e., over-referrals should occur with greater frequency than do under-referrals. Information regarding the validity and reliability of a screening instrument is of first order priority in its selection as an appropriate screening test for office practice. A test's ease of administration, stimulus materials, and manpower and time requirements are of obvious importance as well.

A WORD ABOUT SCREENING SCHOOL CHILDREN FOR SPEECH DISORDERS

Classroom teachers are in a most appropriate position to screen the typical speech and language abilities of school-aged children. The physician in office practice might utilize an instrument such as *The Classroom Teacher's Quick Screen For Speech Disorders* (Kulig and Baker, 1973b) (Fig. 83–7) by forwarding it to a patient's classroom teacher for completion. Should a student's speech and language abilities be found to be at risk, the physician, in cooperation with the classroom teacher, can arrange for a school-based speech pathologist to undertake further evaluation and treatment.

CONCLUSION

This chapter has been concerned with screening children for disorders of speech and language. Techniques have been presented that are designed to enable others besides speech pathologists to identify these problems with at least 90 per cent accuracy (Kulig and Baker, 1973; 1976). Inculcating a willingness among health professionals to adopt speech and language screening as a routine health maintenance procedure remains a most challenging objective at this time when one of every ten Americans is considered to exhibit a disorder of speech, language, or hearing (ASHA, 1974).

THE CLASSROOM TEACHER'S QUICK SCREEN FOR SPEECH DISORDERS
Experimental Edition

CHILD'S NAME: _____ RACE: _____ SEX: _____ DATE: _____

GRADE: _____ CLASSROOM TEACHER: _____ EXAMINER: _____

DATE OF BIRTH: _____ CURRENT AGE: _____ (mos.)

I. **LANGUAGE**

Directions: Indicate with a checkmark the presence of any of the following behaviors thought to be associated with possible language disabilities. To be significant, a behavior must be viewed as typical of the youngster being evaluated.

Yes	No	
( )	( )	1. Difficulty with spelling in contrast to most classmates
( )	( )	2. Difficulty with copying, printing or cursive skills in contrast to most classmates
( )	( )	3. Difficulty with numbers in contrast to most classmates
( )	( )	4. Difficulty reading in contrast to most classmates
( )	( )	5. Difficulty sequencing in contrast to most classmates
( )	( )	6. Difficulty categorizing in contrast to most classmates
( )	( )	7. Difficulty with memorization in contrast to most classmates
( )	( )	8. Difficulty with opposites (up/down, in/out, etc.) in contrast to most classmates
( )	( )	9. Receptive vocabulary poor in contrast to most classmates
( )	( )	10. Difficulty following instructions in contrast to most classmates
( )	( )	11. Difficulty describing a picture or object in contrast to most classmates
( )	( )	12. Expressive vocabulary poor in contrast to most classmates
( )	( )	13. Delayed responses to questions in contrast to most classmates
( )	( )	14. Average sentence length poor in contrast to most classmates
( )	( )	15. Oral grammar poor in contrast to most classmates
( )	( )	16. Difficulty relating a story in contrast to most classmates

I suspect this child's typical classroom performance to be compromised by difficulties with language in light of my observations as indicated by checkmark above.

Yes   No
( )   ( )
If the answer to the above question is yes, the patient fails this section of the screening test.

SCORE: Pass   Fail   (circle one)

II. **RHYTHM OF SPEECH**

Based on classroom observation of the child's speech, note the presence of any of the following characteristics commonly associated with stuttering.

Yes   No
( )   ( )   frequent hesitations
( )   ( )   frequent repetitions (may occur on words or sounds)

Please describe any mannerisms associated with the above (eye blinks, finger-snapping, facial tics, etc.): _____ _____

_____

_____

Please describe any behaviors associated with fear or avoidance of speaking situations: _____

_____

_____

Comments: _____

_____

I suspect this child's speaking abilities to be compromised by stuttering in light of my observations as discussed above.

Yes   No
( )   ( )
If the answer to the above question is yes, the patient fails this section of the screening test.

SCORE: Pass   Fail   (circle one)

Figure 83–7   The Classroom Teacher's Quick Screen for Speech Disorders.

Illustration continued on the opposite page

III. ARTICULATION

Directions: Have the child imitate your production of each of the following words, <u>watching</u> as well as <u>listening</u> to his production. Circle any word in which the underlined sound is mispronounced or absent. Record the number of circled words from each word group in the indicated space. <u>Important</u>: Remember to watch the child as he imitates your models.

No. of words circled	Word Group For Children 6 - 7 Years			No. of words circled	Word Group For Children Above 7 Years of Age		
_____	1. cheese	teacher	much	_____	1. drink	clue	blue
_____	2. red	carry	bear	_____		gleam	crack
_____	3. no	money	pin	_____	2.	singing	song
_____	4. bed	baby	tab	_____	3. skunk	show	tusk
_____	5. coat	cookie	walk	_____		best	
_____	6. day	daddy	bad	_____	4. foot	coffee	off
_____	7. shell	bushel	dish	_____	5. red	carry	bear
_____	8. happy	beehive		_____	6. jello	major	fudge
_____	9. foot	coffee	off	_____	7. pie	puppy	nap
_____	10.	singing	song	_____	8. the	other	smooth
_____	11. pie	puppy	nap	_____	9. sat	lesson	pass
_____	12. ten	mitten	hit	_____	10. shell	bushel	dish
_____	13. yes	yo yo		_____	11. yes	yo yo	
_____	14. go	doggie	egg	_____	12. walk	away	
_____	15. drink	clue	blue	_____	13. zoo	dizzy	buzz
		gleam	crack	_____	14. bed	baby	tab
_____	16. walk	away		_____	15. truck	stop	slow
_____	17. man	mommy	game			sweet	spank
_____	18. land	hello	doll	_____	16. cheese	teacher	much
				_____	17. day	daddy	bad
				_____	18. ten	mitten	hit
				_____	19. man	mommy	game
				_____	20. no	money	pin
				_____	21. land	hello	doll
				_____	22. happy	beehive	
				_____	23. go	doggie	egg
				_____	24. coat	cookie	walk
				_____	25. think	anything	bath
				_____	26. vacation	oven	move

Yes   No
(   )   (   ) In my opinion, this child's speech would be intelligible to strangers.
(The child fails this section of the screening test if two or more words of ANY word group are circled; or if you do not believe that the child's speech would be intelligible to strangers.)

SCORE: Pass   Fail   (circle one)

IV. SPEAKING MECHANISM

I believe the child's speaking ability is compromised by the structure or function of his speaking mechanism (palatal, breathing, or tongue problems etc. suspected).

Yes   No
(   )   (   )
If the answer to the above question is yes, the patient fails this section of the screening test.

SCORE: Pass   Fail   (circle one)

V. VOICE

Directions: Based on your observations of the child's voice as he verbalizes in the classroom, indicate by a checkmark your description of the child's voice.

1. Typical Quality   normal_____ hoarse_____ (in absence of "a cold") history of chronic hoarseness _____
                       hypernasal (sounds as though he's "talking through his nose") _____
                       hyponasal (sounds as though he always "has a cold") ___
2. Typical Pitch   normal_____ unusually low_____ unusually high_____
3. Typical Loudness   normal_____ unusually weak_____ unusually loud_____

(If patient exhibits a significant voice deviation, he fails this section of the screening test. If the patient presently appears to have a "cold", a statement regarding typical voice quality must be deferred until resolution of symptoms occurs.)

SCORE: Pass   Fail   (circle one)

Summary of Impressions

If the child has failed ANY of the above sections, he should be referred to the school pathologist for further evaluation.

Referred to: _____ Date: _____

Referred for further evaluation of: Language_____ Rhythm of Speech_____ Articulation_____ Speaking Mechanism_____ Voice _____

Comments: _____

Figure 83–7 *Continued*

SELECTED REFERENCES

Myklebust, H. R. 1954. Auditory Disorders In Children: A Manual For Differential Diagnosis. New York, Grune & Stratton, (367 pp.).

Designed for use by physicians, psychologists, and communicative disorders specialists, this text is concerned with differential diagnosis of communicative disorders in children. Various clinical approaches to in-depth evaluation of patients at risk for deafness, aphasia, emotional disturbance, and mental retardation are considered. Illustrative cases and recommendations for management are presented.

Travis, L. E. 1971. Handbook for Speech Pathology and Audiology. New York, Appleton-Century-Crofts, (1300 pp.).

This basic reference presents concepts relating to the evaluation and treatment of the numerous possible disorders of speech, language, and hearing. Contributing authors are well-known authorities in the field of communicative disorders. Terminology and nomenclature, differential diagnosis, and varied therapeutic approaches are presented in some detail.

Wilson, D. K. 1972. Voice Problems of Children. Baltimore, The Williams and Wilkins Co., (185 pp.).

This manual presents useful information relating to the differential diagnosis of voice problems in children. Material relating to remedial procedures likely to be employed by speech clinicians in the treatment of voice problems should be particularly interesting and of assistance to physicians.

REFERENCES

American Speech and Hearing Association. 1974. Communication disorders specialist. (A public information narrative text produced by the office of recruitment).

American Speech and Hearing Association. 1978a. Annual Directory. Danville, Il, Interstate Printers and Publishers.

American Speech and Hearing Association. 1978b. Intracommittee Communications of the Standing Committee on Language.

Anderson, R. M., Miles, M., and Matheny, P. A. 1963. Communicative Evaluation Chart from Infancy to Five Years. Cambridge, MA, Educators Publishing Services, Inc.

Asbed, R. A., Masland, M. W., Sever, J. L., et al. 1970. Early case finding of children with communication problems, part I. The Volta Review, 72:23–50.

Davis, I. P. 1938. The speech aspects of reading readiness. 17th Yearbook of the Department of Elementary School Principals, NEA, 17(7):282–289.

Drumwright, A. F. 1971. The Denver Articulation Screening Exam. The University of Colorado Medical Center.

Eisenson, J. 1972. Aphasia in Children, New York, Harper & Row.

Frankenburg, W. K., and Dodds, J. B. 1969. Denver Development Screening Test. The University of Colorado Medical Center.

Froeschels, E. 1948. Twentieth Century Speech and Voice Correction. New York, Philosophical Library.

Hejna, R. 1955. Developmental Articulation Test. Madison, WI, College Printing and Typing.

Houston, S. 1976. Personal communication.

Irwin, O. 1947. Infant speech: Variability and the problem of diagnosis. J. Speech Disord., 12:287–289.

Johnson, W. (Ed.) 1950. Speech Problems of Children. New York, Grune & Stratton.

Kulig, S. G., and Baker, K. A. 1973a. The Physician's Developmental Quick Screen for Speech Disorders (PDQ). Galveston, University of Texas Medical Branch.

Kulig, S. G., and Baker, K. A. 1973b. The Classroom Teacher's Quick Screen for Speech Disorders (CTQ). Galveston, University of Texas Medical Branch.

Kulig, S. G., and Baker, K. A. 1973c. The V-P Competency for Speech Screening Test (VPC). Galveston, University of Texas Medical Branch.

Kulig, S. G., Baker, K. A., and Levine, H. G. 1975. Screening for speech and language disorders: A training program for physicians and allied health professionals. J. Am. Speech Hear. Assoc., 17(8):507–512.

Kulig, S. G., and Baker, K. A. 1976. The Physician's Developmental Quick Screen for Speech Disorders: A preliminary report concerning a 5 minute procedure for testing children aged 6 months to 6 years. Clin. Pediatr., 15(12):1146–1150.

Lass, N. J., Gasparini, R. M., and Overberger, J. E. 1973. The exposure of medical and dental students to the disorder of cleft palate. Cleft Palate J., 10:306–311.

Light, G. S., and Walski, N. 1969. The physician and differential diagnosis of communicative disorders in children. Mich. Med., 68:357–358.

McCarthy, D. 1954. Language development in children. *In* Carmichael, L. (Ed.) Manual of Child Psychology, New York.

Mullendore, J. M. 1965. Communicative disorders of children: Classification and criteria for referral. E. Va. Med. J., 61:143–146.

Myklebust, H. R. 1954. Auditory Disorders in Children: A Manual For Differential Diagnosis. New York, Grune & Stratton.

Poole, I. 1934. Genetic development in articulation of consonant sounds in speech. Elem. Eng., 11:159–161.

Richardson, S. O. 1964. Pediatric evaluation of speech and hearing disorders. J. Clin. Pediatr., 3:150–152.

Schaye, G. F., and Ruben, R. J. 1971. Identification of communication disorders by resident physicians, N. Y. State J. Med., 7:1941–1942.

Shearer, W. M. 1972. Diagnosis and treatment of voice disorders in school children. J. Speech Hear. Disord., 37:215–221.

Templin, M. 1952. Speech development in the young child; The development of certain language skills in children. J. Speech Hear. Disord., 17:280–285.

Templin, M. 1957. Certain language skills in children, their development and interrelationships. Institute of Child Welfare Monograph Series, 26:54, Minneapolis, University of Minnesota Press.

Travis, L. E. 1971. Handbook for Speech Pathology and Audiology. New York, Appleton-Century-Crofts.

West, R., Kennedy, L., and Carr, A. 1947. Rehabilitation of Speech, revised ed. New York, Harper and Row.

Wilson, D. K. 1972. Voice Problems of Children. Baltimore, The Williams and Wilkins Co.

Zimmerman, I. L., Steiner, V. G., and Evatt, R. L. 1969. Preschool Language Scale. Columbus, Ohio, Charles E. Merrill Publ. Co.

Chapter 84

DISORDERS OF LANGUAGE

Jack Matthews, Ph.D., D.Sc.

Section VII deals with communication disorders, which are usually treated by speech pathologists, language pathologists, communicologists, and audiologists. No detailed discussion is presented of communication disorders related to reading, writing, spelling, or other specific learning disabilities. An overall survey of these communication disorders can be found in Tina E. Bangs' Language and Learning Disorders of the Pre-Academic Child (Bangs, 1968). Communication Disorders: Remedial Principles and Practices, edited by Stanley Dickson (1974) provides an introduction to the entire field of speech pathology and audiology. Handbook of Speech Pathology and Audiology, edited by L. E. Travis (1971) provides the most extensive coverage of speech pathology and audiology available in any single volume. Burgi and Matthews (1963) present a brief orientation to the area of communication disorders in childhood. Clevenger and Matthews (1971) cover the larger field of human communication with an emphasis on the processes involved. Table 84–1 presents a glossary of terms used in this chapter.

THE NATURE OF LANGUAGE

Language is a system of symbols that produces similar responses from a group of people. The symbols designate such things as objects, activities, or relationships. Berry (1969) has combined these concepts into the following definition of language.

Language from another point of view is a system of symbols containing socially shared meanings which must be learned and providing categories for classifying experience.

In our culture we learn to accept the color red as a symbol for *stop* and the color green as a symbol for *go*. We learn that the index finger raised to cover the lips or the prolonged forcing of air through clenched teeth to make the /sh/ sound are both symbols that by common agreement in our culture we take to mean *be quiet*.

The relationship between the symbol and that for which the symbol stands is purely arbitrary. The sequencing of symbols is also arbitrary and will differ among languages. German frequently places the verb at the end of a sentence after the subject and object. In English the conventional place for the verb is between the subject and object. In English we place the adjective before the noun it modifies, for example, *red apple*. In French the adjective is placed after the noun.

We take it for granted that there is a symbol (name) for every object, quality, or act in the world. In the process of development, children learn the agreed-upon symbols in their culture that "stand for" or represent various parts of their world. They learn not only appropriate symbols but also the agreed-upon sequence in the arrangement of the symbols.

Among the profoundly deaf, symbols do not involve sound but instead involve various movements of fingers and hands, sometimes with movements of the lips. In our culture a red light or flag is recognized as a symbol to represent *stop* or *danger*. Two crossed lines on a highway sign are the symbol to represent a crossroad. American musicians communicate

Table 84–1 GLOSSARY OF TERMS IN THE STUDY OF LANGUAGE

Articulation—the process of shaping the sounds generated by the vocal tract in order to produce the phonemes of the language.

Communication disorder—a defect in a person's ability to understand or to express information, feelings, wants, or ideas. It may involve problems in hearing, voice production and quality, articulation, speech rhythm, or language.

Communicologist—a specialist in disorders of speech or language.

Consonant—any speech sound articulated either by interrupting the outgoing breath stream or by severely restricting its flow.

Dysgraphia—a disorder of writing.

Dyslexia—impaired reading ability.

Jargon—sound production of young children in which a variety of sounds are put together in nonsense syllables but with the inflectional pattern (melody) of meaningful speech.

Labials—consonants that are articulated by movement of the lips.

Language—a system of symbols containing shared meanings that are arbitrary and learned. The system provides categories that are employed by users of the language to classify their experiences as well as to express them.

Language pathologist—sometimes used to designate those communicologists who concentrate on treating language disorders.

Phoneme—the briefest unit of sound in a language that can be recognized as being distinct from other sounds in the language.

Prosody—speech melody that is produced by changes in pitch, quality, volume, and duration and that carries meaning in addition to the meaning of the word symbols.

Semantic—the aspect of language concerned with the meanings associated with symbols.

Speech pathologist—a specialist in the diagnosis and treatment of speech and language disorders, sometimes used synonymously with communicologist.

Syntax—rules concerned with the appropriate combination, ordering, and relationships among various words in an utterance.

(Based in part on Nicolosi, L., Harryman, E., and Kresheck, J. 1978. Terminology of Communication Disorders. Baltimore, Williams & Wilkins.)

effectively with Russian musicians by means of the symbols of music notation. Again, the association of the symbols and what they stand for is arbitrary and must be learned.

The process by which *oral* symbols are perceived and produced is known as speech (Bangs, 1968). Chapters 85, 86, and 88 treat various disorders of this process of reception and production of oral symbols. The child who says "wed wabbit" rather than "red rabbit" has a speech defect. The child who has no symbol to designate this animal or this color is considered to have a *language disorder*.

We will focus on oral language, which Carroll (1961) has defined as a "structured system of arbitrary vocal sounds and sequences of sounds that is used in interpersonal communication and which rather exhaustively catalogues the things, events, and processes of human communication." Our concern is with disorders of oral language.

LANGUAGE DISORDERS

We use the term "disorders of language" to include two different kinds of language behavior. One is seen in children who do not follow the normal orderly patterns and sequences in learning the language code. The other (often referred to as delayed language) is seen in the child who follows an orderly pattern of language acquisition but at a rate much slower than is appropriate for the child's chronologic age.

VARIATION IN EXPLANATIONS OF CAUSES OF LANGUAGE DISORDERS

The reader should be prepared for a wide variety of explanations of causes of language disorders and rationales for treatment. Part of this variety stems from widespread differences in the explanations of the process of language acquisition and development. A clinician whose orientation to language acquisition is based on learning theory is likely to see the etiology of language disorders differently from one who is trained in the biological–developmental tradition of Lenneberg (1967).

It can be confusing to the parents of a three year old child who is not speaking to receive different and often conflicting opinions concerning the etiology of delayed language. The otolaryngologist may stress the role of hearing loss. The psychologist may attribute the problem to mental retardation. The psychiatrist may give major importance to emotional problems in the home. Other specialists may blame an environment lacking adequate language stimulation or confusion growing out of a bilingual background. The presence of one of these factors does not rule out the possible influences that may be exerted by the others. The incidence of hearing loss is, indeed, higher in the mentally retarded than in the nonretarded population (Birch and Matthews, 1951), and hearing loss can result in frustration and emotional problems. A physical disability can result in parents overly protecting a child so the child finds little need to learn to talk. The task of differential diagnosis in the child with a language disorder is difficult and goes beyond the scope of training of most pediatricians and otolaryngologists, even though the contributions of these physicians are important in the diagnosis and treatment of the disorders. Chapter 83 provides a more detailed discussion of examination techniques for speech and language disorders and describes office screening procedures that can be carried out by clinicians without in-depth training in communication disorders.

LANGUAGE TESTING

Even when used by experienced specialists, our most widely accepted language testing procedures have limitations. Language examinations are carried out on a limited sample of a child's language behavior. We know there is a great variability in a child's language performance from time to time and from situation to situation. We take into consideration normal variations in blood pressure by measuring it under somewhat standardized conditions — at rest, after running in place for a given time, and so forth — but we do not have equivalent "standardized" language situations other than the stimuli employed in "standardized" language tests. Norms for these tests are based largely on white, middle-class populations, and dialect differences may be incorrectly interpreted as language defects. In addition, the testing situation may not elicit the best language performance the child is able to produce.

In spite of all these limitations, the skillful clinician is helped considerably by the fact that, in general, the order of development in language acquisition is fairly stable and cuts across a variety of languages and cultures. We know that language comprehension precedes language production. We also know that language is more highly correlated with motor development than with chronologic age.

Given the present "state of the art" and the pressure of concerned parents, we often begin our remedial procedures before we are able to define the etiology of the problem clearly. We frequently use diagnostic teaching, which involves various language teaching techniques, to provide additional insights into the etiology of the child's language problem. In some instances we are able to use intervention strategies that minimize or eliminate the language disorder even though we are not always able to establish its cause.

RECEPTIVE LANGUAGE DEVELOPMENT

A good developmental history helps to put language development in a broader context. The very early development of receptive language can be seen in the first few weeks of life in the infant's reflexive response to sudden and loud sounds. Shortly after, the infant begins to differentiate among various emotional values in the voices of parents. The six month old infant has learned to move his or her eyes to locate sound. About this same time the infant often vocalizes in response to the intonations of parents' voices. These vocalizations for the most part are vowels but are sometimes combined with the easily produced consonants /m/ and /b/. At about six months of age the infant begins to show evidence that speech sounds are beginning to take on meaning, and by the age of one year the young child can respond to simple instructions, such as "show me your ear," although at this age the infant is not yet ready to *produce* language of such complexity. Indeed, at this age his or her understanding is a global understanding of the instructions rather than of each of the individual verbal components in the instructions. By the age of two years the child enjoys listening to the rhythmic patterns of nursery rhymes without much understanding of the individual words of the rhymes, and such prosodic aspects of language are imitated in jargon even earlier than age two. By the time the child has reached the age of three he or she is following simple stories and ongoing conversation.

The ages cited for each of these stages of receptive language development represent averages in the same way that "norms" for the ages of sitting, standing, and walking represent averages. The sequence in which these receptive language developmental landmarks occur is predictable in the same way that we can predict walking will occur after and not before sitting.

EXPRESSIVE LANGUAGE DEVELOPMENT

McConnell and colleagues (1974) present a brief treatment of expressive language development under the headings of *phonemic, syntactic,* and *semantic* development. Vowels and labials (lip-formed consonants, such as /m/ and /b/), develop early. The correct articulation of the /r/ sound may not be mastered until sometime between the ages of six and seven years. Mastery of the rules for converting singular to plural, present to past tense, and other grammatical concepts is a developmental process that results in most children learning to employ the grammar of the English language before they study grammatical rules in school. Unlike the development of phonemic and syntactic accuracy, which is largely completed by age seven, semantic development — the ascribing of meaning to word symbols — is an ongoing process that continues throughout life as the vocabulary grows.

As is true for receptive language development, there are milestones in expressive language development. An early milestone that occurs during the first year of infancy is vocal play, often referred to as cooing or babbling. Somewhere around the age of one year, the child will produce the first word. Many children will produce spontaneously two or three single words by the time they are a year old. During the second year, voice inflection develops and conveys meaning beyond that of any sounds in the child's jargon. Halfway through the second year of life, the child will be able to produce nearly 25 single words, and by the age of two this vocabulary will have grown to approximately 200 words (Gesell, 1940). By age three the child is describing experiences by means of simple, connected sentences. At this time the child is also producing an almost constant series of "What's that?" questions. By the time the average child reaches four and a half years, he or she will have developed most of the syntactic elements of language and will say "I want cookie" rather than "cookie want I," and

the child is saying that the cookie is *on* the plate, not *in* the plate. Although additional sounds will be mastered up to approximately age seven, "the basic foundations of spoken language are well laid by the age of four and one-half" (McConnell et al., 1974).

ETIOLOGY OF LANGUAGE DISORDERS

Language disorders can include deficits in any or all of the previously mentioned areas — phonemic, syntactic, or semantic. The deficit may be in either the receptive or expressive realm or in a combination of both. The language disorder may go beyond deficits of verbal functioning. Zigmond and Cicci (1968) have described auditory processing deficits that resulted from faulty auditory discrimination, sequencing, and memory. A child may be unable to distinguish between the ring of the bell at the end of a class period and the ring of a telephone. The child who has difficulty with the sequencing of auditory events may have problems learning the numbers from one to ten or the days of the week. Communication problems can be associated with specific learning disabilities, such as problems in reading, writing, or spelling.

Because language reception precedes language production, hearing impairment is an important etiologic factor in many language disorders. Chapters 88 and 89 are concerned with aural rehabilitation and education of the deaf.

Hearing loss may be only one of several etiologic factors that may include mental retardation, neurologic damage, and emotional disturbance, which account for language deficit. Neurologic impairment alone or in conjunction with hearing loss, mental retardation, emotional disturbance, and other etiologic factors can result in a variety of language disorders, including dyslexia and dysgraphia. Frequently children with neurologic impairment have difficulty understanding language. In some children the problem is encountered only with somewhat abstract language, but others may be so impaired that they are not able to associate the spoken word *ball* with the round, bouncy object the symbol represents.

There are some neurologically impaired children who have little or no difficulty *understanding* language but who do have problems of oral *expression*. Johnson and Myklebust (1967) have enumerated the problems of these children in three general categories: (1) problems in reauditorization and word selection, (2) problems in learning to say words, and (3) problems in defective syntax. Children in the first group recognize and attribute correct meaning to individual words, but they are not able to recall the words for spontaneous use. In the second group are children whose problems are not in the areas of comprehension or reauditorization; rather, their difficulty is in performing the motor acts needed for speech. The tongue may perform quite adequately for chewing and other nonspeech acts but not for saying words containing sounds requiring tongue action (such as /t/ or /d/). In the third group are children who have problems organizing words and phrases into sentences with correct word order. These children can use single words and simple phrases but often omit or distort words and phrases when they attempt to produce more complex sentences.

In our own clinical experience we have found that mental retardation has been one of the most frequently encountered factors associated with language and speech retardation. Matthews (1971b) summarized the studies that investigated the relationship between intelligence and language and speech retardation.

The studies concerned with time of speech and language acquisition in mentally retarded children do not provide us with normative data we can accept with confidence. Various indices of speech and language acquisition have been employed by different investigators. Definitions of intellectual levels of subjects are not always presented nor are they comparable from study to study. The sampling procedures and statistical treatment are subject to question. In spite of these limitations, the studies do point out clearly that on the average the mentally retarded child acquires language and speech considerably later than the child of normal intelligence.

Not only is language frequently delayed in the mentally retarded child, but when it does emerge it is often accompanied by speech defects. A summary of approximately 50 studies carried out from 1911 to 1971 clearly demonstrates that the incidence of speech disorders among the mentally retarded is considerably higher than in a nonretarded population (Matthews, 1971b). There is no evidence, however, to suggest that the com-munication disorders of the mentally retarded differ in kind from those of nonretarded children with communication disorders.

As early as 1951, Birch and Matthews demonstrated that it is possible to secure reliable audiometric thresholds from mentally retarded subjects. After summarizing 12 studies of hearing loss in mentally retarded populations, Matthews (1971b) draws the following conclusions.

Although there is not complete agreement among all the investigators as to the incidence of hearing loss in mentally retarded cases, there is a clear cut indication that the incidence of hearing loss among the mentally retarded is considerably greater than that in a non-retarded population.

The role of emotional disturbance in the development of language disorders is extremely difficult to assess. Some children with severe emotional disturbances may give the impression of being deaf. They may ignore sounds bordering in intensity on pain-threshold levels. Morrow (1959) suggests that mentally retarded children can be differentiated from psychotic children on the basis of (1) signs of slow motor development, such as late sitting or walking, (2) physical stigmata of retardation, and (3) presumptive evidence of additional congenital deformities. He also suggests that the retarded child relates more quickly and warmly than does the psychotic child. Matthews (1971b) has cautioned against ruling out mental retardation as an etiologic factor in the language-disordered child who has been labeled psychotic. He stresses the need to recognize the roles of the pediatrician, otologist, audiologist, psychologist, neurologist, and psychiatrist as well as the speech and language pathologist in making a differential diagnosis (Matthews, 1971b).

The child with a handicap may be "hidden" from the world at large and so be deprived of the stimulation necessary for language development. Parents may also overprotect or "baby" the child to such an extent that there is reduced motivation for the child to develop normal expressive language. Occasionally siblings may provide so much language competition that the child with delayed language doesn't have a chance to "get a word in edgewise."

With the advent of the "war on poverty" and programs such as Headstart, there has been much written to suggest that children from low socioeconomic backgrounds are "culturally deprived" and deficient in language development. Matthews (1971a) points out that we must recognize the important distinction between *defective* and *different* language found in children from various minorities. We accept the Bostonian accent of Senator Kennedy or the Georgia accent of former President Carter as *different* rather than *defective.* The Black child expressing himself or herself in Black English is more likely to be labeled *defective* rather than *different.* Racial differences may account for some language differences in spoken English in the United States, but language disorders of children who come from a background of poverty occur across racial lines; poverty and deprivation appear to be more significant than race in the development of language disorders. It must be recognized that clinicians coming largely from white, middle-class backgrounds may perceive deprivation and pathologic signs in environments that are not well-known to them. Differences in language are often equated with deficiencies, and a value judgment is made that the "deficiencies" must be corrected.

Taylor (1971) has pointed out that little information is available to identify legitimate pathologic language patterns among Blacks.

Given the absence of appropriate normative data and tests for blacks, little is known about what a legitimate pathology actually is especially at various ages during childhood. For example, no one knows when to expect the acquisition of the use of the copula to express the continuative aspect of verbs, as in "I be hungry every morning." Until such data are available, it is virtually impossible to determine legitimate language pathologies for blacks, except when deviations are so gross as to make them obvious.

PRINCIPLES AND PROCEDURES IN LANGUAGE TESTING

The communicologist not only assesses the child's level of language development but also often can suggest needed additional tests, such as those provided by psychologists, social workers, and neurologists to evaluate a child's language problems effectively.

In many language disorders there will be dysfunction in auditory comprehension, verbal expression, or both. McConnell and colleagues (1974) describe principles and procedures employed in assessing children with no language development as well as those with deviations in receptive–expressive language. The purpose of these procedures is to arrive at a differential diagnosis, which in turn determines the use of remedial strategies. McConnell and colleagues (1974) describe eleven developmental language scales and five comprehensive tests of language.

Such scales and tests supplement parental reports and observations of behavior. Because parents are with their children many hours each day they can provide much information that might be missed by a clinician with limited time to observe the child. Lenneberg (1967) believes that the developmental milestones of both receptive and expressive language (age of onset of first word, first two word phrase, and so forth) are better indicators of the capacity to develop language than are the results of standardized tests of articulation, vocabulary size, or syntactic complexity. At this stage in our knowledge, both approaches, plus systematic observation by clinicians and family members, will often have to be combined in order to arrive at a differential diagnosis. Chapter 83 treats this topic in greater detail.

Although the physician should not be expected to make a diagnosis of language disorder, she or he must sometimes decide if a child should be seen by another specialist to determine if there is a language problem. The decision to refer a child to a communicologist will be based on the otologist's assessment that the level of language development appears to be lagging considerably behind what is normal. It is highly unlikely that the otologist will administer any standardized language tests. It is, however, very reasonable for the otologist to seek information about the language behavior of his or her young patients. This information can come in part by questioning parents and in part by observing the child's behavior. In general, it would not be considered normal for a nine month old child to fail to move his or her eyes or head to locate sounds. Nor would it be normal for a 2 year old not to respond to a simple instruction, such as "show me your nose," providing time is taken to secure the child's attention and cooperation. This can best be accomplished in a playlike situation rather than on an examining table and is often best carried out when the otologist observes the response the child makes to stimuli provided by the parents. A few toys or attractive pictures can often help the otologist "break the ice" with a young child in order to elicit language responses; such responses are often difficult to elicit in a hurried, pressured examination. If the otologist routinely seeks to determine how his or her young patients' language behavior compares with the developmental language landmarks described earlier in this chapter, he or she will soon develop a sense of what is abnormal in language development. By carefully comparing early impressions with the more complete testing results of the communications disorders specialist, the otologist in time can calibrate his or her clinical judgments concerning possible language disorders. As is true with most suspected problems, it is better to err on the side of over-referral and at an earlier rather than a later age. It is also good to remember that language development generally is more highly correlated with developmental age than with chronologic age.

REMEDIATION

In some instances a program of remedial language training may be initiated without a definitive origin of the problem having been established. The speech and language pathologist is trained to measure growth in language behavior as the remedial program progresses and to shift the emphasis of the intervention strategies if they do not appear to modify language behavior.

There is a wide variety of approaches to the remediation of language disorders. Each approach is partly the result of employing a particular theory to explain the process of language acquisition and development. Some indication of this variety can be seen in Table 84–2.

Although there is considerable variation in method among different investigators, as can be seen from the previous table, there is agreement among most clinicians on several general guidelines. Early intervention is generally accepted as a basic principle of language remediation. The work of Lenneberg (1967) and McNeill (1970) suggests that in the process of language acquisition there are certain critical periods. The most important of these critical periods occurs in the early preschool years. There is also agreement on the desirability of involving parents in the remedial activities designed to stimulate language development during these early critical periods.

Many of the remedial procedures appear to be complete systems of instruction. Most clinicians would agree that effective language remediation does not involve teaching a *system* but should involve teaching a *child.* The individual needs, abilities, and interests of each child will shape the intervention program and modify any general system that is being followed. The language remediation procedures must not only focus on immediate language performance but must also be coordinated with short-term and long-term educational planning.

Although it would be highly desirable to have a clear diagnosis of and etiology for the disorder prior to embarking on a remedial program, there are times when this is impossible, as the diagnosis and etiology often change as various intervention strategies are introduced. For all practical purposes, diagnosis should be an ongoing process, which may shift the emphasis of a given intervention or in some instances lead to dropping one approach or sensory modality in favor of another. The treatment for most language disorders is quite lengthy, and the results of treatment as a rule are seen gradually. The otolaryngologist and the pediatrician can help the speech pathologist by encouraging parents to begin treatment early, to view the treatment program realistically, and to avoid the search for dramatic or spectacular "cures."

Neither the pediatrician nor the otolaryngologist is likely to be directly involved in remedial language procedures. Table 84–2 lists some of the rationales for and goals of remedial procedures. Having this information available will assist the otologist in providing maximal reinforcement to parents and child. The necessity of involving specialists from speech pathology, audiology, special education, psychology, social work, neurology, psychiatry, and other related medical specialties should also be evident. The involvement and the coordination of such a team can be complicated and time-consuming, but clinical experience demonstrates that such multiprofessional efforts provide the best possibilities for the successful treatment of language disorders. No single specialty has the expertise to handle this problem alone.

Table 84–2 SELECTED SOURCES FOR METHODS AND MATERIALS
FOR LANGUAGE REMEDIATION

Author(s)	Reference Source	Brief Description
Bangs, T. E.	Language and Learning Disorders of the Pre-Academic Child: With Curriculum Guide. New York, Appleton-Century-Crofts, Inc. (1968)	A preacademic curriculum guide for ages from six months through kindergarten.
Developmental Language and Speech Center Staff, Grand Rapids, MI	Teach Your Child to Talk: A Parent Handbook. New York, CEBCO/Standard Publishing Company (copyright claimed until December, 1975).	Offers guidance for parents concerning their child's speech and language development.
Dunn, L., Horton, K., and Smith, J.	Peabody Language Development Kits, Level P (Mental ages 3–5). Circle Pines, MN, American Guidance Service, Inc. (1968).	Four items designed to stimulate oral language and verbal intelligence through use of a teacher's manual and a wide number of pictures, color chips, puppets, records, and tapes. For preschool to intermediate grade levels.
Dunn, L., and Smith, J.	Peabody Language Development Kits Level I (Mental ages 4½–6½) (1965); Level 2 (Mental ages 6–8) (1966); Level 3 (Mental ages 7½–9½) (1967). Circle Pines, MN, American Guidance Service, Inc.	
Engelmann, S., Osborn, J., and Engelmann, T.	Distar Language — An Instructional System. Chicago, Science Research Associates (1969).	An instructional program in which a wide range of concepts and stories is included for the teaching of language concepts. For preschool to primary grade levels.
Fitzgerald, E.	Straight Language for the Deaf: A System of Instruction for Deaf Children. Washington, D.C., The Volta Bureau (1949).	A method of structuring language for the deaf that has also been found useful in dealing with other language handicaps. The system is essentially a key consisting of headings such as "who, what (verb), where, and when," which help the child organize language concepts. For preschool to intermediate levels.
Goldman, R., and Lynch, M.	Goldman-Lynch Sounds and Symbols Development Kit. Circle Pines, MN, American Guidance Service, Inc. (1971).	A phonetically oriented program with one symbol for each sound. Uses a manual of lessons and stories, pictures, symbol cards, and puppets for teaching speech production. For preschool to primary levels.
Herr, S.	Perceptual Communication Skills: Developing Auditory Awareness and Insight. 1415 Westwood Blvd., Los Angeles, CA 90024, Instructional Materials and Equipment Distributors (1969).	Presents a broad range of activities designed to develop auditory awareness, concepts, and vocabulary. Teacher's manual and student workbooks. Eighty eight lessons for each of three levels: preschool–third grade; fourth–sixth grade; and junior high–adulthood.

Table 84–2 SELECTED SOURCES FOR METHODS AND MATERIALS
FOR LANGUAGE REMEDIATION (*Continued*)

Author(s)	Reference Source	Brief Description
Johnson, D., and Myklebust, H.	Learning Disabilities — Educational Principles and Practices. New York, Grune and Stratton, Inc. (1967), Chaps. 4–6.	Detailed description of procedures used for teaching children with auditory, reading, and writing language disorders.
Karnes, M.	Helping Young Children Develop Language Skills. Washington, DC, The Council for Exceptional Children (1968).	Activities designed to strengthen language skills in preschool disadvantaged children, based on a model provided by the various subtests of the Illinois Test of Psycholinguistic Abilities
Lindamood, C., and Lindamood, P.	Auditory Discrimination in Depth (A.D.D.). 100 Boylston St., Boston, MA 02116, Teaching Resources Corporation (1969).	Development program in auditory perception which provides "in-depth" experiences in auditory discrimination through training at three levels. Emphasizes the visual, auditory, and kinesthetic modalities as the phonologic structure of language is taught. For preschool to adult levels.
PESO Institute	Handbook of Remedial Techniques for Children and Young Adolescents. Canyon, TX, West Texas State University (1967).	A wide variety of grade-by-grade activities for each subtest of the Experimental Edition (1968) of the Illinois Test of Psycholinguistic Abilities. For primary through intermediate levels.
Sayre, J., and Mack, J.	Think, Listen and Say. Jamaica, N.Y. 11435, Eye Gate House (1967).	An audiovisual kit designed to improve listening abilities for auditory discrimination and comprehension through use of records and filmstrips. For preschool to primary levels.
Watson, D. T.	Listen and Learn with Phonics. Mudelein, IL, American Interstate Corporation (1964).	A series of records and workbooks designed primarily for individual training. For preschool to primary levels.
Woodcock, R., and Clark, C.	The Peabody Rebus Reading Program. Circle Pines, MN, American Guidance Service, Inc. (1967).	Picture–word approach to teaching reading. Uses individual workbooks and readers to introduce and develop an understanding of the semantic and syntactic systems of language. For preschool to primary levels.
Zigmond, N. D., and Cicci, R.	Auditory Learning, San Rafael, CA, Dimensions Publishing Company (1968).	Detailed information on procedures for teaching preschool and school-age children with auditory learning disabilities.

(From McConnell, F. 1974. Language remediation in children. *In* Dickson, S. (ed.): Communication Disorders: Remedial Principles and Practices. Glenview, IL, Scott, Foresman, pp. 87–89.)

SELECTED REFERENCES

Burgi, E. J., and Matthews, J. 1963. Disorders of speech. J. Pediatr., 62(1):15–19.

This brief paper is intended to orient the pediatrician to the subject of communication disorders in childhood and to provide the interest and motivation for further investigation in this area by the pediatrician.

Clevenger, T., and Matthews, J. 1971. The Speech Communication Process. Glenview, IL, Scott, Foresman.

Although this book was written for the college student in the first course in speech communication, it treats a number of concepts previously reserved for graduate study in speech. It is not a text on disorders of speech but is intended to provide an understanding of the larger field of human communication with an emphasis on the processes involved.

Nicolosi, L., Harryman, E., and Kresheck, J. 1978. Terminology of Communication Disorders. Baltimore, Williams and Wilkins.

Of the 273 pages of this volume, 231 constitute a dictionary of terms dealing with communication disorders. The balance of the book presents in tabular form developmental sequences of language behavior as well as descriptions of various tests employed in the diagnosis of communication disorders.

Travis, L. E. (Ed.) 1971. Handbook of Speech Pathology and Audiology. New York, Appleton-Century-Crofts.

This 1312 page handbook consists of 50 chapters prepared by 44 authorities. It provides the most extensive coverage of speech pathology and audiology available in any single volume.

REFERENCES

Bangs, T. D. 1968. Languages and Learning Disorders of the Pre-Academic Child. Englewood Cliffs, N.J., Prentice-Hall.

Berry, M. 1969. Language Disorders of Children. New York, Appleton-Century-Crofts.

Birch, J., and Matthews, J. 1951. The hearing of mental defectives; its measurement and characteristics. Am. J. Ment. Defec., 55:384–393.

Burgi, E. J., and Matthews, J. 1963. Disorders of speech. J. Pediatr., 62(1):15–19.

Carroll, J. B. 1961. Language acquisition, bilingualism and language change. *In* Saporta, S. (Ed.) Psycholinguistics: A Book of Readings. New York, Holt, Rinehart and Winston.

Clevenger, T., and Matthews, J. 1971. The Speech Communication Process. Glenview, IL, Scott, Foresman.

Developmental Language and Speech Center Staff, Grand Rapids, MI, 1975. Teach Your Child to Talk: A Parent Handbook. New York, CEBCO/Standard Publ. Co.

Dickson, S. 1974. Communication Disorders: Remedial Principles and Practices. Glenview, IL, Scott, Foresman.

Dunn, L., Horton, K., and Smith, J. 1968. Peabody Language Development Kits, Level P (Mental ages 3–5). Circle Pines, MN, American Guidance Service, Inc.

Dunn, L., and Smith, J. 1965, 1966, 1967. Peabody Language Development Kits, Level 1 (Mental ages 4½–6½), Level 2 (Mental ages 6–8), Level 3 (Mental ages 7½–9½). Circle Pines, MN, American Guidance Service, Inc.

Engelmann, N. S., Osborn, J., and Engelmann, T. 1969. Distar Language — An Instructional System. Chicago, Science Research Associates.

Fitzgerald, E. 1949. Straight Language for the Deaf: A System of Instruction for Deaf Children. Washington, DC, The Volta Bureau.

Gesell, A., et al. 1940. The First Five Years of Life. New York, Harper Bros.

Johnson, D., and Myklebust, H. 1967. Learning Disabilities — Educational Principles and Practices. New York, Grune and Stratton.

Lenneberg, E. 1967. Biological Foundations of Language. New York, John Wiley and Sons.

McConnell, F., Love, R. J., and Clark, B. S. 1974. Language remediation in children. *In* Dickson, S. (Ed.) Communication Disorders. Glenview, IL, Scott, Foresman.

McNeill, D. 1970. The Acquisition of Language. New York, Harper and Row.

Matthews, J. 1971a. Personal and professional responsibility related to current social problems. ASHA, 13:331–333.

Matthews, J. 1971b. Communication disorders in the mentally retarded. *In* Travis, L. E. (Ed.) Handbook of Speech Pathology and Audiology. New York, Appleton-Century-Crofts.

Morrow, J. 1959. A psychiatrist looks at the nonverbal child. J. Except. Child., 25:348–349.

Nicolosi, L., Harryman, E., and Kresheck, J. 1978. Terminology of Communication Disorders. Baltimore, Williams and Wilkins.

Taylor, O. 1971. Recent developments in sociolinguistics: Some implications for ASHA. *In* Matthews, J. (Ed.) Personal and Professional Responsibility Related to Current Social Problems. ASHA.

Travis, L. E. (Ed.) 1971. Handbook of Speech Pathology and Audiology, New York, Appleton-Century-Crofts.

Zigmond, N. K., and Cicci, R. (Eds.) 1968. Auditory Learning. San Rafael, CA Dimensions Publ.

Chapter 85

DISORDERS OF ARTICULATION, VOICE, AND FLUENCY

Richard F. Curlee, Ph.D.
Ralph L. Shelton, Ph.D.

GLOSSARY

Articulation—the production of speech sounds and the sequencing of those sounds according to the sound pattern of the speaker's language.

Apraxia of speech—impairment of the ability to make voluntary speech movements even though involuntary movements of the articulators are not impaired. Apraxia reflects damage to the central nervous system.

Dysphonia—impairment of the voice.

Fluency—the flow of speech related to how smoothly sounds, syllables, and words are initiated and joined.

Loudness—perception of an aspect of the voice related to its intensity.

Morphology—the study of the formation of words and word inflections, such as plurals and past tense.

Phoneme—a class of speech sounds; for example, all /s/ sounds are members of the /s/ category or phoneme. *Phoneme* is sometimes used synonymously with the term speech *sound*.

Phonetics—the study of the production and perception of speech.

Phonology—the structure and function of speech sounds in a language. Phonology is concerned in part with the child's acquisition of the sound pattern of language.

Pitch—perception of an aspect of the voice related to its fundamental frequency.

Prosody—the melody of speech related to patterns of stress, inflection, and rhythm.

Quality—perception of an aspect of the voice related to the frequency distribution of acoustic energy that can be categorized as breathy, harsh, hoarse, or hypernasal.

Semantics—the study of the communication of meaning through language.

Speech—oral expression of a language.

Syntax—the study of phrase, clause, and sentence structure.

Voice—sound produced by vibration of the vocal folds.

Speech pathologists are concerned with the understanding, assessment, and habilitation of persons presenting with disorders of articulation, voice, fluency, and language. This chapter introduces articulation and voice disorders that are not associated with malformations or neurogenic defects and the disorder of stuttering. Each disorder will be highlighted in terms of its characteristics, evaluation, and treatment.

DISORDERS OF ARTICULATION

Normal and Disordered Articulation. Articulation can be described in terms of phonetics, which is concerned with the production of speech sounds, and phonology, which involves the patterns or rules whereby sounds are organized or distributed in a language. Thus, articulation is the use of the speech mechanism to produce consonants and vowels and also to organize and sequence those sounds into patterns that characterize adults' use of the language. The process is more complex than the assembly of strings of isolated sounds in that articulators move simultaneously for the production of sounds we perceive sequentially — a process termed *coarticulation.* Thus, in the word *construe,* the lips start to round for /u/ while the tongue is producing /s/.

Normal articulatory development has been described in terms of the age at which most children produce various sounds correctly. In English many sounds including /m/, /p/, /t/, /k/, and /f/ are usually produced correctly by most three year olds, whereas other sounds are acquired later. /l/ and /s/, for example, are not consistently articulated by some speakers until about eight years of age. Information of this sort is somewhat misleading in that it suggests that development involves the simple addition of new sounds to a child's sound repertoire. Some writers contend that speech sounds are composed of binary characteristics, such as high-low, front-back, and nasal-oral, which are called distinctive features. Distinctive features are described physiologically and acoustically; for example, the sounds /p/ and /t/ differ from one another in terms of where they are produced in the mouth as well as in their acoustic characteristics. A speaker's development of a mature phonologic pattern may involve the development of rules that allow the speaker to combine a new feature with sounds already in use; in this manner, the addition of new features and rules results in the appearance of new sounds in a child's speech. The ability to produce sounds precedes the incorporation of those sounds into a child's spontaneous speech patterns; thus, a child's ability to imitate a particular sound does not mean he or she uses the sound in conversation.

Articulatory disorders are sometimes described as omissions of speech sounds, substitutions of one sound for another, and as distortions of sounds. A lateral lisp, which is a distortion, involves the use of a deviant /s/ in place of a standard one; the sound produced resembles the target sound, /s/, more than any other sound of the language. Phonologic analysis of the speech of an individual who misarticulates sounds from many phonemes classifies those articulation errors into subsets that follow different rules or patterns (Ingram, 1976). For example, deletion of final consonants or failure to voice voiced consonants will affect sounds from several phonemes. In planning therapy, speech pathologists often go beyond an inventory of the sounds misarticulated to consider how the speaker's misarticulations are patterned. In that way, therapy can be conducted to resolve rules underlying the misarticulation of several sounds.

Severity of disordered articulation is related to the number of different phonemes involved in the problem and to the consistency of the errors. That is, other things being equal, an individual who misarticulates several sounds, perhaps /s/, /r/, and /l/, has a more severe problem than does the person who misarticulates only one sound, perhaps presenting a frontal lisp of /s/. Similarly, the person who always misarticulates /r/ presents a more severe problem than does the person who sometimes misarticulates /r/ and who sometimes articulates it correctly. Since articulatory development is age-related, age is considered in determining whether or not a child has an articulatory problem. However, the error pattern is usually more informative than the age norm as an index to an articulation disorder. Young children developing speech do not immediately use the articulatory patterns of the adult community, and their failure to use adult patterns can be described in terms of phonologic processes that result in simplification of developing articulation. Deletion of final consonants is one such process, and reduction of clusters, for example, the use of /p/ in place of /spl/, is another. The child who uses unique or rare simplification processes is thought to present an especially severe articulation disorder. Such speech is usually classified as deviant and can be contrasted with the delayed articulation development of a child who persists in the use of simplification processes commonly employed by young children. Articulation problems are also especially severe when they interfere with the intelligibility of speech.

The prevalence of articulation problems varies with the age of the children observed and with how the disorder is defined. Recently, 9.5 per cent of a sample of first-grade children were reported to present moderately or severely deviated articulation, and those percentages fell to 4.5, 2.0, and 0.5 per cent for children in the second, third, and twelfth grades, respectively (Hull et al., 1976). Many additional children were classified as presenting mild articulation deviations. There are two conditions that should not be confused with disordered articulation. One is the mispronunciation of words, and the other is dialectal variation. Speech patterns vary geographically and ethnically, and these dialectal differences do not constitute disordered communication.

Variables Related to Disordered Articulation. Many variables have been studied to discover their relationships with measures of disordered articulation in a search for causal hypotheses and for generation of ideas for possible forms of treatment (Winitz, 1969). We will consider only three such variables here: (1) speech sound discrimination, which many studies have shown to be related to misarticulation; (2) language — the phonologic aspect of articulation is a component of language; and (3) tongue thrust, which is a particularly controversial problem for which the child may be taken to the physician for examination and advice.

Any child with a speech disorder should be given a hearing test because of the possibility that a hearing loss may be present; even fluctuating conductive losses may influence articulation development. Except for the study of articulation itself, hearing tests are probably the only observations routinely recommended for all misarticulating children. Some clinicians evaluate speech sound discrimination among children who respond normally to pure tone and speech audiometry. Statistically significant correlations between speech sound discrimination and articulation measures have been reported in many investigations involving children under nine years of age; however, the correlations have not been of sufficient magnitude to allow satisfactory prediction of one score from another. Originally speech sound discrimination testing involved assessing the child's ability to discriminate between two syllables or words that differed in only one sound. Clinicians have also explored children's ability to evaluate the correctness of speech sounds, and recently investigators have been especially interested in children's assessment of

their own speech rather than the correctness of sounds produced by someone else. Evaluation of a child's discrimination pattern should use procedures that are tailored to the individual child; however, an even greater need exists for data that relate discrimination measures or observations to treatment effectiveness. It seems unlikely that most children who present with articulation difficulties have defective discrimination abilities that require remediation.

Phonology is one of four variables used to describe language — the others are morphology, syntax, and semantics. Within this conceptual framework, disordered articulation may be one part of a communication problem that involves all four aspects of language. Descriptive data do show a correspondence between articulation and language impairment in some children with multiple articulation errors, particularly those who omit consonants at the ends of words. Some children whose misarticulations involve only one or two phonemes may also perform poorly on language and reading tests. Investigators have speculated that articulation errors may result from memory defects, verbal apraxia, or undefined neurologic deficits in a chain-like series of unfortunate events and that the articulation disorder in turn interferes with language development. Such speculations require further investigation. In testing the language of articulation-impaired children, it is important to remember that a child may be reluctant to display poor speech, and the language sample obtained may not represent the child's language abilities.

Tongue thrust has been defined as placement of the tongue against or between the teeth during swallowing and perhaps when the individual is talking or at rest. This behavior has been blamed as the cause of malocclusion, relapse to malocclusion following orthodontic treatment, and misarticulation problems. Some persons contend that tongue thrust swallow is a habit acquired as a result of bottle feeding and that it needs to be corrected by training in order to avoid problems with dental occlusion and speech. This issue is controversial because many orthodontists and speech pathologists do not consider swallow training to be of value, whereas others have established an organization to foster myofunctional therapies. It is currently recommended by the Joint Committee on Dentistry and Speech Pathology of the American Association of Dental Schools and the

American Speech-Language-Hearing Association that tongue thrust treatment be considered an experimental procedure.

Infants and young children do use a tongue thrust pattern when swallowing, probably because the tongue fills the oral cavity and the hyoid bone and larynx are positioned high relative to the cranium. With growth and development those structures are displaced to a lower positon, and the patterns of tongue and hyoid cartilage movement in swallowing change. Tongue protrusion has also been associated with macroglossia, enlarged tonsils, and obstructions of the nasal airway. Thus, both advocates and critics of oral myofunctional therapy agree that oral and nasal pathologic conditions should be ruled out in persons who protrude their tongues excessively. We have yet to see evidence that myofunctional therapy benefits speech development, but airway obstruction may be an issue in some persons with articulation disorders, and it may influence speech prosody and also voice quality.

Causation of Functional Articulation Disorders. The etiology of nonorganic articulatory disorders is unknown but is thought to be influenced by environment. Numerous variables probably influence articulation development, and some articulatory errors may reflect a child's developmental location on the low side of a bell-shaped distribution of normal development, but family acceptance of immature articulation may slow the developmental process. That is, stimulus and reinforcement variables that influence learning may operate in the home in a way that slows a child's speech development and perhaps causes other behavioral immaturity, such as slowness in toilet training or in assuming responsibility for dressing and care of toys. Intelligence is not highly correlated with disordered articulation throughout a wide range of ability, but children with very low intellectual development are at high risk for an articulatory disorder. We have already noted that hearing loss can influence articulation development.

Speech pathologists speculate that some articulatory errors classified as "functional" actually reflect an apraxia. This concept may apply to the individual who misarticulates sounds from many phonemes and who shows signs of poor coordination, such as a slow rate of repetition of strings of syllables (diadochokinesis) and inconsistent velopharyngeal closure during syllable strings as determined by measurement of nasal airflow during the production of those syllables. Such children may also display language and school achievement deficits.

The apraxia concept does not apply to the many children whose speech is indistinguishable from that of normal children except for the oral articulation errors themselves. It is seldom possible to identify the cause of functional articulation problems, and speech pathologists have tended to replace the search for causation with efforts to describe the child's articulation and to identify relationships between the articulation problem and remedial procedures that are likely to be effective with the individual child.

Referral Guidelines. Many preschool children who misarticulate will make sufficient spontaneous progress in improving their articulation so that no speech training is needed. Others will not, and they should be evaluated carefully and considered for remedial services. Misarticulating children who especially need referrals for speech pathology evaluation include: (1) children as young as three or four years who misarticulate sounds from several different phonemes (Often the speech of these children is unintelligible, and they may use poor syntax and poor vocabulary. They may also be reluctant to talk.); (2) preschool and early elementary school children who consistently misarticulate /r/ sounds or who distort /s/ sounds laterally; and (3) those misarticulating children who have passed their eighth birthdays.

Thus, as a general rule, younger children should be referred if their speech is difficult to understand, and older children should be referred as they exceed the age at which articulatory development is normally complete. Disordered articulation probably may warrant special attention if school achievement problems or language deficiencies are also present. Some clinicians believe a referral should be made if the parents are concerned about speech even if the problem appears to be mild.

Evaluation of Articulation Disorders. The evaluation process includes the use of screening procedures to identify children who need further assessment, diagnostic evaluation of the articulation of those identified in screening, and measurement of pertinent related variables, such as hearing. Space does not permit a consideration of all the related variables that might be considered in the evaluation process. Speech pathologists working in school settings are responsible for the identification of individuals with communication disorders. While referrals from teachers and others help in the identification process, school programs usually screen all children at two or more grade levels. The screening procedure usually includes observation of hearing, voice, language, and fluency as well as articulation. The articulation portion of the screening procedure typically samples the child's production of speech sounds — especially those such as /s/ and /r/ that are likely to be misarticulated. One screening test (Van Riper and Erickson, 1975) is available that helps speech pathologists to predict articulation at the third grade level from observations of articulation in the first grade.

Diagnostic articulation testing usually requires (1) stimuli for use in eliciting articulation responses, (2) record sheets to record the clinician's evaluation of the sounds produced, (3) directions for extracting a description of the child's articulation pattern, and perhaps (4) normative data against which a child's performance can be compared. Different articulation tests have different features. For example, some tests sample most consonants and some vowels to obtain an overview of a child's articulation to determine if errors fit patterns wherein the misarticulated sounds are phonetically similar. Other tests are constructed to examine the consistency of a child's production of a particular sound in a number of different phonetic contexts. Conversational articulation may be tested as well as articulation of single words and syllables. Also, articulation produced in imitation of the examiner is often compared to that which is uttered spontaneously. Children whose articulation patterns are inconsistent or whose articulation is better imitatively than spontaneously are thought to have a favorable prognosis for spontaneous improvement, especially if they are under nine years of age. However, the prediction of spontaneous improvement is imprecise, and articulation should always be retested to check the predictions. A key feature of articulation testing is the reliability of the observer's assessment of the correctness of a child's sound productions. It is sometimes difficult to distinguish between sounds on a right or wrong basis, especially when a child in training is beginning to approximate correct production, and reliability decreases as the examiner attempts

to make finer descriptions of the nature of any error produced.

Articulation test results are used to plan speech training when it is decided that a child needs remedial training. By considering the phonetic similarities of the different sounds involved in an articulation problem, it is possible to organize therapy so that a child will improve not only the sound taught but also other misarticulated sounds that share distinctive features with the sound taught. Thus, training directed to the /s/ sound may result in improvement of /z/ as well as /s/, presumably because the two sounds are so similar phonetically (they differ only in that one is voiced and the other is not). The potential value of identifying a phonologic pattern was discussed earlier.

Articulation Training. The terms speech *training* and *therapy* are used synonymously in this chapter. They usually refer to procedures wherein a clinician teaches speech behavior to a patient; speech pathologists seldom use exercises to strengthen muscles of clients, even those with paresis, in the hope that better articulation will ensue. Speech therapy for articulation, voice, and fluency disorders is usually directed to the development of skills rather than to increasing the physiologic capacity to produce speech. For example, in working with persons with repaired cleft palates, we are experimenting with the use of television endoscopic displays and pressure-flow pen traces in biofeedback training to teach improved use of the velopharyngeal mechanism, but the emphasis is on improving speech, not muscular strength. Some clinicians may also teach sound discrimination or may provide memory exercises in attempts to develop a child's capacity for good articulation. However, little evidence is now available to support the benefits of such practices.

In teaching articulation to children with functional articulation problems, we use information regarding a child's ability to produce a sound in different production units (isolation, syllables, words, sentences, reading material, and conversation), under different stimulus conditions (imitation, picture naming, sentence completion, written material, and conversational setting), and in different environments (different listeners, clinic, school, and home). Training is often started with syllables, and the target sound is practiced so that it precedes and follows many other sounds (Shelton, 1978). The syllables may also be arranged so that neighboring sounds facilitate production of the target sound. For example, an /s/ sound might follow other frontal consonants, especially for a child who distorts the /s/ by producing it too far back in the mouth. Syllables may be practiced at different rates, pitches, and levels of loudness. Proficiency at the syllable level often facilitates use of the target sound in words, sentences, and conversation. It is believed that phonetic proficiency may facilitate phonologic patterning of sound usage (Ling, 1976). Initially, stimuli are used that carry a high probability of eliciting correct responses, and with increased success in producing the desired response, stimuli that initially would probably have resulted in misarticulations are presented. When success has been achieved in the clinic, techniques are used to encourage generalization of the correct responses to other settings. Reinforcement (reward) is used at each of these steps. In sum, articulation training is compatible with principles of learning.

Improved articulation training effectiveness is one goal of applied research, and several universities are conducting continuing applied research on this topic. Several studies have demonstrated the effectiveness of articulation therapy (for example, Sommers et al., 1967), but success rate data are not available. Some centers now advocate organizing articulation and other therapy so that a child is presented with a problem to be solved. Presumably a child's active participation in planning and evaluating responses may be more effective than stimulus-response-reinforcement sequences by themselves. Programmed instruction has been applied to articulation training, and programmed materials are commercially available that are designed to advance the child's articulation through contextual, stimulus, and environmental steps to correct conversational speech. Some of the programs may be administered by paraprofessional aides under the supervision of speech pathologists. Therapy is often delivered in small groups, and attempts are made to teach one child to assist another or to involve parents in the remedial process by teaching them to reward correct responses. While the relationship between the clinician and the patient is always important, it is especially important when the patient is a preschool child. The younger child is often not ready to participate in the training activities that are used with older children but may benefit from speech activities presented indirectly in a structured play format.

DISORDERS OF VOICE

Voices are usually characterized in terms of three perceptual dimensions: pitch, loudness, and quality. Vocal pitch is directly related to the frequency of glottal pulses generated in the larynx and corresponds to the fundamental frequency measured in hertz (Hz). The higher the fundamental frequency of a complex tone, the higher the pitch heard. Differences in vocal fold length and thickness account for most of the pitch differences among men and women and between adults and children. It has been found that speakers increase their vocal pitch by decreasing the cross-sectional mass of the vocal folds and increasing the tension of the folds while increasing subglottal pressure. Conversely, increases in mass and decreases in tension and subglottal pressure decrease the pitch of the voice.

Loudness is directly related to the intensity of the voice, which is often measured in decibels (dB) of acoustic sound pressure. The way in which speakers modify vocal intensity is not as well understood as the way they modify pitch. It is known that increases in subglottal air pressure, airflow, and glottal resistance typically accompany increases in vocal intensity. However, the relative contributions of each of these factors to the intensity of voice varies substantially from speaker to speaker and across the intensity range within speakers.

Voice quality, unlike pitch and loudness, is not a unidimensional phenomenon. Perkins (1977) views quality as a multidimensional perceptual category that results from interactions among the size and shape of the vocal tract, the coupling effects of resonators, and the vibratory patterns of the glottis. From this perspective, all adjustments of the vocal mechanism contribute to quality, and the patterns of energy distribution across various frequencies of the acoustic spectrum form the physical bases for perceptual judgments of quality. To date, however, research has not been able to relate patterns of vocal behavior or acoustic energy to judgments of voice quality in a satisfactory manner. The literature is filled with dozens of terms to characterize both normal and abnormal vocal quality. Unfortunately, these terms connote different characteristics to different listeners and are often employed inconsistently by the same listener. In short, judgments of vocal quality lack satisfactory reliability and have led to problems in classifying voice disorders and measuring their change.

Characteristics of Disordered Voice. There are no clear-cut, objective standards for differentiating normal and abnormal voices. Indeed, a number of prominent entertainers are identified with highly unusual vocal characteristics, a fact that probably encourages greater tolerance of deviant voices. In any event, the identification of a voice disorder, or dysphonia, is based on the subjective evaluation of one or more listeners. Speech pathologists often describe dysphonias in terms of the perceptual dimensions that are impaired (for example, pitch and loudness or voice quality deviations, such as breathiness, harshness, and hoarseness). Although judgments of vocal quality are not as reliable as is desirable, there is some consistency among speech pathologists in describing the following voice quality deviations. Harshness is used to describe the vocal quality accompanying excessive tension of the laryngeal musculature, abrupt voice onsets, and a constricted vocal tract. This quality is often associated with hyperfunctional vocal behavior. Breathiness results when the vocal folds are not fully approximated and when unvibrated air accompanies the glottal pulse. If phonation is absent so that the voice is a whisper, the term aphonia is used. Hoarseness has been described as a combination of harshness and breathiness; it frequently accompanies common colds, episodes of laryngitis, and other pathologic conditions of the larynx. Just as there is disagreement about what constitutes disordered voice, so there is uncertainty about the prevalence of voice disorders. Nevertheless, among school-aged children estimates range from less than 1 per cent to more than 9 per cent. The most recent, large-scale, nationwide study found that 3 per cent of the children among this population were dysphonic (Hull et al., 1976).

Types of Voice Disorders. There are a number of ways in which voice disorders may be categorized. We have grouped them into three categories: (1) misuse and abuse of the larynx; (2) disease, injury, or malformation of the larynx; and (3) psychogenic dysphonias.

MISUSE AND ABUSE OF THE LARYNX. Inappropriate use of the larynx may damage the larynx, alter the voice, or both, and may occur during phonation or nonspeech acts, such as coughing and throat clearing. Two factors are significant in misuse of the larynx during phonation: the relative efficiency of a person's vocal behavior and patterns of use.

An efficient voice yields maximal acoustic output, flexibility, and pleasant tonal qualities with minimal effort in phonation (Perkins, 1977). Some people appear to use their vocal mechanisms optimally. They can speak frequently and loudly, sing all night, and cheer at football games with no apparent untoward effect on the voice or larynx. Some evidently acquire this ability naturally, others with training. Most people, however, do not use their voices optimally and in stressful speaking situations may abuse their vocal mechanisms. The less efficient an individual's habitual manner of phonation is, the more likely he or she will be to abuse the voice and larynx. Many people probably experience transitory vocal dysfunction some time in their lives. Most, however, are able to use their voices sufficiently efficiently to accommodate the demands of everyday living and do not evidence voice problems of clinical significance.

In general, the larynx seems to be quite resilient to occasional episodes of abuse or misuse: Once the abusive behavior is eliminated, normal phonation returns. Once there is tissue damage, however, the dysphonia will probably become worse, although some people may be dysphonic for years with no observable effects on the larynx or worsening of the dysphonia. Patients with tissue damage always need voice training to learn more efficient voice production, in addition to whatever medical treatment is required.

Abuse of the larynx during voice production usually involves hyperadduction of the vocal folds. Vocal fold approximation can be viewed as a continuum from abducted aphonia through normal vocal fold closure for phonation to hyperfunctional phonation in which the folds are brought together with excessive force (Brackett, 1971). When the folds are completely abducted, laryngeal resistance to airflow is quite low, and no voice is produced. As the folds are gradually adducted to midline, a whisper will be produced, then vocal fold vibration will begin, and vocal quality will gradually decrease in breathiness until vocal fold approximation yields normal phonation. Thus, in the middle of this continuum, minimal laryngeal tension maintains an optimal balance between glottal resistance and subglottal air pressure. The result is efficient voice production with little variation in the duration of opening and closing phases of the vibratory cycle from one cycle to another. In hyperfunctional phonation, however, the vocal folds are tightly approximated and the closed phase of the vibratory cycle increases in duration, which requires an increase in subglottal air pressure to push open the tightly approximated folds and produce vocal sounds. The term "hard glottal attack" refers to the forceful, abrupt closure of the folds that accompanies hyperfunctional phonation. Sometimes discomfort or pain is the complaint of the patient rather than an abnormal-sounding voice. With chronic hyperfunctional misuse, laryngeal membranous tissue may become irritated and develop lesions. When laryngeal abuse causes vocal fold thickening, nodules, or polyps, they may appear on one or both folds (Boone, 1977), and typically occur at the juncture of the anterior and middle thirds of the folds, which is the site of their maximum vibratory excursion (Wilson, 1972). These lesions interfere with satisfactory approximation of the vocal folds and increase their mass. Consequently, the resulting dysphonia is often characterized by breathiness, lowered pitch, hoarseness, and occasional breaks in phonation.

Other types of voice problems associated with vocal abuse that are seen in children include hyperkeratosis and ventricular phonation (Wilson, 1972). Hyperkeratosis in children is believed to result from vocal abuse, inspiration of dust and pollutants, or chronic sinus or pharyngeal infections and appears as an irregular thickening of the mucosa along the anterior or middle thirds of the fold. Ventricular phonation, as the name implies, involves the use of the false vocal folds instead of the true folds for phonation and is rarely observed in children. Its etiology is unknown, but it has been reported to follow laryngeal surgery and severe attacks of laryngitis (Brodnitz, 1965). Vocal pitch is usually substantially lowered, pitch range is restricted, and the child may complain of throat pain and fatigue with this problem. Normal phonation may often accompany the child's cough, laugh, and cry, however. It is interesting to note that ventricular phonation is extraordinarily difficult to teach to those patients who could profit from an alternative sound-generating mechanism.

Misuse of the voice may result from speaking too loudly or at an inappropriate pitch, as well as from faulty approximation of the vocal folds. Frequent episodes of prolonged shouting are commonly noted in the case histories of children with vocal nodules. Also, the amount of time spent talking in noisy situations may be a factor in some cases. Loud speech is likely to be harmful over time if it is accomplished primarily by increasing laryngeal tension. Increases in loudness achieved by balanced increases in airflow, subglottal air pressure, and laryngeal tension may not be harmful, however. The use of an inappropriate pitch is seen relatively frequently among adult dysphonics but much less often in children. Among children, inappropriately high pitches seem to be encountered more often than excessively low pitches, but among adults the opposite is true. Another pitch problem occasionally found among male adolescents is continued use of a high-frequency, falsetto voice after completion of laryngeal growth at puberty. Typically, these clients present no laryngeal or endocrine abnormalities and are amenable to voice therapy.

Children also may abuse their larynges through nonspeech acts. For example, excessive coughing and throat clearing are believed to be two of the more frequent vocal abuses in children. When these behaviors accompany chronic upper respiratory tract conditions and allergies that irritate the mucosal linings of the vocal tract, the probability of laryngeal damage would appear to be substantially increased. Other abusive activities found in children include phonation on inhalation and strained vocal imitations of animals and engines.

DISEASE, INJURY, OR MALFORMATION OF THE LARYNX. As was noted earlier, severe dysphonias may occur and persist in normal laryngeal mechanisms. In addition, a dysphonia that occurs in a normal mechanism may not sound different from one clearly related to an organic pathologic condition. Still, if an organic pathologic process interferes with normal laryngeal function, an obvious dysphonia will occur. Pathologic conditions that disrupt normal phonation include those that restrict vocal fold adduction (such as paralyses and interarytenoid growth); disrupt approximation of the folds and their synchronous vibration (such as papillomas, other growths, and edema of the vocal folds); change the tonus of the vocal folds (such as paralysis); affect the mucosa (such as scarring); result in laryngeal tissue destruction (such as accident or surgery); or modify the size and shape of the larynx (such as congenital malformations (Moore, 1971).

Dysphonias resulting from organic pathologic conditions are first a medical problem. In some cases medical or surgical treatment may eliminate accompanying dysphonias, and there is no need for voice therapy. Other patients may relapse following successful medical treatment without voice therapy. If the larynx is structurally and functionally intact after medical management, restoration of normal phonation is often possible, but if there has been extensive damage to the larynx or if there is a permanent paralysis, voice therapy can only help the child to use the impaired mechanism as effectively as possible.

PSYCHOGENIC DYSPHONIAS. The voice has long been thought to reflect the emotions or personality of the speaker. Clinical reports of hysterical, or functional, aphonia often contain a number of common features (Boone, 1977). The onset of the disorder is usually quite sudden and often follows a major disappointment in life, an emotionally traumatizing experience, or an illness that resulted in a temporary loss of voice. Occasionally, the voice problem appears to "benefit" a child by allowing him or her to avoid a feared situation or to obtain more attention. Brodnitz (1965) has observed that many psychogenic dysphonias appear to exceed the severity of the organic disability and persist long after evidence of the organic impairment disappears. Typically, in aphonias not attributable to adductor paralysis, observation of the glottis during phonation attempts reveals grossly inadequate approximation of the folds. Yet, satisfactory approximation usually occurs during laughing or coughing (Wilson, 1972). Only rarely do dysphonias appear to reflect serious psychopathology that requires psychiatric or psychologic intervention.

Even though the suspected connection between voice disorders and personality is a long-standing clinical impression, there is little research to support this view. After an extensive review of the available literature, Bloch and Goodstein (1971) concluded that little is known about the relationship, if any, of personality to voice disorders. It is possible that widespread clinical acceptance of a relationship between psychoneurosis and some dysphonias has discouraged its scientific study. In addition, small available patient populations and the lack of reliable measures of voice and personality may also have contributed to the dearth of research. With our present level of knowledge it is difficult at times to make a meaningful distinction between functional and organic voice disorders. To distinguish further between functional dysphonias that are psychogenic in nature and those that are not exceeds our empirically based skills of assessment.

Referral Guidelines. Children with deviant-sounding voices should be referred to speech pathologists for evaluation and possible treatment if there are no medical contraindications. During the course of the voice evaluation, the speech pathologist will be able to determine whether or not voice therapy is likely to be successful. In general, (1) children whose dysphonias result from vocal abuse and misuse require behavioral management. Some clinicians believe voice therapy can be effective in reducing vocal nodules as long as the nodules extend less than one third of the length of the vocal folds, and indirect management can begin as early as three to four years of age; (2) children whose dysphonias appear to be psychogenically based usually respond well to voice therapy and rarely need psychotherapeutic intervention; (3) children whose dysphonias require them to learn rather subtle ways of modifying their vocal behavior must be sufficiently mature to understand the task and willing to cooperate actively in learning it; hence, these direct vocal management procedures may not be effective until children are in the third or fourth grade.

Assessment. In evaluating a dysphonic child, a speech pathologist will obtain a case history and will identify vocal behaviors that appear to contribute to the disorder. Information from a physician skilled at laryngoscopy is essential to understand a child's voice disorder. Because dysphonias may result from pathologic conditions of the larynx and vocal tract that require medical management, speech pathologists do not complete voice evaluations or begin treatment until the needed medical information has been received. Once information about the child's vocal folds and vocal tract and physical readiness for voice rehabilitation are available, plans for initiating any needed voice training may proceed.

The case history interview explores potential etiologic and maintenance factors in the child's dysphonia. The interviewer asks when and how the problem began and if this is the first time it has occurred. If the dysphonia is a recurrence of a problem previously resolved, detailed inquiries may reveal recurring patterns of abuse or emotional upset. Precipitating factors can often be determined if the onset was sudden. It is not unusual for dysphonias to be better in some situations and worse in others, and these situations need to be identified. Potential sources of vocal abuse should be covered thoroughly, particularly with children. Is there a lot of loud talking, yelling, or screaming during the day? Under what circumstances? Is there a sensitivity to dust or other allergies? Does the child cough or clear the throat a lot? Once sufficient background information has been obtained, direct examination and observation of the child begins.

The speech pathologist's examination of the child includes audiologic screening, an assessment of the peripheral speech mechanism in terms of its adequacy for speech, an evaluation of vocal performance on selected speech and phonatory tasks, identification of sites of excessive muscle tension during phonation, and observation of pitch, loudness, resonance, and vocal quality. Those dimensions of voice that are affected are then studied in greater detail, often with sophisticated instrumentation. In general, the speech pathologist attempts to identify (1) situations in which vocal abuses occur, (2) vocal behaviors that misuse the larynx, (3) the child's ability to modify those behaviors with assistance and encouragement, and (4) conditions that facilitate production of a better-sounding, more efficient voice. On the basis of the physician's report, the child's history and problem, and direct observation of the child's vocal behavior, the decision of whether or not to initiate voice therapy is made. Often a period of trial therapy is begun to see if laryngeal pathologic conditions can be alleviated without resorting to other treatment alternatives. In the absence of pathologic states in the larynx and in all cases of vocal misuse and abuse, voice therapy is the procedure of choice, and it has often been coordinated effectively with medical, surgical, or psychotherapeutic management. Voice therapy may help even those patients who present permanent laryngeal disabilities to adapt more successfully to the limitations of their vocal mechanisms.

Therapy. The goal of therapy is to facilitate comfortable production of a voice that is more satisfactory to patients and listeners than the impaired one and that does not abuse the voice or larynx. Thus, the treatment plan is designed to restore optimal vocal balance as completely as individual needs and capabilities permit (Perkins, 1977). For most children who present dysphonias that result from vocal hyperfunction, this can be accomplished by substantially reducing daily occurrences of vocal abuse.

Boone (1977) contends that children may maintain their dysphonias by brief, daily periods of abusive vocal behavior. He recommends that clinicians identify those situations at home and at school in which the child abuses the vocal mechanism and have the child tally and chart daily occurrences of abuse. Often, no other form of therapy may be needed. Indeed, young preschool and first and second grade children may not respond effectively to more direct vocal management techniques until they are somewhat older.

With older children and adolescents, remedial techniques can be selected that assist the patient in acquiring more efficient vocal behavior. Boone (1977) has described a number of voice therapy techniques applicable to the range of dysphonias encountered clinically. The techniques embody a strategy for searching for behaviors the patient can accomplish that will improve the voice. Those patients who evidence hyperfunctional voice behavior are taught to use less forceful vocal fold approximation. In some instances, general relaxation with or without biofeedback, chewing while phonating, and yawn/sigh techniques may be used to facilitate more efficient, less tense vocal productions. Wilson (1972) reports considerable improvement among children with vocal nodules by reducing vocal abuse and loudness and changing their habitual pitch. Also, those who do not approximate their folds adequately are assisted in bringing their folds together more forcefully. Often such techniques as pushing while phonating may help them to achieve this.

Treatment of dysphonia caused by laryngeal disease, trauma, or malformation must take under consideration the nature of the disability and its course. The strategy of therapy is to help patients produce the best, most efficient voice their mechanisms are capable of. In some cases voice therapy may be of no benefit, but in most instances speech pathologists can assist patients to improve their vocal functions. When necessary, patients will be encouraged to accept their limited vocal abilities.

Psychogenic dysphonias can usually be handled effectively by direct, symptomatic therapy (Aronson, 1973). Typically, psychogenically dysphonic patients produce a relatively normal-sounding voice while laughing, grunting, and coughing even though they may be aphonic in their speech attempts. With careful encouragement and positive suggestion, most patients rapidly recover normal voice with no evidence of symptom substitution or other adverse psychologic effects. A few patients may need referrals to psychologists or psychiatrists, but most of these can still profit from concurrent voice therapy of relatively brief duration.

Vocal rest is indicated only during severe episodes of acute laryngitis or after surgery involving the larynx. It is probably of little benefit to those patients who misuse their vocal mechanisms. As soon as the period of voice rest ends and the patient resumes old patterns of vocal misuse, the dysphonia and any associated pathologic laryngeal conditions quickly return.

The prognosis for voice improvement in children presenting dysphonias caused by laryngeal abuse and psychogenic dysphonia is believed to be good. The outlook for children with dysphonias resulting from permanent structural and functional disabilities of the vocal mechanism is largely determined by the nature and severity of the residual disability. Their prognosis is occasionally uncertain, often poor. In any event, remedial treatment should be demonstrably effective in a relatively short period of time — perhaps two months.

DISORDERS OF FLUENCY

To the casual listener, the speech of normal speakers seems to flow in a smooth, unbroken manner. This is an illusion. Take a few minutes during a conversation to count the pauses, interjections, repetitions, and prolongations that interrupt the flow of speech. It is likely you will find the speech of most ordinary speakers characterized by relatively frequent breaks in fluency. Consequently, normal fluency does not mean speech free from interruptions.

It should not be surprising that normal speech is not perfectly fluent. Indeed, it is remarkable that a motor act so complex is usually so fluent. In order for speech to proceed without disruption, adjustments of the lips, tongue, pharyngeal and laryngeal structures, and the respiratory mechanism must be successively integrated. This sequence of movements occurs at such a rapid rate during normal speech that the nervous system must be organized in such a manner that there can be parallel processing and coordination of the interdependent elements of speech. Yet, most young children speak quite fluently at an early age with no apparent problems.

Most listeners are quite tolerant of the breaks in fluency of most speakers, and speech pathologists usually refer to these types of disruptions as "normal disfluencies." Some children and adults stumble and repeat "er" and "uh" so frequently that they may be readily identified as disfluent speakers but still not considered to have a fluency disorder. The disruptions in fluency of a few speakers, however, are not accepted as normal by their listeners or themselves. A small proportion of these abnormally disfluent speakers have neurological impairments that result in a dyspraxia of speech or in dysarthria (Chapter 86). Our discussion will be limited to those abnormally disfluent speakers who are identified as stutterers.

Characteristics of Disordered Fluency. The distinction between normal and abnormal disfluency is not as clear-cut or straightforward as it may seem at first glance. There are no objective standards of fluency that are completely satisfactory. Usually, there is good agreement about who is a stutterer and who is not, particularly when the disorder has persisted for many years or is severe. Experts and nonexperts alike can readily identify people who are abnormally disfluent. However, there is substantially less agreement if one attempts to determine if a specific interruption in the flow of speech was abnormal or not. Experienced judges with explicit instructions frequently do not agree when they are asked to identify instances of stuttering. It should be recognized that not all disfluencies are abnormal and that the identification of stutterers during early stages of development or when the disorder is very mild can pose diagnostic problems.

Disfluencies have been described as hesitations, prolongations, repetitions, interjections, broken words, blocks, revisions, incomplete phrases, and dysrhythmic phonation. A number of investigators have attempted to discover the essential characteristics of those disfluencies judged as abnormal. While agreement is not complete, the following types of disfluencies tend to be judged as stuttering.

1. Part-word repetitions: Repetitions of sounds or syllables, the types of disfluencies most frequently labeled as stuttering, usually occur on the first sound or syllable or on the stressed syllable in a multisyllable word. One-syllable words that are repeated are more likely to be judged as stuttered the more times they are repeated.

2. Prolongations: Prolongations that are labeled as stuttering typically occur on initial sounds of words or stressed syllables. The longer the sound is prolonged, the more likely it is to be judged as stuttering.

3. Hesitations: Silent, inappropriate breaks in the flow of speech are more likely to be judged as stuttering as they increase in duration and when they occur within word and linguistic phrase boundaries.

4. Interjections: Interjections of "uhs," "ers," words, or phrases are not likely to be judged as stuttering unless part-word repetitions, prolongations, and hesitations are also present. Once a listener has identified a speaker as a stutterer, however, injections are often viewed as instances of stuttering.

Several other characteristics may accompany these types of disfluencies and are commonly observed in stutterers. Signs of struggle during disfluencies are often seen in chronic stutterers and occasionally in beginning stutterers. These signs may include sudden shifts in pitch or loudness, abrupt stoppages or releases of phonation or the breath stream, cessation of lip and jaw movements, rapid eye blinks, facial grimaces, repeating stereotyped verbal phrases, jerks of the head and other parts of the body, or averting the eyes from the listener. Instances of stuttering can range in duration from a fraction of a second to several minutes. From the stutterer's viewpoint, these speech disfluencies are involuntary and beyond his or her control. Struggling behavior is usually described as an attempt "to get the word out." The longer stuttering persists the more likely a child will be to fear speaking and to try to avoid situations which he or she fears will provoke stuttering. In spite of these general patterns that occur with some regularity among stutterers, it is important to remember that stuttering is a highly variable phenomenon. The only commonality now known to exist among all stutterers is the presence of the same general class of disfluent speech, which varies in the same stutterer from situation to situation, listener to listener, and time to time. This extraordinary intra-stutterer and inter-stutterer variability has intrigued and perplexed many clinicians, patients, and scholars for several thousand years.

Incidence and Prevalence of Stuttering. A number of studies have been completed that provide estimates of the prevalence, incidence, and remission of stuttering (Wingate, 1976). The evidence has been gathered in three ways. First, there are cross-sectional studies with trained examiners that provide direct information on the prevalence of stuttering observed among a given population at a certain point in time. These studies have usually been limited to groups from kindergarten to college age. Second, longitudinal studies with trained examiners provide direct information on how many people will stutter at some time in their lives. Finally, interviews or questionnaires have provided information about prevalence and incidence, but because these data are not based on direct observation of stuttering by a trained examiner, their reliability and validity are questionable.

Information from this research can be summarized as follows.

1. The prevalence of stuttering is generally accepted to be 0.7 per cent and is three to four times higher in boys than in girls. The prevalence is probably highest during preschool years and gradually decreases during elementary school years to slightly less than 1 per cent through college age.

2. The onset of stuttering usually occurs prior to age five or six with increasingly fewer onsets as the population nears puberty. Only isolated reports of new cases of stuttering after puberty are reported, and some of these may be recurrences.

3. Most stutterers stop stuttering whether or not they receive treatment. The recovery rate may be as high as 80 per cent, and most of those who stop stuttering will do so before or during puberty.

4. Recovery is usually reported to be gradual, and a greater percentage of mild stutterers may recover than severe stutterers. Further, among those who report they have recovered, a substantial proportion report that occasional stuttering problems persist from time to time.

Characteristics of Onset. Most children do not appear to pass through a "disfluency stage" after they begin combining words. Among preschoolers, word and phrase repetitions decrease in frequency of occurrence with age, but syllable repetitions do not, and boys evidence more syllable repetitions than do girls. Some children appear to begin stuttering as soon as they begin combining words. Others begin somewhat later, but most of those who stutter will have begun by the time they enter first grade. The most frequent type of disfluency beginning stutterers evidence is repetition of syllables, and this usually occurs on initial words of utterances. Stuttering is often episodic and varies substantially with the communicative task or situation. Usually beginning stutterers display little evidence of fear or embarrassment about stuttering. Occasionally, however, a child begins stuttering quite severely and evidences struggling and emotional reactions typically encountered only in older, chronic stutterers.

Referral Guidelines. It is always appropriate to refer children whose parents have become concerned about their disfluent speech to a qualified speech pathologist. It is probably wise to refer them even if the disfluent speech episodes have been occurring for only a few weeks, because excessive parental concern may contribute to the development of a clinically significant problem. Only rarely does disfluent speech require neurologic or psychiatric assistance, and speech pathologists can be helpful in identifying those children who warrant such referrals. Some general guidelines that may indicate that a child is at risk include the following (Van Riper, 1971).

1. Part-word repetitions on more than 2 per cent of the words spoken. Additional danger signs include increased tempo of repetition, audible vocal tension, and interrupted airflow.
2. Prolongations of one second or longer on more than 1 per cent of the words spoken. Additional danger signs are rises in pitch or increases in loudness during prolongations or interruptions of airflow or phonation.
3. Signs of struggling behavior during disfluencies.
4. Substantial changes in the fluency or severity of disfluencies as speaking situations change.

Explanations of Stuttering. It is not known why people stutter. Despite several decades of scientific investigation that followed centuries of speculative theorizing, it is still not possible to describe the act of stuttering in a definitive manner or to specify the conditions under which someone becomes a stutterer. This frustrating state of affairs has not resulted from lack of attempts to explain stuttering. There is an abundance of explanations. To date, however, none has proved satisfactory. Most theorists have attempted to explain stuttering as learned behavior, as a psychoneurotic symptom, or as a breakdown of normal physiologic functioning.

STUTTERING AS LEARNED BEHAVIOR. Stuttering has been described by various writers as resulting from operant conditioning, instrumental conditioning, a combination of classical and instrumental conditioning, approach-avoidance conflicts, and an attempt not to stutter. Although these explanations differ from each other in a number of ways, they have at least two common features. First, all presume that stuttering is a behavior that develops according to principles of learning. The essential nature of stuttering, therefore, is no different from any other form of learned behavior. Second, all presume that stutterers are no different constitutionally or emotionally from people who do not stutter.

The fact that learning theory explanations are quite popular currently attests to their plausibility. Also, research has not been able to identify reliable biogenic or psychogenic differences between people who stutter and people who do not, which provides some tangential support. Nevertheless, research findings that clearly demonstrate that stuttering is learned are also lacking. Careful analyses of findings interpreted to support these positions often reveal compelling alternative interpretations not consistent with theories of learning. Although it is likely that some aspects of stuttering may be learned, such as the struggling and reported avoidance behaviors often found in long-term stutterers, it is not clear that all aspects of stuttering or all stutterers fit the learning paradigm. In fact, much evidence suggests they do not.

STUTTERING AS A PSYCHONEUROTIC SYMPTOM. Because stuttering appears to occur in anatomically and physiologically normal people and because its occurrence usually varies so much from one speaking situation or from one time to another, many writers have conjectured that stuttering has psychogenic origins. The nature of the psychodynamic conflicts described have varied from writer to writer. All view stuttering as a symptomatic expression of psychologic conflict and assume the stutterer, the parents, or both are somewhat maladjusted.

Research to date has not been able to identify any consistent personality or emotional patterns associated with stuttering (Bloch and Goodstein, 1971). While it is not unusual for isolated studies to find small differences between groups of stutterers and nonstutterers from time to time, these differences have not held up when replicated elsewhere. The bulk of the evidence now available indicates that stutterers are usually within normal limits on standardized tests, do not differ reliably from nonstutterers, and are significantly different from control groups of known psychoneurotics. Further, mild stutterers are not differentiated from severe stutterers on tests of personality, and older stutterers do not appear to be substantially more maladjusted than younger stutterers. Finally, parents of stutterers are not more maladjusted than parents of children who do not stutter, although there is some evidence that they may be somewhat more perfectionistic than other parents. In spite of the lack of research findings to support the psychogenic origins of stuttering, many clinicians who see children and adults who stutter believe there are subtle psychogenic factors involved in the development and maintenance of the problem of stuttering among many of their clients. Whether or not these clinical impressions will ever be validated by scientific observation is problematic but seems unlikely at present.

STUTTERING AS A BREAKDOWN OF NORMAL PHYSIOLOGIC FUNCTIONING. The earliest explanations of stuttering focused on suspected biologic causes. It is known that substantially more males than females stutter and that stuttering tends to run in families. Yet, it is clear that familial incidence does not follow simple mendelian patterns of dominant or recessive inheritance. Reliable biochemical and physiologic differences between stutterers and nonstutterers have not been found, and no biophysical differences between stuttering and fluent speech that are not attributable to the act of stuttering have been identified. Still, the notion persists that some differences must exist in areas such as cerebral dominance, perseveration, or coordination of respiratory, phonatory, and articulatory processes during speech. In recent years there has been a renewed interest in looking for breakdowns in normal physiologic functioning among stutterers, particularly in laryngeal function.

Although current research is furthering our understanding of the biologic bases of stuttering, it is premature to draw definitive conclusions at present. Several models of genetic inheritance of stuttering are being explored and are consistent with preliminary data on familial incidence. It is also possible that a threshold model that incorporates genetic and environmental factors will account for the onset of stuttering. To date, we are not able to exclude with any confidence learning, personality, or physiologic factors as lacking significance in the development of stuttering.

Assessment. Assessment of children who stutter characteristically entails acquiring a detailed case history and making careful observations of the child's speech. We try to answer the following questions: Does the child stutter? When and under what circumstances did the problem begin? What are the major characteristics of stuttering? Under what circumstances is speech improved or worsened? How concerned or upset are the parents about the stuttering? What treatment approach would likely be most successful with this child and family?

When possible, through two-way mirror observations, we try to observe the child in relatively unstructured interactions with each parent, both parents, and clinicians under several speaking situations. We observe the child's speech and analyze it in terms of frequency and type of disfluences and their relationship to the speaking task and situation. We look for signs of struggling, excessive speaking effort, breaks in phonation, and airflow. We ask the parents if what we have observed is representative of the problem they are concerned about. With older children we talk to teachers in school and observe the children's speech as unobtrusively as possible in class and on the playground.

Treatment. Although there is substantial variability in viewpoints and beliefs about the causes of stuttering, treatment practices evidence a number of common denominators. Among preschoolers, the focus is on early identification of children who show incipient signs of stuttering. Treatment usually involves parent counseling designed to decrease the occurrence of fluency disruptors in the child's environment, to eliminate unnecessary parental demands or conditions that are associated with heightened disfluency, and to increase parental emotional support for the child. The essential strategy here is to prevent, arrest, or reverse the development of stuttering by manipulating those elements of the environment that appear to promote the child's fluency and self-esteem.

With older children or with preschool-age children who evidence excessive speaking effort during disfluencies, more direct approaches are often taken. The clinician may contrast "hard" vs. "easy" talking, model and practice speech tasks that facilitate coordination of phonatory and articulatory processes, and discuss feelings and attitudes about stuttering to decrease emotionalism and assist the child in reducing his or her speaking effort and in adopting more fluent speaking patterns. Currently, researchers using conditioning approaches to treating stutterers have reported relatively high rates of improvement. These procedures include rate control with and without delayed auditory feedback, modification of breath stream and airflow during speech, and contingent stimulus techniques. Also, biofeedback techniques have been used with reported success to assist older stutterers. These procedures are still too new to estimate their ultimate value in treating stuttering, however. Systemic treatment programs are employed to facilitate the transfer of fluent speaking behavior learned in therapy to everyday speaking situations. Usually, treatment is gradually discontinued to increase the probability that gains accomplished in therapy will be maintained. It is not unusual for some clients to be seen occasionally, even though they may not have stuttered for several months. Unfortunately, some clients who have stopped stuttering during treatment suffer a complete relapse after therapy is terminated.

It should not be surprising that we cannot predict how successful or unsuccessful treatment will be with an individual stutterer. Our understanding of the nature of stuttering and its causes is limited. Consequently, periods of trial therapy are always necessary to determine if a particular technique will be effective. Likewise, the ultimate·degree of success is usually not known until it has been attained. We know that most people who begin to stutter will stop. Some will continue throughout their lives to stutter some of the time, although it will not constitute a problem for them much of the time. Still others will continue to stutter — sometimes more often, sometimes less often — and will continue to experience their speech as a handicap for as long as they live regardless of the treatment they receive.

REFERENCES

Aronson, A. E. 1973. Psychogenic Voice Disorders. Philadelphia, W. B. Saunders Co., p. 41.

Bloch, E. L., and Goodstein, L. D. 1971. Functional speech disorders and personality. J. Speech Hear. Dis., 36:295–314, 1971.

Boone, D. R. 1977. The Voice and Voice Therapy, 2nd ed. Englewood Cliffs, NJ, Prentice-Hall, Inc.

Brackett, I. P. 1971. Parameters of voice quality. In Travis, L. E. (Ed.) Handbook of Speech Pathology and Audiology. New York, Appleton-Century-Crofts.

Brodnitz, F. S. 1965. Vocal Rehabilitation, 3rd ed. Rochester, American Academy of Ophthalmology and Otolaryngology.

Hull, F. M., Mielke, P. W., Willefore, J. A., et al. 1976. National Speech and Hearing Survey. Fort Collins, Final Report, Project No. 50978, Office of Education, Bureau of Education for the Handicapped, U.S. Department of Health, Education, and Welfare.

Ingram, D. 1976. Phonological Disability in Children. New York, Elsevier North-Holland, Inc.

Ling, D., 1976. Speech and the Hearing-Impaired Child: Theory and Practice. Washington, DC, Alexander Graham Bell Association for the Deaf.

Moore, P. 1971. Voice disorders organically based. In Travis, L. E. (Ed.) Handbook of Speech Pathology and Audiology. New York, Appleton-Century-Crofts.

Perkins, W. H. 1977. Speech Pathology: An Applied Behavioral Science, 2nd ed. St. Louis, The C. V. Mosby Co., Chaps. 13 and 14.

Shelton, R. L. 1978. Disorders of articulation. In Skinner, P., and Shelton, R. (Eds.): Speech, Language, and Hearing: Normal Processes and Disorders. Reading, MA, Addison-Wesley.

Sommers. R. K., Leiss, R. H., Delp, M. A., et al. 1967. Factors related to the effectiveness of articulation therapy for kindergarten, first, and second grade children. J. Speech Hear. Res., 10:428–437.

Van Riper, C. 1971. The Nature of Stuttering. Englewood Cliffs, NJ, Prentice-Hall, Inc.

Van Riper, C., and Erickson, R. L. 1975. Predictive Screening Test of Articulation, 4th ed. Kalamazoo, MI. Continuing Education Office, Western Michigan University.

Wilson, D. K. 1972. Voice Problems of Children. Baltimore, The Williams and Wilkins Co.

Wingate, M. E. 1976. Stuttering: Theory and Treatment. New York, Irvington Publ., Inc.

Winitz, H. 1969. Articulatory Acquisition and Behavior. New York, Appleton-Century-Crofts, Inc.

Chapter 86

MULTIPLE SPEECH DISORDERS
(Cleft Palate and Cerebral Palsy Speech)

Betty Jane McWilliams, Ph.D.

This orientation to multiple speech disorders is addressed primarily to otolaryngologists who are likely to encounter such problems in their practices. The goal is to provide background for diagnosis and management and to suggest that the speech pathologist can frequently play a decisive role on treatment teams or, indeed, by collaborating with the otolaryngologist on an individual basis.

Communication is, even in normal individuals, complex behavior involving sensation, integration of experience, language, thought processes, and the fine motor organization necessary for verbal expression. It is not surprising, therefore, that disruptions in the language and speech system often occur. These disorders may involve only a part of the system, or they may cut across the entire system and affect communication in a global way. These "multiple speech disorders" are always the most difficult to diagnose and treat, the most time-consuming and complicated, and the least promising as far as outcome is concerned. In short, they are likely to require the services of several professional people pooling their knowledge and experience over a relatively long period of time. The speech pathologist can almost never handle these problems alone, and that is true also for the otolaryngologist. Patients with multiple speech disorders are invariably better served if there is professional interaction in an atmosphere of mutual respect.

It should be noted that there are many

"multiple speech disorders" — aphasia, those problems associated with learning disabilities, minimal brain dysfunction, mental retardation, and emotional disturbance, some forms of voice disorder, hearing loss, cerebral palsy, and cleft palate. While this chapter deals only with cleft palate and cerebral palsy, otolaryngologists should be aware that these other areas of communication problems are also worthy of their concern on an interdisciplinary basis.

GLOSSARY

affricate — a consonant produced when a quick plosive is followed by forcing the airstream through a narrow aperture, as in *ch*ip.

aperiodicity (in relationship to voice) — a coming and going of voice.

aphasia — disturbance in symbolic functioning on a receptive and/or expressive level as the result of impairment to central nervous system function.

aphonia — absence of voice resulting from faulty vocal cord vibration rather than from absence of cords.

articulation — the production of speech sounds.

ataxia — a form of cerebral palsy associated with poor spatial orientation.

athetosis — a form of cerebral palsy associated with involuntary movements, usually of a slow, writhing nature.

1508

cerebral palsy — motor impairment of various types resulting from damage to the central nervous system before, during, or just after birth.

consonant — a speech sound, varying from one language to another, that is produced when the expired airstream, with or without voice, is altered, interrupted, or obstructed by the action of the muscles of articulation. An example of a consonant is the first sound in *boy* or *soy*.

fricative — a consonant produced when the airstream is forced through a narrow aperture, as in the first sound in *see*.

glottal stop — a plosive sound produced by the sudden release of subglottic air pressure. While this sound occurs normally in some languages, it is also often used as an alternative plosive by those who cannot impound intraoral pressure because of a defective velopharyngeal valve.

glottis — the opening between the vocal cords.

hypernasality — excessive nasal resonance resulting from the coupling of the oral and nasal airways during the production of non-nasal speech sounds, especially vowels.

hyponasality — speech marked by reduced nasal resonance and oralized characteristics on *m, n,* and *ng* (as in si*ng*).

language — symbols, verbal or nonverbal, which stand for objects, ideas, feelings, and so forth and which are used for communication.

nasal escape — loss of air through the nose on speech sounds other than *m, n,* and *ng* (as in si*ng*) in the English language.

pharyngeal fricative — a fricative produced by constriction of the pharyngeal walls and the posterior elevation of the tongue.

plosive — a consonant produced when the airstream is obstructed and then released, as in *bee*.

resonance — the vibratory response of an air-filled cavity to a frequency imposed upon it.

rhythm — the flow of connected discourse, including stress, inflection, pausing, and movement from one speech sound to another.

rigidity — hyperextension of muscles, which respond with "cogwheel"-like movements or small jerks when moved passively.

spasticity — a form of cerebral palsy characterized by hypertonicity and exaggerated stretch reflex.

speech — the oral expression of language.

tremor — a form of cerebral palsy characterized by fine, involuntary movements that increase during volitional movement.

voiced consonants — speech sounds produced with the vocal cords in vibration (*z* is voiced).

voiceless consonants — speech sounds produced in the absence of vocal cord vibration (*s* is voiceless).

vowel — a speech sound produced when the expired airstream is slightly altered by changes in the vocal tract, primarily the oral cavity, but is not obstructed. An example of a vowel is the first sound in *it*.

CLEFT PALATE

Nature of the Disorder

Embryology and Etiology. Clefts of the lip and palate are congenital malformations of structures that are normally developed by the end of the ninth week of intrauterine life. The reader is referred to Chapter 38 for an in-depth discussion of both the embryology and anatomy of this area. While many explanations for this group of defects have been suggested, the most widely accepted theory today is that clefts result from multifactorial inheritance, usually interacting with the environment. Thus, such teratogens as valium (diazepam) (Safra and Oakley, 1976) and anticonvulsant drugs (South, 1972) may, in the presence of the appropriate genetic background, increase the likelihood of some form of clefting being expressed. Since the genetic predisposition is only rarely known or suspected, the Federal Food and Drug Administration (1975) has suggested that the use of things such as the minor tranquilizers be avoided during the first trimester of pregnancy. The same caution should be exercised in regard to diagnostic roentgenograms and unnecessary exposure to viral infections. Burdi (1977) states:

... A blend of experimental, epidemiological, and genetic studies continue to generate a variety of hypotheses on the underlying causes of these orofacial cleft types. Yet, actual primary cause-and-effect relations still remain elusive ...

Readers who are especially interested in exploring etiology in depth may wish to begin with the work of F. C. Fraser (1971, 1973).

Incidence. There are many studies of the frequency with which some form of clefting occurs, but there is far from universal agreement on the most accurate estimate. A conservative figure, based on many studies, suggests an incidence of approximately 1 in every 750 live births. Clefts are, therefore, one of the most frequently seen major birth defects.

Drillien, Ingram, and Wilkinson (1966) estimate that 20 to 30 per cent of all clefts will involve only the lip on one or both sides with the hard and soft palates being intact. Both the lip and the palate will be defective in 35 to 55 per cent of all clefts, while only the palate will be cleft 30 to 45 per cent of the time.

Clefts of both the lip and palate are found more often in males than in females with the ratio often estimated to be as high as three to one. On the other hand, clefts of the palate only are more commonly seen in girls than in boys by a ratio of about three to two.

Incidence data are often compounded by racial factors. Orientals have an incidence that may be as high as 1 in 400 births, while Negroes, for whom information is not extensive, may have an occurrence rate as low as 1 in 2500. The incidence for Caucasians falls between those for Orientals and Negroes. The reasons for these variations are not clear.

It is also important to be aware that clefts tend to occur in families, although the exact pattern of inheritance has yet to be determined. If unaffected parents have one child with a cleft lip or cleft lip and palate, there is about a 3.8 per cent chance that each future child may be affected. If they have two children with the defect, the risk increases to 9 per cent. If one parent has a cleft, the risk of having one affected child is also about 4 per cent, but it increases to 16.7 per cent after the birth of a baby with a cleft. Figures vary slightly for isolated cleft palate (see Curtis, Fraser, and Warburton, 1961). It is of interest, especially to concerned families, that the chances of having a normal child are always greater than are the chances of having a child with a cleft.

Classification.   There is no universally accepted system of classification. The Veau (1931) system was widely used for many years and is still found in the literature. However, this is a simple system that does not provide for the many variations commonly seen. Kernahan and Stark (1958) proposed a different approach, which they based on embryologic development. Structures anterior to the incisive foramen, which develop separately from those posterior to it, are referred to as clefts of the *primary palate*. Structures posterior to that landmark are called clefts of the *secondary palate*. Those deformities that include both the lip and other structures anterior to the incisive foramen as well as those posterior to it are called clefts of the *primary and secondary palates*. Clefts of the primary or of the primary and secondary palates may be further designated as right or left unilateral, median, or bilateral; complete, incomplete, or submucous. Clefts of the secondary palate only are usually described as complete, incomplete, or submucous, the latter meaning that a mucosal covering conceals the defect in the underlying bone, muscle, or both.

Related Disorders

Associated Malformations.   Cleft lip and cleft palate, alone or in combination, are often present as parts of various syndromes. Examples of some of these conditions include acrocephalosyndactyly, Pierre Robin, and D1 Trisomy. For details on this subject, see Chapter 4. Infants with clefts are also at increased risk for other malformations, which do not necessarily conform to the characteristics of any particular syndrome. These include, among others, syndactyly, club foot, heart malformations, aural defects, various malformations of the eye, and disorders of the central nervous system.

Feeding Problems.   Clefts involving the soft palate are likely to be accompanied by early feeding distress, a subject that still has not been well-studied but that undoubtedly influences early growth and may account in part for slow linguistic and social development. This is usually not a difficult problem to handle (Paradise and McWilliams, 1974), but it is one that is often not addressed clinically and so is never solved. Fortunately, the natural processes of development serve to improve feeding as the baby gets older.

Otitis Media.   There can be no doubt that essentially all infants with palatal clefts have bilateral otitis media. It is reasonable to assume, from what is known of older age groups, that they also have conductive hearing losses (Stool and Randall, 1967; Paradise and Bluestone, 1969; Stool, 1971). Lupovich and colleagues (1971) indicate that sterile, inflammatory effusions are the rule in these cases, but suppuration is also found (Paradise, 1973).

Bluestone (1971) and Bluestone and others (1972) have demonstrated roentgenographically that children with unrepaired cleft palates have obstruction of the normal retrograde flow of instilled radiopaque contrast medium from the nasopharynx into the nasopharyngeal end of the eustachian tube. While there is a decided decrease in ear disease following palatal repair (Paradise and Bluestone, 1971), hearing impairment remains a major concern in all age groups, and surveillance is recommended through the teenage years or beyond when problems persist.

There is still disagreement about the management of these ear problems. While most otolaryngologists recognize the efficacy of myringotomy with tympanostomy tubes in older children with persistent otitis media, there is still confusion over the management of young infants with clefts. Paradise and Bluestone (1971) have maintained that otitis media can usually be controlled and middle ear aeration maintained by early myringotomy with aspiration of fluid and insertion of tympanostomy tubes, repetition of the procedure as needed, and prompt treatment of otorrhea. Others seem more inclined to accept the middle ear condition as it is and not to intervene unless the child experiences an episode of infection and all that it entails. More data in this area should be forthcoming in the near future. In the meantime, it is elementary to warn that hearing and speech are closely related and that even mild conductive hearing losses may be detrimental to speech development (Holm and Kunze, 1969).

Mental Development. Many studies (Irwin and Means, 1954; Goodstein, 1961, 1968) have suggested that children with clefts have a significantly lower mean IQ than is true for noncleft children and that they tend to have higher performance than verbal IQs, suggesting a relationship among defective speech, verbal intelligence, and overall IQ. However, Musgrave and his colleagues (1975) found little evidence to support the conclusion that any observed differences are of sufficient magnitude to account for any communicative disorders that may be present. This is not to imply that mental retardation does not exist among children with clefts. It does sometimes offer a better explanation for speech and language problems than does the cleft *per se*. However, children with clefts are also often gifted or of average abilities.

We can make no assumptions about mental capacities in children with clefts, with or without speech problems.

Social Development. Parents of children born with obvious malformations require time to come to terms with their grief (Tisza and Gumpertz, 1962) but are usually able to do so. Since parental behavior as well as other environmental factors are important to the child's ultimate acceptance of himself (MacGregor et al., 1953), the coping abilities of parents become relevant to the expectations we have for the child.

To date, no one has been able to show conclusively that children with clefts have serious emotional problems. However, they tend to mature more slowly socially and in communication skills and to be less verbal than children without clefts of similar ages (McWilliams and Smith, 1973). These problems appear to lie in the psychosocial sphere rather than in anatomic or physiologic areas. They also suggest the need for early parent counseling and programs such as nursery school for the children.

The Role of Interdisciplinary Care

Since the care of the child with a cleft is complicated, it seems efficient to provide a setting where the many disciplines concerned can work closely together in both planning and executing treatment. Initial concerns are likely to be those of the pediatrician and the social worker or someone else whose responsibility it is to help the parents adjust to the cleft problem and to begin to deal with it.

The plastic surgeon is essential in the early weeks because he or she can help the parents understand that the deformity can be corrected and can begin to plan with them for the child's eventual surgery. Thus, the plastic surgeon also sees the family as early as possible although, on the average, lip repair is not done until about three months of age, and palate repair is not done until the second year of life. There is some variation in this; but many surgeons like the baby to weigh at least ten pounds, be at least ten weeks of age, and have a normal blood count and hemoglobin before undertaking lip repair. Postponing palatal repair until the second year provides the surgeon with greater and more mature tissue mass, which may be desirable in getting an adequate, functional repair. The importance of surgical closure of the palate, which results in the ability to achieve velopharyngeal closure, cannot be overemphasized. Without this, speech will be seriously hypernasal with air escaping into the nasal passages, thus reducing the intraoral pressure necessary for the production of speech sounds. The reader interested in a detailed overview of surgical procedures, both primary and secondary, is referred to Grabb, Rosenstein, and Bzoch (1971), Randall (1973), and Fletcher et al. (1977).

All aspects of dentistry (Spriestersbach et al., 1973; Fletcher et al., 1977) are extremely important in cleft management because teeth are so often missing, malaligned, or defective. In addition, midfacial deficiency may occur. Many of these problems can be handled by the pedodontist, prosthodontist, orthodontist, or oral surgeon; but it is desirable for these specialists to work closely with the other disciplines so that treatment can be well coordinated and one individual does not carry out any procedure that might endanger the plans of another.

The otolaryngologist enters the picture when the child is born and plays many roles in the years that follow. Since the needs of patients with clefts change over time in all areas, it is always necessary to remember the longitudinal nature of treatment. The otolaryngologist's first concerns are likely to be otitis media, maintenance of hearing levels sufficient for the development of communication skills and social behavior, and prevention of complications from ear disease. The otolaryngologist may eventually be faced with the problem of removing the tonsils and adenoids of a child with a cleft. Whether or not to perform such surgery is a difficult decision to make, and the temptation is to say that it should not be done under any circumstances since there is real danger of speech deterioration following the removal of adenoids, which may have been providing the vital extra bit of tissue that made the difference between essentially normal and seriously defective speech. However, since there are few "nevers," a better course is for the otolaryngologist to have such a close relationship with the other members of the cleft palate team that he or she would not make that decision without consultation. Interaction with the speech pathologist is of vital necessity in decisions of this kind.

Since the so-called "cleft-lip nose" is often complicated by septal deviation and other conditions that occlude the nasal airway either partially or completely, the otolaryngologist must be in constant communication with many others, including the plastic surgeon and the speech pathologist, to determine the best time to intervene and how the work may influence subsequent speech performance. The otolaryngologist also has an important role in the assessment and treatment of certain voice disorders, again in conjunction with the speech pathologist and other members of the cleft palate team. These relationships will be expanded upon later.

The speech pathologist and audiologist are also important members of the diagnostic and treatment teams. Both work from the birth of the child until treatment is completed, usually in the late teens but often not until later in adult life, particularly if dental appliances are worn to replace teeth, to obturate a palatal defect, or to elevate a soft palate with motor impairment. The speech pathologist can contribute most in a setting where his or her special skills are valued and where he or she occupies a peer position on the team. This professional person should, after all, know more about speech and language than any of the other specialists — just as each of the others is most knowledgeable about his or her particular field.

Other professions enter the program as they are required. Of great help are the psychiatrist and the clinical psychologist, both necessary in the habilitation of many children. The radiologist is indispensable and has the responsibility for the assessment of the adequacy of the velopharyngeal valving mechanism by radiography, again in conjunction with other team members (Skolnick, 1977).

The Nature and Causes of Speech Problems

If the repair of the palate has achieved the goal of creating a velopharyngeal valve capable of separating the oral and nasal cavities during speech and if there are no other complicating factors, speech should be essentially normal. At least, it should be free of the hypernasality that is characteristic of the open airway. This is the major goal of surgical repair as well as of management by a prosthetic speech aid constructed by a prosthodontist. This goal is almost never achieved in some settings and is usually accomplished in others. The highest success rate to date, 98 per cent, has been reported by Braithwaite (1964) and Morley (1966). Surgeons or prosthodontists who have less than an 80 per cent success rate should attempt to determine the cause and correct it.

Hypernasality. Too much nasal resonance occurs in approximately 20 to 25 per cent of cleft cases. The usual explanation for this is that the velopharyngeal valve is not closing. Hypernasality *per se* is largely a vowel phenomenon, but reduced intelligibility of speech results from disruption in consonant production. Consonants require varying degrees of intraoral pressure. The inability to impound pressure in the oral cavity thus affects consonant sounds differently. The most serious disturbance will occur on those consonants requiring high intraoral pressure over time. These include the fricatives, such as /s/ (as in *s*ee) and /z/ (as in *z*oo) and the affricates /šh/ (as in *sh*oe). The next most difficult are the plosives, such as /p/ in *p*ie, /b/ in *b*oy, /k/ in *k*ey, and /g/ in *g*o, among others. Voiceless consonants (such as /s/ and /p/) will sound more distorted than will those that are voiced. Sounds that are affected by velopharyngeal incompetency tend to be weak, nasally distorted, and often accompanied by nasal escape capable of clouding a mirror placed beneath the nostrils during the speech act. Nasal escape is normal on /n/ as in *n*o, /m/ as in *m*e, and /ng/ as in ki*ng*. The absence of air on these sounds indicates some obstruction in the nasal airways.

It is the human ear that is the decisive instrument in detecting that speech is defective, and the educated ear can reliably determine the probable cause of the differences that are heard. Thus, it is helpful to learn to listen and to make accurate judgments. The speech pathologist should be expert at this. A place to begin is to listen to short speech samples loaded first with vowels and consonants *least* likely to be defective and to end with those at highest risk if the valving mechanism is faulty. "Mama may mail a mop," may sound almost normal even if closure is not obtained since most of the sounds in the sentence require an open nasal airway. "Sissy sees the sky," on the other hand, is loaded with highly demanding sounds and may reveal the presence of a problem. "Kindly give Kate cake," is less difficult than the "sissy" sentence but more revealing of valving inadequacy than the "mama" sentence.

Hypernasality associated with true velopharyngeal inadequacy is usually not treatable by speech therapy (McWilliams et al., 1973). Instead, either the valve must be corrected or certain deficits in speech must be accepted as irreversible.

Hyponasality. Some individuals with clefts are hyponasal or have too little nasal resonance because of obstruction of the nasal airways. Their speech resembles that of children with very large adenoids. The nasal consonants, /m/, /n/, and /ng/, are not accompanied by nasal escape and approach /b/, /d/, and /g/. Therefore, listening to these sounds often helps to reduce the confusion. that commonly exists between hyponasality and hypernasality. When hyponasality is present, opening up the airway will improve speech, provided that velopharyngeal closure is adequate. If the velopharyngeal valve does not close during speech, speech is likely to deteriorate seriously following such a procedure. Thus, it is always desirable to have a complete evaluation of that important valve and to have all the information that the speech pathologist can provide before undertaking procedures on the nasal airway.

Hypo-Hypernasality. In a few cases, both hyponasality and hypernasality will be present in speech. Although this seems like a contradiction, it is possible when nasal airway patency is so reduced as to alter nasal consonants but is associated with velopharyngeal inadequacy leading to emission of air during the production of consonants requiring high intraoral pressure over time, as in /s/. Vowels such as the ones in m*e* and m*oo* may also have somewhat more nasal resonance than is usual. Management usually involves correction of both the nasal airway anomalies and the defective valve, the latter often by pharyngeal flap or, in very minimal degrees of inadequacy, a procedure such as Teflon injection.

Nasal Turbulence. Some speakers with both velopharyngeal inadequacy and partial obstruction of the nasal airways will have what sounds like "noise" in the nose when they are producing high-pressure sounds. This results from loss of air through the velopharyngeal portal and the vibration of that airstream as it passes through the airways. In these cases, correction of both the airway and the valve is usually required.

Hoarseness. Individuals with velopharyngeal valving of only borderline competency appear sometimes to compensate by increasing laryngeal tension in an effort to avoid being hypernasal. Some of them eventually develop bilateral vocal cord nodules (McWilliams et al., 1969; McWilliams et al., 1973a). When hoarseness is present, both the valving mechanism and the larynx should be evaluated. Neither removal of the nodules nor speech therapy has been very successful in the treatment of these problems. Again, improving the valve appears to be the treatment of choice. In the absence of treatment, children with clefts appear to retain their nodules longer than do children without clefts and remain hoarse even after the nodules are no longer present.

Articulation. Faulty production of speech sounds may result from inadequate hearing, although these defects will not usually include hypernasality if only a conductive hearing loss is present. As has already been demonstrated, articulation errors may be caused by faulty velopharyngeal valving. In extreme cases, there may be efforts to compensate for the loss of air by substituting glottal stops for plosives and pharyngeal fricatives for such sounds as /s/ and /z/. A glottal stop uses the vocal cords in a valve-like action, thus producing the consonant well before air can be lost at the velopharyngeal portal into the nose. Needless to say, consonants produced either glottally or pharyngeally are not likely to be associated with nasal escape, and this can lead the uninitiated to believe that the valve is intact.

Speech sounds may also be defective when the tongue assumes unusual postures in attempting their production. These problems may be functional and may reflect immaturity or faulty learning as in the case of any other articulation disorder. However, persons with a cleft face the added hazard of missing or malaligned teeth, sometimes in combination with underdevelopment of the midface. These structural deviations are very often responsible for articulation errors in that the tongue's housing may be too small or the tongue seeks to occlude openings when such sounds as /s/ are produced. These deficits are alterations in the direction of the airstream and so are easily confused with errors caused by velopharyngeal valving problems. Orthodontic intervention is the treatment of choice in these cases.

Another source of confusion is the articulation related to an anterior oronasal fistula. If such an opening is situated where the tongue uses it as an articulator in the production of sibilants (fricatives such as /s/ and /z/), air may be forced into the nose to exit in the form of nasal escape. The articulation errors then seem to relate to the all-important velopharyngeal valve when, in reality, the valve is intact, and the errors are at least partially frontal in nature. A simple test is to evaluate the change in /s/ production when the fistula is closed with dental wax. Obviously closure of the fistula, either surgically or prosthetically, is essential if speech is to improve. Once physical conditions have been corrected to the extent possible, the speech pathologist may suggest and carry out short-term speech therapy designed to help the patient use the speech mechanism at the optimal level — or speech therapy may not be necessary if the patient makes these adaptations without assistance.

Complex Speech Problems

Discussing the various aspects of the speech problems of individuals with clefts is to simplify a complex topic. The characteristics described above are rarely found in isolation. Rather, they exist in combination, interacting to alter each other and to confuse the examiner, experienced as well as inexperienced. Hoarseness, always a highly variable phenomenon even in the same patient, may be obscured by hypernasality, by alteration in the nasal passages, and articulation errors of functional origin, or by errors related to the anatomy and physiology of the entire vocal tract, of which the velopharyngeal complex is only a part. Since these interrelationships exist at every level of the cleft problem, the case for interdisciplinary decision-making and management is clear. In addition, the special skills that the speech pathologist brings to the treatment team are of paramount importance in making reasonable management decisions. Some children with clefts may require speech or language therapy because of problems either unrelated to the cleft or tangential to it. This therapy may be only short-term in nature or it may continue through several years of life. Other children may have seriously disordered speech but may not be candidates for therapy because the speech pattern is compatible with the mechanism. Still others may speak normally and have little need of direct therapy. The speech pathologist is often the person best qualified to assess the situation and to understand what therapy can and cannot accomplish in a given case. It is vital to recognize in this regard that, from birth through adolescence, the child with a cleft is a growing, changing human being and that the clinical situation is not a static one. Thus, the speech pathologist, along with other specialists, must review and reassess clinical needs from birth until adulthood and, sometimes, when problems persist or when prosthetic appliances are involved, throughout the life of the patient. This long-term involvement will usually not include speech therapy *per se* except for specific periods of time and under specific circumstances. Nevertheless, the contribution of the speech pathologist to both diagnosis and treatment cannot be overemphasized.

CEREBRAL PALSY

Nature of the Disorder

Definition. It has been difficult to get general agreement on a definition of cerebral palsy because of the widely diversified nature of the symptoms. However, most writers would agree that it is a neuromotor problem resulting from damage to the brain before, during, or shortly after birth and that the neurologic impairment is nonprogressive. Perlstein (1950) defined it as "paralysis, weakness, incoordination, or any other aberration of motor function due to pathology of the *motor control centers of the brain*." However, since cerebral palsy almost always involves much more than the motor system, Cruickshank (1976) leans toward definitions that include the motor, emotional, sensory, and developmental conditions caused by the neurologic impairment. Nonetheless, the common denominator among cerebral palsied individuals is the neuromotor dysfunction. Of particular interest is the view of Bobaths (1967): ". . . cerebral palsy reveals itself both in a developmental and a pathological deviation from normal motor behavior. The child's motor difficulties are seen as arising from persistence of infantile motor patterns and from abnormal patterning of muscle function with a poverty of motor patterns."

It should be noted that the disorder was first described by William Little in 1853 (Little, 1958). However, little was done to treat such children until Winthrop Morgan Phelps began his pioneering work in this country in the 1930s.

Incidence. There are many, many studies of incidence. Of course, since there is disagreement about the definition of the problem, there is also lack of agreement about how frequently it occurs. Phelps once estimated that there would be approximately 7 cerebral palsied persons in every 100,000 of the population. His figures have been widely quoted. However, since then, estimates have been as high as 3 per 1000 population (McDonald and Chance, 1964).

Types. Cerebral palsy has been classified in many different ways, but most classification systems are based upon the type and degree of motor impairment. The types most often referred to include spasticity, athetosis, ataxia, rigidity, and tremor. Spasticity is the most common of these, accounting for nearly half of all cases of cerebral palsy. Some studies (Illingsworth, 1958) place this figure even higher. Athetosis is the second most frequently diagnosed disorder with 25 per cent of all individuals with cerebral palsy being a fairly representative estimate. Tremor is almost always found to be the least prevalent.

Classification is also made on the basis of motor involvement. Thus, the terms quadriplegia, triplegia, right or left hemiplegia, paraplegia, and monoplegia are also used even though some specialists object to this descriptive classification on the basis that it suggests paralysis rather than impaired function. Most studies agree that athetoids are almost always quadriplegics while spasticity is about equally divided between quadriplegia and hemiplegia. Monoplegia and triplegia are relatively rare in all types.

Related Disorders

Since cerebral palsy is the result of neurologic impairment, it is not unusual for there to be many problems in addition to the damage to the motor system. These deficits include mental retardation, generalized developmental delay, convulsive disorders, speech and language disorders, a wide variety of visual and auditory impairments, learning disabilities, and emotional disturbances, among others. Needless to say, any one of these conditions may be severe enough to render the cerebral palsied child's life extremely difficult. Since well over half of all cerebral palsied children suffer from some degree of mental retardation, disordered communication, or both, it is clear that these children should be viewed as multiply handicapped and that their treatment should include attention to as many of their needs as possible.

The Role of Interdisciplinary Care

Like the child with cleft palate, care for the cerebral palsied infant is best begun in a center with access to many different disciplines, including pediatrics, orthopedics, neurology, otolaryngology, ophthalmology, developmental specialties, speech pathology, audiology, physical therapy, occupational therapy, social work, psychology, and education. Individuals in these fields should plan and act in concert in order to prevent the tragic confusion that so often confronts parents of children with complex problems. Unlike the child with a cleft whose defect is very likely to be diagnosed at birth, it is rare that cerebral palsy is diagnosed until after parents painfully wonder why their child fails to reach developmental landmarks at appropriate ages. Very often, they are told not to worry, that the child will "outgrow" his or her problems. When this does not occur, the frantic search for help begins and is frequently frustrated when physicians do not take the time or are reluctant to deal with the evidence that the baby presents.

Fortunately, this condition is changing, and more and more attention is being given to the management of "high-risk" infants from birth on. For many years, preschool programs have been used as a means of intervening early in the lives of cerebral palsied children. However, it is now recognized that much valuable time may be lost during the early months when an infant is failing to develop well. This has resulted in early intervention programs, which aim to teach parents to assist their child at home long before he or she is old enough for a preschool. United Cerebral Palsy has done a great deal of work in this area, and many local chapters have active programs of this nature. It is important to point out that there are no really conclusive data to support the contention that such programs are helpful. On the other hand, it does appear reasonable to assume that intervention in these early months, when development is taking place so rapidly, is important to eventual outcome. Lencione (1976) reports Köng's claim that, ten years ago, a "large proportion" of the cerebral palsied children

seen in her center were severely involved while, at present, after having undergone treatment based on Bobath's neurodevelopmental method (Bobath, 1959; Semans, 1958), the majority have only slight or minimal impairment.

The Nature and Causes of Speech Problems

Knowing only that an individual has cerebral palsy is insufficient information to decide what his or her speech will be like. Thus, the discussion that follows will be applicable to cerebral palsy *per se* but not to any patient in particular. Diagnostic evaluation is nowhere as important as it is in cerebral palsy — nor as confusing. One part of the speech system influences another, and the cerebral palsied child is likely to have a number of interacting disabilities.

Language. Cerebral palsied children often have both motor and sensory problems, which lead to experiential deprivation, accounting in part for slow speech and language development. When that situation is complicated by mental retardation, the results may be serious problems with the development of a linguistic system. The problem may be further confused by severe hearing losses of a sensorineural nature or by what appears to be central auditory impairment — although this is still debatable. In addition, such children are prone to all other types of hearing problems, including poor attention to auditory stimuli. Estimates of incidence of hearing problems vary from 10 to 30 per cent (McDonald and Chance, 1964).

When auditory disorders are present, the otolaryngologist will be involved actively in diagnosis. It is clear that this physician cannot make a diagnosis in many cases without the input of the audiologist, the speech pathologist, and the clinical psychologist. What appears at the outset to be deafness may not be a peripheral disorder, and certain educational tactics, together with maturation, may assist the child to function on a higher level. This will not be the case if he or she does not have appropriate help, however.

Cerebral palsied children, overall, have long been known to have slow onset of speech. Denhoff (1976) found that the average age for use of single words was 27.1 months. Byrne (1959) found relatively greater delay for the use of longer sentences than for the use of shorter ones. Two-word sentences were delayed by one year, but four-word sentences were delayed by four years. *All* children in this study showed delay, although their language development paralleled that of normal children but at a slower rate. These findings are not surprising when it is remembered that the motor impairment itself makes longer sentences more difficult than shorter ones.

Athetoids appear to have a higher incidence of hearing impairment than do spastics, with ataxics falling between (Hopkins et al., 1954). Mental retardation has essentially the same effect as does hearing loss. In addition, the brain damage may result in aphasia-like symptoms, which add another dimension to the confusion. For the same reasons, verbal output may remain limited throughout life for some of the more seriously affected. It is for this reason that it has been suggested that alternative forms of communication be taught, including the use of such things as language boards (McDonald and Schultz, 1973). These devices should not replace verbal expression but should augment it or serve the needs of those who cannot acquire verbal skills.

Respiration. A common problem in cerebral palsy is with breathing. Respiration is often irregular, immature in that abdominal excursion continues to be a major element long after thoracic patterns should have been developed, improperly coordinated with the rest of the speech process, too rapid, or too slow. This results in defects in voice, resonance, articulation and rhythm. These will be discussed under the appropriate headings.

Voice and Resonance. It has long been recognized that cerebral palsied children have voice disorders, such as breathiness, hoarseness, harsh glottal attacks, low or erratic volume or loudness, aphonia, aperiodicity, speaking on residual air or during inspiration, and inability to initiate voice without delay or to maintain voice as long as required.

Mysak (1971) has suggested that persistence of the primitive glottic-closing reflex may account in part for voice disorders "associated with involuntary, open-close or over-close activity of the glottis." Voice problems that could result from this would include interruption of voicing, intermittent and forced voicing, delay in initiation of voicing, short duration, paucity of phonation, weak phonation, and speaking on inspiration — all voice deviations commonly heard in the cerebral palsied. It should be pointed out that similar voice disturbances can also have their origins in the breathing cycle itself and in the control thereof.

Other writers (McDonald and Chance, 1964; Lencione, 1976) have attributed many of these problems to such things as laryngeal spasms, adductor spasms, abductor spasms, laryngeal tension, and even to involvement of the velopharyngeal valving mechanism (Hardy, 1961). This latter condition results in hypernasal speech because the portal remains open during speech or behaves erratically. It also reduces intraoral pressure and renders already inefficient respiratory and voicing systems even less effective.

The best possible treatment is dependent upon learning why the voice problem exists. Thus, the otolaryngologist can be extremely helpful in providing information about laryngeal function and in contributing to decisions about clinical management. Again, however, this physician will be wise to act in concert with the speech pathologist.

Articulation. The manner in which cerebral palsied individuals produce consonants is also complicated. Irwin (1961, 1963) has reported, as might be expected, that sounds that are less complex are easier for the cerebral palsied to produce and that cerebral palsied children do less well articulating consonants than do retarded children who do not have cerebral palsy. Thus, voiced consonants are more often correct than are the unvoiced. Nasals, which do not require coordinated velopharyngeal behavior, are easier than non-nasals. Sounds produced by the lips seemed simpler than those requiring activity including the teeth, tongue, and palate. His cerebral palsied group also tended to omit many consonants. This latter conclusion supported the work of Lencione (1976), who in 1953 found that consonants occurring in the middle or final position of the word were the most difficult. This finding suggests that the control of the breath stream may be of major significance in articulation skills. It is interesting to note that articulation ability is seriously retarded in cerebral palsied children and may, in fact, never reach the accepted standards for normals. However, as in language, the sequence of development parallels that of normal children.

Consonant articulation may also be defective because of the marked motor incapacities that may be present in structures in the oral cavity. The individual so afflicted may be unable to elevate the tongue, the mandible, or the soft palate, may have trouble compressing the lips, and may have none of the fine motor skills necessary for intelligible speech. This appears to apply to all types of cerebral palsy, but the disorders may manifest themselves in different ways depending upon the type. For example, a spastic may be unable to execute a given movement of the tongue, while an athetoid may be able to execute the movement but may be unable to control extraneous movements sufficiently to arrive at the desired target, and an ataxic may fail to reach his or her goal because of poor orientation in space. The speech that results, however, does not sound particularly unique — although many writers have attempted to make such differentiations.

When articulation disorders are influenced by poor motor capacities, it is essential to investigate all vegetative functions as well (Westlake and Rutherford, 1961). Many of these children drool, cannot suck through a straw or chew food, and have difficulty with swallowing. Any therapeutic approach now in general use takes into account the developmental nature of the disability and the wide spectrum of problems to be treated. Articulation can rarely be attacked as an isolated entity unless the problems are the result of immaturity rather than of the cerebral palsy and its many complicating elements.

Rhythmic Disturbances. As might be expected in a disorder as all-inclusive as cerebral palsy, some of these patients will have disorders of rhythm. Literally all who have breathing problems will demonstrate breaks in the free flow of speech. Sounding "slow and labored" is a description that often appears in the literature. Others will have what sounds a great deal like stuttering. This stuttering-like behavior may result from the breathing deficits noted earlier; from laryngeal spasms, from the inability to coordinate breathing, phonation, and articulation; and, perhaps, from faulty auditory and proprioceptive feedback as suggested by Mysak (1971). Sometimes, as with all other aspects of this problem, the nonfluency will be the result of immaturity coupled with social response to what is really a normal developmental stage for a child who may be experiencing a slow growth rate. Again, differential diagnosis is essential.

Complex Speech Problems

Like cleft palate, cerebral palsy will probably encompass many aspects of the speech system with the resulting speech being an interaction among these different components of the speech tract. Respiration will influence vocalization, resonance, rhythm, and articulation. Vocalization will influence resonance, rhythm, and articulation, and all will interact to create severe disorders of communication that can be understood only by the cooperative diagnostic endeavors of many specialists working together and exchanging information. Even treatment does not rest in the hands of the speech pathologist alone. It may well begin with the physical and occupational therapists with the speech pathologist cooperating in a parallel treatment program. The otolaryngologist will help to unwind many of the mysteries of both hearing and voice and will treat the child for any other problems appropriate to the field. While this last statement seems too obvious to make, cerebral palsied children even today sometimes go untreated for routine illnesses because they are difficult to handle and to communicate with. All professional people need to learn to manage such patients and to do so willingly.

The speech pathologist often begins actual therapy with these children when they are only a few months old and may continue such work well into adulthood if progress is being made or if regression occurs when therapy is stopped. The extent to which speech therapy will be required will depend upon the degree of involvement, as will the eventual outcome for the patient. In many cases, there is no known way to develop "normal" speech. The goal is to help the patient become a communicating person and to realize his or her own best potential, limited though that may be.

The child with cleft palate in today's programs has an excellent prognosis for taking an eventual place in society as a fully participating member. The outlook for the cerebral palsied is highly variable depending upon the complexity and life ramifications of the disorder. Both individuals with clefts and those with cerebral palsy are likely to achieve the highest possible level of *habilitation* when diagnosis and treatment are carried out in an interdisciplinary setting where there is access to experienced professionals who are well-qualified to treat children with these disorders.

SELECTED REFERENCES

Bobath, K. 1959. The neuropathology of cerebral palsy and its importance in treatment and diagnosis. Cerebral Palsy Bulletin, *8*:13.

The Bobath approach to diagnosis and treatment represents, in this writer's view, the most significant advance in the past quarter century.

Cruickshank, W. M. (Ed.). 1976. Cerebral Palsy, a Developmental Disability. Syracuse, Syracuse University Press.

This book provides an excellent overview of cerebral palsy and includes valuable references for additional reading.

Fletcher, S. G., Berkowitz, S., Bradley, D. P., et al. 1977. Cleft lip and palate research: An updated state of the art. Cleft Palate J., *14*:261–330.

This work summarizes research in cleft palate over the past four years.

Grabb, W. C., Rosenstein, S. W., and Bzoch, K. R. 1971. Cleft Lip and Palate. Boston, Little, Brown and Co.

This multi-authored text presents chapters on a wide variety of topics and summarizes information available at the time of publication. The work is detailed and well-documented.

Little, W. J. 1958. On the influence of abnormal parturition, difficult labours, premature birth, and asphyxia neonatorum, on the mental and physical condition of the child, especially in relation to deformities Trans. Obstetr. Soc. Lond. 1861–62, 3, 293). Cerebral Palsy Bulletin, *1*:5.

This paper has historical significance to those interested in exploring the vast literature in cerebral palsy.

McDonald, E. T., and Chance, B. 1964. Cerebral Palsy. Englewood Cliffs, NJ, Prentice-Hall, Inc.

This is a small volume that presents a brief overview with extensive documentation.

McWilliams, B. J., Morris, H. L., Shelton, R. L., et al. 1973. Speech, language, and psychosocial aspects of cleft lip and palate: The state of the art. ASHA Reports No. 9, Washington, DC, American Speech and Hearing Association.

This is a detailed summary of research conducted in the speech, language, and psychosocial aspects of cleft palate up to 1973. It is the complete text of the material summarized in the next paper.

Spriestersbach, D. C., Dickson, D. R., Fraser, F. C., et al. 1973. Clinical research in cleft lip and cleft palate: The state of the art. Cleft Palate J., *10*:113.

This "state of the art" is a skeleton for a number of more detailed papers that grew out of this work. It provides a fine bibliography.

Westlake, H., and Rutherford, D. 1961. Speech therapy for the Cerebral Palsied. Chicago, National Society for Crippled Children and Adults.

This presents a fine picture of speech therapy for the cerebral palsied as it was practiced prior to the Bobath approach.

REFERENCES

Bluestone, C. D. 1971. Eustachian-tube obstruction in the infant with cleft palate. Ann. Otol., Rhinol., Laryngol., Suppl. 2, *80*:1.

Bluestone, C. D., Wittel, R. A., and Paradise, J. L. 1972. Roentgenographic evaluation of Eustachian tube function in infants with cleft and normal palates. Cleft Palate J., *9*:93.

Bobath, K. 1959. The neuropathology of cerebral palsy and its importance in treatment and diagnosis. Cerebral Palsy Bull., *8*:13.

Bobath, K., and Bobath, R. 1967. The neurodevelopmental treatment of cerebral palsy. Physical Therapy, *47*:1039.

Braithwaite, F. 1964. Cleft palate repair. *In* Gibson, T. (ed.). Modern Trends in Plastic Surgery. London, Butterworth.

Burdi, A. R. 1977. Epidemiology, etiology, and pathogenesis of cleft lip and palate. Cleft Palate J., *14*:262–269.

Byrne, M. 1959. Speech and language development of athetoid and spastic children. J. Speech Hear. Disord., *24*:231.

Cruickshank, W. M. (ed.). 1976. Cerebral Palsy, a Developmental Disability. Syracuse, Syracuse University Press.

Curtis, E. J., Fraser, F. C., and Warburton, D. 1961. Congenital cleft lip and palate. Am. J. Dis. Child., *102*:853.

Denhoff, E. 1976. Medical aspects. *In* Cruickshank, W. M. (ed.). Cerebral Palsy, a Developmental Disability. Syracuse, Syracuse University Press, p. 29.

Drillien, C. M., Ingram, T. T. S., and Wilkinson, E. M. 1966. The Causes and Natural History of Cleft Lip and Palate. Edinburgh, Livingstone.

Federal Food and Drug Administration. 1975. Drug Bull., *5*:14.

Fletcher, S. G., Berkowitz, S., Bradley, D. P., et al. 1977. Cleft lip and palate research. An updated state of the art. Cleft Palate J., *14*:261–330.

Fraser, F. C. 1971. Etiology of cleft lip and palate. *In* Grabb, W. C., Rosenstein, S. W., and Bzoch, K. R. (eds.) Cleft Lip and Palate. Boston, Little, Brown and Co., p. 54.

Fraser, F. C. 1973. Aspects of etiology and pathogenesis. *In* Clinical research in cleft lip and cleft palate: The state of the art. Cleft Palate J., *10*:115.

Goodstein, L. D. 1961. Intellectual impairment in children with cleft palates. J. Speech Hear. Res., *4*:287.

Goodstein, L. D. 1968. Psychosocial aspects of cleft palate. *In* Spriestersbach, D. C., and Sherman, D. (eds.) Cleft Palate and Communication. New York, Academic Press, p. 201.

Grabb, W. C., Rosenstein, S. W., and Bzoch, K. R. 1971. Cleft Lip and Palate. Boston, Little, Brown and Co.

Hardy, J. 1961. Intraoral breath pressure. J. Speech Hear. Dis., *26*:309.

Holm, V. A., and Kunze, L. H. 1969. Effect of chronic otitis media in language and speech development. Pediatrics, *43*:833.

Hopkins, T., Bice, H., and Colton, K. 1954. Evaluation and Education of the Cerebral Palsied Child. Washington, DC, International Council for Exceptional Children, p. 13.

Illingsworth, R. S. (Ed.) 1958. Recent Advances in Cerebral Palsy. Boston, Little, Brown and Co.

Irwin, J. V., and Means, B. J. 1954. An analysis of certain measures of intelligence and hearing in a sample of the Wisconsin cleft palate population (abstract). Cleft Palate Bull., *4*:4.

Irwin, O. C. 1961. Comparison of articulation scores of

children with cerebral palsy and mentally retarded children. Cerebral Palsy Rev., *22*:10.

Irwin, O. C. 1963. Difficulties of consonant sounds in terms of manner and place of articulation and of voicing in the speech of cerebral palsied children. Cerebral Palsy Rev., *24*:13.

Kernahan, D. A., and Stark, R. B. 1958. A new classification for cleft lip and cleft palate. Plast. Reconstr. Surg., *22*:435.

Lencione, R. 1976. The development of communication skills. *In* Cruickshank, W. M. 1976. Cerebral Palsy, a Developmental Disability. Syracuse, Syracuse University Press, p. 175.

Little, W. J. 1958. On the influence of abnormal parturition, difficult labours, premature birth, and asphyxia neonatorum, on the mental and physical condition of the child, especially in relation to deformities (Trans. Obstetr. Soc. Lond. 1861–62, 3, 293). Cerebral Palsy Bull., *1*:5.

Lupovich, P., Bluestone, C. D., Paradise, J. L., et al. 1971. Middle ear effusions: Preliminary viscometric, histologic and biochemical studies. Ann. Otol. Rhinol., Laryngol., *80*:342.

MacGregor, F. C., Abel, T. M., Bryt, A., et al. 1953. Facial Deformities and Plastic Surgery: A Psychosocial Study. Springfield, IL, Charles C Thomas.

McDonald, E. T., and Chance, B. 1964. Cerebral Palsy. Englewood Cliffs, NJ, Prentice-Hall, Inc.

McDonald, E. T., and Schultz, A. R. 1973. Communication boards for cerebral palsied children. J. Speech Hear. Dis., *38*:73.

McWilliams, B. J., Bluestone, C. D., and Musgrave, R. H. 1969. Diagnostic implications of vocal cord nodules in children with cleft palate. Laryngoscope, *79*:2072.

McWilliams, B. J., and Musgrave, R. H. 1972. Psychological implications of articulation disorders in cleft palate children. Cleft Palate J., *9*:294.

McWilliams, B. J., Lavorato, A. S., and Bluestone, C. D. 1973a. Vocal cord abnormalities in children with velopharyngeal valving problems. Laryngoscope, *83*:1745.

McWilliams, B. J., Morris, H. L., Shelton, R. L., et al. 1973b. Speech, language, and psychosocial aspects of cleft lip and palate: The state of the art. ASHA Reports No. 9, Washington, DC, American Speech and Hearing Association.

McWilliams, B. J., and Smith, R. M. 1973. Psychosocial considerations. In ASHA Reports No. 9, Washington, DC, American Speech and Hearing Association, p. 43.

Morley, M. E. 1966. Speech and speech therapy in cleft palate. *In* Gibson, T. (Ed.) Modern Trends in Plastic Surgery. Washington, Butterworth, p. 255.

Musgrave, R. H., McWilliams, B. J., and Matthews, H. P. 1975. A review of the results of two different surgical procedures for the repair of clefts of the soft palate only. Cleft Palate J., *12*:281.

Mysak, E. D. 1971. Cerebral palsy speech syndromes. *In* Travis, L. E. (Ed.) Handbook of Speech Pathology. New York, Appleton-Century-Crofts, p. 673.

Paradise, J. L. 1973. Pediatric and otologic aspects. Clinical research in cleft lip and cleft palate: The state of the art. Cleft Palate J., *10*:122.

Paradise, J. L., and Bluestone, C. D. 1969. Diagnosis and management of ear disease in cleft palate infants. Trans. Am. Acad. Ophthalmol. Otolaryngol., *73*:709.

Paradise, J. L., and Bluestone, C. D. 1971. More on the universal occurrence of otitis media in infants with cleft palate, and a preliminary evaluation of its treatment. Presented at the 29th Annual Meeting of the American Cleft Palate Association, Pittsburgh, PA, April 23, 1971.

Paradise, J. L., and McWilliams, B. J. 1974. Simplified feeder for infants with cleft palate. Pediatrics, *53*:566.

Perlstein, M. A. 1950. Medical aspects of cerebral palsy, incidence, etiology, pathogenesis. Am. J. Occup. Ther., *4*:47.

Randall, P. 1973. Surgical aspects. *In* Clinical Research in Cleft Lip and Cleft Palate: The State of the Art. Cleft Palate J., *10*:130.

Safra, M. J., and Oakley, G. P. 1976. Valium: An oral cleft teratogen? Cleft Palate J., *13*:198.

Semans, S. 1958. A neurophysiological approach to treatment of cerebral palsy. Introduction to the Bobath method. Phys. Ther. Rev., *38*:598.

Skolnick, M. L. 1977. A plea for an interdisciplinary approach to the radiological study of the velopharyngeal portal. Cleft Palate J., *14*:329–330.

South, J. 1972. Teratogenic effect of anticonvulsants. Lancet, *2*:1154.

Spriestersbach, D. C., Dickson, D. R., Fraser, F. C., et al. 1973. Clinical research in cleft lip and cleft palate: The state of the art. Cleft Palate J., *10*:113.

Stool, S. E. 1971. Diagnosis and treatment of ear disease in cleft palate children. *In* Grabb, W. C., Rosenstein, S. W., and Bzoch, K. R. (eds.) Cleft Lip and Palate. Boston, Little, Brown and Co., p. 868.

Stool, S. E., and Randall, P. 1967. Unexpected ear disease in infants with cleft palate. Cleft Palate J., *4*:99.

Tisza, V., and Gumpertz, E. 1962. The parents' reaction to the birth and early care of children with cleft palate. Pediatrics, *30*:86.

Veau, V. 1971. Division palatine. Paris, Masson, 1931. *In* Berlin, A. Classification of cleft lip and palate. *In* Grabb, W. C., Rosenstein, S. W., and Bzoch, K. R. (eds.). Cleft Lip and Palate. Boston, Little, Brown and Co., p. 66.

Westlake, H., and Rutherford, D. 1961. Speech Therapy for the Cerebral Palsied. Chicago, National Society for Crippled Children and Adults.

Chapter 87

VELOPHARYNGEAL INSUFFICIENCY

Robin Cotton, M.D.

Nizar S. Nuwayhid, M.D.

This chapter is designed to orient the otolaryngologist, pediatrician, and primary physician to the problems of diagnosing and managing velopharyngeal insufficiency (VPI). These clinicians will see VPI in their practices from time to time and must be able to distinguish this from other speech disorders. The otolaryngologist must develop an educated ear to detect VPI and should regard himself or herself as part of a team in the evaluation of the child's problem so that each child may be managed optimally.

VPI is the inability of the velopharyngeal (VP) sphincter to function effectively during connected speech. This results in varying degrees of hypernasality and, in more severe cases, nasal escape. Hypernasality is the conspicuous amount of perceived nasal cavity resonance that results when acoustic coupling of the nasopharynx and oropharynx, through an incompetent VP sphincter, occurs for sounds other than *m, n,* and *ng*. Nasal escape is the audible passage of air through an incompetent sphincter, producing an aperiodic noise that is perceived by the listener as a consonant distortion. With a competent sphincter there is an air pressure build-up in the oropharynx and oral cavity for the production of certain consonants; with an incompetent sphincter, air is not impounded but escapes via the open VP port into the nose.

ANATOMY

The normal palate has five muscles (Fig. 87–1): the levator and tensor veli palatini,

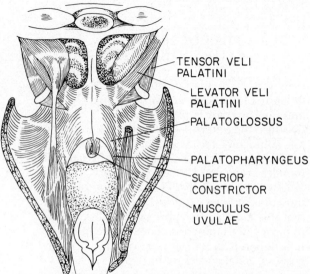

TENSOR VELI PALATINI

LEVATOR VELI PALATINI

PALATOGLOSSUS

PALATOPHARYNGEUS

SUPERIOR CONSTRICTOR

MUSCULUS UVULAE

Figure 83–1   Anatomy of palate and VP area as seen from behind.

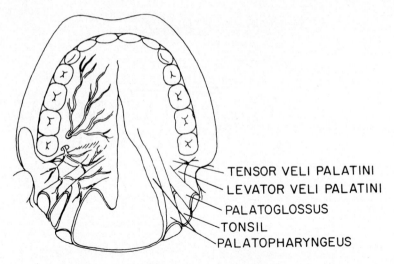

TENSOR VELI PALATINI

LEVATOR VELI PALATINI

PALATOGLOSSUS

TONSIL

PALATOPHARYNGEUS

Figure 87–2 Normal palate muscles and vessels are shown on the left of the diagram. On the right, the cleft anatomy is depicted, showing abnormal muscle insertion reaching the anterior limit of the cleft.

palatoglossus, palatopharyngeus, and musculus uvulae. Dickson (1975) has published an excellent account of the anatomy of the normal VP mechanism, and Kriens (1975) has published a similarly excellent study of the anatomy of the VP area in cleft palate patients.

All these muscles arise from fixed points, either from the base of the skull or from the pharynx, and insert into either the median raphe of the soft palate to form a sling or into the anterior aponeurosis of the soft palate.

In cases of cleft palate or submucous clefts, these muscles, especially the levators, arise from the same point but insert onto the posterior edge of the palatine bone and into the hard palate cleft instead of forming a sling in the soft palate (Fig. 87–2). Muscle fibers will insert as far as the most anterior portion of the cleft allows.

PHYSIOLOGY AND PATHOPHYSIOLOGY

At rest the uvula lies on or just above the dorsum of the tongue. During speech, the anterior two thirds of the palate elevates to decrease the anteroposterior diameter of the VP sphincter, creating a levator eminence due to the bunching of active levator palatini muscles (Fig. 87–3). Azzam and Kuehn (1977) have studied the morphology of the musculus uvulae, and their study suggests that this muscle also contributes substantially to the levator eminence. The degree of elevation depends upon the type of speech (nonnasal vs. nasal speech). Short palates, however, may show excellent elevation without producing VP closure.

In normal children, the Passavant ridge probably plays a relatively unimportant role in VP closure. Synchronous with the palatal elevation, there is a medial movement of the lateral pharyngeal wall to create a tight VP closure (Fig. 87–4). This constrictive action of the portal is probably mediated by upper fibers of the superior constrictor muscle, although levator muscle action may also be important. It has been speculated that both velar and lateral pharyngeal motion during closure for speech could be a function solely of the levator veli palatini (Bosma, 1953; Dickson and Dickson, 1972; Ruding, 1964).

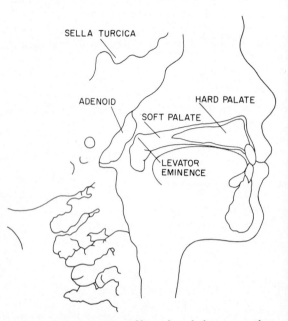

SELLA TURCICA

ADENOID

HARD PALATE

SOFT PALATE

LEVATOR EMINENCE

Figure 87–3 Tracing of lateral cephalometric radiograph with the palate in midposition between quiet breathing and VP closure to show important structures.

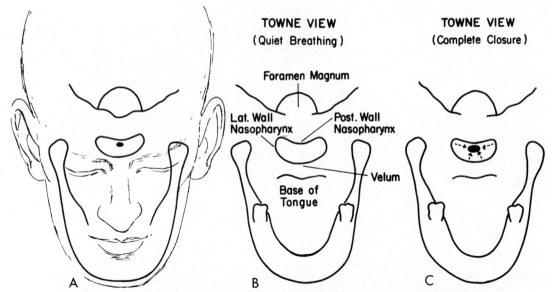

Figure 87–4 *A*, VP sphincter as seen in the Towne projection, looking "straight down the barrel," i.e., at right angles to plane of VP closure. *B*, Landmarks of VP sphincter in quiet breathing. *C*, In complete closure, note importance of soft palate and lateral pharyngeal walls, with minimal movement of posterior pharyngeal wall. (From Cotton, R. T. 1977. Lateral defects in VPI. Arch. Otolaryngol., *103*:90.)

Thus, closure of the VP port during phonation is the result of two types of motion: a midsagittal VP contact and medial motion of localized regions of both lateral pharyngeal walls against the palate, thus closing the lateral aspects of the VP port. Both motions are synchronous, and, thus, the port acts as a sphincter (Fig. 87–4*C*). The important role of lateral pharyngeal wall movement has been emphasized by several authors (Astley, 1958; Skolnick, 1969; Kelsey et al., 1972; Cotton and Quattromani, 1977).

Hynes (1967) has emphasized the importance of the lateral pharyngeal recesses. The width of the oropharynx is greater than it appears on simple inspection of the posterior pharyngeal wall through the mouth. The pharynx extends laterally as a recess on either side behind the posterior tonsillar pillar for a variable distance from patient to patient. These recesses, communicating below via the hypopharynx with the larynx and above via the fossa of Rosenmüller with the nasal cavity, are obliterated during speech in a normal child by this lateral pharyngeal wall movement. Following obliteration, all the air in the larynx ascends via the central portion of the oropharynx and is thus directed into the region controlled by the soft palate. It is important to recognize that the level of maximal lateral pharyngeal wall movement is approximately at the level of the hard palate (Fig. 87–5), varying slightly from individual

to individual. The level of this lateral pharyngeal wall movement is an important factor in planning surgical remediation.

In cases of "failed cleft palate" speech, the inadequacy of the VP mechanism may be due to deficiency in either or both of the parameters of VP motion described before. First, midsaggital closure may be deficient. In children with cleft and submucous cleft palates, the levator muscles are attached to the posterior palatine bone, and the sling is absent. Since the points of origin and insertion of the levator muscles are fixed, there is a resultant decrease in the mobility of the soft palate. After surgical repair, the soft palate may still be short, and the levator eminence is often too anterior, thus creating a defect in anteroposterior closure (Fig. 87–6). During nonnasal speech, there is limited elevation of the soft palate with no adequate levator eminence and a resultant VPI. In some children with repaired clefts, the Passavant ridge may contribute to adequate VP closure. Skolnick and colleagues (1975), using multiview fluoroscopy, reported that 33 per cent of 30 children with repaired palatal clefts and normal speech had a Passavant ridge during speech and that this ridge was used in all cases as a point of closure, in addition to the adenoid tissue.

Secondly, poor lateral pharyngeal wall movement also contributes in some cases to VPI. In cleft palate patients, the pharynx is

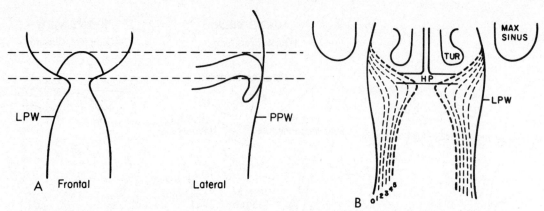

Figure 87–5 *A*, Schematic of VP closure in frontal and lateral projections. Notice the level of lateral pharyngeal wall (LPW) closure at approximately the level of the hard palate and the firm contact of the soft palate against the posterior pharyngeal wall (PPW). *B*, Frontal view schematic to show varying degrees of lateral pharyngeal wall (LPW) movement rated from 0 (no LPW movement) to 5 (normal LPW movement). Hard palate (HP), inferior turbinate (TUR), maxillary sinus (MAX SINUS). (After Kelsey, C. A., et al. 1972. Lateral pharyngeal wall motion as predictor of surgical success in velopharyngeal insufficiency. N. Engl. J. Med., 287:64. From Cotton, R. T. 1977. Lateral defects in VPI. Arch. Otolaryngol., 103:90.)

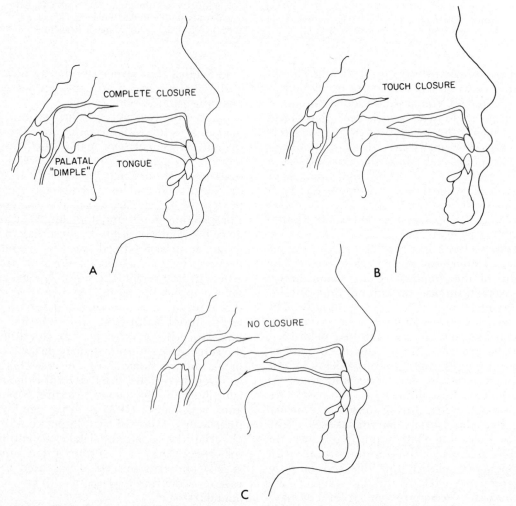

Figure 87–6 Tracings of lateral cephalometric radiographs. *A*, complete VP closure. *B*, touch VP closure. *C*, no VP closure. Palatal dimple is the point on the oral aspect of the soft palate corresponding to the levator eminence on nasal surface, both caused by contraction of levator palatini muscle.

not always normal. The oropharyngeal width is often greater than normal, giving the appearance of a "megapharynx." The anatomic basis for this is the widening of the bony cranial base documented in cleft palate patients. Subtelny's (1955) data indicate a greater than normal interhamular width in cleft palate patients. During speech the lateral pharyngeal movement may be poor to absent, so that large lateral pharyngeal recesses cannot be obliterated during speech. Air can thus bypass the palatopharyngeal region and escape via the nose even if the palatopharyngeal portion of the mechanism is adequate.

NORMAL SPEECH AND SPEECH DEFECTS IN VPI

Normal speech sounds are either voiced (vocal cords vibrate during phonation) or voiceless (no vocal cord vibration). All vowels are voiced, while consonants may be voiced or voiceless: /b/ and /p/ are produced in the same manner, with the exception that /b/ is voiced and /p/ is voiceless. The voiceless consonants, in the case of VPI, are more nasally distorted than the voiced consonants, as described by Arkebauer and colleagues (1967).

There are four consonant classifications. First, the glides, which are composed of the /w/, /y/, /r/, and the lateral consonant /l/ sounds, are voiced and produced with minimal oral obstruction of the airstream. In VPI, their production would be perceived as hypernasal, of a degree of hypernasality similar to that present during vowel production.

Secondly, the plosives (Fig. 87–7A) are either voiced or voiceless and are produced by the complete blockage of the airstream. Air pressure builds up behind two contracting articulators, and as the air is released, an explosive sound results. These sounds are the /p/, /b/, /t/, /d/, /k/, and /g/ consonants; their production requires a moderate degree of VP

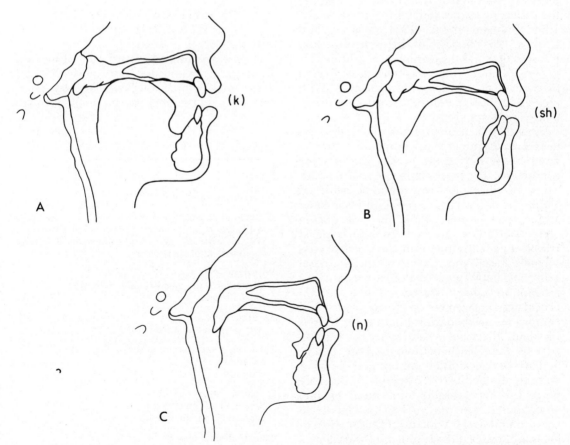

Figure 87–7 *A*, Tracings of lateral cephalometric radiographs of normal child showing plosive consonant with good VP closure and complete blockage of air stream. *B*, Fricative consonant with tight VP closure and constricted oral opening. *C*, Nasal consonants with open VP port.

closure, as compared to the fricatives (Arkebauer et al., 1967).

Thirdly, fricatives (Fig. 87–7B) are also either voiced or voiceless and are produced by the slow, forceful release of air through a constricted oral opening. These require tight VP closure owing to the constriction of the airstream for a longer time. The fricatives are the /f/, /v/, /th/, /s/, /z/, and /sh/ sounds. The affricates, /ch/ and /j/, are plosive-fricative combinations.

Fourthly, nasals (Fig. 87–7C) are all voiced. They are composed of the /m/, /n/, and /ng/ sounds. The pharyngeal wall does not contract, and the soft palate does not fully extend to touch the posterior pharyngeal wall during their production, so that the VP sphincter remains open.

The primary speech defects of VPI are hypernasality and nasal escape. Hypernasality, the result of excessive nasal resonance during phonation, may be evident only during the production of vowels and glides. Fricatives require tighter VP closure than do plosives. Although it is difficult to compare the results of studies (Subtelny and Subtelny, 1959; Subtelny et al., 1961; Warren and DuBois, 1964) because of differences in subject selection and measurement methods, it is generally agreed that fricatives are affected by a smaller nasal leak than plosives. With increasing incompetence, distortion becomes increasingly apparent.

Secondary articulatory disorders develop in the child's attempt to compensate for the nasal escape during the production of some consonants. The necessary air pressure build-up to produce plosives cannot be achieved within the oral cavity, so the sound is created at the level of the larynx, thus producing glottal stops. For similar reasons pharyngeal fricatives are substituted for the fricative consonants. Facial and, more specifically, nasal grimacing habits may develop as yet a further attempt to achieve closure. These deviant articulatory placement patterns and facial contortions are behaviors that create serious problems that can be addressed at least in part by the speech pathologist both before and after surgical intervention. Harshness of voice occurs because of attempts to decrease perceived hypernasality and nasal escape, and about 15 per cent of VPI patients have vocal nodules. McWilliams (1966), McWilliams and colleagues (1969), and McWilliams and others (1973) have written extensively on this subject.

Cleft palate children may have factors other than VPI contributing to their speech and language problems. Hearing loss, especially during the early years of life, when the child is at the stage of listening and familiarizing himself or herself with the language spoken, affects speech and language development. Unfortunately, cleft palate children have a high incidence of middle ear effusion, and if this is not attended to early, it will contribute to the development of speech problems. Stool and Randall (1967) have emphasized that the onset of middle ear effusion is often in infancy. Major dental problems secondary to cleft alveolus may interfere with normal movement of the tongue and lip and may secondarily affect speech.

Emotional and behavioral problems secondary to problems arising from the cleft may cause delay of receptive speech. Often parents or siblings may have cleft problems with poor speech, which may be mimicked by the patient.

CLASSIFICATION OF THE ETIOLOGY OF VPI

There are several causes for VPI (Table 87–1), and in any one case more than one factor may be operant. Following cleft palate repair, hypernasality is the most frequent

Table 87–1   CLASSIFICATION OF VPI

Cleft palate
   primary
   postsurgical repair

Congenital palatal incompetence
   with stigmata, e.g., submucous cleft palate
   without stigmata, e.g., occult submucous cleft palate
     or congenital short palate

Postsurgical
   adenoidectomy, tonsillectomy, or both
   palatal resection

Post-traumatic
   with severe loss of palatal tissue

Palatopharyngeal neuromuscular dysfunction
   congenital
   acquired

Congenital large pharynx
   base of skull abnormality
   cervical spine abnormality

Combination of above factors

Miscellaneous, e.g., posterior tonsillar pillar webbing

residual problem. Data from 46 surgical papers on secondary palatal surgery reviewed by Yules and colleagues (1971) showed that hypernasality was a chief complaint in 38 per cent of patients.

Classic submucous cleft palate is identified by the triad of bifid uvula, a midline furrow along the length of the soft palate due to abnormal levator muscle insertion, and a notch in the posterior margin of the hard palate. In a prospective study of 10,836 children, Weatherley-White and colleagues (1972) found an incidence of one submucous cleft palate per 1200 children. In this condition defective fusion of the palatal structure occurs without overt cleft formation, produc-

ing a submucous cleft of the palate. This is a less severe expression of the clefting process, which may be regarded as a continuum from overt cleft lip and palate to occult submucous cleft palate. In submucous cleft palate there is a bony and muscular deficiency in the midline, often, but by no means always, resulting in a functionally defective soft palate. Certainly in this condition, where VP competence may be barely adequate, adenoidectomy is strongly contraindicated because of the likelihood of creating a VPI.

Occult submucous cleft palate (Fig. 87–8) is another, presumably related, entity in which there appears to be a functional deficiency without any obvious morphologic change

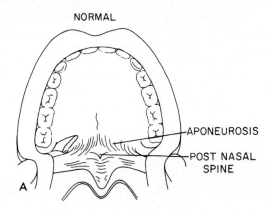

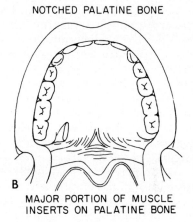

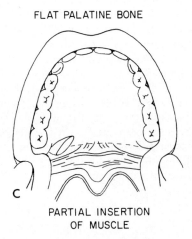

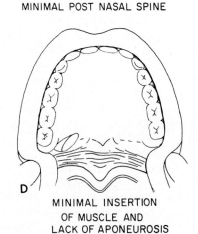

Figure 87–8 Illustration of the continuum of submucous cleft palate to congenital short palate. *A*, Normal hard and soft palate anatomy with palpable posterior nasal spine, aponeurosis, and intact levator sling. *B*, Absent posterior nasal spine with a notched palatine bone with major portion of muscle inserting onto posterior border of palatine bone. Note that the uvula may or may not be cleft. *C*, Absent posterior nasal spine creating a flat posterior border of palatine bone, with only partial insertion of muscle onto posterior border of palatine bone. *D*, Posterior nasal spine present with lack of aponeurosis but minimal insertion of muscle onto posterior border of palatine bone creating an anteriorly positioned levator sling.

(congenital palatal incompetence). Kaplan (1975a) described this entity as a continuum of anatomic abnormalities from the obvious submucous cleft palate (Fig. 87–8B) through abnormal levator muscle insertion onto the hard palate (without visible stigmata) as shown in Figure 87–8C, to the situation in which a full levator sling is present but without an aponeurosis (Fig. 87–8D), creating the anatomic basis for a short soft palate, also called by some authors congenital palatal incompetence.

Pruzansky and colleagues (1977) have classified congenital palatal incompetence into two types: in type I, patients show one or more visible stigmata associated with submucous cleft palate; in type II, patients have VPI in the absence of such stigmata. The same authors stress, however, that the final classification of these disorders must await the outcome of further studies. It is interesting to speculate that whether or not such patients demonstrate competency or incompetency of the VP mechanism may be to some degree dependent on the amount of adenoid tissue present. Such patients, with a marginal VP mechanism and little or no intraoral stigmata of submucous cleft palate, may become frankly incompetent after adenoidectomy.

Kaplan (1975a) has emphasized the characteristic facial features seen in patients with classic submucous cleft, occult submucous cleft, and in some patients with clefts of the secondary palate. These features should alert the otolaryngologist to the diagnosis of occult submucous cleft palate. The features are related to mesodermal deficiencies of the maxillary process of the first branchial arch, just as the muscle of the soft palate has the same embryologic derivation. These deformities are not specific to submucous cleft but are characteristic of maxillary hypoplasia and, as such, may be seen in other cranial or branchial arch syndromes.

The features to look for include maxillary hypoplasia; lip contour deformity at the vermilion border ("gull wing"); drooping of the oral commissure; hypoanimation of the facial muscles, creating a dull expression; and alveolar arch deformities. Fara and Weatherley-White (1977) also emphasize the unique physiognomy of these patients: a wide root of the nose, narrow palpebral fissures, narrow external auditory canals and nasal airways, and a vertically shortened upper lip with a poorly defined philtrum.

Unfortunately, some patients develop persistent hypernasality after adenoidectomy (Gibb, 1958). Certainly, many of these cases occur in that group of patients with occult submucous cleft palate who have no visible stigmata. Mason (1973) has stressed the value of a good preoperative intraoral examination, which looks for anomalies such as cleft uvula, absent posterior nasal spine, notching of the palatine bone, short palate, and abnormal levator muscle insertion with midline translucency. In the presence of all or one of these signs, the physician should be cautioned against performing adenoidectomy and should evaluate the VP closure with fluorography with the patient's head in the normal position and hyperextended, which may reveal borderline VPI (McWilliams et al., 1968). The physician should consider requesting a speech assessment and obtaining cephalometric radiographs in such cases prior to deciding to perform an adenoidectomy.

VPI may occur following severe palatal trauma or resection, for instance, after removal of a rhabdomyosarcoma of the palate.

Paresis of the soft palate due to neurologic defects, both congenital and acquired, may produce VPI either temporarily or permanently.

Calnan (1971) described VPI in patients with congenitally large pharynges, in whom clinical and cephalometric techniques showed the pharynx to be deeper and wider than usual, often with a small volume of adenoid tissue, but with a soft palate of normal length and mobility. Some cases may be secondary to cervical spine or skull base abnormalities.

Posterior tonsillar pillar webbing and palatopharyngeus muscle displacement have recently been described. Warren and others (1978) reported three cases of congenital palatal incompetence in the absence of the usual stigmata associated with hypernasality. In two cases, mucosal webbing of the posterior tonsillar pillars was noted, and in one case the palatopharyngeus muscle was displaced.

EVALUATION

A careful history is taken for every child with VPI, including prenatal, perinatal, and family histories, other congenital anomalies, neurologic problems, and previous operations (e.g., cleft palate repair, adenoidectomy, or palate reconstruction).

A complete ear, nose, and throat examination should be performed. It is known that a very high percentage of children with cleft palate or submucous cleft palate have middle ear effusions. A persistent middle ear effusion in an infant should raise the possibility of an overt or occult submucous cleft.

Occlusion should be inspected since it is known that occlusive abnormalities can interfere with lip and tongue movements during speech and secondary speech defects will arise. The condition of the alveolus, whether intact or clefted, is also important for the same reasons.

When examining the hard and soft palate and pharynx, the examiner should constantly be on the alert for signs of overt or occult submucous cleft palate. The hard palate should be examined for open cleft, palpable bony submucous cleft, fistulae, a posterior notch, absence of a posterior nasal spine, and also for shape, whether contracted or high arched.

The soft palate should be examined for open clefts, congenital short palate, overt submucous cleft, bifid uvula, and mobility of the soft palate. The bifid uvula may very easily be overlooked unless it is delicately touched with the tongue blade in an effort to tease the two halves apart.

The pharynx should be evaluated for depth and mobility of the lateral pharyngeal walls since these contribute to VP closure. Mobility of the lateral pharyngeal walls during speech can be assessed only by radiographic studies or nasal endoscopy, however. Lateral pharyngeal wall closure on gagging or swallowing is a different neurologic mechanism than closure for speech.

Fox and Johns (1970) have described a simple clinical test to predict adequacy of the valving mechanism that may be used as a guide for referral of patients for complete evaluation of the VP sphincter. Although the educated ear is an excellent tool in the diagnosis of VPI, such cases should be evaluated in the following manner.

A speech diagnostic evaluation will not only assess the degree of perceived hypernasality, nasal escape, consonant distortion, and other secondary defects but will also evaluate the patient's linguistic skills. Younger children with cleft palate are generally delayed in their language development (Spriestersbach et al., 1958; Morris, 1962; Smith and McWilliams, 1968). At the time of the diagnostic session, a recording should be obtained for future evaluation of the efficacy of treatment, whether it be speech therapy or surgical correction.

It is important to obtain a radiograph of the cervical spine to detect possible spine anomalies. Since surgical repair of VPI is in the hyperextended position, it is reassuring to the surgeon to know that the cervical spine is normal.

Lateral radiographs at rest and with phonation are of limited value since they are a two-dimensional representation of a three-dimensional sphincter mechanism. If done with standard cephalometric techniques, a lateral view can give information on the length of the hard and soft palate and the depth of the pharynx, and sequential films will give information on structural growth. Similarly, the effective soft palatal length may be measured on phonation, and the amount of adenoid tissue may be verified. Although Ricketts (1954) and Owsley and colleagues (1967) reported on these measurements, there is discrepancy between the two reports. Cephalometric radiographs show the relation of the soft palate to the posterior pharyngeal wall and give some indication of the approximation of the soft palate to that structure. They yield no information concerning lateral pharyngeal wall movement or mobility of the soft palate, however. For such information, multiview fluoroscopy is necessary.

Fluoroscopy is an accurate and physiologic study of the movement of the soft palate and lateral pharyngeal walls during speech. As is emphasized in the section on physiology, VP closure is basically a sphincteric mechanism with simultaneous movements in three planes. The portal can be shown only by a multiview fluoroscopic procedure. A minimum of three fluoroscopic views is recommended, namely, lateral, frontal, and basal (Skolnick, 1969 and 1970), or Towne views may be used (Quattromani et al., 1977). These examinations are better performed with a transnasal injection of a very thin layer of contrast medium sniffed or placed on the nasal surface of the palate through a flexible pediatric feeding tube. This better defines the margins of the soft palate and posterior and lateral pharyngeal walls.

The lateral view, projecting the sagittal plane, shows palatal elevation and posterior elongation, as well as anterior movement of the posterior pharyngeal wall. Palatal mobility, a most important parameter of palatal function, is assessed well in this view. If a pharyngeal flap is present, then its position of attachment to the palate and pharyngeal wall is outlined.

The frontal view, projecting the coronal plane, shows medial movement of the lateral pharyngeal wall; both the degree and the vertical extent of the movement are shown as well as its relation to the level of the hard palate (Fig. 87–5B). Kelsey and colleagues (1972) have suggested a 0 to 5 scale for rating this movement. If a pharyngeal flap is present, then its width and relation to the medial excursion of the lateral pharyngeal walls is outlined.

The base view, projecting the transverse plane, demonstrates an *en face* view of the VP portal, that is, a view "looking down the barrel." Simultaneous movements of palate and pharyngeal walls are demonstrated. If a flap is present, the width of it is shown as well as the adequacy of closure of the lateral portals by medial movement of the lateral pharyngeal walls.

Occasionally the base view cannot be done because the patient's neck is too short or because the plane of the portal cannot be brought to the horizontal position, as occurs when there is a large adenoid pad. Under these circumstances supine fluorography in the Towne projection may be valuable (Quattromani et al., 1977).

The aim of the study is to evaluate the dynamics of VP closure during continuous speech. Hence, simultaneous motion recordings of the radiographic image and the patient's speech are necessary, either with cinefluorography or videofluorography. The latter technique is preferred because the advantages of greater sensitivity of the television recording system (with reduction in total radiation dosage) together with its easier recording techniques outweigh the disadvantage of some decrease in clarity of the picture when compared with cinefluorography.

Nasal endoscopy in the sitting position is a recent valuable adjunct to the evaluation of the VP area. It is quick and easy to perform and is tolerated by most children four years of age and over. In the initial evaluation this examination should be regarded as complementary to videofluoroscopic studies rather than as an alternative, since the information obtained from endoscopy lacks the vertical depth of lateral pharyngeal wall closure obtained on the frontal view of fluoroscopic studies (Skolnick, 1975). Since endoscopy requires no radiation exposure, however, it is an excellent means of following patients dur-

ing speech therapy or after pharyngeal flap surgery.

There are several methods of endoscopy presently available. The oral panendoscope of Taub (1966) shows an *en face* view of the velopharyngeal portal from below, but the bulkiness of the instrument when placed in the oral cavity precludes examination during connected speech. The same objection may be raised for the Berci-Ward indirect scope (Zwitman et al., 1976). Piggott (1969) and Piggott and others (1969) introduced the use of the 3.4 mm Storz fiberoptic rigid telescope with a 70 degree angle of view, while more recently fiberoptic nasal endoscopes have been developed and their uses have been described (Matsuya et al., 1974; Silberman et al., 1976; Croft et al., 1978). The flexible Machida nasopharyngoscope has an outside diameter of 3.9 mm and has the advantage over the rigid scope that the distal tip can be rotated from forward viewing to a 90 degree downward view. Since the plane of the *en face* view of the VP portal varies from patient to patient, the flexible scope does allow a look straight down the barrel in all patients.

With the use of either of these instruments, the defective VP mechanism may be viewed directly during connected speech with little or no interference with normal physiology. Defective palatal movement (Fig. 87–9A) or defects in movement of one or both lateral walls (Fig. 87–9), or a combination of problems may readily be assessed. In particular, careful attention should be given to the lateral pharyngeal recesses on each side to see whether or not they are both fully obliterated during speech.

During phonation it is possible to measure the size of the gap in the VP sphincter by inserting catheters of known diameter into the area of closure of the VP sphincter via the opposite nasal cavity, thus deriving the area of the defect.

The use of these transnasal instruments has strongly suggested the functional importance of the musculus uvulae in normal VP valving by producing a large ridge occupying the central one third of the soft palate rising to a height almost equal to its width. A recent study on the morphology of the musculus uvulae (Azzam and Kuehn, 1977) shows it to be a paired muscle running dorsal to the levator sling, contributing substantially to the levator eminence and upon contraction adding bulk to the nasal surface of the palate. Absence of this ridge when viewed endoscop-

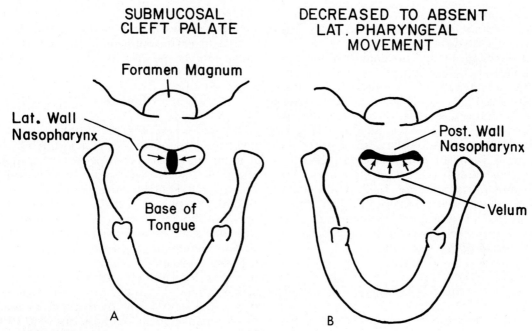

SUBMUCOSAL
CLEFT PALATE

DECREASED TO ABSENT
LAT. PHARYNGEAL
MOVEMENT

Foramen Magnum

Lat. Wall
Nasopharynx

Base of
Tongue

A

Post. Wall
Nasopharynx

Velum

B

Figure 87–9 Diagram emphasizing the defects in different parameters of VP function as seen by fluoroscopy or nasal endoscopy. *A,* Decreased palate movement with adequate lateral pharyngeal wall motion. *B,* Defect in lateral pharyngeal wall movement with adequate palate motion. Often the two defects are combined along a continuum.

ically is thought to contribute to VPI in both repaired cleft patients (Piggott et al., 1969) and in some cases of occult submucous cleft palate (Croft et al., 1978).

Because of the high incidence of middle ear problems in cases of cleft palate and submucous cleft, audiometry is very important in the evaluation of these patients, especially in infants and small children. This should be supplemented routinely with a tympanogram to measure the middle ear pressures and the compliance of the tympanic membrane.

Clinical photographs are important for the record and to detect the abnormal facial features mentioned in the previous section.

Psychologic, neurologic, and intelligence assessments may be necessary. A child of limited intelligence is likely to have limited speech ability, and it may be particularly difficult for such children to compensate for an anatomic defect. Many authors (Hardy et al., 1961; Hardy et al., 1969; Moll et al., 1963; Schulz et al., 1973) feel that the results of surgical treatment of VPI in children with neurologic, emotional, or mental disorders are disappointing, and many surgeons are reluctant to operate on children with multiple handicaps because of the higher risks (Schulz et al., 1973). Some authors (Hardy et al.,

1969; Gonzalez and Aronson, 1970) have reported favorable results with a palatal lift prosthesis for the management of mild to moderate neurologic VPI. Heller and colleagues (1974) are more optimistic, however, and conclude that the pharyngeal flap is an effective procedure in reducing hypernasality in patients with VPI, even if the problem is coupled with mental or neuropsychiatric handicaps. Certainly caution should be exercised before advising surgery in this group of patients. If VPI is clearly demonstrable and there is adequate language development, then factors such as parental and patient cooperation, psychologic and social readiness for speech improvement, degree of intellectual impairment, and the extent of neurologic impairment affecting other oral or respiratory mechanisms are important factors in selecting patients for pharyngeal flap procedures.

TREATMENT

There is no established method for selecting an individual patient with VPI for a given mode of therapy or a given operation. The methods available are speech therapy, surgical repair, retropharyngeal implants, and speech appliances (obturators). A bewildering multitude of surgical procedures has been advocated for the management of VPI, and this suggests that no single method has demonstrated clear superiority. Lack of objective preoperative and postoperative data (Schwartz, 1975) is one factor, and the necessity for future collection of objective data is demonstrated by the fact that the speech failure rate of secondary procedures is variously reported to be between 0 and 34 per cent (Longacre and DeStefano, 1957; Williams and Woolhouse, 1962; Smith et al., 1963; Skoog, 1965; Edgerton, 1965; Bernstein, 1967). Considering the many causes of VPI, it is unlikely that one single procedure will correct all types of VPI.

Speech Therapy

Speech therapy is important in cases where VP escape is minimal or where the patient can be consistently stimulated to close. If, during the diagnostic speech evaluation, the child can be stimulated sufficiently to decrease appreciably the perceived hypernasality, then a period of trial therapy should be started. Even prior to surgery, speech therapy may be able to correct faulty articulatory placement, thus increasing intelligibility and decreasing facial contortion behavior. Even if the period of trial therapy does not yield any appreciable amelioration of the child's speech skills, not all is lost. Often the parents, via the experience, become more accepting of the fact that a further surgical procedure is necessary to achieve more normal speech.

If a significant organic defect is found, its importance lies mainly in the postoperative period to correct previously developed secondary faulty speech patterns.

Obturators

Various types of dental appliances have been used for centuries as a means of obturating unoperated cleft palates. The appliance will consist of an oral segment and a pharyngeal segment connected by means of a palatal strap (Fig. 87–10). The oral segment is analogous to a routine removable denture. It provides fixation and stability of the prosthesis by adaptation to edentulous ridges, by clasping of available, stable teeth, or by both methods. Replacement of missing teeth may also be achieved with this prosthesis. Obturation is no longer a primary method of choice in the management of most cases of VPI. Under some circumstances, however, obturation is still very useful. Indications for obturation include: (1) medical contraindications to surgery, (2) failed surgery, leaving either a badly scarred palate or fistulas in the hard and soft palates with insufficient tissue for surgical repair, (3) surgery refused by the patient, (4) an unoperated cleft in adults, and (5) postsurgical resections.

For control of VPI, an extension is placed on the oral segment of the prosthesis into the area of VPI. A moldable material is built up progressively in the area of greatest muscular activity, most effective just superior to the Passavant ridge. When the appliance is optimally contoured, the patient will be able to

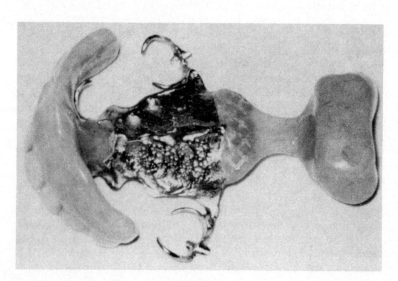

Figure 87–10 Maxillary cleft palate obturator: anterior occlusion, aesthetics, and lip support are restored by acrylic section to the left; metal framework achieves stability and fixation to the remaining dentition; acrylic strap extends across short, immobile soft palate to support the pharyngeal obturator section at the right. (Courtesy of Leroy K. Nakayama.)

effect closure with speech and swallowing but will breathe freely with the muscles at rest. In those patients experiencing discomfort or gagging, the pharyngeal section is initially made small and unobtrusive, then increased in stages to an effective size and contour.

Obturation of a VP defect by prosthetic means will not produce an immediate restoration of normal speech, unless the defect is one that has been surgically acquired, such as by palatal resection for malignancy. The child will need time and practice to learn to speak with the prosthesis and will benefit from a course of speech therapy during this adaptive phase. Older patients who have developed compensatory speech habits without obturation may have greater difficulty in developing normal speech with an obturator when compared to younger patients who develop their speech habits with an obturator in place.

Surgical

Surgical procedures may be classified into four categories: (1) secondary pushback palatoplasty, (2) sphincter pharyngoplasty, (3) posterior pharyngeal wall augmentation, and (4) palatopharyngoplasty (pharyngeal flap).

Secondary Pushback Palatoplasty

These procedures, as described by many authors, including Dorrance (1930) and Wardill (1937), are designed to lengthen the soft palate with or without levator muscle reconstruction by intravelar veloplasty (Kriens, 1970) and have been used as primary procedures for initial palate repair or as secondary procedures for management of VPI. The success or failure of these operations will depend on the size and shape of the VP port preoperatively and on whether or not the pushback effect is maintained. Suitable cases might include those with a short palate with adequate lateral pharyngeal wall movement and a relatively small defect. Local tissue should be used to maintain the pushback; the island flap of Millard (1962, 1963, 1966), "sandwich flap" of Moore and Chong (1967) (Fig. 87–11), and submucosal cheek flaps as described by Ganguli (1971) and Kaplan (1975b) are examples of such techniques. The principle behind the pushback is outlined in Figure 87–12. To date they have not demonstrated their superiority over the pharyngeal flap operation with objective preop-

erative and postoperative measurements, and as scarring occurs the initial effect of the pushback is not always maintained.

Sphincter Pharyngoplasty

Sphincter pharyngoplasty is not widely practiced in the United States, where the superiorly based pharyngeal flap, in one guise or another, is still the cornerstone of surgical management of VPI. It is practiced in Europe and elsewhere, however. Skolnick's (1969) work with videofluoroscopy and Piggott's (1969) work with nasal endoscopy clearly show the sphincteric nature of VP closure. The classic pharyngeal flap operation is not one that attempts to achieve this normal arrangement. Although it works in many patients, most reports of larger series suggest failure to achieve the desired goal in about 20 per cent of cases. Hyponasality and disturbed nasal drainage, which may occur after conventional pharyngoplasty, are additional reasons for considering the sphincter pharyngoplasty approach.

Attempts to narrow the pharynx began with the work of Passavant in the mid-19th century. The two-flap pharyngoplasty of Hynes (1950, 1954, 1967) (Fig. 87–13) is well-known and popular in Europe. In this method the salpingopharyngeal muscles are transferred from lateral insertions to a medial location on the posterior pharyngeal wall, thus providing a ridge on the posterior pharyngeal wall. This reduces both the anteroposterior and transverse dimensions of the velopharyngeal sphincter. Hynes (1954) reported on 30 patients and reported on their long-term follow-up in 1967.

Moore (1960) described a modification of this procedure in which two laterally based flaps are inserted into the nasal aspect of the palate. Orticochea (1968, 1970) reported on 73 patients in whom two lateral pharyngeal flaps containing the palatopharyngeus muscle were sutured into an inferiorly based pharyngeal flap. He claims that this method produces a dynamic sphincter and has published electromyographic recordings (Orticochea, 1968) and photographs (Orticochea, 1970) in support of this contention. In most patients, complete closure of the sphincter occurred on enunciating such sounds as a-a-a.

Jackson and Silverton (1977) have reported excellent results with a modification of the Orticochea technique. Their basic change is

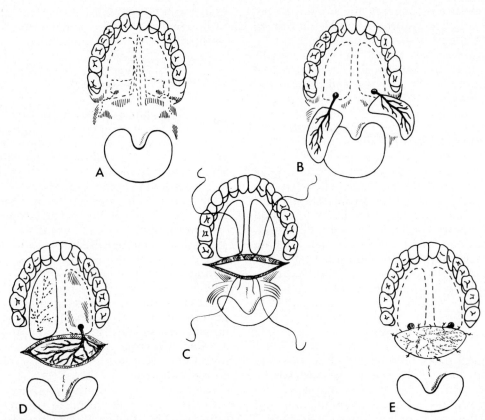

Figure 87–11 *A*, Basal view of palate and wide VP port with two hemipalatal flaps outlined. *B*, Two hemipalatal island flaps developed, each based on a greater palatine artery. *C*, Transverse through-and-through incision at junction of hard and soft palate; the posterior incision of the island flap is part of this incision. *D*, The first hemipalatal island flap, with mucosal surface placed towards the nasal side, is sewn into the defect. *E*, The second hemipalatal island flap is placed raw surface to raw surface, thus producing a sandwich flap mucosally lined on both the nasal and palatal surfaces. (After Moore, F. T., and Chong, J. K. 1967. The "sandwich" technique to lengthen the soft palate. Br. J. Oral Surg., 4:183.)

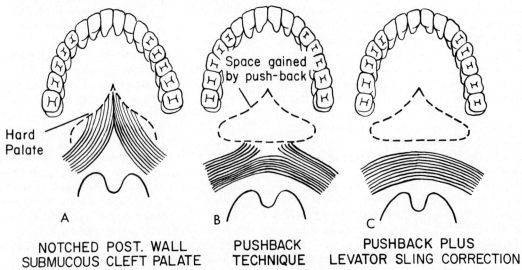

NOTCHED POST. WALL   PUSHBACK   PUSHBACK PLUS
SUBMUCOUS CLEFT PALATE   TECHNIQUE   LEVATOR SLING CORRECTION

Figure 87–12 Illustration of the principle of the palatal pushback procedure. *A*, Abnormal muscle insertion onto posterior border of palatine bone. *B*, Through-and-through incision at junction of hard and soft palate with dissection of muscle from abnormal insertion on posterior border of palatine bone. *C*, Reconstruction of muscle sling; space gained by pushback must be maintained (e.g., by sandwich flaps described by Moore, F. T., and Chong, J. K. 1967. The "sandwich" technique to lengthen the soft palate. Br. J. Oral Surg., 4:183).

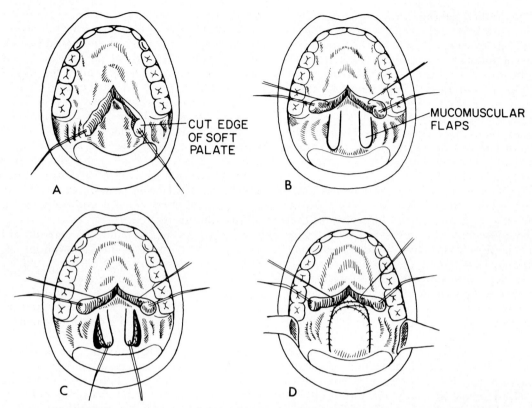

Figure 87–13 Hynes' pharyngoplasty by muscle transplantation. *A*, Soft palate divided in midline to within 5 mm of junction with hard palate. *B*, Incisions of mucomuscular flaps outlined. *C*, Two lateral pharyngeal flaps are raised. *D*, Transverse defect established on posterior pharyngeal wall, with secondary defects closed; flaps transposed to create a horizontal shelf above the region of Passavant's ridge.

to substitute a superiorly based midline pharyngeal flap for the inferiorly based flaps. Cotton and Quattromani (1977) suggested that sphincter pharyngoplasty be considered in those patients in whom poor lateral pharyngeal wall movement does not obliterate the lateral pharyngeal recesses during fluoroscopic or nasal endoscopic examination.

Posterior Pharyngeal Wall Augmentation

Many methods of augmenting the posterior pharyngeal wall using a wide variety of biologic or implant materials embedded in the posterior pharyngeal wall at the level of the second cervical vertebra have been described. Materials have included paraffin (Eckstein, 1904), fascia (Halle, 1925), fatty tissue (Gaza, 1926), autogenous cartilage (Hagerty and Hill, 1961), silastic (Blocksma, 1963), and polytetrafluorethylene (PTFE) paste* (Lewy et al., 1965; Ward et al., 1966,

1967; Bluestone et al., 1968a, 1968b; Ward, 1968; Blocksma, 1971; Sturim and Jacob, 1972; Smith and McCabe, 1977). It is conceivable that increasing the proximity of the newly projected posterior pharyngeal wall to an inert soft palate may stimulate the latter into activity. Hagerty and colleagues (1968) reported on the results of placing a cartilage implant in the posterior pharyngeal walls of 31 patients and noted that the majority had a substantial improvement in palatal lift after implantation. They termed this poor palatal movement in short palates "functional surrender."

Of the variety of materials used to the present, PTFE paste appears to be the most satisfactory in terms of tissue tolerance, degree of resorption, migration from site of placement, and degree of improvement in VP function. Authors reporting on the use of PTFE paste injection pharyngoplasty have reported such favorable results that it would appear it is a viable technique of reducing or eliminating VPI of varying etiologies in selected patients. Kuehn and VanDemark

---

*All reports have used Teflon® paste manufactured by Ethicon Company.

(1978) studied preoperative and postoperative speech and radiograph data on subjects who underwent PTFE paste injection pharyngoplasties. A continuous change in VP competency for speech was observed, resulting in a significant improvement three months or more postoperatively compared to the preoperative assessment. Although some improvement in VP closure was found on the basis of lateral view radiographs, the results were not as consistent as those involving speech ratings.

The technique may be used for primary treatment of VPI or as a secondary procedure following pharyngeal flap surgery that failed to achieve the desired speech result. Suitable cases may include children with congenital palatal incompetence (i.e., non-cleft cases), those with submucous cleft palate who have not had previous surgery, or those cases of cleft palate repair that have failed to achieve an adequate speech result. Careful selection of patients is important. There is general agreement in the literature upon patient selection. Children suitable for consideration for PTFE paste pharyngoplasty should demonstrate only marginal VPI as defined by Morris (1972, 1978), with an anteroposterior aperture of no more than 5 mm as shown on lateral fluorography. Adequate lateral pharyngeal wall movement should be present so that the movement of the walls will reach the pad of PTFE paste. Such patients often demonstrate VP competence during isolated tasks (both speech and nonspeech) but are unable to carry over this competence into connected speech. This phenomenon of marginal VPI is familiar to cleft palate specialists and is described in detail by Morris (1972, 1978). Patients with severe scarring and immobilization or paralysis of the palate are poor candidates for treatment by this method.

As a secondary procedure, PTFE paste can be used successfully after pharyngeal flap surgery in which the flap is not wide enough to prevent nasal escape. PTFE paste injected into one or both ports as necessary may reduce the size of the port sufficiently to achieve a satisfactory speech result.

Careful examination of the fluorographic study and the lateral radiograph is required so that the injection may be placed in the nasopharynx at the optimal point of closure (Fig. 87–14). The Lewy or Brunning gun, familiar to laryngologists, is used to inject 5 to 15 ml of PTFE paste into the submucosal layer (Smith and McCabe, 1977), avoiding the plane of the pharyngobasilar fascia. To minimize further the inferior spread while injecting, a metal tongue depressor should be held firmly against the body of the first or second cervical vertebra. This minimizes the migration of PTFE paste inferiorly. Two to four injection sites are required to raise a transverse ridge across the posterior nasopharyngeal wall at the appropriate level. Since PTFE paste is 50 per cent glycerol, approximately twice as much material is injected than is judged necessary to achieve VP closure. Local anesthesia may be used in adolescents, but for the younger child general anesthesia is required for this procedure.

Postoperatively, the children complain of a mild or moderate stiff neck, although the discomfort is less than that following pharyngeal flap surgery. Complications of injection are infection with localized granuloma and inferior migration of the PTFE paste; caution should be exercised in the use of this material.

The use of PTFE paste for posterior pharyngeal wall injection is still under careful regulation by the U.S. Food and Drug Administration, and final conclusions concerning its long-term efficacy are still awaited.

Palatopharyngoplasty

The origins of pharyngeal flap surgery can be traced to Passavant, but the use of the posterior pharyngeal flap as a secondary procedure was first performed by Schoenborn (1876), who described the use of an inferiorly based flap, and 10 years later (Schoenborn, 1886) described a superiorly based flap. Rosenthal (1924) repopularized the inferiorly based flap, and this technique has been widely used in the United States since Padgett reported on it (1930).

The superiorly based flap was also suggested by Bardenheuer (1892) and popularized by Sanvenero-Rosselli (1935). Although reports of successful results of inferiorly based flaps (Padgett, 1930; Conway and Goulian, 1960; Stark and DeHaan, 1960) cannot be dismissed, the superiorly based flap seems to be more physiologically sound since the vector of palate action that requires enhancement is that of elevation.

In the United States the superiorly based flap is presently the cornerstone of surgical management of VPI, either alone or in combination with other procedures.

The indications for the pharyngeal flap procedure include congenital short palate,

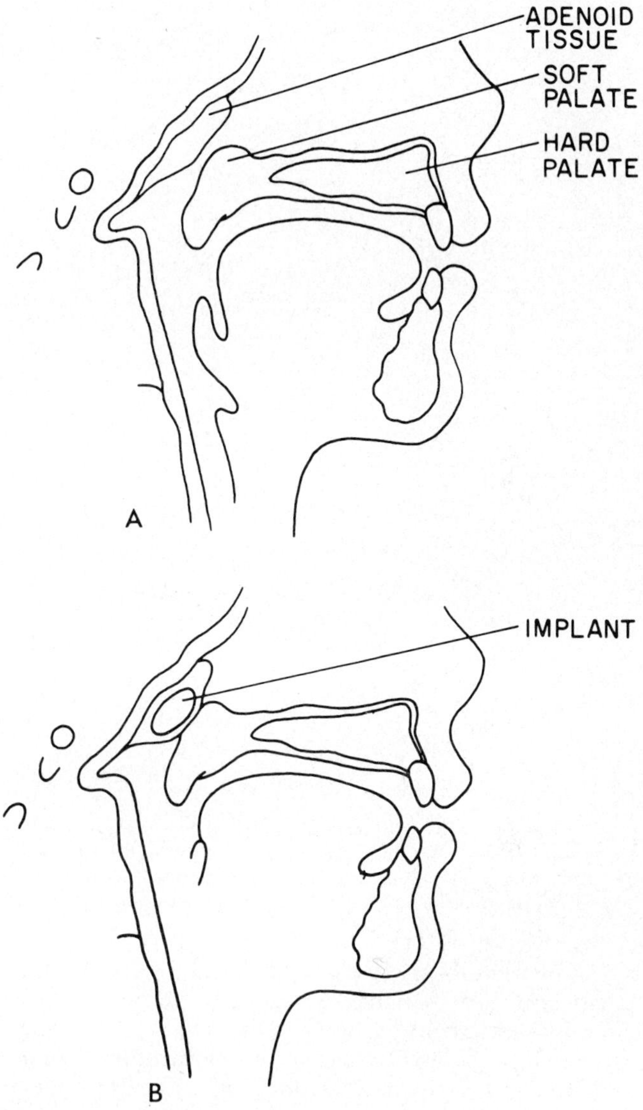

Figure 87–14 Posterior pharyngeal wall augmentation. *A*, Tracing of lateral radiograph of child with marginal VPI and mobile soft palate showing small VP gap despite maximal palate elevation. *B*, Correct site for augmentation of posterior pharyngeal wall, e.g., PTFE paste.

some cases of submucous cleft palate, repaired palatal clefts with residual incompetence, paralysis of the soft palate, recurrent breakdown of the suture line of soft palate clefts, and reconstruction of palate defects after resection of a tumor.

A suitable posterior pharyngeal wall flap is elevated, widely based superiorly, and long enough to reach the soft palate without tension (Fig. 87–15*A* and *B*). The flap is a mucomuscular one, containing the superior constrictor muscle, the plane of dissection being the prevertebral fascia. An incision is made in the central two thirds of the posterior border of the soft palate as far onto the nasal surface as is feasible (Fig. 87–15*A*) to dissect a fishmouth opening into the muscle mass of the soft palate and to create a mucosal flap of

nasal palatal mucosa hinged posteriorly on the free edge of the uvula and soft palate. This may not be possible technically in children with short, immobile palates; it is then necessary to split the palate in the midline to insert the flap. The free end of the pharyngeal flap is led into the fishmouth opening and sutured to the oral palatal mucosa with four 3-0 Dexon sutures (Fig. 87–15*C* and *D*) while the mucosal flap is sutured over the raw surface of the flap (Fig. 87–15*C*). Hogan (1973) claims that control over the port size is important and uses a No. 14 French catheter as his guide to size. To achieve this, the soft palate must be divided in the midline, and his technique has provoked lively debate (JAMA, 1971). Cotton and Quattromani (1977) felt that this was not necessary in all cases but was

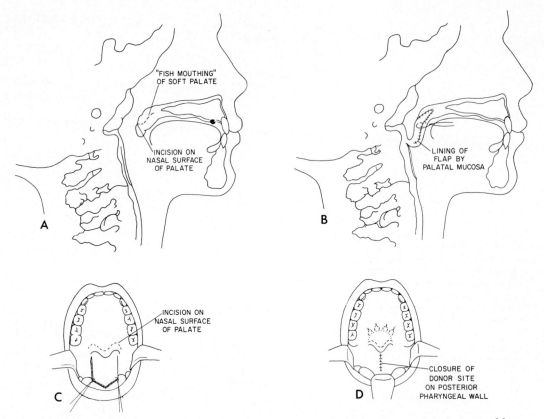

Figure 87–15 Schema of superiorly based pharyngeal flap. *A* and *B*, Incision made as far as possible on nasal surface of palate; soft palate is fishmouthed to accept pharyngeal flap. *C* and *D*, Insertion and suturing of pharyngeal flap into position; note lining of raw surface of flap by palatal mucosa flap dissected from nasal surface of palate and closure of donor site on posterior wall.

a useful adjunct in cases of paralyzed soft palate and those patients with poor or absent lateral pharyngeal wall movement.

The flap essentially acts as an obturator against which active lateral pharyngeal walls may abut during speech (Fig. 87–16*A* and *B*). Although electromyographic activity has been found by some authors in superiorly based flaps (Broadbent and Swinyard, 1959), it is the consensus that these are not dynamic

CLOSURE OF VELOPHARYNGEAL PORTS
AGAINST A CENTRALLY–PLACED
PHARYNGEAL FLAP

INEFFECTIVE MEDIAL MOVEMENT
OF LPW WITH PERSISTENT
VELOPHARYNGEAL INSUFFICIENCY

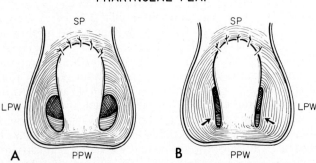
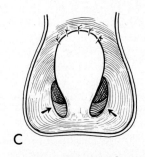

Figure 87–16 Schema of superiorly based pharyngeal flap as seen from below. PPW is post pharyngeal wall, SP is soft palate. *A*, Quiet respiration. *B*, Movement of lateral pharyngeal walls (LPW) closes VP port (arrows). *C*, Inadequate medial movement of lateral pharyngeal walls fails to close VP port (arrows). (From Cotton, R. T. 1977. Lateral defects in VPI. Arch. Otolaryngol., *103*:90.)

flaps. Hence, in those patients with absent lateral pharyngeal wall movement, a superiorly based flap is unlikely to eliminate hypernasality or nasal escape.

Changes in speech after pharyngeal flap surgery depend on certain factors. The flap should be wide enough to contact the lateral pharyngeal walls on their medial excursion (Fig. 87–16B) but must still allow some nasal airway for patient comfort and for normal nasal resonance. Hypernasality and nasal emission should improve spontaneously after surgery, but there is less dramatic improvement in those patients showing several of the compensatory mechanisms, such as glottal stops and pharyngeal fricatives. In such cases, speech therapy is mandatory to aid the normal production of consonants. It has been shown that, provided an adequate flap has been created, the spontaneous response to surgery is influenced more by the type of preoperative speech defect than by any other factor (Hamlen, 1970), although intelligence, age, and hearing are also most important.

The two most important complications of pharyngeal flap surgery are postoperative bleeding and airway obstruction, both fortunately rare if careful hemostasis is achieved during surgery and if there is skillful attention to the airway in the first few postoperative hours. Immediate postoperative bleeding may occur in a small number of patients because of surgical damage to one or both ascending pharyngeal arteries in an effort to make the flap too wide. Airway obstruction in the early postoperative hours may be caused by a combination of retropositioning of the tongue, especially in retrognathic individuals; hypopharyngeal edema; and oozing of blood from the donor site. Tracheotomy may rarely be required for this complication: Yules and colleagues (1971) pooled the results of 19 surgical series and describe an incidence of 15 out of a total of 1149 procedures that required tracheotomy. It is our preference to manage this problem by the placement of a 3.5 mm Portex endotracheal tube as a nasopharyngeal airway under direct vision in the operating room in those cases with the precipitating factors just mentioned. In this way a potential problem is avoided without danger to the VP port, as the 3.5 mm tube is the same size as the No. 14 French catheter used in port construction.

Flap detachment, either partial or complete, may occur at about the fifth to ninth day postoperatively. Yules and others (1971) report the incidence of flap detachment to be 37 out of 1149 cases studied.

A stiff neck occurs transiently in most patients during the second week postoperatively, and snoring is common after pharyngeal flap surgery. Otherwise, late complications are rare. Very seldom is nasal breathing completely eliminated, but occasionally it may be inadequate and may require minor revision of one or both velopharyngeal ports. A single fatal case of meningitis and a case of mediastinitis (Kindler, 1929) have been reported associated with this type of surgery.

SUMMARY

The aim of overall management of VPI is to eliminate hypernasality and nasal escape and any speech problems that have been developed secondary to the VPI. The evaluation and management of this problem should be by a multidisciplinary approach so that all facets of the problem are studied. In this way, the management required may be tailored to the individual problem. Since VPI has many different causes and may present on a continuum from a minimal to a severe problem, each case must be treated individually. Certainly an accurate assessment of the pathophysiology of the sphincter must be obtained. Use of fluoroscopy and nasal endoscopy is essential, with particular attention to lateral pharyngeal wall movement. When the decision for surgery has been made, the most favored operation in North America is the superiorly based pharyngeal flap. Since there are significant failure and complication rates reported with this procedure, there is still a need to explore other techniques such as sphincter pharyngoplasty.

REFERENCES

Arkebauer, H. J., Hixon, T. V., and Hardy, J. C. 1967. Peak intraoral pressure during speech. J. Speech Hear. Res., *10*:196.

Astley, R. 1958. The movements of the lateral walls of the nasopharynx in a cineradiographic study. J. Laryngol. Otol., 72:325.

The authors wish to express special thanks to Ms. Drue Lehmann (speech pathologist) and Dr. Gordon Huntress (prosthodontist) for their generous and helpful comments on this chapter.

Azzam, N. A., and Kuehn, D. P. 1977. The morphology of the musculus uvulae. Cleft Palate J.. *14*:78.

Bardenheuer, D. 1892. Vorschlage zu plastischen Operationen bei Chirurgischen eingriffen in der Mundhohle. Arch. Klin. Chir., *43*:32.

Bernstein, L. 1967. Treatment of velopharyngeal incompetence. Arch. Otolaryngol., *85*:67.

Blocksma, R. 1963. Correction of velopharyngeal insufficiency by Silastic pharyngeal implant. Plast. Reconstr. Surg., *31*:268.

Blocksma, R. 1971. Secondary techniques for correction of palatopharyngeal incompetence: Implants in posterior pharynx. *In* Grabb, W. C., Rosenstein, S. W., and Bzoch, K. R., (Eds.). Cleft Lip and Palate. Bostion, Little Brown and Co., p. 470.

Bluestone, C. D., Musgrave, R. H., and McWilliams, B. J. 1968a. Teflon injection pharyngoplasty — status 1968. Laryngoscope, *78*:558.

Bluestone, C. D., Musgrave, R. H., McWilliams, B. J., et al. 1968b. Teflon injection pharyngoplasty. Cleft Palate J., *5*:19.

Bosma, J. F. 1953. A correlated study of the anatomy and motor activity of the upper pharynx by cadaver dissection and cinematic study of patients after maxillofacial surgery. Ann. Otol. Rhinol. Laryngol., *62*:51.

Broadbent, T. R., and Swinyard, C. A. 1959. The dynamic pharyngeal flap: Its selective use and electromyographic evaluation. Plast. Reconstr. Surg., *23*:301.

Calnan, J. S. 1971. Congenital large pharynx. Br. J. Plast. Surg., *24*:263.

Conway, H., and Goulian, D. 1960. Experiences with the pharyngeal flap in cleft palate surgery. Plast. Reconstr. Surg., *26*:590.

Cotton, R., and Quattromani, F. 1977. Lateral defects in velopharyngeal insufficiency. Arch. Otolaryngol., *103*:90.

Croft, C. B., Shprintzen, R. J., Daniller, A., et al. 1978. The occult submucous cleft palate and the musculus uvulae. Cleft Palate J., *15*:150.

Dickson, D. R., and Dickson, W. M. 1972. Velopharyngeal anatomy. J. Speech Hear. Res., *15*:372.

Dickson, D. R. 1975. Anatomy of the normal velopharyngeal mechanism. Clin. Plast. Surg., 2(2):235.

Dorrance, G. N. 1930. Congenital insufficiency of the palate. Arch. Surg., *21*:185.

Eckstein, H. 1904. Demonstration of paraffin prosthesis in defects of the face and palate. Dermatologica (Basel), *11*:772.

Edgerton, M. T. 1965. The island flap pushback and the suspensory pharyngeal flap in surgical treatment of the cleft palate patient. Plast. Reconstr. Surg., *36*:591.

Fara, M., and Weatherley-White, R. C. A. 1977. Submucous cleft plate. *In* Converse, J. M. (Ed.). Reconstructive Plastic Surgery, Vol. 4. Philadelphia, W. B. Saunders Co., p. 2104.

Fox, D. R., and Johns, D. 1970. Predicting velopharyngeal closure with a modified tongue-anchor technique. J. Speech Hear. Dis., *35*:248.

Ganguli, A. C. 1971. Lengthening the short palate by submucous pedicle cheek flaps. *In* Hueston, J. T. (Ed.). Transaction of the Fifth International Congress of Plastic and Reconstructive Surgeons. Melbourne, Australia, Butterworth.

Gaza, W. V. 1926. Über freie Fettgewebstransplantation in den retropharyngealen Raum bei Gaumenspalate. Arch. Klin. Chir., *142*:590.

Gibb, A. G. 1958. Hypernasality following tonsil and adenoid removal. J. Laryngol. Otol., *72*:433.

Gonzalez, J., and Aronson, A. 1970. Palatal lift prosthesis for treatment of anatomic and neurologic palatopharyngeal insufficiency. Cleft Palate J., *7*:91.

Hagerty, R. F., and Hill, M. J. 1961. Cartilage pharyngoplasty in cleft palate patients. Surg. Gynecol. Obstetr., *112*:350.

Hagerty, R. F., Mylin, W. K., and Hess, D. M. 1968. Velar mobility, velopharyngeal closure and speech proficiency in cartilage pharyngoplasty. The effect of age at surgery. Cleft Palate J., *5*:317.

Halle, H. 1925. Gaumennaht und Gaumenplastik. Arch. Ohr. Nas. Kehlkopfheilk., *12*:377.

Hamlen, M. O. 1970. Speech changes after pharyngeal flap surgery. Plast. Reconstr. Surg., *46*:437.

Hardy, J. C., Rembolt, R., Spriestersbach, D., et al. 1961. Surgical management of palatal paresis and speech problems in cerebral palsy: A preliminary report. J. Speech Hear. Dis., *26*:320.

Hardy, J. C., Netsell, R., Schweiger, J. W., et al. 1969. Management of velopharyngeal dysfunction in cerebral palsy. J. Speech Hear. Dis., *34*:123.

Heller, J. C., Gens, G. W., Moe, D., et al. 1974. Velopharyngeal insufficiency in patients with neurological, emotional, and mental disorders. J. Speech Hear. Dis., *39*:350.

Hogan, V. N. 1973. A clarification of the surgical goals in cleft palate speech and the introduction of the lateral port control (L.P.C.) pharyngeal flap. Cleft Palate J., *10*:331.

Hynes, W. 1950. Pharyngoplasty by muscle transplantation. Br. J. Plast. Surg., *3*:128.

Hynes, W. 1954. The primary repair of clefts of the palate. Br. J. Plast. Surg., *7*:242.

Hynes, W. 1967. Observations on pharyngoplasty. Br. J. Plast. Surg., *20*:244.

Jackson, I. T., and Silverton, J. S. 1977. The sphincter pharyngoplasty as a secondary procedure in cleft palates. Plast. Reconstr. Surg., *59*:518.

J.A.M.A. 1971. Lively debate breaks out over plastic surgery techniques. J.A.M.A., *216*:2075.

Kaplan, E. N. 1975a. The occult submucous cleft. Cleft Palate J., *12*:356.

Kaplan, E. N. 1975b. Soft palate repair by levator muscle reconstruction and a buccal mucosal flap. Plast. Reconstr. Surg., *56*:129.

Kelsey, C. A., Ewanowski, S. J., Crummy, A. B., et al. 1972. Lateral pharyngeal wall motion as a predictor of surgical success in velopharyngeal insufficiency. N. Engl. J. Med., *287*:64.

Kindler, W. 1929. Zur Gefahrlichkeit der Gaumenplastik nach Schoenborn-Rosenthal sowie nach Ernst-Halle und zur Moglichkeit, ihr Vorzubeugen. Beitr. Path. Anat., *27*:187.

Kriens, O. 1970. Fundamental anatomic findings for an intravelar veloplasty. Cleft Palate J., *7*:27.

Kriens, O. 1975. Anatomy of the velopharyngeal area in cleft palate. Clin. Plast. Surg., 2(2):261.

Kuehn, D. P., and VanDemark, D. R. 1978. Assessment of velopharyngeal competency following Teflon pharyngoplasty. Cleft Palate J., *15*:145.

Lewy, R., Cole, R., and Wepman, J. 1965. Teflon injection in the correction of velopharyngeal insufficiency. Ann. Otol. Rhinol. Laryngol., *74*:874.

Longacre, J. J., and DeStefano, G. A. 1957. The role of the posterior pharyngeal flap in rehabilitation of the patient with cleft palate. Am. J. Surg., *94*:882.

Mason, R. M. 1973. Preventing speech disorders following adenoidectomy by preoperative examination. Clin Pediatr., *12*:405.

Matsuya, T., Miyazaki, T., and Yamaoka, M. 1974. Fiberscopic examination of velopharyngeal closure in normal individuals. Cleft Palate J., *11*:286.

McWilliams, B. J. 1966. Speech and language problems in children with cleft palate. J. Am. Med. Wom. Assoc., *21*:1005.

McWilliams, B. J., Musgrave, R. H., and Crozier, P. A. 1968. The influence of head position upon velopharyngeal closure. Cleft Palate J., *5*:117.

McWilliams, B. J., Bluestone, C. D., and Musgrave, R. H. 1969. Diagnostic implications of vocal cord nodules in children with cleft palate. Laryngoscope, *79*:2072.

McWilliams, B. J., Lavorato, A. S., and Bluestone, C. D. 1973. Vocal cord abnormalities in children with velopharyngeal valving problems. Laryngoscope, *83*:1745.

Millard, D. R. 1962. Wide and/or short cleft palate. Plast. Reconstr. Surg., *29*:40.

Millard, D. R. 1963. The island flap in cleft palate surgery. SGO, *116*:297.

Millard, D. R. 1966. A new use of the island flap in wide palate clefts. Plast. Reconstr. Surg., *38*:330.

Moll, K., Huffman, W., Lierle, D., and Smith, J. 1963. Factors related to the success of pharyngeal flap procedures. Plast. Reconstr. Surg., *32*:581.

Moore, F. T. 1960. A new operation to cure nasopharyngeal incompetence. Br. J. Surg., *47*:424.

Moore, F. T., and Chong, J. K. 1967. The "sandwich" technique to lengthen the soft palate. Br. J. Oral Surg., *4*:183.

Morris, H. L. 1962. Communication skills of children with cleft lip and palate. J. Speech Hear. Res., *5*:79.

Morris, H. L. 1972. Cleft Palate. *In* Weston, A. J. (Ed.). Communication Disorders: An Appraisal. Springfield, Ill., Charles C Thomas, p. 128.

Morris, H. L. (Ed.). 1978. Some Results of Cleft Palate Surgery: The Bratislava Project. University of Iowa Press, Iowa City, p. 49.

Orticochea, M. 1968. Construction of a dynamic muscle sphincter in cleft palates. Plast. Reconstr. Surg., *41*:323.

Orticochea, M. 1970. Results of the dynamic muscle sphincter operation in cleft palates. Br. J. Plast. Surg., *23*:108.

Owsley, J. Q., Chierick, G., Miller, E. R., et al. 1967. Cephalometric evaluation of palatal dysfunction in patients without cleft palate. Plast. Reconstr. Surg., *39*:562.

Padgett, E. C. 1930. The repair of cleft palates after unsuccessful operations with special reference to cases with an extensive loss of palatal tissue. Arch. Surg., *20*:453.

Piggott, R. W. 1969. The nasendoscopic appearance of the normal palatopharyngeal valve. Plast. Reconstr. Surg., *43*:19.

Piggott, R. W., Bensen, J. F., and White, R. D. 1969. Nasendoscopy in the diagnosis of velopharyngeal incompetence. Plast. Reconstr. Surg., *43*:141.

Pruzansky, S., Peterson-Falzone, S., Laffer, J., et al. 1977. Hypernasality in the absence of an overt cleft. Commentary on nomenclature, diagnosis, classification and research design. Abstract #60, 3rd International Congress on Cleft Palate and Related Craniofacial Anomalies.

Quattromani, F., Benton, C., and Cotton, R. 1977.

The Towne projection for evaluation of the velopharyngeal sphincter. Radiology, *125*:540.

Ricketts, R. M. 1954. The cranial base and soft structures in cleft palate speech and breathing. Plast. Reconstr. Surg., *14*:47.

Rosenthal, W. 1924. Zur Frage der Gaumenplastik. Zbl. Chir., *51*:1621.

Ruding, R. 1964. Cleft palate: Anatomic and surgical considerations. Plast. Reconstr. Surg., *33*:132.

Sanvenero-Roselli, G. 1935. Divisione palatine e sua cura chirurgica. Atti. Congr. Internatl. Stomatol., p. 391.

Schoenborn, D. 1876. Ueber eine neue Methode der Staphylorrhaphie. Arch. Klin. Chir., *19*:527.

Schoenborn, D. 1886. Vorstelling eines Falles von Staphyloplastik. Ver. Deutsch. Ges. Chir., *15*:57.

Schulz, R., Heller, J., Gens, G., et al. 1973. Pharyngeal flap surgery and voice quality factors related to success and failure. Cleft Palate J., *10*:66.

Schwartz, M. F. 1975. Developing a direct, objective measure of velopharyngeal inadequacy. Clin. Plast. Surg., *2*:305.

Silberman, H. D., Wilf, H., and Tucker, J. A. 1976. Flexible fiberoptic nasopharyngolaryngoscope. Ann. Otol. Rhinol. Laryngol., *85*:640.

Skolnick, M. L. 1969. Video velopharyngography in patients with nasal speech with emphasis on lateral pharyngeal motion in velopharyngeal closure. Radiology, *93*:747.

Skolnick, M. L. 1970. Videofluoroscopic examination of the velopharyngeal portal during phonation in lateral and base projections. Cleft Palate J., *7*:803.

Skolnick, M. L. 1975. Velopharyngeal function in cleft palate. Clin. Plast. Surg., *2*(2):285.

Skolnick, M. L., Shprintzen, R. S., McCall, G. N., et al. 1975. Patterns of velopharyngeal closure in subjects with repaired cleft palate and normal speech. Cleft Palate J., *12*:369.

Skoog, T. 1965. The pharyngeal flap operation in cleft palate: A clinical study of 82 cases. Br. J. Plast. Surg., *18*:265.

Smith, J. K., Huggman, W. C., Lierle, D. M., et al. 1963. Results of pharyngeal flap surgery in patients with velopharyngeal incompetence. Plast. Reconstr. Surg., *32*:493.

Smith, J. K., and McCabe, B. F. 1977. Teflon injection in the nasopharynx to improve velopharyngeal closure. Ann. Otol. Rhinol. Laryngol., *559*:86.

Smith, R. M., and McWilliams, B. J. 1968. Psycholinguistic abilities of children with clefts. Cleft Palate J., *5*:238.

Spriestersbach, D. C., Darley, F. L., and Morris, H. L. 1958. Language skills in children with cleft palate. J. Speech Hear. Res., *1*:279.

Stark, R. B., and DeHaan, D. R. 1960. The addition of a pharyngeal flap to primary palatoplasty. Plast. Reconstr. Surg., *26*:378.

Stool, S. E., and Randall, P. 1967. Unexpected ear disease in infants with cleft palate. Cleft Palate J., *4*:99.

Sturim, H. S., and Jacob, C. T. 1972. Teflon pharyngoplasty. Plast. Reconstr. Surg., *49*:180.

Subtelny, J. D. 1955. Width of the nasopharynx and related anatomic structures in normal and unoperated cleft palate children. Am. J. Orthod., *41*:889.

Subtelny, J. D., and Subtelny, J. D. 1959. Intelligibility and associated physiological factors of cleft palate speakers. J. Speech Hear. Res., *2*:353.

Subtelny, J. D., Koepp-Baker, H., and Subtelny, J. D.

1961. Palatal function and cleft palate speech. J. Speech Hear. Dis., 26:213.

Taub, S. 1966. The Taub oral panendoscope: A new technique. Cleft Palate J., 3:328.

Ward, P. H., Goldman, R., and Stoudt, R. S. 1966. Teflon injection to improve velopharyngeal insufficiency. J. Speech Hear. Dis., 31:267.

Ward, P. H., Stoudt, R. S., and Goldman, R. 1967. Improvement of velopharyngeal insufficiency by Teflon injection. Trans. Am. Acad. Ophthalmol. Otolaryngol., 71:923.

Ward, P. H. 1968. Uses of injectable Teflon in otolaryngology. Arch. Otolaryngol., 87:367.

Wardill, W. E. M. 1937. Technique of operation for cleft palate. Br. J. Surg., 25:117.

Warren, D. W., and Dubois, A. B. 1964. A pressure flow technique for measuring velopharyngeal orifice area during continuous speech. Cleft Palate J., 1:52.

Warren, D. W., Bevin, A. W., and Winslow, R. B. 1978. Posterior pillar webbing and palatopharyngeal displacement: Possible causes of congenital palatal incompetence. Cleft Palate J., 15:68.

Weatherley-White, R. C. A., Sakura, C. Y., et al. 1972. Submucous cleft palate; its incidence, natural history and indications for treatment. Plast. Reconstr. Surg., 49:297.

Williams, H. B., and Woolhouse, F. M. 1962. Comparison of speech improvement in cases of cleft palate after two methods of pharyngoplasty. Plast. Reconstr. Surg., 30:36.

Yules, R. B., Chase, R. A., Blocksma, R., et al., 1971. Secondary techniques for correction of palatopharyngeal incompetence. In Grabb, W. C., Rosenstein, S. W., and Bzoch, K. R. (Eds.). Cleft Lip and Palate. Boston, Little, Brown and Co. p. 451.

Zwitman, D. H., Gyepes, M. T., and Ward, P. H. 1976. Assessment of velar and lateral wall movement by oral telescope and radiographic examination in patients with velopharyngeal inadequacy and in normal subjects. J. Speech Hear. Dis., 41:381.

Chapter 88

HEARING AIDS FOR CHILDREN

Daniel M. Schwartz, Ph.D.

Dan F. Konkle, Ph.D.

One of the most cogent theories of language to emanate in recent years is that children have an innate, maturationally controlled propensity for developing language, given the appropriate environment to foster this potential (Lenneberg, 1967). At about the age of one year, the average child with normal hearing will produce his or her first word. By the age of four years, the child will have acquired a complex set of grammatical rules that serves as the foundation for adult language. These early years are not only the most rapid period for speech and language development but also are critical to the acquisition of normal speech and language skills. It is important to emphasize, however, that this innate propensity is dependent upon the child's ability to abstract the acoustic information received from the environment (Menyuk, 1971). Thus, the auditory channel must be intact if the child is to receive the necessary linguistic input with which to develop the rules of grammar.

In contrast to the child with normal hearing, one deprived of auditory input subsequent to hearing loss will be, albeit endowed with this same innate capacity for developing speech and language, either alinguistic or severely delayed in the acquisition of speech and language. The consequence of a hearing loss on the development of communication skills is dependent upon three important factors: (1) the child's age at onset of the hearing loss, (2) the degree of hearing loss, and (3) the time at which therapeutic intervention is initiated.

The primary objective of early management for the hearing-impaired child is the fostering of speech and language development. If the child's maximal potential for the acquisition of speech and language is to be realized, then exposure to sensory input through the auditory channel must begin during the "critical period" (0 to 3 years of age) for language to develop. Since most hearing-impaired children have sufficient residual hearing to benefit from amplification, the hearing aid represents the primary source of external environmental input to the auditory modality. According to Ross (1975a) ". . . the early and appropriate selection and use of amplification is the single most important habilitative tool available to us."

On the basis of these concepts, the purpose of this chapter is to provide the otolaryngologist with a review of the basic characteristics and acoustic properties of a hearing aid and a discussion of the clinical procedures commonly used for selecting and evaluating appropriate amplification for the hearing-impaired child.

GENERAL CONSIDERATIONS

The process of selecting and fitting hearing-impaired children with effective amplification depends on a basic knowledge of hearing aid operation, design, and function. While it is not the purpose of this chapter to detail technical information about hearing aid mechanics, the scope of subsequent discussions makes it essential that the reader have a basic understanding of the purpose, function, and different types of hearing aids.

Classification of Hearing Aids

Technically, any device that provides a link between the acoustic environment and the hearing-impaired individual may be considered a hearing aid. This generalized definition includes a wide variety of devices that may conveniently be classified into four types: (1) personalized electroacoustic systems that are wearable, (2) group electroacoustic systems commonly found in classroom settings, (3) systems that use electrode implants to stimulate the auditory system directly, and (4) special devices designed to stimulate nonauditory senses (Carhart, 1975). Since instruments defined in the first category (personal electroacoustic systems that are wearable) are most applicable to children, the scope of this chapter will be limited to this type of amplification. The general terms "hearing aid," "hearing aid system," or "amplification system" will be used throughout this chapter to denote such devices. The reader interested in alternative forms of amplification is referred to Ross (1978) for a discussion of classroom systems, to Brackmann and House (1976) for additional information about electrode implants, and to Pickett (1975) for a review of devices designed to stimulate nonauditory senses.

ing aid but also on the handicapping effects imposed by the hearing loss. Oyer (1966) has noted that ". . . there is not a one-to-one relationship between hearing loss and hearing handicap, but rather the hearing handicap varies as a function of the demands that are placed on the person with the loss." This observation has been well documented in studies of adult populations (Davis, 1948; Nett et al., 1960; Dirks and Carhart, 1962; High et al., 1964; Noble and Atherley, 1970; McCartney and Sorenson, 1974; Peters and Hardick, 1974) and, as emphasized in the introduction of this chapter, is of particular concern to children. Stated simply, children with the same degree and type of hearing loss frequently present varied patterns of auditory handicap depending on dissimilarities in the child's age at onset, chronological age, the age at which language intervention was initiated, the child's mental capacity and emotional adjustment, environmental factors, and numerous other variables. Consequently, the effective use of amplification in children depends on an appreciation for the physical and electroacoustic properties associated with various hearing aids in conjunction with an understanding of the relationship between hearing loss and hearing handicap.

Purpose of Hearing Aids

The fundamental purpose of any hearing aid system is to assist the communicative ability to hearing-impaired individuals. Despite recent advancements in microphone design and electronic technology, it should be stressed that modern hearing aids cannot restore normal function to an impaired auditory system. Rather, the hearing aid can only assist the communicative process. The primary objective in providing children with amplification, therefore, is not to restore normal auditory function but to select an amplification system that best suits a child's individual needs. The extent to which this goal is realized, however, depends not only on the physical and electroacoustic properties of the hear-

Function of Hearing Aids

The modern hearing aid assists communication by amplifying environmental sound and directing this sound to the user's ear. This process may be conceptualized as an input–output function and is shown schematically in Figure 88–1. Note that the input to the hearing aid system consists of environmental sound that may originate from a number of sources. For example, the environmental signal at the input of the hearing aid may consist of a primary message in the form of a speaker's voice and several secondary messages, such as the output from a television set, noise from an air conditioner, and classroom or traffic noise. The acoustic energy from these sources summate to pro-

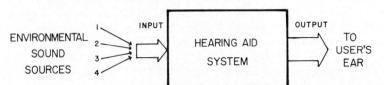

Figure 88–1 Schematic of the hearing aid system representing a simple input–output function.

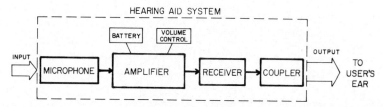

Figure 88–2 Block diagram illustrating the common components of a hearing aid system.

vide a complex input signal to the hearing aid that is amplified without regard to source. Stated differently, the hearing aid system does not selectively amplify the signal from the primary source as compared to signals from secondary sources. The system must be viewed as only changing the acoustic signal delivered to the user's ear and not as altering the sensitivity or acuity of the impaired auditory mechanism.

Components. The hearing aid is a system composed of mechanical, electrical, and acoustical components. As noted previously, recent advancements in microphone and electronic technology have increased the versatility of modern hearing aids. Despite these advancements, however, the basic function of hearing aid components has remained unchanged.

Several components are common to any amplification system. These include a microphone, amplifier, power source, volume control, receiver, and coupler. Although it is beyond the scope of this chapter to consider each component in detail (see Olsen, 1977 for an excellent review of hearing aid technology), it is important to understand the function of each component and how they interact with environmental acoustic stimuli.

Figure 88–2 illustrates the basic components of a hearing aid. Recall that the input to the hearing aid consists of environmental sound that may originate from any number of sources. This signal is picked up by the hearing aid *microphone*, where it is transformed into an electrical analog and conducted to the *amplifier*. Since the electrical signal from the microphone is extremely weak, it is the purpose of the amplifier to make the signal more intense by using additional energy derived from the *power source*, or *battery*. There may be several stages associated with the amplification process. Regardless of its complexity, however, the sole purpose of amplification is to make the signal more intense.

A *volume control* is interfaced with the amplifier and serves to regulate the amount of amplification directed to the *receiver*. The

receiver of the hearing aid may be compared to a miniature loudspeaker in the case of air conduction systems or for bone conduction systems to a bone vibrator similar to that used with a pure tone audiometer. Although the term "receiver" has been used consistently to denote this component, it is actually a poor description since it does not reflect accurately the component's function. The purpose of the receiver is to convert the amplified electrical signal into either acoustic energy for air conduction systems or mechanical energy for bone conduction systems. A term that describes more accurately this process would be "output transducer." Regardless, the receiver (output transducer) is currently the most restricting component in any amplification system. The reason for this relates to the use of magnetic-type receivers in modern instruments. While technology has developed microphones and amplifiers that respond effectively to a broad spectral range, the magnetic-type receiver in comparison is restricted in spectral response. It follows, therefore, that the output from the hearing aid that incorporates a magnetic receiver will also be restricted. Development of wide range receivers (i.e., the electret receiver) should overcome this limitation.

The final component in the hearing aid system is the *coupler*. The coupler functions to direct the amplified signal transduced by the receiver (output transducer) to the user's ear. Bone conduction systems use the same mode of coupling that is employed in pure tone audiometry; that is, the vibrator is placed in contact with the cranial bones, typically the mastoid, and the signal is transduced to the user's ear as mechanical vibrations. Theoretically, this mode of transmission essentially bypasses the external and middle ear and directly stimulates the cochlea. In air conduction systems the signal is delivered to the user's external auditory meatus by way of a length of polyurethane tubing held in place by an earmold.

The individual components of a hearing aid form a system that functions to amplify and direct environmental sound by a series of

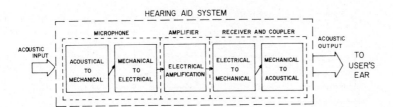

Figure 88–3 Hearing aid system functions as a series of sequential energy transformations.

sequential energy transformations, as shown in Figure 88–3. The microphone of the hearing aid system serves to transform acoustic environmental energy (environmental sound) into mechanical energy represented by the vibration of the microphone's diaphragm. In turn, the mechanical displacement of the diaphragm results in changes in electrical resistance in the microphone, thereby generating electrical energy, or voltage. This electrical energy is then amplified (i.e., increased voltage) and used to drive the diaphragm of the receiver, or output transducer. Thus, electrical energy is transformed into mechanical energy. Finally, the mechanical energy represented by vibration of the receiver diaphragm is either directed to the cranial bones (bone conduction) or converted into acoustical energy (air conduction) and directed to the user's ear.

Electroacoustic Characteristics. Changes in environmental sound that result from this sequential series of energy transformations are known as the electroacoustic characteristics of the hearing aid system. These characteristics are specified in terms of differences between the output and the input acoustic signals: The amount of amplification (electroacoustic characteristics) is calculated by subtracting the input from the output.

Several terms have been used to describe specific parameters associated with the electroacoustic characteristics of hearing aids. Those terms important to the selecting and fitting of hearing aids for children will be discussed next. Readers seeking a more comprehensive discussion of this topic are referred to Kasten (1978).

The amount of *gain* supplied by a hearing aid system is specified as the decibel (dB) difference between the input and output acoustic intensities. For example, if the input to the hearing aid was 60 dB and the output was 110 dB, the gain of the hearing aid would be 50 dB (110 dB − 60 dB = 50 dB). Hearing aids, however, are not equally sensitive to the various frequencies within the spectral range they are able to amplify. The gain at certain frequencies will be greater than that at other

frequencies, depending on the mechanical, electrical, and acoustic properties specific to the system.

The relationship of gain to frequency in Hertz (Hz) is termed the *frequency response* of the hearing aid. The frequency response is obtained by measuring the gain at various frequencies within the spectral range of amplification. It is convenient to plot the frequency response as a gain versus frequency function, as shown in Figure 88–4. Since the amount of gain varies as a function of frequency, the gain of a hearing aid is frequently expressed as *average gain*. The frequencies used to compute average gain include 1000 Hz, 1600 Hz, and 2500 Hz (American National Standards Institute, 1976). The example in Figure 88–4 illustrates the computation of average gain. Note that the individual gain values are derived from the frequency response shown above the example.

The maximal intensity that a hearing aid is able to generate is called the *saturation sound pressure level* (SSPL). SSPL refers to the maximal intensity output, which cannot be exceeded regardless of the extent of volume control rotation or the intensity of the input. For the purposes of standardization, however, SSPL is measured as the intensity output with a 90 dB input and the volume control rotated to full-on. Like gain, SSPL will also vary as a function of frequency, and the *average SSPL* is computed in the same manner as average gain, that is, the average of the output at 1000 Hz, 1600 Hz, and 2500 Hz. The difference between gain and SSPL is that gain is defined relative to output minus input, whereas SSPL is specified only in terms of output.

Manufacturers are required to publish the electroacoustic characteristics associated with their particular hearing aids (Food and Drug Administration, 1977). While this information is often useful in the selection and fitting process, caution should be used when generalizing such data to hearing-impaired children. For example, published specifications are based on the average performance expected from a certain brand and model of hearing aid. They do not represent the specific characteristics of a particular instrument. Moreover, published data are obtained from measurements made with the hearing aid output directed to a "hard-walled" acoustic cavity. Although the dimensions and configuration of this cavity are specified for standardization (American National Standards Institute, 1976), the electroacoustic results obtained with such a device do not reflect accurately the electroacoustic performance when the hearing aid is coupled to a "real" ear. This situation is complicated further by variability in shape, size, and tissue factors among individual ears. Thus, the electroacoustic characteristics published by manufacturers should be used as general guides in the selection and fitting process, rather than being considered representative or predictive of specific performance for a particular individual.

As a final note, the reader should be aware that the measurement of electroacoustic characteristics is a complex task. A knowledge of acoustics, electronics, and physics is necessary in order to obtain valid results. Although the American National Standards Institute (ANSI) has published specifications for the measurement of electroacoustic hearing aid characteristics (ANSI 1976), research has shown that even under highly controlled conditions, substantial differences are noted with

repeated measurements on the same hearing aid (Konkle et al., 1976; Townsend and Schwartz, 1977). These comments are not meant to discourage individuals from making their own electroacoustic measurements. Rather, such a practice is strongly recommended and can provide valuable information about hearing aid performance. Individuals performing this task, however, should be knowledgeable and thoroughly experienced in the techniques of electroacoustic hearing aid assessment.

Types of Hearing Aids

The wearable amplification systems discussed in this chapter may be divided into two groups depending on how they transduce amplified sound to the user's ear. These two groups are composed of bone conduction and air conduction systems, respectively.

There are two types of bone conduction systems: the body type and the eyeglass type. Figure 88–5 illustrates that the body system is characterized by a case that contains all components except the receiver. The case is usually worn on the body attached to an article of clothing or in a special "pocket" harness. A cord connects the case to the bone conduction receiver positioned at the mastoid and secured by a headband. The eyeglass

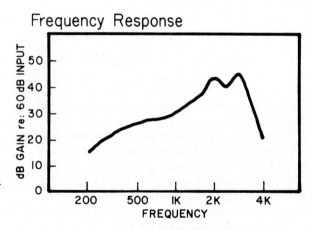

Figure 88–4 Frequency response (gain as a function of frequency) of a hearing aid system and an example of average gain computation.

Example of Average Gain:

Gain at: 1000 Hz = 30 dB

1600 Hz = 35 dB

2500 Hz = 40 dB

Thus, $\dfrac{30\,dB + 35\,dB + 40\,dB}{3} = 35\,dB$ Average Gain

BONE CONDUCTION SYSTEMS

1. Body Type

2. Eyeglass Type

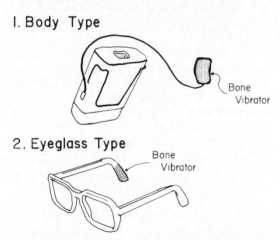

Figure 88–5   Bone conduction hearing aid systems.

system differs from the body unit in that it contains all components in the temple piece with the receiver located in the area of the arm; when the glasses are worn the vibrator rests on the mastoid. Bone conduction systems are seldom recommended unless a physical deformity precludes the use of air conduction aids. For example, children with malformed pinnae, absent external canals, or both may be considered candidates for bone conduction systems.

Air conduction systems may be grouped into four types, as noted in Figure 88–6. The body-type air conduction system is essentially the same as that for the bone conduction body system except that the vibrator is replaced with a "button" air conduction receiver that is held in place by an earmold that directs sound to the user's ear. Characteristic of the hearing aid worn on the body is the distance between the input (microphone) and the output (receiver). Although the receiver is located at ear level, the microphone is typically located at some point other than the ear (e.g., in a shirt pocket, harness, or attached to undergarments). Thus, it is important to realize that the point of acoustic input for body-type instruments does not approximate a natural listening condition where the point of input is at ear level.

The other three types of air conduction systems are all worn on the head. The behind-the-ear, or postauricular, hearing aid is situated on the pinna so that the case of the hearing aid rests behind the ear. These instruments are also referred to as ear-level units. The ear-level system is completed by a

coupler that consists of a length of polyurethane tubing and an earmold. The eyeglass air conduction aid houses components in the temple piece with amplified sound conducted to the user's ear via a coupler of the same configuration as the behind-the-ear system. An in-the-ear hearing aid contains components in a shell that has been fabricated to conform to the dimensions and configuration of the user's individual external ear. Although in-the-ear instruments were originally developed for cosmetic purposes, experience has revealed that these units may also have several functional advantages compared to other types of air conduction systems. The most notable advantage relates to the location of the input microphone at a point that approximates closely the normal listening condition, that is, at ear level in a position and direction that corresponds to the orifice of the external auditory canal. Placement of the hearing aid microphone in close proximity to the ear canal has been shown to improve sound localization, to enhance acoustic gain in the mid and high frequencies, and to improve speech discrimination ability.

An additional approach to amplification that has gained wide clinical acceptance for

AIR CONDUCTION SYSTEMS

1. Body Type

2. Behind-the-ear Type

3. Eyeglass Type

4. In-the-ear Type

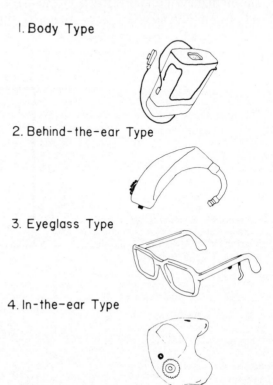

Figure 88–6   Air conduction hearing aid systems.

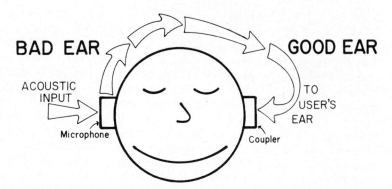

Figure 88–7 Contralateral routing of offside signal (CROS) with the environmental signal directed toward the user's bad ear (microphone) and routed by the hearing aid system to the user's good ear (coupler).

assisting children with unilateral hearing loss is the CROS-type hearing aid. CROS is an acronym for *C*ontralateral *R*outing of *O*ffside *S*ignals and is demonstrated in Figure 88–7. The basic principle of the CROS system is to locate the input microphone at the impaired ear and to direct the output signal via the receiver and coupler to the good ear. Thus, in a listening situation where the primary message (speech) originates on the same side as the impaired ear, the signal is "picked up" by the microphone on that side, amplified, and directed to the user's good (contralateral) ear. Although the CROS hearing aid may not provide assistance in all situations, it can be of benefit in those conditions where orientation of environmental sound sources results in an adverse listening environment (that is, speech directed to the poor ear with environmental noise to the good ear). Consequently, children with one normal ear and one impaired ear should also be considered potential hearing aid candidates.

Table 88–1 presents information on the percentage of hearing aid sales in the United States as a function of hearing aid type for the years 1963, 1973, and 1977, respectively (Endicott, 1978). These data illustrate several trends that reflect both advanced technology and altered philosophy. The decrease in the use of body-worn instruments during this

period of time was almost 15 per cent. Conversely, sales for postauricular instruments increased by 17 per cent. These data clearly reflect a trend toward replacing body-worn aids with ear-level instruments. The reason for this trend probably resulted from the rapid development of microcircuitry that allowed manufacturers to build powerful (high-gain) hearing aids into behind-the-ear models. Since professionals recognized the advantage of having the microphone located at or near the ear, it was logical that high-gain ear-level instruments would replace their body-worn counterparts. A similar trend is observed when the data for eyeglass and in-the-ear hearing aids are examined. In this case, the trend toward the use of ear-level aids probably reflects cosmetic factors more than actual changes in the philosophy of selecting and fitting hearing aids. Current in-the-ear systems should continue to increase in popularity because of their convenience and microphone location, which enhances amplification in the high frequencies and assists in sound localization. It is expected that future data will reveal a decrease in the use of postauricular instruments as in-the-ear models become more popular. Finally, bone conduction systems currently account for only 0.2 per cent of all hearing aid sales, thus reflecting the restricted versatility of bone conduction units.

SPECIFIC CONSIDERATIONS

The preceding discussion has provided general information about the purpose of amplification, the function and components of hearing aids, electroacoustic parameters, and types of hearing aids. This general information serves as a basis for considering several specific concepts important to amplification in children.

Table 88–1 PERCENTAGE OF HEARING AID SALES AS A FUNCTION OF TYPE FOR THE YEARS 1963, 1973, AND 1977

Type of Aid	Year		
	1963	*1973*	*1977*
Body	20.0	8.6	4.8
Behind-the-ear	44.0	65.5	61.2
Eyeglass	34.6	32.5	6.2
In-the-ear	2.1	2.2	27.6
Bone conduction	0.5	0.2	0.2

Candidacy

Hearing aid candidacy in children is frequently approached as an "all-or-none" proposition based on the presence or absence of hearing impairment. That is, if a sensorineural hearing loss can be documented, the child should be considered to be a hearing aid candidate. Although we concur with this practice, such an approach does not provide guidance in situations in which a hearing impairment is suspected but has not been documented. For this reason, previous attempts to categorize hearing aid candidacy based on pure tone threshold data have not been completely acceptable. Despite audiologic procedures that can identify effectively the presence, degree, type, and often the configuration of most hearing losses (see Chapter 8), there are many children who are suspected to have hearing losses that cannot be assessed adequately with current audiologic techniques. Unfortunately, the majority of children included in this group are those for whom amplification is vital for linguistic development (i.e., those younger than age four years). In the absence of audiologic data that document a hearing loss, many physicians and audiologists have been reluctant to recommend amplification even though they were highly suspicious that a hearing loss was present. Instead, they frequently counseled parents to wait until the child was more "mature" and until audiologic data defined the "real" level of hearing. This approach appears to ignore the potential handicapping effects of auditory impairment and probably reflects an overdependence on the need for exact audiologic data prior to considering the use of a hearing aid. Without question, thorough audiologic assessment is essential in the management of hearing-impaired children, but the absence of exact data that define threshold sensitivity should not preclude a child from being considered a candidate for amplification. Rather, when the case history, observations of the child's responses to auditory stimuli, or medical examination strongly suggest the presence of auditory impairment, amplification should be considered, and the use of a hearing aid should be explored. It is of particular importance to realize that use of a hearing aid is not limited to children with a specific type or degree of hearing loss. Instead, amplification should be considered for any child having a hearing loss that may affect the development of normal speech and language whether the hearing impairment be conductive, mixed, or sensorineural.

The Child with Unilateral Hearing Loss. Until recently, a child with no usable hearing in one ear and near normal hearing in the opposite ear (Figure 88–8) was not considered to have a serious communication handicap. The basis for this assumption was that the good ear provided the necessary auditory input for most communication situations. Moreover, these children tended to develop normal speech and language skills despite the deprivation of sensory input to one ear. Consequently, such children were not felt to be candidates for amplification or auditory habilitation. Rather, the traditional recommendation for the child with unilateral hearing loss was that of preferential classroom seating.

Although there is a dearth of longitudinal data related to the linguistic skills, educational achievement, and psychosocial development of children with unilateral deafness, these children are often confronted with a variety of complex listening situations that could potentially interfere with the reception of speech. This is particularly evident in the open classroom, which emphasizes freedom of student mobility, and where the teacher moves about during a lecture. Consequently,

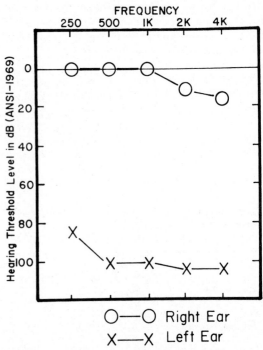

Figure 88–8 Audiogram of a child with a unilateral (left ear) sensorineural hearing loss.

the student with seating "preference" is often in an unfavorable listening situation.

The problems encountered by these children can be explained readily by a phenomenon known as the "head shadow effect." Studies have shown that there is a 6.4 dB reduction of speech intensity as the signal progresses from one ear to the other (Tillman et al., 1963). That is, the head serves to attenuate or reduce the intensity of sounds arriving to the ear farthest from the sound source. This effect is greatest for high frequency sounds, the frequency domain of many voiced and unvoiced consonants (such as, /s/, /sh/, /f/, /t/, and /th/). The importance of this frequency region as it relates to speech perception is that approximately 60 per cent of speech intelligibility is provided by these speech sounds (Gerber, 1974). Moreover, the intensity of the weakest consonant, /th/, is approximately 30 dB below that of the strongest vowel, /aw/, (Whetnall and Fry, 1964; Fletcher, 1970). Consequently, any reduction in the intensity of these important high frequency phonemes due to "head shadow" can result in reduced speech discrimination ability. For example, if the primary speech signal is directed to the impaired ear and a competing classroom noise is directed to the normal ear, the child will experience an unfavorable listening situation. Not only is the noise reaching the good ear at full impact, but the primary speech message is reduced in intensity as it crosses from one side of the head to the other. Hence, it is difficult for the child to perceive the softer primary message embedded in the background noise.

The "head shadow effect" can also result in a favorable listening condition. This occurs if the primary signal is directed to the normal ear and competing speech or noise is transmitted to the impaired ear. The result is a 6 dB reduction in the competing message when it arrives at the good ear, thus minimizing its interference with the primary speech signal.

Although many children with unilateral deafness are able to compensate for this handicap, others are not. Of particular concern is the child with unilateral hearing loss who has concomitant otitis media with effusion (OME) in the ear with otherwise normal hearing. For this child, pathologic conditions in the middle ear can further compromise educational achievement as well as the ability to perceive speech under adverse listening conditions.

Children with unilateral hearing losses who appear to experience problems in school may benefit from the CROS-type hearing aid described earlier (Fig. 88–7). Recall that this special hearing aid serves to route the signal from the impaired ear to the normal ear. When coupled to the normal ear with a non-occluding earmold (see page 1549), which attenuates the low frequencies and emphasizes the high frequencies, this alternative form of amplification transmits sounds emanating towards the poor ear and directs them to the normal ear, thus circumventing the effects of head shadow.

Our experience with CROS amplification in addition to that of others (Matkin and Thomas, 1971; Navarro and Vogelson, 1974; Shapiro, 1977) suggests that the child with unilateral deafness who experiences difficulty in school can benefit from this alternative form of amplification.

The Child with Minimal Conductive Hearing Loss. During the past several years, there has been considerable concern among audiologists, otolaryngologists, and pediatricians relative to the possible consequential effects that persistent middle ear effusion may have on speech and language development. Children with persistent middle ear effusion often present with only slight to mild, fluctuant, conductive-type hearing losses and do not typically experience significant difficulty understanding conversational speech. Since the incidence of middle ear effusion is greatest during the "critical period" for language acquisition, it is entirely possible that even a slight hearing loss can compromise the development of normal speech and language skills.

Unfortunately, few studies have reported the effects of middle ear effusion on speech, language, and cognitive development. A recurrent theme in each of these studies, however, is that children with a history of persistent middle ear effusion from early childhood perform significantly poorer than do their counterparts with normal hearing on speech, language, or educational achievement tests that require auditory processing or the production of a verbal response (Wishik et al., 1958; Ling, 1959; Holm and Kunze, 1969; Lewis, 1976; Needleman, 1977).

Although a careful examination of these studies reveals several deficiencies in experimental design, one cannot ignore the general conclusions that support the hypothesis that "otitis-prone" children demonstrate decreased communicative skills. Whether these differences are due to fluctuant conductive hearing loss associated with this disease and whether these differences are compensated for by most children in later years has not yet been determined.

Despite the paucity of longitudinal data, there remains a large population of children already "at risk" for language delay for whom even a slight conductive hearing loss could possibly be synergistic with the inherent lag in both cognitive and communicative skills. Among these children are (1) the mentally impaired, particularly children with Down syndrome, (2) the learning disabled, (3) the culturally disadvantaged child (that is, a child reared in an impoverished language environment), and (4) the child with a cleft palate.

In an effort to maximize the linguistic and educational potential of these children, it seems reasonable to recommend that they be considered candidates for mild-gain, low-output amplification during the course of medical treatment and until there is complete resolution of pathologic conditions in the middle ear. With the recent impetus toward early detection of middle ear effusion through the use of pneumatic otoscopy and acoustic immittance measures, in association with aggressive surgical treatment, it would seem equally important to recognize the need for audiologic intervention and continuous monitoring of hearing sensitivity. Advocation of a combined medical and audiologic approach to the management of these children should not be considered a universal recommendation for fitting hearing aids on all children with recurrent middle ear effusion. Rather, it is our contention that although a direct cause and effect relationship between middle ear effusion and impaired language development has not been clearly established, mild-gain amplification may assist this special population of children to capitalize on the auditory input from their environment and, thus, will help foster the acquisition of speech and language.

Binaural Versus Monaural Amplification

Probably no other area within the overall realm of hearing aid technology has received as much controversy as the concept of binaural versus monaural amplification. In fact, it would be relatively easy to provide considerable evidence to support both sides of the controversy. Unfortunately, much of the literature consists of case reports or experimental studies that have compared monaural/binaural functioning with normal hearers. Moreover, and perhaps most critical, is that there has been only limited objective research designed to evaluate the merits of binaural versus monaural hearing aids with young hearing-impaired children.

Despite the lack of scientific evidence to support such a practice, there is growing acceptance to fit young hearing-impaired children, whenever possible, with binaural hearing aids. The basic premise for this recommendation is that during the critical language acquisition period the child is in need of as much auditory stimulation as possible in order to facilitate language learning. This maximal input can best be achieved by stimulating two ears independently. The expected advantages from binaural hearing aids include (1) superior ability to localize a sound source in space, (2) enhanced differentiation between foreground and background noise (extracting a speech signal from a competing background of noise), (3) the same intensity level of sound applied to two ears is perceived louder than that delivered monaurally (binaural summation), and (4) with a separate microphone on each ear, the individual is always favorably situated relative to detecting speech originating from various locations (Ross, 1976).

Recently, Ross (1977) and Ross and Giolas (1978) presented a comprehensive review of those studies that compared monaural and binaural hearing aid performance in hearing-impaired adults. He stated that ". . . whatever auditory factors are involved in the binaural and monaural comparisons with hearing-impaired adults also pertain to congenitally hearing-impaired children, particularly those who have experienced early binaural amplification" (Ross, 1977). In general, the majority of studies suggest that the use of binaural hearing aids resulted in significantly greater improvement in word recognition ability than did monaural amplification. Significantly, no study has ever shown binaural inferiority.

Based on these findings and on the recognized need for maximal auditory stimulation to help foster speech and language development, children with bilateral sensorineural hearing losses should be fitted with binaural hearing aids. For those children who have acquired hearing loss postlingually, the decision to fit the child with one or two hearing aids should be made on the basis of individual needs and communicative demands.

Hopefully, future investigations with

young children will lend scientific support to these assumptions. As McConnell (1977) has stated, "This area poses an important challenge for the future, namely, more research conducted with the very young child, and perhaps, as well, the avoidance of locked-in positions that deny benefit to those whom we purport to help."

One additional factor that deserves consideration is the use of binaural amplification for children with asymmetric bilateral hearing loss. If binaural amplification is to be of any value for these children, then it is necessary to compensate for the unique deficits of the two distinct auditory systems through the selection of two different hearing aids having electroacoustic characteristics that compensate appropriately for the hearing loss in each ear.

An alternative approach to binaural amplification for the child with bilateral asymmetric hearing loss is the BICROS (*Bi*lateral *C*ontralateral *R*outing of *O*ffside *S*ignals) arrangement described by Harford (1966). BICROS is applicable to individuals with bilateral hearing losses when one ear is "unaidable." This system is simply a modification of the CROS that consists of placing an extra microphone on the side of the "unaidable" ear in addition to that already placed on the better ear. This "offside" microphone picks up signals originating near the poorer ear and transmits them to the better ear. At the same time, amplification is provided directly to the good ear by the hearing aid fitted to that side.

Couplers

Recall that the fundamental purpose of the coupler is to direct amplified sound to the user's ear. This is accomplished by a length of polyurethane tubing, an associated earmold, or both. Consequently, the specific term "earmold" that has been used frequently to describe this hearing aid component is not an accurate description. Rather, the term "coupler" is preferred since it denotes function that is not restricted solely to the earmold.

There are several variables associated with the coupler that can influence substantially the electroacoustic characteristics of the amplification system. For example, the length and diameter of tubing, depth of eartip penetration into the external meatus, the size of the earmold bore, and the acoustic seal provided by the earmold have all been shown to influence hearing aid amplification (see Lybarger, 1978, for a specific review of this material). In general, the cumulative effects of these variables can result in amplitude (i.e., gain fluctuations) as great as 15 to 20 dB, especially in the lower frequencies (300 Hz to 800 Hz). Moreover, these fluctuations have been associated with changes in behavioral responses, such as speech recognition, comfort levels, and subjective preference ratings for specific systems (Green and Ross, 1968; Jetty and Rintelmann, 1970; Konkle and Bess, 1974). Consequently, special consideration should be given to the coupler when selecting and fitting hearing aids with children.

In 1974, Konkle and Bess reported that differences in hearing aid performance resulted when either a custom or a stock coupler was used in the hearing aid evaluation. Based on these findings, they strongly recommended that custom-made couplers be used in the hearing aid evaluation. We especially endorse this procedure with children since the evaluation process may be extended over a period of several months. In addition, it may be necessary to have a custom earmold fabricated for each ear for maximal versatility in evaluation procedures.

A common problem related to the coupler in the pediatric population is the phenomenon of "acoustic feedback." This results when the earmold does not fit properly and amplified sound "leaks" out of the external meatus and causes a high-pitched "squeal." Acoustic feedback can be eliminated by ensuring an adequate seal between the earmold and the orifice of the external meatus. Unfortunately, feedback is often controlled by decreasing the volume control, resulting in less amplification. The problem of acoustic feedback is a common one in children since anatomic maturation of the external ear will result in an inadequate acoustic seal to a previously well-fitted earmold. Thus, it is important that the coupler be examined frequently and replaced whenever it is found to be inadequate. Inspection of the coupler should be a routine part of the otologic and audiologic follow-up evaluation. Parents should be instructed to examine the coupler when acoustic feedback results and to seek professional assistance from the audiologist to alleviate the problem.

Intentional alterations of the coupler are frequently employed in special circumstances. For example, venting the earmold by drilling a hole from the lateral to the medial surface equalizes pressure between the atmosphere and the external meatus, resulting in increased comfort. Moreover, venting the mold can cause a decrease in amplification of lower frequencies that may be beneficial for certain types of hearing loss (such as high-frequency precipitous hearing loss configurations). An open-type earmold can be used to accomplish this same reduction in low-frequency amplification. This earmold consists of a shell structured to hold the tubing at the external orifice of the ear canal without concurrent occlusion. When a powerful ear level hearing aid is used with the open mold, however, feedback typically results because of the close proximity between the microphone of the hearing aid and the amplified signal directed through the open earmold. To circumvent this problem, the CROS principle is applied, separating the microphone from the sound inlet tube. This hearing aid/earmold configuration has proved useful in providing amplification for asymmetric hearing loss characterized by mild reduction in sensitivity in the better ear.

An additional application of the open-type earmold relates to the child with a chronic draining ear. Appropriate amplification may be provided for such children by using a mild-gain hearing aid with a low SSPL coupled to an open earmold. One final caveat relative to ear couplers: All children should use earmolds fabricated of soft material that is nonallergenic.

ELECTROACOUSTIC CONSIDERATIONS FOR SELECTING APPROPRIATE AMPLIFICATION

The primary purpose of a hearing aid is to provide the child with sufficient acoustic cues with which to develop or maintain speech perception ability. Our goal is to maximize auditory information through amplification, thus permitting perception of as many of the phonemic elements of speech as possible. Because complete audiologic data relative to the degree of hearing loss are often incomplete with infants and young children, ". . . the basic premise of the initial hearing aid selection is that all electroacoustic recommendations are tentative" (Ross, 1975a). Hence, it is essential that the hearing aid be versatile. That is, the instrument should have external controls that will permit the audiologist to

adjust acoustic gain, frequency range, and SSPL as more complete audiologic information becomes available.

Acoustic Gain

It may be recalled from the discussion about the acoustic properties of a hearing aid that gain represents the amount of amplification that the instrument is producing at a specified volume control setting. Although it seems reasonable to assume that one can simply compensate for the degree of auditory deficit by selecting a hearing aid having an acoustic gain equal to the degree of hearing-loss, this is not how the impaired ear functions. If a child with an average hearing loss of 70 dB Hearing Threshold Level (HTL) were fitted with a hearing aid having an acoustic gain of 70 dB, a speech signal of 65 dB would be received at the child's ear at a sound pressure level (SPL) of 135 dB. This intensity level is probably not only above the child's tolerance threshold for intense sound (Hood and Poole, 1966; Morgan et al., 1974) but is also a level that is a potential hazard to residual hearing. Research has shown that most hearing-impaired adults and children subjectively set the gain of their hearing aid to approximately 50 per cent of threshold sensitivity (Brooks, 1973; Martin, 1973; Byrne and Fifield, 1974). For example, a child with a 70 dB hearing loss tends to set the "use gain" of the hearing aid to only 35 dB.

Byrne and Fifield (1974), McCandless (1976), Schwartz and Larson (1977a) and Byrne and Tonnison (1976) have all calculated that an increase of approximately 4.6 dB of gain is needed for every 10 dB of hearing loss. This method provides a simple calculation procedure for determining "use gain" requirements for hearing aid candidates, especially children. An alternative procedure for determining optimal "use gain" requirements had been introduced by Byrne and Tonnison (1976). They carefully developed a series of tables related to hearing aid gain requirements as a function of hearing loss. In order to determine "real ear" gain requirements, they compensated for the differences in loudness at various frequencies and accounted for differences in the intensity level of the various frequency components of average speech. These researchers reasoned that these adjustments (compensation for loudness differences across frequency, and differences in the intensity of various frequency components of speech) in the preferred gain/HTL function would allow all frequency components of speech to be presented with approximately equal loudness, thus minimizing the amount of amplification required to hear speech at a comfortable listening level.

Consider, for example, the child whose audiogram is shown in Figure 88–9. By referring to the data provided by Byrne and Tonnison (1976), one can determine the amount of "operating gain" necessary for this child to receive speech maximally. These predicted gain requirements, in decibels (dB) at each frequency, are shown numerically at the bottom of the audiogram. Improvement with amplification, estimated by subtracting the predicted "use gain" values from the child's pure tone thresholds at each frequency, is illustrated by the dashed line. Hence, for this child, the audiologist will select a series of hearing aids for further evaluation that approximate most closely the gain-by-frequency values shown in Figure 88–7. Of course, different "operating gain" values would be required for different hearing losses; however, the reader can easily obtain such values by

referring to the Byrne and Tonnison (1976) data. It is essential that we caution the reader that this procedure must not be considered a panacea for prescribing optimal amplification. Rather, it provides the audiologist with a set of guidelines with which to begin the search for the most appropriate amplification system.

Saturation Sound Pressure Level

Recall that the SSPL of a hearing aid refers to the greatest sound pressure level that the hearing aid amplifier is capable of producing regardless of the intensity of the input signal. Although SSPL is perhaps the most critical electroacoustic parameter for successful hearing aid use, it typically receives the least attention in the fitting of hearing aids to young children. The reason for this is based on the common misconception that a 1:1 relationship exists between SSPL and acoustic gain; that is, high-gain levels require the instrument to have excessively high output limits (greater than 130 dB SPL). On the contrary, these two parameters are mutually independent. It is entirely possible to reduce SSPL while maintaining high acoustic gain levels. A second misconception is that the threshold of discomfort for hearing-impaired listeners is approximately 130 dB SPL.

Implicit in this discussion is that the most common problem in fitting hearing aids to young children is that of overamplification. In fact, there is a plethora of evidence to suggest that most children fitted with amplification wear their hearing aids at gain settings that are insufficient to deliver speech at both an optimal and comfortable intensity level (Gaeth and Lounsbury, 1966; Brooks, 1973; Byrne and Fifield, 1974; Bess, 1976). Overamplification can be attributed to two primary factors: (1) SSPLs that exceed the child's threshold of tolerance for loud sounds and (2) the physical volume of the child's ear canal.

Recall that a common belief among many professionals in the hearing health field is that the loudness discomfort threshold approximates 130 dB SPL for the ear with sensorineural hearing loss. This universal misconception is based on an early study of tolerance limits reported by Silverman (1947). The results of this investigation indicated that the threshold of discomfort for pure tones was 120 dB SPL for normal

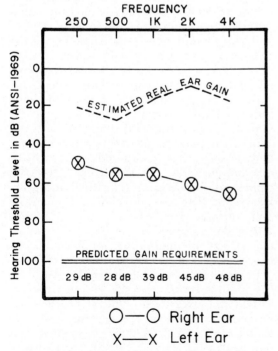

Figure 88–9 Example for predicting "real ear" gain requirements using the Byrne and Tonnison (1976) data for a child with a moderate bilateral sensorineural hearing loss.

hearers and 129 dB SPL for hearing-impaired listeners.

For many years following this investigation, hearing aids have been fitted with the belief that 130 dB SPL was a SSPL that would not permit amplified sounds to exceed the user's tolerance threshold. In 1966, however, Hood and Poole reported results of a classic study that demonstrated that loudness discomfort levels (LDLs) for both normal and hearing-impaired ears had been previously overestimated. They indicated that the loudness discomfort level for 90 per cent of 200 normal hearers ranged from only 90 to 105 dB SPL, whereas that for 200 subjects with cochlear hearing loss approximated 100 dB SPL. Since that time, numerous investigators (Bosatra, 1969; Schmitz, 1969; Stephans and Anderson, 1971; McCandless and Miller, 1972; Morgan et al., 1974) have supported the findings of Hood and Poole (1966) suggesting that the LDL for both normal and cochlearly impaired ears ranges between 90 and 110 dB SPL and not 130 dB SPL as was reported originally by Silverman (1947).

The second factor that contributes to overamplification is the relationship between ear canal volume and sound pressure measured in a closed cavity. Typically, the SSPL of a hearing aid is measured in a hearing aid test box with the instrument coupled to a "hard-walled" cavity that has a volume of approximately 2 cc and that presumably simulates the impedance characteristics of the average adult human ear.

Based on the principle of acoustic impedance, we know that the intensity of a sound trapped in a closed cavity is a direct function of the size of the cavity. Hence, when a signal of a specified intensity is introduced into both a large and a small cavity, the SPL measured in each cavity will be distinctly different: In general, the larger cavity will show a lower SPL than the smaller cavity.

Studies on the clinical measurement of acoustic impedance at the plane of the tympanic membrane have indicated that the volume of a hermetically sealed ear canal will be approximately 1.0 to 1.4 cc for an adult and 0.8 to 1.0 cc for a child, although the physical volume of an infant's ear canal may be as small as 0.5 cc (Northern, 1978).

When the output of a hearing aid is measured in both a 2 cc coupler and directly in the cavity formed by an earmold and a real ear canal, the SPLs developed in these two different cavities are found to differ by approximately 1 to 4 dB for frequencies below 1000 Hz and by as much as 12 dB from 1500 to 2000 Hz (Sachs and Burkhard, 1972; Larson and Studebaker, 1973). Although most audiologists are aware of this difference between coupler and real ear sound pressure measurements, others involved in the fitting of hearing aids to young children usually are not. In addition to the increase in maximal sound pressure that can be expected when generalizing from the hearing aid specification sheet to the real ear, it is equally important to consider that there will be an additional increase in sound pressure when an earmold is coupled to an ear canal having a volume less than 2 cc. In fact, each time the volume of the cavity is reduced by one half, sound pressure increases by approximately 6 dB. That is, the sound pressure generated by a hearing aid measured in a 2 cc cavity will be delivered to a 1 cc ear canal with about 6 dB more intensity than that shown on the hearing aid specification sheet (Cole, 1975).

On the basis of this discussion, it can easily be seen why children are often overamplified and wear their hearing aids at less than optimal volume control settings. Consider, for example, that for a child whose threshold of tolerance was 120 dB SPL, a hearing aid was selected with a SSPL of 130 dB and a gain setting of 50 dB. Since many environmental sounds, such as doors slamming, loud speech, and playground noise, often exceed 70 dB SPL, and SPLs measured in real ear canals may be greater than 12 dB above that reported on the hearing aid specification sheet, this child will receive amplified sound well above his or her threshold of discomfort. To compensate for this, the child simply reduces the gain of the instrument. Moreover, the possibility exists that continued exposure to overamplification may adversely affect the child's residual hearing (Hartford and Markle, 1955; Macrae and Farrant, 1965; Ross and Lerman, 1967; Kasten and Braunlin, 1970). For an excellent review of the potential effects of high-level amplification on hearing, see Rintelmann and Bess (1977).

In view of the possible damaging effects of overamplification, the SSPL of a hearing aid should not exceed the child's threshold of discomfort. Based on the existing evidence, Rintelmann and Bess (1977) have proposed that SSPLs not exceed 120 dB for children with mild to moderate hearing losses and 130 dB for children with severe to profound hearing losses. Children with conductive or mixed-type hearing losses are probably less susceptible to hearing aid trauma owing to the attenuating effect of the conductive pathologic condition.

Unfortunately, the U.S. Food and Drug Administration's recent document (1976) concerning the sale of hearing aids states that instruments with SSPLs exceeding 132 dB should contain a warning statement indicating that such hearing aids are potentially hazardous to residual hearing. Obviously, this excessively high output level was selected on the basis of the early data, which suggested that tolerance levels for individuals with sensorineural hearing loss approach 130 dB SPL. Based on the preceding discussion, it is our contention that for the prelingually deaf child, the SSPL should not exceed 120 dB for the initial hearing aid recommendation. Those children with less severe sensorineural hearing losses should be fitted with hearing aids having the least SSPL possible while maintaining appropriate acoustic gain.

Frequency Response

The final electroacoustic characteristic that requires consideration in the preselection process is the frequency range or bandwidth. The effective bandwidth of a hearing aid represents the lower and upper frequency limits of amplification, that is, the portion of the sound spectrum amplified at an intensity level sufficient to provide usable auditory information to the child.

The importance of selecting a hearing aid having a frequency range appropriate for a given hearing loss configuration can be un-derstood best by relating it to the acoustics of speech. The overall intensity of speech at a distance of one meter from the talker's lips is approximately 65 to 70 dB SPL. With each doubling of distance between the sound source and the receiver's ear, however, the SPL of speech decreases 6 dB.

The sounds of speech contain acoustic energy between about 100 and 8000 Hz. This frequency range is determined by measuring the long-term average speech spectrum, which is shown graphically in Figure 88–10. As illustrated, most of the energy of speech is below 1000 Hz with the greatest acoustic energy occurring between 500 and 600 Hz. If we now describe the frequency characteristics of individual speech sounds, we find that most of the vowel sounds are distributed in the lower frequencies (below 1000 Hz), whereas consonant sounds are reflected in the high frequencies, above 1000 Hz. Hence, it is readily apparent that vowels have considerably more intensity than consonants. In fact, the strongest vowel sound, /aw/, is 30 dB more intense than the weakest unvoiced consonant, /th/ (Fletcher, 1970).

Although low frequency vowels contribute more acoustic energy than do high frequency consonants, the consonants contribute 60 per cent to the intelligibility of speech. Thus, in practical terms, these data indicate that the more intense, low frequency vowels are considerably less important for speech intelligibility than are the weaker, high frequency consonants (Fletcher, 1970). Clearly, these concepts are of considerable importance in the selection of a hearing aid that will provide the greatest amplification in the frequency region most critical to speech intelligibility.

Figure 88–10 Graphic representation of the long-term average speech spectrum.

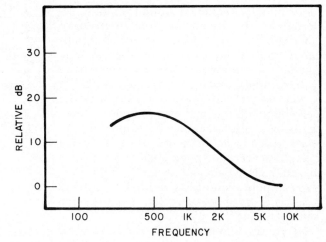

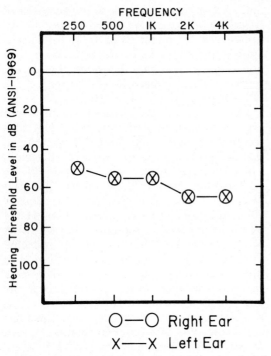

Figure 88–11 Audiogram of a child with a broad frequency hearing loss bilaterally.

Most standard commercially available hearing aids have a bandwidth from 300 Hz to 4000 Hz, although recent technological advancements in the hearing aid industry have resulted in an extension of this upper frequency limit to 7000 Hz and of the lower limit to 100 Hz. When considering amplification for a child having a broad-frequency hearing loss, that is, residual hearing in both the low and high frequencies, as shown in Figure 88–11, it is preferable to select a hearing aid having a frequency response characterized by suppression of low frequencies and emphasis of high frequencies. The importance of extended high frequency amplification is reflected by the frequency domain of most consonant sounds, which contribute significantly to the intelligibility of speech. The rationale for suppressing the low frequencies is that amplification of low frequency speech sounds has been shown to interfere with the perception of the higher frequency consonants by a phenomenon known as the "upward spread of masking," thus reducing overall speech perception ability (Danaher et al., 1973; Danaher and Pickett, 1975). Further, amplification of low frequency ambient noise is a common cause for dissatisfaction with a hearing aid.

In contrast to the child who has some residual hearing across the sound spectrum, many deaf children exhibit residual hearing only in the low frequencies (below 1000 Hz). For the child whose audiogram is shown in Figure 88–12, extended low frequency amplification may enhance perception of the more subtle features of speech, for example, timing, stress, and intonation patterns. The ability to perceive these acoustic cues is particularly important when the profoundly deaf child is attempting to learn speech and language patterns through amplified sound. As the child learns to discriminate among these perceptual cues, greater emphasis can be placed on improving consonant recognition through extended high frequency amplification. Hence, the need for a versatile hearing aid becomes clearly evident.

In summary, the preselection of hearing aids to be used for clinical evaluation with young children requires an understanding of the various interactions that can occur between the physical characteristics of a hearing aid and the perception of speech. It cannot be overemphasized that the selection of amplification for a young child with a sensorineural hearing loss is critically important to optimize the child's ability to receive speech and develop language. "The fitting of a hearing aid to a young child cannot be casually relegated to

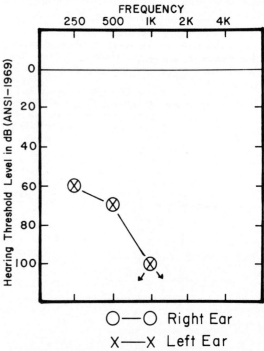

Figure 88–12 Audiogram of a child with residual hearing only in the low frequencies (250 to 500 Hz).

either a technician or any other individual who does not have a sophisticated appreciation of auditory physiology, auditory tests and measurements, the electroacoustic dimensions of hearing aid performance, the acoustics of speech, and current developments in psycholinguistics" (Ross, 1975b).

HEARING AID EVALUATION PROCEDURES

The primary purpose of a hearing aid is to provide the child with maximal auditory information, particularly speech, consistent with the hearing loss. The preceding section discussed the electroacoustic parameters that are critical to achieving this goal. From this information the audiologist will select a series of electroacoustic systems that are considered appropriate for the communicative needs of the child. The final question to be answered, however, is which of these instruments will provide the most optimal amplification? Consequently, it becomes necessary to compare and evaluate each of these instruments more formally prior to making a final recommendation.

It is important to understand that the evaluation and selection of hearing aids for the young child is an ongoing process. That is, because audiologic information relative to threshold sensitivity often is incomplete and since most children have a limited attention span, it usually is necessary to evaluate the child with amplification on several occasions. This, of course, does not imply that the prelingually deaf child cannot be fitted with a hearing aid. Rather, the recommendation of a specific amplification system must be considered tentative and subject to alteration subsequent to trial amplification and close parental and audiologic monitoring to assess changes in auditory behavior with various amplification systems.

The Prelingual Child

Although it is recognized that hearing aids facilitate auditory learning, the evaluation of different hearing aid systems with the prelingually hearing-impaired child is, at best, frustrating. The language deficit exhibited by these children precludes the use of procedures that depend on speech recognition scores to assess the merits of different hearing aids. Consequently, performance with amplification is evaluated with test stimuli that do not require a verbal response.

The Sound Field Audiogram. The most widely accepted procedure for evaluating hearing aids for the nonverbal hearing-impaired child is a comparison of unaided and aided responses to warble tone stimuli presented in a sound field at the octave frequencies 250 to 4000 Hz and the half-octaves 1500, 3000, and 6000 Hz. The relative differences between the unaided and aided response levels provide an estimate of "real ear" gain and frequency range of the hearing aid when coupled to the ear by an earmold. These measurements are made with each of a series of hearing aids, adjustment settings, or earmold configurations in an effort to determine which instrument or adjustment setting produces the greatest improvement from the unaided response levels with the least degree of irregularity across frequencies.

A comparison of the unaided and aided responses to warble tone stimuli for a child with a moderate sensorineural hearing loss is illustrated in Figure 88–13. According to the criteria used for selecting amplification with this procedure, hearing aid 1 provides the most "real ear gain" with the least irregularity across frequency. Results for hearing aid 2 indicated substantial threshold gain only at 2000 Hz, while hearing aid 3 is found not to provide any usable amplification.

Implicit in this procedure is that the child must be capable of responding appropriately to warble tone stimuli. Obtaining detailed and reliable information requires, therefore, an appreciation of the types of responses that are appropriate developmentally for a given age group. Research has shown that reliable minimal response levels can be obtained with infants five months of age and older with Visual Reinforcement Audiometry (Moore et al., 1977). Briefly, for this procedure the stimuli are presented to one of two loudspeakers with the expected response being that of localization to the sound source. If a response is obtained, it is reinforced by the activation of an automated toy or flashing light. Through the use of an operant conditioning paradigm, it is possible to evaluate relative improvement in response levels for infants as young as five months of age. We emphasize the term relative improvement for the young infant because research has shown that minimal response levels increase as a function of age (Matkin, 1977). Obviously, as

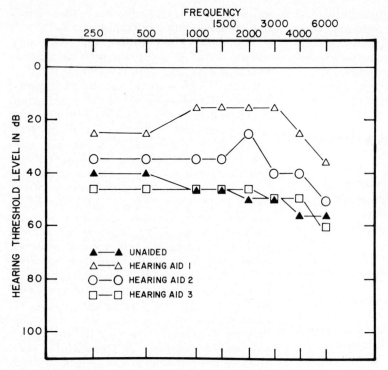

Figure 88–13 Comparison of unaided and aided responses to warble tone stimuli in a sound field for a child with a moderate bilateral sensorineural hearing loss.

the child approaches two years of age there is closer agreement between the expected maturational level of response and the actual sensitivity threshold to a particular stimulus, although improvement in response levels can continue until approximately age four. While these age-related differences in response levels must be recognized, they do not preclude the use of Visual Reinforcement Audiometry for assessing hearing aid performance with young infants.

The Acoustic Reflex Method. Acoustic reflex measurements have proved to be an integral part of the audiologic diagnostic test battery. In addition, however, acoustic reflex measurements provide an alternative objective procedure for evaluating differences among amplification systems with the prelingual hearing-impaired child for whom conventional sound field procedures are not applicable. Specifically, the acoustic reflex method can be used to compare "real ear" gain and frequency response at suprathreshold levels, to estimate threshold of discomfort, and to determine appropriate gain settings for hearing aids.

McCandless and Miller (1972) were among the first to suggest that measurement of the acoustic reflex threshold in a sound field could be used to set hearing aid gain and determine appropriate SSPLs for hearing aids. For this procedure, the child is seated in a sound field approximately 1.5 meters from a loudspeaker. The probe assembly of an acoustic immittance instrument is sealed hermetically into one ear while a hearing aid is coupled to the contralateral ear. Using a constant 60 to 70 dB SPL input signal of speech spectrum noise (Schwartz and Larson, 1977a), environmental sounds or conventional speech (Weber and Northern, 1978), or a speech vowel of low frequency content (Tato and Rainville, 1976), the volume control of the hearing aid is slowly raised until a reflex response is elicited, as illustrated by the strip chart recording shown in Figure 88–14. Hearing aid gain is set just below the point that induced a reflex response. According to Weber and Northern (1978), setting hearing aid gain just below the reflex threshold should avoid overamplification.

In 1976, Rappaport and Tait examined whether setting hearing aid gain via the acoustic reflex method yielded word recognition scores similar to those obtained when the hearing aid was adjusted to levels of +10 dB and −10 dB relative to the reflex threshold or to a subjective, most-comfortable-listening level as set by the patient. Results revealed that when hearing aid gain was adjusted to the reflex threshold, word recognition in noise was six to seven per cent higher than

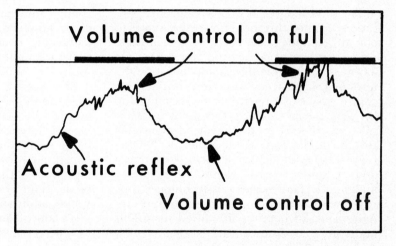

Figure 88–14 Strip chart record-ing illustrating the use of the acou-stic reflex method for adjusting the volume control of a hearing aid.

that achieved when gain was set by the patient or at +10 dB and −10 dB relative to the reflex threshold. These researchers conclud-ed, therefore, that this technique has impor-tant implications for determining a gain set-ting that will enhance speech intelligibility for young children.

More recently, Keith (1979) suggested guidelines for using the acoustic reflex threshold to determine hearing aid gain based on the results of a comprehensive study with 40 cochlearly impaired listeners. Keith reported that when the acoustic reflex thresh-olds under earphones are 95 dB HTL or less, the most satisfactory gain setting is *just below* the aided sound field reflex threshold. If, however, the reflex thresholds under ear-phones are greater than 95 dB HTL, then gain should be set *at* reflex threshold. He went on to state that these guidelines resulted in a gain setting approximating the most comfortable listening level for 75 per cent of the subjects tested.

An additional application of the acoustic reflex threshold method is its use as an objec-tive index of "real ear" gain and frequency response. Consistent with the sound field audiogram discussed previously, this proce-dure involves a comparison between unaided and aided acoustic reflex thresholds to warble tones or narrow bands of noise transduced through a loudspeaker, as shown in Figure 88–15. Here again, the hearing aid that pro-vides the greatest improvement in acoustic reflex threshold with the least degree of ir-regularity across frequencies is presumed to be the one that will be of maximal benefit to the child. Based on these criteria, the infor-mation in Figure 88–15 suggests that hearing aid B yielded the most improvement relative

to the unaided acoustic reflex threshold. The amount of suprathreshold "real ear gain" represents the difference between the unaid-ed and aided reflex thresholds at each fre-quency. In contrast to the sound field audio-gram, this objective procedure is of particular value for evaluating hearing aid performance with infants less than five months of age. In fact, Tonnison (1975) concluded that the acoustic reflex method should be part of every hearing aid evaluation procedure since it permits a more realistic assessment of hear-ing aid performance than that obtained from electroacoustic measurements made with a hearing aid test system (i.e., 2 cc coupler).

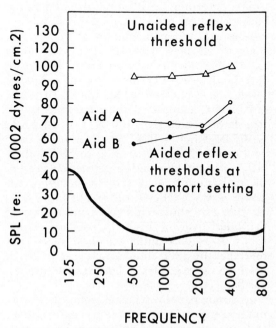

Figure 88–15 Comparison of unaided and aided acoustic reflex thresholds in a sound reflex.

The final and perhaps most valuable application of reflex threshold measurements is to obtain an index of maximal permissible power output of a hearing aid when the loudness discomfort threshold cannot be determined subjectively. Although considerable controversy exists regarding the relationship between the psychologic threshold of loudness discomfort and the acoustic reflex threshold (McCandless and Miller, 1972; Niemeyer, 1971; Dudich et al., 1975; Denenberg and Altshuler, 1976; Keith, 1979), many audiologists have found this technique to be extremely useful for estimating output requirements of hearing aids fitted to infants and young children (for an excellent review of loudness discomfort and the acoustic reflex, see Northern, 1978).

Horning (1975), for example, reported that the determination of SSPL requirements via acoustic reflex threshold levels at 500, 1000, and 2000 Hz has resulted in improved fitting of hearing aids to adults and children who were previously not satisfied with amplification. She stated that "... an increasing number of mild to moderate hearing-impaired youngsters who previously would have been unaidable ... are successfully wearing and benefiting from aids selected on the basis of acoustic reflex measurement." Similar success has been reported more recently by McCandless (1976), Rainville (1976), and Bragg (1977).

To determine SSPL requirements for young children, acoustic reflex thresholds are established under earphones at octave frequencies of 500 to 4000 Hz. These threshold values are then converted from a hearing threshold level reference to sound pressure level (American National Standards Institute, 1970). For example, if the earphone reflex threshold at 1000 Hz is 100 dB HTL, the SPL is 107 dB when a TDH-39 earphone is used as the transducer. According to McCandless (1975), the aided sound pressure delivered to the ear should not exceed the unaided earphone acoustic reflex threshold by more than 10 dB. For those children with severe to profound hearing losses that do not exhibit reflex thresholds under earphones, we contend that the SSPL should not exceed 120 dB until tolerance levels can be assessed audiologically.

In summary, the acoustic reflex threshold method may prove valuable for determining appropriate gain and SSPL requirements of hearing aids and for assessing the performance of different amplification systems with young children. This technique cannot be used, however, with children who exhibit pathologic conditions of the middle ear, which will either alter or negate the reflex response.

The Speech Spectrum Procedure. Despite the value of both the sound field audiogram and acoustic reflex methods for assessing differences in peformance among hearing aids, they often present limited information about the child's potential for receiving speech with amplification. A modification of the sound field procedure that may contribute additional information relative to the reception of amplified speech was reported by Gengel and colleagues (1971) and reviewed more recently by Schwartz and Larson (1977a).

Similar to the sound field audiogram, the test procedure consists of establishing aided thresholds or minimal response levels (in SPL) to warble tones or narrow bands of noise in a sound field with the hearing aid volume adjusted to a comfort level setting or just below the acoustic reflex threshold. To estimate the average level above threshold at which each frequency band of speech will be perceived during normal conversation, the aided threshold SPLs are subtracted from precalculated average speech levels. These average speech levels represent the amplitudes of corresponding segments in normal conversational speech within the frequency range 500 to 4000 Hz. The aid of choice is that which is capable of amplifying the widest region of the speech spectrum 10 to 20 dB above the child's sound field aided response levels.

Sample data from a child with a moderate to moderately severe sensorineural hearing loss are illustrated in Figure 88–16 with specific data depicted in the inserted table. Recall that threshold values are in SPL and not in hearing threshold level. From these data, an estimate of the potential for receiving speech with each hearing aid can be derived by subtracting the aided warble tone or narrow band noise thresholds from the precalculated average speech levels at each frequency. Accordingly, hearing aid 2 is more appropriate since it delivered greater amplification over a wider area of the speech spectrum. Here, the difference between the aided threshold and the average speech levels exceeded 15 dB from 500 to 2000 Hz and 10 dB at 4000 Hz. Conversely, the amplified average speech levels produced by hearing aid 1 approached 10 dB at only 250 and 500 Hz,

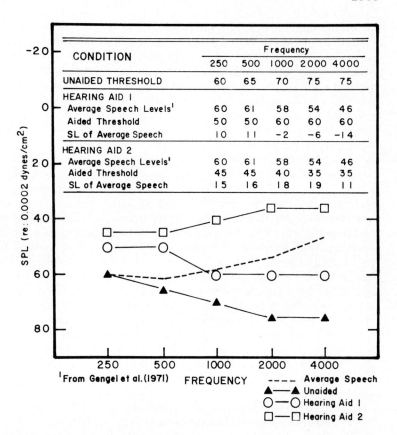

Figure 88–16 Example of the speech spectrum procedure (Gengel et al., 1971) for assessing differences in performance between two hearing aids for a child with a moderate to moderately severe sensorineural hearing loss.

CONDITION	Frequency				
	250	500	1000	2000	4000
UNAIDED THRESHOLD	60	65	70	75	75
HEARING AID 1					
Average Speech Levels[1]	60	61	58	54	46
Aided Threshold	50	50	60	60	60
SL of Average Speech	10	11	−2	−6	−14
HEARING AID 2					
Average Speech Levels[1]	60	61	58	54	46
Aided Threshold	45	45	40	35	35
SL of Average Speech	15	16	18	19	11

[1] From Gengel et al. (1971)   FREQUENCY   ---- Average Speech
▲——▲ Unaided
○——○ Hearing Aid 1
□——□ Hearing Aid 2

suggesting that the various frequency components of average speech above 500 Hz would be potentially inaudible to the child with this instrument.

Schwartz and Larson (1977b) compared results obtained from the traditional sound field procedure to those derived from the speech spectrum method. In general, results for ten hearing-impaired children indicated that for children with severe to profound hearing losses, the sound field audiogram tended to overestimate the amount of usable amplification afforded by a particular hearing aid. That is, while a substantial threshold improvement was demonstrated, the amount of "real ear" gain was still not sufficient to permit any area of the speech spectrum to be perceived with amplification. Differences between procedures did not exist, however, for those with mild or moderate hearing losses. On the basis of these findings, Schwartz and Larson (1977b) concluded that for children with severe to profound hearing losses, the speech spectrum method may provide more information than the unaided versus aided threshold procedure for estimating the child's potential to receive speech with amplification.

The Formula Approach. During the past

several years, a number of investigators have developed simple formulas for prescribing hearing aids (Wallenfels, 1967; Byrne and Tonnison, 1976; Shapiro, 1976; Berger, 1976). Recall that Byrne and Tonnison developed a series of tables that can be used to determine appropriate "operating gain" for a given hearing loss. A similar "prescriptive procedure" that has received attention in recent years is that advocated by Berger. He proposed a gain/frequency response formula for predicting optimal amplification based on the following postulates:

1. The amplified signal reaching the impaired ear should improve speech intelligibility over that unaided for typical conversational levels;
2. The desired gain will have an average magnitude slightly greater than one half of the client's pure tone threshold;
3. Amplification of low frequency ambient noise is detrimental;
4. Less intensity is required at 500 Hz and below than at frequencies more important to understanding speech;
5. Speech sounds above 4000 Hz are extremely weak and relatively unimportant to intelligibility.

Berger (1976) presented several formulas

for predicting hearing aid gain requirements at each frequency based on the air conduction pure tone audiogram. The specific denominators in each weighted formula were chosen to mirror the long-term average spectrum of speech between 500 and 3000 Hz. Included in each formula is an arbitrary reserve gain of 10 dB above the predicted "operating gain" similar to that described by Byrne and Tonnison (1976). To avoid the mathematical computation of the gain/frequency response formula, Berger has also developed a series of tables for use as an easy reference for determining the maximal gain requirements necessary at each frequency to provide optimal amplification for a specific hearing loss.

Subsequent to computing the required gain/frequency specifications, a series of hearing aids that have electroacoustic characteristics consistent with these criteria are selected for evaluation. The objective is to select the instrument that will result in aided sound field thresholds that approximate most closely those predicted from the formula or table.

In addition to the gain/frequency formula, Berger (1976) also recommended guidelines for determining maximal permissible SSPLs based on the individual's loudness discomfort level (LDL) obtained under earphones. According to Berger (1976), the maximal SSPLs at each frequency are:

250 Hz — 6 dB or more below that at 500 Hz

500 Hz — LDL +8 dB, or 110 dB SPL, whichever is lower

1000 Hz — LDL +4 dB

2000 Hz — LDL +6 dB

4000 Hz — LDL +6 dB

If the LDL is not achieved at the limits of the audiometer or if the clinician is unable to assess the LDL, Berger (1976) suggested that an approximate range of minimal acceptable output levels can be estimated by the following formula:

[78 dB (SPL) + operating gain of the hearing aid]

The value of 78 dB is derived from the representative intensity of loud speech, 75 dB SPL, and a 3 dB margin of error. The 3 dB margin of error is added since the current hearing aid standard (American National Standards Institute, 1976) permits SSPL accuracy to vary ±4 dB from 500 to 4000 Hz from that reported on the manufacturer's specification sheet for a given hearing aid. Although the use of this "prescriptive procedure" appears encouraging, it has not received sufficient clinical trial to permit an evaluation of its efficacy in fitting hearing aids in young children.

The Older Child

The evaluation of hearing aid performance with children who have developed speech and language represents a modification of procedures used with adults. For these children hearing aids are compared relative to scores obtained on tests designed to assess word recognition ability.

The most common procedure is to administer monosyllabic word recognition tests in a sound field at a constant intensity level, usually 50 dB HTL, both in quiet and in the presence of a competing noise or speech. The difference in word recognition scores obtained with a hearing aid from those achieved in an unaided condition reflects the magnitude of improvement in speech intelligibility afforded by amplification. The recommended hearing aid, therefore, is that which provides the most substantial improvement in word recognition, particularly in the presence of competing noise or speech.

Hood (1970) recommended that word recognition tests be administered at several intensity levels representing soft, average, and loud conversational speech. This additional step, although time-consuming, enables the audiologist to assess performance of different hearing aids under a variety of listening conditions. For example, if the speech signal was presented to the child at 80 dB HTL, a level representing loud speech, and the child complained that the speech level was "too loud" with a given hearing aid, then some form of output limiting should be recommended, or a different hearing aid should be evaluated. This should avoid overamplification and, ultimately, rejection of the hearing aid.

One important factor to consider when evaluating the merits of a specific hearing aid on the basis of word recognition scores is that the speech testing materials must be appropriate for the child's receptive vocabulary age. If receptive vocabulary age is not considered, it becomes difficult to determine if the discrimination score reflects accurately the child's ability to hear and understand speech or is related to a language deficit. For the nonverbal child or one having a vocabulary age between four and five years, it may be necessary to assess word recognition ability using a picture identification test that does not require a verbal response and is composed of stimulus words that are within the child's recognition vocabulary. Presently, the best standardized test for these children is the *Word Intelligibility by Picture Identification* (WIPI) test developed by Ross and Lerman (1970).

A second step in the hearing aid evaluation procedure is the determination of "real ear" gain/frequency response. As with the prelingual child, this information is obtained by comparing aided and unaided thresholds to warble tone stimuli presented in a sound field at octave frequencies 500 to 4000 Hz and half-octave frequencies 1500, 3000, and 6000 Hz.

Finally, and most critical, is the measurement of tolerance for loud sounds. The usual procedure is to instruct the child to respond when loudness reaches a level that would be intolerable for listening during an extended period of time. A speech signal is presented through earphones, and the intensity is increased slowly until that level is reached. This value is then converted from HTL to SPL. In addition, tolerance thresholds are also determined for pure tone stimuli from 250 to 4000 Hz, thus providing information that will assist in selecting an amplification system having SSPLs across frequencies that do not exceed the child's loudness discomfort level.

To summarize, the evaluation of hearing aid performance with the nonverbal child traditionally consists of a comparison of unaided and aided response levels to warble tones presented in a sound field. An alternative procedure for the young infant, the acoustic reflex method, has the advantage of providing an objective assessment of real ear gain/frequency response, appropriate gain setting of the hearing aid, and permissible maximal power output levels. Although these two procedures contribute valuable clinical information, the speech spectrum method permits the audiologist to define the area of the speech spectrum that may potentially be audible to the child with amplification. The formula approach appears to simplify the selection procedure, but research to date is limited relative to the use of "prescriptive amplification" for fitting hearing aids to young children. The results reported for adults, however, are encouraging. The evaluation of hearing aid performance with the older child represents a modification of those procedures used for adults, which consist of a comparison of aided and unaided word recognition scores in quiet and in the presence of competing noise or speech, as well as a determination of the loudness discomfort level.

Regardless of the procedure used to evaluate differences among amplification systems, the recommendation of any hearing aid must be considered tentative and subject to alteration following a trial period, which will permit close observation and monitoring of changes in the child's auditory behavior with amplification. Significantly, the recommendation of a hearing aid must not be viewed as an end product but rather the initial step toward maximizing the child's potential for developing speech and language.

HEARING AID MANAGEMENT

For the hearing-impaired child, the hearing aid represents a means to minimize the consequential effects of auditory deprivation. In order to insure that the child receives maximal auditory input with amplification, it is essential that the hearing aid perform satisfactorily on a continual basis. Without this, the primary objective of enhancing the child's potential for acquiring speech and language through auditory stimulation will not be realized. Hence, whenever a hearing aid is recommended for a child, regardless of his or her age and degree of hearing loss, a follow-up monitoring program is mandatory if the hearing aid is to maximize auditory learning.

Unfortunately, most studies indicate that the majority of children's hearing aids used in the classroom are either grossly inadequate or inoperable (Gaeth and Lounsbury, 1966; Porter, 1973; Zink, 1972; Northern et al., 1972; Coleman, 1972; Bess, 1976). In fact, these studies have estimated that as many as 40 to 50 per cent of children's hearing aids worn in the classroom perform unsatisfactorily. Such findings are, at best, discouraging when one considers the amount of time and effort spent to provide the child with optimal amplification.

Insuring consistent and adequate performance of children's hearing aids can be accomplished only by a daily hearing aid check performed by the parents and teachers coupled with periodic electroacoustic analysis of the hearing aid by the audiologist. Continual inquiry by the audiologist, otolaryngologist, and pediatrician to insure that the child's parents have taken the responsibility for managing the hearing aid and earmold is essential.

One encouraging technical advancement has been the development of a Hearing Aid Malfunction Detection Unit (Roeser et al., 1977). This instrument is capable of monitoring hearing aids "in situ," producing an easily detected signal in the event of malfunction (such as low battery voltage, broken cords, cracked receivers, or volume control turned off). Although such a device shows a great potential for monitoring hearing aid function, the current cost of manufacturing this instrument precludes large-scale purchase. Hence, at present the least expensive, albeit sensitive, method for performing a daily hearing aid check is the use of a pocket-size battery tester and a personal earmold for the parent. It cannot be overemphasized that without a properly functioning hearing aid, ". . . effective use of residual hearing is a myth shrouded with good intentions" (Ross, 1975a).

CONCLUSIONS

A recurrent theme throughout this chapter has been that oral communication is acquired early in life through auditory experiences. Whetnall and Fry (1964) indicated that many of the severe speech and language deficits resulting from congenital hearing loss can be minimized by capitalizing on residual hearing through wearable amplification during the first 18 months of life. The selection of appropriate amplification, therefore, is considered critical to the acquisition of speech and language for the prelingually hearing-impaired child and to the maintenance of communicative skills for children with acquired hearing losses.

The selection of appropriate, usable amplification for the young child requires the cooperative efforts of an audiologist, otolaryngologist, pediatrician, and educator. Failure to recognize the need for aggressive *audiologic* intervention is apt to result in continued depression of speech and language skills and the eventual inability of the child to interact with his or her environment.

Since the physician is often the first professional to see these children, it is imperative that he or she appreciate the need for auditory habilitation. As stated previously, "The fitting of a hearing aid to a young child cannot be casually relegated to a technician or dismissed as a trivial affair" (Ross, 1975b). Hence, nonmedical management of the hearing-impaired child must be provided by the audiologist who is familiar with the various methods and procedures used for selecting, evaluating, and monitoring amplification systems. All efforts shoud be directed toward providing maximal auditory information consistent with the child's hearing loss. The hearing aid represents only the initial step of a long-term habilitative program designed to integrate these children into an auditory society.

Hearing aid selection with young children requires extensive knowledge and appreciation of the interacting effects that various acoustic characteristics of amplification systems have on the potential for receiving speech. "If we are to consider the habilitative process of these children to be a continually emerging one, leading ultimately to complete integration into our society," then total commitment of all professionals involved ". . . is mandatory. Truly, . . . we can afford to do no less." (McConnell, 1977).

REFERENCES

American National Standards Institute. 1970. Specification for audiometers. ANSI S3.6–1969. New York, American National Standards Institute.

American National Standards Institute/Acoustical Society of America. 1976. Specifications for hearing aid characteristics. ANSI/ASA S3.22–1976, New York, American National Standards Institute.

Berger, K. W. 1976. Prescription of hearing aids: A rationale. J. Am. Aud. Soc. 2(3):71.

Bess, F. H. 1976. Characteristics of children's hearing aids in the public school. Final Report, Dept. Health, Education and Welfare, U.S. Office of Education, Grant and Procurement Management Division, 41, USC 252 (c) (d).

Bosatra, A. 1969. On the semeiological value of loudness discomfort level. Int. Audiol., 8:164.

Brackmann, D. E., and House, W. F. 1976. Direct stimulation of the auditory nerve. In Northern, J. L. Hearing Disorders. Boston, Little, Brown and Co., pp. 257–268.

Bragg, V. C. 1977. Toward a more objective hearing aid fitting procedure. Hear. Instruments, Sept. 6.

Brooks, D. 1973. Gain requirements for hearing aid users. Scand. Audiol., 2:199.

Byrne, D., and Fifield, D. 1974. Evaluation of hearing aid fittings for infants. Br. J. Audiol., 8:47.

Byrne, D., and Tonnison, W. 1976. Selecting the gain of hearing aids for persons with sensorineural hearing impairments. Scand. Audiol., 5:51.

Carhart, R. 1975. Amplification for the hearing impaired. In Tower, D. The Nervous System 3: Human Communication and Its Disorders. New York, Raven Press, pp. 291–298.

Cole, W. A. 1975. Hearing aid gain: A functional approach. Hear. Instruments, 26(10):22.

Coleman, R. F. 1972. Stability of children's hearing aids in acoustic preschool. Final Report, Dept. Health, Education and Welfare, U.S. Office of Education, National Center for Educational Research and Development, 522466.

Danaher, E. M., Osberger, M. J., and Pickett, J. J. 1973. Discrimination of formant frequency transitions in synthetic vowels. J. Speech Hear. Res., 16:439.

Danaher, E. M., and Pickett, J. J. 1975. Some masking effects produced by low frequency vowel formants in persons with sensorineural hearing loss. J. Speech Hear. Res., 18:261.

Davis, H. 1948. The articulation area and the social adequacy index for hearing. Laryngoscope, 58:761.

Denenberg, L. J., and Altshuler, M. W. 1976. The clinical relationship between the acoustic reflexes and loudness perception. J. Am. Audiol. Soc., 2(3):79.

Dirks, D., and Carhart, R. 1962. A survey of reactions from users of binaural and monaural hearing aids. J. Speech Hear. Disord., 27:311.

Dudich, T. M., Keiser, M., and Keith, R. W. 1975. Some relationships between loudness and the acoustic reflex. Impedance Newsletters, American Electromedics Corp., 4;12.

Endicott, J. 1978. Personal communication, Radioear Corp.

Fletcher, S. 1970. Acoustic phonetics. In Berg, F., and Fletcher, S. The Hard of Hearing Child. New York, Grune & Stratton, pp. 57–84.

Food and Drug Administration. 1977. Hearing aid devices. Professional and patient labeling and conditions for sale. Federal Register, 41:78.

Gaeth, J. H., and Lounsbury, E. 1966. Hearing aids and children in elementary schools. J. Speech Hear. Disord., 31:289.

Gengel, R. W., Pascoe, D., and Shore, I. 1971. A frequency response procedure for evaluating and selecting hearing aids for severely hearing impaired children. J. Speech Hear. Disord. 36:341.

Gerber, S. E. 1974. The intelligibility of speech. In Gerber, S. E. 1974. Introductory Hearing Science — Physical and Psychological Concepts, Philadelphia, W. B. Saunders Co., pp. 238–260.

Green, D. S., and Ross, M. 1968. The effect of a conventional versus a nonoccluding (CROS-Type) earmold upon the response of a hearing aid. J. Speech Hear. Res., 11:638.

Harford, E. R., and Markle, D. 1955. The atypical effect of a hearing aid on one patient with congenital deafness. Laryngoscope, 65:970.

Harford, E. R. 1966. Bilateral CROS: Two-sided listening with one hearing aid. Arch. Otolaryngol., 84:426.

High, W., Fairbanks, G., and Glorig, A. 1964. Scales of self-assessment of hearing handicap. J. Speech Hear. Dis., 29:215.

Holm, V., and Kunze, L. 1969. Effects of chronic otitis media on language and speech development. Pediatrics, 43:833.

Hood, J. D., and Poole, J. P. 1966. Tolerable limits of loudness: Its clinical and psychological significance. J. Acoust. Soc. Am., 40:47.

Hood, R. B. 1970. Modifications in hearing aid selection procedures. Acad. Rehabil. Audiol. Newsletter, 3:7.

Horning, J. 1975. Tympanometry and hearing aid selection. National Hear. Aid J., April, (8):50.

Jetty, A., and Rintelmann, W. F. 1970. Acoustic coupler effects on speech audiometric scores using a CROS hearing aid. J. Speech Hear. Res., 13:101.

Kasten, R. N., and Braunlin, R. J. 1970. Traumatic hearing aid usage: A case study. Presented at the annual convention of the American Speech and Hearing Association, New York.

Kasten, R. N. 1978. Standards and standard hearing aids. In Katz, J. 1978. Handbook of Clinical Audiology, 2nd ed. Baltimore, The Williams and Wilkins Co., pp. 485–500.

Keith, R. W. 1979. An acoustic reflex technique of establishing hearing aid settings. J. Am. Aud. Soc., 5:71.

Konkle, D. F., and Bess, F. H. 1974. Custom-made vs. stock earmolds in hearing aid evaluations. Arch. Otolaryngol., 99:140.

Konkle, D. F., Rintelmann, W. F., and Freeman, B. A. 1976. A comparison of electroacoustic hearing aid measurements from three commercial test instruments. Presented at the Annual Convention of the American Speech and Hearing Association, Houston.

Larson, V. D., and Studebaker, G. A. 1973. Sound pressure levels in ear canals and couplers. Presented at the American Convention of the American Speech and Hearing Association, Detroit.

Lenneberg, E. H. 1967. Biological Foundations of Language. New York, John Wiley & Sons, Inc.

Lewis, N. 1976. Otitis media and linguistic incompetence. Arch. Otolaryngol., 102:387.

Ling, D. 1959. The education and general background of children with defective hearing. Unpublished Research Associateship Thesis, Cambridge University, Cambridge, United Kingdom.

Lybarger, S. F. 1978. Earmolds. In Katz, J. Handbook of Clinical Audiology. Baltimore, The Williams and Wilkins Co., pp. 508–523.

Macrae, J., and Farrant, R. 1965. Effect of hearing aid use on the residual hearing of children with sensorineural deafness. Ann. Otol. Rhinol. Laryngol., 74;409.

Martin, M. C. 1973. Hearing aid requirements in sensorineural hearing loss. Br. J. Audiol., 7:21.

Matkin, N. D., and Thomas, J. 1972. The utilization of CROS hearing aids by children. Maico Audiological Library Series, X:8.

Matkin, N. D. 1977. Assessment of hearing sensitivity during the preschool years. In Bess, F. H. Childhood Deafness: Causation, Assessment & Management. New York, Grune & Stratton, pp. 127–134.

McCandless, G., and Miller, D. 1972. Loudness discomfort and hearing aids. Nat. Hear. Aid J., June, 7, 18, 32.

McCandless, G. A. 1975. Future directions. In Jerger, J. Handbook of Clinical Impedance Audiometry. New York, American Electromedics Corp., pp. 186–187.

McCandless, G. A. 1976. Special considerations in evaluating children and the aging for hearing aids. In Rubin, M. Hearing Aids — Current Developments and Concepts, Baltimore, University Park Press, pp. 171–182.

McCartney, J., and Sorenson, F. 1974. A comparison of a self-assessment scale of hearing impairment and selected audiometric population. Presented at the Annual Convention of the American Speech and Hearing Association, Las Vegas.

McConnell, F. E. 1977. Childhood deafness: A prospective. In Bess, F. H. Childhood Deafness: Causation, Assessment and Management. New York, Grune & Stratton, pp. xx–xxi.

Menyuk, P. 1971. The Acquisition and Development of Language. Englewood Cliffs, N.J., Prentice-Hall, Inc.

Moore, J. M., Wilson, W. R., and Thompson, G. 1977. Visual reinforcement of head-turn responses in infants under 12 months of age. J. Speech Hear. Disord., 42:328.

Morgan, D. E., Wilson, R. H., and Dirks, D. D. 1974. Loudness discomfort level: Selected methods and stimuli. J. Acoust. Soc. Am., 56;577.

Navarro, M. R.,and Vogelson, D. O. 1974. An objective assessment of a CROS hearing aid. Arch. Otolaryngol., 100:58.

Needleman, H. 1977. Effects of hearing loss from early recurrent otitis media on speech and language development. In Jaffe, B. F. Hearing Loss in Children. Baltimore, University Park Press, pp. 640–649.

Nett, E., Doerfler, L., and Matthews, J. 1960. The relationships betwen audiological measures and handicap. Unpublished manuscript. Vocational Rehabilitation Project No. 167.

Niemeyer, W. 1971. Relations between the discomfort level and the reflex threshold of the middle ear muscles. Audiology, 10:172.

Nobel, W., and Atherley, G. 1970. The hearing measurement scale: A questionnaire for the assessment of auditory disability. J. Aud. Res., 10;193.

Northern, J. L., McChord, W., Fisher, E., et al., 1972. Hearing services in residential schools for the deaf. Maico Audiological Library Series, XI:4.

Northern, J. L. 1978. Hearing aids and acoustic impedance measurements. Monographs in Contemporary Audiology, Minneapolis, MAICO Hearing Instruments Inc., 1(2).

Olsen, W. 1977. Physical characteristics of hearing aids. In Hodgson, W. R., and Skinner, P. H. Hearing Aid Assessment and Use in Audiologic Habilitation. Baltimore, The Williams and Wilkins Co., pp. 17–41.

Oyer, H. 1966. Auditory Communication for the Hard of Hearing. Englewood Cliffs, N.J., Prentice-Hall, Inc., p. 14.

Peters, G., and Hardick, E. 1974. The relationship between some measures of hearing loss and self-assessment of hearing handicap. Presented at the Annual Convention of the American Speech and Hearing Association, Las Vegas.

Pickett, J. M. 1975. Speech processing aids for communication handicaps: Some research problems. In Tower, D. The Nervous System 3: Human Communication and Its Disorders. New York, Raven Press, pp. 299–304.

Porter, T. A. 1973. Hearing aids in a residential school. Am. Ann. Deaf., 118:31.

Rainville, M. 1976. Hearing aid fitting using stapedial reflex measurement. Proceedings of III International Symposium on Impedance Audiometry. Acton, MA, American Electromedics Corp., pp. 49–50.

Rappaport, B. Z., and Tait, C. A. 1976. Acoustic reflex threshold measurement in hearing aid selection. Arch. Otolaryngol., 102:129.

Rintelmann, W. F., and Bess, F. H. 1977. High-level amplification and potential hearing loss in children. In Bess, F. H. Childhood Deafness: Causation, Assessment and Management, New York, Grune & Stratton, pp. 267–293.

Roeser, R. J., Glorig, A., Gerkin, G. M., et al. 1977. A hearing aid malfunction detection unit. J. Speech Hear. Disord., 42:351.

Ross, M. 1975a. Hearing aid selection for children. In Pollack, M. C. Amplification for the Hearing Impaired. New York, Grune & Stratton, pp. 207–242.

Ross, M. 1975b. Hearing aids for young children. In Glasscock, M. E. Otolaryngol. Clin. North Am., 8(1):121.

Ross, M. 1976. Amplification systems. In Lloyd, L. Communication Assessment and Intervention Strategies. Baltimore, University Park Press, pp. 295–324.

Ross, M. 1977. Binaural versus monaural amplification for hearing impaired individuals. In Bess, F. H. Childhood Deafness: Causation, Assessment and Management, New York, Grune & Stratton, pp. 235–249.

Ross, M. 1978. Classroom acoustics and speech intelligibility. In Katz, J. Handbook of Clinical Audiology. Baltimore, The Williams and Wilkins Co., pp. 469–478.

Ross, M., and Giolas, T. G. 1978. Auditory Management of Hearing Impaired Children. Baltimore, University Park Press.

Ross, M., and Lerman, J. 1967. Hearing aid usage and its effect upon residual hearing. Arch. Otolaryngol., 86:639.

Ross, M., and Lerman, J. 1970. A picture identification test for hearing impaired children. J. Speech Hear. Res., 13:44.

Sachs, R., and Burkhard, M. 1972. Earphone pressure response in ears and couplers. Presented at the 83rd Annual Meeting of the Acoustical Society of America, April.

Schmitz, H. 1969. Loudness discomfort level modification. J. Speech Hear. Res., 12:807.

Schwartz, D. M., and Larson, V. D. 1977a. Hearing aid selection and evaluation procedures in children. In Bess, F. H. Childhood Deafness: Causation, Assessment and Management. New York, Grune & Stratton, pp. 217–233.

Schwartz, D. M., and Larson, V. D. 1977b. A comparison of three hearing aid evaluation procedures for young children. Arch. Otolaryngol., 103:401.

Shapiro, I. 1976. Hearing aid fitting by prescription. Audiol., 15:163.

Shapiro, I. 1977. Children's use of CROS hearing aids. Arch. Otolaryngol., 103:712.

Silverman, S. 1947. Tolerance for pure tones and speech in normal and defective hearing. Ann. Otol. Rhinol. Laryngol., 56:658.

Stephans, S. D., and Anderson, C. M. 1971. Experimental studies on the uncomfortable loudness level. J. Speech Hear. Res., 14:262.

Tato, J. M., and Rainville, M. J. 1976. Utilisation du reflexe stapedien pour l'adaption des protheses. Audiology, 15:428.

Tillman, T., Kasten, R., and Horner, J. 1963. The effect of head shadow on the reception of speech. Presented at the Annual Convention of the American Speech and Hearing Association.

Tonnison, W. 1975. Measuring in-the-ear gain of hearing aids by the acoustic reflex method. J. Speech Hear. Res., 18;5.

Townsend, T. H., and Schwartz, D. M. 1977. A comparison of four hearing aid measurement systems. J. Speech Hear. Res., 20:718.

Wallenfels, H. G. 1967. Hearing Aids on Prescription. Springfield, IL., Charles C Thomas.

Weber, H. J., and Northern, J. L. 1978. Selection of children's hearing aids: Unpublished report, Colorado Department of Health program.

Whetnall, E., and Fry, D. 1964. The Deaf Child. Springfield, IL. Charles C Thomas.

Wishik, S., Kramm, E., and Koch, E. 1958. Audiometric testing of school children. Public Health Reports, 73:265.

Zink, G. D. 1972. Hearing aids children wear: A longitudinal study of performance. Volta Review, 74:41.

Chapter 89

EDUCATION OF THE DEAF

William N. Craig, Ph.D.

Deafness, particularly when sustained prior to the age when normal children begin to utter their first words, produces a set of conditions that alter a person's perception of and adjustment to his or her environment. Although hearing loss can be measured, and certain medical and acoustic corrections may be possible, the hearing-impaired child still must make significant adjustments to the hearing society in which he or she lives. Children with very mild hearing losses will benefit considerably from otologic procedures, a hearing aid, or both, but the adjustment becomes more difficult as the hearing loss increases. When the loss becomes marked, or more than 55 dB in the speech range, the combined skills of the otolaryngologist, pediatrician, educator, audiologist, and others must be brought to bear upon the interwoven set of problems that result — hearing loss, measured loss of auditory discrimination, delayed or nonexistent speech production, delayed or nondeveloping language patterns, and modified social behavior and understanding. Deafness becomes more than a hearing problem; it becomes a communication problem affecting social interactions and lifelong social and personal adjustments. Perhaps the amazing paradox, as a young deaf child matures, is that he or she can learn to make these adjustments and to become a productive citizen.

In June of 1976, the National Advisory Committee on the Handicapped estimated that there were 49,000 deaf children, 328,000 hard-of-hearing children, and 40,000 deaf and blind and other multihandicapped hearing-impaired children of school age in the United States. They also estimated that well over 90 per cent of deaf students were being afforded special education services, whereas only 20 per cent of the hard-of-hearing students and only 40 per cent of the deaf multihandicapped were being offered such services or programs. With the enactment of P.L. 94–142, the Education of All Handicapped Children Act, the federal role in providing services for hearing-impaired children has been increased substantially, prompting an increase in attention to these children. The aid which this federal emphasis provides has been further delineated by Section 504 of the 1973 Vocational Rehabilitation Act, signed by the Secretary of Health, Education and Welfare in April of 1977.

DEFINITION OF HEARING IMPAIRMENT

Various definitions of hearing impairment are available, but perhaps the most comprehensive and useful is that approved by the Conference of Executives of American Schools for the Deaf (CEASD) in 1975. This statement, replacing an earlier and less precise definition (CEASD, 1938), focuses upon both the parameters and the educational ramifications of hearing impairment. A portion of this definition is presented in Table 89–1, which outlines the relations among (1) threshold levels of hearing, (2) the probable

1569

Table 89–1   EDUCATIONAL IMPLICATIONS FOR HEARING-IMPAIRED CHILDREN

Hearing Threshold Levels (ISO)	Portable Impact on Communication and Language	Present-Day Implications for Educational Settings	
		Type[1]	Probable Need
Level I,[2] 35–54 dB	Mild	Full Integration	Most Frequent
		Partial Integration	Frequent
		Self-Contained	Infrequent
Level II, 55–69 dB	Moderate	Full Integration	Frequent
		Partial Integration	Most Frequent
		Self-Contained	Infrequent
Level III, 70–89 dB	Severe	Full Integration	Infrequent
		Partial Integration	Most Frequent
		Self-Contained	Frequent
Level IV, 90 dB and above	Profound	Full Integration	Infrequent
		Partial Integration	Frequent
		Self-Contained	Most Frequent

1. *Full integration* means total integration into regular classes for hearing students with special services provided under direction of specialists in educational programs for deaf and hard of hearing. *Partial integration* means taking all classes in a regular school, some on an integrated basis and some on a self-contained basis. *Self-contained* means attending classes exclusively with other deaf and/or hard of hearing classmates in regular schools, special day schools or special residential schools.
2. It is assumed that these decibel scores were obtained by a qualified audiologist using an average of scores within the frequency range commonly considered necessary to process linguistic information.

*Courtesy of Conference of Executives of American Schools for the Deaf[CEASD], 1975. Report of the ad hoc committee to define deaf and hard of hearing. Am. Ann. Deaf, *120*:509.

impact of these thresholds on communication and language, and (3) implications of hearing thresholds for educational settings. Other parts of the statement deal with a more general division of hearing loss (into "deaf" and "hard-of-hearing"), with "age-of-onset" factors, and with other variables that can be critical for determining placement alternatives.

Basically, the term "hearing impairment" is used in a generic sense to indicate losses ranging from mild to profound. The "deaf" person, then, is "one whose hearing disability precludes successful processing of linguistic information through audition" (CEASD, 1975, p. 509) even with the use of currently available amplification. The "hard-of-

hearing" person, on the other hand, is able to understand and to process spoken language — at least under ideal listening conditions — through audition. From an educational perspective, this dichotomy serves as a starting point for the selection of both a school placement and an instructional approach to the hearing-impaired child. Thus, children with hearing losses at Levels I and II in the Conference definition (hearing losses less than 70 dB) might well be termed "hard-of-hearing," and those in Levels III and IV might be termed "deaf." However, the audiogram gives only a part of the information relevant to hearing impairment. Also specified in the 1975 definition is the age at which the hearing loss was sustained (prelingual or postlingual). If the child has acquired speech and language prior to becoming deaf, he or she will be able to process new spoken and written input based upon a linguistic foundation established through hearing. The child who is born deaf or becomes deaf before approximately 18 months of age, however, will not have the advantage of this auditory language base. The prelingually deaf child must learn by alternate and inferior means not only the meanings of words but also the various syntactic rules and transformations that govern their use. This is an infinitely more difficult task.

The severity of the hearing loss and the age of onset thus are factors that interrelate to determine what language concepts have been acquired prior to the child's deafness and what language learning potential remains. For example, a child who has a profound hearing loss sustained at or about age 10 or 11 years will have the language background necessary to succeed in a regular school program with the addition of tutoring aid to the program. The same child with a profound loss that occurred at birth or shortly thereafter would need an intense program of instruction beginning at an early age.

In addition to this basic assessment of hearing, the Conference definition (1975) recognizes several other decisions that must be made for each child. The educational recommendations may differ when "psychological, personal, and/or social problems exist in addition to hearing impairment"; when the "appropriateness of a given educational setting or methodology" changes as the child progresses from one age level to the next (CEASD, 1975, p. 509); or when changes in language proficiency, communication skills, advancement in instructional levels, and development of personal and social competencies indicate that it is time for reevaluation. As can be seen, this definition attempts to relate the different components of a hearing loss as well as to indicate what the graphs that assess hearing levels may mean. For the professional team, each of these components must be given a value and must be related to the hearing-impaired child's prospects for the future. Table 89–1 is presented with these cautions in mind, and it is intended to serve only as a starting point for relating hearing loss to the current indications for appropriate educational settings. It does not fully account for the processing of information through audition, which, in the general definition, is the significant dividing point for differentiating the deaf from the hard-of-hearing person. The intensive work necessary to instruct a deaf child is in very sharp contrast to the corrective work that can be effective with hard-of-hearing children. This basic concept of language processing potential should not be minimized for children with severe hearing losses sustained at an early age.

INITIAL EVALUATION

Early assessment of hearing loss can be vital for optimal educational intervention as well as for medical correction. The otolaryngologist, pediatrician, educator, audiologist, psychologist, and others that compose the initial evaluation team must, of course, evaluate each child within that specialist's area of competency, and certain immediate choices must be made.

The general roles of the otolaryngologist and the audiologist have been discussed in detail in previous chapters. For the child with hearing impairment, these roles take on an added significance that must be recognized for that child to benefit maximally from their services. The initial objective is to determine the possibility of correcting the hearing impairment through medical procedures. If a sensorineural loss precludes total correction, the possibilities should next be considered for reducing the severity of the loss whenever a conductive component is present in conjunction with the sensorineural. Even with young school-age children, the combination of conductive and sensorineural hearing loss is much more prevalent than was previously suspected. Svitko (1976), for example, studied children with moderately severe to profound losses, combining data from pure tone audiograms, tympanograms, and otoscopic examinations, and reported a high incidence of otherwise undetected middle ear problems. Prevalence data on middle ear pathology in children have been reported by Jerger (1970) and by Berry, Bluestone, Andrus, and Cantekin (1975), who utilized similar procedures. Even though the sensorineural component may stabilize, this attention to the additional possibility of a conductive hearing loss should continue throughout the school years and must involve coordination among the otolaryngologist, the audiologist, and the educator.

The psychologist performs a number of

diagnostic functions at this early stage of the child's development. One of the first is to rule out nonorganic possibilities, a task that for young children will require both experience and intuition. A second role is to assess the child's range of intellectual performance in order to establish a base for recommending a treatment or educational program. Frequently, case history records, parent reports, and direct observation are the only tools available here; however, some formal testing may be possible. Vernon and Brown (1964) present a useful summary of intelligence measures most commonly used with deaf and hard-of-hearing children. However, they caution that scores on preschool and early school-age deaf and hard-of-hearing children tend to be extremely unreliable, especially if the score for intelligence is low. Interpretation errors can also be caused by determining language potential from nonverbal tests, poor performance of a child in a given test situation, administration of tests by psychologists who are not familiar with deaf children, lack of recognition of the fact that tests and test procedures may be modified for deaf children, inattention to the meaning of the time constraints of some tests, and the highly questionable use of any group test. However, tests are useful when an experienced psychologist selects the instrument, knows the patterns that are "normal" for deaf children, and combines these scores knowledgeably with other data.

The psychologist's familiarity with educational programs and with the students they serve is one of the essential components of the decision-making process. The psychologist can provide a point of contact with the educator and a resource to which the otolaryngologist and audiologist can first turn for specialized services dealing with more than hearing loss *per se*.

At this point, we have offered a broad-based definition of the deaf and the hard-of-hearing child, a definition that begins to become useful within the parameters just reviewed — the evaluation procedures and information that are collectively assembled by the otolaryngologist, audiologist, and psychologist. This relationship between the definition of deafness and the alternatives available for dealing with it from the fields of medicine, audiology, and psychology provide an initial base for understanding an individual deaf child. Once the hearing-impaired child is evaluated, he or she may be referred to one of a number of educational alternatives.

EDUCATIONAL PLACEMENT OPTIONS

Very briefly, the alternatives for educational placement of the hearing-impaired child may include the following (CEASD, 1975): (1) self-contained classes within regular schools, within special day schools, or within special residential schools; or (2) integrated classes, either with full integration in regular school classes or partial integration in regular school classes. In addition, for severely involved multihandicapped students, there are also day and residential facilities specifically geared to deal with multiple problems, for example, with children who are blind and/or severely mentally retarded as well as deaf.

A listing of the schools and classes for the deaf in the United States is provided annually in the Reference Issue of the American Annals of the Deaf, which also includes information on the type of programs offered, the number and range of students served, the educational staff employed, and the status of recent graduates (Craig and Craig, 1981).

LEVEL I — THE HARD-OF-HEARING CHILD (Mild Loss)

A child whose hearing loss places him or her in the Level I category (a hearing threshold of 35 to 54 dB) and who is within the normal intelligence range will probably be identified to the local school district for future reference and then will be referred to a local tutor, clinic, or hearing and speech organization. This is the "hard-of-hearing child" who can benefit significantly from amplification, can learn language auditorily, and can be expected to learn to cope rather well in his or her own neighborhood of hearing friends. A local school system will serve the child later and will provide supportive services. As with all handicapped children, the local educational agency will write an individual educational plan for him or her, with the parents participating in the development of this plan. It will be necessary, however, to provide specific instruction in the use of a hearing aid and to pay close attention to language patterns, speech skills, and interrelationships with teachers and hearing friends. To the general public, this child represents the "uncomplicated" problem of deafness where success seems assured. This may, in fact, be the case. However, this is also the child who may seem inattentive, may feel left out of activities, and may experience some learning problems due directly to the hearing loss.

Some years ago, Myerson (1963) wrote a psychology text on hearing-impaired persons in which he discussed adjustment patterns of the hard-of-hearing. Essential to his approach is that the hard-of-hearing person may frequently find himself or herself in overlapping role situations as he or she changes from one experience to another, such as from home to school. He described three basic adjustment patterns: withdrawal to the relatively restricted but safe life with other hearing-impaired people, rejection of the hearing-impaired group in favor of a hearing society, or the balanced scheme of associations with both hearing and hearing-impaired groups. At issue is not the absolute endorsement of one of these three patterns for an individual but the determination of patterns that fit an individual at a given time. Each pattern, under certain circumstances, may be beneficial or at least rewarding to a hearing-impaired student. The concepts of conflict, insecurity, and frustration in some interactions with hearing people must be balanced for each individual with the friendship status and success he or she may experience in a more restricted environment. In short, what effect does "marginal" status have on the individual? Any plan for educating a hard-of-hearing child must account for these psychological parameters. To the extent that a hearing impairment alters normal adjustments, techniques must be developed for coping with society within the three patterns described.

For the hard-of-hearing child, the usual focus of education would begin in a nursery school with hearing students. The elementary school years of the hearing-impaired child's life may be spent in a class with hearing students and with supportive services or in a class with hearing-impaired pupils in which part of the instruction is in regular classrooms. In fact, Public Law 93–380, Title VI-B, Section 612, states that school systems must employ their resources as follows:

... to the maximum extent appropriate, handicapped children, including children in public or private institutions or other care facilities are educated with children who are not handicapped, and that special classes, separate schooling, or other removal of handicapped children from the regular education environment occurs only when the nature or the severity of the handicap is such that education in regular classes with the use of supplementary aids and services cannot be achieved satisfactorily.

The group of students included in the Level I category would certainly benefit from this approach, assuming that the supplementary resources were available and that other multiple handicapping conditions were not present. The local education agency has the basic responsibility for these programs by law, but it is important that the otolaryngologist, special educator, audiologist, psychologist, and others involved in evaluation present a clear picture of the hearing-impaired child's potential and indicate a professional judgment on appropriate placement.

LEVEL II — THE HARD-OF-HEARING CHILD (Moderate Loss)

When the hearing loss moves into the moderate range (hearing thresholds from 55 to 69 dB), the current definition refers to this loss as "Level II." Within this range, a hearing aid is frequently a useful but not adequate instrument for hearing speech, developing language skills, mastering academic subject matter, and participating in normal social interactions. These skills may be developed in a variety of educational settings, but the instructors or supportive personnel need to include in their programs teachers of deaf children rather than speech and hearing therapists alone. The distinction between levels I and II is twofold: The acquisition of speech becomes significantly affected and must be taught systematically along with a carefully developed language program; and the rate of academic learning and the techniques for effective social interactions must be adjusted to the learning of basic language skills. Should the hearing loss have occurred prior to age one or two years, the combined speech and language problems may be considerable.

At this hearing level, differences among individual students become more pronounced. Griffing (1970) has organized a review of plans for educational programs and services for hard-of-hearing children that are pertinent for this group of students. He draws a distinction between students being "eligible" for placement in a program and programs being "suitable" for such a placement. Eligibility is often determined merely by a school-age child's place of residence, while suitability is determined by the needs and abilities of individual children and may change from time to time as the child becomes older. Running the continuum from full integration to full-time special education are some 10 alternatives, including tutoring, partial integration, special classes, and special schools. In some instances, school systems refer children to a special assessment class to provide an appropriate diagnostic and evaluative situation for the preschool and kindergarten years before an initial academic decision is made. This procedure has much to recommend it since early evaluation instruments, as previously noted, provide neither the reliability nor the necessary time that are possible in a special assessment class. The teacher and the supportive personnel working together during these first few years have an unusual opportunity to continue the evaluation of a child's performance over time, to initiate language and speech training experiences, and to observe the child's interactions with other students. The case history, clinical evaluations, and early unstructured experiences can be observed in the more realistic training setting.

Should the child respond well in this setting, curriculum planning may well be organized along the same lines as those used with hearing students, although with considerable attention to communication skills such as reading, writing, speaking, speech reading, and auditory training. In some instances, sign language and finger spelling may be used with Level II children, but the auditory channel is still quite useful. (The manual modes of communication will be discussed in more detail for children in Level IV, where their use is more frequent). If parent cooperation is enlisted, much of the early work with these children can be encouraged at home, often with considerable success. A talented group of teachers who are academically prepared to work with hearing-impaired children and their parents is essential. For children with losses in the Level II range, various instructional procedures for speech, language instruction, and speech reading have a specific

structure, have proponents and detractors, and are abundantly reported in professional journals. However, the major requirements for programs serving children with moderate hearing losses are that they have a number of consistent options and that the professional educators be well trained and competent.

The concept of "mainstreaming" is probably most effective with children falling into the Level I and Level II categories, although some of its advocates would extend this concept to those with greater hearing loss. Mainstreaming is a method of management that involves both an educational placement and an instructional process based on keeping the child in the regular school program ("least restrictive environment") as long as his or her needs can be met satisfactorily there. It does recognize that deaf students have a wide variety of special educational needs and recognizes that a "continuum of educational settings" may be needed from time to time. Basically, the question is whether or not special education services can be brought successfully to the regular school program or whether special classes, a separate school, or home tutoring may be most appropriate. As a deaf child's communication skills and educational achievement levels begin to vary significantly from those of students in the regular classroom, this continuum of services should be explored. Birch (1975) and Northcott (1973) have summarized a number of these approaches to mainstreaming of deaf children, and Aiello (1975) has assembled a teacher training workshop packet on individualized instruction. This latter reference has materials designed for four levels, to focus on items such as the initial exclusion and frustration felt by some children in the regular class, informal diagnostic techniques to be used by the teacher, development of individual modes for teaching, and what are termed "learning games." Although it is beyond the scope of this report to describe or evaluate fully the mainstreaming possibilities, it is important to recognize this effort both from the point of view of the federal incentive for developing a continuum of instructional opportunities for deaf children and because of the rapidly increasing volume of information on the subject. There is general agreement that individual educational plans should be organized in a usable form by special educators at all points along the educational continuum.

LEVEL III — THE DEAF CHILD
(Severe Loss)

Beginning with Level III (hearing threshold of 70 to 89 dB), even for deaf children with no additional handicaps, the situation becomes more complicated. Although the full continuum of placements may be possible in some locations, the number and type of supportive services needed increase rapidly. Early tutoring and family counseling is important to adjust the child to the home and community. Full integration in preschool or early grade school may be possible, but only with the help of some very determined parents and a very alert child. Partial integration under well-staffed and well-organized conditions can be effected, and some variations for integration in selected classes or for out-of-class activities are frequently effective. However, a normal child with a Level III hearing threshold is no longer able to learn speech, language, use of residual hearing, reading, or other skills without intensive work by a qualified and specially trained teacher of the deaf. Should a second handicap in addition to deafness augment the educational problem, the teacher's skills and techniques in a special school or class will be fully challenged. The sensorineural hearing loss at this point will be sufficient to distort speech sounds regardless of the hearing aid recommended, and excessive amplification may even add to the distortion of the sound, particularly in classrooms not treated for ambient noise. Large school systems with well-organized classes — classes with five or more children with similar hearing losses and at approximately the same age level — can serve these children well. A smaller school system, where the special classes are not organized by age groups, intellectual potential, and academic level, will be severely handicapped in its program planning for children at either a Level III or Level IV hearing threshold. Such a program can succeed only where the staff-to-student ratio is about one to two, and since the supportive services in smaller districts are likely to be limited, the program still cannot provide the optimal educational or social experience for the child.

Another approach for these districts and perhaps for some larger school districts is to use the resources of a residential school for deaf children or a day school for deaf students as the instructional base. In fact, both residential schools and day schools may offer a variety of opportunities for integration with hearing students under carefully designed programs. Frequently, arrangements can be made for work with the parents as soon as the deaf infant is identified, and many of the facilities run well-developed preschool programs. These preschool programs, as well as those in later years, may provide for partial integration of deaf with hearing students in neighboring schools. Craig and Salem (1975) have reviewed partial integration of deaf and hearing students, with particular emphasis on the techniques used by residential schools and their relationships with cooperating local school districts. In particular, this study reviews the selection of deaf students for partial integration, the use of supportive personnel, program evaluation, and administrative arrangements necessary to initiate a partial integration program. Included, also, are short selected descriptions of model programs from various parts of the country. Of the 75 residential schools surveyed, 39 schools reported some form of partial integration with local schools, and seven schools for deaf children reported having hearing students enrolled — an apparent reversal of the usual integration trend. Essentially, partial integration has two thrusts: It can be accomplished either by the local special classroom assigned in a local school district or by residential schools and day schools specifically designed for deaf children. This aspect of the continuum of services for deaf children has been formally recognized by the Conference of Executives of American Schools for the Deaf (1977) in an endorsement of four statements that develop the concept of high-quality programs for deaf students combined with a least restrictive placement. Such an emphasis provides for a recognition of the "pervasive nature of deafness and the severity of a handicapping condition which seriously affects the organization of language, speech and auditory information, as well as the satisfaction of the human need to communicate." The statement concludes by asserting that "the right to 'least restrictive' placement must not result in a 'most restrictive' situation in terms of opportunity for educational and social development" (CEASD, 1977, p. 70) for the deaf child. In the final analysis, the placement of children with Level III audiograms is most dependent on the professional interpretation of this statement. The emphasis is placed on identification and enrollment of deaf students with a hearing threshold level of 70 dB or greater in settings where professionally qualified teachers of deaf children are employed; where homogeneous groups of students in terms of hearing loss, intellectual potential, academic level, and social adjustment are programmed; and where the supportive services of otolaryngologists, psychologists, audiologists, and related professionals are readily available. For most children with this hearing threshold, these are minimal requirements.

It should be noted that these services will offer a better educational opportunity for the capable deaf student to reach his or her fullest potential as well as for the multihandicapped student to reach a level of independent living. In many instances, the intensive work with the deaf child suggested here enhances later opportunities to attend college, technical school, or another postsecondary facility. Listings of the postsecondary placements of deaf students are published annually (Craig and Craig, 1981), and in a number of schools, this record is impressive. An interesting account of deaf persons who have succeeded in professional employment has been compiled by Crammattee (1968), who has explored the communication problems, education, career selection, and various job-related experiences of successful deaf adults. Two thirds of the respondents in his study had received most of their elementary and secondary education in schools for the deaf. The main point of interest here is that residential schools and day schools for deaf students at this hearing threshold level can and do provide programs for very bright students, as well as for those with average intelligence or those having additional handicapping conditions.

LEVEL IV — THE DEAF CHILD
(Profound Loss)

At Level IV (hearing thresholds of 90 dB and above), deafness may be considered profound, and self-contained classes for these students are most frequently needed. As with Level III (70 to 89 dB threshold), which is sometimes referred to as severe deafness, full integration may occur in selected cases, but the complexities of language through audition alone, or even with ideal amplification

combined with part-time hearing, speech, and reading tutoring, would indicate that a more comprehensive approach is necessary.

Communication Methodology

In a number of schools the use of finger spelling and sign language is encouraged. Both of these are manual techniques. Finger spelling, or "dactology," involves the use of manual equivalents for each letter of the alphabet, as shown in Figure 89–1. "Sign" language involves use of specific hand configurations to correspond with whole words or whole ideas. The term "total communication," which is currently applied to an overall use of these techniques, has been defined in 1976 by the Conference of Executives of American Schools for the Deaf as a "philosophy incorporating appropriate aural, manual and oral modes of communication in order to ensure effective communication with and among hearing-impaired persons." As a philosophy dealing only with communication modes, it does not endorse any specific curriculum approach; rather, curriculum planning is based on the incorporation of total communication into a number of teaching systems. Quite possibly, the same school may offer a total communication system at one age level and not another or for one hearing threshold group but not another. Currently, there are few school systems that do not offer total communication as an alternative at some point. Mindel and Vernon (1971) present a rationale for the use of total communication based on the premise that it is the only system "that can be introduced at a very early age that is effective, because it conveys critical non-ambiguous language formation as it is needed." Schlesinger and Meadow (1972) also discuss a wide range of possibilities for the use of total communication, stating that "optimal conditions would include an early input of manual communication, associated with excellent oral/aural training wherein both signs and speech are equally valued by parent (and subsequently, by child)," and therefore would be free of stress. The proponents of total communication have established a logical basis for their encouragement of combining spelling and sign language, and, in fact, a number of revised sign language systems have evolved. At the preschool and elementary levels, a dictionary of signed English (Bornstein et al., 1975) has been

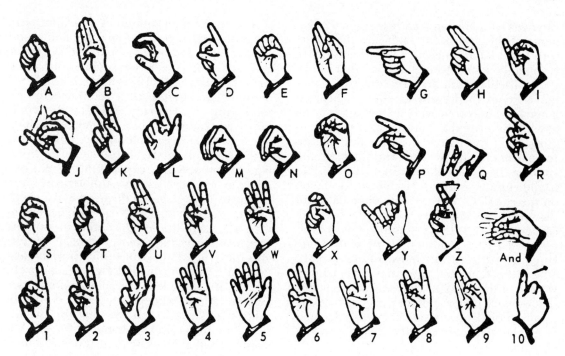

American Manual Alphabet of the Deaf.

Figure 89–1

published, and among books used to learn sign language, one of the more popular has been that edited by Riekehof (1979). A journal devoted to sign language studies is edited by Stokoe (1981) and appears quarterly.

The major advantage of a total communication approach is that signs are highly visual and deaf students can learn the system rather rapidly. As used by most deaf adults, however, simple conversational situations do not require adherence to English syntax, and, in a sense, sign language, such as Ameslan (Fant, 1976), can serve as a language of its own with its own set of rules. For use with children in schools, various modifications have been made to set up a closer correspondence between sign and English, such as adding English components and changing word order. Since these changes are rarely required to communicate with other deaf people, the additional signs are frequently dropped in informal conversation. In short, sign language is a natural and useful communication tool among deaf people and with hearing people who know the language. As Schlesinger and Meadow (1972) have suggested, under optimal conditions where speech and listening skills are successfully combined with sign language, the grammatical problems of total communication may be

avoided. There is little question that a signed vocabulary of objects (nouns) and selected action verbs and adjectives can be conveyed through the normal use of sign language. Whether speech skills or English grammatical forms will develop concurrently is still a question. The use of finger spelling alone or in combination with signs is also a helpful adjunct, but this skill requires a reading comprehension level adequate to spell the words and to keep up with changes in word forms (the difference between "fair" and "fare," for example), verb changes (the irregular verbs such as "go," "went," "gone"), and other language components. If sign language were a word-by-word translation of English, this problem might be minimal; however, the correlation between sign and spoken language is more of an interpretation than a translation of English into common usage. Nevertheless, total communication is widely employed, has popular appeal with many parents, and is a valuable tool for a number of students in the Level III and IV hearing threshold groups.

There are schools or departments within schools that prefer to encourage an oral option, especially for younger children, rather than to adopt a universal total communication mode. There are advantages and disadvantages with this approach as well. Proponents of this approach emphasize that, even with Level III and Level IV thresholds, there is generally some residual hearing that can be used. Tactile vibrators are sometimes employed both to present a sense of hearing language and to provide a feeling for the rhythm or prosodic features of spoken language, and speech reading provides vital information from the lips and face of the speaker. Basically, the residual hearing and tactile clues give the deaf child information on the vowels and overall language patterns; the speech-reading clues help to identify critical consonants. If these stimuli are effectively integrated, the combination of words into language patterns can move rather rapidly. The tradeoff is that signs may give a faster word-by-word recognition manually but that the auditory patterns of language, which are significant in learning syntactic relations, may be established more rapidly through oral instruction.

A program with an oral emphasis usually employs a very specific method of teaching speech that is strictly adhered to year by year. Integration with hearing students is encouraged to provide models for oral skills and social interactions. At the same time, the oral approach is likely to be not only a philosophic basis for teaching but also a pragmatic development of techniques. Visual cues are abundantly used, including speech reading, reading, and pictured information, but formal sign language either is delayed until the child is older or is not encouraged at all. Most "oral" programs emphasize the complimentary use of auditory and visual information; some place more emphasis on the auditory, others on the visual (oral) only. In practice, there are few strictly oral programs for children, beyond the elementary school level, when the children's hearing losses fall into the Level III and IV range. The older children either are integrated more fully into the local school districts or are shifted to total communication after the oral language base is established. Although an emphasis on early speech and auditory skills may seem futile at first, many children at this earlier age level do respond, and some remarkable results have been attained. The ideal, of course, would be to identify children at a very early age who could benefit maximally from either a total communication approach or an oral-aural approach; however, because of the number of variables involved, this is beyond the present state of the art.

As with the total communication approach, the oral-aural system has its proponents, and considerable literature about the system is available. The Alexander Graham Bell Association for the Deaf (1971) has published a set of guidelines to use as a reference for establishing oral programs for hearing-impaired children. These guidelines include items such as organization and philosophy, administration, staff, enrollment, facilities, equipment, services, curriculum, parent orientation, and evaluation. Although it is not exhaustive, this manual does serve as a check list for program quality. Nix (1975) has examined research studies that tend to support total communication as a system of preference but found the conclusions to lack appropriate support owing to test design problems, uncontrolled variables, improper generalizations, and poorly selected control groups. His conclusion was that the profession should not seek "a panacea for all children but rather to work toward development of quality programming which includes alternative approaches" for individual students. Lane (1976) looked at severely and profoundly deaf graduates from an oral-aural school program over a period of 55 years and found that oral education had been successful (in terms of after-school placement) for a majority of this group. Her data provide one example of the studies that support an oral-aural education of Level III and Level IV children.

There are numerous references on speech teaching approaches and speech reading methods that develop teaching techniques. Calvert and Silverman (1975) have developed a test for the teacher that is intended to encourage skills in speech analysis and speech teaching. Although it is different in approach from Calvert and Silverman's test, many educators would be familiar with a volume on speech instruction by Ling (1976), which organizes theory, assessment, and teaching procedures. Jeffers and Barley (1971) have produced one of the more complete texts on speech reading, covering the development of this skill, materials necessary for teaching, and evaluation of the student's progress.

Instructional Options

Although the modes of communication used with young deaf children vary from one setting to another or from one child to the next, the more critical components may be the consistency of usage and the skill of the teacher. This suggests that an educational plan must be adopted, but that each child be considered separately within this framework. The term "curriculum" is undergoing some changes as a result of the federally mandated need for individual educational plans, but the capability of the instructional setting must still be considered. The more comprehensive the setting, the larger the number of options; and it is in this context that the larger residential schools have certain advantages. For example, Craig, Craig, and Burke (1974) describe one approach that includes the use of Verbotonal instruction for deaf children as part of the program. This particular option is an activity-oriented, auditory approach in which the preschool child is encouraged to develop language through systematic activities or games rather than through formal tutoring sessions. Short drills, nursery rhymes, and stories provide the basis for new language. Placed in this context, both receptive and expressive language have a high probability of repetition, and thus for the learning of language patterns from memory. Within the system, careful provision is made for teacher orientations, student evaluations, and language modification and development. The issue in this example is that an auditory system is placed into a set of preselected activities that maximally enhance the basic approach. Similar systematic organizations could, of course, be described for a program initiated from a total communication base.

It is quite possible, as well, to use other organizing concepts, and a number of these have been summarized by Craig (1976) in a discussion of curriculum perspectives and prospects within school systems. Open classroom organization (Craig and Holman, 1973) or instructional technology such as computer-assisted instruction may be part of the classroom organization. Many schools can provide a basic curriculum indicating the options available, but most schools have not reduced these volumes to an easily manageable size. A presentation by Kopp (1968) is a useful review of curriculum as process.

The capabilities of residential schools and day schools for serving a wider range of children at Levels III and IV should be recognized. In addition to classroom organization by age, hearing loss, and academic ability, the development of curricular options has been mentioned. Not discussed to this point are the capabilities for initiation of new programs and for extended-day programming. A language laboratory for specific groups of children can be organized after school, for example, to encourage role playing, project-centered language, and student interactions. Computer-assisted instruction is motivating and effective and can readily be employed during the evening hours. Project LIFE (Pfau, 1974) materials and the Computer Curriculum Corporation (1977) programs are examples of this capability since they can be operated by the students themselves. Clubs, sports, social activities, and other organized events are part of the social and developmental obligations of these schools. Special medical needs, physical rehabilitation needs, and attention to other handicapping conditions can be coordinated centrally. The list is quite expansive, but central to the concept is that a facility specifically devoted to deaf children has the instructional, supportive-services, and social potentials that must be considered when children at Level III and Level IV are considered for placement.

SUMMARY

The deaf child is not a single entity, but rather is a combination of many factors contributing to his or her hearing loss and adjustment patterns. Hearing impairment alone is not the only criterion for medical assessment, nor is it the sole determiner of instructional planning. If this were the case, the otolaryngologist and audiologist could merely combine their findings into a single index number, consult a chart, and recommend one particular placement, one communication system, and a single curricular plan. However, this shortcut has never been implemented successfully; somehow the children involved never fit the system.

This summary of education for deaf children has tried to focus selectively on a definition of deafness, on the instructional implications, and on the diversity among hearing-impaired children. The Conference definition adopted in 1975 has served as an organizational point for this discussion of deafness. The instructional implications have been expanded from this definition to include alternatives to instruction and placement, variations in communications systems, and resources available for gaining additional information. Particularly, the individual hearing-impaired child has been discussed in terms of hearing threshold, psychosocial background, instructional potential, and optimal educational opportunities. The education of deaf children is a reflection, first, of a great number of decisions before school begins and, later, of a particular school system's ability and resources to meet the child's needs. Cooperative professional efforts can make the educational potential for deaf children an encouraging reality.

REFERENCES

Aiello, B. 1975. Mainstreaming, Teacher Training Workshops on Individualized Instruction. Reston, Va., The Council for Exceptional Children.

Alexander Graham Bell Association for the Deaf. 1971. Guidelines for Oral Programs for Hearing Impaired Children. Washington, D.C., The Volta Bureau.

Berry, Q., Bluestone, C., Andrus, W., et al. 1975. Tympanic pattern classification in relation to middle ear effusion. Ann. Otol. Rhinol. Laryngol., 84:56.

Birch, J. W. 1975. Hearing Impaired Children in the Mainstream. Reston, Va., The Council for Exceptional Children.

Bornstein, H., Hamilton, L., Saulnier, K., et al. 1975. The Signed English Dictionary. Washington, Gallaudet College Press.

Calvert, D., and Silverman, S. 1975. Speech and Deafness. Washington, D.C., Alexander Graham Bell Association for the Deaf.

Computer Curriculum Corporation. 1977. Report by Instructional Systems, Inc., 119 Hudson Ave., Tenafly, NJ, 07670.

Conference of Executives of American Schools for the Deaf (CEASD). 1938. Report of the Conference Committee on nomenclature. Am. Ann. Deaf, 83:3.

Conference of Executives of American Schools for the Deaf (CEASD). 1975. Report of the Ad Hoc Committee to define deaf and hard of hearing. Am. Ann. Deaf, 120:509.

Conference of Executives of American Schools for the Deaf (CEASD): 1977. Statement of 'least restrictive' placements for deaf students. Am. Ann. Deaf, 122:70.

Craig, H. B., and Holman, G. 1973. The open classroom in a school for the deaf. Am. Ann. Deaf, 118:685.

Craig, W. 1976. Curriculum, its perspectives and prospects. Volta Rev., 78:52.

Craig, W., and Craig, H. (Eds.). 1981. Reference Issue. Am. Ann. Deaf, Washington, D.C.

Craig, W., and Salem, J. 1975. Partial integration of deaf with hearing students: Residential school perspectives. Am. Ann. Deaf. 120:28.

Craig, W., Craig, H., and Burke, R. 1974. Components of verbotonal instruction for deaf children. Lang. Speech Hearing Serv. Schools, 5:38.

Crammattee, A. 1968. Deaf People in Professional Employment. Chicago, Charles C Thomas.

Fant, L. 1976. AMESLAN. Northridge, CA, Joyce Motion Picture Co.

Griffing, B. 1970. Planning educational programs and services for the hard of hearing children. In Berg, F., and Fletcher, S. (Eds.) The Hard of Hearing Child. New York, Grune and Stratton, p. 233.

Jeffers, J., and Barley, M. 1971. Speechreading (Lipreading). Springfield, IL, Charles C Thomas.

Jerger, J. 1970. Clinical experience with impedance audiometry. Arch. Otolaryngol., 92:311.

Kopp, H. 1968. Curriculum, cognition and content. Volta Rev., 70:1.

Lane, H. 1976. The profoundly deaf. Has oral education succeeded? Volta Rev., 78:329.

Ling, D. 1976. Speech and the Hearing Impaired Child. Theory and Practice. Washington, D.C., Alexander Graham Bell Association for the Deaf.

Mindel, E., and Vernon, M. 1971. They Grow in Silence. Silver Spring, MD, National Association of the Deaf, p. 85.

Myerson, L. 1963. A psychology of impaired hearing. In Cruickshank, W. (Ed.) Psychology of Exceptional Children and Youth. Englewood Cliffs, NJ, Prentice-Hall, p. 145.

National Advisory Committee on the Handicapped. 1976. Education of the handicapped today. Am. Educ., June.

Nix, G. 1975. Total communication: A review of the studies offered in its support. Volta Rev. 77:470.

Northcott, W. H. (Ed.) 1973. The Hearing Impaired Child in a Regular Classroom. Washington, D.C., The Alexander Graham Bell Association of the Deaf

Pfau, G. S. 1974. Instructional manual for the General Electric Project LIFE program. Ballston Lake, NY, Industrial Industries.

Riekehof, L. 1979. The Joy of Signing. Springfield, MO, Gospel Publishing House.

Schlesinger, H., and Meadow, K. 1972. Sound and Sign. Berkeley, University of California Press, p. 44.

Stokoe, W. 1981. Sign Language Studies. Washington, D.C. Gallaudet College Press.

Svitko, C. 1976. Objective evaluations of middle ear mechanisms for a school-age deaf population utilizing a Grason-Stadler otoadmittance meter. University of Pittsburgh, Faculty of Arts and Sciences (thesis).

Vernon, M., and Brown, D. 1964. A guide to psychological tests and testing procedures in the evaluation of deaf and hard of hearing children. J. Speech Hear. Disord., 29:414.

INDEX

Page numbers in *italics* indicate illustrations. Page numbers followed by t indicate tables.

Airway (*Continued*)
　examination of, patient's history and, 1152
　　pulmonary function tests in, 1158, 1158t
　　radiography in, 1158–1159
　　respiration and, 1153
　　visualization of, 1156–1158
　　　by endoscopy, 1157, 1159–1168
　facial injury and trauma to, 807–808
　function of, 1143–1146, *1144–1145*
　humidification of inspired air by, 1146
　innervation of, 1143
　obstruction of, 58–64, 1146, 1190–1203. See also
　　Stridor and *Tracheotomy*.
　　chronic, 61
　　craniofacial surgery and, 62
　　dysphagia and, 904, 909
　　esophageal burn and, 1092
　　in Pierre Robin syndrome, 926, 927
　　malocclusion and, 967
　　neonatal, 59
　structure of, 1143
Albers-Schönberg disease, 324, 608
Alkaptonuria, 354
Allergens
　defined, 850
　identification and avoidance of, 858
　interaction with IgE, *852*
Allergic rhinitis, 849–861
　compared to vasomotor rhinitis, 857t
　differential diagnosis of, 856–858, 857t
　etiology of, 850–851
　immunopathology of, 851–854, 852t, *852*
　immunotherapy for, 860
　laboratory studies for, 855, 856t
　nasal obstruction and, 712
　symptoms and signs of, 854
　therapy for, 858, 859t
　　pharmacologic, 859, 859t
Allergy
　defined, 850
　eustachian tube function and, 398, *399*
　nasal, sinusitis and, 784
　otitis media with effusion and, 417
　parotid gland dysfunction and, 1028
　tonsil or adenoid surgery and, 1002
Allergy testing, middle ear effusions and, 432
Alport disease, 589, 589t, 590t
Alveolar bone, abscess of, 939, *939–940*. See also *Teeth, disorders of*.
Alveolar hypoventilation, surgical treatment of, 1001
Alveolar macrophage, 1150
Alveolar-arterial gradient for oxygen, 1341
Alveoli. See also *Pulmonary parenchyma*.
　compliance of, 1147
　development of, 1139
　pulmonary microlithiasis of, 1276
　pulmonary proteinosis of, 1276
　smoke inhalation and, 1267
　structure of, 1147
　surfactant in, 1147
Amelogenesis imperfecta, 943, *943, 944*
American Indians, cholesteatoma in, 534
American Manual Alphabet of the Deaf, *1577*
Amino acid(s), embryology and, 15
Amniotic fluid, decreases of, 48, *49*, 50
Amyotonia congenita, swallowing and, 1070

Anaerobic bacteria, otitis media and, 405
Anatomic defect, acquired, dysphagia and, 905, 909
Anemia
　hypoplastic, congenital anomalies and, 323
　tonsil or adenoid surgery and, 1002
Anencephaly, 316
Anesthesia
　craniofacial surgery and, 62
　general, nasal examination and, 689
　in tracheotomy, 1325
Angina, Ludwig, 977
Angiofibroma, nasopharyngeal, 845, *845*
　epistaxis and, 721
　management of, 845–846
　nasal obstruction and, 715
　treatment of, 846–848
　　surgical, 846–847
Angiokeratoma corporis diffusum, 1123
Angioma, subglottic, 1314
Angioneurotic edema, 1254
Angle's classification of malocclusion, 959–962, *960–961*
Angular stomatitis, 1046
Animal bites, 1115
Ankyloglossia, congenital mandibular, 919, *921*
Anomalous carotid artery in middle ear, 312
Anomaly(ies)
　acquired, dysphagia, 905, 909
　anthelix, 328
　auricular, 328
　congenital. See *Congenital anomalies*.
　craniofacial. See *Craniofacial anomalies*.
　genital, recessive, 325
　hearing loss related to, 234t–239t
　helix, 328
　lobular, 328
　minor
　　frequency of, *46*
　　significance of, 45t
　recessive renal, genital and middle ear, 325
Anotia, surgical repair of, 338
Anoxia, sensorineural hearing loss and, 594
Anterior nares, 679
Anterior neuropore, in embryo, *6, 7*
Anthelix anomalies, 328
Antibiotic agents
　infectious eczematoid dermatitis treated by, 560t
　orbital complications of sinusitis and, 793
　septal hematoma treated with, 792
　topical, otitis media and, 520t
　use in sinusitis, 788
Antibody(ies)
　immunoglobulin, allergic rhinitis and, 851
　role in otitis media, 414–416, 415t
Antigens, bacterial, identification in otitis media, 406
Antihistamines, for treatment of allergic rhinitis, 859, 859t
Antimicrobial agents
　brain abscess treated by, 571
　clinical pharmacology of, 445–454
　diffusion into middle ear fluids, 454–457, 455t, 457t
　for prophylaxis, 467, 467t
　intracranial suppurative complications of otitis media and, 566, 574
　intravenous vs. intramuscular administration of, 464
　meningitis treated by, 568
　oral preparations of, 463

Deaf children (*Continued*)
  education of, severe hearing loss and, 1575
  otologic examination of, 430
Deafness. See also *Hearing loss.*
  congenital heart disease and, 319
  genetic causes of, 233
  leukonychia and, 322
  sensorineural. See *Sensorineural deafness.*
Decannulation, following tracheotomy, 1328–1329, *1329*
Decongestants
  use of, in nasopharyngitis, 783
    in sinusitis, 789
Defect, genetic, transmission of, *15*
Deformation
  defined, 47
  vs. malformations, 48, 48t
Deformation complex
  defined, 48
  vs. malformation complex, *43*
Deformation syndromes, 47, 50
Degranulation, immunologic, 687
Dental disease. See also *Teeth, disorders of.*
  headache and, 734
  otalgia and, 216
Dental disorders. See *Teeth, disorders of.*
Dental studies, for craniofacial surgery, 69
Dentinogenesis imperfecta, 943, *944*
Dentition, 937. See also *Teeth* and *Orthodontic problems.*
  development of, 931, 946
  mandibular growth and, 24, *24*
  nasomaxillary configuration and, 26, *26*
Deoxyribonucleic acid (DNA), embryology and, 15, *15*
Deposition, bone growth and, 22, *23*
Depression, facial paralysis and, 297
Dermal anomalies of neck, 1389–1391
  cutis hyperelastica, 1390
  cutis laxa, 1390
  dyskeratosis congenita, 1390
  multiple lentigines syndrome, 1389
  multiple pterygium syndrome, 1390
  Noonan syndrome, 1390
  pseudoxanthoma elasticum, 1390
  pterygium colli, 1389
  XO syndrome, 1389
Dermatitis, infectious eczematoid, 560, 560t
Dermatomyositis, 1130
Dermatoses, pinna affected by, 354
Dermoid cysts
  congenital nasal, 773–775, *773–774*
  neck mass and, 1381
Descending auditory pathway, *134*, 135
Desquamative interstitial pneumonitis, 1276
Deviated nasal septum, eustachian tube dysfunction and, 401
Dexamethasone phosphate, croup treated with, 1253
Diagnosis
  facial configuration and, 3
  of syndromes, 52
Diaphragm
  congenital hernia of, 1212
  neonatal paralysis of, 1213
Diaphysis, *21*, 22
Difference limen for frequency, *115*
Differential growth. See *Growth, differential.*
Diffusion, physiology of, 1149
DiGeorge syndrome, 325

DiGeorge syndrome (*Continued*)
  oropharyngeal manifestations of, 1008
Dilantin (diphenylhydantoin sodium), gingival hyperplasia induced by, 950, *950*
Diphenhydramine, herpetic stomatitis treated with, 975
Diphtheria, 984–987, 1253–1254
  bacterial rhinitis and, 784
  clinical features of, 985t
  nasal, 711
  therapy for, 986
    effect of delay in, 986t
Diphtheritic otitis, 408
Diphtheritic rhinitis, 711
Diphtheroids, otitis media and, 405
Diplegia, congenital facial, 319, 916
Diplopia, orbit fracture and, 825
Disease, systemic. See *Systemic disease.*
Displacement
  craniofacial growth and, 22
  of nasomaxillary complex, 26
  of orbit, 26
Dizziness, 261–269. See also *Vertigo.*
  etiology of, 262
  patient history and, 261
DNA (deoxyribonucleic acid), embryology and, 15, *15*
Dog bites, facial, 809. See also *Facial injuries.*
Doll's eye phenomenon, 205, *206*
Dominant proximal symphalangism, hearing loss and, 320
Down syndrome, 315, 914, *914*
Drugs
  for allergic rhinitis, 859, 859t
  saliva production and, 1025
  sensorineural hearing loss caused by, 596
  tinnitus caused by, 276t
Duane syndrome, 320, 1128
Dwarfism, 916
  perichondritis of pinna and, 353, *353*
Dysautonomia, familial, 1127
Dyschondroplasia, craniofacial growth and, 22
Dyshistogenesis, 40–41
Dyskeratosis congenita, 1390
Dysmetabolic syndromes, *37*, 40
Dysmorphia, facial, *42*, 43
Dysostosis
  cleidocranial, 318, 916
  craniofacial. See *Crouzon disease* and *Crouzon syndrome.*
  mandibulofacial. See *Treacher-Collins syndrome.*
Dysphagia, 903–910
  acquired anatomic defect and, 905
  airway obstruction and, 904
  congenital defects and, 904
  defined, 903
  differential diagnosis in, 904t
  etiology of, 903–905, 904t, 909–910
  examination for, 908
  patient's history and, 907
  prematurity and, 903
  symptoms of, 907
Dysphonia, neonatal, 1184
Dysplasia
  bronchopulmonary (BPD), 1273
  cleidocranial, 916
  craniometaphyseal, 609, *610*
  fibrous, 611, *612*
    in temporal bone, 638
    of paranasal sinus, 843, *843*

Dysplasia (*Continued*)
frontometaphyseal, *610*, 611
nasal, 776
oculoauriculovertebral, 917
white folded, 1020
Dysrhythmia, cerebral, headaches and, 732

Ear
acoustic impedance of, 118–121, *119, 120*
disease of, headache and, 734
embryology and developmental anatomy of, 85–111
examination of in otalgia, 214
external. See *External ear.*
general function of, 112
growth and development of, postnatal, 18
injuries of, 614–634. See also *Temporal bone, fractures of.*
external auditory canal, 614
middle ear, 615–620
otitic barotrauma, 620
inner. See *Inner ear.*
middle. See *Middle ear* and *Tympanic membrane.*
physiology of, 112–137
prominent, otoplasty for, 755, *757*
Ear canal
effect of on sound conduction, 116, *116, 117*
stenotic lesions of, 354
systemic diseases and, 354
Ear disease
diagnosis of, 139–151. See also *Otoscopy.*
examination of head in, 140
external examination of ear in, 140, *141*
signs and symptoms of, 139–140
Ear piercing, inflammation from, 353
Ear pit, *44*
Ear tag, 42, *44*
Ear wax. See *Cerumen.*
Eardrum, development of, 89. See also *Tympanic cavity.*
ECOCHG (electrocochleography), 174
Eczematous otitis externa, 351
Edema
angioneurotic, 1254
pulmonary, following tracheotomy, 1331
Edward syndrome, 314
Ehlers-Danlos syndrome, 1390
EKG (electrocardiogram), hearing loss and, 239
Ekman syndrome, 915
Electrical potentials, cochlear, 125–127
Electroacoustic impedance bridge, 162, *163, 164*
Electrocardiogram (EKG), hearing loss and, 239
Electrocochleography (ECOCHG), 174
Electrodermal audiometry, 178
Electromyography (EMG), facial paralysis and, 291
Electroneurography (ENoG), facial paralysis and, 291
Electronystagmography (ENG), 209, 209t
hearing loss and, 240
vertigo and, 262, *263, 264*
Electroretinography, retinitis pigmentosa diagnosis with, 583
ELISA (enzyme linked immunosorbent assay), 406–407
Embryo
artery development in, 12, *13*
craniofacial bones of, origin of, 10
craniofacial complex of, cell differentiation in, 16
differential growth of, 7

Embryo (*Continued*)
facial development in, *6, 7*
muscle development in, *13*, 14
nerve development in, *13*, 14
Embryology
of craniofacial complex, 3–17
subcellular, 14–17
Embryonic pleiotropy, 46
EMG (electromyography), facial paralysis and, 291
Emphysema, 1260–1261, *1261*
lobar, neonatal, 1211
Enamel hypoplasia, localized, *945*
Encephalitis, focal otitic, 569
Encephaloceles, basal and sincipital, 772t
surgery for, *78*
Endemic cretinism, 327
Endochondral ossification, 20, *21*
Endolymphatic duct and sac, development of, 105
Endoscopic procedures, in airway examination, 1157, *1157,* 1159–1168
bronchoscopy, 1162–1168
direct laryngoscopy, 1160–1162, *1160*
Endoscopy, 1099–1100
in removal of foreign bodies, 1309, 1309t, *1310*
preparation of patient for, 1105
stridor and, 1202
velopharyngeal insufficiency and, 1530
Endotracheal intubation. See also *Tracheotomy.*
complications of, 1269–1273
injury from, 1287, 1287t
nasal route for, 1351–1353
ENG (electronystagmography), hearing loss and, 240
ENoG (electroneurography), facial paralysis and, 291
Enteric bacilli, gram-negative, otitis media and, 404
Enzyme(s)
dysmetabolic syndromes and, *37*, 40
otitis media and, 413
Enzyme linked immunosorbent assay (ELISA), 406, 407
Eosinophil(s), in nasal mucosa, 686
Eosinophilic granuloma, 639
Epidemiology, middle ear disease and, 359
Epidermoid
of middle ear, 313
of temporal bone, 641
Epidermoid carcinoma of mouth, 1049
Epidermolysis bullosa, 1018
Epiglottis
absence of, 1218
bifid, 1218
development of, 1137
laryngeal muscles and, 1141
visualization of, 1156
Epiglottitis, acute, 1250
Epilepsy, temporal lobe, dizziness and, 267
Epiphysis, *21, 22*
Epistaxis, 719–727
etiology of, 720–722, 721t
management of, 722–725, *723–726*
nasal anatomy and, 719
prevention of, 726, *726, 727*
Epithelial tumors
of tongue and floor of mouth, 1043
oral, 1041
Epitympanic recess, embryology and development of, 93
Epitympanum, embryology and development of, 93